OPERATIVE GYNECOLOGY

OPERATIVE GYNECOLOGY

Richard W. Te Linde, M.D.

*Professor Emeritus of Gynecology and
Emeritus Gynecologist-in-Chief,
Johns Hopkins Hospital*

and

Richard F. Mattingly, M.D.

*Professor and Chairman,
Department of Gynecology and Obstetrics,
Marquette School of Medicine*

FOURTH EDITION

440 Figures and 12 Color Plates

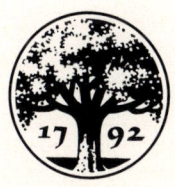

J. B. Lippincott Company

Philadelphia and Toronto

FOURTH EDITION

Copyright © 1970, by J. B. Lippincott Company

Copyright © 1962, by J. B. Lippincott Company

Copyright, 1946, 1953
By J. B. Lippincott Company

This book is fully protected by copyright and, with the exception of brief excerpts for review, no part of it may be reproduced in any form by print, photoprint, microfilm or any other means without written permission from the publisher.

Distributed in Great Britain by
 Blackwell Scientific Publications,
 Oxford and Edinburgh

Library of Congress Catalog Card No. 79-97124

Printed in the United States of America

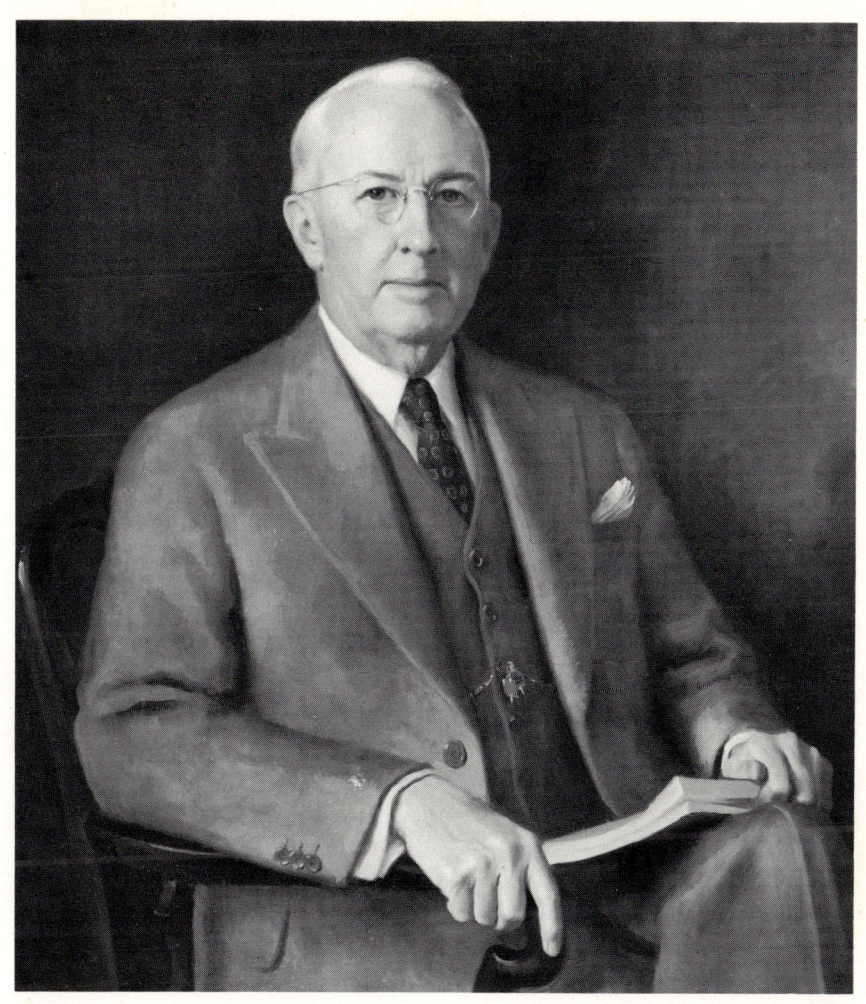

This book is dedicated to
DR. EDWARD H. RICHARDSON
friend and counselor
in whom are combined the rare qualities of excellent surgical judgment and an appreciation of fine surgical technic.

Preface to the Fourth Edition

When compiling the third edition of this book, the senior author believed that it would be his last revision. But time has treated him kindly, and the book has continued to be in great demand—by practicing obstetricians, gynecologists, and, especially, men in the various residency training programs throughout the United States and abroad. It is evident, therefore, that there is need of an up-to-date version of this book. The senior author is in the twilight of his career and would like to cast a shadow beyond his physical lifetime. As stated in the preface to the third edition, a sound surgical philosophy is perhaps more important than technic. Therefore, in addition to the technical aspects of pelvic surgery, the author has set forth his views on indications and contraindications for the various procedures. The perfectly performed operation done without a proper indication may be more detrimental to the woman's total health, both physiological and emotional, than a clumsily performed indicated procedure. Nature may compensate and heal trauma from a technically poor operation, but no one today can replace a uterus which has been unnecessarily removed.

To assure the continuity of this work for future generations, it seemed wise to bring in a younger gynecologist as co-author, who will continue with subsequent revisions when the senior author no longer can. Dr. Richard F. Mattingly, Professor and Chairman of the Department of Gynecology and Obstetrics at Marquette School of Medicine and a former student of the senior author, consented to assume this task. In addition, I have asked a few who served on my residency staff to revise some chapters in the field in which they have a special interest. Dr. Lawrence Wharton, who has continued animal experimental work on endometriosis following that of Dr. Roger Scott and the author, has brought that chapter up to date. Dr. John Ridley of the Emory University faculty has had vast experience with surgery in more complicated cases of urinary incontinence and has brought that chapter up to date in the light of recent experience.

Dr. Eleanor Delfs, Professor of Gynecology and Obstetrics at Marquette School of Medicine, was for many years our chief consultant on borderline conditions between gynecology and obstetrics at Hopkins. One of her special interests is the subject of reproductive failure. She has modernized the chapter on abortions, as well as the one on sterilization. The other chapters have been updated by Dr. Mattingly and the senior author. The subject of cervical cancer has become quite a different problem from that of several years ago. Dr. Mattingly has completely rewritten the chapters on this subject, which has become so broad that it was necessary to treat it in four separate chapters under the titles of The Epidemiology of Cancer of the Cervix, Carcinoma in Situ of the Cervix, Invasive Carcinoma of the Cervix, and Pelvic Exenteration.

Because radical surgery has come into the picture and been made safer by the use of antibiotics and by our current understanding of fluid and electrolyte balance, the well-trained pelvic surgeon must be knowledgeable in electrolytic metabolism. It was therefore thought advisable to include a chapter on that subject by the experts. Drs. Edward Lennon and Jack Lemann from the Department of Medicine at Marquette consented to contribute this chapter, which should be educational and of practical value to the reader. Dr. Peter Safar and Dr. David Torpey from the University of Pittsburgh have completely rewritten the chapter on anesthesia and resuscitation.

Several new illustrations have been added, most of them by Mr. Robert H. Albertin, Chairman of the Department of Medical Illustrations at Marquette. They are of the same high quality as those of the earlier editions. Although all the chapters have been carefully checked for possible modernization, changes have been made only when, in the opinion of the authors, they constitute an improvement.

A short history of pelvic surgery has been added to this edition. Although necessarily brief, it covers the important contributions to modern pelvic surgery. It should be both interesting and inspiring.

With this, his final effort, the senior author wishes to express his thanks to the many readers, past and future, who have shown their confidence and continued interest in successive editions. Also, both Dr. Mattingly and I are grateful to the J. B. Lippincott Company. Working with its staff has been more of a pleasure than a task.

RICHARD W. TE LINDE, M.D.

The decision to accept the challenge to continue the authorship of this recognized textbook was not an easy one. It is evident that such a responsibility must include a major commitment of one's future academic career toward this effort. The joint authorship of the fourth edition of *Operative Gynecology* acknowledges this commitment.

The reader is entitled to know the motivating forces that have entered into this decision. The faithful followers of each edition of this textbook will clearly recognize that one of the major contributions of this work of a lifetime has been the development of the senior author's time-honored philosophy of pelvic surgery. It is essential that these principles be maintained by his students who share the same surgical and medical approach toward problems of the female reproductive tract.

While the entire faculty at Marquette take pride in the coauthorship of this edition, there is a clear understanding that this work is a Hopkins tradition, and regardless of its future contributors, it will always serve to unite the hearts and minds of students the world over who recognize the major contributions to our specialty from its Hopkins heritage. If the new author makes no other contribution to the textbook than the acknowledgment that the Hopkins approach toward pelvic surgery shall continue to serve as a guideline in our specialty, he will consider his efforts richly rewarded.

Although the present explosion in scientific knowledge prohibits the inclusion of every known detail of gynecologic interest in a single textbook, the approach of the present and future editions will be to "sift out" the important advances for the reader and incorporate such new information into our basic understanding of the pathophysiology and treatment of pelvic disease. In the present era of superspecialization, it is essential that the gynecologist-obstetrician have a broad *education* in the entire background of pelvic disease, as well as adequate *training* in surgical technics if he is to be successful in his therapeutic efforts. It is important, therefore, that a textbook such as *Operative Gynecology* include more than the surgical approach to gynecologic disease. This fact is well documented in previous editions.

RICHARD F. MATTINGLY, M.D.

Preface to the First Edition

Gynecology has become a many-sided specialty. No longer is it simply a branch of general surgery. In order to practice this specialty in its broad sense, the gynecologist must be trained in a comprehensive field. He must be a surgeon, expert in his special field; he must be trained in the fundamentals of obstetrics; he must have the technical skill to investigate female urologic conditions; he must have an understanding of endocrinology as it applies to gynecology; he should be well grounded in gynecologic pathology; finally, he must be able to recognize and deal successfully with minor psychiatric problems which arise so commonly among gynecologic patients. With this concept of the specialty in mind this book has been written. It then becomes apparent, when one seeks training in gynecology beyond the simplest fundamentals such as are taught to undergraduates, that special works are necessary for training those who intend to practice it.

More and more this modern conception of gynecology is becoming apparent in the newer works that are appearing in the subject. Within the past decade books on gynecologic endocrinology, medical gynecology, as well as general textbooks on gynecology, have made their appearance. These volumes have been eagerly received, but there seemed to be a void in the books available for training young men in the field of gynecologic surgery. The author has attempted to fill this void with the present volume.

In the early days of the development of gynecology, progress in surgery was rapid and brilliant. Much of this has been recorded in Kelly's "Operative Gynecology." Since these pioneer days, progress has been slow, but there has been advance in surgical technic, in the development of new operations, in the improvement in anesthesia, and in the pre- and the postoperative care of patients. Within the surgical lifetime of the author, which extends for a quarter of a century, operative mortality and morbidity have been greatly reduced as a result of improvements in these fields. Brilliant discoveries have been few, but the sum total of the minor advances add up to surprising progress.

The present volume attempts to bring the subject of operative gynecology up to date and to make recent information on that subject available in a single volume. The views expressed are those of the author and, in general, those which are put into practice on the gynecologic house service at the Johns Hopkins Hospital. On a service where many attending gynecologists work, differences of opinion are inevitable, and the author's views in this book are not held uniformly by all the attending gynecologists. Indeed, the differences in point of view expressed by the visiting staff are of value to the members of the house staff, causing them to realize early in their careers that all is not forever settled in medicine.

The author is a firm believer in the system of long hospital residencies for training young men in the various surgical specialties when their minds are quick to grasp ideas and their fingers are nimble. This volume has been written particularly for this group of men. Unfortunately, there is a paucity of good gynecologic residencies in the United States in the sense that the author has in mind. Many positions bear the name of residency but fail to give the resident sufficient operative work to justify the name. Another excellent method of development of the young gynecologist is an active assistantship to a well-trained, mature gynecologist. If the assistant is permitted to stand at the operating table opposite his chief, day after day, eventually he will acquire skill and judgment which he himself will be able to utilize as an operator. When such a preceptor system is practiced, it is important that the assistant be given some surgery of his own to do while he is still young. If a man is forced to think of himself only as a perennial assistant, this frame of mind will kill his ability to accept responsibility of his own. However, many must learn their operative gynecology under less favorable circumstances than those of the fortunate resident or assistant. This volume should be of value to those who, by self-instruction, must acquire a certain degree of operative skill. Finally, it must be admitted that more gynecology is practiced today by general surgeons in this country than by gynecologists. Although this is not ideal, circumstances make it necessary, and much of this gynecologic surgery is well done. It is hoped that many general surgeons will use this volume as a reference book.

In connection with general surgery, it is only fair to say that much has come to gynecology by way of general surgeons of the old school, who practiced general surgery in the broadest sense. Now that gynecology and/or obstetrics has become a specialty unto itself, it is well in our training of men not to swing too far from general abdominal surgery. In spite of the most careful preoperative investigation, mistakes in diagnosis will be made, and at times the gynecologist will be called upon to take care of general surgical conditions in the region of the lower abdomen and the rectum. With this in mind, the author has included in this volume a consideration of a few of the commoner general surgical conditions occasionally encountered incidentally with gynecology or by mistaken diagnosis.

Operative Gynecology is written with the primary purpose of describing the technic of the usual and some of the rarer operative procedures. It also includes indications for and against operations as well as pre- and postoperative care of patients. Although gynecology is divided into several fields, these fields interlock so that it has been found impossible to compose a volume on gynecologic surgery to the exclusion of the other divisions of the specialty. Gynecologic pathology, for instance, is the bedrock upon which good gynecologic surgery is practiced. Without an understanding of it, surgery becomes merely a mechanical job, and errors in surgical judgment are inevitable. Hence, it has become necessary to include in this volume a minimum of gross and microscopic pathology, as it applies directly to the surgical subject under consideration. Also, some consideration is given to psychology and psychiatry in relation to gynecologic surgery. The author believes that getting the young woman on whom a hysterectomy must be done into the proper frame of mind to accept it is as important as possessing the technical skill to perform the operation.

The nature of this book has made it essential that it be well illustrated. With few exceptions, the illustrations were sketched at the operating table. The principal illustrator is James Didusch. Without the use of his talents the book could not have been produced. In addition, other excellent medical illustrators have contributed to the volume. These are the late Max Brödel, P. D. Malone, Mrs. Elinor Widmont Bodian, Miss Ranice Birch, William Didusch and Mrs. Grace Elam. The author is grateful to all of them, and the illustrations themselves speak for the quality of their work.

The author is grateful to Dr. Houston S. Everett, who has read the manuscript and made many valuable suggestions. This volume was written during the period of World War II, when the added burden of work caused by a reduced staff would have made the writing of the book impossible except for the co-operation of the resident staff. The resident gynecologists during that period, Dr. Donald Woodruff, Dr. Edward H. Richardson, Jr., Dr. Roger B. Scott, Dr. Gerald A. Galvin, Dr. Constantino Manahan and Dr. David Cheek, have performed several of the operations portrayed and have been helpful in criticizing the sketches. Dr. Charles B. Brack and Dr. George Farber prepared the sections relating to irradiation.

Mrs. Christine Nisbet has read the manuscript and given innumerable valuable suggestions in respect to literary style.

Much of the typing was done by Mrs. Gerald Hopkins, one of the many volunteers during the war period who have made it possible to keep the hospital open. I am grateful to my secretaries, Miss Margaret A. King, Miss Elizabeth Wood, Miss Grace F. Koppelman and Miss Bertha M. Scroggs, for their assistance in typing and looking up references. Dr. Lois Fess has also been helpful in searching the literature.

Finally, E. W. Bacon at the J. B. Lippincott Company has contributed generously from his store of practical knowledge acquired by a lifetime of experience in publishing medical works.

Baltimore, Maryland, 1946

RICHARD W. TE LINDE

Contents

1. **Historical Development of Pelvic Surgery** 1

   PART ONE: PREOPERATIVE AND POSTOPERATIVE MANAGEMENT

2. **Preoperative Care and Complications** 15

    History-Taking 15
    Gynecologic Examination... 17
    Laboratory Examinations 19
    Preoperative Evaluation 22
       Age as a Factor in Pelvic Surgery 22
    Discussion of the Necessary Operative Procedure 23
    Preparation of the Patient for Operation 25
    Preoperative Medical Complications 25
    Preoperative Procedures in the Operating Room 26
    Armamentarium 27
       Instruments for Pelvic Laparotomies 27
       Instruments for Major Vaginal Operative Procedures ... 27
       Instruments for Dilatation and Curettage 28
       Instruments for Rubin's Test 28
       Instruments for Insertion of Radium 28
       Instruments for Therapeutic Abortion or Completion of Abortion . 28
       Instruments for Posterior Colpotomy 28
       Instruments for Radical Pelvic Surgery 28

3. **Anesthesia and Resuscitation** 36
   By Peter Safar, M.D., and David Torpey, M.D.

    Introduction 36
    Mortality 36
    The Preanesthetic Visit.. 37
    Preanesthetic Medication 38
    Posture 39
    General Anesthesia.. 40
    Spinal Anesthesia 42
    Paracervical Block 46
    Choice of Anesthetic Agents and Technics 46
    Complications During Anesthesia............................. 49
    Monitoring of Vital Signs 51
    The Postanesthetic Period 52
       Most Common Life-Threatening Complications ... 53

3. Anesthesia and Resuscitation (*Continued*)

Resuscitation 55
    Introduction 55
    Hypoxemia, Airway Obstruction, and Hypoventilation 57
    Cardiac Arrest 62
    When To Start and When To Discontinue Efforts 64
    Complications of Resuscitation 64
    Postresuscitation Care 64
    Inhalation of Foreign Matter 65
    Respiratory Insufficiency in Shock 65
    Cardiac Arrest From Exsanguination 66

4. Postoperative Care and Complications 68

Immediate Postoperative Care 68
Shock 71
    Pathophysiology of Hemorrhagic Shock 71
    Treatment 72
Pulmonary Complications 75
    Etiology and Incidence 75
    Symptoms 77
    Treatment 78
Urinary Output and Postoperative Fluid Needs 79
Routine Orders 80
Care of the Gastrointestinal Tract 80
Paralytic Ileus and Distention 80
Postoperative Care of the Urinary Bladder 82
Postoperative Urinary Tract Infections 83
Venous Thrombosis and Thrombophlebitis 85
    Pathophysiology 86
    Etiologic Factors 86
    Symptoms and Signs 87
    Treatment 88
Pulmonary Embolism 91
    Symptoms 91
    Pathophysiology 92
    Treatment 92
    Prognosis 93

5. Fluid and Electrolyte Balance 97
By Edward J. Lennon, M.D., and Jacob Lemann, Jr., M.D.

Introduction 97
    Caloric Requirements 97
Water 98
    Normal Body Content and Distribution 98
    Water Turnover 99
    Hormonal Regulation of Body Water Losses 101
    Manifestations and Therapy of Water Deficits 102
Sodium 104
    Body Content and Distribution 104
    Normal Sodium Turnover 104
    Adjustments to Variation in Sodium Intake 105
    Clinical Evaluation of Sodium Deficits or Excesses 106
    Maintenance and Replacement of Sodium Requirements 107
Potassium 107

5. **Fluid and Electrolyte Balance** (*Continued*)
   - Body Content and Distribution ... 107
   - Adaptations to Variations in Potassium Intake ... 108
   - Clinical Evaluation of Potassium Deficits or Surpluses ... 109
   - Replacement Therapy ... 109
   - Acid-Base Metabolism ... 110
     - Definitions ... 110
     - Normal Body Content and Distribution ... 110
     - Hydrogen Ion Turnover ... 111
     - Renal Acid Excretion ... 111
     - Evaluation of Acid-Base Balance ... 112
     - Clinical Recognition and Therapy ... 113
   - Other Mineral Requirements ... 114
   - Appendix ... 114
     - Concentration Units ... 114
     - Conversion of pH to Hydrogen Ion Concentration ... 115
     - Illustrative Cases ... 115

6. **Estrogen Replacement Therapy** ... 118

PART TWO: ABDOMINAL OPERATIONS FOR BENIGN DISEASE

7. **Opening and Closing the Abdomen** ... 125
   - Opening the Abdomen ... 125
     - Midline Incision ... 125
     - Transverse Incision ... 128
     - Gridiron (Muscle-Splitting) Incision ... 131
   - Closing the Abdomen ... 132
     - Midline Incision ... 133
     - Transverse Incision ... 136
     - Gridiron Incision ... 136
   - Complications ... 137
     - Wound Infection ... 137
     - Wound Dehiscence and Evisceration ... 138
     - Etiologic Factors ... 139
     - Diagnosis ... 140
     - Treatment ... 141

8. **Myomata Uteri** ... 143
   - General Considerations ... 143
   - Asymptomatic Myomata ... 145
   - Signs and Symptoms Indicating Treatment ... 148
   - Choice of Treatment ... 151
     - Surgical Treatment ... 151
     - Irradiation Treatment ... 151
   - Total vs. Subtotal Abdominal Hysterectomy for Benign Conditions of the Uterus ... 152
   - Ovarian Management at Hysterectomy for Benign Disease ... 154
   - Technic: Subtotal Abdominal Hysterectomy ... 156
   - Total Abdominal Hysterectomy for Benign Uterine Disease (Richardson Technic) ... 163
   - Comments on and Modifications of Richardson Technic of Total Abdominal Hysterectomy ... 173

Contents

8. Myomata Uteri (*Continued*)
    Technic: Total Hysterectomy for Cervical Myoma 175
    Injury to the Bladder 177
    Posthysterectomy Hemorrhage 177
    Vaginal Hysterectomy for the Myomatous Uterus................ 179
    Abdominal Myomectomy.. 180
        Indications and Contraindications 181
        Technic: Abdominal Myomectomy 183
    Vaginal Myomectomy 186
        Vaginal Myomectomy for Cervical Myoma 189

9. Endometriosis **193**
    By Lawrence R. Wharton, Jr., M.D.
    Adenomyosis 192
        Symptoms 194
        Pelvic Findings 194
        Differential Diagnosis 194
        Treatment 195
    External Endometriosis...................................... 196
        Distribution and Gross Pathology 197
        Histology 203
        Histogenesis... 204
        Symptoms 214
        Diagnosis 215
        Treatment 217
    Malignancy in Endometriosis................................ 220

10. Presacral Neurectomy **225**
    General Considerations...................................... 225
    Anatomy.. 227
    Technic: Presacral Neurectomy 227
    Ovarian Denervation 229

11. Pelvic Inflammatory Disease and Its Complications............ **230**
    Gonorrhea 230
        Epidemiology.. 230
    Gonorrheal Disease of the Lower Tract 231
        Methods of Culture..................................... 231
        Clinical Evidence of Infection 231
        Treatment of Gonococcal Infection of the Lower Tract 232
        Treatment of Residual Infections in the Lower Tract 233
    Gonorrheal Disease of the Upper Genital Tract (Above the Internal
        Os) 234
        Differentiation of Acute Salpingitis From Appendicitis 234
        Treatment of Acute Salpingitis 235
        Indications for Surgery During the Acute Stage of Salpingitis... 237
    Surgery for the Residue of Gonococcal Tubal Disease 238
        Selection of Operation.................................. 238
        Ruptured Tubo-ovarian Abscess 242
        Cornual Resection 244
        Technic: Salpingectomy 246
        Technic: Salpingo-oophorectomy for Chronic Salpingitis........ 247

11. Pelvic Inflammatory Disease and Its Complications (*Continued*)

- Technic: Bisection Operation 249
- Drainage at Laparotomy for Salpingitis 253
- Septic Shock 256
  - Gram-Negative Endotoxic Shock 257
  - Pathophysiology of Endotoxic Shock 257
  - Metabolic Effects of Septic Shock 258
  - Bacteriology 258
  - Clinical Features 258
  - Treatment 259
  - Mortality 263
- Tuberculosis of the Female Genital Tract 263
  - Clinical Features 264
  - Pathogenesis 265
  - Diagnosis 266
  - Treatment 266
  - Results of Treatment 267

12. Operative Injury of the Ureters 270

- Causes 270
- Treatment of Operative Ureteral Injuries 272
  - Technic: Ureteroureteral Anastomosis 276
  - Technic: Implantation of the Ureter into the Bladder 277

13. Surgery of the Double Uterus 281

- Indications for Surgery 281
- Surgery for Hematometra 282
- Surgery for Pyometra 283
- Surgery for History of Habitual Abortion 285
  - Technic 287

14. Infertility 293

- General Considerations 293
- Diagnostic Evaluation 293
- Special Diagnostic Studies 298
  - Tubal Insufflation 298
  - Hysterosalpingography 299
  - Culdoscopy; Laparoscopy 301
- Operative Treatment 302
  - Treatments To Be Considered Prior to Major Surgery 302
  - Salpingolysis 303
  - Cornual Implantation 303
  - Technic: Reimplantation of Distal Portion of Tube into Uterus 303
  - Salpingostomy 305
  - Technic: Cuff Salpingostomy (Sovak's Method) 307
  - Estes Procedure 307
  - Summation of Experience 308

15. Culdoscopy 311

- Instrument 311
- Procedure 312
- Indications 316

15. Culdoscopy (Continued)

- Failures 320
- Complications and Morbidity 321
- Outcome of Concurrent Intra-uterine Pregnancy 322
- Evaluation of Culdoscopy and Contraindications 322

16. Ectopic Pregnancy 323

- Etiology 323
- Pathophysiology 324
- Symptoms 325
- Clinical Findings 326
- Diagnostic Procedures 326
- Treatment 330
  - General Considerations 330
  - Extent of Operative Procedure 331
  - Technic: Simple Salpingectomy for Tubal Pregnancy 332
  - Conservative Procedures in Tubal Pregnancy 334
- Interstitial Pregnancy 335
  - Treatment 335
  - Technic: Excision of Interstitial Pregnancy With Salpingo-oophorectomy 336
- Abdominal Pregnancy 337
- Ovarian Pregnancy 340
- Other Forms of Ectopic Pregnancy 341

17. The Intestinal Tract in Relation to Gynecology 344
By Larry C. Carey, M.D.

- Intestinal Obstruction 344
- Regional Enteritis 347
- Meckel's Diverticulum 347
- Intestinal Fistula 347
- Obstruction of the Large Bowel 348
  - Technic 350
- Surgery of the Anus and Rectum 359

18. The Vermiform Appendix in Relation to Gynecology 364

- Treatment of Acute Appendicitis 365
- Appendicitis in Pregnancy 367
  - Differential Diagnosis 367
  - Perinatal Mortality 368
  - Treatment 369
  - Incidental Appendectomy following Cesarean Section 369
- Technic of Appendectomy 369

19. Sterilization 374
By Eleanor Delfs, M.D.

- General Considerations 374
- Indications 375
- Optimum Time for Sterilization 377
- Methods and Efficacy 378
  - Technic: Pomeroy Operation for Tubal Sterilization 380
  - Technic: Modified Irving Sterilization 381

PART THREE: VAGINAL OPERATIONS FOR BENIGN DISEASE

20. Nonmalignant Cervical Lesions and Their Treatment 387

- Congenital Pseudo-erosion 387
- Cervical Lacerations 388
- Cervicitis 388
- Stricture of the Cervix 392
- Cervical Polyps 393
- Leukoplakia of the Cervix 395
- Operative Procedures 396
- Cauterization of the Cervix 396
  - Technic: Cervical Cauterization 399
- Conization of the Cervix 400
  - Technic 401
- Amputation of the Cervix 401
  - Technic: Low Amputation of the Cervix 403
  - Technic: High Amputation of the Cervix 405
  - Technic: Sturmdorf Tracheloplasty 406
- Schröder Amputation 407
- Trachelorrhaphy 407
  - Technic: Trachelorrhaphy 408

21. Dilatation of the Cervix and Curettage of the Uterus 410

- Dilatation of the Cervix 410
  - Indications 410
  - Technic: Cervical Dilatation 411
- Curettage of the Uterus 412
  - Indications, Contraindications, and Anesthesia 412
  - Technic: Curettage of Uterus 414
  - Perforation of the Uterus 416
- Dysfunctional Uterine Bleeding 417
  - Symptoms 418
  - Pathophysiology 418
  - Pathology of Endometrial Hyperplasia 419
  - Etiology 420
  - Treatment of Dysfunctional Uterine Bleeding 420

22. Abortions 425
By Eleanor Delfs, M.D.

- Terminology 426
- Therapeutic Abortion 426
  - Legal and Medical Considerations 426
  - Methods of Therapeutic Abortion 430
- Habitual Abortion 437
  - Investigation of Recurrent Abortion 438
- Treatment of Uninfected, Afebrile Abortions—Threatened, Inevitable, Complete, and Incomplete 444
- Treatment of Infected Abortions 446
- Extra-uterine Septic Infection 448
  - Pathology 449
  - Treatment 450
- Perforation of the Pregnant Uterus 452

23. Congenital Absence of the Vagina ... 457

 Frank Nonsurgical Method of Making an Artificial Vagina ... 458
  Technic ... 458
 Wharton Operation for Construction of a Vagina ... 459
 McIndoe Operation ... 460
  Technic ... 461
  Complications and Results ... 466
 Partial Absence of the Vagina ... 466

24. Malpositions of the Uterus, Cervical Stump and Vagina ... 469

 Retrodisplacement of Uterus ... 469
  History ... 469
  Anatomical Considerations ... 470
  Symptomatology in Relations to Treatment ... 472
  Indications for Suspension ... 474
  Choice of Operations ... 474
  Ventrofixation in Relation to Retrodisplacement ... 479
 Prolapse of Uterus ... 479
  General Considerations ... 479
  Anatomical Considerations ... 480
  The Manchester (Donald or Fothergill) Operation ... 482
  The Watkins Transposition Operation ... 485
  The Vaginal Hysterectomy ... 489
  Te Linde-Mattingly Technic of Suspension of Vaginal Vault ... 500
  Technic of Anterior Colporrhapy ... 504
  The Spalding-Richardson Composite Operation for Uterine Prolapse and Allied Conditions ... 505
  Vaginal Plastic Operations Combined With Modified Gilliam Suspension of Uterus ... 512
  Ventral Fixation of Uterus or Cervical Stump for Prolapse ... 513
  The Le Fort Operation ... 513
  Goodall-Power Modification of Le Fort Operation ... 514
 Prolapse of the Vagina, With or Without Cervix, following Hysterectomy ... 518
  General Considerations ... 518
  Treatment ... 519
 The Use of Pessaries ... 527
  The Smith-Hodge Pessary ... 527
  The Ring and the Menge Pessaries ... 531

25. Urethrocele, Cystocele, and Stress Incontinence of Urine ... 534

 Urethrocele and Cystocele ... 534
  Treatment ... 536
  Technic: Repair of Cystocele ... 536
 Repair of Cystocele With Vaginal Hysterectomy ... 540
 Stress Incontinence of Urine ... 540
  Technic: Operation for Urethrocele and Plication of Vesical Sphincter for Stress Incontinence of Urine ... 544
  Results ... 547

26. Urinary Incontinence Not Curable by Sphincter Plication 548
By John H. Ridley, M.D.

    Historical Development of Operative Procedures 549
    Choice of Operation 551
    Preoperative Evaluation of the Bladder 553
    Operative Procedures 555
        Technic: The Goebell-Frangenheim-Stoeckel Procedure Using the Fascia Lata Strap 555
        Technic: Aldridge Modification of the Sling Operation 557
        Technic: Goebell-Frangenheim-Stoeckel Procedure (Original Technic)... 559
        Technic: The Transected Sling Modification 563
        Technic: The Marshall-Marchetti-Krantz Operation 565
    Postoperative Care 567
    Results 568
    Analysis of Failures 569

27. Surgical Conditions of the Urethra 572

    Urethral Caruncle 572
    Urethral Prolapse 573
    Cysts of Skene's Ducts 574
    Suburethral Cyst.. 576
    Diverticulum of the Urethra 577
    Carcinoma of the Urethra 581

28. Vesicovaginal and Urethrovaginal Fistulas 584

    History 584
    Etiology 585
    Symptoms and Diagnosis.. 586
    Treatment 588
        General Principles 588
        Technic: Closure of Small Vesicovaginal Fistula 592
        Technic: Standard Operation for Closure of Simple Vesicovaginal Fistula 594
        Technic: Operation for Large Vesicovaginal and Rectovaginal Fistulas, Following Irradiation for Advanced Carcinoma of the Cervix 599
        Technic: Operation for Restoration of Urethra and Urinary Incontinence 600
        Another Operation for Formation of Urethra and Restoration of Urinary Continence..................................... 600
        Technic: Operation for Urethrovesicovaginal Fistula 604
        Technic: Another Type of Operation for Repair of Urethrovesicovaginal Fistula, Involving Sphincter 607
        Technic: Latzko Operation for Vesicovaginal Fistula Following Total Hysterectomy 608
        Technic: Utilization of Latzko Method for Closure of Large Postirradiation Vesicovaginal Fistula 608
        Technic: Transabdominal Closure of Vesicovaginal Fistula 610
    Urinary Diversion 611
        Choice of Technic 611

28. Vesicovaginal and Urethrovaginal Fistulas (*Continued*)

- Transplantation of Ureters into the Sigmoid 612
  - Technic: Modified Coffey II Method 616
  - Technic: Cordonnier-Leadbetter Ureterosigmoid Anastomosis .. 617
  - Technic: Bricker's Ileal Loop Bladder Substitution 620

29. Relaxed Vaginal Outlet, Rectocele, and Enterocele 624

- Anatomic Considerations 624
- Symptoms of Relaxed Vaginal Outlet and Rectocele 625
- Repair of Relaxed Vaginal Outlet and Rectocele 626
  - Technic: The Most Conservative Perineal Repair 626
  - Technic: Simple Perineal Repair for Relaxed Vaginal Outlet Without Rectocele 626
  - Technic: Repair of Relaxed Vaginal Outlet and Moderate-Sized Rectocele 627
  - Technic: Repair of Large Rectocele 632
  - Technic: Repair of High Rectocele 634
- Enterocele 635
  - Technic: Repair of Enterocele 638
  - Technic: Repair of Enterocele From Within Abdomen (Moschowitz) 638
- Prevention and Repair of Enterocele in Connection With Vaginal Hysterectomy 639

30. Complete Perineal Lacerations and Rectovaginal Fistulas 641

- Complete Perineal Lacerations 641
  - General Considerations 641
  - Treatment 642
- Rectovaginal Fistulas 646
  - Causes and Symptoms 646
  - Diagnosis and Treatment 648
- Congenital Rectovaginal Fistulas 655
  - Treatment 657

PART FOUR: TREATMENT OF PELVIC TUMORS — BENIGN AND MALIGNANT

31. Surgical Conditions of the Vulva 665

- Fibroma and Fibromyoma of the Vulva 665
- Lipoma of the Vulva 665
- Hidradenoma (Sweat-Gland Tumor) of the Vulva 666
- Papillomata of the Vulva 669
- Cysts of the Vulva 671
  - Bartholin's-Gland Cysts 671
  - Other Cysts 673
- Kraurosis of the Vulva 674
- Leukoplakia of the Vulva 675
  - Clinical Characteristics 676
  - Treatment 676
- Paget's Disease of the Vulva 679
- Carcinoma in Situ of the Vulva 681
  - Diagnosis 682
  - Treatment 682

31. Surgical Conditions of the Vulva (*Continued*)

- Invasive Carcinoma of the Vulva 682
  - Symptoms and Diagnosis 683
  - Treatment 683
  - Complications 693
  - Mortality and Cure Rate 694
- Basal Cell Carcinoma of the Vulva 695
- Unusual Malignancies of the Vulvourethral Region 696
  - Melanoma of the Vulva 696
  - Carcinoma of Bartholin's Gland 697

32. The Epidemiology of Cancer of the Cervix 701

- Presymptomatic Diagnosis 702
- Etiology 705

33. Carcinoma in Situ of the Cervix 708

- The Microscopic Picture 708
- The Relation of Dysplasia to Carcinoma in Situ 713
- The Relation of Carcinoma in Situ to Invasive Cancer 715
- Diagnosis 719
- Colposcopy   *By Hugh J. Davis*, M.D. 722
- Treatment 723
- Treatment of Recurrences 724
- Microinvasive Carcinoma 724
  - Treatment 726
  - Technic: Modified Wertheim Hysterectomy for Microinvasive (Stage I A) Cervical Carcinoma 726

34. Invasive Carcinoma of the Cervix 732

- Classification 732
  - International Classification 732
  - Microscopic Classification 732
- The Diagnosis 736
- Choice of Treatment 737
  - Operative Results 738
  - Our Current Views on Treatment 741
  - Irradiation Results 741
- Technic of Irradiation 745
- Irradiation Therapy 747
- Dosimetry of Irradiation Therapy 749
- Radical Wertheim Hysterectomy 750
  - Preparation 750
  - Technic: Radical Wertheim Hysterectomy 751
- Complications of Radical Hysterectomy 764
- Adenocarcinoma 765
- Carcinoma of Cervix in Pregnancy 765
  - Diagnosis 766
  - Treatment 766

35. Pelvic Exenteration 771

- Indications 771
  - As Related to Stage of the Disease 772

35. Pelvic Exenteration (*Continued*)

- Contraindications ... 772
- Operative Procedure: Total Pelvic Exenteration ... 773
  - Urinary Diversion ... 774
  - Pelvic Lymphadenectomy ... 778
  - Deep Pelvic Dissection ... 780
  - Closure of the Pelvic Peritoneum ... 783
- Anterior Pelvic Exenteration ... 785
- Complications ... 785
- Cure Rate ... 786

36. Carcinoma of the Corpus Uteri ... 789

- General Considerations ... 789
- Histopathology in Relation to Prognosis ... 790
  - Histologic Grading ... 790
  - Histologic Types ... 792
- Associated Clinical Conditions ... 793
- Symptoms ... 794
- Diagnosis ... 795
- Clinical Staging and Factors Influencing Prognosis ... 796
- Treatment and Evaluation of Treatment ... 797
  - Plan of Therapy in Our Clinic ... 801
  - Technic: Total Hysterectomy for Carcinoma of the Corpus Uteri ... 803
- Treatment of Recurrent Endometrial Carcinoma ... 804
  - Radiation Therapy ... 804
  - Radical Surgery ... 805
  - Chemotherapy ... 805

37. Sarcoma of the Uterus ... 811

- Histology ... 812
- Diagnosis ... 813
- Treatment ... 813
- The Mixed Mesodermal Tumor ... 815

38. Adnexal Tumors ... 817

- General Considerations ... 817
- Gross Pathology in Relation to Treatment ... 818
- Physiologic (Retention) Cysts of the Ovary ... 818
- Neoplastic Cysts of the Ovary ... 820
- Benign Solid Tumors of the Ovary ... 826
- Meigs's Syndrome ... 828
- Primary Solid Carcinoma of the Ovary ... 829
- Primary Cystic Carcinoma of the Ovary ... 831
- Carcinoma in Dermoid Cysts ... 833
- Metastatic Ovarian Cancer ... 833
- Sarcoma ... 834
- Teratomas ... 834
- Dysgerminomas ... 834
- Functioning Tumors of the Ovary ... 835
  - Feminizing Group ... 835
  - Masculinizing Group ... 837

38. Adnexal Tumors (*Continued*)

- Gynandroblastoma 838
- Parovarian Cysts 838
- Bilateral Polycystic Ovaries: Stein-Leventhal Syndrome 839
    - Treatment 840
- Treatment of Ovarian Cancer 842
    - General Considerations 842
    - Classical Staging 843
    - Primary Surgery 843
    - Irradiation Therapy 845
    - Chemotherapy 846
    - Special Considerations 848
- Prognosis in Ovarian Carcinoma 848
- Technical Points in Ovarian Surgery 849
- Carcinoma of the Fallopian Tube 850
    - General Considerations 850
    - Pathology 851
    - Diagnostic Difficulties 851
    - Treatment 853

1

Historical Development of Pelvic Surgery

All specialties in medicine have evolved gradually. New specialties are still coming into existence as we learn more and more about each field. In the early days of medicine in the United States it was customary for one man to hold a chair of anatomy and surgery, obstetrics and gynecology being included with surgery. Philip Syng Physick, often considered the father of American surgery, held the first chair of surgery in the United States divorced from anatomy. This was at the University of Pennsylvania in 1805. At this time John Warren, the founder of Harvard Medical School, was its first professor of anatomy and surgery. Obstetrics was divorced from the chair of surgery during the first part of the 19th century. Although gynecology began to be identified as a specialty during this period, its separation from general surgery was more gradual. In fact, gynecology has not yet been completely divorced from general surgery in practice, although in almost all medical schools it is combined with obstetrics.

Oophorectomy—McDowell. Abdominal surgery may authentically be said to have begun in the back woods of Kentucky when Ephraim McDowell successfully removed a large ovarian tumor. He had studied under John Bell of London, who suggested the operation to McDowell, who carried it out in 1809. The operation was done without the benefit of anesthesia or asepsis. McDowell considered the operation an experiment, as it truly was, and frankly told the patient so. She agreed to accept the risk and demonstrated her faith in her doctor and the Lord by singing hymns during the operation. While McDowell was performing the operation, his house was surrounded by a crowd of the patient's friends, who intended to shoot or hang him if the patient died. Fortunately, she made a rapid recovery and lived for 32 years, to die at the age of 78. McDowells publication of his first three successful cases of "ovariotomy" (oophorectomy) marks the beginning of abdominal surgery. The operation fell into disrepute shortly after this, but was popularized by the brothers Atlee of Lancaster, Pennsylvania, about the middle of the 19th century.

Myomectomy. Amussat of France performed the first recorded myomectomy in 1840. In the United States the operation was done shortly thereafter by Washington Atlee. In 1850 Professor Mussey wrote: "Of all the achievements of modern surgery we meet with, none [is] more striking or extraordinary than the operation performed by Professor Atlee for the removal of fibrous tumors." A generation later J. Marian Sims wrote: "The name of Atlee stands without a rival in connection with uterine fibroids. His operations were so heroic that no man has as yet dared to imitate him." In more modern times Victor Bonney in England and Isadore Rubin in this country were the greatest advocates of myomectomy. Their enthusiasm exceeded that of most more recent gynecologists, but myo-

Hysterectomy. It was not until many years after "ovariotomy" was being done rather frequently and had met with some success that anyone successfully performed a hysterectomy. Myomectomy, as indicated above, was done before hysterectomy was attempted. In 1843 Charles Clay of Manchester removed a fibroid uterus. On the 12th day the patient was thought to be doing well, but on the 13th day, while the nurse was turning her in bed to arrange the bedding, she fell on the floor somewhat violently and died on the morning of the 15th day. The first completely successful removal of a fibroid uterus took place in Massachusetts in 1853. Dr. Walter Burnham of Lowell, while operating, was forced to remove the uterus without intending to do so. The abdomen had been opened to remove what was thought to be an ovarian cyst. Suddenly the patient vomited and extruded the fibroid uterus through the incision. The operator could not replace it and was forced to remove it. The patient survived, and Burnham was encouraged to attempt further hysterectomies. Of his next 15 cases, only 3 survived. It is no wonder that medical opinion of the day, as expressed by the editor of the *London Medico-Chirurgical Review,* was as follows: "We consider extirpation of the uterus, not previously protruded or inverted, one of the most cruel and unfeasible operations that ever was projected or executed by the head or hand of man." Professor Charles Meigs said in 1848 that it was hopeless to do anything with fibroids extending into the abdomen. Sir J. Y. Simpson, considered a daring surgeon at the middle of the 19th century, said that the idea of removing uterine fibroids should be rejected "as an utterly unjustifiable operation in surgery." Lawson Tait attempted to solve the fibroid problem by castration, by means of bilateral oophorectomy.

Vesicovaginal Fistulas — Sims. The history of vesicovaginal fistulas dates from antiquity. That they existed in ancient times is proven by the discovery of a large fistula in the mummy of Queen Henhenit, one of the wives of King Menuhotep, who reigned about 2050 B.C. Avicenna, an Arabo-Persian physician who died in 1037, was said to be the first to recognize that incontinence of urine in women may be due to a fistula resulting from difficult labor. He considered the condition incurable and advocated contraception in the very young as a preventative. Until the time of Sims in the mid-19th century there had been a long period during which attempts at cure had extremely limited success. Roonhuyse of Holland was one of the most ardent experimentors, and Lamelle of France reported some successes; but failures were much more frequent than successes. Mettauer of Virginia also struggled with the problem during this time.

During these preanesthesia and preasepsis days, a Southerner, Marion Sims, began his experiments on the cure of vesicovaginal fistulas. The term "experiments" is used advisedly, since 4 years of experimentation elapsed before his first success. Sims had had a successful career in surgery as practiced in those days in Montgomery, Alabama. He had had no experience in pelvic surgery. In fact, he disliked it. It was his custom to turn away patients with pelvic disorders, referring them to doctors whom he considered more competent in this field. His slave-holding planter friends owned female slaves who had been delivered by incompetent midwives, and some of these slaves suffered from huge vesicovaginal fistulas, then considered incurable. With this disturbing condition, the slaves were unacceptable as house servants. Whether motivated by selfish interests to rehabilitate valuable slaves or by human compassion, one cannot be sure, but one of Sims's planter friends pled with him to attempt to cure the women. At first Sims declined the task, believing it to be hopeless, but finally his compassion for the unfortunate women convinced him to undertake it. He worked on a group of these Negro women from 1845 to 1849 before attaining his first cure. During these years he housed and boarded the patients at his own expense in a small hospital that he constructed for this purpose on his own property. His many failures only stimulated his determination and efforts. The colleagues who at first assisted him at the operations forsook him, and his friends begged him to give up what appeared to be a hopeless effort; so he trained other slave patients to assist him in operating. His ultimate success he attributed to the use of the lateral position (now known as Sims's position), the use of silver wire sutures, and the use of special instruments which he devised. The most important and lasting of these instruments was Sims's speculum, which evolved from a pewter spoon he had used in earlier cases. His success in his small private hospital in Montgomery soon became known and took him to New York City, where he became one of the founders of the Woman's Hospital. From there his fame spread to the capitals of Europe, where he was received with the greatest esteem, and where he demonstrated his operative technic on several women with fistulas, which had been considered incurable. All his operations were done without asepsis and without anesthesia. During the 20th century Mahfouz of Egypt has reported on his vast experience with vesicovaginal fistulas utilizing the principles of Sims, with the great advantage of general anesthesia.

Anesthesia. Soporifics had been used from time immemorial to lessen the pain of surgery, but none was very successful. The discovery of general anesthesia by chloroform and ether is one of the most fascinating stories in medicine. It introduced a new era in surgery, and progress thereafter was rapid.

There is much discussion as to who first used chloroform as an anesthetic (discovered by the great German chemist Justus von Liebig in 1831), but it is certain that after a number of personal experiments with it, Simpson administered its beneficent fumes to a woman in the pangs of labor on November 4, 1847. He was the first to apply it in just this way and probably the first to use it for the relief of pain.

The discovery of ether as a general anesthetic was undoubtedly America's greatest contribution to medicine up to that time. A detailed account of the struggle for priority in this great discovery is not in order in this short review, but a few salient points may be of interest.

There is little doubt that Crawford Long, a practitioner in a rural community in Georgia, first used ether an an anesthetic in surgery. He was a simple, modest practitioner who did only such surgery as came his way in his general practice; the discovery was somewhat accidental. It was the custom in Long's rural community to hold "ether frolics." The participants would inhale the fumes and become quite intoxicated. During the cavorting about, the merrymakers often fell and bruised themselves. On questioning them, Long was surprised to learn that they had no recollection of falling and suffered no pain at the time of the injury. From this experience he conceived the idea that surgery might be made painless by the use of this drug. It was in 1842 that he first used it, though he did not publish his results until 1849.

While Long was using ether as a surgical anesthetic in Georgia, Horace Wells, a dentist, was experimenting with nitrous oxide and had some of his own teeth extracted under "laughing gas." After an untoward result, however, he abandoned its use. A chemist suggested to Morton, who was Wells's partner, that he use ether, and Morton persuaded John Collins Warren to use it in surgery at the Massachusetts General Hospital—which he did successfully in 1846. A month later this was reported by an observer of the operation, H. J. Bigelow. Thus the Massachusetts group was the first to publicize the use of ether anesthesia, although Crawford Long was the first to use it. Long would probably never have received recognition had it not been for Marion Sims' bringing it to the attention of the medical public in an article published in 1877. As a result of this, Long's statue now stands in the Hall of Fame in New York. In passing, it is of interest to note that Oliver Wendell Holmes suggested the name "anesthesia."

Asepsis, Antisepsis. The discovery of

general anesthesia opened the door to rapid progress in pelvic surgery, but other discoveries also stimulated its development. One of these was the proof by Semmelweis of the contagiousness of puerperal fever in the Vienna Krankenhaus. His work was published from Budapest, where he became professor in 1845. His insistence upon asepsis in the delivery room was responsible for a new era in obstetrics, but his principles were also adopted for surgery. Like many revolutionary discoveries, his ideas were rejected by his colleagues, who ridiculed and persecuted him, eventually forcing him to an insane asylum, where he died prematurely at the age of 47.

Another event that had a profound effect on the development of surgery was the work of Joseph Lord Lister, who explored the possibility of sterilizing the operating field to prevent the growth of pathogenic bacteria. His method of sterilizing not only the operative field but also the operating room by a carbolic spray was first used in 1865. His results were published 2 years later, and his ideas were widely adopted. It is noteworthy that whereas Lister's was the principle of antisepsis, Semmelweis' principle was one of asepsis by thorough scrubbing to sterilize the hands of the operator. So, not only did Semmelweis' work precede Lister's by 20 years, but his ideas were more advanced than those of Lister and corresponded more nearly to the customs of modern surgery. Pasteur further advanced the principles of surgical asepsis by advocating passage of the scalpel blade through a flame before using it.

With the adoption of general anesthesia and asepsis, the way was cleared for rapid progress in all fields of surgery.

Other Advances in Operative Gynecology, 1850–1900. T. A. Emmett, a Virginian who had migrated to New York, was Sims's illustrious pupil at the Woman's Hospital. He devised operations for the repair of the vagina and cervix. The Emmett vaginal repair has persisted, with some modifications, though the cervical repairs as done by Emmett are seldom used today. Emmett did not follow his master, Sims, as chief surgeon at the Woman's Hospital—not from lack of ability but because of personality clashes between him and the governing boards of the hospital.

During this era, progress was also being made in England in operative gynecology. Sir Thomas Spencer Wells performed many "ovariotomies" and published his ideas on the subject in his book *Diseases of the Ovaries*. He was one of the first in England to insist on the greatest cleanliness of the operator's hands and instruments. A little later a Scot, Robert Lawson Tait, transferred to London and Birmingham, made these cities the center of gynecologic surgery in England. He was a violent opponent of antisepsis and antagonistic in his personal relations to the profession.

In the United States, leadership in pelvic surgery was transferred from New York to Baltimore. Howard A. Kelly graduated from the University of Pennsylvania in 1882, the year before Sims died. He spent several years in postgraduate work in Germany when that country led the world in teaching pathology under Virchow and bacteriology under Koch. He was brought to Johns Hopkins as the head of gynecology and obstetrics in 1889, at the age of 31, by Welch and Osler, who had known him in Philadelphia. He was a bold and aggressive surgeon and was given carte blanche to develop his ideas at the new medical school. After several years, realizing that his real interest was in pelvic surgery, he turned the Department of Obstetrics over to J. Whitridge Williams, whose illustrious career in that specialty justified Kelly's decision. Kelly had great interest in the female urinary system, realizing that symptomatology of urinary tract disease is often intertwined with that of the reproductive organs. As a means of investigating these symptoms, Kelly invented the air cystoscope and devised ureteral catheters. He was the first to plicate the vesical sphincter for stress incontinence of urine. He also devised many technics and refinements of pelvic surgery, which were published in his *Operative Gynecology,*

Historical Development of Pelvic Surgery 5

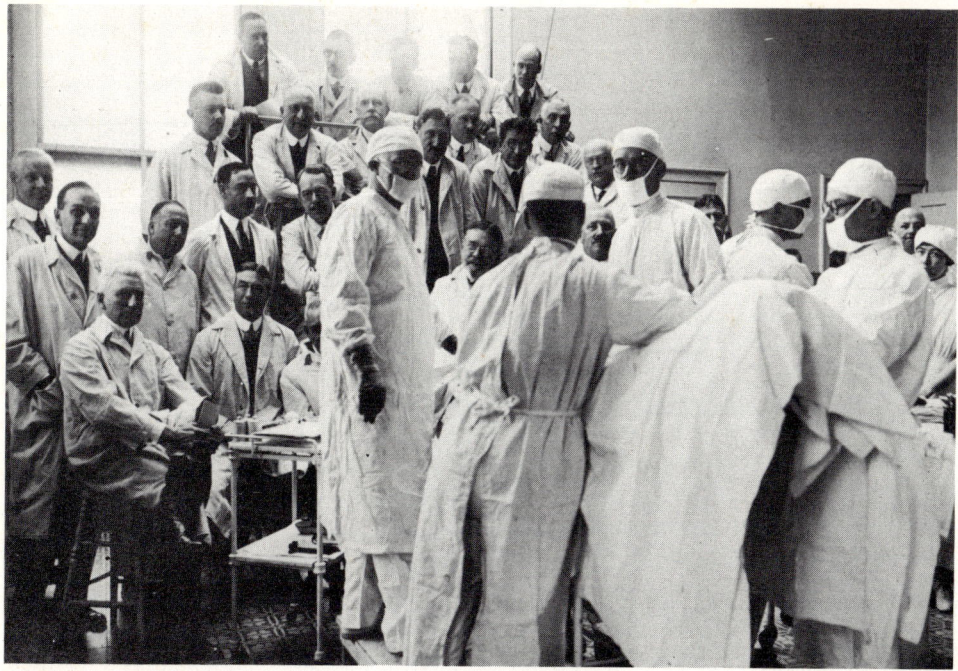

FIG. 1-1. Howard A. Kelly, operating before the American Gynecological Club in 1922.

the classic on that subject for many years. It was beautifully illustrated by Max Broedel, whom Kelly brought to the United States from Germany as a very young man. Broedel's contribution to operative gynecology was tremendous in his portrayal of operative technics and pathologic specimens. His contribution was great not only to gynecology but to all medicine. He set a standard for medical illustrating never before attained and unsurpassed since. His school for medical illustrators supplied medical artists to many medical centers throughout the United States.

Great as were Kelly's contributions to pelvic surgery, perhaps the most enduring results of his professorship at Johns Hopkins was his establishment of the long-term residency training program, which has been copied generally throughout the United States and to some extent in foreign countries. This plan for training pelvic surgeons has done more to elevate the quality of gynecology than any other factor.

Radium Therapy. Kelly's other great contribution was his pioneer work in radium therapy in gynecology in association with Curtis Burnam. In 1898 Marie Curie, born in Poland and then living in France, announced the discovery of a new element found in pitchblende which was radioactive. In this work she was assisted by her husband, Pierre, also an eminent scientist. Burnam, whom Kelly sent to France, obtained some radium from Madame Curie; Kelly eventually owned more radium personally than any other individual in the United States. Because of its great value, Burnam was afraid to permit the radium to be away from his person. He therefore carried it across the Atlantic in his vest pocket, receiving a skin burn on his chest wall that scarred him for life. The technics of administering radium as practiced by Kelly and Burnam have been greatly modified, but their work established a permanent place for irradiation therapy in gynecology.

Rubber Gloves. The use of rubber gloves was, of course, a great step in aseptic surgery. Although Halsted of

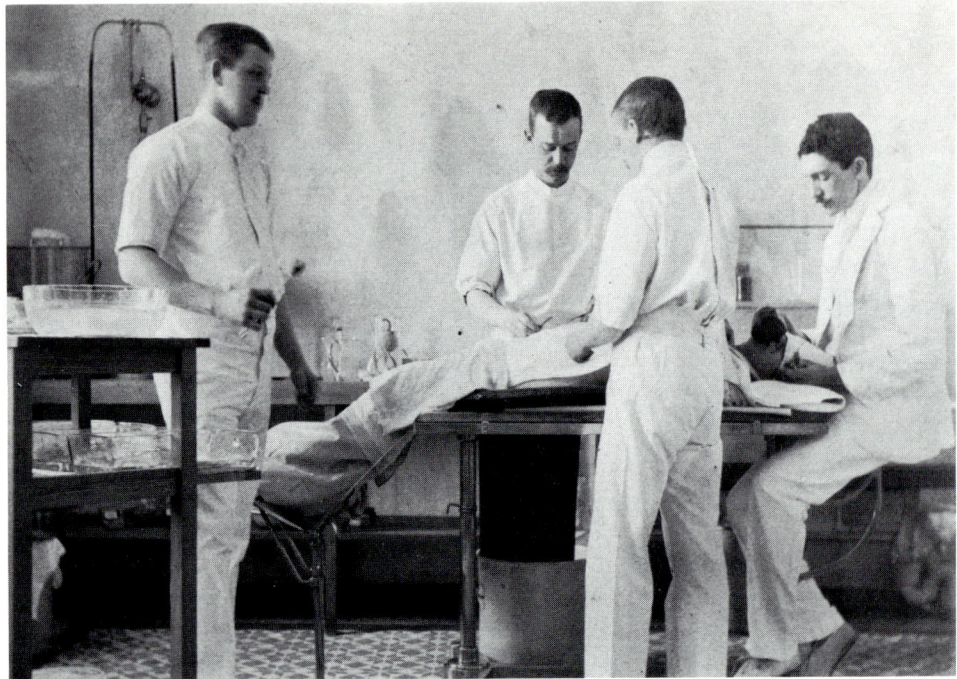

FIG. 1-2. Howard A. Kelly operating. Hunter Robb, his first resident, assisting. Robb was the first to suggest rubber gloves for the operator.

Hopkins is generally credited with the introduction of rubber gloves in surgery, the idea was not solely his. Halsted wrote:

The operating in gloves was an evolution rather than an inspiration or happy thought. In the winter of 1889 and 1890, I cannot recall the month, the nurse in charge of my operating room (later Mrs. Halsted) complained that the solutions of mercuric chloride produced a dermatitis of her arms and hands. As she was an unusually efficient woman, I gave the matter my consideration and one day in New York requested the Goodyear Rubber Company to make as an experiment two pair of thin rubber gloves with gauntlets. In the report which I made of the first year's work at the hospital, written in November and December, 1890, and published in March, 1891, I stated that the assistant who passed instruments wore rubber gloves to protect his hands from the solution of phenol—in which the instruments were submerged—rather than to eliminate him as a source of infection. I do not recall having referred again, in my publications, to the employment of rubber gloves. Dr. Hunter Robb in 1894 in his book on aseptic technique recommended that the operator wear rubber gloves. Dr. Robb was at that time resident gynaecologist of the Johns Hopkins Hospital.

A photograph taken in the Halsted clinic of a breast operation in 1893 shows that gloves were not being worn by him at that time. Halsted states further that it was remarkable that "we could have been so blind as not to have perceived the necessity of wearing them invariably at the operating table." So to Hunter Robb, a gynecologist, belongs the credit of recommending that the *operator* use rubber gloves.

Treatment of Cervical Cancer. The earliest attempts to cure cervical cancer were made by simple amputation of the cervix. Marie Anne Boivin had amputated a cervix which showed cancerous ulceration in the early part of the 19th century. Many others—Osiander, Dupuytren, Recamier, and Lisfranc—had performed the same operation. England was a long way behind France in the diagnosis and treatment of cervical cancer, possibly because of Victorian modesty, which prevented vaginal examinations except in the most desperate cases. Sir J. Y. Simpson attacked the problem in England and stressed the importance of early diagnosis. He wrote of cervical amputation: "It is one which can be employed only in very few cases of cancroid disease of the cervix, seeing that it is only when you can catch the disease, so to speak, before it has reached the line of reflexion between the cervix and the vagina, that you can amputate with any hope or prospect of success."

Following these failures with cervical amputation, simple hysterectomy was done. This, too, was generally unsuccessful, and it became evident that a more radical surgical approach would have to be taken if any measure of success was to be attained. In 1895 Emil Reis of Chicago attacked the problem and developed a radical abdominal operation with pelvic lymph gland dissection which he performed on dogs and cadavers. In that same year John Clark, the resident gynecologist at Johns Hopkins, employed this technic in women. His account of this undertaking in his own words is as follows: "After laying a plan before Dr. Kelly for the more complete extirpation of the uterus, the broad ligaments and a portion of the vagina and receiving his cordial endorsement and encouragment, I was granted the opportunity in April, 1895, to put into effect the principles embodied in the proposed operation." Three years later Wertheim of Vienna began doing the same radical abdominal type of hysterectomy and popularized it in Europe and to a less extent in the United States. His name has been associated with it since, although Clark was the first to perform the operation. Some success was attained with his radical procedure for the disease when limited to the cervix; but when the disease had progressed beyond this stage, the salvage was indeed small. The operation carried with it approximately a 10 per cent mortality, and ureteral, vesical, and rectal fistulas to the vagina were common. Sampson, who was later to become famous for his work on endometriosis, did special work on the blood supply of the ureter with the intention of attempting to preserve it and thus avoid fistulas from the extensive lymph node dissection. In spite of his work, the percentage of ureteral fistulas remained high.

Realizing the shortcomings of operative cure of this disease, Kelly experimented with radium therapy. He and the many gynecologists who followed his early attempts attained greater success in the overall salvage of cervical cancer than had been attained by surgery. Although fistulas and other complications occurred from radium therapy, they occurred most often in the advanced cases in which cure was impossible by surgery or irradiation.

In the 1940's Meigs at the Massachusetts General Hospital revived the Wertheim type of operation and even extended it. He believed that with the modern therapy at his disposal, such as antibiotics and intravenous control of the electrolytes, the operation should be reevaluated. He proved that in expert hands the operation could be done with a mortality rate of not over 1 per cent. He was unable, however, to reduce appreciably the incidence of fistulas.

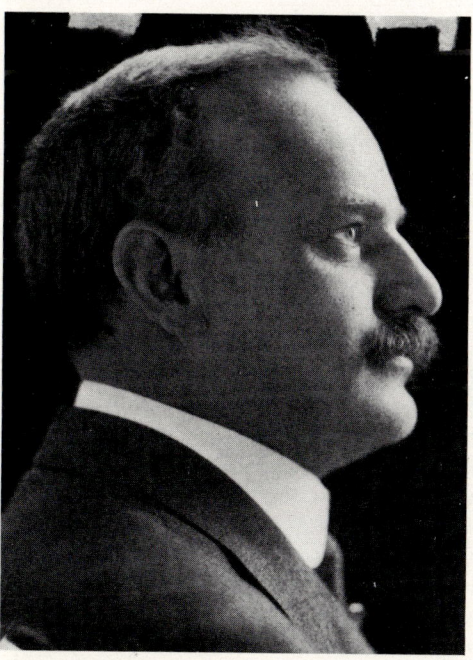

FIG. 1-3. Dr. John G. Clark, who performed the first radical abdominal operation for cervical cancer.

Another surgical approach to the treatment of cervical cancer was made in 1908 by Schauta, who published a volume on an extensive vaginal removal of the uterus and parametrium by the vaginal route, which he had first done in 1901. One of the greatest proponents of this operation was van Bouwdijk Bastiaanse of Amsterdam, but it never attained popularity in the United States. The great disadvantage of the procedure is that it does not permit a complete lymphadenectomy, as does the Wertheim procedure. However, the mortality rate in expert hands was only 3 to 4 per cent, in contrast to several times that percentage with the Wertheim procedure.

In spite of the attempts to eradicate the disease by vaginal and abdominal radical surgery, the salvage was meager when the disease had spread beyond the cervix; so today the therapy for invasive cervical cancer in most clinics is irradiation. At Johns Hopkins, the Wertheim type of operation is reserved for irradiation failures in cases falling into Stage I. The Schauta operation never attained appreciable popularity in the United States, but it is still used in a few European clinics.

More Milestones. Thomas S. Cullen succeeded Kelly to the chair at Hopkins in 1919. His contribution to pelvic surgery was indirect—the establishment of a gynecological pathological laboratory. This was somewhat accidental. He came to Baltimore after an internship in Toronto, intending to work with Kelly in pelvic surgery. But there was no position available on Kelly's surgical staff immediately, and to mark time he was sent to the Department of Pathology to work under William Welch. He established a laboratory of gynecological pathology which remains to this day. Cullen's book *Cancer of the Uterus* (1901) was published from this laboratory and was considered the classic on the subject for many years. Cullen was succeeded in his laboratory by Emil Novak, who published extensively from it, especially in the field of ovarian tumors. Thus, indirectly, with an understanding of the pathology of the pelvic organs, pelvic surgery was placed on a scientific rather than a purely technical level.

Endometriosis, one of the most common conditions requiring pelvic surgery, was first described by Russell in Cullen's laboratory in 1899. The disease was publicized by extensive studies of its histology by Sampson of Albany, who had been one of Kelly's early residents. His publications began in the early 1920's and extended to 1940. His theory of retrograde menstruation was the subject of great controversy during this period. It was greatly strengthened by the experimental work of Scott and Te Linde, who in 1950 created endometriosis artificially in monkeys by permitting them to menstruate into their peritoneal cavities, thus demonstrating the ability of the cast-off endometrium to grow on the serosal surfaces. The effect of hormones on this artificially created endometriosis was studied by Scott and Wharton, and Kistner of Boston has used progesterone therapeutically. However, the backbone of therapy remains surgical.

In the realm of vesicovaginal fistulas, the tenets of Sims still stand; however, Hunner introduced the practice of secondary drainage of the bladder through a catheter placed in a vaginal cystotomy incision. This has contributed greatly to the curability of difficult fistulas. Also, Latzko's contribution in 1914 of partial colpocleisis for high posthysterectomy fistulas was a major step in the curability of fistulas of this type.

Rectovaginal fistulas and third-degree tears are today curable in a much higher percentage of cases than before, due to three important milestones. The first of these dates from 1882, when Warren described his method of turning down a flap of vaginal mucosa. A second advance was made by the use of Sulfasuxidine and neomycin for bowel sterilization. Finally, the cutting of the anal sphincter, as described by Norman Miller in 1939, was a major step. This made possible the release of pressure from gas and feces, thus preventing the tying up of the bowels for several days after the operation. Prompt bowel evacuation is augmented by the use of Sulfasuxidine and mineral oil after operation.

In 1948 Alexander Brunschwig of New York published his radical surgical method of treating advanced and recurrent cervical cancer. It consisted essentially of exenterating adjacent pelvic organs and the generative organs, with diversion of the urine and/or feces, depending on whether the bladder or rectum or both were removed. Naturally, there was a high mortality and morbidity, and small salvage. There was a short-lived flurry of acceptance of this procedure, but it seems apparent at present that much of the former enthusiasm is waning. However, with ample blood replacement, antibiotics, and attention to electrolyte balance, these extensive procedures have found a limited place in the cure of cervical cancer in carefully selected cases.

Cytology and Carcinoma in Situ. The real advance in the cure of cervical cancer came about as the result of cytology and the recognition of carcinoma in situ. These two discoveries have worked hand in hand in the detection of cervical cancer in the microscopic and, hence, curable stage. Without cytology very few microscopic carcinomas would be discovered. Without the recognition and proper interpretation of the microscopic picture known as carcinoma in situ, cytology would be of little value. The first publication of Papanicolaou and Traut appeared in 1941. Subsequent publications by them and others, notably Ruth Graham, demonstrated beyond doubt the almost infallible value of cytology in detecting cervical cancer. In a publication by Walter Schiller of Vienna in 1927, and in many subsequent articles in the 1930's, he described a lesion in the surface epithelium of the cervix which we now recognize as carcinoma in situ. The same microscopic picture had been noted by Cullen, Isador Rubin, Schottlander, and Kermauner shortly after the turn of the century, but its relation to invasive cancer was not understood. This relationship was demonstrated by Galvin and Te Linde in an article published in 1944, and in several subsequent articles. Since then the literature has been replete with confirmation of this relationship, and early cervical cancer has become a curable disease.

Treatment of Uterine Prolapse. After the advent of anesthesia and asepsis, the surgical cure of uterine prolapse was first attempted. Up to that time pessaries of all types had been the vogue. Some of the first surgical attempts were made by ventrofixation, but this proved unsatisfactory, the results often being temporary. Various types of vaginal operations which rarely succeeded were: amputation of the elongated cervix; constriction of the vaginal outlet and reconstruction of the perineum; and operations for diminishing the caliber of the vagina, usually by removing a strip or triangle of mucosa and suturing the edges together. The almost complete union of the labia majora was tried in Germany. Then in 1888 A. Donald of Manchester and his assistant, Fothergill, devised what became known as the Manchester operation. This operation, with various minor modifications, still deservedly maintains a place in the cure of uterine prolapse.

There are still some differences of opinion on the best method of treating uterine prolapse and allied conditions. Vaginal hysterectomy with suitable plastic vaginal repair has gained wide acceptance in the United States. Among the contributors to our present knowledge are Watkins of Chicago (the interposition operation), Spalding of San Francisco and Richardson of Baltimore (the composite operation), Heaney of Chicago (the vaginal hysterectomy) and Le Fort of France. Heaney's greatest contribution was the development of a meticulous technic for the removal of the uterus vaginally, applicable in the removal of the benign uterus even when no prolapse exists.

Total Abdominal Hysterectomy. There has been a gradual change from subtotal to total abdominal hysterectomy for benign disease by most operators during the past 30 years. One of the major advances in technic, which has contributed greatly to the safety of total hysterectomy and subsequent avoidance of fistulas, was the description of the intrafascial removal of the uterus by E. H. Richardson of Baltimore in 1929. Total abdominal hysterectomy is now the most frequently performed of all major gynecologic operations, and it is rare indeed that ureteral or vesical fistulas result.

Treatment of Urinary Incontinence. Great progress has been made in the surgical cure of urinary incontinence in the present century. Simple plication of the sphincter with or without cystourethrocele repair fails to cure the condition in about 10 per cent of the cases. In 1910 Rudolf Goebell of Germany first used the pyramidalis muscles to give continence to a child with congenital incontinence (possibly spina bifida occulta). Frangenheim modified the original procedure by using a strip of rectus sheath attached to the pyramidalis muscles. Further modifications were made by Stoeckel in Germany and Aldridge in the United States, and out of this work there has evolved the so-called sling operation in its various modifications. In 1949 Victor Marshall and Andrew Marchetti of New York published their first results on vesicourethral suspension, which procedure has gained considerable popularity in the United States. The sling and vesicourethral suspensions have resulted in the cure of many cases of stress incontinence heretofore considered incurable.

Treatment of Congenital Malformations. Within the last 30 years great progress has been made in plastic procedures on congenital malformations of the female generative tract. Many ingenious operations have been devised for forming a vagina when it is congenitally absent. Among the originators of procedures now only of historical interest are Baldwin, Frank, Wharton, Graves, and Shirodkar. In 1938 McIndoe devised the simple method of lining the newly formed vaginal cavity with a split-thickness skin graft. The operation has been extremely successful in most hands and has made obsolete other methods, many of which are more complicated and more dangerous.

Paul Strassman of Berlin was the first to unify a double uterus in 1907. His operation was done through a transverse incision in the uterine fundus and merely bisected, without removing, the septum. More recently, an operation characterized by excision of the septum or the inner aspects of the two horns has been frequently and very successfully done. The procedure was described in 1953 by Jones and Jones.

The epochal work on intersexuality by a pediatrician, Lawson Wilkins, dating from 1940, opened the door for surgical work on reconstruction of the genitalia according to the child's physical and emotional instincts. This surgery was carried out chiefly by Howard Jones.

This short review of the development of pelvic surgery makes no pretense of being complete. It does, however, attempt to convey to the pelvic surgeon of today how our present technics—often taken for granted—were developed by the "blood, sweat, and tears" of those who preceded him, some of whom risked their professional reputation and even endangered their lives to take what they believed to be the right step into the unknown.

BIBLIOGRAPHY

Bonney, Victor: Technique and results of myomectomy. Lancet, *220*:171, 1931.

Castiglioni, Arturo: A History of Medicine. New York, Alfred A. Knopf, 1941.

Clark, J. G.: A more radical method of performing hysterectomy for cancer of the uterus. Bull. Johns Hopkins Hosp., 6:120, 1895.

de Lamelle, Jobert: Traite des Fistulas Vesicouterine et Vesico-Uterine Vaginales. Paris, 1892.

Galvin, G. A., and Te Linde, R. W.: The minimal histological changes in biopsies to justify a diagnosis of cervical cancer. Amer. J. Obstet. Gynec., *48*:774, 1944.

Graham, Harvey: Eternal Eve: The History

of Gynecology and Obstetrics. Garden City, N. Y., Doubleday & Co., 1951.

Halsted, W. S.: An Account of the Introduction of Gloves, etc. Menosha, Wis., George Banta Publishing Co., 1939.

Harris, Seale: Woman's Surgeon. New York, Macmillan, 1950.

Kelly, H. A.: Operative Gynecology. New York, Appleton & Co., 1898.

Latzko, William: Behandlung hochsitzender Blasen und Mastdarm Scheiden Fistlen Noch Uterus exterpetion Mit hohem Scheidenverschluss. Zbl. Gynaek., 38:906, 1914.

Mahfouz Bey, N. J.: Urinary and recto-vaginal fistulae in woman. J. Obstet. Gynaec. Brit. Empire., 36:581, 1929.

Mettauer, J. T.: Vesico-vaginal fistula. Boston Med. Surg. J., 22:154, 1840.

Richardson, E. H.: A simplified technique for abdominal panhysterectomy. Surg. Gynec. Obstet., 48:248, 1929.

Robb, Hunter: Aseptic Surgical Technique. Philadelphia, J. B. Lippincott, 1904.

Rubin, I. C.: Progress in myomectomy. Amer. J. Obstet. Gynec., 44:197, 1942.

Schiller, Walter: Untersuchen zur Entstehung der Geschulste, Collumcarzinom des Uterus. Virchow Arch. Path. Anat., 263:279, 1927.

Schottlander, J., and Kermauner, F.: Zur Kenntnis des Uterus Karzinoms. Berlin, Karger, 1912.

Sims, Marion: The Story of My Life. New York, D. Appleton & Co., 1884.

——: On the treatment of vesico-vaginal fistulas. Amer. J. Med. Sci., 23:59, 1852.

Te Linde, R. W., and Scott, R. B.: Experimental endometriosis. Amer. J. Obstet. Gynec., 60:1147, 1950.

Wertheim, E.: Zur Frage der Radical Operation beim Uterus Krebs. Arch. Gynak., 61:627, 1900.

PART ONE

Preoperative and Postoperative Management

2

Preoperative Care and Complications

A surgeon should not be judged solely on his technical skill. His philosophy may be equally and, at times, more important to the patient. It is a delight to see a technically perfect surgeon, but if the operation which he performs is not done on good solid indications, the patient may suffer a loss rather than gain. Too often a patient is subjected to an unnecessary operation or a major procedure when a minor one would have sufficed. Not infrequently the surgeon operates without knowledge of the basic pathologic lesion and without having conducted a proper diagnostic investigation.

Surgery may be indicated on sound grounds, or it may be done without defensible indications. It may be adequate or inadequate. It may be excessive and only add to the patient's misery. Before performing surgery, the surgeon would do well to consider the three indications for surgery laid down by the late J. M. T. Finney. As students we frequently heard them, and they are, in the mind of the authors, worthy of repetition.

1. To save life.
2. To relieve suffering.
3. To correct deformity.

If a surgeon cannot justify his contemplated surgery on the basis of one of these indications, he should take another long look at the problem.

HISTORY-TAKING

The preoperative care of the patient begins in the office or outpatient department with the careful taking of a complete history. Good history-taking, careful preoperative examination, and the preparation of the patient physically and mentally are essential to good surgical results. No matter how busy the gynecologist may be, it is strongly recommended that he take the history personally. Only by this personal contact with the patient can he properly evaluate the symptoms and thus be guided diagnostically as well as at the operating table, where a knowledge of the temperament and symptoms of the patient is often of great value in making decisions. The importance of psychiatry in gynecology has never been sufficiently stressed, and the personal talk between patient and physician, when she comes to him for advice, may result in great benefit to the patient. Personal contact is also of the greatest value to the physician in permitting him to get an overall picture of the patient and to be guided in his evaluation of the case by this, rather than simply by his findings on pelvic examination. The maxim that "the patient will tell you what is wrong with her, if you will only give her time" is too often disregarded by the busy surgeon. Good history-taking requires time and patience, and neither of these is found easily in the busy routine of a surgical career. However, the reward for following such a course is the avoidance of unnecessary operations. Such operations, particularly upon neurotic women or those mentally troubled by some difficult problem of life, are not only useless but tend to concentrate the attention of the patient upon the pelvic organs and to aggravate invalidism.

The history should be concise, but accuracy should not be sacrificed for the sake of brevity. For several years it has been our custom to use the form shown below in obtaining the history. There are objections to such a form, for no one has ever devised a perfect form for every case. However, if one uses records for clinical research, important omissions are much rarer when information is compiled on a form. No form is utilized in recording the present illness, and the greatest freedom is permitted the physician in his notes on the present condition. Often there are events in the patient's history that do not fit into the above form but have an important bearing on the present illness; these, too, may be recorded properly and completely in connection with the present illness.

A few points which should be stressed in taking a gynecologic history are discussed below:

The menstrual history must be accurate and detailed, since the clue to a correct diagnosis of the lesion for which surgery is considered often appears in the menstrual irregularity. This holds true whether there is an organic lesion or a functional menstrual upset. In fact, differentiation between functional and early organic disease is one of the most common and difficult distinctions to make. Of major significance are accurate dates of the latest and the previous menstrual periods. When there is a great discrepancy between the menstrual dates and the pelvic findings in suspected pregnancy, the pregnancy tests are invaluable; but these tests are not infallible, and one may have to overrule the results of the test on the basis of one's pelvic findings and clinical judgment.

The marital history is of great importance in the gynecologic history, with particular reference to pregnancies and their complications—dystocia, postpartum infections, abortions, urinary-tract infections, vaginal tears, embolisms, and so on. A knowledge of these complications aids the surgeon greatly in his evaluation of the patient and in determining the preoperative studies and postoperative measures necessary to obviate com-

---

Name.. Age................ Date ....
Address... Reference.................. Phone ....
Complaint...
General Health ....
Menstrual Age Onset .... L.M.P. .... P.M.P. ....
Interval .... Duration ...... Amount.................... Pain............
Intermenstrual Bleeding... Leukorrhea..................
Married........... yrs. Children .... oldest.............. youngest ...... Abortions......
Urinary...
Rectal...
Operations...
Present Illness ....

plications during and after operation. A well-taken marital history may reveal unsatisfactory sexual relations which may, in turn, explain symptoms resembling those due to organic pelvic disease.

The symptomatology of the urinary tract is so closely related to that of the generative tract that in many instances a more or less complete urologic investigation is necessary before making a diagnosis and a decision as to treatment. All too commonly, women have vaginal plastic and suspension operations for symptoms of frequency, urgency, and dysuria, while the real lesion lies undiagnosed in the urinary tract. It is well to remember that a primary urinary-tract disorder may give rise to symptoms suggestive of generative-tract disease, and vice versa. For this reason we have advocated urologic training for every gynecologist. The gynecologist who is adept at using the cystoscope is far better able to evaluate the case than one who must depend on the urologist's report.

GYNECOLOGIC EXAMINATION

It is incumbent upon the gynecologist to make a complete assessment of the medical as well as the gynecologic diseases in the female. Frequently he is the only physician who has seen the patient, particularly if she seeks medical advice initially about a problem involving the reproductive tract. It is important, therefore, that a complete examination be performed, which must include blood pressure, weight, examination of the thyroid and heart, auscultation of the chest, and examination of the breast, abdomen, and pelvis. Particular importance must be placed on any evidence of abnormal sexual development, including ambiguity of the external and internal female genitalia and abnormal hair growth of the extremities, chest, abdomen, and pubic regions. A critical evaluation of cardiac and pulmonary function must be the responsibility of the gynecologist prior to any proposed surgical procedure; in the event that additional consultation is required, this must be determined prior to administering a general anesthetic. A meticulously collected midstream, "clean catch" or catherterized urine specimen should be examined and cultured in all cases in which the symptoms even remotely suggest the possibility of urinary-tract disease. Although there is a reported 2 to 3 per cent incidence of urinary-tract infection or significant bacteriuria (Kass) following catheterization, recent evidence suggests that most reports of such complication are from patients in whom urinary-tract infections or abnormal bladder function existed prior to the catheterization. Hence we still believe that catheterization of the female bladder, if properly performed, is not a serious hazard to the normal bladder and may provide valuable information in the total appreciation of the patient's gynecologic symptoms.

Breasts are first inspected as to symmetry, size, and the condition of the nipples and the superficial blood vessels. Normal breast tissue, which feels rather shotty with the fingertips, is often erroneously considered to be tumor by patients and even by physicians who are unfamiliar with the proper method of breast palpation. Breasts should be felt with the flat surface of the fingers and the palm; a neoplasm almost always will be detected in this manner. The breasts are then milked gently, and the presence and character of secretion are noted. Papanicolaou smear of breast secretions has recently been reported by Masukawa to reveal very early cases of breast carcinoma prior to a demonstrable gross lesion. The finding of secretion often gives valuable information when pregnancy is suspected, but colostrum-like secretion is not uncommon in parous women many years after the last child, and occasionally it is found in women who have never been pregnant.

Abdomen. Examination of the abdomen includes inspection and palpation; percussion and auscultation are also useful. Bulging of the flanks suggests free abdominal fluid, but thin-walled ovarian cysts and irregularly shaped fibroids may give a similar picture. Although large ovarian cysts and fibroids more commonly cause protrusion anteriorly, there are many confusing exceptions. Palpation for a fluid wave is a useful procedure. Percussion for areas of flatness and tympany may aid in determining whether distention is due to fluid or to gas. Areas of localized tympany can be due to intestine between tumor masses. Auscultation is especially useful in differentiating large tumors from advanced pregnancy and in evaluating intestinal activity.

Pelvis and Rectum. An accurate clinical evaluation of the female reproductive tract is essential in establishing an accurate diagnosis of the underlying pathology of the patient's gynecologic symptoms. While a detailed description of a pelvic examination is not given here, it is important to stress some of the steps in evaluating the female pelvis. The bladder should be emptied either by voiding or catheterization prior to an adequate pelvic examination. If the patient has urinary-tract symptoms, a catheterized specimen should be obtained for complete urinalysis and for culture and sensitivity studies. Should the patient complain of urinary incontinence, she should be examined with a full bladder to demonstrate stress incontinence of the urethral sphincter. On inspecting the vulva for gross lesions, the Bartholin's and Skene's glands should be examined for evidence of cyst formation and purulent exudate as sources of previous gynecologic infection. The outlet should be closely inspected for relaxation of the anterior and posterior vaginal walls, and the vagina mucosa should be observed for infection and estrogen effect. The patient should be encouraged to bear down and cough to demonstrate the degree of uterine descensus, without the use of a tenaculum. The urethra should be milked along its entire length for a possible suburethral diverticulum—often manifested by the expression of purulent material from the urethral meatus or by a suburethral tender mass, found on palpation. The cervix should be grossly evaluated for abnormal pathology, particularly ulceration, eversion, and abnormal discharge. A Papanicolaou smear, combining a sample of posterior vaginal pool material with a sample of cells scraped from the entire circumferential external os and endocervical canal, is essential for every gynecologic patient prior to proposed pelvic surgery. A separate smear, aspirated from the endocervical canal, is extremely valuable in detecting endocervical and endometrial lesions and should always be used in suspect cases. A patient should not undergo pelvic surgery without complete knowledge of the cytologic report of the cervix within the past 6 months. In view of the fact that 70 to 80 per cent of all preclinical malignancies of the cervix demonstrate no significant gross lesion, it is impossible to be certain of the pathologic condition of the cervix without a Pap smear and/or cervical biopsy. The uterus is examined bimanually by the abdominovaginal route for position, size, mobility, regularity, and tenderness to motion. Both adnexal regions are evaluated vaginally and by rectovaginal examination. Rectal examination should never be neglected in the routine pelvic examination: in addition to giving information regarding the anus and rectum, it is confirmatory in detecting pelvic pathology and especially in evaluating the broad and uterosacral ligaments, the cul de sac, the uterus, and the adnexa.

In this procedure the index finger is inserted into the vagina and the middle finger into the rectum (Fig. 2-1). This permits examination of the rectum up to a higher point than when examined with the index finger. When the pelvic findings are doubtful or inconclusive, a more adequate examination should be done under general anesthesia before making a final decision for or against surgery. In fact, an adequate pelvic examination under anesthesia should always precede any gynecologic procedure, whether major or minor. Frequently, suspected pelvic pathology is completely ruled out by an adequate pelvic examination under anesthesia, and a needless laparotomy is avoided. The most common area of con-

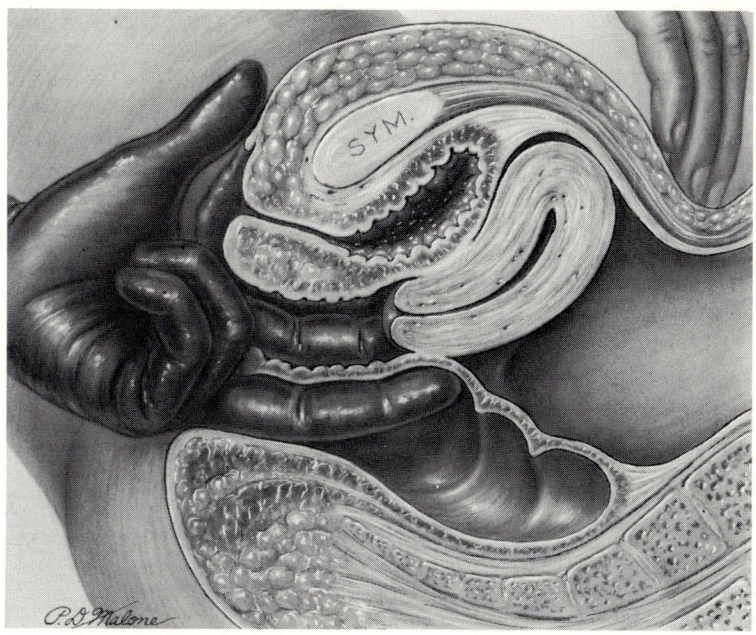

Fig. 2-1. Demonstrating recto-vagino-abdominal examination.

flict is in establishing the presence of an ovarian cyst, which may be mistaken for bowel, bladder, or uterine fibroid. If a normal ovary can be palpated, and a cyst is not identified under anesthesia, the patient has been spared a needless operative procedure. All patients having a dilatation and curettage should be thoroughly examined under anesthesia, and the pelvic organs should be described in detail for future reference.

LABORATORY EXAMINATIONS

A hemoglobin, a hematocrit, a white blood count, a differential white blood count, and a urinalysis should be a part of every preoperative work-up of a gynecologic patient. Patients having extensive pelvic surgery should also have blood-volume studies prior to surgery. A history or symptoms suggestive of hepatic, renal, or metabolic disease should be thoroughly investigated by liver function studies, with fasting and 2-hour postprandial blood sugar levels, total protein with A/G ratio, thymol turbidity, cephalin flocculation, prothrombin time, and total bilirubin. For all patients having extensive pelvic surgery, electrolyte studies are essential as a basis for postoperative fluid and electrolyte replacement. These should include sodium, potassium, chloride, CO_2, blood urea nitrogen, and phenolsulfonphthalein tests. An intravenous pyelogram should be obtained when indicated by renal symptoms. Chest x-ray with anterioposterior and lateral views are routine hospital admission procedures. Patients over the age of 40 should have an electrocardiogram prior to major pelvic surgery. When advanced or recurrent pelvic malignancy is present or suspected, the pelvis and long bones should be x-rayed for possible metastatic disease. When masculinizing or feminizing ovarian tumors are suspected, 24-hour urine for 17-ketosteroids and total urinary estrogens are frequently helpful.

TABLE 2-1. NORMAL VALUES FOR ROUTINE CLINICAL LABORATORY DETERMINATIONS

Constituent	Sample	Normal Range
Amylase	Urine	200-400 U./hr./vol.
Amylase	Serum	50-180 U.
Bilirubin	Serum	Conjugated: up to 0.35 mg./100 ml. Total: up to 1.5 mg./100 ml.
BSP	Serum	Less than 5% retention at 45 min.
Calcium	Serum	9.0-11.0 mg./100 ml.
Calcium	Urine	50-200 mg./24 hr.
CO_2 content	Venous serum	24-32 mEq./L.
Cephalin–cholesterol flocculation	Serum	0-1 + at 24 hr.
Cholesterol	Serum	100-350 mg./100 ml.
Chloride	Serum	96-109 mEq./L.
Chloride	CSF	122-132 mEq./L.
Creatinine	Serum	0.8-1.4 mg./100 ml.
Creatinine	Urine	800-1,900 mg./24 hr.
Electrolytes Na K CO_2 content Cl	Serum	135-148 mEq./L. 3.6-5.5 mEq./L. 24-32 mEq./L. 96-109 mEq./L.
Fibrinogen	Plasma	200-400 mg./100 ml.
Glucose	Serum	65-110 mg./100 ml.
Glucose	CSF	50-75 mg./100 ml.
Hemoglobin	Serum	Up to 5 mg./100 ml.
5-Hydroxyindoleacetic acid	Urine	10 mg./24 hr.
Iron	Serum	50-170 μg./100 ml.
Iron-binding capacity, total		265-425 μg./100 ml.
17-ketosteroids	Urine	6-15 mg./day
LDH (lactic dehydrogenase)	Serum	60-130 Wacker U.
Lipids, total	Serum	533-765 mg./100 ml.
Osmolality	Serum	290 ± 10

TABLE 2-1. NORMAL VALUES FOR ROUTINE CLINICAL LABORATORY DETERMINATIONS—(*Cont.*)

Constituent	Sample	Normal Range	
PBI (protein-bound iodine)	Serum	4-8 µg./100 ml.	
Phosphatase, alkaline	Serum	2-15 King-Armstrong U.	
Phosphorus, inorganic	Serum	2.5-4.8 mg./100 ml.	
pH, blood	Venous	7.32-7.39	
pH, blood	Arterial	7.35-7.42	
Potassium	Serum Urine	3.6-5.5 mEq./L. 40-65 mEq./24 hr.	

Protein
  Total
  Albumin
  Globulin
	Serum	6.2-8.5 gm./100 ml.
		3.5-5.0 gm./100 ml.
		2.5-3.5 gm./100 ml.	

Protein	Serum electrophoresis	*% Total Protein*	*gm./100 ml.*
Albumin		52-67	3.5-5.0
Alpha$_1$ globulin		2.5-4.5	0.1-0.4
Alpha$_2$ globulin		6.5-13.5	0.5-1.0
Beta globulin		9.0-14.5	0.6-1.2
Gamma globulin		9.0-21.0	0.6-1.6
Protein	CSF	15-45 mg./100 ml.	
Protein	Urine	Up to 100 mg./24 hr.	

PSP (phenolsulfonphthalein) excretion (6 mg. dye)
  0-15 min.
  15-30 min.
  30-60 min.
	
	Urine
	Urine
	Urine
		
		25-35% dye excreted
		15-25% dye excreted
		10-15% dye excreted	

Sodium	Serum	135-148 mEq./L.	
Sodium	Urine	130-200 mEq./24 hr.	
Thymol turbidity	Serum	Less than 5 U.	
Transaminase (SGOT)	Serum	0-36 Karmen U.	
Urea nitrogen (SUN) (BUN)	Serum	5-20 mg./100 ml.	
Uric acid	Serum	2.0-7.0 mg./100 ml.	
Uric acid	Urine	250-750 mg./24 hr.	
Urobilinogen	Feces	30-200 mg./100 gm.	
Urobilinogen	Urine	Up to 1.0 Ehrlich U./2 hr.	

PREOPERATIVE EVALUATION

The outcome of pelvic surgery is related to three major factors: (1) the severity and reversibility of coexisting organic disease, (2) the presence of a surgically resectable or medically treatable gynecologic disease, and (3) the skill and judgment of the pelvic surgeon and his knowledge of the disease process. Diminished cardiac, pulmonary, and renal reserve produce an unstable physiologic background for extensive or emergency surgery. Arteriosclerosis with its ischemic and compromising effect on these organs produces myocardial changes detectable by electrocardiogram in more than 75 per cent of such patients. Digitalization should be afforded all patients in whom there is significant disfunction as evidence by right and left ventricular failure. The merits of prophylactic digitalization are debated in academic circles, but when extensive surgery and blood loss is anticipated, it should be used to its fullest advantage.

Dehydration and hypovolemia are serious and frequently critical factors in the surgical risk of the gynecologic patient. Blood-volume studies utilizing radioactive chromium or similar technics are of valuable assistance in replacing the intravascular plasma volume and red cell mass. Without adequate replacement prior to surgery, such patients are unable to tolerate even minor blood loss without serious risk of vasomotor collapse and acute renal tubular nephrosis. In an effort to maintain an adequate urinary output of approximately 50 to 60 cc. per hour, it is necessary to avoid dehydration for any prolonged period of time preoperatively, during the operation, or postoperatively. Proper hydration is assured if approximately 250 to 300 cc. per hour of intravenous fluids is given during surgery. Because of the lack of resilience of the cardiovascular tree in elderly gynecologic patients, adequate blood replacement during surgery is essential and warrants the risk of cardiac decompensation in order to avoid the devitalizing effects of shock and hypoxia.

Chronic pulmonary disease is a frequent respiratory complication, although less so in the female than in the male. Such anatomic changes in the bronchial tree and alveoli produce an excellent environment for chronic respiratory infection, impaired oxygen exchange, and respiratory acidosis. Bronchial pneumonia in such a setting is difficult to control and is one of the major postoperative complications terminating in death.

Particular preoperative attention must be given to the elderly gynecologic patient, whose cardiac-pulmonary-renal reserve requires meticulous evaluation and preoperative correction of any physiologic and pathologic abnormality. In a recent survey of 500 surgical patients 80 years of age or older at Milwaukee County General Hospital, Carey noted the following preoperative complications: (1) nearly one third were malnourished (below 100 pounds), (2) anemia was present in 15 per cent of those cases, and 1 in 4 required preoperative blood transfusions, (3) hypertension, cardiomegaly, or arteriosclerotic heart disease was present in more than 50 per cent of the cases, and the EKG was abnormal in 80 per cent, and (4) acute and/or chronic lung disease was present in over 25 per cent. Of paramount importance is the fact that the mortality rate of such patients is 4 to 5 times higher than the expected rate when emergency surgery prevents the proper evaluation and preparation of such patients.

AGE AS A FACTOR IN PELVIC SURGERY

The chronologic age of a patient is no longer an accurate indicator of biologic function. The female is unique in her ability to maintain an "endocrinologic immunity" to atheromatous changes in the cardiovascular system until she is well past the climacteric. This biologic phenomenon is but one of the many factors which promote increasing longevity in the female. With increased interest in the entire field of geriatrics, the past half-century has witnessed an increase in the average life-span of the female to the age of 70. Since the turn of the 20th century, the number of persons aged 65 or over has quadrupled, whereas the general population has only doubled.

The predictable life expectancy at various ages in the elderly has likewise changed. According to actuarial life tables, an 80-year-old has a life expectancy of 6.5 years; at 85 there is a 5-year expectancy, and at 90 years, a 3.5-year expectancy. It is an acknowledged fact that such changes in longevity have revolutionized the surgical approach toward the aging female.

Many clinics, similar to that reported by Powers, show the current incidence of major surgery to be highest in the 60- to 69-year age group. However, when combined with precise medical control of concurrent disease, physiologic and pharmacologic competence in the fields of anesthesiology, and excellence of surgical skill, pelvic surgery in the aging female has relatively unlimited potential.

DISCUSSION OF THE NECESSARY OPERATIVE PROCEDURE

Once it has been concluded that surgery is necessary, the patient and at least one responsible member of the family should be informed. The manner of doing this is extremely important. No matter how busy the surgeon is, a brief explanation of the situation is greatly appreciated by the patient and her relatives. Apparently some surgeons proceed on the assumption that their valuable time should not be spent in attempting to give the layman an understanding of the surgical situation. We do not subscribe to this thought and believe that every patient and her family are entitled to a simple explanation of the problem involved. During this interview the surgeon may gain or lose the confidence of the patient, and this confidence is an extremely important asset for the surgeon, as well as for the patient, during the convalescent period. One must judge the patient carefully and choose one's words according to her temperament and intelligence. Often it is wise to discuss the situation first with a relative or close friend and to obtain the advice of this person—who knows the patient much better than the surgeon does—on how the patient should be approached. This is particulary true if a question of malignancy is involved. It is our custom always to be perfectly frank with the responsible relative, but only the exceptional patient should be told that she has cancer. Preoperatively, when malignancy is only suspected, it is clearly unwise to terrify the patient by mentioning the possiblity of cancer—unless this becomes necessary in order to convince her that she should submit to the necessary diagnostic or operative procedures.

Since curettage to rule out or establish a diagnosis of malignancy is the commonest gynecologic operation, it is often necessary to provide an adequate reason to operate for what the patient considers a minor symptom. It is our custom to tell the patient that the curettage is to be done for the dual purpose of diagnosing the cause of the bleeding and of stopping it, if possible. If malignancy is discovered, and radical surgery and/or irradiation become necessary, the patient is usually told that a condition has been found which, if neglected and not treated as recommended, might lead to cancer. In almost every instance such a statement is strong enough to persuade the patient to consent to any necessary therapeutic measures.

When a pelvic condition is found which requires surgery but is obviously benign, the patient is told the facts frankly, and the reason for surgery is explained to her in layman's terms. The danger involved in the contemplated surgery is faced squarely, and the truth is told to the patient and/or the family.

When a sterilizing operation is contemplated, such as bilateral salpingectomy, hysterectomy, or a pelvic operation with complete ablation of the ovaries, the possibility should be discussed openly with the patient. The attitude of women toward the loss of any of their sexual organs is quite variable. Not infrequently a woman regards the loss of her uterus as a blessing—if it has been the source of trouble to her for a long time. More often women forfeit any of their pelvic organs very reluctantly, and many young women view a sterilizing operation as a major catastrophy. When radical ovarian surgery becomes necessary, the surgeon should not regard it lightly. It is far better to assume a serious, sympathetic and yet encouraging attitude. The patient may be honestly assured that the symptoms of surgical menopause may be greatly allayed by estrogenic therapy, and the menopause of today is not to be dreaded as it was four decades ago.

Some women attempt to exact a promise from their surgeon that he will not, under any circumstances, remove certain organs. It is our custom never to operate under such restrictions; if one does, sooner or later one will encounter difficulties. Even with the most complete preoperative investigation, unsuspected conditions are occasionally encountered which should be handled according to the best judgment of the surgeon at the operating table, unhampered by preoperative promises of conservatism. The surgeon can safely tell the patient that he is a firm believer in conservative pelvic surgery, when indicated, and that he will be conservative if this is compatible with cure. Further promises should not be made.

Closing the door to the possibility of future pregnancy naturally upsets many otherwise stable young women. This is usually due to real disappointment in being unable to have children, but not infrequently there is confusion in their minds about their ability to carry on satisfactory marital relations following removal of certain pelvic organs. They should be comforted with the thought that matrimony need not be given up and should be told that there is no reason why marital relations may not be normal after most gynecologic operations. The possibility of adopting children should be held out to them; any experienced gynecologist or social worker can cite many homes that have been made happy by successful adoptions.

Little is gained from a technically perfect operation if the patient suffers remorse for the rest of her life on realizing what has been done. It is far better to discuss the situation frankly with the woman before an operation and to encourage a receptive frame of mind for the operation. Subsequently she will be able to adjust herself much more easily, and, incidentally, she will think more kindly of her surgeon for having fully gone into the matter preoperatively, rather than brutally telling her of the accomplished deed.

As soon as the patient has been impressed with the necessity of the operation and has given her consent, it is generally wise to make hospital arrangements without delay. If the operation is an emergency, the patient should be informed of it, and the surgery should be done immediately; even when the condition does not constitute an emergency, it is better not to procrastinate. To some individuals the anticipation of surgery is worse than the realization. If the operation is postponed, the patient will probably discuss it with family and friends, who often unthinkingly tell the patient about all the bad surgical results of which they have heard. A woman in whom only a hysterectomy is contemplated may be told of a friend's tragic artificial menopause, brought on by a "hysterectomy." The fact that a bilateral oophorectomy was involved is probably not even recognized, and the tale does unnecessary damage to the prospective patient's nervous system. Delay only heightens the patient's anxiety; when the job is inevitable, it is better to proceed with it as soon as possible.

Occasionally patients are encountered who, in spite of the urgent necessity of surgical care, flatly refuse an operation. Such patients and their families should be given the facts and the surgeon's recommendations in plain language, although they should not be "talked into" the operation. In our experience, such patients almost always return for the operation after a family conference, and sometimes after having obtained confirmatory surgical opinions from other doctors. If necessary, such cases should be followed up by a social service worker.

PREPARATION OF PATIENT FOR OPERATION

A vaginal suppository of nitrofurazone, inserted in the posterior fornix two or three nights preceding surgery, has been useful in decreasing the frequency of cuff cellulitis postoperatively. Many gynecologists routinely prepare the atrophic vagina of the postmenopausal patient with estrogen vaginal suppositories for 4 to 6 weeks preoperatively. This has been particular useful in vaginal surgery in which thickening the vaginal mucosa makes the tissues easier to dissect.

The evening meal on the day before an operation should be light and easily digestible. Overloading the alimentary tract shortly before the operation is particularly hazardous, not only as an anesthetic risk but also because it increases postoperative discomfort from nausea and gas formation. It is important that the patient have an adequate night's rest prior to the operation. Since the hospital environment usually causes apprehension, a mild sedative is advisable to ensure a good night's sleep. We commonly use Seconal, Nembutal, Doriden or chloral hydrate in moderate dosage.

The patient should be in the fasting state overnight, with nothing by mouth unless the operation is scheduled for late in the day. In such cases a light breakfast of a liquid diet is permissible not later than 6 hours preoperatively. The lower colon should be cleansed by a preoperative enema approximately 2 or 3 hours before the operation is scheduled. It is unrealistic for the patient to be awakened at dawn by an attendant to be given an enema when the operation is posted at noon. Not only is it a discourtesy to the patient, but the lower bowel may become refilled with fecal material due to increased intestinal activity from the anxiety of awaiting the operative procedure. Preoperative sedation is usually requested by the anesthesiologist at the time of his visit with the patient on the night before surgery. The usual medication includes atropine sulfate 0.5 mg. (I.M.) with morphine or meperidine (Demerol) at least 30 minutes prior to the anesthetic. As discussed in the chapter on anesthesiology, it is important that the patient have adequate sedation for any type of an operative procedure, whether major or minor, in order to decrease the amount of the anesthetic required for the operation.

PREOPERATIVE MEDICAL COMPLICATIONS

Secondary anemia is one of the commonest preoperative conditions encountered in gynecology, since many of the gynecologic conditions requiring surgery are associated with bleeding. While adequate iron replacement by oral medication is effective in correcting an iron-deficiency blood-loss anemia, a period of several weeks is required for replenishment of iron stores and erythrocytes. In the event of continued vaginal bleeding, it is usually preferable to replace the blood loss by means of preoperative transfusions and proceed with the indicated operation. It is advisable that the patient's blood volume be within the normal range prior to any major operative procedure, on the basis that it is always better to transfuse the patient when she is awake than when she is asleep, as at the time of an operative procedure. For major pelvic surgery, the hematocrit should be 35 per cent or greater, and blood should always be available in adequate amounts during the operation for replacement when needed.

Cardiovascular evaluation, especially the assessment of cardiac reserve, must be accurate. In patients known to have cardiac disease, an electrocardiogram, venous pressure, circulation time, and pulmonary function studies are frequently required for complete evaluation of the patient as a surgical risk. When there is evidence of cardiomegalia, hepatic enlargement, and left or right-sided heart failure, preoperative digitalization and correction of cardiac decompensation is essential prior to elective pelvic surgery. In case of an emergency operative procedure, such cardiac patients require meticulous preoperative and postoperative attention for the earliest changes of congestive heart failure. Rapid intravenous degitalization and close observation of cardiac reserve by central venous pressure monitoring, as described under postoperative care, is an essential part of the patient's gynecologic treatment.

PREOPERATIVE PROCEDURES ON THE OPERATING ROOM FLOOR

The patient is brought to the operating room floor in her bed. She is transferred to the operating table in the anesthesia room, adjoining the operating room. The operating table is previously prepared for laparotomy by placing a Kelly pad transversely on the table, so that liquids used for the vaginal cleanup will drain into a floor basin. The patient is shaved by a nurse in the anesthesia room after the induction of anesthesia. Since several minutes are required to attain surgical anesthesia, no time is lost as a result of shaving while the patient is unconscious.

The patient is requested to empty her bladder before coming to the operating room, but catheterization is done routinely after she is anesthetized except before the operation of dilatation and curettage. Even in these minor cases catheterization is done frequently in order to perform a satisfactory examination under anesthesia. The technic of catheterization under anesthesia is the simplest. The labia are spread with the fingers of one hand, and the region of the urethral meatus is washed with a gauze sponge saturated with liquid soap. The region is then flushed with 70 per cent alcohol. The urethral meatus and the outer portion of the urethra are swabbed with a toothpick swab saturated with 1 per cent Zephiran. Then the catheter is passed. Gently pressing the base of the bladder per vaginam ensures its complete emptying.

After shaving and catheterization, the patient is usually sufficiently anesthetized for a careful bimanual examination. We make examination under anesthesia a matter of absolute routine. Usually, it is simply confirmatory of the previous examination, but occasionally very valuable data are obtained, useful to the operator.

Following the vaginal examination, the perineum and the vagina are cleaned in the anesthesia room before all pelvic laparotomies. There is always the possibility that the findings at operation may make a total abdominal hysterectomy advisable, even when the preconceived plan in the operator's mind does not call for such an extensive procedure. It is extremely awkward to be caught with the necessity of a total hysterectomy at operation without have the vagina properly prepared. To prevent this, we have made preoperative vaginal cleanup a routine procedure. To clean the perineum and the vagina, the surgical assistant first scrubs the vulva and the perineum with a soapy sponge in his gloved hand. Then the vagina is scrubbed with a soapy sponge held in the fingers. By spreading the fingers, the outlet is enlarged, and the perineum is depressed to permit the soapy water to run out of the vagina. This is flushed away with sterile water poured by the nurse. From this point on, the cleanup is done with a sterile sponge on a sterile sponge stick. As successive sterile sponges are used, they are handed to the surgical assistant by the nurse. After the soap-and-water cleansing, the vagina, the vulva and the perineum are scrubbed with 70 per cent alcohol.

Next, the vagina is swabbed with Scott's solution or a similar tinctured antiseptic solution, and an unfolded sterile sponge is inserted in the vagina. The end of this is left protruding from the outlet, and the sponge stick is left attached to facilitate its removal during the operation. The sponge absorbs any secretions that may come from the cervical canal as the result of operative manipulation. At operation the sponge is removed by a nurse who pulls on the sponge stick just before the vagina is opened.

After the vaginal cleanup, the abdomen is washed with ether, and particular attention is paid to cleansing the umbilicus with a toothpick swab. A clean towel is thrown over the abdomen, and the patient is wheeled into the operating room. This towel is removed after the operating table is in position in the operating room, and the abdomen is cleaned up with a sterile sponge on a sponge stick, first making two applications of 70 per cent alcohol. This is followed with a saturated ether sponge to remove any film of grease on the skin. Next, the dry skin is painted twice with a sterile sponge, saturated with Metaphen (1:200). The painting of the abdomen is done in such a manner as always to progress from the clean to the unclean field. The nurse who is assisting in the cleanup first pours some of the germicidal solution into the umbilical depression to form a small pool. From a central point at the periphery of the umbilical pool, the surgical assistant applies the disinfectant concentrically and finally covers the lowermost pubic region, the upper portions of the vulva, and the thighs. An alternate method, using an iodine skin preparation (Betadine) for 5 minutes, has decreased the incidence of postoperative incisional infections. In recent years Viodrape has been used in many clinics to reduce the possibility of contamination of the incision.

ARMAMENTARIUM

Every experienced surgeon has his own favorite instruments, and equally good work can no doubt be done with different tools by different men. In the course of years of active service in gynecologic surgery we have standardized our instruments for major and minor surgery. With the hope that our experience will be useful to others, and particularly to younger surgeons, we are listing the instruments routinely employed in the usual gynecologic operations.

INSTRUMENTS FOR PELVIC LAPAROTOMIES

- 4 Heaney clamps
- 18 Large curved Ochsner clamps
- 12 Small Kelly clamps
- 8 Straight Ochsner clamps
- 6 Long Kelly clamps
- 24 Halsted clamps
- 4 Long Adson clamps
- 1 Long needle holder
- 3 Mayo needle holders
- 3 Snap or Kelly needle holders
- 2 Crile Murray needle holders
- 1 Long Metzenbaum scissors
- 1 Long suture scissors
- 1 Long Mayo scissors
- 1 Regular Metzenbaum scissors
- 2 Suture scissors
- 6 Allis clamps (mucosa clips)
- 12 Towel clips
- 2 Long ring forceps (Singley)
- 1 Long Ferguson forceps
- 1 Medium mousetooth forceps
- 2 Short mousetooth forceps
- 1 Short smooth forceps
- 1 Straight Mayo scissors
- 3 Curved Vosellum clamps
- 1 Cullen uterine elevator
- 1 Long blunt dissector
- 4 Long Mixter clamps
- 2 Short Mixter clamps
- 3 Assorted spatulae
- 2 Bard-Parker knife handles No. 4
- 1 Edebohls' double retractor
- 6 Appendix retractors—2 small, 2 medium, and 2 large
- 2 Abdominal retractors (self-retaining) —1 medium and 1 large
- 4 Lateral retractors—2 medium and 2 large
- 4 Deavor retractors—2 medium and 2 large
- 10 Laparotomy rings
- 1 Glass retractor
- 2 Suction tips
- 2 Wide rake retractors, shallow
- 8 Large sponge sticks
- 2 Babcock clamps
- 6 Small Kocher clamps

INSTRUMENTS FOR MAJOR VAGINAL OPERATIVE PROCEDURES

- 2 Deaver retractors
- 2 Small lateral retractors
- 2 Heaney retractors
- 1 Pair finger retractors
- 1 Weighted retractor
- 1 Uterine sound
- 2 Jacob's clamps
- 12 Small Kelly clamps
- 12 Halsted clamps
- 12 Allis clamps

Preoperative Care and Complications

12 Kocher clamps
6 Heaney clamps
4 Long Kelly clamps
3 Lahey thyroid clamps
1 Metzenbaum scissors
1 Straight Mayo scissors
4 Ring forceps
12 Towel clips
12 Curved Crile clamps
6 Kocher 8″ clamps
4 Allis 8″ clamps
2 Babcock clamps
2 Tenacula
2 Suture scissors
1 Long Mayo scissors
1 Curved Mayo scissors
2 Small mousetooth forceps
1 Small smooth forceps
2 Ring-tipped forceps
1 Russian forceps
3 Mayo needle holders
3 Heaney needle holders
2 Knife handles

To this set add entire dilatation and curettage set.

Instruments for Dilatation and Curettage

4 Ring forceps
4 Towel clips
4 Hegar dilators
1 Uterine sound
1 8″ forceps
3 Serrated curettes, different sizes
1 Jacob's clamp
1 Long Kelly clamp
2 Tenacula
1 Posterior retractor
1 Anterior retractor
1 Biopsy forceps
1 Kidney stone forceps
1 Uterine-packing forceps

Instruments for Rubin's Test

Dilatation and curettage set plus:
1 York claw holder
2 Rubin's cannulae
1 Small bowl for saline

Instruments for Insertion of Radium

Dilatation and curettage set plus:
1 Long needle holder
1 Long mousetooth forceps
1 Long smooth forceps
1 Long straight scissors
1 No. 18 Foley catheter
1 No. 20 Foley catheter
2 2″ × 60″ vaginal packs
1 Long tissue forceps
1 Teperson intubating forceps

Instruments for Therapeutic Abortion or Completion of Abortion

Dilatation and curettage set plus:
4 Placenta forceps, Kelly's
1 Thomas blunt curette
8 Hegar dilators, up to No. 16
1 Aspiration curettage apparatus

Instruments for Posterior Colpotomy

1 Weighted vaginal retractor
2 Heaney retractors
1 Jacob's clamp
4 Long Kelly clamps
4 Allis 8″ clamps
1 Long Mayo scissors
1 Uterine sound
1 Long forceps
1 Heaney needle holder
1 Culture tube

Instruments for Radical Pelvic Surgery

Pelvic laparotomy set plus:
Abdominal, Part I
18 Towel clips
6 Kocher 6″ clamps
6 Allis 6″ clamps
2 Long needle holders
8 Kelly 10″ clamps
6 Kelly 12″ clamps
6 Rumel clamps
6 Carmalt clamps
2 Adson clamps
4 Long Mixter clamps
8 Mixter clamps
4 Collins intestinal clamps
2 Babcock clamps
4 Allis 8″ clamps
4 Scudder clamps (2 curved, 2 straight)
4 Payer clamps (2 large, 2 small)
6 Wertheim clamps
3 Tissue forceps—8″, 10″, 12″
3 Thumb forceps—8″, 10″, 12″
1 Long fine thumb forceps

Armamentarium 29

2 Vein retractors
  Silver slips and applier
1 Ligature carrier
1 Nerve hook and dissector
4 Bulldog vascular clamps
2 Long deBakey forceps
2 Satinsky clamps
1 Long Metzenbaum scissors
2 Long Mayo scissors

Vaginal Procedure, Part II
1 Weighted retractor
2 Heaney retractors
2 Jackson retractors
2 Langenbeck retractors
4 Ring forceps
12 Towel clips
12 Curved Crile clamps
12 Straight Crile clamps
24 Kelly clamps
12 Allis 8" clamps
12 Long Kocher clamps
1 Uterine sound
2 Russian 6" forceps
3 Tissue 5½" forceps
2 Thumb 5½" forceps
2 Thumb 8" forceps
2 Mayo scissors
1 Metzenbaum scissors
2 Suture scissors
2 Mayo needle holders
2 Heaney needle holders

The following several pages illustrate the instruments we have found most useful.

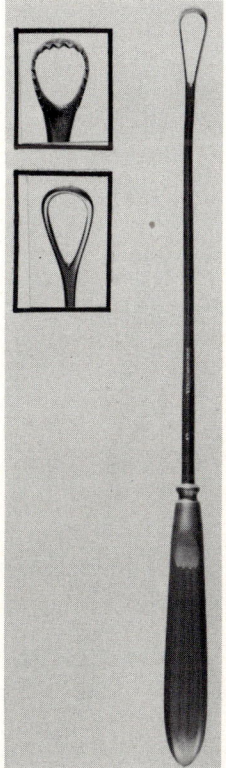

FIG. 2-2. Curette, sharp with serrated and blunt inserts.

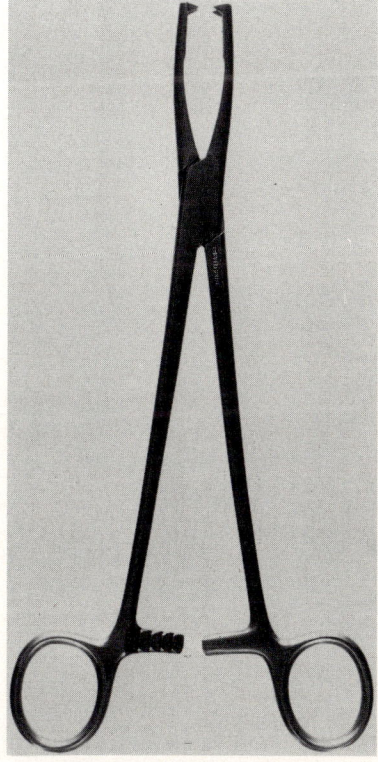

FIG. 2-3. Jacob's clamp.

30 Preoperative Care and Complications

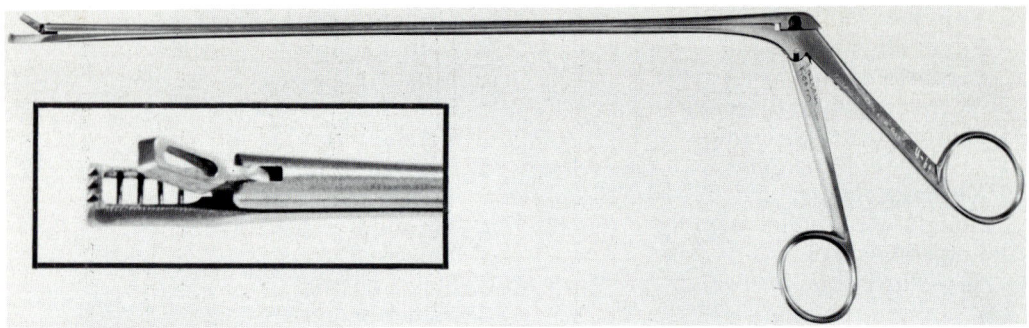

Fig. 2-4. Younge biopsy clamp, a most useful instrument for biopsying cervices in the office and the operating room.

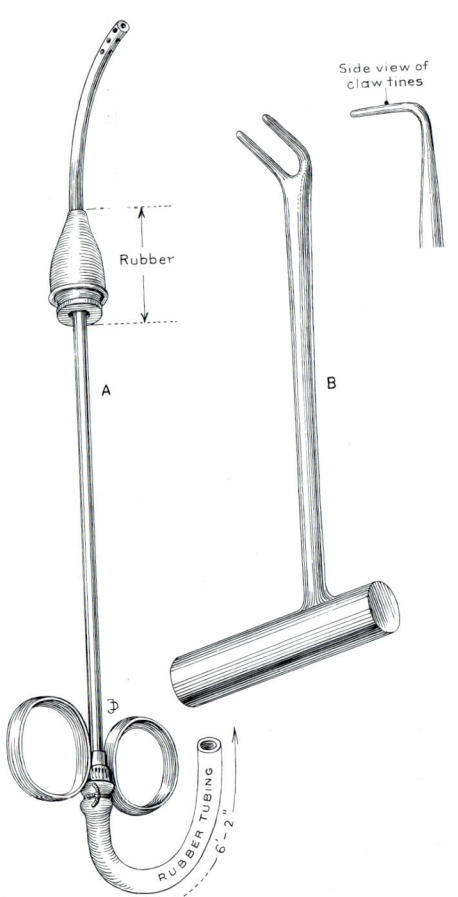

Fig. 2-5. Rubin's cannula, (A) with rubber stopper and (B) York "claw" for holding stopper against cervix.

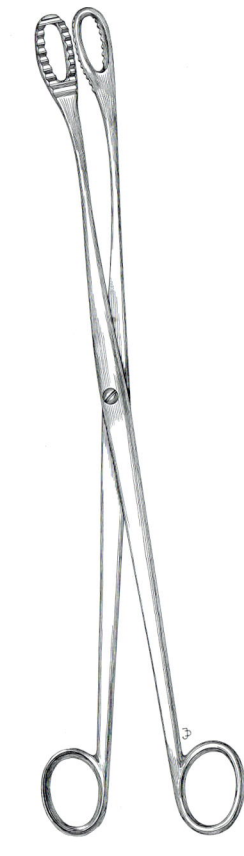

Fig. 2-6. Placenta forceps. Useful for removing the products of conception.

Armamentarium 31

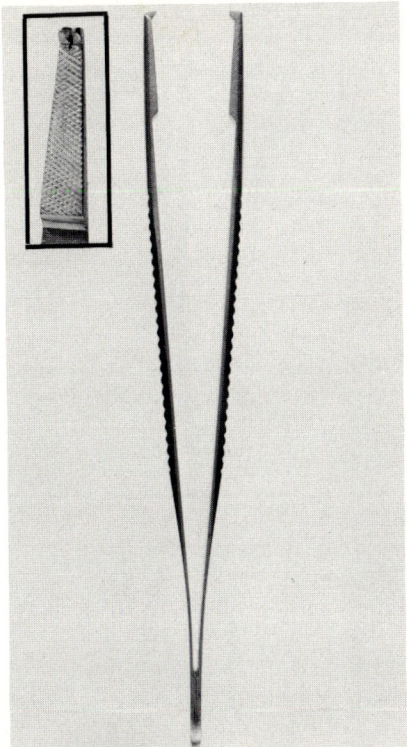

FIG. 2-7. Bonney forceps.

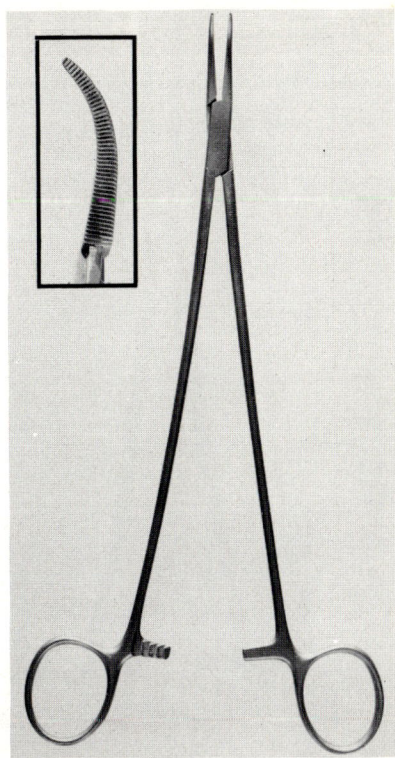

FIG. 2-8. Adson clamp.

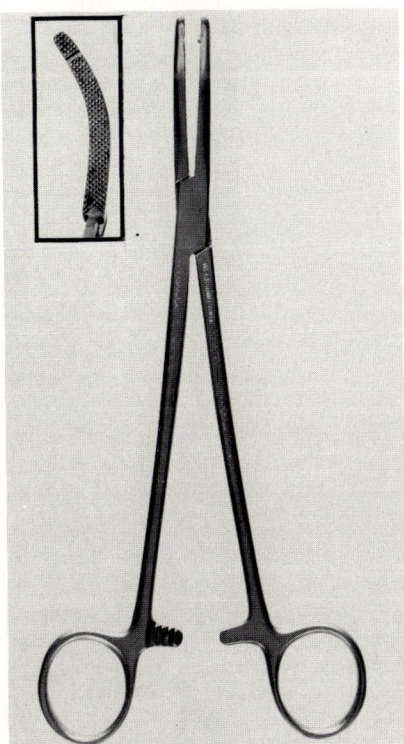

FIG. 2-9. Heaney clamp.

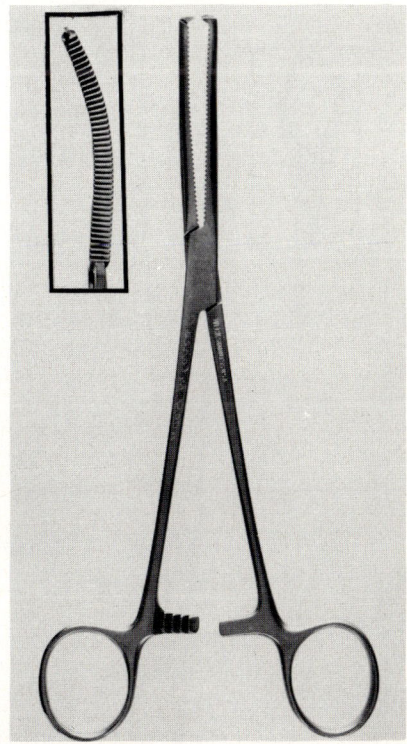

FIG. 2-10. Curved Ochsner clamp with insert.

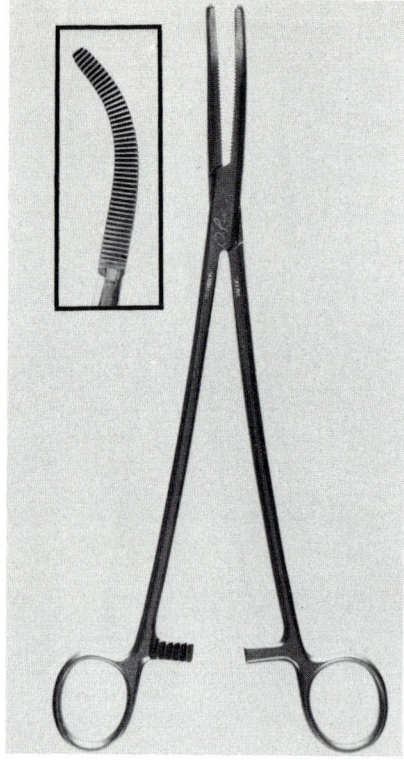

FIG. 2-11. Wertheim clamp.

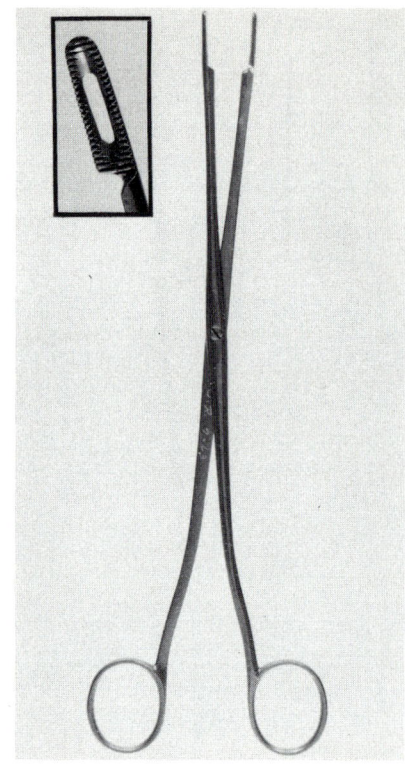

FIG. 2-12. Stone forceps with insert.

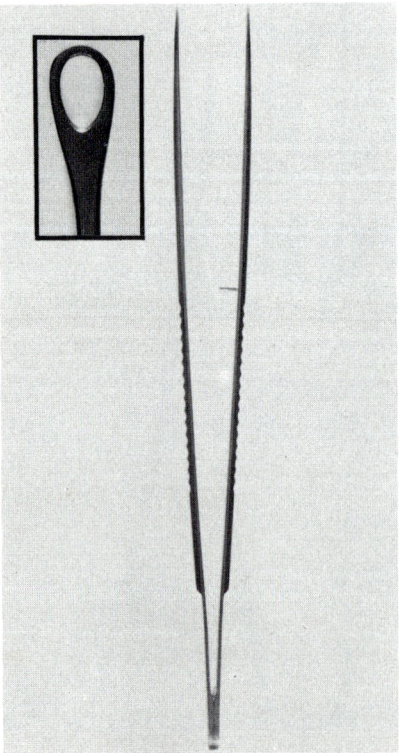

FIG. 2-13. Singley pickup forceps.

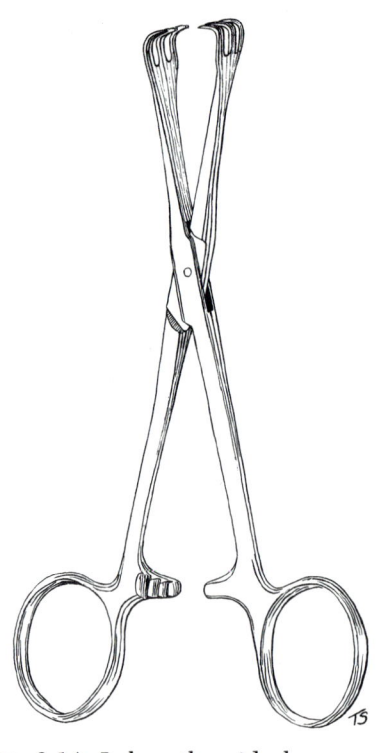

FIG. 2-14. Lahey thyroid clamp, a very useful instrument for delivering the uterus at vaginal hysterectomy.

Armamentarium 33

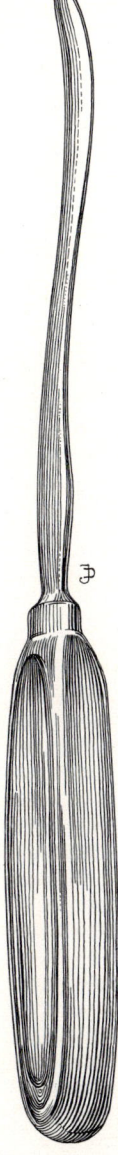

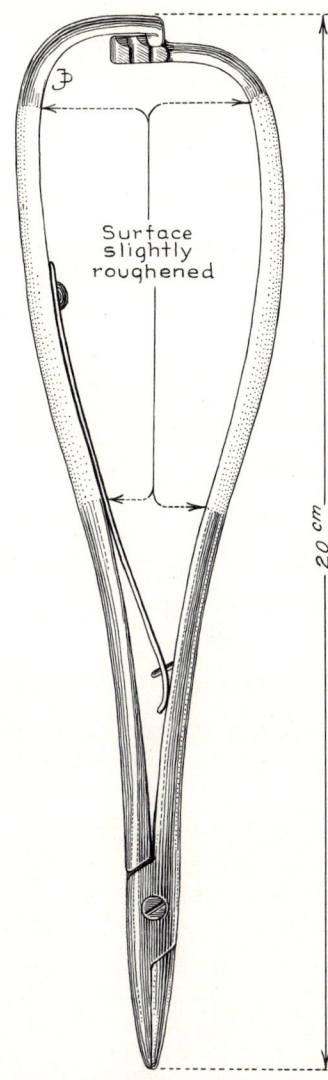

FIG. 2-15. Blunt dissector, useful for dissection in the region of large vessels, as in performing presacral neurectomies and pelvic gland dissections.

FIG. 2-16. Kelly needle holder, more convenient and more quickly manipulated than the usual needle holder.

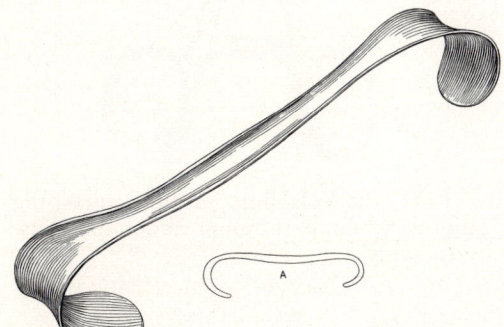

FIG. 2-17. Edebohls' retractor, a very useful instrument for exposing the fascia at the ends of the incision for beginning the fascia closure.

34 Preoperative Care and Complications

FIG. 2-18. Babcock clamp, a most useful instrument for picking up tube or appendix without applying pressure to these tubular structures.

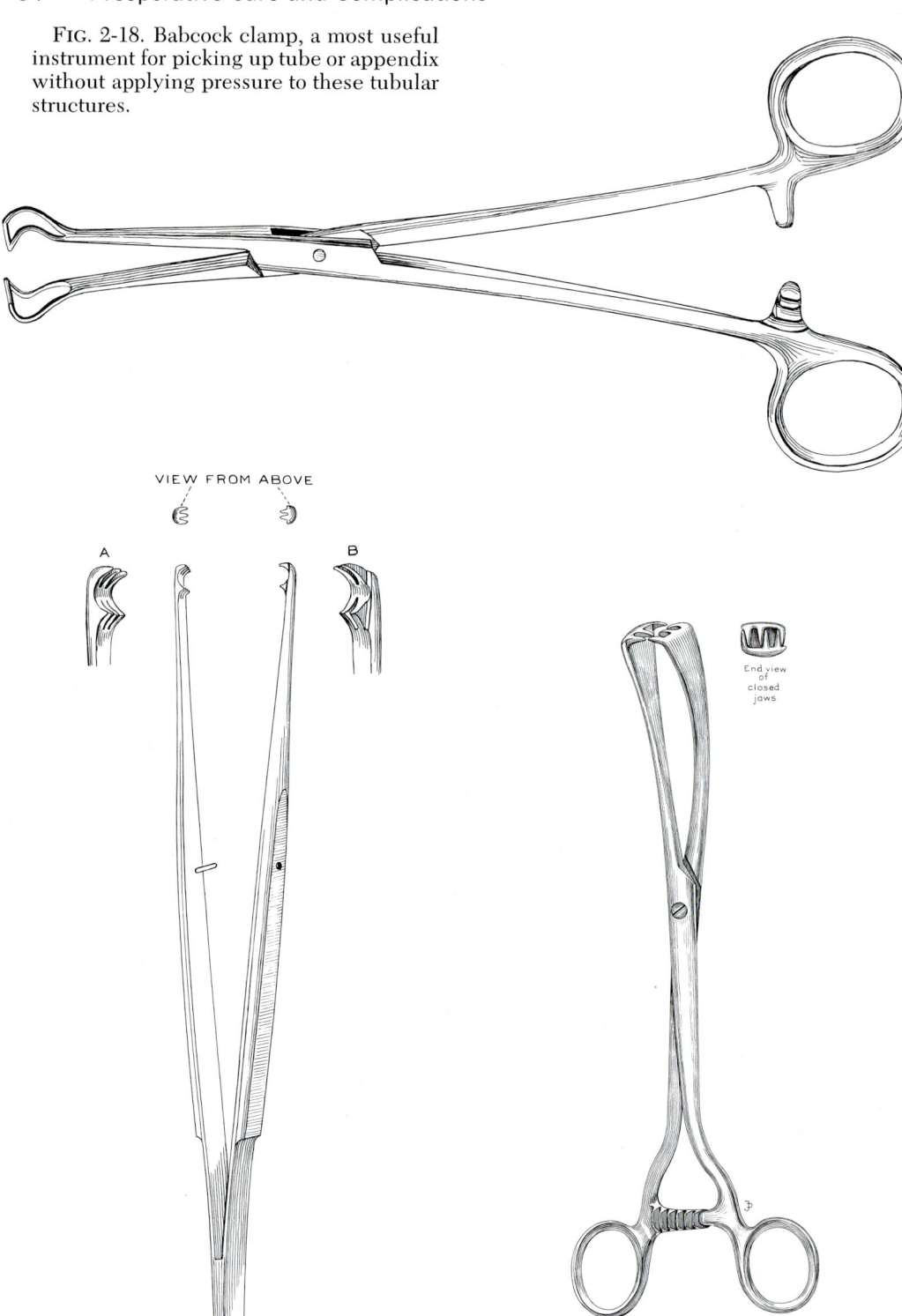

FIG. 2-19. Long Ferguson forceps, especially useful for working on the cervix.

FIG. 2-20. Volsellum, useful for grasping uterus when performing abdominal hysterectomy.

BIBLIOGRAPHY

de Peyster, F. A., and Gilchrist, R. K.: Current principles governing abdominal surgery in the aged. A.M.A. Arch. Surg., 83:138, 1961.

Glenn, F., Moore, S. W., and Beal, J. M. (eds.): Surgery in the Aged. pp. 45-48. New York, McGraw-Hill, 1960.

Henegar, G. C.: The importance of blood volume determination in surgical patients. Surg. Clin. N. Amer., 43:187, 1963.

Jesseph, J. E., and Harkins, H. N.: Geriatric Surgical Emergencies. pp. 1-18. Boston, Little, Brown & Co., 1963.

Masukawa, T., Levinson, E. F., and Frost, J. K.: The cytologic examination of breast secretions. Acta Cytol., *10*:261, 1966.

Mattingly, R. F.: Surgery in the aging female. Clin. Obstet. Gynec., 7:573, 1964.

Powers, J. H.: Geriatric trends in surgery. Surg. Clin. N. Amer., *40*:865, 1960.

Scott, D. L.: Anesthetic experiences in 1,300 major geriatric operations. Brit. J. Anaesth., *33*:354, 1961.

Stahlgren, L. H.: An analysis of factors which influence mortality following extensive abdominal operations upon geriatric patients. Surg. Gynec. Obstet., *113*:283, 1961.

Ziffren, S. E.: Management of the aged surgical patient. Chicago, Year Book Medical Publishers, 1960.

3

Anesthesia and Resuscitation

PETER SAFAR, M.D.,[*] AND DAVID TORPEY, M.D.[†]

INTRODUCTION

Anesthesia for gynecologic surgery presents few problems not also encountered in anesthesia for general surgery. A text on the science and art of anesthesia and on the pharmacology of anesthetic drugs is beyond the scope of this chapter. However, an attempt is made to summarize some basic concepts of anesthesia as they concern both the surgeon and the anesthesiologist, who need to appreciate each other's problems. Those who seek further knowledge of anesthesiology are referred to standard teaching texts.[4, 6, 10, 14, 22] Knowledge gained only by reading does not qualify even a physician to administer an anesthetic. There is no substitute for practical experience obtained under adequate supervision.

A serious shortage in manpower is found in anesthesiology. About 15 million anesthesias are given in the United States every year by fewer than 9,000 physician members of the American Society of Anesthesiologists with the help of 10,000 nurse anesthetists and other personnel. Only about 4,500 physicians are certified by the American Board of Anesthesiology. Ideally, one anesthesiologist can personally administer up to approximately 1,000 anesthesias per year. Therefore anesthesiologists must "extend their hands" in the operating room, in at least some patient care environments, by the use of ancillary personnel. For example, the anesthesiologist may control or supervise the maintenance by nurse anesthetists of 2 to 3 anesthesias simultaneously. However, patients in poor physical status, particularly those with cardiopulmonary disease, should be managed throughout by the anesthesiologist. Ideally, nurse anesthetists working without the direct supervision and professional control of anesthesiologists should not be permitted.

Every anesthesia service should aim for the following: (1) optimal patient safety, (2) optimal working conditions for the surgeon, and (3) optimal patient comfort. Obtaining these goals in any given hospital depends upon the organization of the Department of Anesthesiology, which in turn is dependent on local circumstances.

MORTALITY

Physical Status Classification. Considerations of surgery and anesthesia-related mortality and morbidity are made more meaningful by use of the physical status (PS) classification of the American Society of Anesthesiologists:

PS 1. A normal healthy patient for elective operations.

---

[*] Professor and Chairman, Department of Anesthesiology, University of Pittsburgh School of Medicine.

[†] Assistant Professor, Department of Anesthesiology, University of Pittsburgh School of Medicine.

ACKNOWLEDGMENT: Miss P. Sands helped in the preparation and editing of the manuscript.

PS 2. A patient with a mild systemic disease.

PS 3. A patient with a severe systemic disease that limits activity, but is not incapacitating.

PS 4. A patient with an incapacitating systemic disease that is a constant threat to life.

PS 5. A moribund patient not expected to survive 24 hours with or without operation.

Patients in physical status 1 or 2 can tolerate a great deal of physiologic trespass, whereas even a slight mistake may cause death in patients of physical status 3 to 5. The mortality and the morbidity associated with anesthesia for gynecologic surgery is lower than that associated with anesthesia for general surgery. This may be explained by the fact that most gynecologic patients are in good physical condition. Nevertheless, deaths in which anesthesia is a primary or contributing factor do occur in connection with gynecologic operations.[2, 17]

No particular anesthetic agent or technic appears to be the culprit. The primary cause of death associated with general anesthesia seems to be airway obstruction and/or respiratory depression. Fatal anesthetic overdose has become relatively rare because of the avoidance of deep planes of general anesthesia following the introduction of muscle relaxants, the use of more sophisticated equipment (e.g., calibrated vaporizers), and well-trained personnel. The principal cause of death associated with spinal anesthesia is sudden, uncontrolled hypotension.

Such tragedies, due to asphyxia or hypotension, can be averted by a rapid, skillful, and effective resuscitative approach on the part of the team.

Although the anesthesiologist is personally responsible for anesthetic complications, we believe that the surgeon can help to minimize anesthetic mortality and morbidity as follows: (1) by demanding and supporting a well-trained anesthesia staff with adequate physician control; (2) by requesting the anesthesiologist's participation as early as possible in the preoperative evaluation and preparation, particularly of patients in poor physical status; (3) by accepting the anesthesiologist's judgment and choice of agents and technic; and (4) by considering safe practices rather than personal convenience (e.g., speed), as when slow induction is required in patients with poor physical status.

THE PREANESTHETIC VISIT

Adequate preanesthetic evaluation and preparation can prevent many difficulties in the operating room. This evaluation and preparation is the responsibility of the anesthesiologist.

If at all possible, the anesthesiologist who is to administer or supervise the anesthesia should see the patient the day prior to the operation in order personally to evaluate the physical status, to ask for any additional examinations that he may deem necessary, and to order the preanesthetic medication. He should also establish a rapport with the patient in order to gain her confidence and to alleviate any apprehension.

In reviewing the patient's record the anesthesiologist pays particular attention to the following: (1) evidence of cardiopulmonary disturbances, low circulating blood volume (e.g., recent weight loss, malignancy, dehydration, blood loss), and systemic infection; (2) medications (e.g., insulin, steroids, antihypertensive drugs, digitalis); and (3) laboratory findings.

The surgeon should inform the anesthesiologist about any problem which he thinks might influence the choice of anesthetic and the manner in which it is administered. The anesthesiologist's evaluation of the patient's condition influences the preanesthetic preparation, the final choice of the anesthetic, and the immediate postoperative care.

If the anesthesiologist's final choice of anesthetic differs from that desired by the surgeon, a discussion should resolve the issue. Disagreements that are allowed to go uncorrected until the morning of surgery are detrimental to patients and to physician relationships.

PREANESTHETIC MEDICATION

Preanesthetic orders should be written by the anesthesiologist. The orders should include the discontinuance of food, drink, and medication; additional preanesthetic preparative measures; and the administration of the preanesthetic medication.

Food and drink should be discontinued at least by midnight prior to the day of an elective operation. As pain, fear, or narcotic drugs may delay emptying of the stomach for more than 12 hours, only a soft meal should be permitted the night before the operation. When the operation is scheduled for the afternoon, an early breakfast of clear liquids may be permitted.

The preanesthetic medication should be considered part of the anesthetic, since the choice of one influences the choice and means of administering the other. The preanesthetic medication should be individualized, taking into consideration both the findings obtained during the preanesthetic visit and the planned anesthetic technic.

Large doses of depressant drugs are to be avoided as they may cause hypotension or unconsciousness, the latter sometimes leading to preoperative airway obstruction. Avoiding heavy sedation is particularly important prior to short operations and in ambulatory patients.

Alleviating apprehension by gaining the patient's confidence and by explaining with well-chosen words what is to be expected, even though more time-consuming, is preferred to heavy sedation. An increasing number of anesthesiologists, therefore, prefer to use atropine only.

Premedication for Adults. The drugs employed for preanesthetic medication vary greatly in different institutions. The following medications are recommended for the average adult:

1. A *parasympatholytic* drug such as *atropine* or *scopolamine*, to prevent salivation, is mandatory prior to anesthesia with cyclopropane or ether but is optional with use of halothane, as the former increases salivation whereas the latter depresses it. Atropine or scopolamine, 0.5 mg., is given intramuscularly about 60 minutes (30-120 minutes) prior to induction of anesthesia. If induction of anesthesia is delayed for more than 120 minutes following the injection of the belladonna drug, the injection should be repeated. When in an emergency it is given intravenously, the drying effect should not be expected until 5 to 10 minutes after the injection. A vagal blocking effect must not be expected from this intramuscular dose and is also unnecessary in anesthesia for adults in good physical status.

The advantages of scopolamine over atropine lie in its better drying effect and its ability to produce amnesia—especially helpful when analgesia (e.g., nitrous oxide alone) is used. Before regional anesthesia, however, atropine is to be preferred to scopolamine, as the latter may make the patient uncooperative. A belladonna drug may even be omitted prior to regional anesthesia if the anesthesiologist feels certain that supplementation with general anesthesia will not be required.

2. To alleviate apprehension, a *hypnotic* drug such as *pentobarbital* (Nembutal) or secobarbital (Seconal), 100-150 mg./70 kg. body weight, or an ataractic drug such as hydroxyzine (Vistaril), 50-100 mg./70 kg. body weight, or both are administered by the intramuscular route, together with either atropine or scopolamine. Barbiturates and ataractics in the recommended doses are less depressing to respiration and circulation than narcotics. The use of barbiturates should be avoided in very old, debilitated patients or in patients in shock, as they are prone to develop hypotension and respiratory depression from barbiturates. Ataractics are particular valuable in apprehensive patients.

3. *Narcotic* drugs, such as *morphine* or *meperidine* (Demerol) are not recommended for routine use because of their well-known side-effects, which include respiratory depression, airway obstruction due to unconsciousness, hypotension (particularly postural hypotension), nausea, constipation, and urinary reten-

tion. Circulatory collapse has been described with the use of narcotics, particularly in the aged. Therefore, in all patients over 65 years (physical age) and in patients with low blood volume or severe atherosclerosis, narcotics should either be avoided or, if used, employed with great caution, preferably by intravenous titration in the operation room. As a rule, narcotics should be reserved for patients in pain and those scheduled for regional anesthesia. For reinforcing light anesthesia, a narcotic is best titrated by the intravenous administration of small doses in the operating room under the control of the anesthesiologist.

When used, the preanesthetic dose of *morphine* for a 70-kg. adult is 10 mg. (5-15 mg.) intramuscularly. A comparative dose of meperidine is 75 mg. (50-100 mg.). Either narcotic may be given together with atropine or scopolamine, 0.5 mg. When heavy sedation is desired in a generally healthy adult, pentobarbital or secobarbital may be added to the narcotic and the belladonna drug.

Miscellaneous Drugs. Phenothiazines (e.g., chlorpromazine), antihistaminics (e.g., promethazine), similarly acting new agents, and combinations of narcotics with narcotic antagonists have been recommended for preanesthetic medication. There is little evidence that these drugs provide better preanesthetic conditions with fewer side-effects than the "old-fashioned" medication described above, and, in fact, severe hypotension and excitement have been seen with some of these new drugs.

In the choice of premedicant drugs, experience with the dose-effect relationship of familiar drugs is a practical advantage that is more important than theoretical advantages of new drugs.

Route of Administration. We do not recommend the oral or rectal route for preanesthetic medication, as the variable rate of drug absorption makes the onset, the degree, and the duration of action unpredictable. However, if a hypnotic or analgesic drug is indicated the evening before operation, it may be given by mouth.

In acute pain, intravenous titration with small doses of narcotics is preferable to intramuscular injection, particularly in shock states, when the absorption of intramuscular drugs is unpredictable.

POSTURE

Supine Position. Ulnar or radial nerve paralysis may occur if the arm is positioned carelessly. The arm should be placed on top of the table and held in position with a lifting sheet. Stretch due to abduction of the arm beyond a 90° angle and/or dropping the arm below table level may cause brachial plexus paralysis, a hazardous complication, as the paralysis may be irreversible. The anesthetist can avoid excessive stretch of the brachial plexus by watching to see that the surgeon does not accidentally push the arm board cephalad. This stretch may also be minimized by pronating the arm. Injury of the brachial plexus from abduction of the arm may be avoided when both arms are placed alongside the patient. In this case the intravenous infusion can be secured by insertion of a plastic catheter. If an additional intravenous infusion is required in a patient whose trachea is intubated, the external jugular vein may be used. The needle should be withdrawn before the patient awakens, as movement of the head may cause injury to the neck structures. When central venous or arterial catheterization is necessary or contemplated, one arm should remain free (abducted).

Trendelenburg Position. The Trendelenburg (head-down) position is commonly used during gynecologic operations, particularly during laparotomies, in order to give better exposure of the pelvic organs.

In order to compensate for poor anesthesia, the surgeon often demands the steepest head-down position, which the anesthetist prefers to minimize because of it deleterious effects on respiration and circulation. The degree of head-down tilt required for optimal exposure depends largely upon the degree of abdominal relaxation, and on the smoothness of the respiratory movements provided by the anesthesiologist. Moderate Trendelenburg position should be adequate with good anesthesia.

The deleterious effects of the steep Trendelenburg position are as follows: (1) The abdominal contents push the diaphragm cephalad and thus decrease the functional residual capacity of the lungs, which increases airway resistance, decreases compliance, and increases pulmonary shunting (hypoxemia). Spontaneous diaphragmatic movements may become jerky, which defeats the original purpose of this position, namely, keeping the abdominal contents out of the pelvis. Assisted or controlled ventilation is mandatory, and, as compared with a level position, higher inflation pressures are required.[19] (2) When the body weight of the patient is supported by a shoulder brace, the brachial plexus is prone to injury by direct compression at the neck. When the arm is abducted in addition, the plexus may be unduly stretched over the head of the humerus. Therefore, a shoulder brace should never be used on the side of the abducted arm, and if used, it should be placed over the acromion. (3) Pulmonary congestion may occur and harm a patient who is in borderline heart failure. (4) The increased jugular vein pressure may cause cerebrovascular engorgement, decreased cerebral blood flow, and edema of the conjunctiva and the face.

In the use of regional anesthesia for laparotomies the steep Trendelenburg position should also be avoided because of discomfort and the difficulty of assisting respiration in the awake patient.

Lithotomy Position. The patient should be placed in the lithotomy position after induction of anesthesia. In positioning the legs in the stirrups care should be taken that nerves and veins are not compressed, and that vessels are not kinked by excessive flexion at the knee. Paralysis of the peroneal nerve may be caused by pressure of the knee supports. Stirrups which suspend the legs without touching them are preferable.

If spinal anesthesia is chosen for operations in the lithotomy position, the sensory anesthetic level should be above the first lumbar dermatome, since numbness of the legs is required for patient comfort.

Prone and Culdoscopy Position. In the prone (face-down) and the culdoscopy (knee-chest) positions, the face and the upper airways are poorly accessible, which makes maintenance of a patent airway difficult, if not impossible. Inflation of the lungs is also more difficult in these positions, since more of the patient's weight must be moved with each breath.[19] Observation of the patient's color and vital signs is difficult because of the awkwardness of the position and because the room is usually darkened. Therefore, before placing an anesthetized patient into the culdoscopy position, a tracheal tube should be inserted, and respirations should be assisted or controlled throughout.

Low spinal, caudal, or lumbar epidural anesthesia has proven to be satisfactory for culdoscopies. Some prefer general endotracheal anesthesia for culdoscopies, since it allows for assistance in ventilation and spares the patient the discomfort and the embarrassment associated with this position. Paracervical block[21] plus sedation may be used satisfactorily for culdoscopy when an anesthesiologist is not available.

Injury to the brachial plexus has been seen subsequent to the use of the culdoscopy position. This may be due to excessive elevation of the arms over the head plus the turning of the head sideways. Also, injury to the lateral femoral cutaneous nerve may occur in the prone or culdoscopy positions with improper hip support.

GENERAL ANESTHESIA

It is not the purpose of this chapter to discuss anesthetic technics or the pharmacology of anesthetics, which should be studied with the help of other texts.[4, 6, 10, 22] A few general comments follow.

Induction. The induction of anesthesia with the intravenous injection of thiopental (Pentothal Sodium) is most popular because of its rapidity and pleasantness for the patient. Induction with an inhalation anesthetic may be equally smooth and rapid in skilled hands, and is often safer for the patient in poor physical status.

Maintenance. For extraperitoneal procedures (e.g., D and C, vaginoplasty) light anesthesia which provides unconsciousness, lack of movements, and regular spontaneous breathing is sufficient. Muscular relaxation is not required except for difficult pelvic examinations. In vaginal hysterectomies moderate abdominal wall relaxation is usually required to avoid the extrusion of abdominal viscera through the vaginal incision when the pelvic peritoneum is open.

In abdominal intraperitoneal procedures, maximal muscular relaxation and quiet respiratory movements (by assisted or controlled ventilation) are desirable, to provide optimal working conditions for the surgeon and to permit smooth convalescence by minimal trauma to the abdominal viscera.

Relaxation and quiet respiratory movements are particularly important during the opening and the closing of the peritoneum, during exploration of the abdominal cavity, during packing of the intestines, and during placing of the retractors.

Muscle Relaxants. The proper use of neuromuscular blocking agents avoids the circulatory and metabolic changes associated with the use of high concentrations of potent general anesthetics, which otherwise would be necessary to provide muscular relaxation. The use of muscle relaxants obviously necessitates skillfully assisted or controlled ventilation. More controlled relaxation with the avoidance of unintentional postanesthetic muscular weakness can now be provided with use of a neuromuscular stimulator ("Block-Aid" Monitor).

The intraperitoneal instillation of antibiotics (e.g., neomycin, kanamycin) may lead to prolonged apnea when curariform drugs have been used.

Assisted Respiration and Controlled Ventilation.[18] Assisted respiration is the augmentation of shallow spontaneous breaths, usually by intermittent positive pressure breathing. Controlled ventilation is entirely artificial ventilation, usually in the form of intermittent positive pressure ventilation by manual compression of a breathing bag or by mechanical ventilator.

Exposure during laparotomies is sometimes difficult due to inadequate muscular relaxation. Exaggerated, jerky, spontaneous diaphragmatic movements may increase exposure difficulty and may be more troublesome than the lack of abdominal muscular relaxation. To avoid such diaphragmatic movements, we prefer to use assisted or controlled ventilation during laparotomies. In the case of controlled ventilation the patient is rendered apneic, usually by a combination of hyperventilation, central respiratory depression by anesthetics or narcotics, and peripheral respiratory depression by neuromuscular blocking agents.

Tracheal intubation[18] is merely one of several maneuvers the anesthetist uses for providing a patent airway and ensuring adequate pulmonary ventilation. The advantages of tracheal intubation are: (1) upper airway soft tissue obstruction is bypassed; (2) laryngeal stridor or laryngospasm is prevented; (3) the lungs are protected from aspiration if gastric content is regurgitated; (4) gastric distention with intermittent positive pressure respiration is prevented, and thus the use of a mechanical ventilator is facilitated; and (5) tracheobronchial suctioning is facilitated.

Intubation is desirable for prolonged major intraperitoneal operations and should always be performed in the very obese patient who is to be operated upon in the Trendelenburg position, and in any patient who is to be placed in the knee-chest (culdoscopy) position. Although a tracheal tube facilitates positive pressure ventilation in the curarized patient, a skilled anesthetist should also be able to produce adequate controlled ventilation in the apneic patient with the use of a face mask and a pharyngeal airway.

Complications associated with tracheal intubation are more common in the hands of the inexperienced anesthetist. The choice of a tube with too small a diameter, intubation of a bronchus or the esophagus, or a kink in the tube may produce airway obstruction. Traumatic intubation, the use of too large a tube, or the use of irritating lubricants very occasionally result in obstructive laryngeal edema or laryngeal granuloma. Trauma to lips, tongue, teeth, pharynx, and larynx may occur during attempts at intubation. Transient tachycardia and hypertension, which accompany intubation under light anesthesia, are usually harmless. Prolonged and repeated unsuccessful attempts at tracheal intubation, however, may lead to hypoxia and cardiac arrest; therefore, if an airway can be maintained without the use of a tracheal tube, unsuccessful attempts at intubation should not be pursued. Unrecognized esophageal intubation may lead to death. If there is any doubt about ventilation after intubation, the tracheal tube should be removed and the patient ventilated by bag and mask.

Sore throat and hoarseness are common minor complications following tracheal intubation. The incidence of sore throat is minimized by an atraumatic technic of intubation, by avoidance of coughing and bucking once the tube is placed, and by the inhalation of warm mist immediately after extubation. The prolonged pressure of a face mask during a long-lasting anesthesia may produce edema and dermatitis of the face, a more unpleasant condition than a slightly sore throat. In general, the advantages of tracheal intubation outweigh its disadvantages.

Fire and Explosion Hazards. Death from anesthetic explosions prior to the introduction of halothane was estimated to occur in about 1 of 1 million anesthesias.[15] A fire or explosion may occur whenever there are present both a combustible material (e.g., ether, cyclopropane, ethylene, Vinethene, ethyl chloride) and oxygen or nitrous oxide for the support of combustion. Inhalation anesthetics which may be used safely in the presence of electrical equipment are nitrous oxide, halothane, and trichloroethylene. The introduction of halothane (Fluothane) has greatly reduced the need for flammable anesthetics, and some anesthesiologists feel that the expensive explosion protection in operating room design is no longer necessary.

Whenever a flammable anesthetic is used, the following considerations and precautions are essential: (1) The flammability of ether in anesthetic concentrations is about as great as that of cyclopropane. Cyclopropane merely explodes with greater force. (2) Obvious sources of ignition are open sparks and open flames. (3) A less obvious ignition source is the static spark. If two objects with different electrical potential approximate, a spark may occur. Therefore the grounding of personnel and of objects prevents the development of these different electrical potentials. (4) As important as sparkproof equipment is the discipline of the operating room personnel. Personnel in the anesthetizing area, including the surgeons, should wear conductive shoes and check them for conductivity prior to entering the operating room. Blankets and clothes of wool or nylon should be prohibited in the operating room. The floors, the operating tables, and the mattresses should be conductive or grounded with wet towels before starting anesthesia. Persons other than the anesthetist should not touch the anesthetic machine or the patient at a site close to the airway. Physical contact should be made at a distance from the combustible agent. Cautery and other electrical equipment should not be plugged in or turned on without the permission of the anesthetist. (5) For removal of combustible fumes, the operating room should be adequately ventilated. (6) If during the use of a flammable agent, use of electrocautery becomes essential, surgeon and anesthesiologist must be aware of the hazards involved. These can be minimized by delaying the use of cautery until the flammable agent is washed from the anesthetic system and patient or by confining the flammable agent in a closed system, using a barrier between airway and cautery (e.g., wet towel) and keeping cautery at least 2 feet from the anesthetic gas (apparatus and/or airway).

SPINAL ANESTHESIA

Spinal anesthesia is described here in more detail for the following reasons: (1) Every gynecologic surgeon and obstetrician should be thoroughly trained in this technic. (2) Most gynecologic operations can be performed under spinal anesthesia. (3) Because of the manpower problems in anesthesiology, in some areas in this country and abroad there are still hospitals without anesthesiologists; in this case, the use of spinal anesthesia for gynecologic surgery may be safer than the routine use of general anesthesia, provided that the surgeon who gives the spinal anesthetic is experienced not only in the performance of lumbar puncture but also in the management of the patient following subarachnoid injection.

Some patients seem to be more afraid of paralysis from spinal anesthesia than of death from general anesthesia. Therefore we do not recommend the use of spinal anesthesia in patients who feel strongly against its use. The patient is persuaded to agree to a spinal anesthetic only if a general anesthetic would represent a greater hazard.

The poor reputation which spinal anesthesia has gained in some parts of the world is undeserved and is due primarily to indiscriminate use, which has caused (1) major neurologic complications and (2) sudden death following subarachnoid injection.

Prevention of Major Neurologic Complications. In 1950 Foster Kennedy stated that "paralysis below the waist is too large a price for a patient to pay in order that the surgeon should have a fine, relaxed field." Since then careful follow-up studies by Dripps and Vandam[7, 20] and other investigators of several thousand patients who had spinal anesthesia have shown clearly that serious neurologic sequelae do not occur when equipment is prepared properly, and an atraumatic technic is used.

Cases of adhesive arachnoiditis and myelitis seem to have been due to subarachnoid injection of irritating substances other than the local anesthetic. This can be avoided by meticulous cleaning of the equipment, by careful technic, and by abandoning the habit of soaking ampules in antiseptic solutions, as an invisible crack may permit contamination of an ampule with the antiseptic. During the presence of persistent paresthesia following lumbar puncture the drug should never be injected, since the needle may have been inserted into a nerve root, and intraneural injection may damage the spinal cord.

Prevention of Sudden Death.[9, 14] The subarachnoid injection of a local anesthetic may lead to sudden hypotension and respiratory arrest, a complication which can be avoided with correct technic. Spinal anesthesia is contraindicated in patients in hypovolemic shock.

The spinal anesthetic block causes vasodilation, which in turn leads to pooling of blood in the anesthetized and dependent areas of the body, and thus hampers the venous return to the heart. The resulting hypotension may cause cerebral ischemia and thus respiratory arrest. Apnea caused by a rise of the motor block to the 4th cervical segment (i.e., the phrenic nerves) is very unlikely with the use of conventional technics and dosages.

Since hypoxia and hypotension are the principal hazards of spinal anesthesia, oxygen is given by a light plastic face mask, whenever possible, and the blood pressure is checked frequently. Hypotension occurs most commonly following movement of the patient from the lumbar puncture position to the operating position. Therefore this movement should be performed gradually and cautiously. In an attempt to prevent hypotension the legs should be elevated immediately following subarachnoid injection. A flexed position is obtained when, in addition, the shoulders are elevated to prevent a further rise of the anesthetic. After the anesthetic level has stabilized (see later), the patient may be placed in the desired position. If hypotension occurs, the legs should never be lowered in the mistaken belief that this would counteract hypotension by preventing a rise of the anesthetic level. On the contrary, the legs should be elevated to enhance venous return. Hypotension should be corrected promptly with the intravenous injection of a vasopressor and infusion of fluids.

If the anesthetic level includes the splanchnic segments (T-5), hypotension is more likely to occur. The patient with low blood volume, essential hypertension, or arteriosclerosis is more prone to develop hypotension with spinal anesthesia.

The routine prophylactic intramuscular injection of a vasopressor prior to the subarachnoid injection of an anesthetic is a matter of personal preference. Many feel that prior to performing high spinal anesthesia, a prophylactic intramuscular injection of a vasopressor is advisable. Once hypotension occurs, a vasopressor should be injected intravenously for titration of the blood pressure.

Postspinal-Anesthesia Headache. Although not a life-threatening condition, postspinal-anesthesia headache deters some people from the use of spinal anesthesia. Headache has been shown to be most likely due to loss of cerebrospinal fluid through the puncture hole, as the incidence of postspinal-anesthesia headache is higher following the use of a large-gauge needle than following the use of a small-gauge needle. The incidence of headache is also high in women, in young patients, in patients with increased intra-abdominal pressure (e.g., full-term pregnancy) and with early ambulation. The use of a 24-gauge needle can reduce the incidence of headache to between 1 and 6 per cent. We have been using 24- and 26-gauge lumbar puncture needles satisfactorily without the use of introducer needles.

Once headache occurs, the best treatment is the intravenous infusion of large amounts of fluid and the maintenance of the patient in the level position. Analgesics and narcotics may be given as needed. If this fails, one may inject saline solution into the epidural space in an attempt to increase subarachnoid pressure.

Preparation of the Spinal Tray. Not only sterility but also chemical cleanliness of syringes, needles, and ampules is imperative. Our spinal tray consists of the following: 1 cover towel; 1 drape with hole for the patient's back; 1 glass cup for the skin antiseptic; 1 syringe, 5 ml. plain tip for the subarachnoid injection; 1 syringe, 2 ml., for local anesthesia of the skin and injection of a vasopressor; 1 needle, 20-gauge, 2", for drawing the spinal anesthetic into the syringe, which may also serve as introducer for small-gauge spinal needles; 1 hypodermic needle, 25-gauge, for skin anesthesia; 1 needle, 22-gauge, 2", for I.M. injection; lumbar puncture needles, 3½" with stylette, 1 each 22-, 24- and 26-gauge; 2 sponge forceps and 3 sponges for sterilizing the skin; 1 ampule file; 1 ampule, 2 ml., of tetracaine 1%; 1 ampule, 3 ml., of dextrose, 10%; 1 ampule of epinephrine 1:1000; 1 ampule, 2 ml., of lidocaine 5%/dextrose 7.5%; 1 ampule of procaine 1% for anesthesia of the skin; 1 ampule, 1 ml., of the vasopressor ephedrine 50 mg./ml.

Before autoclaving, needles and syringes are first cleaned with a nondetergent soap and then rinsed thoroughly with distilled water. All drugs should be in sealed ampules, prepared by reputable manufacturers. The anesthetics should not be reautoclaved. The spinal trays are autoclaved for 12 minutes at 270° F. and 32 lbs. pressure. Factory-prepared and sterilized disposable spinal trays may also be satisfactory. They are safe and preferable in hospitals where the meticulous preparation of trays described above is not possible.

Anesthetic Solution. The type and the specific gravity of the anesthetic used depends on personal preference and experience. We are commonly using hyperbaric tetracaine (Pontocaine), i.e., 1 per cent tetracaine plus equal amounts of 10 per cent dextrose, which has a specific gravity of 1.024; the specific gravity of cerebrospinal fluid is 1.004 to 1.007. After injection of the dosages listed in Table 3-1 anesthesia of 2 to 3 hours' duration can be expected. If anesthesia is desired for longer than 2 hours, epinephrine, 0.3 to 0.5 mg., should be added to the tetracaine/dextrose solution. A larger amount of epinephrine should not be used because of the danger of producing ischemia of the spinal cord. Hyperbaric lidocaine (Xylocaine) (lidocaine-dextrose) may be used for operations which can be completed within about 1½ hours. The approximate doses of both drugs are summarized in Table 3-1.

Spinal Anesthetic Level. The level of the autonomic block is higher than that of the sensory block, which in turn is

TABLE 3-1. SPINAL ANESTHESIA WITH HYPERBARIC SOLUTIONS
Lidocaine (Xylocaine) 5% with Dextrose 7.5%, for Anesthesia of up to 1½ Hours;
Tetracaine (Pontocaine) 1%, Plus Dextrose 10% in Equal Amounts for
Anesthesia of up to 2 Hours; Epinephrine, 0.3-0.5 mg., added to
Tetracaine-Dextrose for Anesthesia Over 2 Hours

SITE OF OPERATION	POSITION FOR OPERATION	POSITION FOR INJECTION	ANESTHESIA SENSORY LEVEL REQUIRED*	APPROXIMATE DOSE† LIDO-CAINE	TETRA-CAINE
Anus	Jackknife-prone	Sitting 5 min.	S-1	50 mg.	5 mg.
Anus, vulva	Lithotomy	Sitting 30 sec.	T-12	50 mg.	10 mg.
Uterus, bladder (vaginal, extraperit.)	Lithotomy	Sitting for injection	T-8	75 mg.	12 mg.
Uterus, etc. (vaginal, intraperit.)	Lithotomy	Sitting for injection	T-5	75 mg.	12 mg.
Laparotomy	Supine Trendelenburg	Lateral-horizontal for injection	T-5	100 mg.	14 mg.

* Xyphoid = T-5/6
  Umbilicus = T-10
  Symphysis = T-12/L-1

† For patient 5 ft. 5 in. tall. If shorter, smaller dose. If taller, larger dose. If increased intra-abdominal pressure (e.g., full-term pregnancy) ½ to ⅔ dose.

higher than that of the motor block. The reasons are that the drug is diluted by diffusion, and a higher concentration of the anesthetic is required for blocking myelinated and thicker fibers. For vaginal operations which do not include opening the peritoneal cavity, an anesthetic level at or above T-8 is required, since autonomic afferent impulses from the pelvic organs enter the spinal cord to this level. For intraperitoneal procedures, both vaginal and abdominal, the block should include the splanchnic afferents, i.e., to the level of T-5. For laparotomies the motor block should be higher than for vaginal hysterectomies. Therefore, for laparotomies injection is performed in the lateral position, whereas for vaginal hysterectomies the injection is usually performed in the sitting position.

The spinal anesthetic level is influenced by (1) the dosage of the anesthetic; (2) the specific gravity of the solution; (3) the length of the patient's vertebral column, i.e., the patient's height; (4) the rate of injection; (5) the volume injected; (6) the position of the patient during and immediately following injection; (7) the addition of epinephrine to the solution, which delays fixation of the anesthetic and, thus, "drifting" of the level; and (8) the intra-abdominal pressure. Increased intra-abdominal pressure (ascites, large intraperitoneal tumors, obesity, full-term pregnancy, straining and coughing) may cause engorgement of the epidural veins, and thus narrowing of the subarachnoid space, which results in a higher anesthetic level. In full-term pregnancy the dose should never exceed two thirds of the usual dose.

Technic. The person who has never given a spinal anesthetic should first study a standard text[6, 9, 14] and perform several spinal anesthetics under the close supervision of an experienced anesthesiologist. More difficult than the lumbar puncture itself is prevention of hypotension, retching, and patient discomfort following the subarachnoid injection. Before the subarachnoid injection, a blood pressure cuff should always be applied, and an intravenous infusion should always be started so that a vasopressor may be given rapidly. Also, an anesthetic machine or bag-mask oxygen unit should be at hand for control of respiration.

The anesthetist must wear sterile gloves and use the "no touch" technic, namely, no touching of the barrel of the syringe and the shaft of the lumbar puncture needle. A sterile hand-scrub is not essential. The contamination of syringes and needles with powder from the gloves should be avoided.

The first 2 to 5 minutes following the subarachnoid injection are the most critical. During this time the anesthetic level should be tested and its rise controlled by correct positioning of the patient. The blood pressure should be checked repeatedly and maintained near normal, and the patient should be given oxygen especially when the anesthetic level is high, or the patient is in poor physical status. The anesthetic level is reasonably stabilized approximately 5 minutes after the injection of lidocaine/dextrose; 10 minutes after tetracaine/dextrose; and 15 minutes after pontocaine/dextrose/epinephrine.

A surgeon who injects a spinal anesthetic and leaves the patient unattended in order to perform the operation himself is negligent. If at all possible, the person who injects the anesthetic should attend the patient throughout the operation. If this is not possible, a trained nurse who is experienced with monitoring and resuscitation as well as with the use of vasopressors may attend the patient after the anesthetic level has been established. Consultation with a physician should be immediately available.

Continuous Spinal Anesthesia. This technic is rarely used now, as the addition of epinephrine to a single injection of tetracaine/dextrose provides anesthesia of 3 hours or more. The use of a large-bore needle, which is required for the insertion of a subarachnoid catheter, is associated with a high incidence of postlumbar-puncture headache.

Supplementation With General Anesthesia. Autonomic pain due to visceral stimulation may be controlled by intravenous injections of small amounts of thiopental. Somatic pain occurring when the anesthetic level is too low requires either the intravenous injection of an opiate or full supplementation with general anesthesia.

During major intra-abdominal operations, even the best spinal block often does not prevent patient discomfort and retching movements, apparently due to impulses via vagal afferents. This is more pronounced during upper abdominal than lower abdominal operations. Therefore in major laparotomies, spinal anesthesia should be administered by an anesthesiologist since supplementation usually proves necessary, and may be difficult and hazardous (total autonomic block, vomiting, etc). In these cases, deliberate supplementation from the beginning with light general anesthesia is often preferred. This may provide optimal working conditions, maximal abdominal wall relaxation, quiet spontaneous breathing, and a contracted intestine.

PARACERVICAL BLOCK

Paracervical block[4, 10, 21] may be used for D and C, culdoscopy (with supplementary intravenous sedation) and other operations at the cervix in those cases in which major conduction anesthesia or general anesthesia is unavailable or contraindicated. The dosage of local anesthetic used approximates 20 ml. of lidocaine 1 per cent, i.e., 10 ml. in each lateral fornix. Possible, although rare, complications include hematoma of the broad ligament, sacral neuritis, and parametritis.

CHOICE OF ANESTHETIC AGENTS AND TECHNICS

Most operations can be performed safely and satisfactorily with any of a great number of anesthetic agents and technics. Even with patients in poor physical status, more than one approach is usually satisfactory. The anesthetist with limited experience, who is giving anesthesia without supervision, should use the technic with which he is most familiar. The experienced anesthetist should consider why one approach should be preferred to another. The following should be considered: (1) the physical status and complicating diseases of the patient; (2) the previous experience of the patient with anesthetics and her desire to be awake or asleep; (3) the need for muscular relaxation or controlled ventilation; (4) use of electrocautery or other explosion hazards; (5) the operative technic to be used by the surgeon; and (6) the surgeon's desire to have the patient awake or asleep.

An internist, asked to evaluate the patient preoperatively, should not suggest the anesthetic to be used. The internist rarely has had firsthand experience in the operating room which is necessary to understand the problems of induction, airway obstruction, artificial ventilation, the needs of the surgeon, and the influence of disease and drugs on the conduct of anesthesia. The judgment and the skill of the anesthesiologist are more important in the safe choice of an anesthetic than theoretical considerations.

There are very few contraindications to most anesthetic agents or technics. Spinal anesthesia should be avoided in patients with preexisting neurologic disease,[20] in patients with skin infection over the lumbar puncture area, and in patients who refuse spinal anesthesia, unless a different anesthetic would appear to be more hazardous. High spinal anesthesia should be avoided in impending and frank shock.

Pulmonary Disease. Patients with a history of asthma or suspicion of chronic obstructive lung disease should be evaluated and prepared by a physician experienced in respiratory care.[3, 11, 18] Evaluation may have to include spirometry and blood gas analysis. Complicating infection, heart failure, or allergy (eosinophilia) should be corrected before elective operation. If at all possible, the patient should be made wheeze-free prior to operation. In asthma, which is not amenable to usual bronchial clearing measures including the use of IPPB/mist/bronchodilators, it may prove lifesaving to give large doses of steroids for 3 to 5 days "para-operation."

Asthmatic patients in need of vaginal operations can be managed safely with spinal or caudal anesthesia. For abdominal procedures the high spinal anesthesia which would be required enhances the likelihood of an asthmatic attack because of respiratory depression and block of the pulmonary sympathetics. Therefore general endotracheal anesthesia is preferred for laparotomies in asthmatics. Excessive coughing and bronchial secretions require relaxation and tracheal intubation for traechobronchial clearing. Although ether anesthesia, because of its bronchodilator effect, has been recommended in the past as the agent of choice for asthmatics, recent experience indicates that $N_2O/O_2(50\%/50\%)$, reinforced with halothane and, if necessary, with relaxants, is more satisfactory. Thiopental and cyclopropane may produce or augment bronchoconstriction in asthmatics. The latter may also augment airway secretions. The use of narcotics should be avoided unless respirations are assisted or controlled. Muscle relaxants do not block spasm of the smooth bronchial musculature, but may facilitate control of wheezes during positive pressure inflation of the lungs because of blockage of abdominal wall spasm (i.e., coughing, bucking).

PULMONARY TUBERCULOSIS does not contraindicate any anesthetic technic unless the sputum is positive. In such patients, any general anesthetic may provoke the spread of a tuberculotic process. Therefore elective operation should be postponed until the patient is sputum-negative.

For emergency operations in patients with positive sputum, spinal anesthesia is used whenever possible. Excessive bronchial secretions cause coughing, which may annoy the surgeon; suctioning of the trachea is difficult when the patient is awake under spinal anesthesia but is facilitated with general endotracheal anesthesia.

Cardiovascular Disease. Patients with cardiovascular disease should be anesthetized in a way that will not produce sudden changes in their already precarious circulatory balance. Induction must be slow and cautious. Therefore the surgeon should not be impatient with the anesthetist who performs a gradual induction with inhalation anesthesia, rather than a rapid induction with thiopental, which may be more hazardous.

Patients with congestive heart disease may benefit from the peripheral vasodilation produced by spinal anesthesia (bloodless phlebotomy). In contrast, patients with coronary artery disease may suffer myocardial infarction if a sudden reduction in aortic pressure occurs. Therefore in the latter group, light general anesthesia is preferred.

Obesity. One of the most serious obstacles to the safe management of anesthesia is severe obesity, particularly in abdominal operations in the Trendelenburg position. A short neck often makes tracheal intubation mandatory. When the already overtaxed ventilation of the obese patient is further impaired by the use of narcotics, anesthetics, or relaxants, adequate ventilation can be maintained only with assisted or controlled ventilation.

As peripheral arteries and veins are not easily accessible in obese patients, a plastic catheter should be inserted into a vein prior to the induction of anesthesia. Monitoring with the esophageal stethoscope is recommended during endotracheal anesthesias. Since after major laparotomies, postoperative gastric distention and vomiting seem to be more common in obese than in lean patients, a gastric tube is often used prophylactically during the early postoperative period.

Light inhalation anesthesia with relaxants is not contraindicated, provided that postoperative controlled ventilation via tracheal tube is continued until there is full recovery of consciousness and muscle power, together with proof that the patient can take spontaneous "sighing" breaths of 15-20 ml./kg. of body weight.

Anemia, Low Blood Volume, Shock. In anemia the oxygen-carrying capacity of the blood is reduced, which narrows the margin of safety in case of airway obstruction or apnea. Therefore particular attention must be paid to high inhaled oxygen concentrations. Patients with anemia, low blood volume, or shock require smaller amounts of anesthetics.

In a patient with hypovolemic shock (cold and clammy skin, tachycardia, pallor), cyclopropane may have the advantage in increasing peripheral vascular resistance and cardiac output in light planes of anesthesia and thus protecting cerebral and coronary perfusion pressures. Succinylcholine may be used although positive pressure ventilation should be performed gently and at a slow rate in order to permit filling of the heart. High spinal and epidural anesthesia are contraindicated in patients in shock, unless general anesthesia is not available (e.g., in medically underdeveloped areas).

It should be obvious that in all instances except those in which surgical intervention is considered part of the resuscitative effort, for instance, in intra-abdominal hemorrhage, blood volume and extravascular fluid volume should be restored prior to the induction of anesthesia.

Pregnancy.[4, 10] Elective operations should be avoided, if possible, during the first 3 months of pregnancy. There is as yet an unknown risk of inducing teratologic changes with most drugs. There is no evidence that general anesthetics and narcotics per se may damage the fetus, or may cause abortion when given after the period of organ development. If anesthesia is required during pregnancy, particular attention should be paid to prevent hypoxemia, hypercarbia, hypotension, and oligemia. Induction and emergence of anesthesia should be smooth. Regional anesthesia, when appropriate, is the first choice during pregnancy Halothane/oxygen produces uterine quiescence and permits high concentrations of oxygen to be used. Large amounts of narcotics should be avoided preoperatively and postoperatively to prevent hypoxia and hypotension. When spinal anesthesia is given in full-term pregnancy, two thirds of the regular dose should not be exceeded.

Old Age. There is no evidence that one anesthetic agent or technic is preferable to another in the elderly patient. Naturally, the aged cannot tolerate as much physiologic trespass as the young. Even a brief period of hypoxia or hypotension may result in further deterioration of a senile mind or in the worsening of an existing complicating disease. Preoperative correction of low blood volume and anemia, accurate replacement of blood loss, optimal pulmonary ventilation and oxygenation, and maintenance of a normal blood pressure are all of greater importance in the aged than in the young.

Deep anesthesia should be avoided if possible. Rapidly reversible anesthesia with inhalational drugs is preferred. In the case of hypotension and tachycardia, with anesthetic overdose and blood loss having been ruled out, rapid intravenous digitalization may be helpful.

Hazard of the Full Stomach. Inhalation of gastric content seems to account for about 20 per cent of all deaths due to anesthesia.[8, 17]

Vomiting or regurgitation of gastric content may lead to death by one of the following mechanisms: (1) laryngospasm; (2) acute obstructive asphyxia from aspiration of large amounts of gastric content; (3) inhalation of acid (gastric) or alkaline (duodenal) fluid with acute status asthmaticus/pulmonary-edema type clinical picture (chemical pneumonitis, Mendelson syndrome).[13]

Active vomiting may occur at any time during anesthesia, but it is most likely to occur in light anesthesia during induction or recovery. Passive regurgitation, which is more likely to go unnoticed, occurs usually when fullness of the stomach plus one of the following factors coexist: increased intra-abdominal pressure (e.g., intraperitoneal hemorrhage, intestinal obstruction); a gastric tube, rendering the cardia incompetent; curarization with relaxation of the striated muscles of the cricopharyngeal sphincter and diaphragm; the head-down position. Emptying of the stomach is prolonged by pain, peritoneal irritation (peritonitis, twisted ovarian cyst), serious illness (septicemia, shock), or narcotics; and in a patient with intestinal obstruction or paralytic ileus.

Every attempt must be made to prevent inhalation of gastric content. Patients who presumably have a full stomach should not be anesthetized unless the postponement of operation presents a greater risk. A patient who needs emergency operation and is suspected of having a full stomach should have a gastric tube inserted prior to the induction of anesthesia in order to aspirate as much liquid gastric content and gas as possible. Nevertheless, the presence of a gastric tube does not mean that the stomach is empty, as food particles do not pass into the tube or clog it. The gastric tube may merely decompress the stomach by allowing removal of some of the liquid and air, thus reducing the likelihood of regurgitation.

If a patient with a full stomach requires a perineal procedure, or a limited lower abdominal operation (e.g., uncomplicated appendectomy, or ovarectomy), spinal anesthesia is usually satisfactory. However, if a major laparotomy is required, a regional anesthesia would not necessarily be the best choice for the following reasons: (1) A high level of spinal or epidural anesthesia would be required, which by paralyzing the respiratory muscles would depress the protective cough. (2) Intraperitoneal stimulation often causes pushing or retching. (3) Patients with intestinal obstruction (ileus) are often oligemic, a contraindication for high spinal or epidural anesthesia. (4) Aspiration of vomitus may occur even under regional anesthesia with the patient conscious, particularly when patients are debilitated and when hypotension leads to nausea and vomiting. Therefore, in skilled hands general anesthesia with the use of a cuffed tracheal tube is safer for laparotomies in patients with full stomachs than is regional anesthesia.

COMPLICATIONS DURING ANESTHESIA

Although arterial hypotension may be related to respiratory inadequacy and hypoxemia, it is more commonly due to (1) inadequate blood volume, (2) overdose with anesthetic, (3) pre- and para-anesthetic drugs, and (4) surgical manipulations.

Blood Loss. Even the experienced surgeon may underestimate the amount of blood loss during gynecologic operations. Therefore, in teaching hospitals it is frequently advisable to measure blood loss by weighing sponges and by measuring blood in the suction bottle.[1] This gravimetric technic of blood loss measurement can be applied any time if dry sponges of known weight are routinely used. With the use of moist sponges gravimetric measurement of blood loss, although less accurate, is also possible, if the nurse measures the amount of saline solution used for moistening the sponges, provided that spilling of the solution is avoided. Colorimetric technics of blood loss measurement require special equipment and do not give results as readily as the gravimetric technic.

Measurement of circulating blood volume before, during, and after operation may be helpful. The more reliable technics available at present (measurement of the dilution of injected radioactive chromium-tagged red cells or radioactive-iodine-tagged serum albumin) are technics which require expensive equipment and trained personnel, so that their routine clinical use is hardly justified. They give erroneous results in the presence of bleeding. Arterial hypotension, low central venous pressure, tachycardia, constricted veins, clammy skin, and pallor are considered signs of hypovolemic shock. With impending shock the systolic pressure is less likely to be low than the pulse pressure, particularly in the young and fit person. The pulse rate is not always a reliable sign as tachycardia can also be caused by poor ventilation or anesthetics, and as hemorrhage may be accompanied occasionally by bradycardia, particularly in the aged.

The generally healthy woman undergoing gynecologic surgery does not require transfusion if the blood loss is less than 500 to 800 ml. The risk from blood transfusion (hepatitis, hemolytic transfusion reaction) must be weighed against the possibility of retarding recovery if transfusion is withheld. The patient in poor physical status and the aged should have accurate replacement of blood loss.

During exsanguination hemorrhage with massive blood transfusions, measurement of blood loss and estimation of arterial and venous pressure help to avoid overtransfusion and undertransfusion.

Uncontrollable *oozing* is sometimes observed after extensive pelvic operations. The etiology of this oozing is obscure, although it is known that some organs, such as the uterus, may liberate substances which block coagulation. Also banked blood, when transfused in large quantities, may be responsible for oozing, since it lacks clotting factors. Unusual oozing and unexpected hypotension during anesthesia may be the sign of a hemolytic transfusion reaction. This is best ruled out by inspection of a centrifuged blood sample. Probably the best treatment for uncontrollable oozing is the infusion of fresh whole blood, i.e., blood drawn within 1 to 2 hours. In those patients in whom fibrinolysis is diagnosed (laboratory or bedside observation of blood clotting and lysis in test tube at body temperature), the intravenous administration of epsilon-aminocaproic acid with or without heparin is indicated. Calcium, fibrinogen, and vitamin K should be used when it is specifically indicated.

Overdose With Anesthetics. Thiopental, halothane, or ether is more likely to cause hypotension than cyclopropane or nitrous oxide. If the anesthetist is in doubt as to the cause of hypotension, the concentration of the inhaled anesthetic is reduced immediately, or the injection of the intravenous anesthetic is stopped. The blood level of inhalation anesthetics can be reduced rapidly by "flushing" the lungs with oxygen.

Hypotension with too vigorous a performance of controlled ventilation has been observed in the hypovolemic and debilitated patient. However, positive pressure ventilation can hardly be blamed as a cause of hypotension if performed with a low mean airway pressure (i.e., by allowing the airway pressure to drop to atmospheric pressure during exhalation). Whenever hypotension occurs, the rate of positive pressure ventilation should be reduced in order to permit better filling of the heart.

Pre- and Para-anesthetic Drugs. The frequent use of phenothiazines, imipramine, and MAO inhibitors as tranquilizers or mood-modifiers in the female population, especially during menopausal years, has definite implications when general anesthesia is used. These drugs may produce hypotension (which is poorly controlled by vasopressors) or hypertensive crises with the induction or maintenance of general anesthesia.

Current opinions favor the discontinuance of MAO inhibitors for approximately 10 days preoperatively, if possible. Phenothiazines and imipramine as well as antihypertensive drugs such as reserpine and guanethidine do not have to be discontinued, but the anesthetist must be aware of their use to control properly the hypotensive and other cardiovascular responses which may ensue.

The anesthesiologist should also be made aware of those patients who are receiving steroids, anticonvulsive drugs, anticoagulants, and others.

Hypotension From Surgical Manipulations. If hypotension and bradycardia occur during surgical stimulation of the abdominal viscera, and anesthetic overdose and blood loss have been ruled out, a vagal type reflex, (probably via the celiac plexus) is to be suspected. If, in such a case, atropine (0.5 to 1 mg. I.V.) does not raise the blood pressure promptly, a vasopressor should be injected intravenously. A decrease of vena caval blood flow may cause reduction in cardiac output and hypotension. This has been seen as the result of vena caval compression by surgical retractors, the heavy pregnant uterus, or large heavy tumors when the patient is supine, or by tilting of the liver as in gallbladder operations. Treatment consists of appropriate changes of posture and/or cessation of manipulations.

Treatment of Hypotension. Moderate hypotension which is not due to blood loss is harmless in the young, generally healthy patient, and therefore does not have to be corrected, if it is due to vasodilation. However, in the middle-aged or elderly patient, in the diabetic, and in the patient with cardiovascular disease, even moderate reductions in arterial pressure should be corrected promptly with the judicious use of vasopressors, if necessary. In such cases, even brief periods of hypotension may cause ischemic, myocardial, or cerebral damage.

Therefore, besides appropriate blood volume balance (see later) a vasopressor should be used briefly to combat severe arterial hypotension until the cause of the hypotension is corrected. Examples of pure peripheral vasoconstrictors are methoxamine (Vasoxyl) and phenylephrin (Neo-Synephrine). Examples of vasoconstrictors which also stimulate cardiac contraction are ephedrine, metaraminol (Aramine), and norepinephrine (Levophed). Titrated intravenous infusion of the drugs mentioned is usually more satisfactory in treating vasodilation hypotension than the intermittent injection of individual doses. While metaraminol or phenylephrine usually raise the arterial pressure effectively, specific types of hypotension may respond only to norepinephrine. Raising the arterial pressure above the level considered normal for the individual patient is unsound. Epinephrine (vasoconstrictor/vasodilator and cardiac stimulant) as well as isoproterenol (vasodilator and cardiac stimulant) are reserved for specific indications in cardiac resuscitation and are contraindicated in conjunction with cyclopropane and halothane.

Air embolism is extremely uncommon but must be considered as a possible cause of sudden hypotension or cardiac arrest during operations involving large veins, and during pressure infusion from bottles. Tubal insufflation, performed with CO_2, should not lead to lethal gas embolism. Air embolization must be recognized immediately ("millwheel murmur," arterial hypotension, central venous hypertension) if resuscitation is to be successful.[16]

MONITORING OF VITAL SIGNS

Some general aspects of monitoring respiratory, circulatory, and metabolic parameters are discussed later. Some aspects of monitoring vital signs in the operating room are discussed here. The most reliable, simplest, and least expensive monitors are the anesthesiologist's senses. Sophisticated methods may, however, be indicated in the patient in poor physical status (PS 3 to 5) or during extensive operations, regardless of the patient's physical status.

Monitoring of Ventilation. The adequacy of alveolar ventilation can be determined with certainty only by measuring arterial pCO_2. The next best measure for patients with healthy lungs would be end-expiratory pCO_2. Both of these parameters cannot be monitored continuously at this time with the presently available equipment in a practical form in all anesthetized patients. Therefore, realizing that hypoventilation may be harmful, anesthetists usually aim for moderate hyperventilation by assisted or controlled ventilation when respiratory depressant drugs are used. A ventilation meter, which can be inserted into the anesthetic system, is used to measure tidal volumes and, in the conscious person, vital capacity when respiratory movements remain depressed, particularly after the use of muscle relaxants.

Monitoring of Oxygenation. Because of the notorious unreliability of cyanosis, adequate arterial oxygenation can be determined with certainty only by measuring PaO_2. *Cyanosis* depends upon the total amount of reduced hemoglobin in capillary and venous blood visible in mucous membranes and skin. Therefore, hypoxemia in an anemic person may not produce cyanosis, whereas a polycythemic person may be cyanotic in spite of adequate oxygenation. Sometimes even severe hypoxemia is not associated with visible cyanosis—for instance, when concomitant hypercarbia produces vasodilation.

When the surgeon remarks that the blood is dark, the anesthesiologist should attempt to rule out hypoxemia by checking ventilation and the patient's color at other sites—for instance, the tongue. Dark venous blood may also be due to posture (pooling), or slowed blood flow (regional, e.g., use of local vasoconstrictors; or general, e.g., reduced cardiac output).

While the absence of cyanosis does not rule out hypoxemia, the presence of cyanosis in the absence of polycythemia should be cause for concern. In general, adequate ventilation with at least 50 per cent O_2, the absence of dark blood in the incision, and the absence of peripheral cyanosis in the presence of a near-normal hematocrit would rule out hypoxemia.

Monitoring of Circulation. There is no substitute for continuous palpation of the peripheral pulse. Any accessible artery may be used. Frequent checking of the arterial blood pressure with the Riva-Rocci cuff method is desirable, but it should neither replace continuous palpation of the pulse nor cause interruption of artificial respiration in the apneic patient for more than a few seconds.

Controlled ventilation, by abolishing spontaneous breathing movements (a useful sign of life), must be accompanied by continuous monitoring of the circulation, either by continuous palpation of a pulse or by continuous auscultation of heart sounds. These two parameters are more meaningful in terms of oxygen transport than the EKG.

Heart sounds may be monitored either with a regular stethoscope taped over the precordium or with an esophageal stethoscope. The latter frees the hands of the anesthetist for other tasks—for instance, infusion. Continuous monitoring of heart sounds gives information not only concerning the heart rate but also concerning the quality of cardiac contractions. During shock, when the heart sounds become faint, such information may be important. The esophageal stethoscope also gives valuable information concerning respirations. It enables the anesthesiologist rapidly to detect secretions in the airway, wheezing, pulmonary edema, and air embolization.

Continuous monitoring of the EKG is indicated in patients with cardiovascular disease, particularly those with arrhythmias and those with a history of coronary artery disease, and during operations associated with massive blood transfusions or major electrolyte shifts.

THE POSTANESTHETIC PERIOD

The dangers of the immediate postoperative period cannot be overemphasized. Many deaths have occurred at the conclusion of an operation, when the surgeon is leaving the operating room, the anesthetist is transporting the patient, and the nurses are cleaning the equipment.

Recovery Room/Intensive Care Unit. The value of a recovery room is well-known. The data of the Baltimore Joint Anesthesia Study Committee indicate that the incidence of postoperative deaths is higher when patients are returned to the ward immediately after surgery.[1]

Most hospitals have acquired a postanesthetic recovery room, in which patients remain until they have recovered from anesthesia. It is desirable to have such a room potentially staffed around the clock. One step further has been the establishment of intensive care units to which nonoperative as well as operative patients are admitted. A general multidisciplinary intensive care unit has certain advantages over fragmented, departmental intensive care units.[5] Ideally, recovery room, intensive care unit and coronary surveillance unit should be separate, but located adjacent to each other for easier around-the-clock staffing by physicians and for better utilization of special equipment. Specially trained nurses should be assigned permanently to these units. The establishment of an intensive care unit should follow these steps in order of priority:[5] (1) organization (ICU committee, medical supervisor, nursing supervisor); (2) physical design and equipment; (3) around-the-clock coverage by nurses; (4) around-the-clock coverage by physicians; and (5) research.

Most Common Life-Threatening Complications

The most common life-threatening complications of the early postoperative period are: (1) asphyxia, (2) hypoxemia, (3) postanesthetic hypotension, and (4) hemorrhage or inadequate replacement of surgical blood loss.

Asphyxia is hypoxemia plus hypercarbia. This may occur when the respiratory movements are depressed, or when there is airway obstruction. The unconscious patient breathing adequately should be placed on her side with head tilted backward. Postoperative respiratory complications and their management are described in detail elsewhere.[18]

During closure of the skin, the patient may appear to breathe adequately, while respiratory depression may supervene when the surgical stimulus has ceased. A partially curarized patient may appear to breathe adequately through the tracheal tube, but may become weaker after extubation—for instance, when airway obstruction imposes increased respiratory work. Tracheal extubation and control of postextubation complications (e.g., laryngospasm, vomiting, upper airway soft tissue obstruction) should be according to the anesthesiologist's judgment: he should ascertain the adequacy of ventilatory volumes and respiratory reserve muscle power (an inspiratory capacity of about 1000 ml./70 kg.) prior to extubation.

Hypoxemia may occur when the mask or the tracheal tube is removed, and the high inhaled oxygen concentration used during anesthesia is suddenly reduced to that of air. Hypoxemia may also occur when the anesthetic apparatus is disconnected from the patient at the conclusion of a nitrous oxide anesthetic, without previous hyperoxygenation of the lungs. In this case, nitrous oxide, which is much more soluble and better diffusable than nitrogen, leaves the blood in large quantities and floods the alveoli, which, in combination with the inhaled nitrogen of the air, may dilute the alveolar oxygen to dangerously low levels. This "diffusion hypoxia" is prevented by "flushing" the lungs with oxygen before allowing the patient to breathe air.

Normal PaO_2 values in healthy young or middle-aged adults range between 80 and 100 mm. Hg; those in elderly patients may normally be between 70 and 90 mm. Hg. PaO_2 values below about 70 mm. Hg must be considered abnormal, and those below 50 mm. Hg, life-threatening (at sea level).

The most common cause of hypoxemia is the absence of periodic deep breaths. Most patients with healthy lungs can maintain a normal $PaCO_2$ with tidal volumes of as little as 500 ml./70 kg. body weight, at a rate of 15 to 20 per minute. However, in the absence of periodic deep breaths, progressive miliary atelectasis with right to left shunting of blood through nonrecruited alveoli and resulting hypoxemia will develop.[3] This can be prevented by active or passive lung inflations of 1000-1500 ml./70 kg. sustained for 3 to 5 seconds each, about every 10 to 20 minutes. Oxygen enrichment and periodic deep breaths, therefore, must be part of routine postoperative care.

In the intubated patient, this artificial sighing is best provided by the volume limited technic of manual compression of a self-refilling bag-valve unit. In the patient without a tracheal tube, the best method for preventing postoperative pulmonary complications is a skillful, vigilant, stir-up regime, namely, coached deep-breathing and coughing, frequent change of position to prevent hypostatic atelectasis, and early ambulation.

The adequacy of spontaneous sighing is first ascertained with a ventilation meter and mask. If the patient is unable to sigh himself adequately in spite of coaching and analgesia, he should be sighed passively. One method, satisfactory in the alert patient, is to make him inhale increased concentrations of carbon dioxide with the CO_2 rebreathing technic. This technic, which depends upon the accumulation of endogenous CO_2, is safer than the inhalation of unknown high concentrations of carbon dioxide from a cylinder. CO_2 therapy is contraindicated in obstructive lung disease, heart disease with cardiac arrhythmias or severe hypertension, and when there is increased intracranial pressure. In these cases, skillfully coached intermittent positive pressure breathing via mouthpiece, mask, or tracheal tube may be used.

Prolonged Artificial Ventilation and Oxygenation.[18] Respiratory insufficiency may occur after major abdominal operations, in patients with severe pulmonary disease, or after residual curarization. Incisional pain and abdominal distention augment the respiratory insufficiency, which may necessitate mechanical controlled or assisted ventilation. Prolonged tracheal intubation and mechanical ventilation should not be used as a last resort but rather as a prophylactic, postoperative measure whenever inadequacy of ventilation, increased work of breathing, or hypoxemia during 50 per cent O_2 inhalation is suspected. Skillfully performed, prolonged postanesthetic artificial ventilation via tracheal tube has become one of the leading contributions to the survival of critically ill surgical patients. Tracheal tubes have been left in place without causing serious damage for up to about 72 hours. When there is need for prolonged artificial ventilation beyond 3 days, one should consider switching to tracheostomy. Airway and pulmonary care of the intubated or tracheotomized patient must be by vigilant, aseptic, atraumatic technic.[18]

After general and major regional anesthesia, oxygen enrichment of the inhaled atmosphere is indicated through most of the recovery room period, even in patients with healthy lungs. Among the equipment used for oxygen inhalation in the postoperative period, the plastic, semi-open, oro-nasal, valveless face mask (with large bore tube for mist administration) proved satisfactory. An oxygen flow of at least 10 liters per minute should be used in order to prevent CO_2 accumulation, to provide an inhaled O_2 concentration of 50 to 70 per cent and to deliver adequate mist. Nasal catheters (O_2 flow 4-6 liters/minute, inhaled O_2 concentration 30-40 per cent) are also satisfactory, particularly the nostril "moustache" catheter. Nasal catheters are not suitable for delivery of mist. Oxygen tents hamper nursing care and usually provide lower concentrations of oxygen than the inexpensive equipment mentioned above. Pulmonary oxygen toxicity may occur if oxygen concentrations of over 70 per cent are inhaled for more than 12 hours. Inhalation of 100 per cent O_2 is limited to periods of 10 to 15 minutes preceding arterial pO_2 determinations, and require a tight-fitting, nonrebreathing system.

Dry oxygen rapidly causes drying of the respiratory mucosa, which destroys ciliary activity and thus may lead to lethal tracheobronchial infection, atelectasis, and pneumonitis. Breathing through the nose normally delivers gas with a relative humidity of 100 per cent at body temperature into the trachea. Whenever the nasal air passage is bypassed—for instance, by tracheal tube, tracheostomy tube, or mouth breathing (e.g., nasogastric tube)—heated humidification (water molecules in gas) or nebulization (water droplets in gas) is required. A satisfactory approach is heated nebulization, provided that nebulizers and administration equipment are maintained sterile to avoid iatrogenic infection by droplets. Routine administration of mist following endotracheal anesthesia after extubation seems to reduce the incidence of postintubation sore throat. Maximum mist is delivered by an ultrasonic nebulizer which is of value, in the form of periodic clearing sessions, in patients with lung disease and thick tracheobronchial secretions.[11, 18]

Since respiratory insufficiency is present in essentially all critically ill patients, respiratory care should be given with modern sophisticated technics[3, 18] under the direction of experienced physicians.

Postanesthetic Hypotension. Since during operation the blood pressure has been supported by accumulation of carbon dioxide or by the sympathetic stimulus of the operation or the anesthetic (e.g., cyclopropane), hypotension may ensue when these factors are removed at the conclusion of the operation. This postanesthetic hypotension occurs mainly after deep anesthesia and after periods of inadequate ventilation and is usually associated with a slow pulse rate. Movement of a patient may cause postural hypotension, particularly when his vasomotor control is blocked by spinal anesthesia, deep general anesthesia, or narcotics.

When the patient's legs are lowered after a long operation in the lithotomy position, gravity pooling of blood into the legs may be expected. To prevent this, the patient should be placed in the Trendelenburg position, and her legs lowered slowly. Possibly, wrapping the legs with elastic bandages before lowering them may prevent this complication.

If operative or postoperative blood loss has been ruled out, the treatment of postanesthetic hypotension consists of raising the legs, administering O_2, and giving intravenous solutions at a more rapid rate. If hypotension persists, a vasopressor drug should be injected intravenously. Vasopressor drugs may be used as a therapeutic measure to restore normal arterial pressure while search for the etiology of hypotension continues.

Hemorrhage or inadequate replacement of surgical blood loss must always be suspected when postoperative hypotension is observed. With low blood volume, the skin is cold and clammy, the veins and the arteries are contracted, the pulse pressure is narrow, the central venous pressure is decreased, and there is oliguria. Tachycardia is usually but not always observed during blood loss. In retroperitoneal hemorrhage, persistence of hypotension has been seen even after blood has been given much in excess of the amount found in the retroperitoneal space. This can possibly be explained by paravertebral sympathetic blockade caused by the hematoma. Also, continued retroperitoneal bleeding provokes consumption of clotting factors and perpetuates the bleeding through a state of hypocoagulability.

If operative blood loss has been replaced, and the signs of shock persist without evidence of external hemorrhage, internal bleeding should be ruled out by physical examination, aspiration of the cul-de-sac, or re-exploration of the abdomen. Normal hemoglobin or hematocrit values are obviously meaningless since hemorrhage leads to hemodilution of varying degrees and at varying rates.

A generally healthy patient who has lost less than 500 to 800 ml. of blood during operation does not require transfusion. On the other hand, a woman who has been anemic or hypovolemic before operation may require more blood than she has lost during operation, particularly if she is elderly or has cardiovascular disease. Patients who have had anemia due to chronic loss of small amounts of blood (metromenorrhagia) may have a normal circulating blood volume due to compensatory elevation of their plasma volume, and therefore should be transfused with packed red cells to avoid pulmonary edema.

RESUSCITATION

INTRODUCTION

Irreversible brain damage occurs when severe hypoxemia remains uncorrected or when cessation of circulation lasts longer than 3 to 5 minutes. Immediate application of modern cardiopulmonary resuscitation (Fig. 3-1) is capable of preventing biologic death and can be applied anywhere without the use of equipment by trained individuals. Clinical results depend, among other factors, upon the effectiveness of training,[23, 30] uniformity of teaching the details of technic, logistics of hospital resuscitation team function,[24] and an appreciation of the importance of the time factor.

EMERGENCY MEASURES
Oxygenate

IF UNCONSCIOUS

Airway

Tilt head back

IF NOT BREATHING

Breathe

Inflate lungs rapidly 3–5 times
mouth-to-mouth, mouth-to-nose,
mouth-to-adjunct, bag-mask

MAINTAIN HEAD TILT
- Feel carotid pulse
- If pulse present, continue 12 lung inflations per minute

IF PULSE ABSENT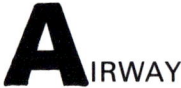
pupils dilated and deathlike appearance,

Circulate

Depress sternum once per second.

ONE OPERATOR:
Alternate 2 quick lung inflations with 15 sternal compressions ⟶

TWO OPERATORS:
Interpose one inflation after every fifth compression ⟶

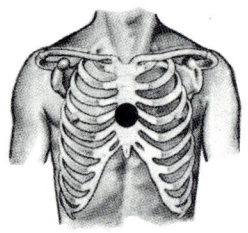 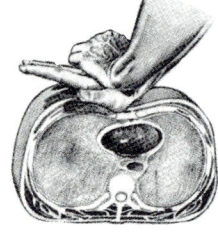 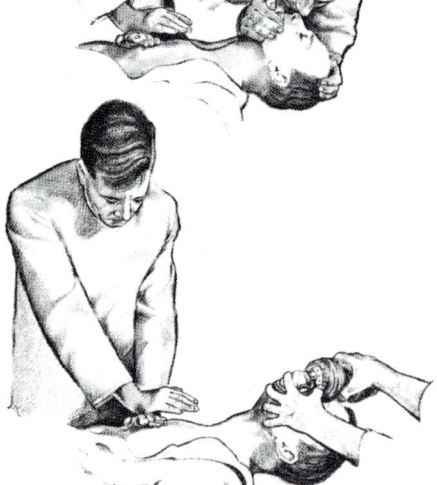

Depress lower sternum 1½–2″ (4–5 cm)
CONTINUE RESUSCITATION until spontaneous pulse returns

Fig. 3-1. Phases and steps of cardiopulmonary resuscitation. (Safar, P.: Cardiopulmonary Resuscitation: A Manula for Physicians and Paramedical Instructors. Published by the World Federation of Societies of Anaesthesiologists, 1968)

Hypoxemia, Airway Obstruction, and Hypoventilation

Causes

Asphyxia (hypoxemia plus hypercarbia) is usually caused by airway obstruction, hypoventilation, or apnea.

Hypoxemia without hypercarbia may be caused by oxygen-deprived atmosphere, carbon monoxide, and lung disease. Obstruction of bronchi, pulmonary edema, or pneumonia first cause increased right to left shunting of blood through unventilated alveoli and/or ven-

DEFINITIVE THERAPY
Restart Circulation—Support Recovery

DO NOT INTERRUPT CARDIAC COMPRESSIONS AND LUNG VENTILATION
INTUBATE TRACHEA WHEN POSSIBLE

DRUGS
EPINEPHRINE:
0.5–1.0 mg i.v. or i.c., repeat larger dose as necessary

SODIUM BICARBONATE:
1–2 mEq/kg i.v.
Repeat dose every 10 minutes until pulse returns or give sodium bicarbonate infusion

I.V. FLUIDS as indicated

EK.G. Ventricular fibrillation? Asystole? Bizarre complexes?

FIBRILLATION TREATMENT
EXTERNAL DEFIBRILLATION:
A.C. 440–880 V; D.C. 100–400 W/sec.
Repeat shock as necessary

LIDOCAINE or PROCAINE AMIDE:
1–2 mg/kg i.v. if necessary

IF ASYSTOLE,
repeat step **D**—calcium and vasopressors as needed
CONTINUE RESUSCITATION until good pulse is maintained

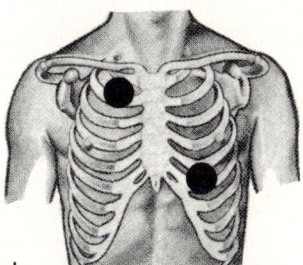

A.C. 440–880 V; D.C. 100–400 W/sec.

GAUGE Evaluate and treat cause of arrest

HYPOTHERMIA Start immediately if no CNS recovery, 30–32° C

INTENSIVE CARE
SUPPORT VENTILATION:
Tracheostomy, prolonged controlled ventilation, gastric tube, control of arterial PO_2, PCO_2, pH—as necessary
SUPPORT CIRCULATION – CONTROL CONVULSIONS – MONITOR

FIG. 3-1 (*Continued*). Phases and steps of cardiopulmonary resuscitation. (Safar, P.: *Ibid.*)

tilation/perfusion mismatching in the presence of relative hyperventilation. These conditions call for inhalation of oxygen.

Hypercarbia without hypoxemia occurs during shallow or partially obstructed breathing of high concentrations of oxygen.

Airway obstruction may be partial or complete. It is important to point out that partial airway obstruction and/or hypoventilation, even without cessation of circulation, may result in hypoxic brain damage, cerebral and pulmonary edema, or secondary apnea from exhaustion.

Unconsciousness (coma) per se causes hypopharyngeal obstruction because when the muscles relax and the patient's neck is flexed, the base of the tongue is pressed against the posterior pharyngeal wall (Fig. 3-1). This type of obstruction is the most common cause of asphyxia in the unconscious patient. Holding the head tilted backward is, therefore, the most important step in resuscitation, since it moves the mandible forward, and this stretches the anterior neck structures and lifts the base of the tongue from the posterior pharyngeal wall (Fig. 3-1). Sometimes additional forward displacement of the mandible and opening of the mouth are required.

The nose may be blocked by congestion or mucus. In a number of unconscious patients the nasal passage is open during inhalation, but obstructed during exhalation because of a valve-like behavior of the soft palate.

Another cause of airway obstruction is the presence of foreign matter such as vomitus or blood, which the unconscious patient cannot eliminate by swallowing or coughing. Laryngospasm is usually caused by upper airway stimulation in the stuporous or lightly comatose patient. Lower airway obstruction may be the result of bronchospasm, bronchial secretions, inhaled gastric contents, or foreign matter.

Recognition

Hypoxemia is suspected when there is restlessness, tachycardia, sweating, and cyanosis. Absence of cyanosis is not proof of adequate oxygenation since anemia or cutaneous vasodilation may give a pink color in spite of profound hypoxemia. Hypoxemia is *proven* by the determination of arterial pO_2, which can be performed—in conjunction with arterial pCO_2 and pH—within 5 minutes.

In order to differentiate the causes of hypoxemia, it is desirable to take arterial blood samples (1) during spontaneous breathing of air; (2) after at least 10 minutes of spontaneous breathing of 100 per cent O_2 (this requires a nonrebreathing system with tight fitting face-mask or tube), which overcomes hypoxemia from hypoventilation and ventilation/perfusion mismatching without shunting; and (3) intermittent positive-pressure assisted or controlled ventilation with 100 per cent oxygen, which may partially reverse hypoxemia from shunting (Table 3-2).

If the patient is already in need of oxygen when the blood sample is drawn, then Step 1 above (breathing air) is eliminated, and the sample is drawn during breathing of 100 per cent O_2. Decreased cardiac output reduces venous O_2 content and thus increases the degree of venous admixture through any existing shunt channels. Arterial pO_2 values, therefore, reflect the status of the lungs; whereas mixed venous (or central venous) pO_2 values (or, better, oxygen content values) reflect the status of the circulation, provided that arterial hemoglobin is fully saturated.

Hypercarbia is suspected when progressive somnolence is observed. Hypercarbia is *proven* by an increase in arterial pCO_2. With the use of nomograms, ventilation volumes may be helpful in assessing the adequacy of ventilation in individuals with healthy lungs under resting conditions. The important value is alveolar ventilation, which equals minute volume minus (dead space times respiratory frequency). In healthy lungs dead space is approximately 2 ml./kg. of body weight. Ventilation volumes are meaningless in determining the adequacy of ventilation in patients with abnormal lungs.

TABLE 3-2. INTERPRETATION OF ARTERIAL BLOOD GASES

PULMONARY STATUS PaO_2 mm. Hg	NORMAL	VENTILATION/PERFUSION MISMATCHING WITHOUT SHUNTING	INCREASED PHYSIOLOGIC SHUNTING	REDUCED CARDIAC OUTPUT
1. Spontaneous breathing/air	75-100	<75	<75	<75
2. Spontaneous breathing/100% O_2	500-650	High	Slightly improved, remains low	Remains low
3. IPPV or IPPB/100% O_2	600-650	High	Improved further, partial reversal of shunt	Not improved or reduced
VENTILATORY STATUS $PaCO_2$ mm. Hg	NORMAL	HYPOVENTILATION		HYPERVENTILATION
	35-45	>45		<35
ACID BASE STATUS pHa	NORMAL	ACIDEMIA		ALKALEMIA
	7.35-7.45	<7.35		>7.45

Treatment

1. **Steps of Emergency Airway Care.**[18, 30, 31, 33] In the unconscious patient the following steps should be carried out in rapid sequence until an open airway is established: (1) positioning; (2) backward tilt of the head; (3) positive-pressure inflation attempt; (4) forward displacement of the mandible; (5) clearing of the pharynx; (6) insertion of a pharyngeal tube; (7) tracheal intubation and tracheobronchial suctioning (or cricothyreotomy); and (8) treatment of bronchospasm.

POSITIONING. The unconscious patient in need of resuscitation should be placed supine with her head tilted backward. The unconscious patient not in need of resuscitation (pink, breathing spontaneously) should be placed on her side (to promote drainage from the pharynx) with her head tilted backward. Increased stretching of the neck and the frequent occurrence of partial or complete *nasal* obstruction make closure of the mouth undesirable.

POSITIVE PRESSURE INFLATION ATTEMPTS (Fig. 3-1). Increase the pressure gradient in an attempt to overcome airway obstruction by any of the methods described below under Methods of Artificial Ventilation.

FORWARD DISPLACEMENT OF THE MANDIBLE. If head tilt and positive pressure do not result in ventilation, *the optimal airway is provided by adding forward displacement of the mandible and opening the mouth.*

CLEARING OF THE PHARYNX. If foreign matter is visible or audible, it should be cleared swiftly by wiping or suctioning. For oropharyngeal suctioning the tonsillectomy suction tip is more satisfactory than a rubber catheter. Suction apparatus should deliver high flow rate and vacuum. For *suction via tracheal tube,* use reduced vacuum; pre- and postoxygenation; a curved-tip suction catheter for insertion into the mainstem bronchi; and a Y-tube between catheter and suction delivery tube to permit insertion without suction.

PHARYNGEAL TUBES (Fig. 3-2). Oropharyngeal and nasopharyngeal tubes are used to hold the base of the tongue forward and overcome obstruction of nose and mouth. Even with a pharyngeal tube in place, the patient's head must be maintained in the tilted-backward position. Unnecessary insertion of a pharyngeal tube may cause gagging, laryngospasm, and delay in reoxygenation.

TRACHEAL INTUBATION. If the steps described thus far do not result in prompt reoxygenation, swift orotracheal intubation is mandatory. Tracheal intubation is also indicated when inhalation of gastric contents is suspected. For emergency intubation the orotracheal route is preferred to the nasotracheal route. The technic of tracheal intubation is described elsewhere.[18] Prolonged unsuccessful attempts at tracheal intubation have led to asphyxia and cardiac arrest.

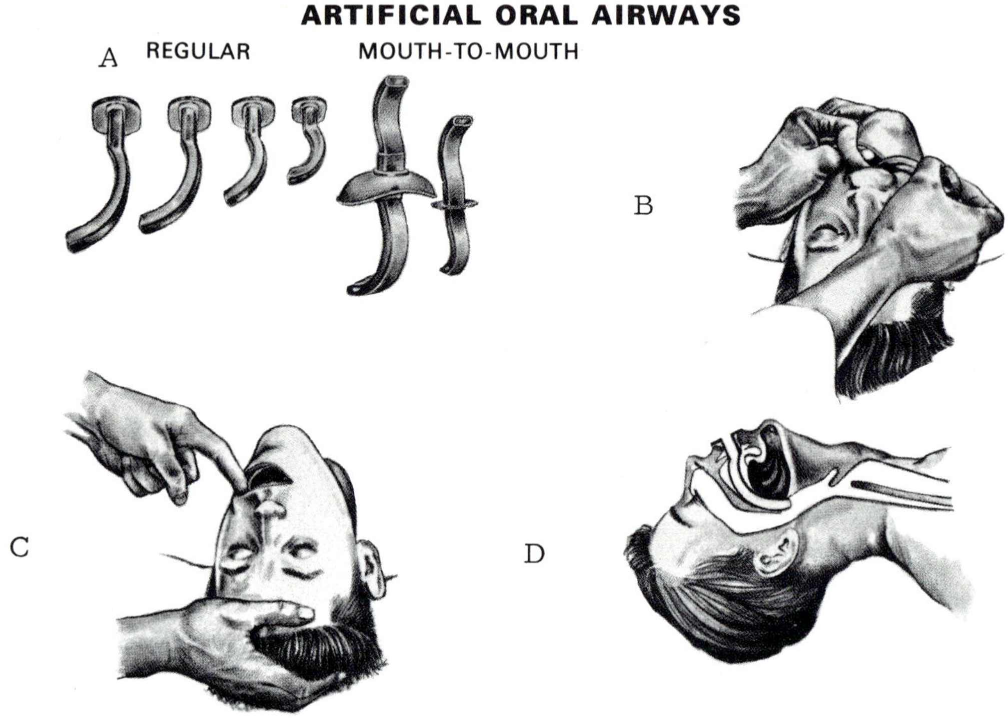

ARTIFICIAL ORAL AIRWAYS

FIG. 3-2. Oropharyngeal airways and their insertion. (A) Oropharyngeal airways, regular (*left*) and mouth-to-mouth S-shaped airways (*right*). (B) Insertion of oropharyngeal airway. Mouth is forced open with thumb and index finger crossed, and airway is inserted over tongue with rotation. (C) Forcing the mouth open when jaws are clenched (for airway insertion or suctioning) by sliding the index finger backward between cheek and teeth and wedging the tip of the index finger behind the last molars. (D) Correct position of airway. (Safar, P.: *Ibid.*)

CRICOTHYREOTOMY. When tracheal intubation is required but either equipment or skilled personnel are not immediately available, puncture of the cricothyroid membrane may have to be performed as a last step in attempting to open the airway.[33]

TRACHEOTOMY[18] is not considered an emergency reoxygenation procedure but rather an operation designed to establish a long-term airway. It should be performed, when possible, under controlled conditions in the well-oxygenated and ventilated patient, if necessary, after preliminary tracheal intubation. In adult patients cuffed tracheostomy tubes are preferred.

2. **Methods of Artificial Ventilation.** Most presently recommended methods of artificial ventilation depend upon intermittent inflation of the lungs with positive pressure applied to the airway (IPPV; controlled ventilation).[18, 32] Ideally, airway pressure should return to atmospheric pressure between positive pressure inflations. The forces opposing inflation which have to be overcome are essentially the elastic resistance of the lungs and thorax and airway resistance. Exhalation is passive. Shallow spontaneous breaths may be augmented with positive pressure (assisted respiration; IPPB). IPPV and IPPB may be performed with exhaled air, air, or oxygen.

MOUTH-TO-MOUTH AND MOUTH-TO-NOSE VENTILATION (Fig. 3-1).[30, 32] When blowing into the mouth, prevent air leakage through the nose either by pinching the nose with one hand or by pressing your cheek against the patient's nostrils while blowing. Backward tilt of the head usually opens the patient's mouth automatically.

When blowing into the *nose*, close the

mouth with your thumb and encircle the nose with your mouth.

Air can be blown into the patient's *stomach*, particularly when the air passage is obstructed or the inflation pressure is excessive. Inflation of the stomach may make lung inflations more difficult and provoke vomiting. Therefore, if you see the patient's stomach bulging, press briefly over the epigastrium to force air out of the stomach. Since this may also cause regurgitation, turn the patient's head and shoulder to one side and be prepared to clear his pharynx.

MOUTH-TO-ADJUNCT VENTILATION. S-tube, mask, or other adjuncts have been recommended to make mouth-to-mouth ventilation more acceptable, but do not make it necessarily more effective. In the hospital, adjuncts are indicated where a bag-mask unit is not available.

BAG-MASK VENTILATION (Fig. 3-3). The use of the Ruben type self-refilling bag-valve-mask unit is simple and effective. The technic is as follows: *Spread* the mask; *mold* it over the patient's mouth and nose; *clamp* it to her face with one hand; *tilt* her head backward; *squeeze* the bag until the chest rises; and *release* the bag for exhalation. Abrupt bag release is necessary for proper valve function. Clamp the mask to the patient's face with your thumb at the nose part and your index finger at the chin part of the mask, while the middle, ring, and little fingers pull the patient's chin upward and backward. This maneuver usually closes the mouth under the mask. If there is nasal obstruction (expiratory nasal obstruction is common), insert a regular pharyngeal tube under the mask.

AUTOMATIC VENTILATORS (RESUSCI-

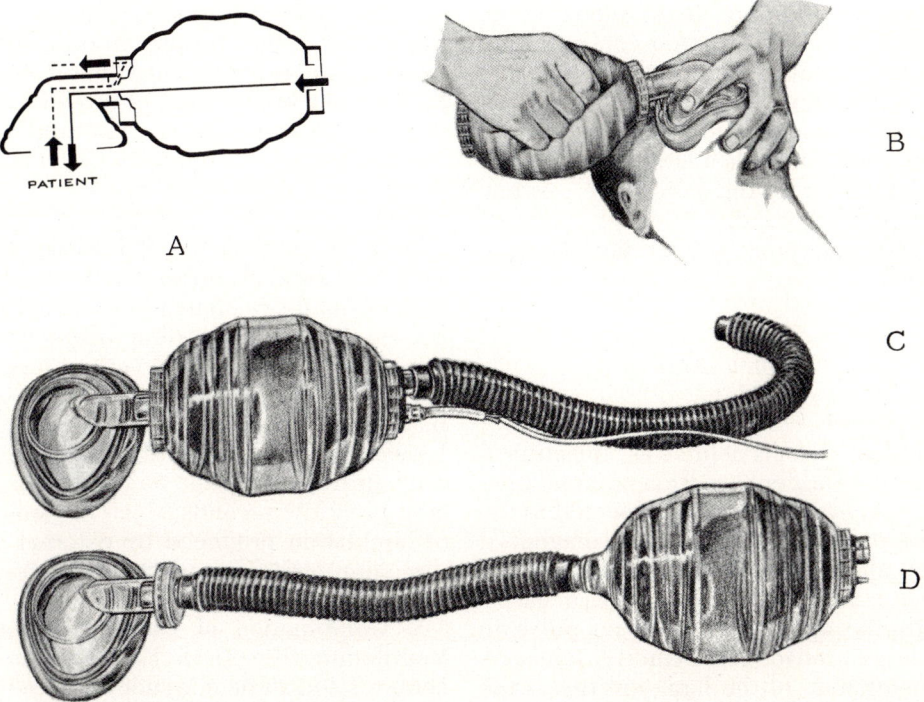

FIG. 3-3. Self-refilling bag-valve-mask unit for artificial ventilation. (A) Diagram of bag-valve-mask unit with inlet valve on right, nonrebreathing valve on left, and face mask; universal adaptor (15 mm. female for tracheal tube/22 mm. male for mask). (B) Ventilation with Resusci-Folding Bag II (Laerdal); mold and clamp mask to face with one hand, tilt head back, squeeze bag rhythmically with other hand. (C) Self-refilling bag-valve-mask unit with oxygen reservoir and delivery tube for 100% inhaled oxygen; mask should be transparent for recognizing color, vomitus, and breathing (clouding). (D) A corrugated reservoir tube can be inserted between nonrebreathing valve and bag for greater mobility. (Safar, P.: *Ibid.*)

TATORS). Pressure-cycled, oxygen-powered automatic ventilators or resuscitators are *not* recommended for *emergency* artificial ventilation in the nonintubated patient.[5, 18, 23, 24] For *prolonged* artificial ventilation of the intubated or tracheotomized patient in the postresuscitation period, suitable automatic ventilators are recommended. They should be capable of producing assisted as well as controlled ventilation with 50 to 100 per cent oxygen, drug aerosols, and warm humidity, with airway pressures and tidal volumes readable.

3. **Oxygen Inhalation.** If the patient is breathing spontaneously, but is cyanotic or dyspneic, she should inhale an oxygen-enriched atmosphere until an acceptable arterial pO_2 value during breathing of air is ascertained.

Semiopen oxygen masks or oxygen bag-mask units, used with 10 to 20 liters of oxygen per minute (continuous flow), deliver an inhaled-oxygen concentration of approximately 50 to 80 per cent and are recommended. For the intubated patient a simple, semiopen technic of oxygen inhalation is a large-bore T-tube. For long-term inhalation of oxygen through the mouth, tracheal tube, or tracheostomy tube, warm humidity is required.

Cardiac Arrest

Causes and Recognition

Cardiac arrest is defined as "the clinical picture of sudden cessation of circulation in a patient who was not expected to die at the time." Cardiac arrest is diagnosed when all of the following conditions are present: unconsciousness, apnea or gasps, death-like appearance, and no pulse in the large arteries (e.g., carotid, femoral). Pulselessness of the large arteries is the most important sign. Absence of heart sounds is an unreliable sign unless there has been continuous monitoring via an esophageal stethoscope prior to and during the arrest. Although dilated pupils are listed as an additional sign, one should not wait for pupils to dilate since this may occur within 1 minute after cessation of circulation, and in some patients the pupils may never dilate. Relative changes in pupil size, however, are valuable in following the efficiency of artificial circulation and the course of postresuscitation recovery.

How the feeling of the pulse fits into the sequence of resuscitative steps is shown in Figure 3-1. While feeling the carotid pulse with one hand, maintain backward tilt of her head with your other hand. Interrupt resuscitation as briefly as possible.

Treatment

1. **External Cardiac Compression** (Fig. 3-1).[26, 28] Artificial circulation is produced by external cardiac compression, i.e., squeezing the heart between the sternum and the spine.[28] In giving external cardiac compression, pressure must be applied with the heel of the hand at exactly the lower half of the sternum in order to be effective and to avoid injury. Rates slower than 60 per minute do not provide sufficient blood flow. In small children compress with one hand only; in infants use the tips of 2 fingers.

Compress the sternum forcefully enough to produce a good artificial carotid or femoral pulse. Have another member of the team monitor one of these pulses. As soon as feasible, place the patient on a solid surface. Do not waste time moving him to the floor. If he is in bed, place a bed board or hospital meal tray between his thorax and the mattress. Do not interrupt rhythmic compressions except for a few seconds, since the amount of circulation produced by external cardiac compression is only 20 to 40 per cent of normal.

2. **Combination of Compression and Ventilation** (Fig. 3-1). External cardiac compression alone does not produce ventilation of the lungs and therefore must be combined with intermittent positive-pressure ventilation. In the nonintubated patient ventilation should be interposed between sternal compressions. After tracheal intubation, however, inflations may be interposed or superimposed ad libitum.

Continue cardiopulmonary resuscitation until a spontaneous pulse returns; then continue artificial ventilation without sternal compression until spontaneous breathing returns. Continue to administer oxygen, perhaps with positive pressure, until the patient regains consciousness.

3. **Definitive Therapy.** This consists of the restoration of spontaneous circulation, treatment of the precipitating causes of cardiac arrest, and postresuscitation care (Fig. 3-1, D to I).[26, 30]

The patient's trachea should be intubated by a person trained in this technic, and controlled ventilation should be started with high concentrations of oxygen. Attempts at intubation should be stopped if there is interruption of ventilation for more than 15 seconds, and external cardiac compression is required.

DRUGS. As soon as possible after initiation of cardiac compression, inject *epinephrine*, 1 mg., intravenously. Repeat this or larger doses about every 2 to 5 minutes, as indicated. Intracardiac injection may produce pneumothorax, injury to a coronary artery, and prolonged interruption of cardiac compression, and it therefore should be used only if a vein is inaccessible. Give epinephrine without waiting for an electrocardiographic diagnosis. In asystole, epinephrine will help to start cardiac action. In ventricular fibrillation, epinephrine will facilitate the resumption of adequate spontaneous circulation after successful countershock. This recommendation is made in spite of the fact that occasionally an asystole may be converted to ventricular fibrillation by the injection of epinephrine.

Vasopressors, such as phenylephrine and norepinephrine, are also effective in supporting the resumption of spontaneous circulation.

Acidosis depresses the circulatory effect of catecholamines and cardiac contractility. Therefore, immediately after the injection of epinephrine, give *sodium bicarbonate* or *THAM* (tris buffer), approximately 1-2 mEq./kg. body weight, intravenously. Repeat this dose every 3 to 5 minutes during cardiopulmonary resuscitation until adequate spontaneous circulation is restored, or until further alkalinization can be controlled by arterial pH determinations.

ELECTROCARDIOGRAPHIC DIAGNOSIS. Sternal compressions may produce EKG artifacts. Therefore compression should be interrupted for a few seconds to allow a clear electrocardiographic diagnosis.

FIBRILLATION TREATMENT (Fig. 3-1). The most effective way of terminating ventricular fibrillation is the use of *electric countershock*. This may be performed by direct or alternating current. Direct current countershock may be more effective in large diseased hearts as well as in hypothermic patients. Consult the manufacturer and the literature when installing a defibrillator on your crash cart. Prior to countershock the heart must be well oxygenated. The recommended energy for direct external countershock is 200 watt seconds or more in adults, and 100 watt seconds in children. Alternating current defibrillation in adults should deliver a shock of 500 to 1,000 volts of 0.1 to 0.25 second's duration. AC defibrillators must be used with heavy duty cords to avoid drops in amperage.

High-energy levels are recommended because failure of the first countershock may delay restarting of spontaneous circulation. External application of high-energy countershocks does not so damage the heart as to impair its resumption of spontaneous contractions.

When several countershocks fail to terminate ventricular fibrillation, epinephrine and bicarbonate administration should be repeated and cardiac compressions resumed prior to repetition of countershock.

In intractable ventricular fibrillation the use of an antiarrhythmic drug is indicated. Lidocaine (Xylocaine) is preferred at present, in individual doses of 1 mg./kg. intravenously. One to 2 minutes later the countershock should be repeated.

Efforts to reverse ventricular fibrillation should be continued until success or the appearance of obvious signs of cerebral death. Some patients have recovered with intact central nervous systems after 1 to 2 hours of ventricular fibrillation.

In patients who develop ventricular fibrillation or ventricular tachycardia while being monitored (coronary surveillance unit, intensive care unit), countershock should be applied at first within seconds, without prior artificial ventilation and external cardiac compressions.

4. Internal Cardiac Compression and Defibrillation. At present there seem to be only four indications for thoracotomy and internal cardiac compression: (1) when one suspects intrathoracic pathology such as pneumothorax or hemorrhage; (2) when one cannot produce a palpable femoral or carotid pulse with external cardiac compression, as occasionally is seen in emphysematous patients with very rigid chests; (3) when repeated external defibrillation attempts have failed (particularly in hypothermia when the heart would have to be rewarmed directly to be defibrillated), and (4) when the thorax is already open at the time of arrest.

When To Start and When To Discontinue Efforts

In the terminal stages of an incurable disease resuscitation should not be attempted. This should be understood by physicians and nurses alike prior to the death of a patient with such a disease. If after restoration of spontaneous circulation the patient has not regained consciousness, the underlying disorder appears incompatible with survival and/or irreversible cerebral destruction is obvious, the physician should not hesitate to discontinue long-term resuscitation.

Judging the salvagability of the nervous system is not easy. Good prognostic signs are rapid recovery of eye and upper airway reflexes. Progressive deterioration of reflexes, continuing unconsciousness, and nonreaction of dilated pupils are poor prognostic signs. The EEG (e.g., cortical silence for over 12 hours) is only one of several signs and should not be considered decisive in itself.

Complications of Resuscitation

If the airway is inadequate or inflations are too forceful, gastric insufflation may occur and may provoke *regurgitation* and inhalation of gastric contents.

Lung rupture with *tension pneumothorax* is possible when excessive volumes are blown into infants or when the patient's lungs are diseased. This must be immediately recognized. Diagnostic findings include: subcutaneous emphysema of the neck, progressive resistance to lung inflation, progressive deterioration of circulation, progressive distention of the chest and abdomen from downward displacement of the diaphragm. Immediate pleural drainage* or, in the case of pulselessness, thoracotomy is indicated.

External cardiac compression results in costochondral separation or *fractured ribs* (especially in elderly patients) even if performed correctly. This is not a serious complication. Should a flail chest result, prolonged controlled ventilation is necessary after resuscitation. Pressure applied too high on the sternum may fracture the *sternum*; pressure applied too low may rupture the *liver,* and pressure applied laterally may contuse the *lungs*. Bone-marrow emboli are possible, but not considered to be serious.

Postresuscitation Care

When resuscitation is successful and cardiac action is restored with a spontaneous blood pressure over 60 mm. Hg, external cardiac compression is discontinued. If the blood pressure falls, cardiac compression should be resumed. There is no need for synchronization. Arterial pressure should be supported with inotropic drugs (e.g., isoproterenol) or vasopressor drugs (e.g., norepinephrine) and intravenous fluids, titrated according to arterial pressure, central venous pressure, urinary output, etc.

In recurrent arrhythmias, a prophylactic infusion of lidocaine (about 2 mg./min./70 kg. body weight) has proved to be effective.

Indications for prolonged mechanical controlled ventilation via tracheal tube

---

* Pleural drainage tray includes knife, trocars, tubes, and 1-way valves.

or tracheostomy tube include: flail chest, hypoventilation, severe hypoxemia, metabolic acidosis, and increased work of breathing. Postresuscitation care is facilitated by using indwelling arterial and central venous catheters.

Hypothermia seems beneficial in supporting recovery of the central nervous system after a hypoxic insult (only when induced soon after the arrest), if the patient fails to awaken immediately. Immobilization and control of convulsions and shivering may require the use of relaxants. Steroids are used to prevent or reduce cerebral edema and following inhalation of gastric content.

INHALATION OF FOREIGN MATTER[13, 25]

In *massive* aspiration of blood, gastrointestinal contents, or other foreign matter with acute major airway obstruction, oxygenation with IPPV/O_2 has priority over clearing attempts and drug treatment. The clinical picture that ensues depends upon the volume and nature of the aspiration.

When aspiration is *suspected*, immediate action is essential to avoid irreversible progressive pulmonary consolidation and chronic pneumonitis with abscess formation. Lengthy contemplation and consultation should not delay the necessary emergency management.

Emergency treatment consists of the following: oxygenation of the lungs with IPPV/O_2. If there is hypoxemia and/or the clinical picture of aspiration syndrome (asthma-like symptoms), the trachea should be intubated (under topical anesthesia or with brief paralysis by succinylcholine) and the tracheobronchial tree suctioned. Some of the suctioned material should be collected for examination of smear, culture, antibiotic sensitivity, and pH. Bronchial irrigation with increments of 5 to 10 ml. of isotonic salt solution, injected via curved-tip catheter into one or the other mainstem bronchus, is carried out until the suctioned material is clear. A broad-spectrum antibiotic is administered intravenously and later changed according to bacteriologic and antibiotic sensitivity reports.

If after reoxygenation and tracheobronchial suctioning there are wheezes and rhonchi, all-out respiratory care should be instituted. This consists of IPPB or IPPV/O_2/warm mist/bronchodilator aerosol; adjustment of inhaled oxygen concentration between 50 and 100 per cent according to PaO_2; control of $PaCO_2$ and pHa; and adjustment of lung inflation volumes and flow rates according to optimal reversal of hypoxemia, which may require stabilization of the patient with curare or narcotics.

Steroid treatment is specific for the chemical pneumonitis of aspiration. For instance, hydrocortisone is administered, 200 mg. I.V., followed by 200 mg. every 6 hours for the first 24 hours, and smaller doses subsequently (or prophylactically). Steroid should be used for a minimum of 2 to 3 days or as long as there are symptoms of "asthma."

Therapeutic bronchoscopy is indicated when suctioning through the tracheal tube suggests inhalation of solid matter, or when there is evidence of atelectasis of one lobe or lung which does not clear with the measures mentioned.

RESPIRATORY INSUFFICIENCY IN SHOCK[29, 34, 35]

Shock states may lead to hypoxemia which may become irreversible because of progressive pulmonary consolidation and hepatization ("shock lung"). These changes are most likely due to decreased pulmonary perfusion, hypoxemia, alveolar hypoxia, toxins, and acidosis, resulting in failure of the capillary alveolar membrane, with pulmonary interstitial edema followed by alveolar edema, hemorrhage, and destruction of parenchyma.

Respiratory changes in shock are complex and usually a combination of several of the following factors: (1) increased physiologic dead space due to lung ischemia and/or embolism; (2) increased ventilation/perfusion ratio; (3) decreased ventilation/perfusion ratio; (4) increased physiologic shunting from alveolar consolidation; (5) reduction in cardiac output per se, which lowers the oxygen content of mixed venous blood and thus increases the degree of venous admixture via existing shunt channels; (6) opening of arteriovenous shunts due to spasm of precapillary sphincters (e.g., hypoxia, acidosis) and/or microcirculatory thrombosis or embolism; and (7) increased metabolic demands of tissues because of increased catecholamine liberation and, later, tissue repair.

Hemorrhage usually results in spontaneous hyperventilation. Therefore oxygen enrichment by openface mask will usually compensate for ventilation/perfusion mismatching. In late stages of shock, PaO_2 should be determined after 15 minutes of breathing 100 per cent oxygen. When the PaO_2 during breathing of 100 per cent O_2 is below 100 mm. Hg or there is hypercarbia, controlled ventilation via tracheal tube with controlled oxygen concentrations is in order.

One hundred per cent oxygen and alkalinization are beneficial in pulmonary vascular occlusive states. When pulmonary thromboembolism is suspected (it is proven only by pulmonary arteriography), heparinization is indicated but must be weighed against the risk of inducing hemorrhage.

Cardiac Arrest From Exsanguination[27]

Exsanguination usually leads to an agonal state (no pulse, gasping) and finally to clinical death with asystole. Ventricular fibrillation may occur during resuscitative efforts.

Resuscitation consists of the simultaneous application of the following: IPPV/ 100% O_2; external cardiac compressions; massive venous infusion through large-bore catheter of salt plus colloid (albumin or dextran) until type specific cross-matched blood is available; epinephrine and bicarbonate I.V.; and hemostasis. As soon as feasible, electrocardiography should be performed and electric defibrillation applied when necessary. When bank blood is infused in large quantities, it should be passed through a blood warmer as soon as possible, since cold blood may induce ventricular fibrillation. Hemostasis in lower abdominal hemorrhage may have to include aortic compression. Arterial infusion with plasma substitutes or banked blood is not superior to venous infusion.

REFERENCES

Anesthesia

1. Baronofsky, I. D., Treloar, A. E., and Wangensteen, O. H.: Blood loss in operations. Statistical comparison of losses, as described by gravimetric and colorimetric methods. Surgery, 20:761, 1946.
2. Beecher, H. K., and Todd, D. T.: A Study of the Deaths Associated with Anesthesia and Surgery. Springfield, Ill., Charles C Thomas, 1954.
3. Bendixen, H., et al.: Respiratory Care. Saint Louis, C. V. Mosby, 1965.
4. Bonica, J. J.: Principles and Practice of Obstetric Analgesia and Anesthesia. Philadelphia, F. A. Davis, 1967.
5. Community-wide emergency medical services. Recommendations by the Committee on Acute Medicine of the American Society of Anesthesiologists. J.A.M.A., 204:595, May 13, 1968.
6. Dripps, R. D., Eckenhoff, J. E., and Vandam, L. D.: Introduction to Anesthesia. Philadelphia, W. B. Saunders, 1967.
7. Dripps, R. D., and Vandam, L. D.: Long-term follow up of patients who received 10,098 Spinal Anesthetics. I. Failure to discover major neurological sequelae. J.A.M.A., 156:1486, 1954.
8. Edwards, G., Morton, H. J. V., Bask, E. A., and Wylie, W. D.: Deaths associated with anesthesia. A report on one thousand cases. Anesthesia (London), 11:194, 1956.
9. Greene, N. M.: Physiology of Spinal Anesthesia. Baltimore, Williams & Wilkins, 1958.
10. Hingson, R. A., and Hellman, L.: Anesthesia for Obstetrics. Philadelphia, J. B. Lippincott, 1956.
11. Holaday, D. A. (ed.): Clinical Anesthesia: Lung Disease. Philadelphia, F. A. Davis, 1967.
12. Lund, P. D.: Peridural Analgesia and Anesthesia. Springfield, Ill., Charles C Thomas, 1966.
13. Mendelson, C. L.: Aspiration of stomach contents into lungs during obstetric anesthesia. Amer. J. Obstet. Gynec., 52:191, 1946.

14. Moore, D. C.: Regional Block. ed. 4. Springfield, Ill., Charles C Thomas, 1965.
15. National Fire Protection Association, 60 Battery March Street, Boston 10, Massachusetts: Recommended Safe Practice for Hospital Operating Rooms, Bulletin 56. Published by the same organization, 1956.
16. Nicholson, M. J., and Crehan, J. P.: Emergency Treatment of Air Embolism. Curr. Res. Anesth. Analg., 35:634, 1956.
17. Phillips, O. C., Frazier, M. S., Graff, T. D., and DeKornfeld, T. J.: The Baltimore Anesthesia Study Committee. Review of 1,024 Postoperative Deaths. J.A.M.A., 174:2015, 1960.
18. Safar, P. (ed.): Respiratory Therapy. Philadelphia, F. A. Davis, 1965, 1970.
19. Safar, P., and Escarraga, L. A.: Lung-thorax compliance of apneic anesthetized adults. Anesthesiology, 20:283, 1959.
20. Vandam, L. D., and Dripps, R. D.: Exacerbation of pre-existing neurologic disease after spinal anesthesia. New Eng. J. Med., 255:843, 1956.
21. Van Praagh, I. G. L., and Povey, W. G.: The use of paracervical block anesthesia for dilatation and curettage. Canad. Med. Assoc. J., 94:267, February 5, 1966.
22. Wylie, W. D., and Churchill-Davidson, H. C.: A Practice of Anesthesia. Chicago, Year Book Medical Publishers, 1960.

Resuscitation

23. AHA Committee on Cardiopulmonary Resuscitation: Cardiopulmonary Resuscitation: A Manual for Instructors. New York, American Heart Association, 1967.
24. AHA Committee on Cardiopulmonary Resuscitation: Emergency Resuscitation Team Manual: A Hospital Plan. New York, American Heart Association, 1968.
25. Cameron, J. L., Anderson, R. P., and Zuidema, G. D.: Aspiration pneumonia: A clinical and experimental review. J. Surg. Res., 7(1):44, 1967.
26. Jude, J. R., and Elam, J. O.: Fundamentals of Cardiopulmonary Resuscitation. Philadelphia, F. A. Davis, 1965.
27. Kirimli, B., Kampschulte, S., and Safar, P.: Resuscitation from cardiac arrest due to exsanguination. Surg. Gynec. Obstet., 129(1):89, July 1969.
28. Kouwenhoven, W. B. J., Jude, J. R., and Knickerbocker, G. G.: Closed-chest cardiac massage. J.A.M.A., 173:1064, 1960.
29. Moore, F. D., et al.: Post-Traumatic Pulmonary Insufficiency. Philadelphia, W. B. Saunders, 1969.
30. Safar, P.: Cardiopulmonary Resuscitation: A Manual for Physicians and Paramedical Instructors. World Federation of Societies of Anaesthesiologists, 1968. May be obtained from American Society of Anesthesiologists, 515 Busse Highway, Park Ridge, Illinois 60068.
31. Safar, P., Escarraga, L., and Chang, F.: A study of upper airway obstruction in the unconscious patient. J. Appl. Physiol., 14:760, 1959.
32. Safar, P., Escarraga, L., and Elam, J.: A comparison of the mouth-to-mouth and mouth-to-airway methods of artificial respiration with the chest-pressure arm-lift methods. New Eng. J. Med., 258:671, 1959.
33. Safar, P., and Penninckx, J.: Cricothyroid membrane puncture with special cannula. Anesthesiology, 28(5):943, September-October 1967.
34. Smith, J., Penninckx, J. J., Kampschulte, S., and Safar, P.: Need for oxygen enrichment in myocardial infarction, shock and following cardiac arrest. Acta Anaesth. Scand., Suppl. 29:127, 1968.
35. Torpey, D., and Safar, P.: Preoperative resuscitation and preparation of the traumatized patient. Int. Anesth. Clin., in press.

4

Postoperative Care and Complications

IMMEDIATE POSTOPERATIVE CARE

Perhaps the most critical period of a patient's postoperative course falls within the first 72 hours following surgery. During this time the most accurate assessment of the patient's physiologic reserve is required. The three parameters which provide the most valuable information concerning the patient's postoperative homeostatic condition include:
1. Cardiac.
2. Renal.
3. Respiratory.

Proper balance of these three vital organ systems assures the surgeon of accurate control of the patient's major physiologic mechanisms and provides the best method of monitoring the patient's postoperative progress.

Cardiac Aspects. While blood pressure is one of the most valid indicators of cardiovascular reserve, there are wide variations in blood pressure recordings that may occur postoperatively. Changes in position of the patient with peripheral vasodilatation or constriction as related to shifts in the intravascular compartment, as well as lability of the recently anesthetized peripheral nerves result in unpredictable blood pressure fluctuations in the immediate postoperative period. Compensatory tachycardia and peripheral vasoconstriction may temporarily mask major blood loss at the time of surgery or from continued bleeding postoperatively. It is not until at least 25 per cent of the total blood volume has been lost that tachycardia persists, and a drop in blood pressure is noted. Only when approximately 40 per cent or more of the blood volume has been lost will blood pressure changes be profound and persistently low. Although the pulse rate is perhaps more sensitive to pressure changes in the great vessels, an increase in pulse rate in itself is not pathognomonic of impending cardiac decompensation. It is true that pressure receptors in the aortic arch and the carotid sinuses stimulate cardioaccelerator response, but acceleration of the heart is frequently seen in many conditions other than a fall of pressure in the aorta or great vessels. Excitement, fear, and anxiety are all among such causes, particularly following surgery. In addition, changes in pulse rates in elderly individuals are frequently delayed and fail accurately to predict impending cardiac failure.

Nonetheless, persistent tachycardia, combined with other clinical signs of cardiac decompensation, such as peripheral vasoconstriction with cold, clammy extremities and pallor, as well as oliguria and hypotension, are all classic evidences of cardiovascular decompensation.

Central Venous Pressure Monitoring. More recently, central venous pressure monitoring has provided the most sensitive clinical method available in the evaluation of four measurable and independent forces:
1. The volume and flow of blood in the central veins.

2. Distensibility and contractility of the right chambers of the heart during filling of the heart.

3. Vasomotor activity in central veins.

4. Intrathoracic pressure.

While all four factors may vary with profound blood loss, one of its primary clinical functions is its accuracy in monitoring the central venous compartment while replacing intravascular fluids. A high central venous pressure (such as 15 cm. of water) may indicate a full intravascular compartment and an adequate circulating blood volume, but it may also indicate impending cardiac decompensation with right-sided heart failure. Consequently, blood volume studies, combined with continuous central venous pressure recordings, provide the most useful information regarding both intravascular and cardiac reserve.

Central venous pressure (CVP) monitoring was first used in the operating room as a guide during extracorporeal circulation during heart surgery. It was later applied to the management of postoperative circulatory failure. In 1962, Wilson and his associates reported on extensive use of CVP monitoring in the management of acute circulatory failure as a guide to massive fluid therapy. Since that time, numerous reports have verified its clinical usefulness in monitoring cardiac output, peripheral vascular tone, and intravascular volume.

The French physicians Aubainac and Villafane were the first to advocate the use of the subclavian vein for intravenous infusions. Wilson cannulated the superior vena cava via a percutaneous puncture of the subclavian vein. He reported a high percentage of successful cannulations and a low incidence of complications. Currently, there are 6 methods for central venous monitoring, namely, the groin, the anticubital fossa, the shoulder, the jugular vein, and the subclavian vein, which are all percutaneous insertions; venous cutdown of the jugular vein is also used.

METHOD OF CVP MONITORING BY SUBCLAVIAN CATHETER. As demonstrated in Figure 4-1 A, insertion of the subclavian catheter is accomplished by placing the patient in a supine position with the foot of the bed elevated 6 to 12 inches to increase the pressure in the subclavian vein and produce venous distention. After proper aseptic preparation of the skin, it is infiltrated with 1% Xylocaine if the patient is awake. The point of injection is approximately 1 cm. below the midportion of the clavicle. A 15-gauge 6" Rochester needle is introduced into the skin with the shaft of the needle held almost parallel with the anterior chest wall. The needle is directed medially toward the junction of the middle and the inner third of the clavicle. The needle is advanced along the undersurface of the clavicle, where it is directed toward a slightly more posterior plane for 2 or 3 cm. By applying suction constantly, the needle enters the vein and immediately aspirates dark red blood, which confirms the successful puncture. If the vein is not entered, the needle is withdrawn from under the clavicle and readvanced in a similar manner but in a slightly more cranial or caudal direction. As soon as the free flow of blood is obtained, the needle is held in place, and the plastic catheter is advanced as far as possible into the innominate vein and superior vena cava. It is important to aspirate the catheter before removal of the needle to make sure there is a free flow of blood for accurate monitoring. The catheter is firmly grasped with a clamp against the skin as the needle is withdrawn over the surface of the catheter to avoid dislodgment of the catheter into the right atrium. The catheter is then sutured to the skin and taped securely in place.

Figure 4-1 B and C demonstrates the cannula in place and taped to the skin.

The zero reference point on the manometer is adjusted to a point approximately 5 cm. posterior to the 4th costochondral junction. Others choose a point 10 cm. anterior to the skin of the back in the plane of the 4th costochondral junction, whereas still others select a point equidistant between the anterior and the posterior chest wall. The point of reference is directed toward the level of the right atrium, but slight variations in position are insignificant in central monitor-

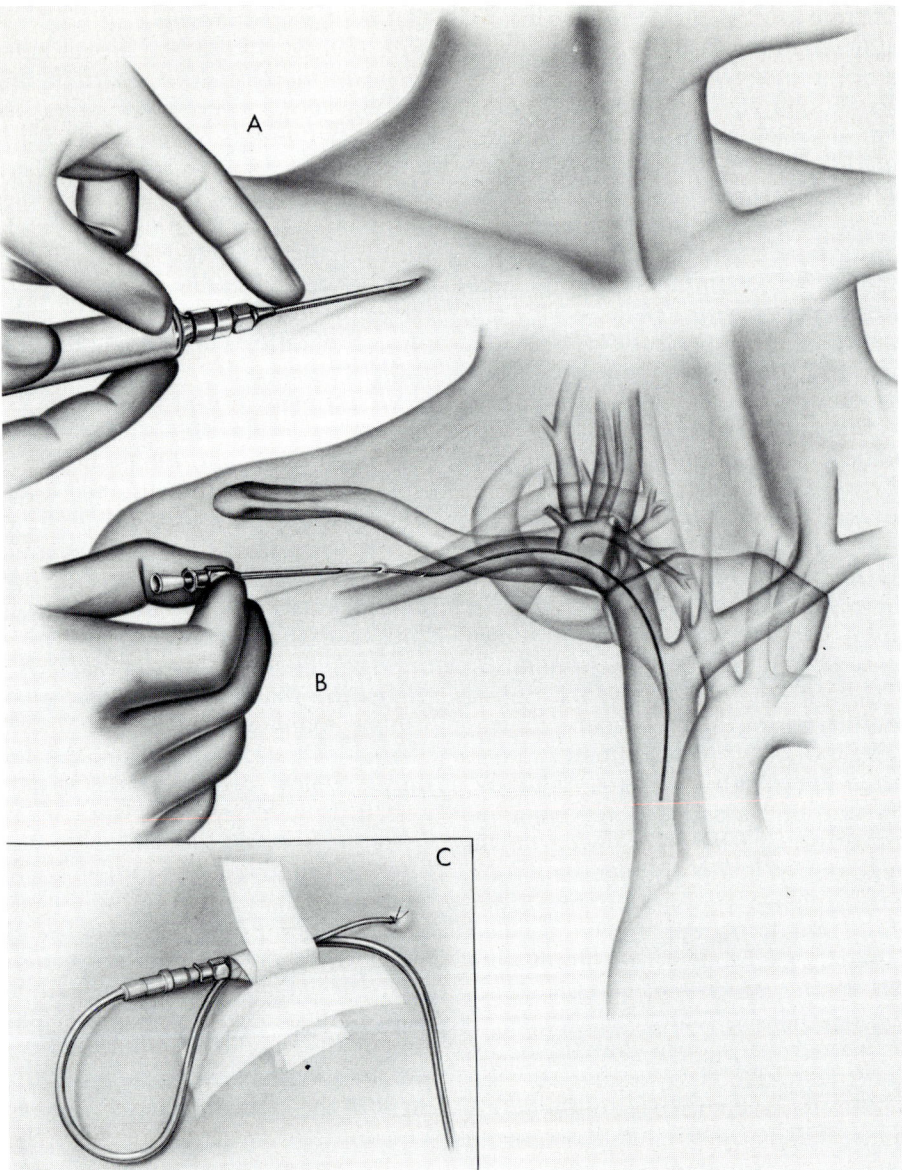

Fig. 4-1. Method of inserting a catheter in the subclavian vein for CVP monitoring. (A) The skin is punctured by the needle with attached syringe 1 cm. below the midpoint of the clavicle. Needle is held parallel to anterior chest wall and pointed medially along surface of clavicle. (B) Catheter is inserted into subclavian vein and superior vena cava at the junction of inner and middle third of the clavicle. Needle is withdrawn over the outside of the catheter. Tip of catheter is removed and replaced with blunt needle. (C) Central venous catheter is connected to polyethylene tubing and attached to water manometer. Catheter is sutured securely to skin to avoid catheter emboli.

ing. Normal venous pressure is considered to be within the range of 5 to 12 cm. of water. However, since pressure readings depend on the integrated effects of blood volume, cardiac output, and vascular tone, there is a wide variation in the CVP level, and it is best interpreted as a continuous monitor of central pressure.

FACTORS WHICH TEND TO ELEVATE CVP include:
1. Cardiac failure.
2. Increased venous return.
   a. Hypervolemia.
   b. Increased venous tone.
   c. Reduced peripheral resistance.

FACTORS WHICH TEND TO LOWER CVP include:
1. Improved cardiac output.
2. Diminished venous return.
   a. Hypovolemic shock.
   b. Increased peripheral resistance.
   c. Venous pooling.

Perhaps the most precise method of monitoring the intravascular effect of fluid replacement including blood, plasma, water, and electrolytes, is the repeated use of CVP levels. This method permits adequate fluid replacement without concern for cardiac overloading. As the central pressure rises to the level of 12 to 15 cm. of water, fluid replacement is restricted until the CVP level is gradually reduced.

As is true with other clinical armamentaria, CVP monitoring cannot be assumed to be infallible, but must be utilized with critical evaluation of other clinical methods of cardiovascular monitoring. In general, we prefer not to leave the subclavian catheter in the vein longer than 3 to 5 days, although we have on specific occasions left it in place for as long as 2 to 3 weeks. The longer the catheter is maintained in the vena cava or great veins, the greater is the risk of seeding the bloodstream with bacteria from the skin, and the greater is the risk of venous thrombosis and possible pulmonary emboli.

THE COMPLICATION RATE of catheterization of the superior vena cava and major veins varies in frequency from less than 1 per cent to 10 per cent of the reported cases. Most of the serious complications of the subclavian puncture, such as pneumothorax, hemothorax, hydrothorax, brachial plexus injury, and subclavian artery puncture result from introducing the needle with too great a posterior angulation. These problems can be prevented by keeping the needle almost parallel to the anterior chest wall as it is introduced, and by directing it between the 1st rib and the clavicle, close to the posterior surface of the clavicle.

SHOCK

Shock may be defined in various ways, but in practical terms it is a state of acute circulatory insufficiency, characterized by cardiac output inadequate to provide normal perfusion of the major organs. Whether the basic underlying factor is one of myocardial failure, obstruction of main arterial pathways (pulmonary embolus), increased peripheral resistance to blood flow, widespread peripheral pooling of blood, or direct blood loss, the end result is still the same—insufficient circulating blood volume to ensure adequate tissue perfusion. Blalock in 1934 proposed a classification for shock according to various causative mechanisms, and although the exact pathophysiologic mechanism of each factor is still not fully understood, the categories are still valid today:

1. Regional loss of blood (oligemic).
2. Toxemic (septic).
3. Neurogenic (decreased vascular resistance).
4. Cardiogenic.
5. Various combinations of these.

While each type of shock is related to a particular pathophysiologic pattern, in practice there is usually a combination of interrelated factors involved in the more serious forms of circulatory collapse. Sepsis, with its adverse effect on cellular metabolism, is a frequent complication of patients with acute blood loss. The end stage of shock is the same, regardless of whether it is initiated by a single factor or a combination of factors—a decreased cardiac output, diminished blood volume with progressive hemoconcentration, irreversible alterations in cell metabolism, peripheral capillary dilatation, and, finally, failure of return of blood to the heart, resulting in cardiac standstill.

PATHOPHYSIOLOGY OF HEMORRHAGIC SHOCK

Hemorrhagic shock is perhaps the best understood of all types of vascular collapse and is the most common cause occurring in the field of gynecology. Septic shock, arising from pelvic infections, is a less frequent entity but a more lethal disease than shock from blood loss alone. A dramatic demonstration of hemorrhagic shock is seen in massive intraperitoneal bleeding from a ruptured ectopic pregnancy. Such cases clearly demonstrate the early stage of shock by a temporary decrease in cardiac output and arterial blood pressure, which is followed by compensatory mechanisms of the sympathetic nervous system and decreased vagal activity. In effect, these adaptive measures tend to restore temporarily cardiac output and arterial pressure by peripheral arterial contractility and inotropic effect on the cardiac muscle, producing more forceful contractions. At this stage the patient with ectopic pregnancy will experience increasing symptoms of abdominal and pelvic pain, but acute vasomotor symptoms will be masked by these normal physiologic responses.

In the past, prior to the modern conveniences of transportation, such patients were frequently delayed in obtaining prompt medical care, and shock would progress to a more critical and frequently irreversible phase. Such changes included ischemic peripheral vascular constriction with sympathetic stimulation of the sweat glands, producing cold, clammy extremities, diminished cardiac output, and impaired cerebral perfusion, manifested by lightheadedness, confusion, and, later, syncope. A decrease in renal blood flow is immediately sensed by the juxtaglomerular apparatus of the afferent arterioles, with the release of renin into the plasma and the subsequent conversion of renin to an inactive polypeptide, angiotensin I, and finally to the vasoactive form, angiotensin II. This is a potent arteriolar constrictor which also induces catecholamine secretion from the adrenal medulla and aldosterone from the adrenal cortex. Aldosterone is only temporarily beneficial in conserving salt and water for the depleted circulating blood volume. Renal ischemia also produces a decrease in glomerular filtration rate, with resultant oliguria or anuria and progressive acidosis and with an elevation of serum lactate and pyruvate. The use of bicarbonate solutions and other alkaline buffers is important in controlling progressive acidosis, although one must recognize the fact that acidosis per se is merely an expression of cellular anoxia caused by inadequate circulation. Unless circulation is restored to normal, changing the blood pH will have no effect on the end result of this condition.

Treatment

1. **Fluid Replacement.** While the most essential requirement in the management of hemorrhagic shock is the immediate control of the source of bleeding, it is first necessary to replace rapidly the patient's blood volume. Adequate volume is more important than the type of fluid administered. Although whole blood has no equal in the treatment of shock, immediate replacement with plasma expanders, including low-molecular-weight dextran, glucose, and saline may be required temporarily, and are very effective in increasing plasma volume. At the present writing, we prefer to avoid the use of lactate in patients in shock due to the presence of existing acidosis and an elevated blood lactate level, although there is increasing evidence in the human that this philosophy may be inaccurate.

The use of dextran has been shown to be most effective as a colloidal, osmotic agent which quickly expands blood volume. As a result, blood flow rapidly improves. In addition to its effect as a plasma expander, dextran reduces the viscosity of blood, breaks up noncirculating aggregations of erythrocytes and restores them to the circulating blood, increases the electronegative charge of the erythrocyte and other elements of the blood, and coats the endothelium of blood vessels. All of these effects tend to prevent thrombosis and to disintegrate clot formation. Because of this influence on the clotting mechanism, dextran may interfere with the clot mechanism and produce bleeding if more than 20 to 25 per cent of the blood volume is replaced with dextran. While the recomended dosage of low-molecular-weight dextran is 7 cc./kg.

as a priming dose, and 3 cc./kg. daily thereafter, our preference is 500 cc. of 10 per cent dextran 40 (Rheomacrodex) per day (approximately 10% of blood volume). Commercial dextran has an average molecular weight of 75,000, and is more effective in preventing thrombosis. Dextran 40, having a low molecular weight of 40,000, is particularly beneficial in establishing blood flow in capillaries and is more effective as a plasma volume expander.

2. **Vasopressors.** There has been recent controversy regarding the time-honored routine of attempting to maintain arterial blood pressure by the use of additional vasopressor substances. The effect would seem to intensify the peripheral vascular resistance and further impair the peripheral perfusion of tissues. Such an effect would aggravate the process of hypoxia and acidosis, and may have little biologic effect on improving circulation. In 1940 Blalock cautioned against the use of vasopressors in treating shock, but throughout the years clinicians have persisted in the use of these pressor substances in an effort to produce an improvement in pulse pressure and, hopefully, visceral perfusion. However, Wilson states that, contrary to animal experiments which indicate the potential deleterious effects of pressor amines in shock, there is strong clinical evidence that these drugs have been lifesaving, either "in spite of" or "because of" their use. Nonetheless, one must be able to determine when the effective clinical end point of a drug has been reached, beyond which no improvement would be anticipated. The two best methods of monitoring such a clinical response are the hourly urine output and continuous recording of the central venous pressure.

Strong clinical evidence suggests that the more potent the vasopressor effect of an agent, the more hazardous is its use in treating shock. A preferable hypertensive agent in our experience has been metaraminol (Aramine). When titrated in a dilute solution of 100 mg. in 500 cc. of normal saline, it is effective in improving cardiac output by a cardiac inotropic effect, producing sufficient rise of the blood pressure to improve renal blood flow and glomerular filtration rate. Its effectiveness in improving venous return is mediated through improvement in venous tone. No attempt should be made to restore the systolic arterial pressure to normal levels but only to a level adequate to perfuse vital organs and peripheral tissues. The most sensitive clinical measurement of this physiologic level is a minimal urinary output of 30 ml./hr. When this clinical response has been achieved, one should make no further demands on the patient's adaptive vascular mechanisms, and one is best guided by urinary flow rather than blood pressure levels. An ideal urinary output of 50-60 ml./hr. may not be achievable during the acute phase of shock.

3. **Vasodilators — Adrenergic Blocking Agents.** The recent use of adrenergic blocking agents is an effort to prevent the irreversible effects of peripheral vasoconstriction in prolonged shock which may result in bypassing of vital organs through the establishment of arteriovenous shunts. In 1948 Wiggers introduced the idea of the use of vasodilators and demonstrated the beneficial effect of an adrenergic blocking agent, Dibenamine, in the shocked dog. More recently, Nicherson, Hardaway, Longerbeam, Lillehei, and Scott, and others have championed the beneficial effects of the antiadrenergic drugs, such as phenoxybenzamine hydrochloride (Dibenzyline) as an effective vasodilator when used in shock.

In our own experience, however, we have found the three distinct pharmacologic properties of isoproterenol (Isuprel) to have far greater advantages to other vasodilators in the treatment of profound shock: (1) beta-adrenergic stimulation, resulting in peripheral vasodilatation; (2) inotropic stimulation, resulting in restoration of cardiac efficiency; and (3) pulmonary vasodilatation, with improvement in pulmonary blood flow. The combined effect of myocardial stimulation and peripheral vasodilatation results in an improved peripheral and renal circulation, producing an improvement in urinary output and blood pressure.

When used in a dilute solution (2 mg. in 500 ml. 5% glucose or normal saline), Isuprel does not produce a significant drop in central venous pressure if the total blood volume has been adequately replaced. The use of Isuprel or any other inotropic drug is contraindicated in the presence of cardiac arrhythmia and extreme tachycardia.

The hypotensive effect of chlorpromazine (Thorazine) has been well recognized since its early clinical use. Collins, Jaffe, and Zahony, using chlorpromazine in doses of 10 to 100 mg. per day, found the drug to be effective in overcoming severe vasoconstriction and allowing perfusion of the kidneys with a marked improvement in oliguria and the reversibility of the shock-like state. The use of chlorpromazine has received widespread clinical trial and has been shown to be effective, particularly in patients with septic shock.

4. **Treatment of Acidosis.** The effect of progressive acidosis from hypoxia and anaerobic glycolysis is cytotoxic, particularly to arteriolar smooth muscle fibers and the myocardium. Such effects contribute to a decrease in peripheral vascular tone and diminished cardiac function. It is therefore important to correct acidosis with adequate amounts of alkali, either sodium bicarbonate or a buffered electrolyte solution, tris(hydroxymethyl)-aminomethane (THAM), which acts as an intracellular hydrogen ion acceptor to buffer the extracellular compartment. Although wide experience has now accumulated with this organic buffer, we prefer the generous use of sodium bicarbonate, using 40 to 60 mEg. per liter of parenteral fluid.

5. **Corticosteroids.** In the absence of adrenal failure, the use of hydrocortisone in the treatment of hemorrhagic shock is of questionable benefit. However, numerous investigators have described the beneficial effects of hydrocortisone in cases of septic or endotoxin shock. Corticosteroids, however, should be given whenever there is evidence of adrenal insufficiency as a result of prolonged shock and visceral ischemia.

Summary Statement on the Treatment of Hemorrhagic Shock. It is important to reemphasize that the successful treatment of shock is primarily dependent on the adequate replacement of the circulating blood volume prior to the irreversible changes of ischemia and hypoxia which result in cell death and circulatory collapse. While no protocol of therapy is applicable to every case of hemorrhagic shock, the essential points of our own treatment are worth summarizing:

1. Immediate replacement of fluid loss, preferably by whole blood, but low-molecular-weight dextran or balanced salt solution may be temporarily used as plasma expanders to support circulating blood volume until whole blood is obtainable.

2. Central venous pressure monitoring, preferably by the subclavian or jugular puncture, with accurate continuous measurement of venous pressure in the superior vena cava, is an essential requirement for the accurate treatment of shock.

3. Hourly monitoring of urinary output with the replacement of sufficient intravenous fluids to provide urine flow of 30-50 ml./hr. Renal perfusion with adeuate urinary output is considered one of the most accurate clinical measurements of effective arterial pressure.

4. Vasopressor agents—pressor amines —should be used only if central venous pressure and urinary output remain low after adequate replacement of circulating blood volume, and in the absence of peripheral constriction. When indicated, Aramine is a preferable vasopressor agent due to the fact that it also produces inotropic cardiac stimulation. The more potent vasoconstrictors may have a deleterious effect on peripheral capillary circulation.

5. The use of alkali for the correction of impending or existing acidosis should be initiated early in the treatment of shock. It is unnecessary to delay the use of bicarbonate until acidosis has become clinically evident as demonstrated by a low blood pH and CO_2. In our experience, bicarbonate is preferable to lactate in the correction of acidosis where the lactate level is already elevated. Liberal use of normal saline is recommended in the treatment of shock to counteract the predictable hyponatremia that occurs with

progressive capillary damage and renal dysfunction.

6. Surgical control of hemorrhage is one of the initial steps to be undertaken to control the circulating blood volume. However, it is mandatory that the blood volume be adequately replaced, and that supportive steps be taken prior to subjecting the patient to a surgical procedure for the control of the hemorrhage. The most expedient method of controlling major pelvic hemorrhage is by ligation of the anterior division of the hypogastric arteries and collateral ovarian circulation.

7. An adequate airway and good ventilation is important in the treatment of shock. While oxygen therapy may be administered, it is generally ineffective in the presence of normal ventilation since the hypoxia is at the cellular level rather than the result of decreased oxygenation of the pulmonary circulation.

8. Finally, the use of vasodilators is restricted to those cases in which there is progression of the physiologic effects of shock, which have so far not responded to all other forms of therapy. Isuprel has the distinct pharmacologic advantage of peripheral vasodilatation (beta-adrenergic stimulation), inotropic cardiac stimulation, and pulmonary vasodilatation. Where cardiac arrythmia and/or tachycardia contraindicate a cardiac stimulant, the alpha-adrenergic blocking agent, chlorpromazine (Thorazine) is useful in producing peripheral vasodilatation and improving renal blood flow.

The Surgical Control of Pelvic Hemorrhage. The most singularly important step in the treatment of hemorrhagic shock in the field of gynecology is the control of hemorrhage. It is superflous to state that exploration of the patient with control of the pelvic bleeding must be undertaken as soon as the patient's vital signs and blood volume have been stabilized. Serious life-threatening pelvic hemorrhage is a more frequent complication of obstetrics, where it is frequently seen with a ruptured uterus, than of gynecology. Uncontrollable gynecologic hemorrhage is seen primarily with extensive or radical pelvic surgery, and postoperatively from retraction of either an ovarian or uterine vessel from its ligature, resulting in retroperitoneal hemorrhage.

Efforts to control hemorrhage from the pelvis by identifying the specific bleeding point may be technically impossible. The anatomy is altered, and the vessels are retroperitoneal and retracted. However, the blood should be rapidly blotted away with large laparotomy pads, and a rapid search should be made for the bleeding vessel. If it is not found promptly, one should not lose valuable time by continuing the search while the patient's condition is deteriorating. One should proceed with ligation of the hypogastric arteries. This becomes necessary more often following difficult dissection from advanced pelvic disease, both benign and malignant, than after more conservative pelvic surgery.

HYPOGASTRIC ARTERY LIGATION. The most effective and rapid method of controlling severe pelvic hemorrhage is hypogastric artery ligation. Because of the major collateral circulation from the internal iliac artery, mainly the lumbar, iliolumbar, middle sacral, lateral sacral, and superior and middle hemorrhoidal, it is important to ligate the internal iliac artery distal to the posterior division, as demonstrated in Figure 4-2. In ligating the hypogastric artery, the peritoneum is opened on the lateral side of the common iliac artery near its bifurcation, with the ureter attached to the medial peritoneal reflection to avoid disturbing its blood supply. The posterior branch of the hypogastric artery must be clearly identified prior to selecting the point of clamping, doubly ligating, and excising the hypogastric artery bilaterally. The hypogastric vein is not ligated as the major control of the blood supply to the pelvis arises from the hypogastric artery. It is essential also to ligate the ovarian vessels to avoid collateral circulation and persistent bleeding from this source.

PULMONARY COMPLICATIONS

ETIOLOGY AND INCIDENCE

Postoperative pulmonary complications are of interest not only to the gynecologist

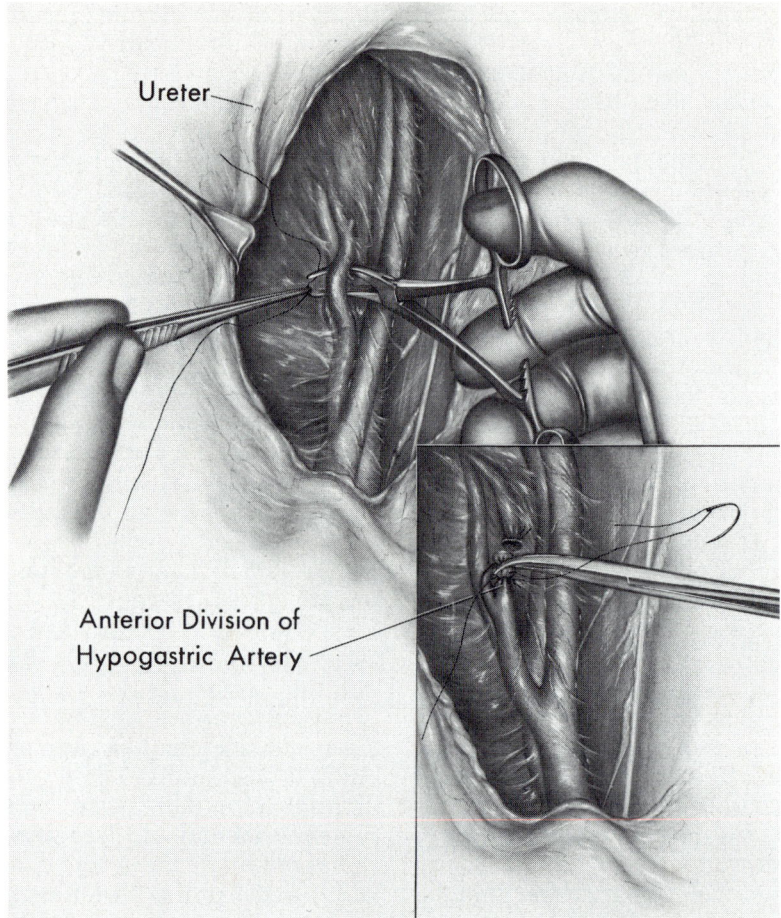

Fig. 4-2. Ligation of hypogastric artery, showing peritoneal reflection with attached ureter from bifurcation of iliac artery, and silk ligature placed around anterior division of hypogastric artery. (*Insert*) Shows anterior division of hypogastric artery ligated and excised, and transfixion ligature placed distal to initial silk tie.

but also to the internist who is frequently called in for aid in diagnosis and treatment. They also concern the roentgenologist, whose interpretation of the film is of greatest importance, and the bronchoscopist, whose skill in removing mucous plugs is often exceedingly valuable as a therapeutic measure. Fortunately, pulmonary complications are not as frequent following gynecologic laparotomies as after surgical operations in the upper abdomen. There appear to be two reasons for this: the patients are operated upon while in the Trendelenburg position, and there is less suppression of respiratory movement with pelvic surgery than with operations nearer the diaphragm.

It is difficult to classify pulmonary complications with accuracy, but the grouping of the various clinical types by King is convenient and as satisfactory as any. Exclusive of massive pulmonary embolism, he has classified pulmonary complications as bronchopneumonia, pneumonitis, and massive collapse (atelectasis). The cases that run the clinical course and present the typical x-ray picture of true bronchopneumonia are relatively few, but most of the fatal cases are included in this group. There is another relatively small group of cases which present the clinical picture and x-ray findings of massive collapse. These cases are due to occlusion of the large bronchus by exudate and get well quickly when the plug is expelled or removed. The third group is numerically larger, but the cases are less clear-cut than those of either of the other two groups. They are not pneumonia in the usual medical sense, since they run a shorter and less toxic course. Whipple has called this group pneumonitis, indicating that the alveolar exudate is caused by relatively less-virulent pneumococci. Some clinicians consider these cases to be the result of multiple small emboli. Attractive as this theory is, it cannot be proved. Certainly this type of pulmonary complication occurs much earlier in the postoperative course than the typical proved cases of massive pulmonary embolism. Another group of clinicians regards the primary cause of this type of pneumonitis as mucous plugs in the lesser bronchi, causing small areas of atelectasis and resultant penumonitis.

The incidence of postoperative pulmonary complications does not appear to be diminishing. Modell and Moya report a recent study of 1,680 patients who died within 6 weeks of surgery, and identified pulmonary complications as the major contributory cause of death in 30 per cent.

Factors Affecting the Incidence. By far the most important factor determining the development of postoperative pulmonary infection is preexisting chronic bronchopulmonary disease. Palmer reports that 65 per cent of patients who develop chest complications after abdominal surgery gave a history of bronchitis. The importance of bronchitis was strikingly demonstrated by Stein, Koota, Simon and Frank (1962), who found that 70 per cent of patients with known bronchitis developed postoperative bronchopneumonia. The diagnosis of even minimal bronchitis is of major importance preoperatively. Spirometry is of great value in detecting minimal airway obstruction and, where indicated, should be combined with other pulmonary function studies including inhalation of 1 per cent Isuprel in the measurement of forced vital capacity. Preoperative bronchodilators and chest physiotherapy should be given to all high-risk cases before surgery, including the use of bronchial expectorants and antibiotics in therapeutic dosages, until all clinical evidence of pulmonary disease has resolved. Positive pressure aerosol inhalation of Isuprel is continued until no sputum is produced. This regime is maintained until normal pulmonary function studies are obtained, which may require several days or weeks prior to elective surgery.

Analysis of the etiologic factors concerned in respiratory complications following surgery indicate that spinal and local anesthesia are not necessarily a safeguard against pulmonary complications. Statistics show that the incidence of pulmonary complications is in direct proportion to the duration of the anesthesia and the medical condition and age of the patient.

Secondary factors which may contribute to the development of obstructive atelectasis include hypoventilation following general anesthesia, aspiration of blood or intestinal contents, preexisting bronchiectasis or chronic lung disease, particularly in the elderly patient, and excess mucous production from bronchi of heavy smokers.

The pathologic physiology associated with those cases in which atelectasis exists is due to plugging of a bronchus or bronchi with mucus. Air is thus prohibited from entering the portion of the lung aerated through them, and soon the trapped air is absorbed from the lobe or lobules. It is probable that the plugged bronchus or bronchi and others go into spasm, which further increases the obstruction. If a large area of lung is involved, a negative pressure is created in the affected half of the chest, and the heart and the mediastinal structures are retracted toward the involved side. The diaphragm is pulled upward, and the intercostal spaces are narrowed. If the bronchus is permitted to remain occluded, the affected lung area becomes invaded with organisms, and an area of pneumonitis develops.

Symptoms

Most pulmonary complications of the types under consideration become manifest within 2 or 3 days after the operation, but occasionally they occur after many days. The nature and the severity of the symptoms are most variable. Massive atelectasis where a whole lobe or a whole lung is involved usually produces sudden alarming symptoms. There is a sudden rise in the temperature, the pulse, and the respiratory rate. The patient attempts to cough and becomes dyspneic and cyanotic. With bronchopneumonia or pneumonitis the onset may be fairly acute, but usually respiratory symptoms develop much more gradually.

The physical signs vary as greatly as do the pathologic processes. Distinguishing between atelectasis due to plugging of the lesser bronchi and true bronchopneumonia may be impossible. Indeed, it is undoubtedly true that the primary lesion in many cases of bronchopneumonia is atelectasis. X-ray evidence is often unconvincing in attempting to distinguish the two processes. With massive collapse the physical signs and the x-ray picture are identified more easily. There is diminished expansion on the affected side; the trachea and the cardiac apex are displaced toward the atelectatic side. The collapsed lung is dull or flat to percussion, and breath sounds and rales are absent. After the mucous plug is expelled, there may be bronchial breathing due to areas of pneumonic consolidation about the bronchi. The x-ray showing the displaced organs and the shadow cast by the collapsed lung is a typical picture and confirmation of the rather characteristic physical signs.

Treatment

Prevention is of the utmost importance in pulmonary complications, and much can be done which is most effective. Elective surgery should be avoided if there is any degree of upper respiratory infection. If acute or chronic bronchitis or tracheitis is present, an active attempt should be made to clear up the condition. Frequent inhalations of benzoin or menthol mixtures are most effective. The Trendelenburg position during the operation permit secretions to run out of the trachea or be aspirated by the anesthetist, and this is without doubt a factor in the decreased incidence of these complications in gynecologic laparotomies. Since this position is used routinely in most gynecologic laparotomies, it is unnecessary to call this fact to the attention of gynecologists, but it is doubtful whether most gynecologists appreciate the value of the Trendelenburg position during the immediate postoperative period when bronchial secretions are often excessive. Some students of these lung conditions advocate the avoidance of atropine preoperatively, believing that it dries the bronchial secretions and makes them more tenacious. We have used atropine routinely for years and hold a contrary view. The reduction in secretions during the operation permits better aeration of the lungs and in our opinion has contributed to our very low incidence of pulmonary complications. Patients should be encouraged to breathe deeply after operation, and when respirations are shallow, they may be increased greatly in depth by using a paper bag for re-breathing. Intermittent positive pressure oxygen inhalation with Isuprel-Alevaire-saline for bronchiolar dilatation should be started immediately after surgery in the high-risk patient.

The active treatment of postoperative pulmonary complications varies with the type of lesion present. If the picture is one of bronchopneumonia or pneumonitis, chemotherapy should be used as in ordinary pneumonia. If the patient is anoxemic, oxygen should be supplied. When the picture is that of a massive plugging of a bronchus by a mucous plug, the bronchial obstruction should be relieved as soon as possible and by the best means available. Coughing should be encouraged, and, as the patient coughs, the affected side of the chest may be compressed by the physician's hands. The abdomen should be splinted tightly with a Scultetus binder during this procedure. Morphia should be avoided to prevent suppression of the cough reflex unless one is in constant attendance with the patient to encourage or stimulate coughing. Deep intratracheal catheter suction is now used routinely, and will effectively clear tracheobronchial secretions. This will also produce active coughing and release mucous plugs, which essentially eliminates the use of bronchoscopy for this condition.

URINARY OUTPUT AND POSTOPERATIVE FLUID NEEDS

Perhaps the most accurate method of evaluating the degree of hydration of the postoperative patient, in the absence of impaired renal function, is the hourly record of urinary output and the serial observation of the urinary specific gravity. In the critically ill patient, these observations are best achieved by an indwelling Foley catheter, even though there is a significant incidence of lower urinary tract infection after 72 hours of bladder drainage. However, accurate monitoring of renal function is difficult to accomplish without access to hourly urinary volumes, which may be difficult to obtain from a recently anesthetized patient.

For the less critical postoperative patient, accurate measurements of voided urines is satisfactory. Fluid intake should include the daily minimum requirement of 70 mEq. of sodium (500 cc. of normal saline). In general, daily fluid replacement of 1,000 cc. of normal saline will compensate for any previous sodium deficit resulting from preoperative limitation of dietary intake and extensive insensible fluid loss from the exposed peritoneal surface at the time of surgery.

Depending on the length of the operative procedure, insensible loss from the peritoneal cavity can amount to 2,000 to 3,000 cc. of water with prolonged surgery, and must be included in the calculation of postoperative fluid needs. While the average daily insensible water loss from the skin and lungs is approximately 1,000 cc., as discussed in Chapter 5, Fluid and Electrolyte Balance, this loss is increased with each degree of temperature rise. An average urinary output of 60 cc. per hour will provide a daily output of at least 1,500 cc.

Therefore, fluid replacement during the first 24 hours following surgery should include at least 2,500 to 3,000 cc. of parenteral fluids to cover both insensible water loss and urinary output. This should include 1,000 cc. of normal saline (140 mEq.) to replace normal daily sodium metabolism and a mild serum sodium deficit which is usually present following surgery. The remaining 2,000 cc. of fluid may be 5 per cent glucose and water. Potassium supplementation is usually withheld during the first 24 to 48 hours until adequate urinary outputs are observed, to avoid the possible complication of oliguria and hyperkalemia. In the event of diminished urinary output with a high specific gravity, the rapid water loading of 500 cc. of 5 per cent G/W in 1 hour will suppress antidiuretic hormone (ADH) temporarily because of an expanded plasma volume, and produce a transient diuresis which will document previous dehydration. However, should the urinary output fail to improve, and in the presence of clinical dehydration, large amounts of fluid replacement are best monitored by continuous central venous pressure observation. The inability of the kidney to concentrate and dilute urine postoperatively, associated with a diminished urinary output and a rising blood urea nitrogen, would strongly suggest the complication of acute tubular nephrosis as a result of prolonged hypotension and renal ischemia during the operative procedure. Blood urea nitrogen levels should be followed closely, and the patient's fluid replacement during the oliguric phase of this complication should be restricted to daily insensible loss and urinary output.

One additional complication of a diminishing urinary output following surgery is a rare occurrence of accidental ligation of the ureter. Although this is usually a unilateral complication, total aneuria can occur from bilateral ligation or hyperangulation of the lower ureter, which may be unrecognized at the time of injury. The clinical symptoms of progressive CVA tenderness, decreased urinary output, and a spiking temperature should encourage the surgeon to obtain an intravenous pyelogram for observation of possible ureteral obstruction and renal shutdown. This complication is discussed in a later chapter on urinary tract injuries.

ROUTINE ORDERS

The above observations of the cardiac, pulmonary, and renal functions of the postoperative patient are ideally observed by trained medical and nursing personnel in the recovery room or intensive care unit, should the patient require constant observation. When the patient has fully recovered from her anesthetic and is suitable for return to the nursing floor for routine postoperative care, the postoperative orders should include the following:
1. Vital signs:
   _____ q. 15 min. × 4
   _____ q. ½ hr. until stable
   _____ q. 2 hr. × 24 hr.
2. Position:
   _____ Low Trendelenburg
   _____ Semi-Fowler
   _____ Flat
   _____ Other
3. Turn, cough, hyperventilate:
   _____ q. 2 hr. × 24 hr.
   _____ q. 4 hr. until ambulatory
4. Suction trachea and aspirate pharynx p.r.n.
5. Input and Output Chart.
6. Sedation:
   _____ Morphine sulphate
   _____ Codeine sulphate
   _____ Demerol
   _____ Other
7. Diet
8. Privileges.
9. Fluid orders.
10. Catheterize q. 6 hr. if unable to void or p.r.n. for discomfort.
11. If Foley catheter is used, connect to straight drainage.

CARE OF THE GASTROINTESTINAL TRACT

Every surgeon of experience has developed confidence in his own routine for feeding the postoperative patient and stimulation of the gastrointestinal tract. The senior author has long adhered to the conservative appproach, which provides only warm tap water for the 1st and 2nd postoperative days (day 1 is the day of surgery); a liquid diet on the 3rd day, exclusive of fruit juices, cocoa and milk; a full liquid diet on the 4th day; a limited soft diet on the 5th day; a full soft diet on the 6th day, and a full diet beginning on the 7th day. The junior author encourages early and progressive use of soft and solid foods postoperatively and initiates a full liquid diet on the 2nd or 3rd postoperative day with the appearance of active bowel sounds and the passage of gas per rectum. Rapid progression to a full soft diet on the following day and a full diet as desired thereafter has stimulated early bowel functions without significant complications. Seriously ill patients, however, remain on parenteral fluids until bowel activity is well established, regardless of the length of time that this might require.

PARALYTIC ILEUS AND DISTENTION

Postoperative ileus and distention associated with peritonitis, bowel surgery, or prolonged packing of the bowel during surgery frequently requires gastric suction and gentle intestinal stimulation in the immediate postoperative period.

Prevention of distention should be the aim of every surgeon, and it can be accomplished to a great degree by bearing in mind some of the causes discussed above. In cases such as ruptured ectopic pregnancy or ruptured tubo-ovarian abscess, where distention is anticipated, a course of Prostigmin or Ilopan, given every 4 hours, beginning immediately postoperatively, may be a valuable preventive measure.

At the first indication of tympanites, treatment should be prompt and vigorous, for the condition is much more easily conquered early than when fully developed. A course of Prostigmin is begun immediately. Our usual order is for 1 cc. of Prostigmin, given hypodermically every hour for 3 doses, unless there is reason to suspect organic obstruction or inflammatory bowel lesions; bowel anastomosis or repair also contraindicates such stimulation. After this initial short vigorous course, the drug is given every 4 hours as long as necessary. A rectal tube is inserted and left in place for sufficient time to permit the gas forced along by the peristaltic stimulants to be expelled. Enemas are given not oftener than twice a day.

Within the first 48 hours after operation we use enemas of small volume composed of 200 cc. of water and 200 cc. of glycerine, or 130 cc. of Fleet's Phosphosoda in disposable containers. Later, enemas of larger volume, such as the soapsuds enema of 1,000 cc. with 8 cc. of turpentine, may be more effective. An enema of 240 cc. of milk and 240 cc. of molasses is particularly effective. It is well to time the giving of an enema a few minutes after the injection of the drug. If the patient is unable to expel the enema after a reasonable time, it is siphoned off with a rectal tube, for a retained enema serves only to increase the patient's discomfort.

The Levin tube should be passed and attached to suction. This is especially effective if gastric dilatation is prominent, and if nausea and vomiting accompany the distention. The intake of fluids by mouth should be reduced, and when the tympanites is marked, and nausea and vomiting are present, they should be stopped temporarily. Body fluids and nourishment should be maintained by intravenous solution composed of glucose and normal saline. In the first 48 hours after operation cathartics are worse than useless. Some time should elapse to permit it to regain tone before administering stimulants to it. On the 3rd postoperative day mild laxatives, such as milk of magnesia or senna granules (Senokot) may be given by mouth. When a mechanical obstruction is seriously suspected, cathartics are contraindicated. Likewise, when the condition of the large bowel is weakened by operative injury or inflammation, enemas and rectal tubes are contraindicated. Often

TABLE 4-1. DIFFERENTIAL DIAGNOSIS BETWEEN POSTOPERATIVE ILEUS AND POSTOPERATIVE OBSTRUCTION

Symptoms and Signs	Postoperative Ileus	Postoperative Obstruction
Abdominal pain	Discomfort from distention but not cramping pains	Cramping, progressively severe
Relationship to previous surgery	Usually within 48-72 hours of surgery	Usually delayed; may be 5-7 days for remote onset
Nausea and vomiting	Nausea and vomiting	Nausea and vomiting
Distention	Distention	Distention
Bowel sounds	Absent or hypoactive	Borborygmi with peristaltic rushes and high pitched tinkles
Fever	Only if related to associated peritonitis	Rarely present unless bowel becomes gangrenous
Abdominal films	Distended loops of small and large bowel; gas usually present in colon	Single or multiple loops of distended bowel, usually small bowel with air fluid levels
Treatment	Conservative, with nasogastric suction; enemas; cholinergic stimulation	Partial: conservative or with nasogastric decompression; or Complete: surgical

a glycerine suppository may be substituted safely and effectively. When a certain degree of chronic distention persists for 5, 6, or more days, we occasionally give a dose of castor oil or oral Fleet's Phospho-soda (30 cc.). It is drastic therapy; but after it has passed through the intestinal tract, usually the patient is relieved permanently of her distention.

It is important to differentiate between postoperative ileus and postoperative obstruction if proper therapy is to be promptly initiated with beneficial results (Table 4-1).

It is obvious from the above review of the clinical manifestations of postoperative ileus and obstruction that there may be difficulty in accurately distinguishing between one entity and the other. This is due to the fact that partial bowel obstruction frequently occurs with a secondary ileus as a part of the clinical picture. Only by close clinical observation, with serial abdominal x-ray films and close observation of the white blood count, can one clearly separate these two postoperative complications. Obviously, the most frequent clinical entity is that of ileus, a fact which may mislead the surgeon into a false sense of security unless he remains acutely aware of the distinguishing features of intestinal obstruction. The most common gynecologic disease associated with both ileus and intestinal obstruction is severe pelvic inflammatory disease. Notoriously, intra-abdominal rupture of a pelvic abscess is associated with prolonged postoperative ileus, but occasionally fibrous adhesions form, and secondary obstruction occurs. Cellulitis resulting from hematoma formation and secondary infection of the vaginal cuff following either abdominal or vaginal hysterectomy is frequently associated with ileus, whereas intestinal obstruction only rarely results from such a complication.

In contrast to pelvic surgery for a benign disease, radical surgery, including exenterations for cervical carcinoma, is frequently complicated by postoperative intestinal obstruction. Bricker recently reported the occurrence of intestinal obstruction in 11 per cent of a large series of pelvic exenterations for the treatment of various pelvic malignancies, including 207 cases of postirradiation carcinoma of the cervix. This problem is related to the difficulty in achieving adequate pelvic peritonization after the extensive en-bloc dissection.

POSTOPERATIVE CARE OF THE URINARY BLADDER

In order to appreciate the many problems related to the postoperative care of the urinary bladder, it is necessary to review the physiologic mechanisms of voiding. The recent development of cinefluoroscopic technics and accurate methods of monitoring intravesical and intra-urethral pressures have provided additional information in our understanding of the mechanisms of voiding. Both voluntary and involuntary components of the act are essential:

1. **Voluntary Components.** The diaphragm is fixed after a short inspiration, following which the lower abdominal musculature is contracted, producing intra-abdominal pressure which is directed toward the bladder. At the same time there is relaxation of the pubococcygeus portion of the levator ani muscle which encircles both the urethra and anus. Definite relaxation of the muscle bundle during voiding may be demonstrated by the occasional release of gas from the rectum with this maneuver.

2. **Involuntary Components.** The combined efforts of the intra-abdominal pressure and relaxation of the pubococcygeus muscle produces a downward displacement of the base of the bladder, which stretches the trigone and stimulates the parasympathetic nerves to the trigone, thus initiating smooth muscle contraction of the bladder.

The most common cause of postoperative atony of the female bladder is the hesitancy to initiate the voluntary phase of voiding. In abdominal surgery, the patient is unwilling to contract the abdominal muscles to produce intra-abdominal pressure against the dome of the bladder. In vaginal surgery, spasm, edema, and tenderness of the pubococcygeus muscle following anterior colporrhaphy produce spasm of the muscle, which acts as an obstruction to the process of voiding. The operative trauma from plication of the pubovesicocervical fascia causes edema of the urethral tube, especially at the urethrovesical junction, thus contributing to obstruction.

Consequently, for spontaneous voiding to occur, it is necessary to await the return of parasympathetic function and coordinated voluntary motor activity of the abdominal wall and the levator muscles. In the past it has been customary to insert an indwelling Foley catheter for 5 days or more following vaginal plastic surgery. The patient is catheterized repeatedly until spontaneous voiding ensues following abdominal surgery.

Avoiding Overdistention of the Bladder. It is our belief that improper handling of the urinary tract contributes more to the patient's postoperative pain than any other single complication during that period. Everyone with considerable surgical experience regards the use of the catheter postoperatively as far from ideal, and recently a technic has been developed for handling the postoperative bladder differently. Since the use of the catheter is still the common method of caring for postoperative urinary retention, it will be described. Later, a more recently developed method will be discussed.

While the usual postoperative orders instruct that the patient be catheterized within 6 hours if unable to void, it is important to have the patient catheterized as often as necessary when symptoms of bladder discomfort are present. With the rapid absorption of intravenous fluids, the normal kidney will excrete urine rapidly and produce bladder distention by more than doubling the usual urinary output of 50 to 60 cc. per hour. Also, a patient does not completely empty the bladder on initiating voiding, and the bladder will contain varying amounts of residual urine after each voiding process. This can accumulate and produce overdistention of the bladder, even though the patient is presumably voiding normally. Therefore, if the patient desires and is unable to void, she should be given the benefit of the doubt and catheterized, regardless of how little time has elapsed since the last voiding, and regardless of any other evidence which would seem to suggest that the bladder is not distended.

POSTOPERATIVE URINARY TRACT INFECTIONS

Since Kass's work the literature is replete with reports on this subject. The major clinical importance in the transient use of the urethral catheter is its effect on persistent symptomatic urinary tract infections. Numerous studies have shown urinary tract infection, varying from 40 per cent to 97 per cent, following pelvic operations and the use of the indwelling catheter postoperatively. There is no doubt that the immediate incidence of urinary infections is high, and any procedure which can avoid it is most desirable. Some of these infections persist, but the incidence of persistence is apparently not great. For example, in the study of Barr and Paterson on 452 patients who were repeatedly catheterized and followed at 8 weeks and 6 months postoperatively, but in whom the urine was not checked unless symptoms indicated, there was microscopic evidence of urinary tract infection in 50 per cent of the patients at 8 weeks. However, all the patients had sterile urine at 6 months when properly treated. Numerous technics have been devised to reduce the incidence of infection, such as closed drainage, the use of a polyethylene foam collar around the Foley catheter fitted tightly against the meatus, and bactericidal irrigating solutions. The benefits from most of these different technics have not been striking.

Recently a technic developed by Mattingly at Marquette-Milwaukee County General Hospital holds great promise. He has abandoned the use of the indwelling urethral catheter in preference to the use of the suprapubic bladder drainage. This idea, although well recognized in urologic circles, was first discussed in the field of gynecology in this country by Mattingly in 1964.

The procedure of initiating suprapubic bladder drainage is easy to perform at the completion of either an abdominal or vaginal operation. It includes inserting a No. 8 French Silastic (silicone) catheter into the bladder through a 9-gauge needle, 4″ in length (Fig. 4-3). The bladder is filled with 150 to 200 cc. of sterile water, and the needle is inserted through the surgically prepared anterior abdominal wall, approximately 2 cm. above the symphysis pubis. The suprapubic tube is attached to a sterile intravenous tubing set (Fig. 4-3), and the opposite end is inserted into a sterile liter bottle or to a regular urinary drainage set. The tubing is kept filled with fluid at all times. The tubing is sutured to the skin or fixed to a silicone body seal (Silastic Cystocath by Dow Corning Corp.) in order to avoid accidental removal (Fig. 4-3), and a two-way stopcock may be inserted between the tubing connections for easy opening and closing of the system when the pa-

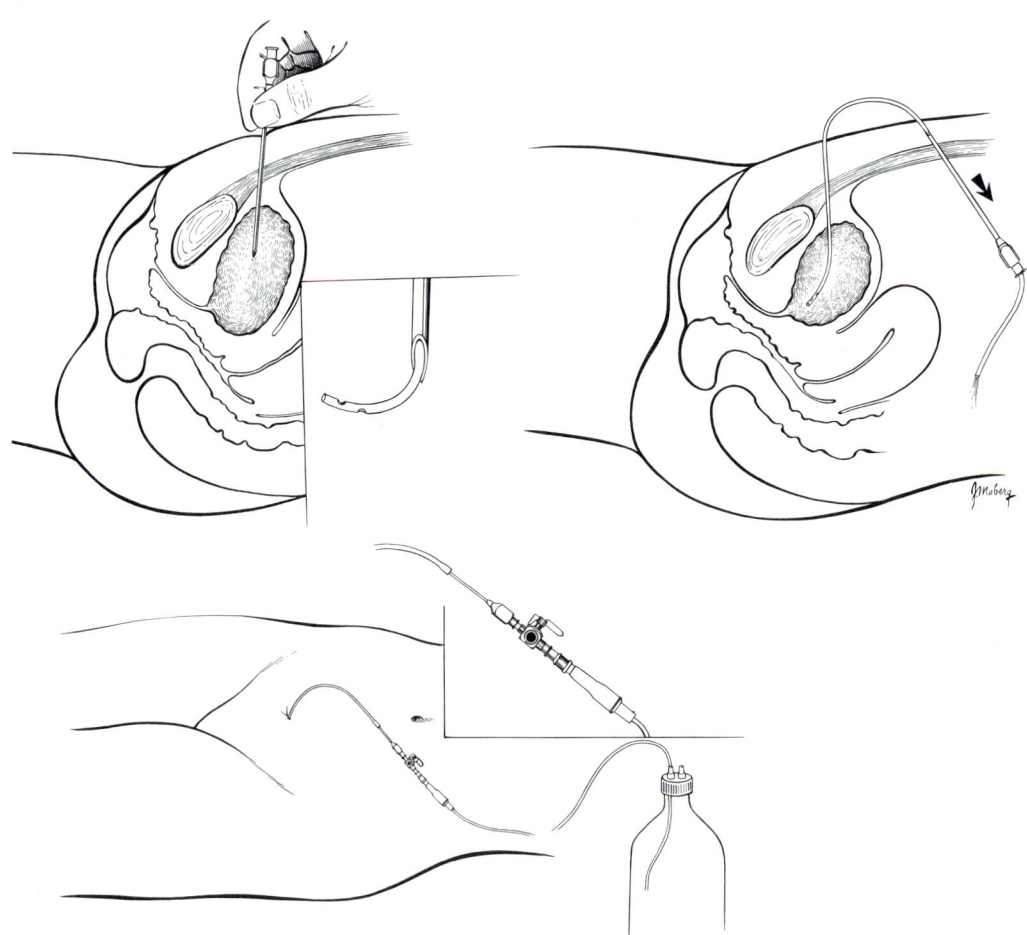

Fig. 4-3. Showing method of inserting suprapubic tube through needle and drainage into bottle. Thus the urethra is not traumatized by repeated catheterization or indwelling catheter.

tient desires. The system is never irrigated unless there is plugging of the catheter in the bladder, and symptoms of bladder distention occur. Consequently, throughout the entire postoperative course it is rare that the drainage tube system is ever irrigated.

Results of Suprapubic Bladder Drainage. In the past 100 cases of vaginal plastic surgery at Milwaukee County General Hospital, where the suprapubic bladder drainage was utilized, approximately 75 per cent of the patients voided spontaneously within the first 5 days postoperatively. We have the patient begin clamping the tube on the 3rd postoperative day, and leave the supracath clamped in place as a method of obtaining a postvoiding residual urine without requiring urethral catheterization. Fifty per cent of the patients were voiding normally with a normal residual urine by the 5th postoperative day. This is the day on which we would ordinarily remove the urethral catheter following vaginal plastic surgery.

In a control series with Foley catheter drainage, appproximately 60 per cent of the patients required reinsertion of urethral catheter for periods of 48 to 72 hours or longer after removal on the 5th postoperative day. Urine cultures obtained preoperatively and prior to removal of the suprapubic catheter clearly demonstrated that there is a reduction in the incidence of bacteriuria and urinary tract infection from 95 per cent to 33 per cent with this technic. There is further reduction in the incidence of urinary tract infection (20%) by this suprapubic technic if both significant bacteriuria and pyuria are included in the definition of urinary tract infection. More recently, meticulous attention to aseptic technic in the management of the suprapubic catheter has reduced the infection rate below 15 per cent.

Aside from the improvement in urinary tract infection by one technic or another, the major advantage of the suprapubic bladder drainage is clearly evident to our nursing service, as 76 per cent of our patients did not require a single catheterization following vaginal hysterectomy and repair. This fact alone, plus the comfort of the suprapubic catheter to the patient, has encouraged us to continue using this method of bladder drainage.

We are in agreement with Hodgkinson, as well as Martin and others, who have clearly demonstrated that prophylactic sulfonamides, when given with the use of an indwelling catheter, are ineffective in preventing urinary tract infection.

VENOUS THROMBOSIS AND THROMBOPHLEBITIS

Of all complications following pelvic surgery, the most sinister and difficult to control is that of venous thrombosis. Whether associated with inflammation of the vein wall, known as thrombophlebitis, with partial or complete venous obstruction, or whether associated with a silent venous thrombus from vascular injury and stasis, the hazard of thromboembolism is a serious and frequently lethal clinical problem. Unfortunately, pelvic surgery is complicated by venous thrombosis more frequently than surgery in other operative fields.

Jeffcoate and Tindall report a study of 12,189 patients admitted to the gynecologic wards of Liverpool Royal Infirmary between 1951 and 1963, where the incidence of newly acquired thromboembolic disease, including either venous thrombosis or embolus, occurred in 1 case for every 112 operations. A recent intensive study of the rate of idiopathic thromboembolism in the United States in nonpregnant hospitalized women, 20 to 44 years of age, is reported as 1 per 1,000 (Searle). The incidence is even greater among gynecologic high-risk patients with one or more of the following known surgical hazards: (1) over the age of 40; (2) obesity, (3) pelvic malignancy, (4) varicose veins, (5) previous thromboembolic disease, (6) severe diabetes, (7) arteriosclerotic cardiovascular disease, (8) cardiac failure, and (9) chronic pulmonary disease. The fact that numerous autopsy studies have demonstrated that approximately 80 per cent of fatal pulmonary emboli arise from thrombosis of the iliac, femoral, and deep veins of the lower venous tree should alert every pelvic surgeon to the realistic fact that each postoperative patient is a possible candidate for venous thrombosis and pulmonary embolism.

Pathophysiology

More than 100 years ago Virchow presented his concept of venous thrombosis and at the same time documented the mechanism of venous embolization. Since that time blood coagulation has advanced in importance until it has become a subspecialty of medicine, and research has been accelerated in this field. Nonetheless, there has been little progress in the advancement of our knowledge of the mechanisms of thrombogenesis until the present day of electron microscopy. Virchow's basic premise of thrombosis included a triad of etiologic factors, namely, (1) an increased tendency to blood clotting, (2) damage to the vessel wall, and (3) stagnation of blood flow. The fact that 70 per cent of a patient's total blood volume is contained within the venous system contributes to the fact that venous thrombosis occurs 3 to 4 times more frequently than arterial thrombosis.

Venous thrombosis may be distinguished from arterial thrombosis in several ways: (1) in the venous circulation the role of intimal damage is a less frequent factor; (2) venous blood flow is more frequently altered than arterial; and (3) fibrin rather than the platelet is the major constituent of the venous thrombus. While the terms "red" and "white" thrombus are convenient terms to differentiate venous and arterial thrombosis, respectively, the components of both "white" and "red" thrombus may occur in the same thrombus. In thrombophlebitis, venous thrombi may have platelet material as a small "white head" attached to the vessel wall, while a larger "red tail" may stream out into the lumen of the vessel. The fragile "red" thrombus is most hazardous and frequently dislodges from the vein wall as a vascular cast or simply breaks away from the "red tail" as a pulmonary embolism.

In contrast, the "white" thrombus represents a platelet mesh which is found predominately in arterial lesions and is more adherent to the vessel wall. Damage to the vessel wall from such causes as inflammation, trauma, or chemicals will produce the following sequence of events which lead to the formation of a venous thrombus: First, platelets attach themselves to the damaged endothelium and produce an adherent aggregate of platelets which may break loose and be carried away in the bloodstream or may continue to build a network for the deposition of thrombin and the formation of fibrin. Red blood cells become trapped in the fibrin network. This process may be repeated several times, with the enlargement of the thrombus and final obstruction of the vessel.

The important difference between arterial and venous thrombi has not been appreciated in the past and bears directly on the value of anticoagulant therapy. While anticoagulant drugs have little effect on platelet aggregation in arteries, their benefit is well recognized in preventing fibrin formation in a typical "red thrombus." Recent evidence suggests that clinical dextran is effective in coating platelets and endothelium, which interferes with the ability of platelets to adhere to the damaged wall.

Etiologic Factors

The major factors associated with venous thrombosis in the gynecologic patient include venous stasis and damage to the vessel wall. Nonetheless, Sharnoff has demonstrated a significant rise in circulating platelets in the immediate postoperative period and later between the 8th to 14th days. In addition, Emmons and Mitchell describe an increase in the rate and intensity of platelet clumping during the first 10 days following surgery.

Sites of predilection for venous thrombi are predominantly characterized by obstacles to blood flow such as vascular overcrossing, uphill flow, and low-pressure gradients. The frequency of thrombi in the femoral and iliac veins is clinical evidence of such obstruction, particularly the left common iliac vein, which has been shown by Calnan *et al.* to be compressed between the right common iliac artery and the vertebral column. Pressure gradients between the left common iliac vein and the inferior vena cava sometimes reach 10 mm. of mercury. While it is convenient to consider venous obstruction as the major contributory factor to thrombosis, it is well to recall that Ashoff (1925) pointed out that the development of thrombosis is due to several different conditions, interrelated to each other, and is "the function of a number of variable factors."

During pelvic surgery several factors are known to impair venous return from the lower extremities and pelvis. Blood pools in the lower extremities under general anesthesia due to loss of the pump action of the calf muscles. There is also a decrease in the negative intrathoracic pressure due to limitation of thoracic expansion during anesthesia and in the postoperative period. Normally, this negative pressure assists the venous return to the heart and is one of the major benefits of early postoperative ambulation. Prolonged pelvic operations, with excessive packing of the intestines in the upper abdomen, produces pressure on the inferior vena cava and partial obstruction of venous return. Injury to the vessel wall during pelvic surgery is conducive to intravascular thrombosis. This is borne out by the fact that operations in the neighborhood of the pelvic veins have the highest instance of thrombosis in the pelvis and the femoral veins.

Postoperatively, the cornerstone for thrombus formation is primarily that of stasis. Although usually associated with other factors, impairment of blood flow from the lower limbs is more marked in the elderly age group, as shown by McLachlin and others. McLachlin further demonstrated that elevation of the legs to 15° from the horizontal produced better venous drainage by dye studies than either active movements or elastic stockings. The two major factors which promote venostasis and are clinically related to an increase of venous thrombosis include immobilization in bed and the sitting position, with the knees and thighs acutely flexed. Sharnoff and Rosenberg have demonstrated that immobilization in bed is more significant than age as a cause of postoperative thrombosis. Early ambulation is of no value in the prevention of venous thrombosis and thrombophlebitis unless the patient is actively walked rather than permitted to sit in a chair. It is far better to exercise the legs in bed than to obstruct the return of blood from the legs by sitting in a chair or dangling at the bedside. Many authors have demonstrated a direct relationship between an increased instance of thrombosis of the lower legs and the length of confinement to bed. As demonstrated by Gibbs, pooling of blood in the calf muscles, particularly the soleus muscle, is one of the major causes of deep vein thrombosis in immobilized patients.

The relation of thromboembolism to specific types of pelvic surgery has been studied by Jeffcoate and Tindall. In their report there was no difference in the incidence of thrombosis for hysterectomy, which carries a 3 to 4 per cent risk of thrombosis, and embolism, irrespective of an abdominal or vaginal procedure. An incidence of thromboembolism of 2 to 5 per cent was found for any type of major pelvic procedure, despite routine physiotherapy, early ambulation, and modern surgical technics. Understandably, their highest rate of thromboembolism was in radical vulvectomy (8.3%). A significant observation of this study was the fact that a decrease in physical activity of patients admitted to the hospital for diagnostic evaluation prior to surgery was associated with a higher rate of postoperative thrombosis than that which occurred in patients admitted directly for surgery the following day.

Symptoms and Signs

Postoperative venous thromboses occur in three major forms.

The first, and most serious, is the acute picture of thrombophlebitis resulting from thrombosis of the deep veins of the lower extremity. Acute massive venous occlusion of the iliac and femoral veins, with progressive ischemia of the entire extremity and gangrene formation, is the most life-threatening and least frequent in occurrence. The most common form of deep venous thrombosis is in the deep popliteal veins of the calf. Such cases represent true thrombophlebitis and are ushered in by fever, sometimes chills, and throbbing pain in the calf and the popliteal space. In the event of iliofemoral venous thrombosis, pain in the groin is a prominent symptom and is difficult to control by analgesics. The leg begins to swell promptly, and within a short time the typical picture of *phlegmasia alba dolens* appears, and is demonstrated by cyanosis for 1 or 2 days, followed by a pale and edematous extremity, suggesting lymphatic obstruction in the inflammatory process. The presence of numerous anastomatic venous channels among the deep veins of the leg usually provide adequate venous drainage and explains the absence of persistent cyanosis.

The diagnosis of deep thrombophlebitis is confirmed by pain in the calf on dorsiflexion of the foot (Homans' sign). Production of pain in the calf on inflation of the blood pressure cuff around the involved part of the extremity (Löwenberg test) is a more sensitive test of venous inflammatory disease than other symptoms and signs. During inflation of the cuff slowly to 200 mm. Hg, discomfort is normally experienced at about 160 mm. Hg. With subclinical thrombophlebitis, pain is acutely noted at a lower level (60-150 mm. Hg).

The second type of spontaneous venous thrombosis occurs as a *superficial thrombophlebitis* in either the greater or lesser saphenous veins. There is reddening of the paravascular tissues and considerable localized induration and tenderness. The adjacent lymphatics become obstructed, and edema develops. This edema is much less than that encountered with deep thrombophlebitis but recurrences of saphenous phlebitis are common, and chronic edema frequently develops. The ultimate condition of the leg is often worse with superficial phlebitis than with the deep variety. Provided that the clotting process does not extend to the deep veins, superficial thrombophlebitis is relatively free of the major sequelae of pulmonary embolus.

The third type of venous thromboses is that associated with preexisting varicose veins. This type is less commonly encountered postoperatively but is seen occasionally. Trauma and infection play a lesser role in this type, which usually represents *phlebothrombosis* resulting from venostasis and an altered venous endothelium. In thromboses of this type there is usually little if any edema or induration.

In the diagnosis of venous obstruction, an unequivocal Homans' sign is pathognomonic, and a Löwenberg blood pressure cuff test is frequently more sensitive and detects the vascular condition earlier than other methods. Comparative leg measurements are useful, but the palpation of tender venous cord is frequently difficult in the acute phase and is usually possible only in the superficial type of phlebitis.

Treatment

The treatment of venous thrombosis may be conveniently divided into three categories: (1) prophylactic, (2) conservative, and (3) operative.

Prophylaxis. Prevention of postoperative venous thrombosis begins at the time the patient is admitted to the hospital. It is essential that patient remain ambulatory, and that encouragement be given to walking and leg exercises prior to surgery. Fitted elastic stockings should be applied *prior to* surgery to improve peripheral venous tone and avoid vascular pooling. Adequate preoperative hydration of the patient and establishment of a normal blood volume is important for maintenance of venous circulation. Avoidance of prolonged compression of the vena cava during pelvic surgery with laparotomy packs is particularly important in prolonged operative procedures. Avoidance of trauma to the pelvic veins by blunt instruments and vascular dissection is of major importance in preventing postoperative thrombosis. Cushioning of the patient's heels during surgery will protect the calf veins from external pressure and possible endothelial damage.

The major debate in prevention concerns the early vs. delayed postoperative ambulation of the patient. In recognition of the fact that blood flow from the calf veins is reduced by about 50 per cent during the first 2 weeks following operation (Browse, 1962), there is much interest in immediate ambulation and active walking, beginning on the day following surgery. Avoidance of sitting either in or out of bed with the knees flexed is the most important issue in maintaining adequate venous circulation. The senior author's preference and experience in delayed ambulation refutes the more current aggressive approach. However, his insistence on active leg (bicycle) exercise while in bed and the avoidance of foot drop is responsible for his personal observation of no greater incidence of postoperative thromboembolism than that reported with early ambulation. Nonetheless, in high-risk patients, including those having the hazards of advanced age, obesity, malignant disease, circulatory disorders, or previous thromboembolic disease, it is important to make every effort to improve venous drainage of the legs, where possible. The foot of the bed should be elevated 15° from the horizontal, and fitted elastic stockings should be used until the patient is discharged from the hospital.

Perhaps the most important prophylactic against venous thrombosis is the constant awareness of the surgeon of the possibility of this condition. Knowledge of the fact that half of the cases of fatal pulmonary embolism occur in patients with silent thrombosis, in whom the embolism is not preceded by pain or swelling of the limbs, should increase the postoperative vigilance of this complication.

ANTICOAGULANT THERAPY. Recent evidence that small pulmonary emboli occur as a continuing process from silent venous thrombi prior to the terminal embolus has encouraged many clinicians to use prophylactic anticoagulants in high-risk patients immediately following pelvic surgery. Much of the current interest began 10 years ago with the report by Sevitt and Gallagher in England, who clearly demonstrated that anticoagulants prevented pulmonary embolism and thrombophlebitis when employed prophylactically in patients with fractured hips. Since that time, additional reports by Sevitt and co-workers and other British investigators have clearly documented the effectiveness of prophylactic anticoagulation in the prevention of pulmonary emboli. The relative ease of oral and intravenous anticoagulation has justified their use in high-risk patients but is associated with postoperative bleeding in up to 14 per cent of the cases.

Although this treatment has been beneficial in preventing emboli from serious injuries of the lower extremities, it is our opinion that it is unnecessary to give anticoagulants to all patients in the older age groups who have major pelvic surgery. If the elderly female is managed following gynecologic surgery in the same manner as that outlined above, we have not found prophylactic anticoagulation to be necessary. However, there is mounting evidence that patients subjected to prolonged radical surgery, particularly radical vulvectomy and groin dissection, may profit by postoperative anticoagulant therapy. In such cases postoperative ambulation is difficult, and trauma to the vascular wall from the dissection is a recognized result of such surgery. When indicated, it is our preference to use intravenous heparin, 10,000 units (100 mg.) every 6 hours, due to its immediate anticoagulant effect and its rapid excretion within 3 to 6 hours, thereby providing an added safety factor. The antithrombin effects of heparin are observed by the clotting time (at least 2 times normal). The patient is gradually converted to the oral administration of bishydroxycoumarin (Dicumarol), which inhibits prothrombin activity. The daily dosage must be sufficient to maintain the prothrombin time between 15 and 30 per cent of normal. If the prothrombin time falls to less than 15 per cent, Hykinone (50-100 mg.) should be administered subcutaneously to increase prothrombin production by the liver.

Because of the frequency of serious postoperative bleeding in fully anticoagulated surgical patients, it is our personal preference to use clinical dextran as a prophylactic measure in the prevention of venous thrombosis and pulmonary emboli. In high-risk patients it is our policy to use clinical dextran 500 ml./day, starting 1 day prior to surgery and continuing 4 to 5 days postoperatively until the patient is completely ambulatory and shows no signs of thrombophlebitis. Patients undergoing radical pelvic surgery receive dextran on the day preceding surgery as a part of their preoperative hydration regime, and the dextran is continued for 5 days postoperatively, or until the patient is fully ambulatory. Our routine is to use 500 cc. of 10 per cent clinical dextran daily.

Conservative Treatment. Superficial thrombophlebitis is easily managed by the use of analgesics, elastic bandage, antibiotics, elevation of the extremity to about 30°, and a heat cradle. It is not our policy to treat such superficial thromboses with anticoagulants; nor is it wise to keep the patient at prolonged bed rest in order to avoid propagation of the clot to the deep veins. Within 48 to 72 hours the acute symptoms will have subsided, and the patient is encouraged to become ambulatory. Broad-spectrum antibiotics are continued until the perivascular cellulitis has subsided, and there is no further tenderness along the course of the vein. The elastic stocking or wrapping is worn until leg measurements are identical bilaterally, suggesting complete resolution of the process.

The major objectives in the early treatment of deep venous thrombosis are:

1. To prevent pulmonary embolism by fragmentation of the "red tail" of a venous thrombus or separation of the thrombus from the vein wall, and

2. To prevent organization and lymphatic scarring of the perivascular tissues with resultant postphlebitic complications.

The usual treatment of bed rest, antibiotics, elevation of the extremity, heat cradle, and anticoagulants are time-honored and effective. Because of its immediate effect on inhibiting thrombin and fibrin formation, heparin is an effective drug in preventing the formation of a fibrin tail on a recent thrombus. Rapid anticoagulation is achieved within 24 hours by the intravenous use of 10,000 units (100 mg.) heparin every 6 hours. While this dosage rarely produces a clotting time of greater than 2 times normal, heparin can be inhibited by protamine sulfate, on a mg.-for-mg. basis, if required. Because of the usual need for prolonged anticoagulation in deep venous thrombosis, the patient is started on oral anticoagulants such as Dicumarol (bishydroxycoumarin), Coumadin (sodium warfarin), Tromexan (ethyl biscoumacetate), or Sintrom (acenocoumarol). When the prothrombin time has decreased to 30 per cent of normal, the intravenous heparin is discontinued. The patient with acute deep thrombophlebitis should be kept in bed for a week after the symptoms of pain and fever have subsided. Until the swelling has disappeared, the foot should remain elevated even when the patient is allowed to ambulate. Activity should be greatly restricted as long as swelling is present, and the use of an elastic bandage should be maintained until the leg measurements are identical bilaterally. The sympathetic ganglia may be blocked by paravertebral injection of procaine to abolish reflex arterial vasospasm, but is used infrequently.

Surgical Treatment. Usually, surgical treatment of acute thrombophlebitis is reserved for massive ileofemoral venous thrombosis. Progression of this massive venous occlusion produces *phlegmasia cerulea dolens*, which is associated with a high mortality and the very serious sequelae of pulmonary embolism, gangrene, and the postphlebitic syndrome. As described by Haller, the femoral vein is opened under local anesthesia, and the clot is removed from the ileofemoral vessel, with aspiration of the vessel to the level of the vena cava to remove the clots completely. Venous ligation is not employed in this procedure, but the patient is rapidly anticoagulated with heparin, followed by an oral anticoagulant. Anticoagulation is maintained for about 6 weeks, and elastic support of the leg is provided as long as there is residual edema. The most recent report by Haller, Wagner and Jackson (1966) of thrombectomy in 50 patients revealed normal postoperative phlebograms in 84 per cent of their patients. While Homans recommends early ligation in superficial phlebitis, the effective use of anticoagulants and antibiotics has minimized the use of surgery in acute thrombophlebitis.

PULMONARY EMBOLISM

Postoperative pulmonary embolism is one of the major tragedies of pelvic surgery. While the true incidence of pulmonary embolism is impossible to assess accurately, the usual rate of 10 per cent of autopsy studies is frequently quoted. However, more recent studies by Freiman at the Beth Israel Hospital revealed a more accurate incidence of pulmonary emboli in 64 per cent of autopsy studies. Other critical autopsy studies reveal this entity to be 5 to 6 times more frequent than was previously diagnosed by routine examination.

The most common site of pulmonary emboli is from the lower extremities, which account for approximately 80 per cent, while thrombi from pelvic veins contribute an additional 15 per cent of such emboli. Unfortunately, more than one half of the cases of fatal pulmonary embolism occur in patients with silent venous thrombosis prior to the pulmonary complication.

Recent studies by Sabbiston and Wagner, using radioactive scanning technics, have demonstrated the incidence of pulmonary embolism in man to be far greater than previously suspected. This technic demonstrates unprofused areas of the lung, which upon resolution shows return of circulation to the affected area. Such information provides radiographic evidence that embolization of the lung is a repetitive phenomenon and represents a continuous balance between embolization and lysis of pulmonary emboli. Allison has demonstrated that a large part of the pulmonary circulation can be occluded by thrombi without such clinical symptoms as change in heart rate, blood pressure, chest x-ray, or electrocardiogram. Unexplained tachypnea may be the only clinical sign available to explain the occurrence of emboli in the pulmonary arterial tree. When there is clinical suspicion of pulmonary emboli, close observation of the respiratory rate every 30 minutes is a far better diagnostic tool than all other vital signs combined. The pathologic changes of nonfatal emboli include infarction and scarring of the pulmonary parenchyma, which may result in pulmonary hypertension, cor pulmonale, and chronic lung disease.

Symptoms

The presence of an obvious thrombophlebitis or of an unexplained fever may warn of the possibility of embolism, but often the patient will have had a totally uneventful convalescence of from 1 to 3 weeks when the embolism occurs with the suddenness of lightning. Since phlebothrombosis, without fever, is the type of intravenous clot which most often becomes dislodged and results in embolism, it is understandable that often there are no premonitory symptoms or signs. However, embolization is usually a continuous process of small embolic episodes, and the only clinical sign which may suggest the embolic process is that of unexplained tachypnea.

Frequently, physical efforts, such as occur with getting out of bed, a bowel movement, or an enema, appears to be the precipitating factor. Suddenly the patient has an excruciating pain in the chest, she becomes cyanotic, respirations become shallow and rapid, the pulse rapid and feeble, there is a sudden fall in blood pressure, beads of perspiration appear on the face, and she lapses into unconsciousness. Gorham studied 100 fatal cases of proven pulmonary embolism and found that 44 per cent of the patients died within the first 30 minutes, while 56 per cent lived from 2 hours to 2 weeks.

Small nonfatal emboli may produce sudden chest pain, or may be relatively asymptomatic until respiratory distress from infarction occurs. The usual symptoms of hemoptysis, elevated temperature, orthopnea, dyspnea, and tachypnea are usually present. A friction rub may make its appearance within 1 or 2 days of the embolization, but the x-ray changes of pneumonic consolidation are late and frequently difficult to identify.

PATHOPHYSIOLOGY

The physiologic effects of massive embolic obstruction of the pulmonary arterial system include:

1. Obstruction of venous return to the left heart with diminished cardiac output.
2. Obstruction of the right ventricle with acute right heart failure.
3. Infarction of the involved segment of the lung.

With massive obstruction of a main pulmonary artery or arteries, there is rapid right heart failure, and cardiac output is diminished by impaired venous return to the left heart. The resultant effect of diminished coronary and cerebral blood flow, hypoxia, and hypotension may lead quickly to irreversible shock and death, depending on the rate of cardiac output. The resultant effects of coronary ischemia and hypoxia produce the acute symptoms of dyspnea and anginal pain. Fortunately, massive embolization, with obstruction of the major pulmonary arterial circulation is the most infrequent type and is seen in about 2 per cent of autopsy series.

Emboli to medium and small arteries occur more frequently and may produce a variety of pathologic effects. There may be no residual pathologic findings if the emboli are quite small. However, the small emboli may produce pulmonary infarction with hemoptysis, pleuritic pain, and x-ray evidence of a wedge-shaped consolidation. Other cases may result in acute symptoms similar to those of massive pulmonary embolism and may produce a reflex vasoconstriction of the pulmonary and coronary vessels with acute heart failure and cardiac arrest. Finally, chronic pulmonary disease from scarring may result from repeated small emboli and may produce pulmonary hypertension and cor pulmonale.

TREATMENT

Acute, massive pulmonary embolism is rapidly fatal in approximately 50 per cent of the cases, while the remainder of the patients live long enough to warrant consideration of pulmonary artery embolectomy. The major problem is related to the decision for or against embolectomy. It has been the experience of Cooley and others that pulmonary emboli involving 50 per cent or less of the pulmonary arterial tree will not be fatal if the patient survives the immediate vasomotor and respiratory effects. Gradual lysis and resorption of the clot will occur over a period of time, although there is a high incidence of residual pulmonary pathology. In cases in which more than 50 per cent of the pulmonary arterial tree has been included, the likelihood of survival by conservative clinical management is extremely remote, and consequently such patients are candidates for cardiopulmonary bypass and embolectomy. Such procedures are far more successful today than when they were originally suggested by Trendelenburg in 1908. The first successful embolectomy was performed by Kirschner in 1924, and the effective use of the operation awaited the introduction of cardiopulmonary bypass before achieving its present-day survival of approximately 50 per cent.

Either emergency pulmonary arteriogram or radioactive scanning of the chest will confirm the presence of pulmonary embolus, while the EKG will show only right heart strain. The diagnosis can be accurately determined by evaluating the signs of right ventricular failure, namely:

1. Circulatory collapse with sinus tachycardia, faint pulse, low blood pressure, and cyanosis of the extremities.
2. Elevation of central venous pressure as visible in the neck.
3. The presence of a right ventricular heart sound or gallop.

The management of smaller pulmonary emboli unassociated with hypotension and cyanosis is best accomplished by conservative medical measures. Recent advances in radioisotope pulmonary scanning as developed by Sabiston and Wagner have greatly improved the diagnostic accuracy of smaller emboli. Rapid anticoagulation with intravenous heparin followed by the continued use of oral anticoagulants will prevent further intravascular clotting and will control further embolization in most of the cases. Broad-spectrum antibiotics are useful in preventing secondary pulmonary disease, and digitalization is indicated in the presence of cardiac failure. Oxygen and vasopresors may be required in more severe cases. Our own preference of metaraminol (Aramine) (100 mg. in 500 cc. of glucose or saline) is based on its known inotropic effect of improving coronary perfusion and myocardial function. The use of intravenous aminophylline, 250 to 500 mg., is of assistance in improving dyspnea.

Vena caval ligation has been reserved for those cases in which recurrent pulmonary emboli have followed adequate anticoagulation. It has also been useful in conditions in which anticoagulation is contraindicated.

While Collins and others have recommended immediate vena caval ligation for pulmonary embolism from femoral or pelvic thrombophlebitis, our own experience would agree with that of Gurewich, Sasahara and Stein, who have shown that such operations are not absolute protection against the development of further pulmonary embolism. In general, vena caval ligation has replaced bilateral femoral or iliac vein ligation.

To date there are 6 reported cases in the American literature of vena caval ligation during pregnancy for pelvic thrombophlebitis and recurrent emboli with a successful outcome of the pregnancy and a live-born infant. The major complication of this procedure during pregnancy is premature separation of the placenta and intra-uterine hypoxia with resultant fetal death in utero.

Prognosis

Approximately one third of all patients experiencing an acute pulmonary embolus will die as a result of the initial embolic episode. However, the death rate is increased with subsequent embolic incidents. These facts necessitate early diagnosis of embolic disease with rapid anticoagulation and medical treatment. The fact that many cases of fatal pulmonary emboli are preceded by clinically detectable symptoms and signs should decrease the mortality rate of this complication if thromboembolic disease is recognized as a potential entity in all patients undergoing pelvic surgery. The success in treatment of this complication is directly related to the early diagnosis of the small nonfatal lesion. However, the major effort of all pelvic surgeons should be directed toward effective methods of preventing venous thrombosis and its lethal embolic sequelae.

BIBLIOGRAPHY

Shock

Berdjis, C. C., and Vick, J. A.: Endotoxin and traumatic shock. J.A.M.A., 204:191, 1968.

Blalock, A.: Acute circulatory failure as exemplified by shock and hemorrhage. Surg. Gynec. Obstet., 58:551, 1934.

——: Consideration of present status of shock problem: Problems on shocks. Surgery, 14:487, 1943.

——: Gordon Wilson lecture: Shock or peripheral circulatory failure. Trans. Amer. Clin. Climatol. Assoc., 57:2, (1941), 1942.

Brooks, D. K., Williams, W. G., Manley, R. W., and Whiteman, P.: Osmolar and electrolyte changes in hemorrhagic shock. Lancet, 1:521, 1963.

Burchell, R. C., and Olson, G.: Internal iliac ligation: aortograms. Amer. J. Obstet. Gynec., 94:117, 1966.

Carey, L.: Personal communication, 1968.

Cohn, J. N.: Central venous pressure as a guide to volume expansion. Ann. Intern. Med., 66:1283, 1967.

Collins, V. J., Jaffe, R., and Zahony, I. Shock: a different approach to therapy. Illinois Med. J., 122:350, 1962.

Elliot, W. C., and Gorlin, R.: Isoproterenol in the treatment of heart disease. J.A.M.A., 197:315, 1966.

Fine, J.: Intestinal circulation in shock. Gastroenterology, 52:454, 1967.

Gordon, M., and Horowitz, A.: Septic shock following vaginal hysterectomy. Obstet. Gynec., 31:208, 1968.

Gowdey, C. W., Kilborn, R. M., and Stevenson, J. A. F.: Treatment of hemorrhagic shock in the dog with chlorpromazine and/or hypothermia. Canad. J. Biochem. Physiol., 35:1241, 1957.

Hamit, H. F.: Current trends of therapy and research in shock. Surg. Gynec. Obstet., 120:835, 1965.

Hardaway, R. M., James, P. M., Jr., Anderson, R. W., Bredenberg, C. E., and West, R. L.: Intensive study and treatment of shock in man. J.A.M.A., *199*:779, 1967.

Hemady, K. T., Hopkins, R. W., and Simeone, F. A.: Effect of vasopressors on renal functions in acute oligemia. Surg. Forum, *12*:85, 1961.

Jacobson, E. D.: A physiologic approach to shock. New Eng. J. Med., *278*:834, 1968.

Kardos, G. G.: Isoproterenol in the treatment of shock due to gram negative pathogens. New Eng. J. Med., *274*:868, 1966.

Lepley, D., Jr., Weisfeldt, M., Close, A. S., Schmidt, R., Bowler, J., Kory, R. C., and Ellison, E. H.: Effect of low molecular weight dextran on hemorrhagic shock. Surgery, *54*:93, 1963.

Longerbeam, J. K., Lillehei, R. C., and Scott, W. R.: The nature of irreversible shock; a hemodynamic study. Surg. Forum, *12*:1, 1962.

MacLean, L. D., Duff, J. H., Scott, H. M., and Peretz, D. I.: Treatment of shock in man based on hemodynamic diagnosis. Surg. Gynec. Obstet., *120*:1, 1965.

MacLean, L. D., Mulligan, W. G., McLean A. P. H., and Duff, J. H.: Patterns of septic shock in man—a detailed study of 56 patients. Ann. Surg., *166*:543, 1967.

Moncrief, J. A., Darin, J. C., Canizaro, P. C., and Sawyer, R. V.: Use of dextran to prevent arterial and venous thrombosis. Ann. Surg., *158*:553, 1963.

Nassif, A. C., Nolan, T. R., and Corcoran, A.C.: Angiotensin II in treatment of hypotensive states. J.A.M.A., *183*:751, 1963.

Nickerson, M.: Drug therapy of shock. *In* Bock, K. D. (ed.): Shock; Pathogenesis and Therapy, an International Symposium, Stockholm, June 27-30, 1961, sponsored by Ciba Foundation. p. 356. Berlin, Springer, 1962.

Ratliff, A. H. C.: Low-molecular weight dextran (Rheomacrodex) in the treatment of severe vascular insufficiencies after trauma. Lancet, *1*:1188, 1963.

Siegel, J. H., and Fabian, M.: Therapeutic advantages of an inotropic vasodilator in endotoxic shock. J.A.M.A., *200*:696, 1967.

Spink, W. W.: Endotoxin shock. Ann. Intern. Med., *57*:538, 1962.

——: The pathogenesis and management of shock due to infection. Arch. Intern. Med., *106*:433, 1960.

Weil, M. H., Shubin, H., and Biddle, M.: Shock caused by gram negative microorganisms; analysis of 169 cases. Ann. Intern. Med., *60*:384, 1964.

Wiggers, H. C., Ingraham, R. C., Roemhild, F., and Goldberg, H.: Vasoconstriction and the development of irreversible hemorrhagic shock. Amer. J. Physiol., *153*:511, 1948.

Wilson, J. N.: The management of acute circulatory failure. Surg. Clin. N. Amer., *43*:469, 1963.

Wilson, J. N., Prevedel, A. E., Demong, C. V., Grow, J. B., Sr., and Dalkowitz, T.: Use and abuse of vasopressor therapy. Amer. Surg., *29*:374, 1963.

Pulmonary Complications

Modell, J. H., and Moya, F.: Postoperative pulmonary complications: incidence and management. Anesth. Analg., *45*:432, 1966.

Palmer, K. N. V.: Postoperative pulmonary complications: postoperative bronchopneumonia. Brit. J. Surg., *54*(Suppl.):479, 1967.

Palmer, K. N. V., Gardiner, A. J. S., and McGregor, M. H.: Hypoxaemia after partial gastrectomy. Thorax, *20*:73, 1965.

Stein, M., Koota, G. M., Simon, M., and Frank, H. A.: Pulmonary evaluation of surgical patients. J.A.M.A., *181*:765, 1962.

Central Venous Pressure and Urinary Tract Infections

Aubaniac, R.: L'injection intraveineuse sousclaviculaire: advantages et technique. Presse Med., *60*:1456, 1952.

Barr, W., and Paterson, M. L.: Urinary infection after colporrhaphy and its effect on subsequent bladder symptomatology. J. Obstet. Gynaec. Brit. Comm., *69*:110, 1962.

Barron, J.: Technique and apparatus for bladder irrigation. Henry Ford Hosp. Med. Bull., *11*:443, 1963.

Corwin, J. H., and Mosely, T.: Sub-clavian venipuncture and central venous pressure technique and application. Amer. Surg., *32*:413, 1966.

Donald, I., Barr, W., and McGarry, J. A.: Postoperative care and complications of repair operations for prolapse. J. Obstet. Gynaec. Brit. Comm., *69*:837, 1962

Everett, H. S.: Gynecological and Obstetrical Urology. Baltimore, Williams & Wilkins, 1944.

Everett, H. S., and Long, J. H.: The treatment of urinary infection. Amer. J. Obstet. Gynec., *67*:916, 1954.

Hannah, W. J.: Prevention of urinary tract infection after vaginal surgery. Canad. Med. Assoc. J., *88*:803, 1963.

Hodgkinson, C. P., and Hodari, A. A.: Trocar suprapubic cystostomy for postoperative bladder drainage in the female. Amer. J. Obstet. Gynec., 96:773, 1966.

Johnson, H. D.: Venous pressure: its physiology and pathology and hemorrhage shock and transfusion. Brit. J. Surg., 51:276, 1964.

Kass, E. H., and Sossen, H. S.: Prevention of infection of urinary tract in presence of indwelling catheters. J.A.M.A., 169:1181, 1959.

Linton, K. B., Gillespie, W. A.: Causes and prevention of postoperative urinary infection in female patients, J. Obstet. Gynaec. Brit. Comm., 69:845, 1962.

Longerbeam, J. K., Vannix, R., Wagner, W., and Joergenson, E.: Central venous pressure monitoring. Amer. J. Surg., 110:220, 1965.

Martin, C. M., and Bookrajian, E. N.: Bacteriuria prevention after indwelling urinary catheterization. Arch. Intern. Med., 110:703, 1962.

Mattingly, R. F.: In discussion of Hodgkinson, C. P., and Hodari, A. A. (above).

Matz, R.: Complications of determining the central venous pressure. New Eng. J. Med., 273:703, 1965.

Maudsley, R. F., and Robertson, E. M.: Common complications of hysterectomy. Canad. Med. Assoc. J., 92:908, 1965.

Prout, W. G.: Relative value of central venous pressure monitoring and blood volume measurement in the management of shock. Lancet, 1:1108, 1968.

Puyo Villafane, E. P.: Tecnica de la transfusion por via clavicular. Prensa Med. Argent., 40:2379, 1953.

Taussig, F. J.: Bladder function after confinement and after gynecological operations. Trans. Amer. Gynec. Soc., 40:351, 1915.

Williams, T. J., and Julian, C. G.: Tidal drainage in the postoperative bladder. Amer. J. Obstet. Gynec., 83:1313, 1962.

Wilson, J. N., Grow, J. B., Demong, C. V., Prevedel, A. E., and Owens, J. C.: Central venous pressure in optimal blood volume maintenance. Arch. Surg., 85:563, 1962.

Woodruff, J. D., and Te Linde, R. W.: The postoperative care of the urinary bladder. J.A.M.A., 113:1451, 1939.

Venous Thrombosis and Pulmonary Embolism

Allison, P. R., Dunnhill, M. S., and Marshall, R.: Pulmonary embolism, Thorax, 15:273, 1960.

Aschoff, L.: Vortrage Über Pathologie. XI. Über Thrombse. pp. 230-252, Jena, Fischer, 1925.

Browse, N. L.: Effective surgery on resting calf blood flow. Brit. Med. J., 1:1721, 1962.

Calnan, J. S., Kountz, S., Pentecost, B. L., Shillingford, J. P., and Steiner, R. E.: Venous obstruction in the aetiology of lymphoedema praecox. Brit. Med. J., 2:221, 1964.

Collins, C. G., Weinstein, B. B., Norton, R. O., and Webster, H. D.: The effects of ligation of the inferior vena cava and ovarian vessels on ovulation and pregnancy in the human being. Amer. J. Obstet. Gynec., 63:351, 1952.

Cooley, D. A., and Beal, A. C., Jr.: Embolectomy for acute massive pulmonary embolism. Surg. Gynec. Obstet., 126:805, 1968.

Cooley, D. A., Beal, A. C., Jr., and Alexander, J. K.: Acute massive pulmonary embolism: successful surgical treatment using temporary cardiopulmonary bypass. J.A.M.A., 177:283, 1961.

Crafoord, C., and Jorpes, E.: Heparin as a prophylactic against thrombosis. J.A.M.A., 116:2831, 1941.

Davidson, C. S., and MacDonald, H.: A critical study of the action of 3-3'-methylenebis (4-hydroxycoumarin) (Dicoumarin). Amer. J. Med. Sci., 205:24, 1943.

Emmons, P. R., and Mitchell, J. R. A.: Postoperative changes in platelet-clumping activity. Lancet, 1:71, 1965.

Freiman, D. G., Sasahara, A. A., and Stein, M.: Pulmonary embolic disease. In Sasahara, A. A., and Stein, M. (eds.): Symposium on Pulmonary Embolic Disease. p. 81. New York, Grune & Stratton, 1965.

Fuller, C. H., Robertson, C. W., and Smithwick, R. H.: Management of thromboembolic disease. New Eng. J. Med., 263:983, 1960.

Gibbs, N. M.: Venous thrombosis of the lower limbs with particular reference to bed rest. Brit. J. Surg., 45:209, 1957.

Gorham, L. W.: A study of pulmonary embolism. Arch. Int. Med., 108:48, 1961.

Gurewich, Z.: Pulmonary embolic disease. In Sasahara, A. A., and Stein, M. (eds.): Symposium on Pulmonary Embolic Disease. p. 162. New York, Grune & Stratton, 1965.

Haller, J. A., Jr.: Thrombectomy for acute ileofemoral venous thrombosis. Arch. Surg., 83:448, 1961.

Haller, J. A., Jr., Wagner, H. N., and Jackson, D. P.: Conjoint clinic on thrombophlebitis. J. Chronic Dis., 19:785, 1966.

Hampton, H. H., and Wharton, L. R.: Venous thrombosis, pulmonary infarction and embolism following gynecological operations. Bull. Johns Hopkins Hosp., 31:95, 1920.

Hanlon, C. R.: Ileofemoral venous thrombec-

tomy. Surg. Gynec. Obstet., 122:833, 1966.
Henry, G. A.: Bronchoscopy in the management of massive collapse. Canad. Med. Assoc. J., 49:305, 1943.
Homans, J.: Thrombophlebitis of the lower extremities. Ann. Surg., 87:641, 1928.
———: Exploration and division of the femoral and iliac veins in the treatment of thrombophlebitis of the leg. New Eng. J. Med., 224:179, 1941.
Jeffcoate, T. N. A., and Tindall, V. R.: Venous thrombosis and embolism in obstetrics and gynecology. Aust. New Zeal. J. Obstet. Gynaec., 5:119, 1965.
Kirschner, M.: Embolectomy of pulmonary artery. Arch. klin. Chir., 133:312, 1924.
———: Ein durch die Trendelenburgische operation geheilter fallen von emboli der art. pulmonalis. Arch. klin. Chir., 133:312, 1924.
Leriche, R., and Kunlin, J.: Traitement immédiat des phlebites post-opératoires par l'infiltration novocainique du sympathique lombaire. Presse Med., 42:1481, 1934.
Lowenberg, E. L.: Femoral vein ligation in the treatment of pulmonary embolism due to femoral thrombophlebitis. Virginia Med. Monthly, 71:288, 1944.
Lowenberg, R. I.: Early diagnosis of phlebothrombosis with aid of a new clinical test. J.A.M.A., 155:1566, 1954.
McLachlin, A. D., McLachlin, J. A., Jory, T. A., and Rawlings, E. G.: Venostasis in the lower extremities. Ann. Surg., 152:678, 1960.
Meyerowitz, B. R.: Pulmonary embolism in surgical patients; is embolectomy superior to prophylaxis? Surgery, 60:521, 1966.
———: Venous thrombosis in surgical patients. Amer. J. Surg., 113:520, 1967.
Ochsner, A., and DeBakey, M.: Treatment of thrombophlebitis by novocaine block of sympathetics. Surgery, 5:491, 1939.
Paneth, M.: The treatment of pulmonary embolism. Brit. J. Surg., 54:468, 1967.
Pizarro, A. R., and Roth, O.: Inferior vena cava ligation in early pregnancy. Amer. J. Obstet. Gynec., 101:265, May 1968.
Poole, J. C. F.: The pathogenesis of venous thrombosis. Brit. J. Surg., 54:463, 1967.
Roberts, G. H.: Venous thrombosis in hospital patients; a post mortem study. Scot. Med. J., 8:11, 1963.
Rossi, N., Lawrence, M. S., and Ehrenhaft, J. L.: Surgical treatment of massive ileofemoral venous thrombosis. Amer. J. Surg., 113:533, 1967.
Rubin, H.: Ligation of the inferior vena cava in early pregnancy. Amer. J. Obstet. Gynec., 80:542, 1960.
Sabiston, D. C., Jr., and Wagner, H. N., Jr.: The diagnosis of pulmonary embolism by radioisotope scanning. Ann. Surg., 160:575, 1964.
Salzman, E. W., Harris, W. H., and de Santis, R. W.: Anticoagulation for prevention of thromboembolism following fractures of the hip. New Eng. J. Med., 275:122, 1966.
Sautter, R. D., Fletcher, F. W., and Lewis, R. F.: Inferior vena caval and ovarian vein ligation for antepartum pulmonary thromboembolism. J.A.M.A., 196:290, 1966.
Sevitt, S.: Anticoagulant prophylaxis against venous thrombosis and pulmonary embolism after injury. In Koller, R., Duckert, F., and Strueli, F. (eds.): Pathogenesis and Treatment of Thromboembolic Diseases. Stuttgart, F. K. Schattauer-Verlag, 1966.
Sevitt, S., and Gallagher, N. C.: Prevention of venous thrombosis and pulmonary embolism in injured patients. Lancet, 2:981, 1959.
Sharnoff, J. G.: Results in the prophylaxis of postoperative thromboembolism. Surg. Gynec. Obstet., 123:303, 1966.
Sharnoff, J. G., Bagg, J. F., Breen, S. R., Rogliano, A. G., Walsh, A. R., and Scardino, V.: The possible indication of postoperative thromboembolism by platelet counts and blood coagulation studies in the patient undergoing extensive surgery. Surg. Gynec. Obstet., 111:469, 1960.
Sharnoff, J. G., and Rosenberg, M.: Effects of age and immobilisation on the incidence of postpartum thromboembolism. Lancet, 1:845, 1964.
Sharp, E. H.: Pulmonary embolectomy: successful removal of a massive pulmonary embolus with support of cardiopulmonary bypass: case report. Ann. Surg., 156:1, 1962.
Stone, S. R., Whalley, P. J., and Pritchard, J. A.: Inferior vena cava and ovarian vein ligation during late pregnancy. Obstet. Gynec., 32:267, 1968.
Thromboembolic Phenomena in Women. Proceedings of a Conference at the A.M.A. headquarters, Chicago, on September 10, 1962, sponsored by G. D. Searle & Co. Chicago, G. D. Searle & Co., 1962.
Trendelenburg, F.: Ueber bie operative behaudlung der emboli der lungenarterie, Arch. klin. Chir., 86:686, 1908.
———: Zur operation der embolie der lungenarterien, Zbl. Chir., 35:92, 1908.
Virchow, R.: Gesammelte Abhandlungen zur. wissenschaftlichen Medicin. p. 219. Frankfurt, Meidinger Sohn, 1856.
———: Handb. spec. Pathol. u. Therapie. Bd. I, s. 1958. Erlangen, Enke, 1854.
Young, R. L., and Derbyshire, R. C.: Ligation of the inferior vena cava during pregnancy. Ann. Surg., 131:252, 1950.

5

Fluid and Electrolyte Balance

EDWARD J. LENNON, M.D.,[*] AND JACOB LEMANN, JR., M.D.[†]

INTRODUCTION

The body composition of healthy adults remains remarkably constant from day to day. Water, nitrogen, and minerals ingested in the diet are quantitatively excreted. Energy arising from the catabolism of foodstuffs is quantitatively expended. In health, mechanisms are operative which lead to adjustments of both intake (hunger, thirst) and excretion (antidiuretic hormone, aldosterone, etc.). During illnesses or after surgical operations, oral intake may be curtailed or eliminated, abnormal losses of water and minerals may occur, and the control mechanisms regulating excretion may be impaired. The parenteral administration of water and electrolytes is intended to compensate for these abnormalities.

An orderly approach to the repair of disorders of fluid and electrolyte metabolism requires that three questions be answered:

1. What quantities of calories, water, and electrolytes would the patient require each day in health?
2. How should these estimates be adjusted to take into account the effects of the patient's illness or operation?
3. What deficits had already been incurred when the patient first presented for care?

The answers to these questions permit a reasonable estimate of parenteral fluid requirements. The correctness of the estimate can then be evaluated during therapy by relatively simple bedside and laboratory observations, and appropriate adjustments can be made.

Those units of measurement employed in the biochemical laboratory which are indispensable to an understanding of these topics are defined in the Appendix to the chapter.

CALORIC REQUIREMENTS

The degradative metabolism of dietary protein, carbohydrate, and fat yields both mechanical and heat energy necessary for the maintenance of life. Energy requirements vary with body size, state of nutrition, activity, catabolic stimuli (fever, trauma, etc.), and hormonal influences, and are obviously increased during growth, pregnancy, and lactation.

Considerable variations in prior nutritional status as well as activities and stresses in hospital are to be expected from patient to patient. Table 5-1 provides a generous but safe estimate of caloric expenditure based on body weight.

TABLE 5-1. ESTIMATED CALORIC EXPENDITURE BASED ON BODY WEIGHT

BODY WEIGHT, KG.	CALORIES/KG./DAY
60 and over	35
40–59	40
25–39	50

---

[*] Professor of Medicine, Marquette School of Medicine, and Chief of Renal Service, Milwaukee County General Hospital.
[†] Associate Professor of Medicine and Chief of Renal Section of the Department of Medicine, Boston University School of Medicine.

For patients who are significantly obese, caloric expenditure should be calculated from ideal rather than actual body weight. A nonobese 60-kg. woman would thus be estimated to expend 60 kg. × 35 cal./kg. or 2,100 calories per day in the hospital in the absence of fever or other abnormal stresses. Smaller individuals expend larger number of calories/kg./day. The special problems of small children and infants are beyond the scope of this chapter.

With fever, the estimate of caloric expenditure should be increased by 10 per cent for each degree Fahrenheit above 99°. Thus, if the 60-kg. woman considered above developed an infection, and her rectal temperature rose to 103° F., she would increase her caloric expenditure by 40 per cent to a total of 2,100 + .40(2,100) or 2,940 calories/day. The impact of other influences on caloric expenditure cannot be predicted accurately. Careful clinical observation of body weight, subcutaneous fat stores, and muscle mass will dictate adjustments in the provision of caloric needs.

It is seldom possible to satisfy caloric needs completely with parenteral fluids. Over relatively short periods, and in the absence of massive catabolic stimuli (such as occurs with severe burns or sepsis), this is unimportant. Body tissue stores can easily make up short-term caloric deficits. The rate of breakdown of tissue protein and fat can be minimized by providing 150 to 200 gm. of carbohydrate per day. Long-term parenteral nutrition is never satisfactory, but the addition of protein hydrolysates and fat emulsions may be of help. When a patient is unable to eat for protracted periods, it is far preferable when possible to initiate feeding via gastric tube, gastrostomy or jejunostomy.

WATER

Normal Body Content and Distribution

The water content of the body accounts for 50 to 70 per cent of the total body weight. Since fat cells contain relatively little water, the per cent of body weight attributable to water is lowest in obese individuals and highest in lean, muscular individuals.

Water diffuses freely across cell membranes and is distributed passively throughout the body in response to osmotic forces. The content of osmotically active particles within cells and outside of cells determines the relative volumes of the intra- and extracellular fluid compartments. Living cells actively extrude sodium (Na) and accumulate potassium (K). Potassium and its accompanying (chiefly organic) anions comprise the major quantity of osmotically active particles within cells, while Na and its accompanying anions (principally chloride and bicarbonate) comprise the major quantity of osmotically active particles in the extracellular fluids (ECF).

A 60-kg. woman would be estimated to contain 33 liters of water (55% of body weight). Because the total quantity of K in solution within cells exceeds the total quantity of Na in solution in ECF, about two thirds of the total body water is intracellular (22 liters), while the remaining one third is extracellular (11 liters). About one fifth of the ECF volume is confined to the vascular tree by the oncotic pressure of the plasma proteins, contributed chiefly by albumin.

If water alone is lost from or added to the body, the losses or gains are distributed between cells and ECF in the same 2 to 1 ratio. If, on the other hand, Na or K salts alone are lost from or added to the body, the relative volumes of water within cells and ECF are altered by passive shifts of water. For example, if NaCl were added to the body, the concentration of Na and Cl ions would increase in the ECF, increasing the osmotic pressure in this compartment. Water would then diffuse passively from cells to ECF until osmotic equilibrium across the cell membranes was again restored. At equilibrium the volume of the ECF compartment would be expanded at the expense of an identical reduction in the volume of cell water. The concentrations of Na in ECF and K in cell water would be identically increased. Note that although all of the added Na would remain in the extracellular compartment, the increase in the concentration of Na in the ECF at equilibrium would be predicted by dividing the quantity of Na added by total body water volume. Clearly, the reason is that water is free to diffuse between compartments in response to the transient osmotic gradient created.

WATER TURNOVER

In health, some 6 per cent of the total body water content is eliminated and replaced each day. As will be discussed below, physiologic mechanisms exist to minimize water losses during water deprivation. However, significant obligatory losses of water occur each day in urine formation, by evaporation from the skin and lungs, and in the feces. These obligatory losses may be increased and additional routes of water loss created during illness. Since a 20 per cent reduction in total body water content may be lethal, it is clear that these losses must be replaced.

Urinary Water Losses. Some 150 liters of fluid are filtered through the glomeruli of the kidneys each day in the adult. The majority of this filtrate, containing all needed minerals and useful organic compounds (glucose, amino acids, etc.), is reabsorbed by the tubules. Since the kidneys defend both the volume and osmolarity of the body fluids, the final volume of urine excreted will reflect (1) the need to expand or reduce the volume of body fluids, (2) the need to conserve or excrete solute, and (3) the ability of the kidney to concentrate osmotically active waste particles. The minimum urine volume required to maintain constant body composition is a function of the solute load requiring excretion and the renal concentrating capacity. All end products of metabolism (urea, uric acid, etc.) and any quantities of ingested minerals (Na, K, Cl, etc.) not excreted in the stools or lost in dermal secretions must be eliminated in the urine. The composition of the diet determines the magnitude of the solute load requiring renal excretion. The number of biologically nondegradable waste particles generated during metabolism depends chiefly on the diet protein content. Each gram of protein in natural foods yields on metabolism approximately 8 milliosmoles of solute (as urea, K, phosphorus, etc.). Normal North American diets yield about 0.35 milliosmoles of urinary solute per calorie of caloric intake. Patients receiving only maintenance parenteral fluids usually have urinary solute contents in the range of 0.2 milliosmoles per calorie of caloric expenditure.

When urinary water losses need to be minimized, the solute particles to be excreted must exist in the final urine at higher concentration (i.e., in a lesser volume of water) than was present in the glomerular filtrate. The ability to concentrate the urine is frequently impaired in patients who are ill, elderly, or who have specific acute or chronic renal diseases. The kidneys of healthy young adults can vary the concentration of the urine from 50 to 1,200 milliosmoles per liter. Since the normal osmolarity of the serum is approximately 285 milliosmoles per liter (range 275-295), final urine solute concentration can be about fivefold increased or decreased from that of the serum, thus allowing the excretion of water excesses and water conservation.

Table 5-2 compares the urinary water needs of a 60-kg. woman in hospital when receiving a normal diet and when receiving only maintenance intravenous fluids, under circumstances in which final urine concentration is maximal (1,200 mosm./L.) or estimated at a more reasonable value for an ill patient (600 mosm./L.). Her caloric expenditure would be estimated as 60 kg. × 35 cal./kg. or 2,100 calories. If she ingested a normal diet providing 2,100 calories per day, the estimated solute load requiring renal excretion would be 2,100 cal. × 0.35 mosm./cal. or 735 milliosmoles per day. At a urine concentration of 1,200 mosm./L., this would require about 600 milliliters of water, while at a more realistic concentration of 600 mosm./L., about 1,200 ml. of water would be required. If she received only maintenance intravenous fluids providing 0.2 mosm. of waste solute per calorie, her solute load

TABLE 5-2. EFFECT OF SOLUTE LOAD AND URINE
CONCENTRATION ON RENAL WATER LOSSES

SOLUTE LOAD	ML. URINE REQUIRED AT CONCENTRATION OF	
	1200 mosm./L.	600 mosm./L.
Normal diet = 735 mosm.	612	1,224
Maintenance I.V. fluids = 420 mosm.	350	700

would be 420 mosm. and could be excreted in 350 ml. of urine at 1200 mosm./L., or 700 ml. of urine at a safer estimate of 600 mosm./L. If the patient had renal disease and could not achieve a urine concentration greater than that of the glomerular filtrate (285 mosm./L.), still larger urine volumes would be required. Obligatory urinary water losses would also be increased if abnormal solute loads had to be excreted, as, for example, during diabetic ketoacidosis (glucose and organic acids) or with high protein intake.

Water Losses From the Skin and Lungs. The loss of water by evaporation from the surfaces of the skin and lungs ("insensible" water loss) is an obligatory mechanism in the regulation of body temperature. Under conditions of minimal activity in hospital, virtually all of the energy produced each day from metabolism appears as heat. Approximately 70 per cent of the heat generated is dissipated by radiation to cooler objects in the environment. A small amount of heat is lost with the excreta (no more than 5%). The remaining heat energy (25% or more of the total) is eliminated by evaporating water from the moist surfaces of the skin and lungs. At normal body temperature, 0.6 calorie is consumed in the evaporation of one milliliter of water.

Let us consider again a 60-kg. female in hospital with an estimated caloric expenditure of 2,100 calories; about 25 per cent of this heat energy (or 520 calories) would be eliminated by evaporating water from lungs and skin. This would obligate the loss of 520/0.6 or about 870 milliliters of water.

With fever, evaporative water losses increase by about 10 per cent for each degree Fahrenheit above normal body temperature. Hyperventilation increases water losses from the lungs. Doubling the respiratory rate increases total insensible water losses by 50 per cent or more. In a hot environment less heat can be dissipated by radiation, and evaporative water loss will rise. Overt sweating constitutes a partial failure of the contribution of water evaporation to heat regulation (i.e., water is secreted to the surface of the skin faster than it can be evaporated) and may result in the loss of liters of water per day. The exposure of additional moist or denuded areas will also increase evaporative water losses. For example, 2 or 3 liters of water may be lost by evaporation from the exposed peritoneal contents during a prolonged operation.

Gastrointestinal Water Losses. The gastrointestinal tract normally absorbs not only ingested fluids, but also substantial quantities of fluid secreted into upper segments of the alimentary tract. In health, this includes some 800 ml. of saliva, 1,200 ml. of gastric juice, 800 ml. of bile, 1,000 ml. of pancreatic juice, and 1,500 ml. of small intestinal secretions, for a total of about 5 liters. With normal formed stools, only about 150 ml. of water is lost each day in the feces, an indication of the efficiency of water reabsorption by the colon. With vomiting, gastric suction, or diarrhea, the secretions of the gut, as well as ingested fluids, are lost. With intestinal inflammation, the secretions of the gut may be increased. Thus in bacterial diarrheas (such as cholera), 10 or more liters of stool water may be lost daily.

Endogenous Water Production. A small quantity of water arises *de novo* during metabolism each day when dietary hydrogen atoms are combined with oxygen. This amounts to approximately 0.1 ml. per calorie of caloric expenditure, or some 210 milliliters per day for a 60-kg. woman.

Summary of Normal Water Turnover. Figure 5-1 depicts the approximate values for the components of normal daily water turnover which might be expected in a 60-kg. woman in hospital eating a calorically adequate diet and expending 2,100 calories per day. Such a patient would lose 150 ml. of water per day in formed stools. With a diet of normal composition, she would produce 730 mosm. of solute, which could be excreted in 1,200 ml. of urine at a concentration of 600 mosm./L. About 25 per cent of her caloric energy would be dissipated by evaporating water from the skin and lungs, with the loss of 900 ml. of water. Some 210 ml. of water would be formed *de novo* during metabolism. Thus her total water losses would equal 2,040 ml. The provision of an intake of 1 ml. of water per calorie of caloric expenditure would thus meet her water needs. With normal diets, some 1,000 ml. would be contained in the foods provided and only 1,100 ml. would be ingested as water *per se* or other liquid beverages. Although the solute load requiring renal excretion would be reduced if the patient were receiving only maintenance I.V. fluids, the provision of 1 ml. of water per calorie of caloric expenditure in this situation would place even less strain on the renal concentrating mechanism (i.e., it would allow elimination of the solute load at a concentration of 300 mosm./L.) and thus allow flexibility if other minor fluid losses should occur.

HORMONAL REGULATION OF BODY WATER LOSSES

Evaporative losses of water are obligatory, and, in health, the quantities of water formed endogenously and lost in the feces are too small to have an important impact on overall water balance. Variations in the amount of water excreted by the kidneys thus constitute the major adjustment to varying water intake.

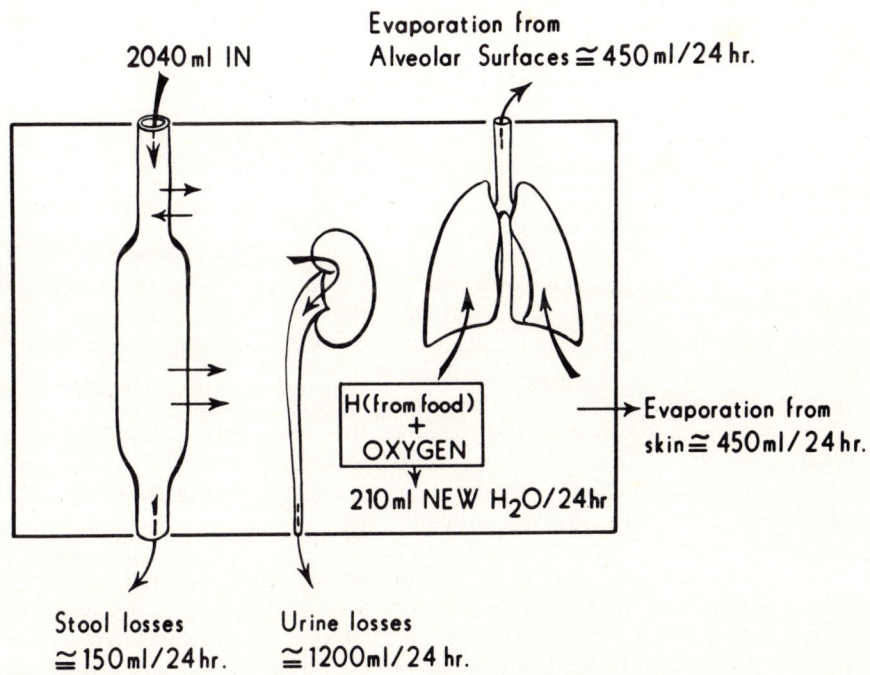

FIG. 5-1. Normal daily water turnover (60-kg. female).

Variations in the rate of secretion of antidiuretic hormone (ADH) regulate urinary water losses. A sensing system located in cells in the hypothalamus monitors the osmolarity of the ECF. A 2 per cent increase in osmolarity is sufficient to cause increased release of ADH from the posterior pituitary gland. The fundamental action of ADH is to increase the permeability of the cells of the renal collecting ducts to water. The collecting ducts traverse the renal medulla, where water is reabsorbed passively from the urine into the hyperosmotic medullary interstitial fluids. Increasing the permeability of the collecting ducts increases water reabsorption, thus again lowering ECF osmolarity to normal and restoring ADH secretion to basal levels.

ADH release is also regulated by a volume-sensitive system monitored by stretch receptors in the atria of the heart. When ECF volume falls by 15 per cent or more, ADH secretion increases regardless of the osmolarity of body fluids, and renal water reabsorption is increased in the defense of body fluid volume. Thus, the urine may be "paradoxically" concentrated despite body fluid hypo-osmolarity in volume-depleted patients who are given only water. In such patients, volume depletion will be obvious on clinical examination, and the urinary Na concentration will be low (less than 20 mEq./L.), since aldosterone secretion is also activated by volume depletion (see below).

The maximum achievable urine concentration is reduced below that of normal subjects in all forms of chronic renal disease. This must be considered in planning fluid therapy for such patients.

Prompt elimination of a water load depends upon the inhibition of ADH secretion, as body fluids are made hypo-osmolar, and the excretion of a dilute urine. In order to make the final urine more dilute than the filtered plasma water, solute (chiefly sodium salts) must be reabsorbed without water in distal tubular segments. This function, too, is impaired in chronic renal diseases, as well as in situations in which less than the normal amount of glomerular filtrate is delivered to the distal tubules (as with congestive heart failure or hepatic cirrhosis), or when tubular Na reabsorption is impaired (adrenal insufficiency). In such circumstances the administration of excessive amounts of water will lead to pronounced dilution of body fluids, neuromuscular irritability, convulsions, and even death (so-called "water intoxication").

Manifestations and Therapy of Water Deficits

If water intake is inadequate to meet obligatory water losses, the total body water content will fall. Any losses of water without solute will be identified by a rise in the osmolarity of the body fluids, reflected in an increase in the serum Na concentration. If the concentration of Na (and its anions) in the ECF is increased by 20 mEq./L., this means that the concentration of K (and its anions) within cells has also increased by 20 mEq./L., since water diffuses freely between the two compartments. Thus the quantity of water required to lower serum Na concentration by 20 mEq./L. is that needed to lower the concentration of *both* Na in ECF and K in cell water by 20 mEq./L. For example, the quantity of water lost in excess of solute losses in a 60-kg. woman presenting with volume depletion and a serum Na concentration of 160 mEq./L. would be calculated as follows: Na concentration in the ECF is $\frac{160}{140}$ above normal. Potassium concentration within cells (although not measured) would be increased according to the same ratio. To correct this, her total body water content would have to be increased to $\frac{160}{140}$ of its present volume. On the assumption that there is an initial total body water of 30 liters (50% of body weight), it would be necessary to increase this to a value of $30 \times \frac{160}{140}$, or about 34 liters. Thus, water losses without solute would equal 34 − 30, or 4 liters. Clearly, losses of fluids having the same osmolarity as that of body fluids in general would not alter serum Na concentration.

The total water deficit will be indicated by an equivalent weight loss and the signs and symptoms of volume depletion (see section on Sodium). Sodium and K losses will also have occurred in almost all cases. The magnitude of the weight loss will accurately reflect the magnitude of the water losses, and knowledge of the patient's body weight shortly before the onset of illness and at the time of initiation of therapy provides the most reliable guide to the quantity of water which must be replaced. Body tissue losses seldom exceed 200 to 300 gm. per day if patients do not eat but are able to drink and retain water. Accurate daily (or more frequent) weighing provides the single most valuable guide in accessing the adequacy of the replacement of water needs. A good bed scale is the *sine qua non* of adequate fluid management in difficult cases.

One circumstance must be considered in translating weight changes to changing water needs. In addition to the water contained in cells and in the effective extracellular fluid volume, relatively unavailable "third spaces" may develop when fluid becomes sequestered in edematous, burned or crushed tissues, in the atonic gut, or in effusions or exudates within serous cavities. For example, in acute pancreatitis, the fluid trapped in the edematous retroperitoneal tissues, within the peritoneum, and in the lumen of the intestine accumulates at the expense of the effective extracellular fluid volume. This fluid must be replaced, and a weight gain is required to restore the volume of the effective extracellular fluids. When the pancreatitis subsides, the trapped fluid will again be mobilized and excreted, and weight loss is expected during the recovery phase.

The special problems of shock due to blood loss or sepsis are discussed elsewhere in the text. In the absence of these phenomena, patients with a clinical history indicating body fluid losses who have (1) diminished tissue turgor but (2) a good peripheral circulation and (3) can maintain a normal blood pressure when both supine and seated on the side of the bed with legs dangling, are apt to have water deficits of the order of 10 per cent of total body water or less (i.e., about 5% of total body weight or 50 ml. of water per kilogram of body weight). Patients who manifest, in addition, poor peripheral circulation and hypotension when either supine or with legs dangled, are apt to have body water deficits closer to 20 per cent of total body water (i.e., about 10% of body weight or 100 ml. per kilogram of body weight). Evaluation of blood pressure in a supine patient may be deceptive, since vasoconstrictor reflexes may maintain blood pressure despite significant volume depletion. Rechecking the blood pressure with the patient seated and challenged by gravitational force may unmask this. The numerical value of the blood pressure may also be misleading unless the patient's normal blood pressure is known; a patient with a normal blood pressure of 180/110 may be in frank shock with a blood pressure of 130/80.

A 60-kg. woman presenting with a history of several days of diarrhea and poor food and fluid intake, whose tissue turgor was diminished but blood pressure normal (for her) both lying and seated, would be estimated to have a water deficit of 60 kg. × 50 ml./kg. or 3 liters. If her disease had been more severe or persisted for a longer time, so that she now also had cool extremities and hypotension, her water deficit would be estimated to be 60 kg. × 100 ml./kg. or 6 liters. These estimates, while admittedly crude, are nonetheless serviceable, since only half of these estimated deficits (in addition to estimated basal needs and ongoing losses) would be administered in the first 12 to 24 hours of therapy. Thereafter, adjustments would be made on the basis of the patient's responses. When fluid losses of the order of 10 per cent of body weight are expected, and circulatory impairment is present, central venous pressure monitoring is mandatory. The measured level of central venous pressure before therapy is not of itself a guide or a contraindication to fluid administration. In the absence of other signs of congestive failure, an initial venous pressure of 15 or even 20 cm. of water need not contradict fluid administration to a patient with clear evidence of volume depletion. A *rise* in venous pressure above these levels as fluids are administered indicates either too rapid administration or a physiologic end point.

The cumulative errors of intake-output sheets in patients who may be losing fluid simultaneously from gastric suction, drains, diarrhea, and sweat, and have insensible losses difficult to estimate accurately because of fever and hyperpnea, are substantial indeed. We find changes in body weight, with allowance for "third spaces" and expected losses of tissue mass, a far safer guide to fluid administration. Approximate measures of fluid losses from the intestine are useful in estimating Na, K, and acid or base losses.

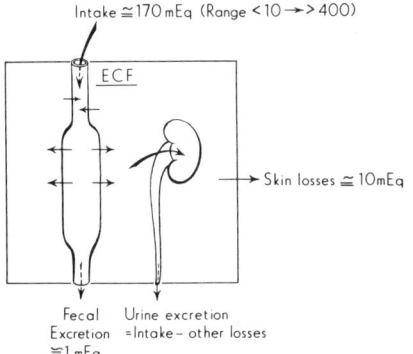

FIG. 5-2. Normal daily sodium turnover.

SODIUM

Body Content and Distribution

Total body Na averages about 60 mEq./kg. of body weight in adults or approximately 3,600 mEq. in a 60-kg. individual. Over one half of total body Na is present in the extracellular fluid, where normally it exists at a concentration of 140 mEq./L. and represents over 90 per cent of the total extracellular cations. Sodium, together with the major accompanying anions, Cl and bicarbonate, thus constitute the osmotic skeleton of the plasma and interstitial fluid. The remaining Na is contained chiefly in bone (30% of total body Na), with only small quantities present in other connective tissues and in cells.

Normal Sodium Turnover

The average American diet provides about 170 mEq. of Na per day, which is equivalent to about 10 gm. of NaCl, and thus about 4 per cent of the Na contained in a 60-kg. adult is turned over each day. Figure 5-2 diagrams normal daily Na turnover. Sodium is actively absorbed by the intestine, and normal formed stools contain less than 2 mEq. of Na per day. The intestine absorbs not only the Na ingested with the diet, but also the Na secreted into the gut in saliva, bile, gastric juice, etc. Skin losses of Na (in the absence of visible sweating) average only 5 to 10 mEq./day. In health, the quantity of Na ingested and not eliminated via the gut and skin is excreted in the urine. The kidneys thus regulate body Na stores and hence the volume of the ECF.

In the average adult about 150 liters of ECF containing 21,000 mEq. of Na are filtered each day through the glomeruli. Approximately 85 per cent of the filtered Na is actively reabsorbed in the proximal tubules. The proximal tubules are freely permeable to water. Thus, water follows passively, and the reabsorbed fluid has a Na concentration of about 140 mEq./L. The more distal tubular segments are less permeable to water, and additional quantities of Na are reabsorbed at these sites without water. Finally, Na is also reabsorbed in exchange for hydrogen or K ions in the distal tubules and collecting ducts by a transport process that is stimulated by aldosterone. Of the 21,000 mEq. of Na filtered through the glomeruli each day, more than 99 per cent is reabsorbed by these tubular transport mechanisms, and only about 150 mEq. of Na is excreted in the final urine by subjects eating usual diets. In contrast to water metabolism, in which substantial extrarenal losses occur in all circumstances, Na balance is maintained in health almost exclusively by adjustments of renal

diarrhea, losses of up to 160 mEq. of K daily have been observed. Osmotic diuresis, diuretic drugs, aldosterone or other steroids that stimulate tubular Na reabsorption in exchange for K, as well as some unusual kinds of intrinsic kidney disease, such as renal tubular acidosis, may result in abnormal urinary K losses.

Clinical Evaluation of Potassium Deficits or Surpluses

Evaluation of body stores of K are dependent primarily upon assessment of the clinical history and upon laboratory studies.

Potassium Deficits. Patients who have experienced marked anorexia, vomiting, diarrhea, osmotic diuresis, or prior diuretic drug therapy are apt to be K-depleted. Such patients often complain of muscular weakness or, rarely, if the deficiency of K is severe, of paralysis. Smooth muscle hypotonia with consequent constipation may also occur. Nocturia or frequency occasionally is noted, because K depletion impairs the renal capacity to concentrate the urine. Because the quantity of K contained in the ECF constitutes only about 2 per cent of the total body K in health, the concentration of K in plasma does not provide a precise estimate of body K stores. Furthermore, plasma K concentration may be low even when body K stores are normal. This may occur during metabolic alkalosis, when ECF potassium enters cells in exchange for hydrogen ions, or as a result of glucose metabolism when ECF potassium is taken into cells during glycogen deposition. Despite these limitations, measurements of serum K can provide a rough estimate of body K stores.

Serum K concentrations in the range of 3.0 to 3.4 mEq./L. suggest that body stores are reduced by about 4 to 5 mEq./kg., or approximately 300 mEq. in a 60-kg. individual. Serum K levels of less than 3 mEq./L. generally indicate deficits of 5 to 10 mEq. per kg. of body weight, or 300 to 600 mEq. in a 60-kg. patient. If K depletion has occurred because of extrarenal losses, urinary K excretion is usually less than 15 mEq./day.

Potassium Surplus. Potassium excess is most likely to occur in patients with oliguria due to acute renal failure, who have a continuing dietary K intake or accelerated rates of tissue breakdown, causing release of K into the ECF. These patients may complain of paresthesias, weakness, and even paralysis. As serum K levels rise, progressive changes in the electrocardiogram occur. At serum K levels of 6 to 7 mEq./L., high and peaked T-waves are seen, followed by prolongation of the P-R interval, atrial arrest, and prolonged QRS, with ventricular arrest occurring at serum K levels of 8 to 9 mEq./L.

Replacement Therapy

Because of the hazards of hyperkalemia, two general rules should always be followed in ordering K administration. First, the patient must be known to have an adequate urine flow if the actual serum K level is not known. Second, intravenous injections of K salts should not be given at concentrations of greater than 40 mEq./L. or at rates exceeding 40 mEq. per hour. Most preparations of K for intravenous injection are available in ampules containing KCl at concentrations of 1500 to 2000 mEq./L. These *must* be diluted in other fluids before injection.

Ongoing Normal Needs. Potassium, like Na, should be supplied in amounts approximating those contained in normal diets. Usually, .02 mEq. per calorie of estimated caloric expenditure is provided. Thus, a 60-kg. female would be given .02 × 2,100 or about 40 mEq. of K. This is given as KCl and is distributed in the parenteral fluids so that the concentration is not greater than 40 mEq./L.

Ongoing Losses. Continuing losses occur primarily from the gut. External losses of K from nasogastric suction, biliary tract or intestinal fistula drainage are replaced at rates of 10 mEq. per liter of fluid lost. Losses in diarrheal stools are initially replaced at the same rate, but in these circumstances additional K replacement may be required.

Replacement of Preexisting Deficits. Potassium deficits should be replaced gradually. Generally, about one third of estimated deficits are given on the 1st day of treatment in addition to providing for basal requirements and ongoing losses. For example, a 60-kg. patient estimated to have sustained losses of 5 mEq./kg. would be given 100 mEq. of K during the first 24 hours of therapy. Serial measurements of serum K levels are required to monitor the therapy.

ACID-BASE METABOLISM

Definitions

An *acid* is a substance which in solution can liberate 1 or more hydrogen ions, whereas a *base* is a substance which in solution can combine with 1 or more hydrogen ions. Table 5-3 gives a few examples of acids and bases. On dissociation in solution, each acid yields not only hydrogen ions, but also a base (the "conjugate base" of the acid). As shown, acids or bases may be cations, anions, or uncharged. Note also that the "strength" of an acid (i.e., its tendency to liberate hydrogen ions in solution) is determined by the hydrogen ion affinity of its conjugate base. For example, hydrochloric acid is a very strong acid because its conjugate base (the chloride ion) has only a very slight tendency to recombine with hydrogen ions in solution. By contrast, carbonic acid is a weak acid because the bicarbonate anion has a strong affinity for hydrogen ions. Some substances may behave as either an acid or a base, depending upon the concentration of hydrogen ions in solution. For example, $H_2PO_4^-$, shown in Table 5-3 as an acid, can also behave as a base, reacting as $H_2PO_4^- + H^+ \rightarrow H_3PO_4$, when in solution containing higher concentrations of hydrogen ions.

The central concern of acid-base metabolism is maintaining the balance of forces resulting in gains and losses of hydrogen ions from body fluids.

Normal Body Content and Distribution

Few hydrogen ions are ingested as such, arising instead from the dissociation of acids generated during the catabolism of neutral dietary precursors. These acids are produced by metabolic reactions within cells and diffuse freely into the ECF. In the ECF the normal concentration of hydrogen ions is about 40 nanoequivalents/L. (0.000040 milliequivalents/L.). Because of the important influences of hydrogen ion concentration on many enzymatic reactions, this tiny quantity is nevertheless of critical physiologic importance.

There is no meaningful way to define the total body hydrogen ion content. At a given instant, a healthy 60-kg. woman might contain approximately 0.004 milliequivalents of hydrogen ion in solution in body waters (on the assumption that there is a hydrogen ion concentration of 40 nanoEq./L. in ECF and 160 nanoEq./L. in cell water). However, far larger quantities of hydrogen ions are available when needed from the dissociation of substances existing partially as undissociated acids in body fluids ($H_2PO_4^-$, H_2CO_3, etc.), and far greater numbers of hydrogen ions can be removed from body fluids when required by reacting with available bases (such as $HPO_4^=$ or HCO_3^-). This capacity of body fluids to liberate or bind hydrogen ions as the situation demands is referred to as "buffering." The buffering capacity of the body prevents large changes in hydrogen ion concentration in body fluids by removing the major quantity of hydrogen ions from solution when hydrogen ions are added, and by releasing hydrogen ions when hydrogen ion concentration falls below normal. The total physiologic buffer capacity of the human organism (i.e., the total quantity of acid which can be buffered before hydrogen ion concentration rises to lethal

Table 5-3. A Few Examples of Acids and Bases

Acids		Bases
HCl ⇌	H^+ +	Cl^-
H_2SO_4 ⇌	$2H^+$ +	$SO_4^=$
H_2CO_3 ⇌	H^+ +	HCO_3^-
$H_2PO_4^-$ ⇌	H^+ +	$HPO_4^=$
NH_4^+ ⇌	H^+ +	NH_3
NH_3^+—R—NH_3^+ ⇌	H^+ +	NH_2—R—NH_3^+

Acid-Base Metabolism

TABLE 5-4. PRINCIPAL ENDOGENOUS REACTIONS CONTRIBUTING TO NONVOLATILE ACID FORMATION

Methionine or Cysteine	$\xrightarrow{O_2}$	Urea + CO_2 + H_2O + $SO_4^=$ + $2H^+$
Glucose	$\xrightarrow{O_2}$	2 Lactate$^-$ + $2H^+$
Triglyceride	$\xrightarrow{O_2}$	Acetoacetate + H^+
Nucleoprotein	$\xrightarrow{O_2}$	Urate$^=$ + $2H^+$

levels) has been estimated to be about 15 mEq. per kilogram of body weight.

HYDROGEN ION TURNOVER

As discussed above, the addition of hydrogen ions to body fluids is a consequence of metabolism rather than of acid ingestion. The acids which arise endogenously can be divided into two classes, depending upon the routes available for their excretion. Volatile acids can be excreted by the lung, whereas nonvolatile acids can be excreted only by the kidneys.

The single volatile "acid" of quantitative significance in health is carbon dioxide. Carbon dioxide can react with water to form carbonic acid (CO_2 + H_2O → H_2CO_3) and is transported in part in this form from sites of metabolic production to the lungs. At the alveolar membranes the reaction is reversed, and the CO_2 gas is liberated and expelled in the expired air. Some 20,000 millimoles of CO_2 are produced each day in the adult. The unique role of the carbonic acid-bicarbonate buffer pair in acid-base metabolism is discussed below.

All nonvolatile acids are ultimately excreted by the kidneys. If an acid, such as HCl, is added to body fluids, the great majority of the dissociating hydrogen ions immediately react with body buffers and are removed from solution. Those hydrogen ions which react with extracellular bicarbonate ions to form carbonic acid are transported to the lungs, where carbonic acid dissociates into CO_2 and water, and the CO_2 is exhaled. This transient buffering reaction must not be confused with ultimate elimination of the added hydrogen ions, since the bicarbonate consumed in the reaction must ultimately be regenerated by the kidney (see below).

The principal endogenous reactions contributing to nonvolatile acid formation are shown in Table 5-4. Neutral sulfur contained in amino acids, such as methionine, is oxidized by steps to inorganic sulfate. During these steps, 2 hydrogen ions are added to body fluids for each millimole of sulfur oxidized. Organic acids are generated during the degradation of protein, fats, and carbohydrate. While the great majority of these are further combusted to carbon dioxide and water, and the carbon dioxide then excreted by the lungs, a small but significant fraction of the organic acid anions are lost in the urine, deserting hydrogen ions in body fluids. Approximately 0.02 milliequivalents of nonvolatile acid per calorie of caloric expenditure is added to body fluids each day in health. Thus a 60-kg. woman would produce a net amount of about 46 mEq. of nonvolatile acid each day. The kidneys would be obligated to excrete the same quantity if body composition were to be held constant.

RENAL ACID EXCRETION

Figure 5-7 illustrates the mechanisms involved in renal acid excretion. The kidney can be viewed as a bicarbonate-generating organ, since the source of the hydrogen ions excreted is from metabolically produced CO_2, which reacts with water to yield carbonic acid. The reaction is catalyzed by the enzyme carbonic anhydrase. The carbonic acid generated dissociates into a hydrogen ion, which is

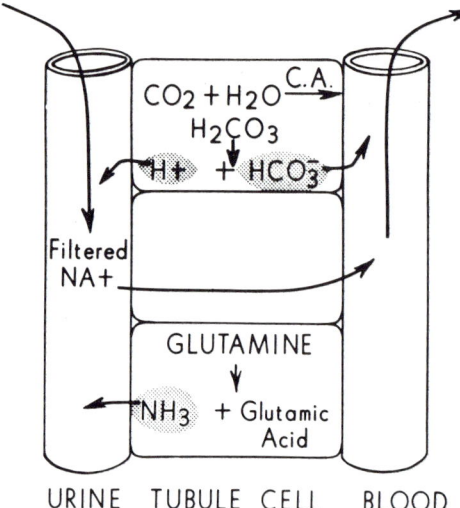

FIG. 5-7. Renal acid excretion.

actively secreted into the tubular urine, and bicarbonate, which is secreted into the peritubular blood. The kidney can concentrate hydrogen ions in the urine to a level that is 800 times as great as that existing in the blood. The hydrogen ions secreted by the kidney react with filtered bicarbonate, ultimately yielding CO_2 and water. This process accomplishes in its net form the reabsorption of filtered bicarbonate.

Other filtered buffers are also titrated. For example, phosphate exists normally in blood (and glomerular filtrate) in a state such that 4 of each 5 millimoles can take up a hydrogen ion when the hydrogen ion concentration of the urine is raised above that existing in the blood. Finally, renal cells generate an additional buffer, ammonia, by deamination of the amino acid glutamine. Ammonia gas diffuses into the urine, reacting with hydrogen ions to form ammonium. The ammonium ion cannot easily penetrate cell membranes and is excreted in the urine. Thus, net renal acid excretion can be taken as the sum of the filtered buffers titrated ("titratable acid"), plus ammonium, minus any filtered bicarbonate which escapes in the final urine. In health, this quantity equals the quantity of nonvolatile acid produced endogenously.

EVALUATION OF ACID-BASE BALANCE

As indicated, the rate of metabolic production of acid must be equal to the rate at which acid is removed from the body in the normal steady state. Whenever a disparity exists between these two processes, the hydrogen ion concentration of body fluids will be altered, and the body buffers will either take up or release hydrogen ions. Since the actual rates of production and excretion of acid are not easily measurable, measurements of the hydrogen ion concentration and state of the buffers in body fluids must be employed. In practice, such measurements are limited to the blood. The major buffer in blood and ECF is bicarbonate. Studies of the acute effects of large exogenous acid loads have indicated that extracellular bicarbonate is in rapid equilibrium with another buffer pool of approximately equal size, much of which is presumed to be within cells. Thus measurement of serum bicarbonate provides useful information about the state of titration of rapidly available body buffers.

Moreover, the carbonic acid/bicarbonate buffer pair is unique in other regards. Carbonic acid concentration in body fluids is a function of the partial pressure of CO_2 gas, such that (H_2CO_3) mM./L. = 0.03 (pCO_2 mm. Hg). The lungs regulate pCO_2. Bicarbonate concentration, as discussed above, is regulated by the kidneys. Thus knowledge of blood hydrogen ion concentration, pCO_2, and bicarbonate concentration can provide sufficient information to define the etiology (metabolic or respiratory), severity, and adequacy of compensation of acid-base disturbances to the physician familiar with the normal relationship among these variables.

L. W. Henderson recognized many years ago that these variables could be related by the following equation:

$$[H^+] = K' \frac{[H_2CO_3]}{[HCO_3^-]}$$

The dissociation constant for carbonic acid (K') has a value of approximately 794 when H^+ is expressed in nanoEq./L., and

[H_2CO_3] and [HCO_3^-] are expressed in mM./L. The concentration of carbonic acid is a direct function of pCO_2, such that [H_2CO_3] mM./L. = 0.03 (pCO_2 mm. Hg). Most clinical laboratories report values for pH and serum total CO_2 content. Hydrogen ion concentration can be obtained from measured pH by a simple mathematical operation (see Appendix to this chapter). The total CO_2 content of the serum measures the sum of serum carbonic acid and bicarbonate concentrations. The equation can then be rewritten as:

$$[H^+] \text{ nanoEq./L.} = \frac{0.03 \, pCO_2 \text{ (mm. Hg)}}{\text{Total } CO_2 \text{ content (mM./L.)} - 0.03 \, pCO_2 \text{ (mm. Hg)}}$$

The equation can then be solved for pCO_2, and serum bicarbonate can be obtained by subtracting the concentration of carbonic acid from the total CO_2 content.

Acidosis results whenever acid production exceeds acid excretion and is identified by an increase in blood hydrogen ion concentration above the normal level of about 40 nanoEq./L. (pH less than 7.4). The *cause* of the acidosis is disclosed by the values for pCO_2 and bicarbonate concentration. If acidosis results from impaired pulmonary CO_2 excretion, pCO_2 will be elevated (above 40 mm. Hg). In acute respiratory acidosis, hydrogen ion concentration will be considerably elevated, while serum bicarbonate concentration will be little altered (from the normal value of about 28 mM./L.). As the duration of respiratory acidosis increases, the kidneys have time to generate additional quantities of bicarbonate. Thus in chronic respiratory acidosis, serum bicarbonate concentration will be increased above normal, and blood hydrogen ion concentration will not be as high because of this renal compensation. If acidosis results from an increased rate of hydrogen ion production or failure of renal hydrogen ion excretion, blood hydrogen ion concentration will, of course, also be elevated. In this situation, however, the serum bicarbonate concentration will be low. In acute metabolic acidosis, pCO_2 will be markedly depressed as a result of pulmonary compensation, and blood hydrogen ion will be only modestly elevated. As the duration of metabolic acidosis increases, however, the respiratory work required to maintain a low pCO_2 presumably becomes a limiting factor, and the pCO_2 is allowed to rise somewhat with concomitant further rise in blood hydrogen ion concentration.

Alkalosis results whenever acid elimination exceeds acid production and is identified by a reduction in blood hydrogen ion concentration (elevation of blood pH). If alkalosis is caused by overbreathing, pCO_2 will be low. Acutely, only a small reduction in bicarbonate concentration will be present, but with time the kidney will excrete bicarbonate, lowering serum bicarbonate concentration and partially raising blood hydrogen ion concentration back toward normal. If alkalosis results from excessive losses of acid, as during vomiting of acid gastric juice, a low blood hydrogen ion concentration will be accompanied by a high serum bicarbonate concentration. Little change in pCO_2 (respiratory compensation) can be expected either acutely or chronically, since significant depression of respiratory exchange would impair oxygen supplies.

CLINICAL RECOGNITION AND THERAPY

A careful clinical history and bedside observation will usually suggest both the presence and etiology of acid-base disturbances. Blood measurements are then, of course, needed to confirm the impression and to assess the severity of the problem.

Respiratory acidosis is anticipated in a clinical setting of ineffective respiration, airway obstruction, or large pulmonary deadspace (as in emphysema). The only effective therapy of respiratory acidosis is improvement of ventilation by providing an adequate airway and, when necessary, supporting respiration mechanically.

Respiratory alkalosis would be anticipated in patients who have some other primary drive to overventilation (such as brain tumor or a low blood oxygen content because of pulmonary interstitial fibrosis). This can be treated (if treatment is indeed required) by having the patient breathe a CO_2-containing gas mixture, or rebreathing in a paper bag.

Metabolic acidosis occurs in subjects who have unusual acid loads of endogenous (diabetic ketoacidosis, spontaneous lactic acidosis) or exogenous (ammonium chloride administration) origin, or who lose large quantities of alkali (in diarrheal stools, small bowel drainage, or vomiting in achlorhydric patients). Alternatively, this may result from impaired renal acid excretion, as occurs in chronic renal diseases. This is treated by administering bicarbonate salts or bicarbonate precursors (such as lactate salts). It is important to remember that bicarbonate behaves as if distributed in a volume equal to 40 per cent of body weight. Thus to increase the serum bicarbonate concentration by 10 mEq./L., a 60-kg. woman would require 60 kg. × 0.40 × 10 mEq./L. or 240 mEq. of sodium bicarbonate. An important clue to the presence of an acidosis caused by accumulation of organic acids (such as in diabetic acidosis or lactic acidosis) is provided by comparing the serum Na concentration to the sum of the serum chloride and total CO_2 content concentrations. Normally, serum Na concentration exceeds the sum of chloride and total CO_2 by 6 to 12 mEq./L. The "unmeasured anions" which fill this gap normally consist of the negative charges on albumin along with small quantities of sulfate and phosphate anions. When organic acids accumulate in the blood, the "unmeasured anion" content increases considerably.

Metabolic alkalosis is expected with vomiting (if the patient is not achlorhydric), when renal acid excretion is inappropriately increased (as by some diuretic drugs), or when the patient has been given sizeable quantities of alkali (such as sodium bicarbonate). This is best treated by correcting the cause of the vomiting or stopping the drugs or alkali. Treatment with acidifying salts (such as ammonium chloride) is seldom indicated, since the body normally produces acid endogenously each day and, given time, will correct the alkalosis.

OTHER MINERAL REQUIREMENTS

Chloride. Since chloride is added as NaCl to most normal diets and is given as NaCl in most parenteral fluids, the factors involved in chloride metabolism are essentially the same as those for Na, and, in general, chloride needs are automatically taken care of when Na is provided.
Calcium, Magnesium, and Phosphorus. Bone and soft tissue stores of these inorganic elements are large, and generally it is not necessary to consider their replacement during short periods of parenteral fluid therapy.

APPENDIX

CONCENTRATION UNITS

The clinical laboratory reports the concentrations of many substances in body fluids in mass/volume units (i.e., milligrams per 100 ml., grams per 100 ml., etc.). Many of the fundamental properties of the body fluids, however, depend not on the *mass* of substances in solution, but rather on the *number* of *particles* of the substance in solution and on the *electrical charge* of the particles. Three units of concentration are employed to take these important properties into account.

A *mole* of any substance is equal to the sum of the atomic weights of its constituents, expressed in grams. This expression is useful because a mole of any substance contains the same number of molecules as a mole of any other substance. Table 5-5 lists the atomic weights of those substances pertinent to the present discussion.

TABLE 5-5. ATOMIC WEIGHTS OF SUBSTANCES PERTINENT TO THE DISCUSSION

Substance	Chemical Symbol and Charge	Atomic Weight
Sodium	Na+	23
Potassium	K+	39
Chloride	Cl-	35.5
Hydrogen	H+	1
Carbon	C	12
Oxygen	O	16
Nitrogen	N	14

One mole of NaCl would thus equal 23 + 35.5 or 58.5 grams. One mole of sodium bicarbonate (NaHCO$_3$) would equal 23 + 1 + 12 + 3(16) or 84 grams. A millimole = 1/1000 of a mole. A molar solution contains 1 mole of the solute per liter. For example, a molar solution of NaCl would contain one mole (58.5 grams) of NaCl per liter.

An *osmole* of any substance *in solution* contains the same number of particles as does an osmole of any other substance. This unit takes into account the fact that some compounds dissociate in solution. For example, NaCl when dissolved in water undergoes the reaction: NaCl → Na+ + Cl-. Thus, 1 mole of NaCl, when dissolved in water, would yield 2 osmoles. For substances which do not dissociate (glucose, for example) 1 mole = 1 osmole. A milliosmole = 1/1000 of an osmole.

The *equivalent* or combining weight of an element or ion is equal to its atomic weight divided by its valence. Chemical reactions between elements or ions take place on an equivalent basis. For example, Na has a valence of 1 and an atomic weight of 23. One equivalent of Na thus equals 23 grams, and 1 milliequivalent (mEq.) equals 23 milligrams. For divalent ions, for example, sulfate (SO$_4^=$, molecular weight = 96), the equivalent weight is obtained by dividing the formula weight by 2. Thus 96 milligrams equals 1 millimole of sulfate, while 96/2 or 48 milligrams equals 1 milliequivalent. Note that each milliequivalent of sulfate reacts with a milliequivalent of Na to yield Na$_2$SO$_4$ (2 mEq. of Na + 2 mEq. of SO$_4$).

CONVERSION OF pH TO HYDROGEN ION CONCENTRATION

By definition, the hydrogen ion activity in a solution equals 10^{-pH}. The activity of an ion is not necessarily identical to its concentration. The relationship between activity and concentration is altered by the presence of other ions, temperature, etc. For clinical purposes this small potential error can be neglected, and 10^{-pH} can be taken as equivalent to hydrogen ion concentration. Table 5-6 gives the hydrogen ion concentrations equivalent to pH values between pH 6.90 and 7.68.

TABLE 5-6. CONVERSION OF pH TO [H+] NANOEQ./L.

pH	.00	.02	.04	.06	.08
6.9	126	120	115	110	105
7.0	100	96	91	87	83
7.1	79	76	72	69	66
7.2	63	60	58	55	52
7.3	50	48	46	44	42
7.4	40	38	36	35	33
7.5	32	30	29	28	26
7.6	25	24	23	22	21

ILLUSTRATIVE CASES

Case 1

A 43-year-old housewife is admitted for elective vaginal hysterectomy because of uterine myomata with intermittent bleeding. Otherwise, her general health has been good, weight stable at 110 pounds (50 kg.), and she has been eating a normal diet. The physician caring for her does not want her to eat on the day of surgery but wishes to provide for basal water and electrolyte needs. What and how much should be given?

Basal Water and Electrolyte Needs on Day of Surgery. WATER: Estimated caloric expenditures = 50 kg. × 40 calories/kg./day or 2,000 calories. Since approximately 1 ml. water is required per calorie of estimated expenditure, 2,000 ml. of water is needed.

SODIUM: .03 mEq./calorie of estimated expenditure = .03 × 2,000 = about 60 mEq.

POTASSIUM: .02 mEq./calorie of estimated expenditure = .02 × 2,100 = about 40 mEq.

Thus we could give either 1,500 ml. 5% G/W plus 500 ml. 5% G/S, adding 20 mEq. KCl to each liter, *or* 1 liter 5% G/W and 1 liter 0.45% (75 mEq./L.) saline with 20 mEq. KCl added to each liter.

Case 2

A 24-year-old moderately obese woman in previous good health is admitted to the hospital because of chills, fever, and left lower abdominal pain for 3 days. She had been unable to eat for 2 days and had repeatedly vomited. On examination there was marked lower abdominal tenderness and a left adnexal mass thought to represent acute salpingitis. Her weight was 158 pounds (72 kg.), whereas she recalled having weighed 165 pounds (75 kg.) about 5 days earlier. Height 5'6" (168 cm.); T 101.6° orally, BP 115/75 supine and unchanged on sitting, p 100, and R = 18. The hands and feet were cool.

Laboratory Studies. Hgb 15.6 gm.%, HCT 46%, WBC 14,300, 24 stabs, 62 segs, 12 lymphs and 2 monos. Creatinine 1.3 mg.% and BUN 20 mg.%. Na 132, K 3.5 and Cl 92 mEq./L. CO_2 content 32 mM./L. H^+ = 33 nEq./L. (pH 7.48), and pCO_2 42 mm. Hg. The urine obtained on admission had a Na concentration of only 2 mEq./L.

The physician caring for the patient wishes to replace existing deficits of fluid and electrolytes and provide for ongoing losses and basal needs by the parenteral route to avoid oral intake. What is required?

Basal Needs. Her estimated ideal body weight for her height is about 60 kg., so that her estimated basal needs are identical to those required for the preceding example (Case 1) — water 2,000 ml., Na 60 mEq., and K 40 mEq.

Abnormal Losses. Because of fever, which increases basal water needs by 10 per cent per degree F. above normal, she would need 3 × 10% = 30% × 2,000 ml. = roughly 600 ml. additional water.

Deficits. WATER: The weight loss of 3 kg. indicates a loss of about 3 liters of water.

SODIUM: The history, along with the weight loss, cool extremities, postural hypotension, slightly raised Hgb and HCT and low urine Na concentration, indicates moderate Na depletion of about 5 mEq./kg. or 300 to 400 mEq.

POTASSIUM: The history and slightly low serum K suggest mild K deficits of less than 5 mEq./kg., or less than 300 mEq.

ACID-BASE DISTURBANCE: The mild metabolic alkalosis due to vomiting is neglected in therapy since it is expected that it will be spontaneously corrected.

Replacement of Deficits. These deficits could be approximately replaced by providing 3 liters of 5% glucose in saline with 40 mEq. KCl added to each liter. About one half the deficits would be made up during the 1st day of treatment in addition to providing for basal needs and expected abnormal losses.

Thus the fluids for the 1st day might consist of:

FOR BASAL NEEDS: 500 ml. 5% G/S + 10 mEq. KCl
1500 ml. 5% G/W + 30 mEq. KCl

FOR EXPECTED ABNORMAL LOSSES: 500 ml. 5% G/W

FOR ONE HALF OF TOTAL DEFICITS: 1500 ml. 5% G/S + 60 mEq./KCl

OR

2 liters 5% G/W
  with 25 mEq. KCl in each liter, plus
2 liters 5% G/S

Fluid orders for the next day would be determined by the rate of improvement as judged by weight gain, peripheral circulation, and laboratory findings.

Case 3

A 62-year-old woman in previous good health was found to have an adenocarcinoma of the uterus and is admitted for a total hysterectomy after previous intracavitary radium treatment. Prior to operation her weight was 50 kg., BP 130/85, and there was no evidence of cardiovascular or renal disease. Hgb 13 gm.%, HCT 39%, Na 138, K 4.2, and Cl 102 mEq./L.; CO_2 content 26 mM./L. Creatinine 0.8 mg.% and BUN 14 mg.%. A random urine has a specific gravity of 1.021, pH 5.5, and negative tests for protein and glucose. The sediment contains only a few epithelial cells. An intravenous urogram and barium enema, chest film, and EKG were within normal limits. During the operation the patient was transiently hypotensive (90/60) for about 45 minutes despite transfusion of 2 units of whole blood to replace estimated losses. Postoperatively, her BP was steady at 120/75. On the day of operation she was given 1,500 ml. 5% G/W and 500 ml. 5% G/S together with 40 mEq. KCl to provide for basal needs. Less than 200 ml. of fluid was aspirated from the nasogastric tube inserted before operation and was not replaced. During this 24-hour period her urine output was only 300 ml.

The following morning after operation her weight was 50.5 kg., blood pressure unchanged, and urine output only 10 ml. during a 2-hour period. This urine had a specific gravity of 1.012, pH 5.0, protein 3+, and no glucose. The sediment contained 5-15 RBC and 3-8 WBC/hpf together with occasional muddy-brown pigmented granular casts. The Na concentration in this specimen was 40 mEq./L.

Although the history of transient hypotension, oliguria, and the results of the examinations of the urine suggested acute tubular damage, ureteral catheterization was carried out on one side only to exclude obstruction, and none was found.

Other laboratory studies the same morning showed Hgb 12.1 gm.%, HCT 37%, BUN 22 mg.%, creatinine 1.2 mg.%, Na 135, K 5.2, Cl 98 mEq./L., CO_2 content 23 mM./L.

A central venous catheter was inserted, and a rapid infusion of 500 ml. of isosmotic saline resulted in a rise in venous pressure from 8 to 16 cm. of water, weight gain, and no increase in urine flow rate. Thus it appeared clear that the patient had suffered significant renal damage, and that oliguria was not secondary to unrecognized volume depletion.

What fluid orders would be appropriate for the next 24-hour period?

Basic Needs. WATER: Since no significant volume of urine is expected, water losses would occur only from the skin and lungs. Since her weight is 50 kg., her estimated caloric expenditure would be 2,000 calories. Twenty-five per cent of this heat energy would be lost by evaporation (i.e., 500 calories), and this would require the evaporation from the skin and lungs of 500/0.6 = about 800 ml. water. Endogenous water formation would supply 200 ml. of this water requirement, so that only about 500 to 600 ml. would be given to meet insensible losses.

SODIUM: The sole source of Na loss would be via the skin, and this need not be replaced.

POTASSIUM must not be given because of the hazards of hyperkalemia in the presence of oliguria.

Abnormal Losses. Since 200 ml. of fluid was lost via nasogastric suction the preceding day, about 200 ml. of water would be added to the basic fluid allotment.

In summary, about 700 to 800 ml. of water would be given intravenously as 10% or 15% G/W to provide some caloric intake. The patient would be expected to lose 0.2 to 0.3 kg. per day because caloric intake is, of necessity, inadequate.

On subsequent days fluids would be provided to meet insensible losses and the urine volumes and nasogastric suction losses of the preceding day.

BIBLIOGRAPHY

Christensen, H. N.: Diagnostic Biochemistry. New York, Oxford University Press, 1959.

Dittmer, D. S. (ed.): Blood and Other Body Fluids. Washington, D.C., Federation of American Societies for Experimental Biology, 1961.

Duncan, G. G. (ed.): Diseases of Metabolism. ed. 5. Philadelphia, W. B. Saunders, 1964.

Elkinton, J. R., and Danowski, T. S.: The Body Fluids. Baltimore, Williams & Wilkins, 1955.

Moore, F. D., Olesen, K. H., McMurrey, J. D., Parker, H. V., Ball, M. R., and Boyden, C. M.: The Body Cell Mass and Its Supporting Environment. Philadelphia, W. B. Saunders, 1963.

Ussing, H. H., Kruhoffer, P., Hess Thaysen, J., and Thorn, N. A.: The Alkali Metal Ions in Biology. *In* Handbuch der Experimentellen Pharmakologie. vol. 13. Berlin, Springer-Verlag, 1960.

6

Estrogen Replacement Therapy

Since the pelvic surgeon is frequently responsible for castration, he is often called upon to consider the treatment of the resultant menopausal symptoms. It is therefore appropriate to consider this subject in this volume on operative gynecology.

Many women cease menstruating, either naturally or as the result of surgery, without any unpleasant symptoms. Others have a very disagreeable time. Women who are inclined to be unstable nervously are apt to have more symptoms at the climacteric, but many a woman who considered herself quite tranquil becomes greatly disturbed when ovarian function fails. Hot flushes, often accompanied by drenching sweats, headaches, palpitation, emotional instability, and mental depression are frequent. One of the major factors in the menopausal syndrome is fear based on old wive's tales from mothers and older women. It is especially depressing to vain women to know that they have "turned the corner," and that physical changes indicative of old age are imminent. Their future sex life and particularly the possibility of losing attractiveness to their husbands worry them greatly.

Most physicians today agree on the desirability of estrogen replacement therapy in the natural and artificial menopause. However, there is great disagreement concerning the indications for treatment. The difference of opinion lies between those who believe that all women should have replacement therapy from the menopausal years to their graves and those who believe therapy should be used for the relief of symptoms only. Unfortunately, the evidence pro and con is not all clear-cut. Therefore in this chapter we shall briefly present the evidence and then give our own interpretation of the evidence and our practice.

Are Estrogens Carcinogenic? Perhaps the question which should be considered first is whether estrogens are carcinogenic. Some breast surgeons apparently think they are and consequently oppose estrogen therapy in women who have had benign cysts or tumors, and especially in women who have had a mastectomy for malignancy.

What is the origin of this belief? In 1932 a French scientist showed that spaying mice early in life prevented the development of cancer in female mice. Conversely, breast cancer was produced in *male* mice belonging to a cancer-susceptible strain by administering huge amounts of estrogen to them over a long period of time. He was unable to produce such cancer in mice belonging to a strain in which spontaneous breast cancer seldom occurred in females. The amount of estrogen in proportion to body weight was tremendous as compared to that given to women. Experiments on dogs, rabbits, and monkeys have failed to produce cancer even when the animals were subjected to estrogen for prolonged periods of time.

In our experience with estrogen therapy over many years, we have failed to see any evidence that estrogen-treated women were more than normally susceptible to malignancy. Furthermore, women appear to be more susceptible to breast cancer in the later years of their life when there is less estrogen in the body than in their earlier years.

Our clinical experience is substantiated by that of many other reliable observers. Albright *et al.* found that among 200 women treated for approximately 1,100 patient years there were only 4 instances of genital cancer. They were as follows: endometrial, 1; breast, 0; invasive cervical cancer, 0; carcinoma in situ of the cervix, 1; and ovary, 2. They concluded that there is no evidence that prolonged estrogen therapy is carcinogenic. Rhoades reported a compilation of 5 separate studies comprising more than 1,400 women who took estrogen for as long as 25 years. Although the projected expectancy of pelvic malignancy was 96 cases in the general population, only 5 genital cancers occurred. So, in making a decision regarding estrogen therapy, it is our belief that the fear of producing cancer should not be a consideration.

Being Honest With the Patient About Treatment. When discussing estrogen therapy, one should give the patient an honest opinion on what may be expected from the treatment. It is our duty as conscientious physicians to correct some of the misconceptions which most women have gleaned from popular magazines and books carrying false statements regarding eternal youth. It is far better to attempt to prepare the women psychologically for old age than to promise them falsely that they will be feminine forever in the sense of retaining sexual charm, which inevitably will diminish.

It is not uncommon today for women to request a vaginal smear as an evaluation of their estrogen level. From magazine articles they have gotten the idea that femininity can be gauged by a vaginal smear. A few minutes spent in explaining to them that the vaginal smear is not a measure of their sex appeal usually satisfies them. Actually, we have found the smear of no practical value in judging estrogen therapy. There is one exception to this statement. It is of value in judging estrogenic response to estrogen suppositories in elderly women being treated for dyspareunia and senile vaginitis. One can honestly tell the patient that flushes are usually abolished or greatly reduced by the administration of estrogen. Headaches, if dependent on the menopause, are often cured, and in most cases emotions are quieted, and the patient has a sense of well-being. When estrogens are given by suppository or vaginal cream, there is often great improvement of the dyspareunia.

The Blood Vessels and Prolonged Estrogen Therapy. One of the arguments used in favor of universal estrogen therapy for women over 45 is that there is a beneficial effect of prolonged therapy on the blood vessels, particularly the coronary vessels. The evidence is conflicting on this point. Davis *et al.* in 1961 concluded that estrogen therapy taken over a long period of time reduces the incidence of atherosclerosis in postmenopausal women. It is well recognized that premenopausal women have a much lower incidence of atherosclerosis than their age-matched male counterparts. Wuest, Dry, and Edwards studied 49 women at autopsy who had undergone hysterectomy and bilateral oophorectomy. They compared them with 600 men and women of comparable ages. In general they found that there was less sclerosis in women who had their ovaries than in the castrated women and men. The time interval between the time of oophorectomy and death was in all instances greater than 2 years. Higano, Robinson, and Cohen showed an increase in atherosclerosis in women castrated before 45 as compared with a group of noncastrated women who had had hysterectomy with preservation of their ovaries. Davis *et al.* also showed a greater incidence of abnormal electrocardiograms in the castrated group of women than in a noncastrated group of comparable age. In addition they found less hypertension in a group of castrated women who had been treated with stilbestrol than in an untreated group.

These statistics sound rather convincing, but there are studies which do not confirm these observations. Novak and Williams studied the autopsy records of 85 women who had been surgically castrated and compared them with the records of 250 controls. The autopsies had been conducted by several different pathologists on the Johns Hopkins staff who had no interest in this subject and who had no knowledge that the records would subsequently be used for this study. In other words, the study was totally objective. No significant difference was found in the blood vessels of the castrated and controlled groups. They concluded that estrogen therapy was indicated for relief of symptoms, but there was no evidence that estrogen deficiency was a factor in atherosclerosis.

Osteoporosis and Estrogen Therapy. One of the other principal arguments presented by the advocates of universal therapy concerns the prevention of osteoporosis. Let us examine the evidence. Albright gave to the orthopedists the first nosologic and etiologic description of the disease. He also found in approximately 200 postmenopausal women treated with estrogen for a period of 1 to 20 years that the progress of osteoporosis was arrested in nearly all instances as judged by total height and radiographic examination of the spine. But he also found that careful radiographic studies done at intervals on osteoporotic women after 5 to 20 years of estrogen therapy failed to demonstrate a single incidence of increased bone density. He concluded that estrogen therapy might stop the progress of the disease but does not restore bone density. Saville and Nilsson came to similar conclusions and drew attention to the fact that only a small proportion of the female population seeks medical advice for symptomatic osteoporosis. They also pointed out that underweight women have a tendency to osteoporosis. Hunt states that "the problem of effective therapy in osteoporosis has not been solved," and that no theraputic agent has been found that produces a reversal of the process as far as can be ascertained by x-ray. He further concludes that an increased incidence of osteoporosis in postmenopausal women is hardly evidence enough to establish hormonal imbalance as the cause. Bones of women are less dense than those of men throughout life, and it is impossible to demonstrate greater hormonal imbalance in osteoporotic women than in nonosteoporotic women. Many claim relief from estrogen therapy, but Soloman *et al.* in a double blind study showed that the symptomatic relief was largely a placebo effect. Finally, Hurxthal and Vose studied the density of the 3rd lumbar vertebra and found, by the method employed, no effect on bone density as the result of spontaneous menopause or surgical castration. He concluded that there is identical regression of bone structure in males and females. Further studies could be cited, but a more complete review of the literature only substantiates the confusion and disagreement among orthopedists on the effect of the menopause and estrogen therapy on osteoporosis.

Treatment Based on Symptoms. If it be granted that the evidence for the prevention of osteoporosis and atherosclerosis may not be conclusive, the question might be asked: Why not give the patient the benefit of the doubt, and treat all menopausal and postmenopausal women indefinitely with estrogen? Since we have stated that it is our belief that its carcinogenic action may be disregarded, that is a fair question. The answer is that there may be side-effects of estrogen therapy which outweigh the possible benefits. Therefore we have not practiced universal therapy but believe it is better to base our treatment on the patient's symptoms. A certain proportion of the recipients of estrogen become nauseated; others have painful breasts. Some have a sense of heaviness in the pelvis and lose their sense of well-being. But these symptoms do not constitute our main objection to universal and perpetual therapy. The frequent occurrence of uterine bleeding is sufficient reason for barring its universal use. Contrary to what is published by some authors, bleeding does occur not infrequently when estrogen is given in conjunction with methyltestosterone, as well as when given alone.

Curettage is then necessary to exclude bleeding from malignancy, although in most instances the chances are greatly in favor of the bleeding being due to the hormonal therapy.

After all, osteoporosis and coronary diseases are not universal illnesses, and the above disadvantages seem to outweigh the possible advantages of prolonged estrogen therapy in the asymptomatic woman. There is evidence to believe that estrogen is of value in arresting and relieving symptoms of osteoporosis, but that does not justify its universal use in all postmenopausal women in whom there is the possibility of a small proportion developing the disease. To be sure, the same bleeding may, and sometimes does occur when the hormone is given for the symptomatic menopause, but it is worth the risk in a woman who is miserable and can be made comfortable by such therapy. It is our policy to tell the complaining woman the probable benefits of estrogen therapy and allow her to make her choice about treatment.

Many women have no symptoms of any kind during the menopause; in fact, some feel exceptionally well. They are often free of the responsibility of raising small children; they need no longer worry about further pregnancies; often their economic situation is better than earlier in life, and their increased leisure makes the future look bright. Why rock the boat and insist on medication?

In contrast to these women, at the other extreme is the woman who is really miserable from hot flushes, headaches, lack of sleep, and general irritability. Between these two extremes are the women with less marked symptoms. Menopausal symptoms may last only a few months, or they may persist for years. When they do, we have no hesitancy in continuing therapy as long as necessary to relieve symptoms. We do not believe that there is any substantial evidence that estrogen therapy prolongs menopausal symptoms. We can recall many old women in the past who have never taken estrogen who had menopausal symptoms extending into the 8th decade.

How Shall Estrogens Be Given? In previous editions of this book, the implantation of 50 mg. of estrone through a 12-gauge needle was advocated. We still use this procedure and believe it to be a superior method of administering the hormone. Unfortunately, the estrone pellets have not been made available to the profession; hence there is no point in continuing to advocate this method until such pellets are marketed.

Oral administration is the most practical method of giving estrogen and is quite effective. Several potent products are on the market, and it is not our desire to express a preference for any brand. There is no doubt, however, that some women obtain relief from one product, whereas others seem to prefer another. Therefore some individualization of treatment is often desirable, but this is usually discovered only by trial and error. In short, it is our policy to treat those patients who consider their symptoms sufficiently severe to request treatment. If one brand does not give relief, we try another. Almost always a product can be found which gives relief. We have no objection to continuing therapy as long as the symptoms persist, and the patient requests treatment. It must be admitted, however, that there is a very rare patient whose menopausal symptoms are not relieved by estrogen therapy. In such case, one must do the best he can with sedatives and tranquilizers.

Estrogens may be given on a cyclic monthly basis, but regardless of how they are given, it is advisable to stop therapy at intervals to determine whether menopausal symptoms recur. If they recur, treatment may be resumed. If they do not, treatment may be stopped.

BIBLIOGRAPHY

Albright, F., Bloanberg, E., and Smith, P. H.: Postmenopausal osteoporosis. Trans. Amer. Physicians, 55:298, 1940.

Albright, F., Smith, P. H., and Richardson, A. M.: Postmenopausal osteoporosis; its clinical features. J.A.M.A., *116*:2465, 1941.

Bennett, H. G., Biskind, G., and Mark, J.: Subcutaneous implantations of compressed crystalline theelin pellets in the treatment of menopausal cases. Amer. J. Obstet. Gynec., 39:504, 1940.

Bennett, H. G., and Te Linde, R. W.: The menopausal syndrome: Treatment with implantation of crystalline estrone pellets. J.A.M.A., 118:1041, 1942.

Davis, M. E., Jones, R. J., and Jarolim, C.: Long-term estrogen substitution and atherosclerosis. Amer. J. Obstet. Gynec., 82:1003, 1961.

Deanesly, R., and Parks, A. S.: Factors influencing the effectiveness of administered hormones. Proc. Roy. Soc. Med., ser. B., 124:279, 1937–38.

Higano, N., Robinson, R. W., and Cohen, W. D.: Atherosclerosis in castrate women. New Eng. J. Med., 268:1123, 1963.

Hunt, D. D.: Changing concepts in osteoporosis. J. Iowa Med. Soc., 55:563, 1965.

Hurxthal, L. M., and Vose, G. P.: Radiographic bone density in the late postmenopausal state and after surgical castration. Lahey Clin. Found. Bull., 14:15, 1965.

Kaufman, S. A.: The Ageless Woman. Edgewood Cliffs, N. J., Hall, 1968.

Novak, E. R., and Williams, T. J.: Autopsy comparison of cardiovascular changes in castrated and normal women Amer. J. Obstet. Gynec., 80:863, 1960.

Saville, P. D., and Nilsson, Bo E. R.: Height and weight in symptomatic postmenopausal osteoporosis. Clin. Orthop., 45:49, 1966.

Soloman, G. F., Dickersen, W. J., and Eisengerg, E.: Psychologic and osteometabolic responses to sex hormones in elderly osteoporatic women. Geriatrics, 15:46, 1960.

Soule, S. D., and Burnstein, R.: Prophylaxis of the postsurgical menopause. J. Clin. Endocr., 3:417, 1943.

Wuest, J. H., Dry, T. J., and Edwards, J. E.: The degree of coronary atherosclerosis in bilateral oophorectomized women. Circulation, 7:801, 1953.

PART TWO

Abdominal Operations for Benign Disease

7

Opening and Closing the Abdomen

OPENING THE ABDOMEN

It is frequently stated that the credentials of a surgeon are enclosed within the indelible scar of his incision. In selecting the location and type of abdominal incision, the pelvic surgeon is concerned with many important requirements: (1) adequate operative exposure, (2) strength of the healing scar, (3) postoperative comfort of the patient, and (4) simplicity and speed of the procedure. While many other factors enter into the choice of an abdominal incision, such as cosmetic considerations, abdominal contour, previous scars, and the pelvic pathology, the requirement for adequate exposure of the underlying pelvic organs far exceeds all others. Every surgeon must be completely familiar with the anatomy of the anterior abdominal wall before he can make an intelligent decision on a particular type of incision. The distribution and course of the nerves and blood vessels of the abdominal wall bear directly on the postoperative healing and function of the abdominal wall. The quality of the tissues, including the abdominal fascia and muscles, as well as the lines of elasticity and the direction of muscular contractility, are factors which influence healing and provide strength to the resultant scar.

The anterior abdominal wall has an excellent blood supply except at the linea alba, where the limited blood supply accounts for the increased incidence of impairment of healing from midline incisions and the occurrence of incisional hernias and evisceration.

There are three major incisions through which practically all pelvic surgery is done: (1) the midline, (2) the transverse incision, and (3) the muscle-splitting gridiron incision.

MIDLINE INCISION

Most abdominal operations on the female reproductive tract are performed through a low midline incision. It can be done rapidly and easily and can be extended above the umbilicus when necessary. Consequently, it has the greatest advantage of operative exposure with the least time requirement. The length of the incision is important in the healing process, even though it is frequently stated that "the incision heals from side to side." As measured by Sloan, tension on a midline incision is roughly proportional to the square of the length of the incision; i.e., a 30-lb. force was found necessary to approximate a 3-inch incision, while an 80-lb. force was necessary to approximate a 5-inch incision. The incision is carried down through the fat to the linea alba with a clean knife separate from the skin incision (Fig. 7-1 A). Bleeders are clamped with Halsted clamps and tied with No. 000 plain or chromic catgut.

The aponeurosis is incised at the linea alba for the full length of the incision (Fig. 7-1). The adherent fat is not separated extensively from the fascial margin, only sufficiently to permit adequate

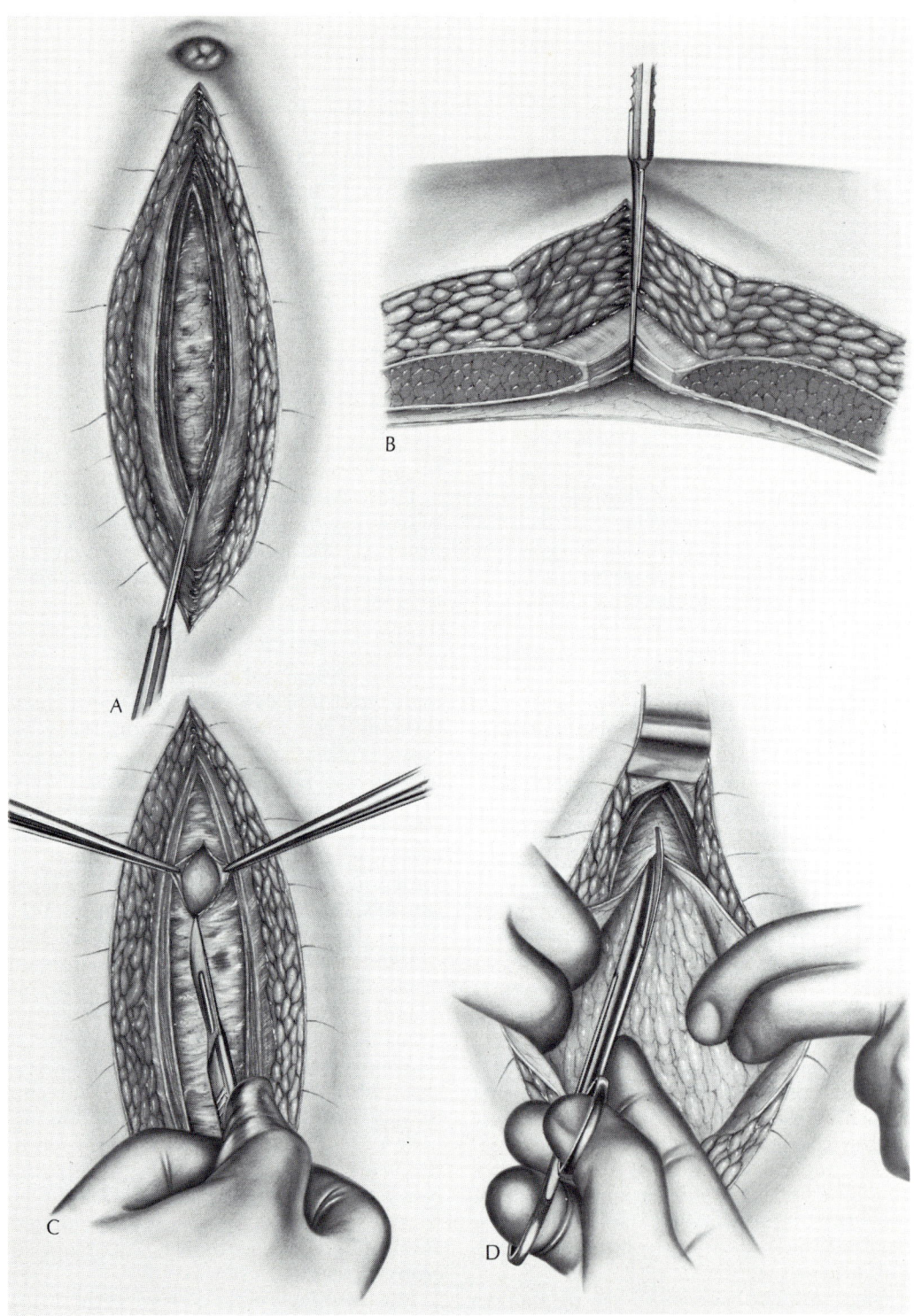

Fig. 7-1. (A) Cutting of linea alba in low midline incision with scalpel. (B) Cross section of abdominal wall showing skin, subcutaneous fat, anterior and posterior rectus sheaths, and underlying peritoneum. (C) Opening of peritoneum with knife and demonstrating small bowel protruding into peritoneal opening. (D) Enlargement of peritoneal opening with Mayo scissors to the region of the umbilicus.

closure. In parous women there is usually no difficulty in finding the midline of the underlying rectus muscles for separation, but in nulliparous women the midline may not be immediately evident. The pyramidalis muscles which arise from the symphysis pubis are the most useful landmark in directing the surgeon to the midline. Although there is great variation in the development of the pyramidalis muscles, the medial border of the muscles is found to pass upward and inward and to insert in the linea alba on the midline. Near the umbilicus the rectus muscles are usually widely separated and can be further divided by using the handle of the scalpel. At this point the skin edges are covered with towels before entering the peritoneal cavity.

The peritoneal fat is incised, and the peritoneum becomes visible beneath. The urachus is frequently seen and identifies the midline of the lower abdomen as it courses from the dome of the bladder to the umbilicus. The peritoneum is picked up with mouse-tooth forceps by the operator and his assistant and is carefully incised to avoid accidental laceration of bowel which may be adherent beneath the peritoneum (Fig. 7-1 C). Pushing the bowel away with the knife handle before incising the peritoneum is an excellent precaution. The cut edges of the peritoneum are grasped with Kelly clamps, and the peritoneal incision is enlarged with the scissors while the assistant and the operator lift up the abdominal wall (Fig. 7-1 D). Enlargement of the peritoneal incision downward is done under direct vision, care being exercised to avoid injury to the bladder.

Special care must be taken in entering the peritoneal cavity, particularly when there has been a previous laparatomy; when the bladder is distended or possibly displaced upward by a tumor; when there is a large tumor such as a fibroid or an ovarian cyst pressing tightly against the parietal peritoneum, and when the history suggests previous pelvic inflammatory disease. In entering the abdomen through a previous scar, it is advisable to enter the peritoneal cavity at a higher point than the scar of the former operation. When a large tumor presses against the parietal peritoneum, it is best to attempt entrance above the tumor by nicking the peritoneum slightly and listening for the inrush of air into the peritoneal cavity. Injury to the bladder occurs more frequently at the time of entry into the peritoneal cavity, in the experience of Everett and Mattingly, than at any other time. It is, therefore, important for the gynecologist to observe the thickness of the tissues that he is incising, and if it appears muscular or vascular, it is well to abandon entrance at that point and attempt an opening of the peritoneum at a higher level. Adherent bowel from previous surgery or pelvic inflammatory disease must be identified by gently opening the thin layer of peritoneum, and if muscle appears beneath this incision, it is well to attempt an entrance elsewhere.

After the peritoneal cavity has been entered, the walls are retracted with either self-retaining or wide-bladed retractors. It is advisable, in cases in which prolonged surgery is anticipated, to protect the incision with moist laparotomy packs placed beneath the retractor blades. Although the Trendelenburg position is helpful in displacing the intestines in the upper abdomen, steep Trendelenburg is not necessary with the use of modern methods of anesthesia and smooth muscle relaxants. As a matter of fact, the elderly patient whose circulatory system is borderline should not be subjected to steep Trendelenburg position. This will frequently lead to cardiac failure and compromises the adequacy of pulmonary ventilation during surgery.

The intestines may be gently held in the upper abdomen with a moist laparotomy pack, but it is unnecessary to place undue pressure on the bowel with multiple packs. If the bowel does not remain out of the operative field with 1 or 2 laparotomy packs placed carefully over the small intestines and anchored well in the lateral corners of the abdomen, it is probable that the anesthesia is inadequate, and that the bowel needs further relaxation. It is well to remember also that the average moist laparotomy pack when formed into a sphere occupies approximately 240 cc. of available intra-abdominal space; consequently, excessive packs will reduce the amount of exposure available to the surgeon and may interfere with the operative procedure. In addition, excessive compression of the small bowel between laparotomy packs will produce temporary damage to the terminal motor nerves, which results in postoperative adynamic ileus.

Transverse Incision

Pfannenstiel is reported to have first recommended a transverse low abdominal incision in 1900, but the initial use of this surgical approach was advocated by Baudelocque, a French obstetrician, in 1823. Although this incision has been championed by a number of authors, it has been less popular in the United States than the low midline incision. The critics of this approach emphasize the longer time required for entry into the abdomen as well as the increased amount of bleeding that occurs from dissecting the fat from the rectus fascia. In addition, exposure is somewhat less than that with a midline incision as the margins are limited by the lateral pelvic walls; consequently, it is not advised for large pelvic tumors.

The advantages cited for the transverse incisions include the well-known fact that incisional hernias are rare, while much more frequent in vertical incisions. This fact is undoubtedly the strongest point in favor of the transverse incision, but it also has a cosmetic advantage, with the scar hidden near the margin of the pubic hairline and a reported increase in postoperative comfort for the patient. It is contradicted in cases in which only light anesthesia can be used with poor muscle relaxation, as well as for the removal of large pelvic tumors. In the event that bowel surgery is contemplated, the transverse incision limits access to the upper abdomen and interferes with the location of the colostomy site.

Pfannenstiel Incision. The original Pfannenstiel incision is described as a transverse incision which is slightly curved (concavity upwards) and may be made at any level suitable to the surgeon. It is usually 10 to 15 cm. in length and extends through the skin and subcutaneous fat to the level of the rectus sheath. The rectus sheath is incised transversely on either side of the linea alba, which is cut separately, joining the two lateral incisions. The rectus sheath is manually separated from the underlying muscle by inserting the fingers on either side of the cut edge of the rectus sheath and pulling the fascia in opposite directions with one hand toward the head and the other hand toward the feet. This maneuver should free the sheath from the anterior surface of the rectus muscle as far as desired. The rectus muscles are separated in the midline, and the peritoneal cavity is entered. This procedure avoids the necessity of dissecting the subcutaneous fat away from the anterior rectus sheath, as is done in the modified Pfannenstiel incision.

THE MODIFIED PFANNENSTIEL INCISION is shown in Figure 7-2. The slightly curved transverse incision begins at the level of the anterior superior iliac spine and extends just below the pubic hairline, through subcutaneous fat, down to the aponeurosis of the external oblique muscle and the anterior sheath of the recti. The superficial inferior epigastric vessels may be encountered at the lateral margin of the incision and are ligated. The fascia is cleaned upwards and downwards until a sufficient area is exposed to the region of the umbilicus and symphysis to permit a longitudinal incision in the linea alba (Fig. 7-2 B). Separation of rectus muscles and entrance into the peritoneum is made in the ordinary midline incision. Because of the importance of obtaining adequate hemostasis in the attached subcutaneous fat of the skin flaps, the modified procedure is definitely more time-consuming than the low midline incision or the original Pfannenstiel incision, which incises the fascia transversely.

Transverse Muscle-Cutting Incision. The limitation of operative exposure encountered with the Pfannenstiel incision can be overcome by utilizing the transverse muscle-cutting incision as advo-

FIG. 7-2. Modified Pfannenstiel incision. (A) Skin incision just below hairline. (B) Midline incision has been made through fascia, exposing rectus and pyramidalis muscles.

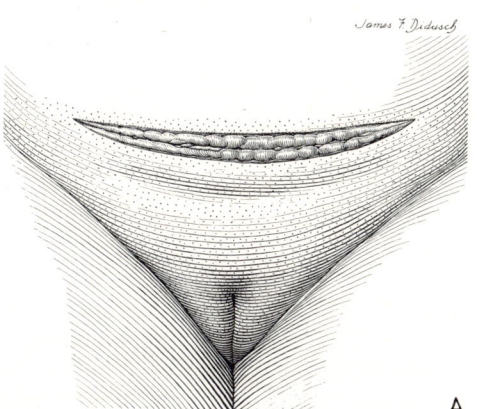

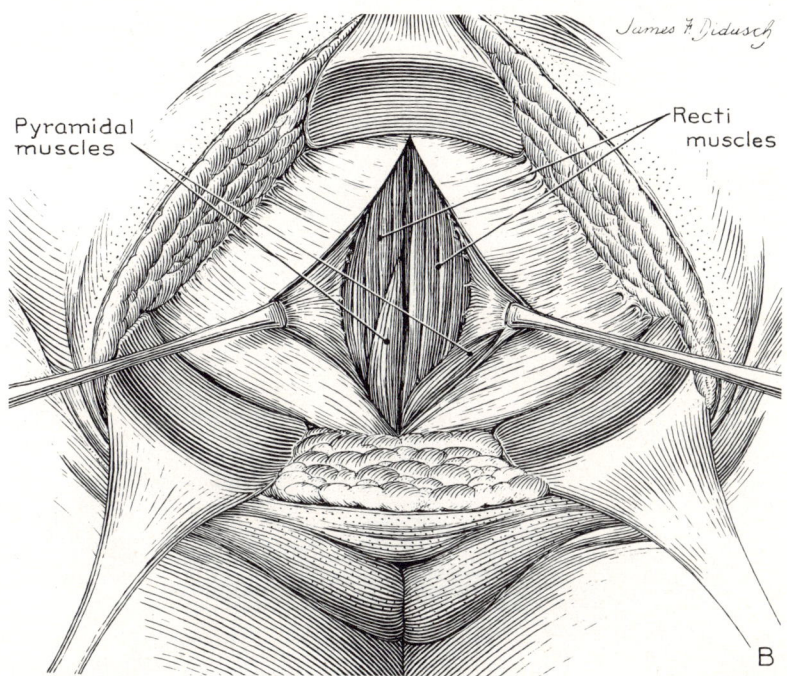

cated by Maylard. By cutting the rectus and abdominal muscles transversely, excellent exposure is obtained for any type of procedure. The incision is illustrated in Figure 7-3 and requires identification and ligation of the inferior epigastric vessels to avoid retraction and hematoma formations in the incision. Anatomically, this incision produces the least injury to the nerves and blood vessels which enter the abdominal muscles in the same direction as the incision; consequently, it does not cut across nerve endings or devitalize segments of the abdominal wall, as occurs in the right and left rectus incisions. In closing the incision it is preferable to include the fascia with the muscle stitch since the sutures will pull through muscle tissue when closed separately. No. 1 chromic catgut is used for this closure. While this incision produces a firm scar, its major disadvantage is the time required for incising and reapproximating the abdominal muscles.

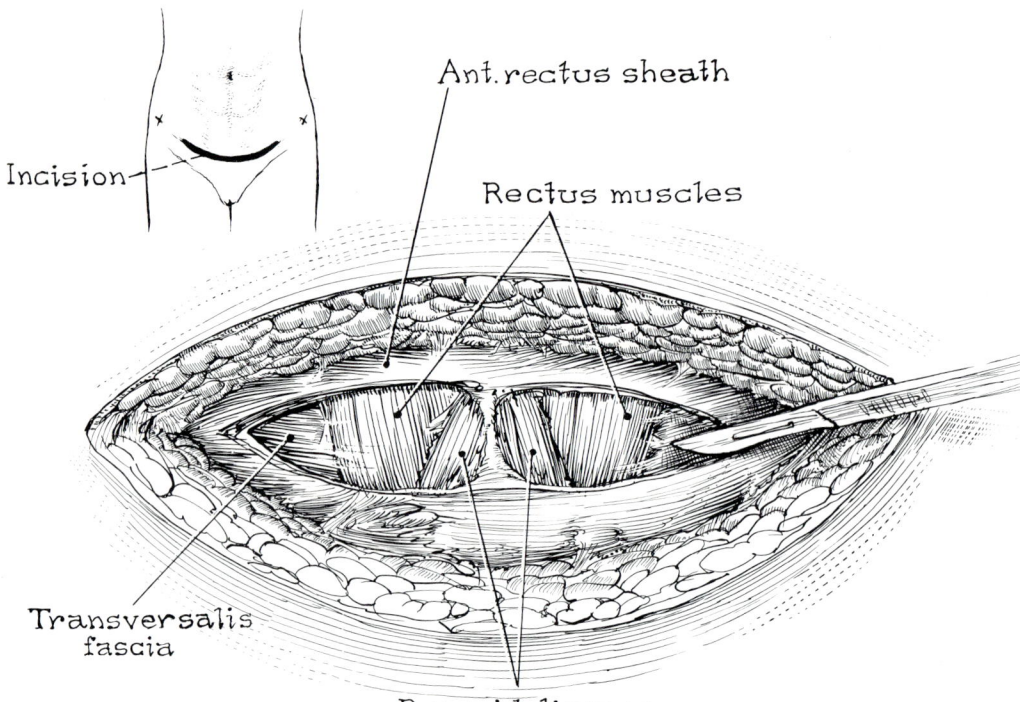
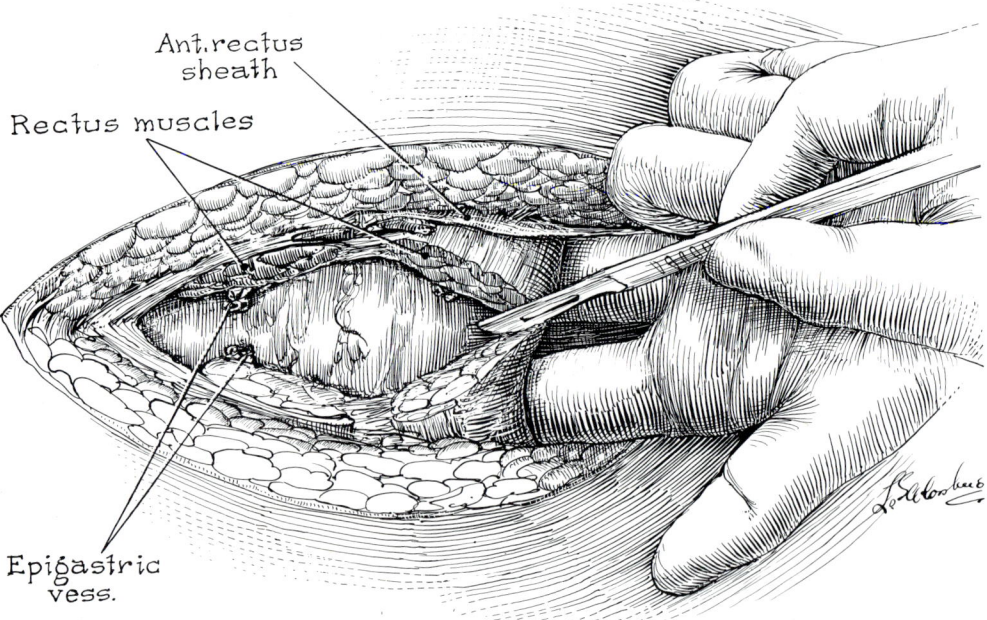

Fig. 7-3. (*Top*) Transverse muscle-cutting incision. The inset shows the incision which may be carried as far laterally as desired. The fascia is cut transversely, exposing the rectus and the pyramidalis muscles. (*Bottom*) The rectus muscles are cut transversely. The deep epigastric vessels are ligated and cut. Transversalis fascia is exposed.

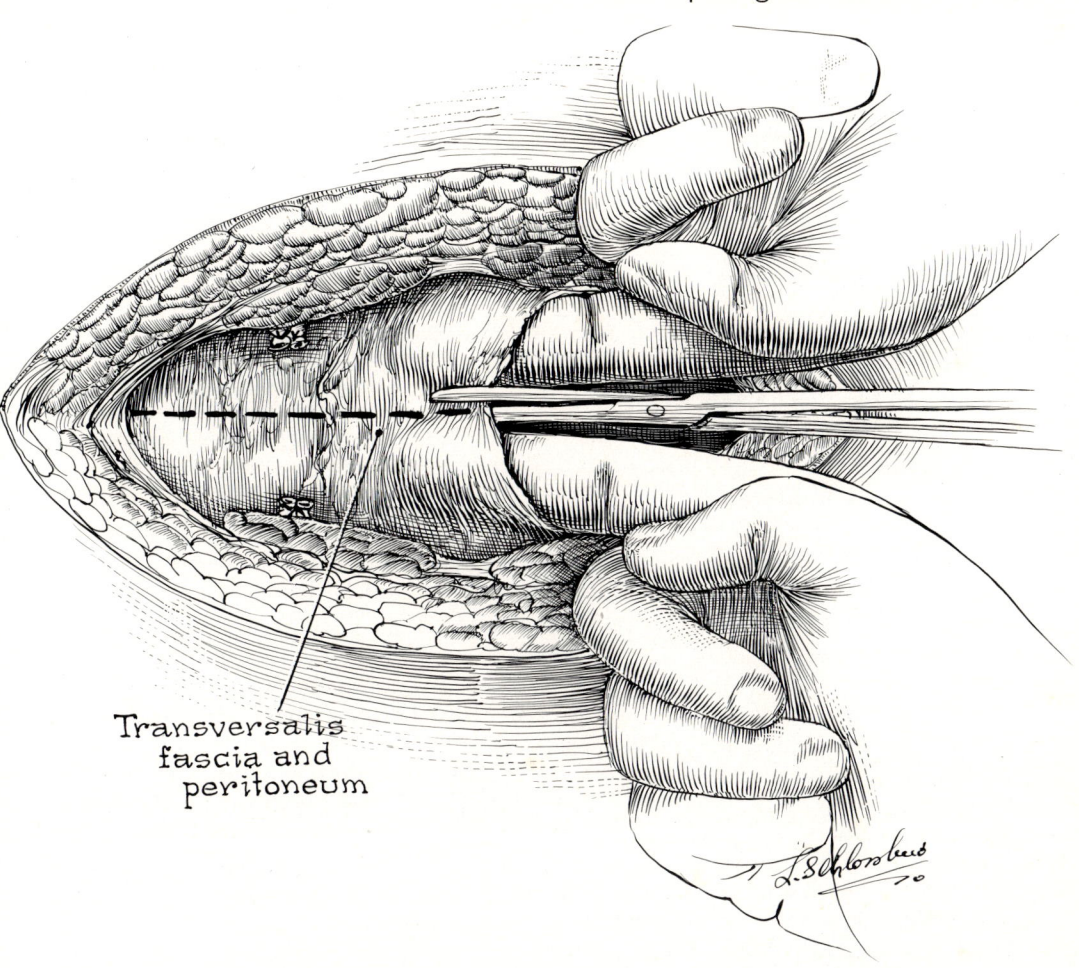

Fig. 7-3 (*Continued*). The transversalis fascia and peritoneum are cut transversely.

Gridiron (Muscle-Splitting) Incision

The gridiron incision is our choice for appendectomy and may be used for extraperitoneal drainage of broad ligament abscesses from pelvic inflammatory disease. In such cases, when drainage becomes necessary for an indolent broad ligament abscess that does not point into the cul-de-sac, drainage through a gridiron incision is most effective. The incision is made as for an appendectomy except that it is made a little lower, and the peritoneal cavity is not entered. Similarly, should drainage of the pelvis be required during a pelvic laparotomy, we prefer to avoid drainage through a midline incision and use a small gridiron (stab wound) incision in placing cigarette drains in the pelvis. In treating large tubo-ovarian abscesses, which extend high out of the pelvis and do not respond to chemotherapy or diathermy, such a "frozen" pelvis may require drainlarge. Abdominal drainage of such an abscess through a muscle-splitting incision made directly over the abscess permits entrance into the center of the abscess without soiling the general peritoneal cavity. This procedure may be followed

132 Opening and Closing the Abdomen

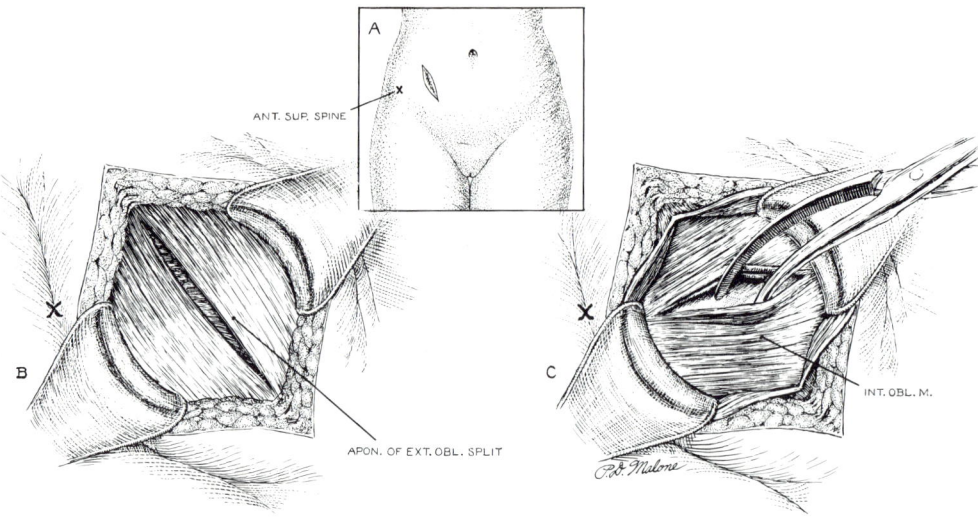

FIG. 7-4. Gridiron incision, opening. (A) Position of incision. (B) Aponeurosis of external oblique has been split. (C) Internal oblique muscles being split with Kelly clamp.

by a pelvic laparotomy several weeks after the pelvic inflammatory disease has subsided, depending on the patient's symptoms.

The gridiron incision is made obliquely downward and inward over McBurney's point (Fig. 7-4 A). Variations in the location of the incision may be made when it is done for appendectomy during pregnancy or when it is used for abscess drainage, as mentioned above. The incision is carried down through the skin and subcutaneous fat to the external oblique aponeurosis. The fibers of the aponeurosis are separated in the direction in which they run (Fig. 7-4 B). The internal oblique fibers and those of the transverse abdominis are separated in the line of their fibers (Fig. 7-4 C). At this point the internal oblique fibers and the transversus abdominis course in the same direction, and no attempt is made to separate the internal oblique layer from the transversus. The retractors are placed to retract these muscles, and the preperitoneal fat is exposed. This is incised, and the peritoneal cavity is entered. The cecum lies very close to the peritoneum at this point, and more care must be taken to avoid injury of the bowel here than in the midline.

CLOSING THE ABDOMEN

After completion of the pelvic operation the sigmoid is thrown over the field of pelvic operation to prevent the small

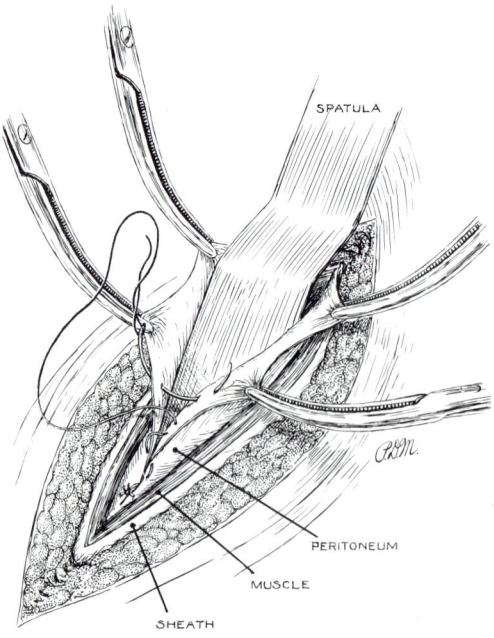

FIG. 7-5. Demonstrating method of closure of peritoneum which results in everted peritoneal edges.

intestines from becoming adherent to the recently traumatized operative field. The omentum is drawn down over the viscera, and the peritoneum is closed.

Midline Incision

In closing the midline incision the peritoneal closure is begun at the upper end; both the peritoneum and the posterior sheath of the rectus muscles are sutured together with a continuous suture of No. 00 plain catgut. Nonchromatized catgut is used on the peritoneum because it is more pliable, there is less tissue reaction, and possibly there is less adhesion formation. The stitch used should evert the cut peritoneal edges to make the intraperitoneal suture line as smooth as possible (Fig. 7-5). To improve the exposure of the peritoneal edge, the peritoneum is grasped with Kelly clamps which exteriorize the edges for the operator to suture. If the intestines should interfere with the closure, they may be retracted with a malleable spatula, or, if great difficulty is experienced, a Mikulicz pad may be inserted over the intestines and withdrawn just before completion of the closure. The senior author routinely places 2 or 3 tension sutures of braided silk (Fig. 7-6 A). These silk sutures pass through the skin, fat, and anterior rectus sheath, but, to prevent bleeding, they avoid the muscles (Fig. 7-6 B). Small pieces of fine rubber tubing are placed on each suture to prevent cutting of the skin by the sutures when tied (Fig. 7-6 C).

It is important to qualify our routine use of tension sutures as we ordinarily tie them loosely enough to permit 1 or 2 fingers to pass beneath the suture and the skin. They are used primarily to hold the incision together in the event of abdominal distention. Constricting tension sutures can impair circulation to the incision and produce local ischemia,

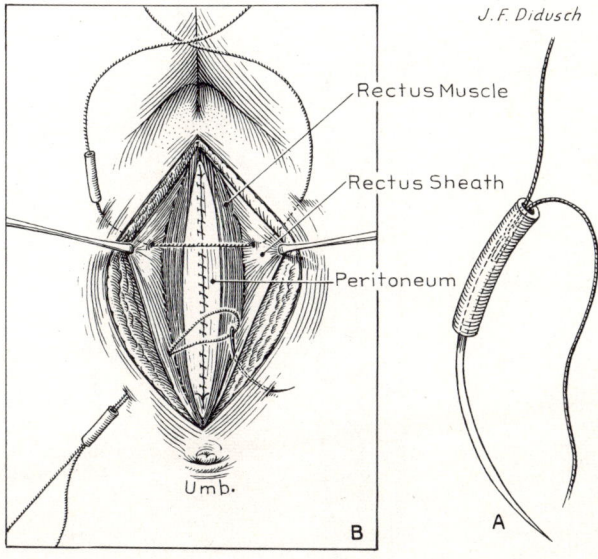

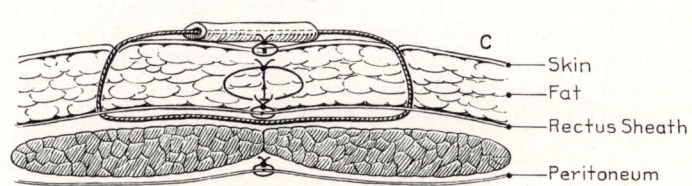

Fig. 7-6. Method of placing tension sutures. (A) Long cutting needle threaded with braided silk and shod with rubber tubing. (B) Method of placing sutures through skin, fat and fascia. (C) Layer-for-layer closure of abdomen and position of tension suture.

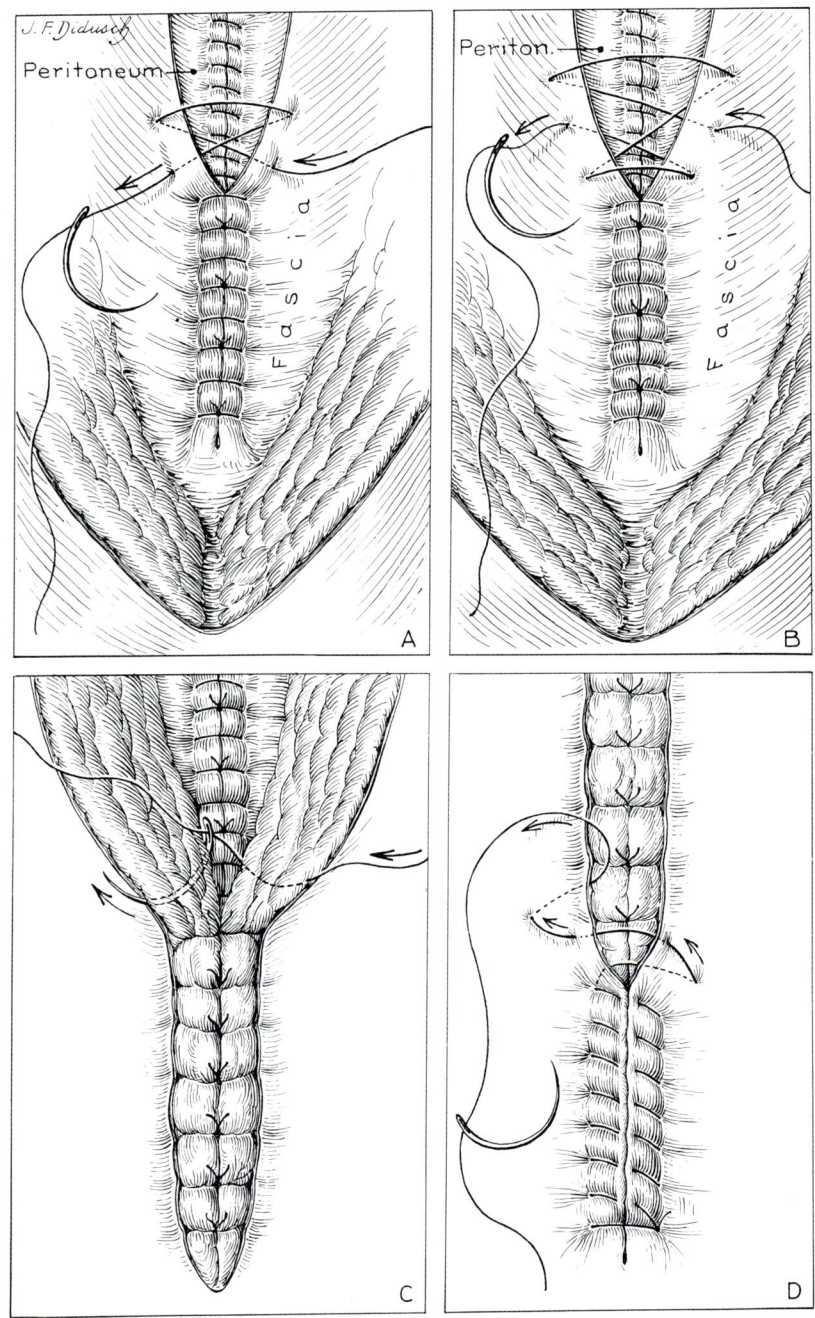

FIG. 7-7. Layer-for-layer closure of abdomen. (A) The peritoneum has been closed with a continuous catgut suture. The fascia is being closed with horizontal figure-of-eight sutures. (B) Double horizontal figure-of-eight suture. (C) Fat is approximated with interrupted sutures of fine catgut. (D) Skin is approximated with a continuous on-end mattress suture of fine silk.

Closing the Abdomen   135

which may result in poor healing. Healing of the incision is more effective when the skin edges fall together without tension and without undue pressure from deep tension sutures.

The muscles are not sutured together in the midline incision unless there is sufficient diastasis to cause symptoms. In that case a special closure is used similar to a ventral hernia repair. In the routine closure fascia edges are approximated with single or double horizontal figure-of-eight sutures of No. 1 chromic catgut. If speed is essential because of the condition of the patient, closure can be done more quickly with the double figure-of-eight stitch than with the single. These stitches are shown in Figure 7-7.

After closure of the fascia, the subcutaneous fat is approximated with interrupted sutures of No. 000 chromic catgut, and the skin is closed with silk in the stitch preferred by the operator (Fig. 7-8). Figure 7-8 A demonstrates skin closure with a continuous on-end mattress suture. This favorite skin suture of ours requires a little more time than the simple continuous suture, but it makes an excellent closure and is particularly useful when one is dealing with the lax skin of a parous woman, since it prevents inversion. Figure 7-8 B shows a horizontal mattress stitch. Figure 7-8 C shows the method of closing the skin with a lock stitch. We prefer the lock stitch when hemostasis is desired because of bleeders in the skin which are too superficial to lend themselves to buried ligatures and are usually controlled by pressure on the skin margins. The lock stitch also has the

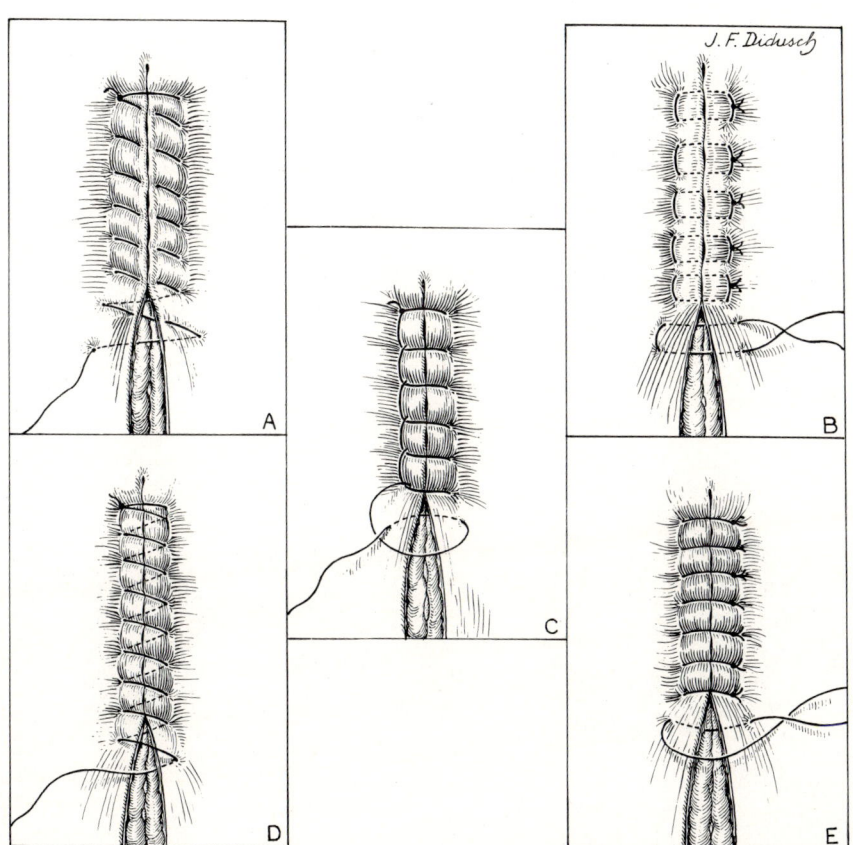

Fig. 7-8. Skin sutures (silk). (A) Continuous on-end mattress suture. (B) Interrupted mattress sutures. (C) Lock suture. (D) Plain continuous suture. (E) Plain interrupted sutures.

advantage of being removed easily. Figure 7-8 D demonstrates the continuous suture, which is quite satisfactory when the texture of the skin is firm. Figure 7-8 E demonstrates the simple interrupted stitch. The interrupted stitches, particularly the vertical mattress, are placed with straight Keith needles instead of the usual skin needle. They make an ideal skin closure although they are more time-consuming than the continuous suture.

TRANSVERSE INCISION

In closing the original Pfannenstiel incision, the peritoneum and rectus fascia are closed separately, as in the midline incision, but tension sutures are not used. In closing the modified Pfannenstiel incision, special attention must be directed toward obliterating the dead space by anchoring the subcutaneous fat to the underlying fascia with sutures of No. 000 chromic catgut. Additional sutures of No. 000 chromic catgut are used to approximate the opposing margins of subcutaneous fat. Occasionally, the skin margins are closed with a subcuticular suture of No. 0 plain catgut.

The transverse muscle-splitting incision is closed by suturing the peritoneum transversely and approximating the abdominal wall muscle with horizontal figure-of-eight sutures that incorporate both fascia and muscle in the stitch. A separate layer of fascia stitches is placed for reinforcement of the muscle closure even though the incision is anatomically stronger than a midline incision. Contraction of the oblique muscles of the abdomen or strain on the incision tends to draw the muscles and aponeurosis edges tighter together. The edges of the subcutaneous fat are approximated with No. 000 chromic catgut, with the skin closure according to the preference of the surgeon.

GRIDIRON INCISION

The gridiron incision may be closed with lighter catgut than the midline incision since there is less strain on the suture line. Similar to the transverse incision, tension on the incision from contraction of the abdominal muscles tends to draw the edges of the muscle and fascia closer together. The peritoneum is closed with a continuous suture of No. 00 plain catgut. The internal oblique and the transversus abdominis are closed as a single layer with horizontal figure-of-eight mattress sutures of No. 0 chromic catgut (Fig. 7-9 A). The fibers of the aponeurosis of the external oblique are closed with a continuous suture of No. 0 chromic catgut (Fig. 7-9 B). The fat and

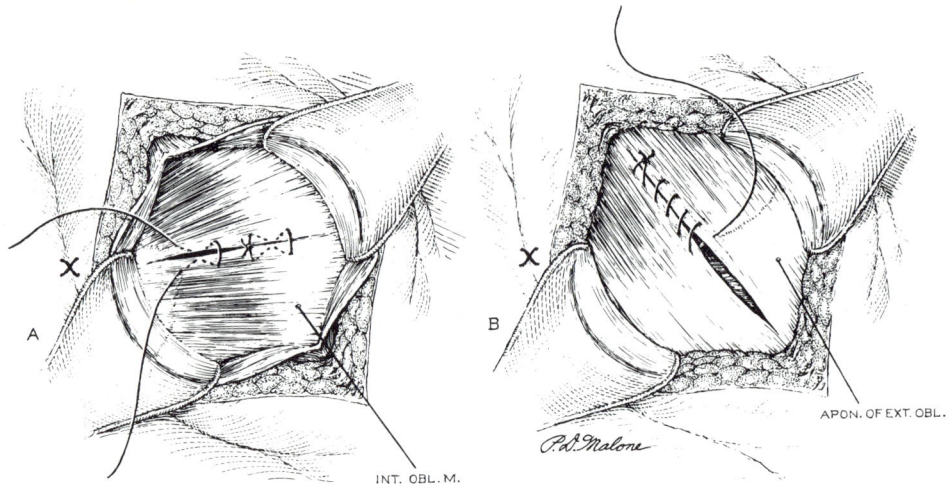

FIG. 7-9. Gridiron incision, closing. (A) Internal oblique fibers approximated with figure-of-eight sutures of No. 0 chromic catgut. (B) Aponeurosis of external oblique is closed with continuous sutures of No. 0 chromic catgut.

the skin are closed as usual. We usually close the skin of this incision with interrupted sutures of fine silk, by which a beautiful approximation can be obtained.

COMPLICATIONS

The major early complications of abdominal wall incisions are wound infections and dehiscence or evisceration. Incisional hernias are a late complication and are omitted from the present discussion.

WOUND INFECTION

The frequency of postoperative wound infections varies from one clinic to another and is related to many factors, including the experience of the surgeon, the type of procedure performed, the clinic population operated upon, and the surgical condition of the patient. At Bellevue Hospital, Douglas noted that wound infections were responsible for 38 per cent of the major postoperative infections. While this rate is admittedly above the usual 5 to 10 per cent, it demonstrates the result of operating on indigent patients with a high rate of pelvic inflammatory disease.

The most frequent cause of wound infection is probably the direct implantation of bacteria at the operating table. Although sterile supplies may possibly be a factor in surgical contamination, it is indeed a rare cause of postoperative infection. More commonly, an inoculum of bacteria reaches the incision from either the skin of the patient or from the skin of the operator. During a recent study at Barnes Hospital at Washington University, Bernard and Cole determined that 20 to 40 per cent of all surgical gloves are punctured during the course of an average operation, and that such a puncture site could contaminate the wound with 4,000 to 18,000 staphylococci in 20 minutes. Many studies are in agreement with the findings of Price that 5 to 40 per cent of surgeons scrubbing with hexachlorophene-containing compounds actually shed more bacteria on a fingertip impression plate culture after the scrub had been completed than they did prior to the scrub. Consequently, newer antiseptic scrubs have been developed, including iodine-containing compounds which are quite effective against the most resistant organisms.

More importantly, the most frequent site of infection is the patient's skin since many studies have demonstrated that the patient's own skin is a carrier of *Staphylococcus aureus* and coliform bacteria into and out of the operating room, regardless of the surgical preparations. Preoperative scrubbing of the patient's skin the night before surgery with an iodine-containing compound, with a proven decrease in the bacterial count of the skin, has greatly reduced the frequency of postoperative infection in many clinics operating primarily on charity patients. At operation the skin of the patient is inadequately isolated from the incision with skin towels or plastic drapes, although the latter technic is considered to be more effective than loose skin towels.

In addition, although fewer than 5 per cent of the surgical personnel were found to be persistent skin carriers of *Staphylococcus aureus,* 28 per cent of the surgeons in the Barnes Hospital study carried *Staphylococcus aureus* on their hands at least once after their surgical scrub with hexachlorophene-containing compounds. When the surgeon's gown is saturated with blood or serum, there is direct contamination of the operative site with the bacteria from the operator's skin.

Airborne bacterial contamination is an unlikely source of significant wound contamination leading to postoperative infection, provided that the operating room is kept in a reasonably hygienic state by proper housekeeping technics. The use of proper air filtration with approximately 20 air changes per hour, the maintenance of relative humidity between 50 and 55 per cent, and a reduction of human occupants in the operating room have greatly reduced the possibility of the external environment being a source of operative infection. Whenever a bacterial-containing organ is opened, mainly the bowel, gallbladder, or urinary tract, there is a marked increase in the infection rate of the incision.

Frequently, small areas of infection occur in low midline incisions, particularly at the lower end of the incision, where the hair follicles may harbor bacteria which are not sterilized by the surgical scrub. Such cases are benefited by the scrubbing of the abdomen for 20 minutes the evening before surgery. The number of such infections vary directly with the obesity of the patient. An incision through a large panniculus is a favorite place for bacteria to multiply. The fact that folds in the skin, moistened by perspiration, harbor more bacteria than the dry skin is the basis of the current rationale used by many surgeons for leaving the incision exposed postoperatively. When the operative procedure has been unusually long, and particularly when the abdominal wall is obese, the incision should be thoroughly irrigated with saline prior to closure of the subcutaneous tissues in order to make certain that a hematoma is not overlooked in the operative site. Prophylactic antibiotics are useful in controlling wound infections when infection has been encountered in the pelvis, particularly when a stab wound is required for drainage.

Coliform bacilli, particularly *E. coli* and *A. aerogenes,* are the most frequent contaminants of the incision in postoperative patients, along with *Staphylococcus aureus*. Isolation technics for linen, clothing, and dressings are employed, primarily for *Staphylococcus aureus* coagulase-positive infections, since most of the other infections are initiated in the operating room and not in the postoperative healing period.

Clinically, the wound may show evidence of infection almost immediately after operation. In the majority of cases, however, the wound infection develops to the stage of clinical recognition within 5 to 6 days postoperatively. Usually the temperature remains slightly elevated, and the patient may frequently complain of tenderness in the incisional area, although this symptom is not consistently present. In most instances the wound infection is discovered in a routine search for the cause of a temperature elevation and is noted by the presence of reddening of the skin with fluctuation or induration of the subcutaneous tissues.

In general, the wound is not opened until it is somewhat fluctuant, at which time wide drainage and evacuation of the abscess is usually associated with clinical improvement in the temperature and the symptoms. The wound should be cultured and bacterial sensitivities obtained in order to treat the patient with appropriate antibiotics. The wound is cleaned daily with hydrogen peroxide, and occasionally antibiotic solutions of bacitracin (500 U./cc.) or Wynn's solution (1 gm. Chloromycetin, 1 gm. neomycin sulfate, 50 mg. polymyxin B dissolved in 1,000 cc. isotonic saline solution) are used to irrigate the wound. There have been good reports with the use of streptokinase-streptodornase enzymatic débridement, although we have not personally used this method. Hot compresses are used if there is considerable induration of the adjacent tissue, as it is the authors' opinion that moist heat is superior to dry heat in aiding evacuation of the abscessed cavity. The incisional cavity should be stimulated to granulate from the base upward by the use of iodoform wick, urea crystals, and the like. After healing has been initiated, the skin edges may be drawn together by narrow strips of sterile adhesive tape, or, if necessary, secondary closure may be required.

Wound Dehiscence and Evisceration

In the broadest sense, the term *dehiscence* includes the separation of any of the suture layers of the abdominal wall, although it is frequently used synonymously with the terms *evisceration, wound disruption* and *burst abdomen*. In the latter definitions the implication includes disruption of all layers of the abdominal wall and protrusion of the intestines through the incision.

Complete disruption and evisceration is one of the most serious of all wound complications, and at Massachusetts General Hospital it is accompanied by a mortality rate of 15 per cent, whereas others report rates from 11 to 50 per cent. The frequency of actual dehiscence and evisceration varies considerably in the surgical literature, and was found to be 0.26 per cent by Hull and Hankins or 5 of 1,810 gynecologic operations. Tweedie and Long reported an incidence of 0.71 per cent of 5,166 gynecologic incisions and 0.14 per cent of 1,434 caesarean section incisions in comparison to an incidence of dehiscence of 0.47 per cent in general surgical cases. In a recent report from the Mayo Clinic, the incidence of dehiscence after gynecologic operations was 1 in 500 cases or 0.2 per cent. As noted by Rollins et al. in patients with serious wound complications, approximately 50 per cent had had prior abdominal and/or pelvic surgery. In all series the largest percentage of incisions was low midline or paramedian, with a very rare disruption of a transverse incision.

Etiologic Factors

The various reported factors associated with wound dehiscence may be summarized in four general categories: (1) the type and location of the incision, (2) the specific type of suture, (3) the inherent strength of the tissues, and (4) mechanical factors.

The importance of the type of incision has been previously discussed. It is well recognized that low midline incisions have a higher rate of wound dehiscence than transverse or gridiron incisions. In addition, the strength of the incision is inversely proportional to its length.

The choice of a permanent or absorbable suture in the closure of an incision has been long debated as a factor contributing to wound healing. However, a recent study of wound dehiscence at Massachusetts General Hospital is in agreement with Hampton and our experience that there is no greater instance of wound disruption in those cases in which the fascial closure was accomplished by nonabsorbable suture than in those cases in which chromic catgut was used. The amount of tension on the suture line is more important than the type of suture used in the fascial closure.

The inherent strength of the tissue has been related to various factors, including vitamin C deficiency, protein deficiency, anemia, wound infection, and the age of the patient. Unquestionably, major surgical wounds have a higher disruption rate in the elderly patient than in the young—a finding that has been observed by many surgeons. In addition, inflammation disrupts collagen deposition in a wound, with separation of tissue by the accumulation of purulent exudate. Such inflammatory response weakens the fascial suture line and produces necrosis of the absorbable suture in addition to allowing the permanent suture to pull through the fascial edge of the incision. As the inflammatory reaction spreads along the fascial plane, more of the suture line is involved, which process may result in fascial separation and wound dehiscence. Patients with a chronic disease, notably an advanced neoplasm, are known to have poor wound healing due to limitation of collagen deposition and fibroblastic activity. Surgery through a previous operative site is known to produce a weaker scar due to limitation of blood supply and diminished fibroblastic activity. Obesity is a common feature in most reports of wound disruption, and is related to the amount of tension on the suture line. There is also an increased frequency of wound infection in such patients with a large panniculus. The thickness of the subcutaneous fat layer undoubtedly has a direct bearing on wound infection and failure of healing. Hematoma formation in the incision is a frequent cause of poor healing and produces an excellent nidus for sepsis. It is frequently associated with wound disruption and evisceration and is one of the preventable factors in such complications.

One of the most striking findings of most large series of wound dehiscence is the association of mechanical factors, including pulmonary complications and abdominal distention. In the study by Guiney and associates, 87 per cent of their cases experienced one or more of such complications in contrast to a 15

140 Opening and Closing the Abdomen

per cent occurrence in a control group. Excessive vomiting and coughing, abdominal distention, and hiccups have been implicated as causative factors in increasing tension on the suture line. In such cases we feel strongly that the use of tension sutures will support the suture line, where there is increased tension and strain. These tension sutures are of special value when such symptoms continue for a prolonged period of time. Without question, the use of tension sutures is a definite asset in wound healing and has played a role in maintaining our very low incidence of wound disruption (0.1%).

Diagnosis

It is important that early recognition and prompt treatment be accomplished to facilitate the chances of recovery since the mortality rate in reported series varies between 10 and 50 per cent. It is true that some eviscerations occur entirely

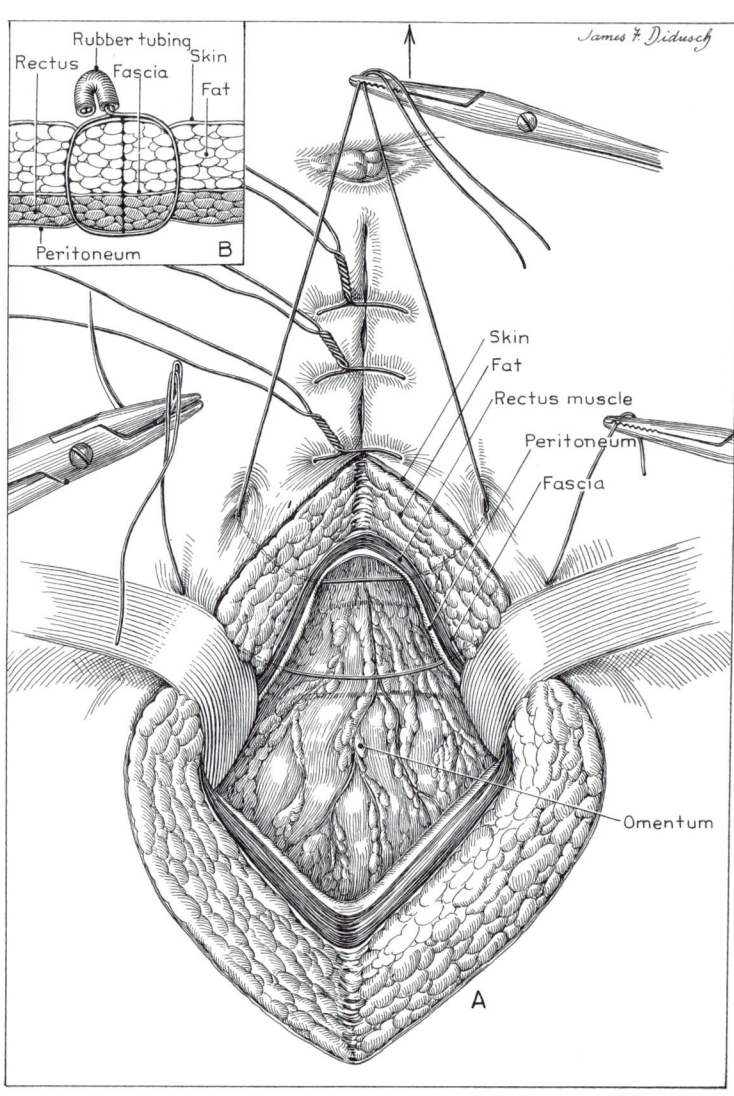

Fig. 7-10. Secondary closure of disrupted wound with through-and-through silver-wire sutures. (A) Method of closure. (B) Showing suture twisted tight and approximating the wound edges.

without symptoms and are discovered on routine inspection of the incision. However, the majority of cases present symptoms and signs which at least call for investigation. Sometimes the patient is conscious of something "giving away." One of the most common signs, in our experience, is the presence of a serosanguineous drainage from the incision, which should alert the astute clinician to the possibility of an impending evisceration. This finding was present in approximately two thirds of the cases of evisceration reported by Wolff. When this occurs in the presence of abdominal discomfort in the region of the incision, disruption should be strongly suspected. When the evisceration is discovered, a sterile towel should be placed over the incision and a tight adhesive bandage applied for temporary control of the protruding bowel through the incisional site.

TREATMENT

Immediate suturing is indicated. Due to the fact that this complication may be life-threatening, delay in secondary closure is not recommended since the patient's condition will not improve until the incision is reapproximated, as demonstrated in Figure 7-10. Secondary closure after evisceration is best accomplished by through-and-through suture of an inert material, preferably silver wire sutures. Prior to closure, the wound should be cleansed thoroughly at the operating table under general anesthesia, and gentle débridement should be accomplished where needed. The intestines are manipulated as little as possible in replacing them into the peritoneal cavity. The wound is cultured, and bacterial sensitivities are obtained. The silver wire sutures are placed through the entire thickness of the abdominal wall, including the peritoneum, as demonstrated in Figure 7-10 B. The statistics show that the percentage of recovery is greater with this technic than when layer-for-layer closure is attempted. We have found fairly heavy silver wire to be the suture material of choice. After inserting the silver wires, these are held up with clamps but are not twisted closed before all the sutures are placed. This precaution pulls the abdominal wall away from the viscera and guards against injury to the bowel. The silver wire sutures are placed about 1 inch apart. When the sutures are closed by twisting, the skin is fairly well approximated, but if more careful approximation is desirable, interrupted silk sutures may be placed between the silver wires. The wires may be loosened gradually on the ward when the wound swells.

A broad-spectrum antibiotic is initiated and adjusted according to the bacteriology report. Postoperatively, the patient is treated with a nasogastric tube for decompression of the bowel, and intravenous fluid replacement is maintained until bowel function returns and oral feedings are well tolerated. The silver wire sutures are left in place until healing appears to be complete, which usually requires approximately 14 to 21 days. We frequently discharge the patient to her home and remove the sutures sometime later when healing is complete.

BIBLIOGRAPHY

Alexander, H. C., and Prudden, J. F.: The causes of abdominal wound disruption. Surg. Gynec. Obstet., 122:1223, 1966.

Bernard, H. R., and Cole, W. R.: The epidemiology of postoperative surgical infection. Surg. Clin. N. Amer., 45:509, 1965.

Cherney, L. S.: A modified transverse incision for low abdominal operations. Surg. Gynec. Obstet., 72:92, 1941.

Cole, W. R., and Bernard, H. R.: Inadequacies of present methods of surgical skin preparation. Arch. Surg., 89:215, 1964.

Daly, J. W., and Rutledge, F.: Experience with wound dehiscence in patients treated for pelvic malignancies. Southern Med. J., 58:308, 1965.

DeVito, R. V.: Healing of wounds. Surg. Clin. N. Amer., 45:441, 1965.

Douglas, G. W.: Postoperative infections. Clin. Obstet. Gynec., 5:501, 1962.

Emmett, J. M., and Cole, F. N., Jr.: Wound disruptions. Virginia Med. Monthly 86:567, 1959.

Everett, H. S., and Mattingly, R. F.: Urinary tract injuries resulting from pelvic surgery. Amer. J. Obstet. Gynec., 71:502, 1956.

Gall, R. J.: Transverse lower abdominal incision in obstetrics and gynecology. Aust. New Zeal. J. Obstet. Gynaec., 5:94, 1965.

Guiney, E. J., Morris, P. J., and Donaldson, G. A.: Wound dehiscence. Arch Surg., 92:47, 1966.

Hampton, J. R.: The burst abdomen. Brit. Med. J., 2:1032, 1963.

Hull, H. C., and Hankins, J. R.: Disruption of abdominal wounds. Amer. Surg., 21:223, 1955.

Hunter, G. W.: Transverse abdominal incisions in pelvic surgery; report of 700 cases. Am. J. Obstet. Gynec., 39:593, 1940.

Keeley, J. L., and Schairer, A. E.: Mechanical methods of improving exposure in abdominal operations. Surg. Clin. N. Amer., 48:91, 1968.

Maylard, A. E.: Direction of abdominal incisions. Brit. Med. J., 2:895, 1907.

Palumbo, L. T., Smith, A. N., and Lulu, D. J.: Nonsuture closure of clean muscle-splitting abdominal wounds; preliminary report of 117 wounds. Surgery, 41:986, 1957.

Pfannenstiel, H. J.: Ueber die Vortheile des suprasymphysären Fascienguerschnitt fur die gynäkologischen Koeliotomien. Samml. klin Vortr, Gyn., Leipzig, n.F., Nr. 268 (Gynäk Nr. 97):1735, 1900.

Price, P. B.: Fallacy of current surgical fad — 3 minute preparation scrub with hexachlorophene soap. Ann. Surg., 134:476, 1951.

Rollins, R. A., Corcoran, J. J., and Gibbs, C. E.: Treatment of gynecologic wound complications. Obstet. Gynec., 28:268, 1966.

Souders, J. C., and Pratt, J. H.: Wound dehiscence and incisional hernia after gynecologic operations. Clin. Obstet. Gynec., 5:522, 1962.

Tweedie, F. J., and Long, R. C.: Abdominal wound disruptions. Surg. Gynec. Obstet., 99:41, 1954.

Wolff, W. I.: Disruption of abdominal wounds. Ann. Surg., 131:534, 1950.

8

Myomata Uteri

GENERAL CONSIDERATIONS

Myomata uteri are the commonest tumors of the uterus, and the commonest of the female pelvis. It is impossible to determine with accuracy the incidence of fibroids in women. The incidence, frequently quoted, of 1 in 5 found at postmortem examinations seems to be too small on the basis of the authors' experience. Certainly in the colored race the incidence is much greater than that. Fibroids occur chiefly during the latter half of the menstrual life, but their occurrence earlier is not uncommon. In the colored race they are commonly seen before 30. Their growth is dependent upon estrogen, and after the cessation of estrogen secretion at the menopause atrophy is the almost invariable rule. In rare instances a fibroid grows after the menopause. When this occurs, one should think first of the possibility of malignant change.

There are rare instances, however, of postmenopausal growth of benign fibroids. This may suggest the possibility of postmenopausal estrogen formation, either in the ovary or elsewhere. In two such instances the senior author has found lutein-like cells distributed through the postmenopausal ovarian stroma, suggesting that the estrogen had been formed there. Further evidence of the relation of estrogen to fibroid growth is the fact that small fibroids have been produced artifically on the serous surfaces of the uteri of guinea pigs by estrogen injections.

The proper treatment of fibroids is not as simple as one might judge when one sees a constant succession of hysterectomies for fibroids in almost any gynecologic operating room. In order to treat fibroids properly, their growth characteristics should be known to the surgeon. They may occur singly, but the vast majority are multiple. They arise in the fibromuscular tissue of the myometrium, and histologically they are fibromyomata. There is great variation in the relative amount of fibrous and muscular tissue, but on the whole smooth muscle exceeds fibrous tissue. Since they arise in the myometrium, they are all, at the onset, interstitial. As they enlarge, they may remain interstitial, but often the growth extends internally or externally, becoming submucous or subserous. In either position they may become pedunculated. The subserous tumors not infrequently become adherent to other structures, especially the omentum. They then obtain some of their blood supply from the omentum and in some cases all of it, as the uterine pedicle disappears completely.

The typical fibroid uterus is a firm multinodular structure of variable size. The largest observed by the authors was 40 pounds, but much larger ones have been reported. Tumors of 8 to 10 pounds are not rare, especially in the colored race, but most are much smaller. At the operating table they appear as nodular tumors of different sizes which distort the uterus in various ways, depending upon their size and direction of growth.

Growth between the leaves of the broad ligament may make surgical removal difficult.

It is an excellent practice to have an assistant open the uterine cavity of all myomatous uteri in the operating room directly after their removal. The endometrium should be inspected in a search for incidental endometrial cancer. In addition to opening the uterine cavity, the larger fibroid nodules should be cut into. In order to interpret the findings at such an examination, the surgeon should be familiar with the various gross changes that take place in fibroids. The normal fibroid, on section, appears pinkish white and glistening. It is firm, and there is a whorl-like arrangement of the muscle and the fibrous tissue. The commonest change is hyaline degeneration. The cut surface of a hyalinized area is smooth and homogeneous and does not show the whorl-like arrangement of the rest of the fibroid. Almost all fibroids, except the smallest, have scattered areas of hyaline degeneration. Eventually, these may become liquefied and form cystic cavities filled with clear liquid or gelatinous material. Sometimes the cystic change is so great that the fibroid becomes a mere shell and is a truly cystic tumor. When such tumors cause symmetrical enlargement of the uterus, they may be taken for a pregnant uterus on bimanual examination; when subserous and pedunculated, they may easily be confused with ovarian cysts. However, softness of a tumor does not necessarily indicate cystic degeneration. Fleshy myomata may be equally soft.

Fibroids may undergo changes due to infection, and in patients in whom salpingitis commonly complicates fibroids, an extension of the infection into the tumor from without is common. Microscopic abscesses are frequently found, and gross abscesses occasionally occur in the tumors. In addition to this route of infection, submucous fibroids may become infected within the uterine cavity or the vagina. The pedunculated submucous fibroid thins out the endometrium as it grows downward, and eventually the surface becomes ulcerated and infected. This is invariably true if the fibroid descends as low as the cervical canal. Such infections are usually due to the streptococcus and may be very virulent. Parametritis, peritonitis, and even septicemia may result.

Necrosis of a fibroid results from interference with the blood supply. Occasionally, a pedunculated subserous fibroid twists, and if operation is not done immediately, gangrene results. Interference with the blood supply of a tumor may also occur as a result of thrombosis of the blood vessels due to infection. Such thromboses are seen commonly in the pedicle of a necrotic submucous fibroid. Necrosis sometimes occurs in the center of a large tumor simply as a result of poor circulation. Necrotic fibroids are dark and hemorrhagic in the interior; eventually, the tissue breaks down completely. So-called red or carneous degeneration is seen occasionally, especially associated with pregnancy. The cause is unknown, but thromboses and extravasation of blood are responsible for the reddish discoloration.

On rare occasions fat occurs in fibroids as true fatty degeneration, to the extent of giving the cut surface a yellowish discoloration. Still more rarely is there a deposit of true fat forming a fibrolipoma

Finally, the most important change, sarcomatous degeneration, should be considered. Fortunately, it is rare. There is much variation in the reported incidence of sarcoma occurring in myomata. The incidence given by Evans of the Mayo Clinic is 0.7 per cent. Novak and Anderson found it in 0.56 per cent in our laboratory. A recent review of 13,000 myomas by Montague, Swartz, and Woodruff at Johns Hopkins during 1930–60, revealed 38 cases of malignant change, the incidence of sarcoma thus being 0.29 per cent.

Corscaden and Singh found the incidence of *lethal* sarcomatous change in fibroids to be 0.13 per cent or 1 in 800 cases. In the literature, however, a reported incidence up to 4 per cent can be found. The reason for the disparity in the statistics is understandable if one is familiar with the histology of fibroids.

Very cellular fibroids are relatively common, and at first glance they suggest sarcoma; however, they lack a significant number of mitotic figures, and patients from whom such tumors are removed all remain well. The misinterpretation of the histologic picture of this type of cellular fibroid undoubtedly accounts for the increased incidence reported by some. On cutting fibroids in the operating room, sarcomatous areas have a characteristic appearance. Sarcoma is apt to occur in rather large fibroids and toward the center of the tumors where the blood supply is poorest. Instead of the firm fibrous tissue which grates when scraped with a knife blade, the tissue is soft and homogeneous. Cullen has described it as simulating raw pork. Later, there is a necrosis of the malignant tissue, and it becomes friable and hemorrhagic.

The possibility of malignancy is, as indicated above, small. However, the consequences resulting from incomplete pelvic surgery when sarcoma is present are so serious that routine cutting of the tumor in the operating room is worth while. Novak and Anderson clearly demonstrated that complete surgery is the backbone of successful treatment. They found that 30 per cent of their traced cases were well 5 years after the operation; Kimbrough found 34 per cent of his series of patients were well after 5 years. Our most recent experience at Hopkins has been unusual, as noted by a total 3-year survival rate of 53 per cent. Hysterectomy with adnexectomy was the treatment of choice, while no therapeutic value was noted with postoperative irradiation. Instead, survival was specifically related to blood vessel involvement and a high mitotic count (greater than 2-5/hPF) where the mortality rate was the greatest. Favorable therapeutic results of postoperative megavoltage irradiation are being reported from various cancer clinics in recent years.

An unusual benign form of myomata uteri – intravenous leiomyomatosis – was first recognized at the turn of the century and was reported sporadically during the following three decades. Marshall and Morris presented the first detailed report of this entity in the American literature in 1959, which has resulted in several publications on the subject since that time. The characteristic feature of this peculiar intravenous smooth muscle tumor is the extension of the polypoid intravascular projections into the veins of the parametria and broad ligament. Although there may be some difficulty in distinguishing such lesions from low-grade sarcoma, they are distinctly different histologically from the entity "stromatosis uteri," as the intravascular plugs are smooth muscle in origin. The important question is whether they arise from the adjacent leiomyomata or from the smooth muscle of the wall of the uterine veins. The former theory is the most prevalent one at the present time. While the possibility of intravenous leiomyomata progressing to distant metastases is unproven to date, there have been two deaths in the history of this disease resulting from extension of the smooth muscle plugs into the right atrium, with mechanical obstruction and subsequent death, even though the tissue was histologically benign. At the present time there are 32 reported cases of this entity, and in roughly 50 per cent of the cases the intravenous tumor was confined to the parametrium and 75 per cent extended no further than the veins of the broad ligament. The observations of Edwards and Peacock suggest that the severed intravenous extensions are probably incapable of independent parasitic existence and remain dormant after removal of the uterus.

ASYMPTOMATIC MYOMATA

Before considering the symptoms that demand treatment of the fibroids, it might be well to regard the large group of fibroids that give no symptoms. Asymptomatic fibroids are encountered much more frequently than tumors which do give rise to symptoms. Untold numbers of such symptomless fibroids have been removed surgically which would have been better left undisturbed. One always should bear in mind that the incidence of malignancy is less than 1 per cent; and in small tumors it is far less than that. This incidence is less than the mortality rate of hysterectomy in the average hospital, so unless there is some surgical reason to suspect malignancy, the danger of the operation exceeds the danger of malignancy. A history of rapid growth, or especially postmenopausal growth, calls for removal even though the tumor is giving no symptoms.

Small tumors that are quite symptomless need only be observed from time to time. It is remarkable how stationary in size such tumors may remain for years. If such small fibroids are discovered late in menstrual life, it is unusual for treatment to be required. Larger tumors may also be watched safely, but if a policy of watchful waiting is adopted, one should be very sure of the nature of the tumors. If there is uncertainty of the uterine or ovarian origin of a tumor, as may well be the case when the tumor fills the whole pelvis, or when a pedunculated tumor is felt in the adnexal region, the uncertainty can usually be cleared up by an examination under anesthesia. If still in doubt, culdoscopy may be of great value in making the differentiation, provided that the cul-de-sac is not blocked by tumor. If uncertainty still exists, a laparotomy should be done.

When asymptomatic fibroids are discovered in young women, the problem of the relation of such tumors to sterility and pregnancy usually arises. With the increase in sterility work that has appeared during recent years, a growing number of asymptomatic fibroids has been discovered in young women. The finding of small fibroids in sterile women is not an indication for immediate myomectomy Both marital partners should be completely investigated for sterility, and the fibroids should be disregarded for at least a while. The ultimate disposal of the fibroids depends on their nature. Usually, small subserous fibroids cannot reasonably be considered a factor in the sterility; even though the woman fails to become pregnant, removal of the fibroids is not justified. When fibroids are intramural and of fair size or submucous, they may well be factors in the sterility, and a myomectomy may be rewarded with a subsequent pregnancy.

The finding of asymptomatic fibroids in women who expect to undergo pregnancy often presents a problem requiring the best of obstetric and gynecologic judgment. Many small subserous and intramural fibroids do not influence the course of pregnancy in the least; nor does the pregnancy influence the fibroids in many instances. On the other hand, intramural and, to a greater degree, submucous fibroids of fair size undoubtedly increase the incidence of abortions and complicate the abortions when they occur. Pedunculated subserous fibroids are more prone to twist during pregnancy; fibroids of reasonable size may become painful in the course of pregnancy, due to pressure and degeneration; finally, large fibroids low in the pelvis may obstruct the birth canal and make vaginal delivery impossible.

The finding of totally unsuspected, asymptomatic fibroids in a young woman who contemplates pregnancy is usually very much of a shock to her. The greatest tact is required in presenting the problem to the patient, and the best of surgical and obstetric judgment is needed to arrive at the right solution. Should she be allowed to attempt the pregnancy with a realization that her chances of complications are greater than in the normal woman? Should a myomectomy be advised before pregnancy is attempted, the risk being taken that the surgeon may be forced to perform a hysterectomy when attempting the myomectomy? Should she be permitted to become pregnant, go to term, and then have a cesarean section, leaving the fibroid uterus, with the hope of more pregnancies? Should she go to term and have a cesarean section and hysterectomy at term? These, and others, are problems that one must attempt to answer. Such questions cannot be answered by any rule. Each case presents its own problem, and the answer is not entirely dependent upon the physical condition of the pelvis. The patient's age, her general physical condition, and, not the least, her mental attitude must all be considered before a final decision is made.

When large asymptomatic fibroids occur in young women who have had their familes or in whom childbearing is not important, they should be removed. Such tumors, with perhaps 15 or 20 years to grow before the menopause, are bound to require surgical removal eventually; hence, it is better to remove them when the patient is relatively young and a good operative risk.

In women approaching the menopause relatively large fibroids are often safely kept under observation, with the hope that after the menopause they will regress. While observing fibroids of this type in recent years, we have made it a rule to make intravenous urograms. Everett and Sturgis have shown that not uncommonly there is evidence of pressure at the pelvic brim, so that hydroureters and hydronephroses develop (Fig. 8-1). Although at times this back pressure results in pain, the process is often quite painless, even when serious damage is done to the kidneys. Evidence of kidney damage seen in the pyelogram may be the deciding factor in making up one's mind to operate on a patient with an entirely asymptomatic fibroid. Furthermore, the incidence of hypertension was found by Everett and Scott to be more than twice as great among those patients who showed x-ray evidence of urinary tract stasis. It was suggested by the authors that this hypertension might be the cause of "myoma heart," about which there was so much discussion in years past.

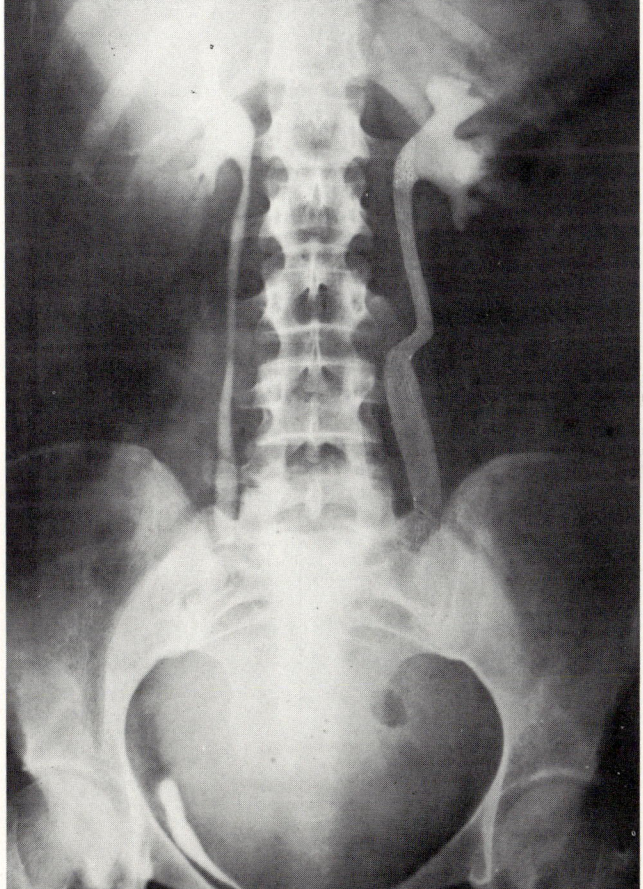

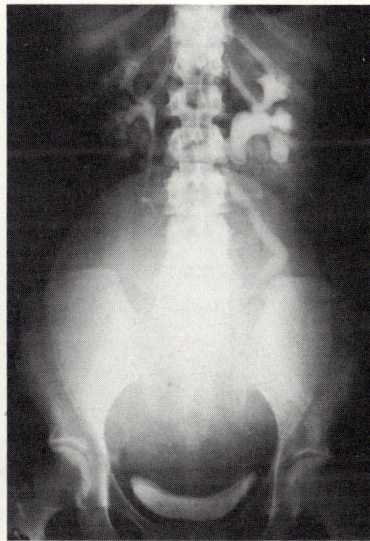

FIG. 8-1. (*Left*) Unilateral ureteral dilatation and distortion of bladder from pressure of large fibroids. (*Right*) Unilateral hydro-ureter and hydronephrosis resulting from pressure of large myoma.

Myomata Uteri

After the menopause, asymptomatic fibroids generally should be left undisturbed. Here again the surgeon must be absolutely certain that he is not dealing with a solid ovarian growth. The appearance of even a little vaginal bleeding should make one suspect cervical malignancy, endometrial malignancy, or sarcomatous change in the myoma. Papanicolaou smear, curettage, and cervical biopsy should be done; if the bleeding is not explained by these procedures, the fibroid uterus should be removed because of the danger of sarcomatous change.

SIGNS AND SYMPTOMS INDICATING TREATMENT

Bleeding is the commonest symptom that indicates the necessity of treatment. The mechanism by which fibroids cause bleeding is not clear in every instance. The pedunculated submucous fibroid (Fig. 8-2) bleeds freely at menstruation as a result of passive congestion, necrosis, and ulceration. With these changes there is usually a constant thin blood-tinged discharge, in addition to the menorrhagia. The intramural tumor, which is just beginning to encroach on the endometrial

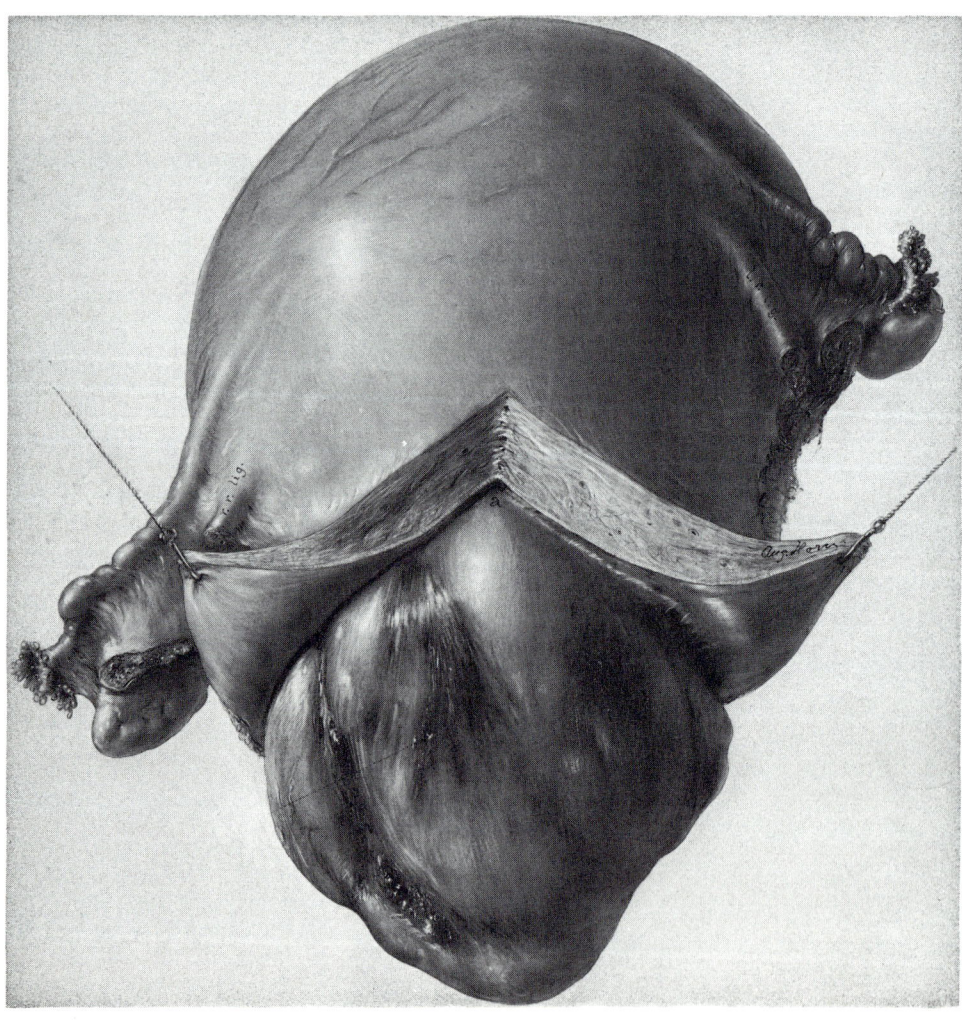

FIG. 8-2. Pedunculated submucous myoma showing necrosis and ulceration.

cavity, can be responsible for menorrhagia by virtue of its pressure on the veins formed by confluence of the endometrial capillaries. Large tumors may greatly increase the size of the uterine cavity and thus give rise to menorrhagia simply because there is an increased bleeding surface. The intramural fibroids near the serosal surface and pedunculated subserous tumors cannot be considered responsible for bleeding; when bleeding occurs with such tumors, one should search for some other lesion to account for it. Indeed, one always should bear in mind that the mere presence of fibroids in a bleeding women is not proof that the fibroid causes the bleeding, for the fibroids may be incidental and the bleeding due to some unrelated lesion. This fact is particularly to be stressed when there is intermenstrual bleeding. It is a rule on our service to curette and to perform a cervical biopsy on all women with fibroids in whom there is intermenstrual bleeding, before proceeding with the treatment of the fibroid.

When bleeding occurs postmenopausally, and fibroids are discovered on bimanual examination, the question arises whether or not the fibroid is responsible for the bleeding. The answer is usually in the negative. In more than half of such instances the bleeding is due to some other lesion, such as cervical or endometrial malignancy, and the fibroids are purely incidental. The next question that naturally arises is whether or not the postmenopausal fibroid *can* be responsible for the bleeding. The answer to that question is in the affirmative. Fibroids that did not bleed during the menstrual life of the patient have been found to migrate to a submucous position after the menopause, become ulcerated, and bleed. Also, we have very rarely observed growth in a fibroid postmenopausally and have found no malignancy in the tumor. However, whenever there is evidence of growth in a fibroid after the menopause, one should consider seriously the possibility of malignant change and treat the patient accordingly. If, in addition, there is bleeding, the chances of malignancy are very high.

Evidence of pressure on nearby pelvic viscera is also an indication for treatment. The urinary bladder is the organ that suffers most often from such pressure, giving rise to frequency of urination (Fig. 8-3). Although this symptom is common with large fibroids, it is remarkable how frequently one sees the pelvis filled with fibroids without any increased frequency of urination. The great ability of the bladder to function normally in spite of extreme distortion by pelvic tumors is truly remarkable. Occasionally, acute retention of urine results from a fibroid and necessitates surgical interference. We have seen this occur as the result of marked growth of the fibroid anteriorly, pressing the superior surface of the bladder against the internal sphincter region. More frequently a tumor of about the size of a 3-months' pregnancy incarcerated in the cul-de-sac pushes the cervix downward and forward and obstructs the flow from the urethra. We have also observed a large pedunculated submucous tumor, filling and distending the vagina, pressing on the urethra, and causing retention. As stated previously, the pressure of the tumor upon the ureters at the pelvic brim, with resultant

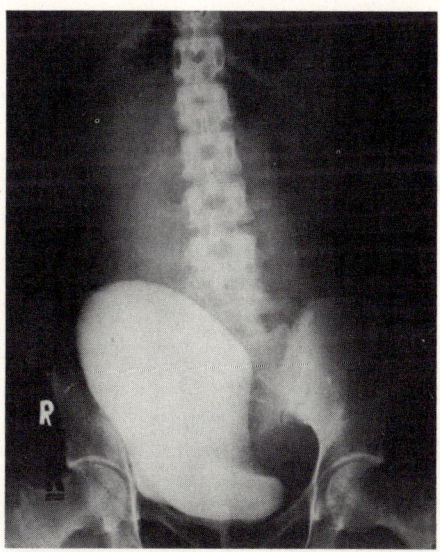

FIG. 8-3. Cystogram, showing distortion of the bladder by pressure from a fibroid.

kidney damage, may indicate the necessity of operative treatment.

The bowel is less apt to show symptoms from pressure than the bladder, but constipation can be caused and aggravated by such pressure; more frequently, one is astounded by the relatively normal function of the bowel in the presence of large fibroids that almost completely fill the pelvis. Very rarely, we have seen acute intestinal obstruction occur from pressure of a large fibroid on the bowel.

Occasionally, treatment is indicated because of edema of the lower extremities caused by pressure of the fibroid on the iliac veins. As a rule, however, even large fibroids cause surprisingly little lower extremity edema; when the edema is great, it is well to think of the possibility of an infiltrating malignant pelvic tumor occluding pelvic veins and/or lymphatics, or to consider cardiac or renal disease.

Abdominal or pelvic pain is a frequent reason for operative interference. There are many causes for pain with fibroids; the pressure of a large but uncomplicated tumor on the pelvic nerves may give rise to pain, and tumors which are the site of extensive necrosis are also sometimes painful. In rare instances pedunculated fibroids twist and give rise to a clinical picture of acute abdominal pain much like that which one sees with a twisted ovarian tumor. In the author's experience fibroids twist on their pedicle more often postmenopausally and during pregnancy. The commonest cause for pain in our public ward experience is a complicating pelvic inflammatory disease, acute or chronic. A long-standing pelvic inflammatory residue that has been asymptomatic for months or years may become painful when the growing fibroid begins to stretch the pelvic adhesions. Circulatory disturbances and edema resulting from pressure of the tumor upon chronically infected tubes sometimes result in acute or subacute painful exacerbations. Such pelvic inflammatory disease seldom responds well to palliation, and surgery is necessary soon or late. Dysmenorrhea, acquired in the 4th or the 5th decade, may be the outstanding symptom of the growth of fibroids. A common symptom complex resulting from fibroids at this time of life is menstrual pain, coupled with increased menstrual flow. Diffuse adenomyosis may also cause these symptoms, and the differentiation of this condition from a symmetrically developed intramural fibroid may be extremely difficult. The differentiation is chiefly academic, for in either case surgery is indicated if the symptoms are of sufficient severity.

Distortion of the abdomen due to large tumors may justify their removal. Tumors of such size frequently give rise to other symptoms also, so that there is ample reason for surgical interference; but when no other symptom is present, one is justified in removing the tumors if the abdominal distortion is of such proportions as to be distasteful to the woman. Occasionally, ascites forms with benign fibroids as a result of pressure on the veins, but when it is discovered, there is always a likelihood of malignancy in the fibroid or an accompanying ovarian malignancy, and operation should not be deferred.

Rapid Growth. Evidence of rapid growth of a fibroid is an indication for surgical interference. It may suggest malignancy in the premenopausal fibroid, but this is not usually the case. In the postmenopausal fibroid, however, growth almost always indicates malignancy. Although this is not an invariable rule, the chances are so great in favor of malignancy that one must proceed on that assumption and resort to immediate removal.

Sterility. Fibroids are not infrequently the cause of sterility, especially in late marriages; pregnancy following myomectomy is often observed. On the other hand, pregnancy occurs innumerable times in myomatous uteri, and we who have a large proportion of colored patients in our clinic are often astounded at the presence of pregnancy in uteri containing huge multiple fibroids. The best obstetric judgment is often needed to decide whether pregnancy should be attempted before surgery is done on the fibroids. Clinical experience teaches us that many times fibroids are responsible for *repeated abortions or premature deliveries,* and yet one is frequently surprised at the smooth course of pregnancy in the presence of even large tumors. Due to increased blood supply and hormonal action, fibroids may grow rapidly during pregnancy. On the other hand, they may become very soft and apparently disappear; they usually again become firm and palpable after involution of the uterus. Pressure of the growing fetus may interfere with the blood supply of the tumor formed in the pelvis, causing painful necrosis and giving rise to tenderness suggesting peritoneal irritation. These complications during pregnancy may call for surgical relief without delay.

CHOICE OF TREATMENT

Fibroids are successfully treated surgically and with irradiation. Both methods have their advantages and disadvantages; both have their indications and contraindications.

Surgical Treatment

Surgery has many advantages over irradiation, and the mortality of hysterectomy for fibroids in the better clinics is very low. We operate on many times as many patients for fibroids as we treat by irradiation, chiefly because surgery offers a flexibility of treatment that is not possible with radium. We refer particularly to the possibility of myomectomy, conservation of one or both ovaries, removal of diseased tubes, and the removal of the chronically infected cervix. It also permits corrective plastic surgery, which is often indicated in women of the myoma age. In this group of patients vaginal hysterectomy is often the operation of choice. Although we do not advocate removal of very large tumors by morcellation by the vaginal route, vaginal hysterectomy is an extremely useful procedure when dealing with small fibroids. The advantages and the contraindications for vaginal hysterectomy in relation to fibroids are discussed later in this chapter.

The advantages of surgery over irradiation are reflected in the contraindications to irradiation that follow.

Since the removal of myomata is the most frequent indication for hysterectomy, the discussion of total versus subtotal hysterectomy is included in this chapter. The technics of total abdominal and subtotal abdominal hysterectomy are also included, as well as a discussion of the question of myomectomy. The technics of abdominal and vaginal myomectomy are also described and illustrated.

Irradiation Treatment

In our clinic irradiation is reserved for those fibroids requiring treatment in which the patient's general condition contraindicates surgery and for small bleeding fibroids occurring in women near the menopause, provided that these bleeding fibroids are not of the pedunculated submucous variety. However, not all of such small bleeding fibroids are irradiated. If the patient is a very nervous woman for whom the artificial menopause would almost certainly be a serious ordeal, we prefer surgery with preservation of ovarian function. It is our clinical impression that the symptoms of the radium menopause are, in general, more severe than those of the natural menopause. There is also an occasional patient who has a fibroid which should be removed surgically, but she steadfastly refuses operation. Such tumors are irradiated as the second best method of treatment. In all patients who are irradiated, preliminary curettage and cervical biopsy are done.

If the patient lives in the city where x-ray equipment is available, we are inclined to treat her with x-rays rather than radium. X-ray treatment has the advantage of not requiring hospitalization, but it is more time-consuming. If the patient lives out of the city, we admit her to the hospital for a few days and treat her with intra-uterine radium. X-ray treatment, preferably Co^{60}, is given in 10 doses at 200 r each day for a total midplevic dosage of 2,000 r in the hormonally active female. In the patient approaching menopause, a total ovarian irradiation dosage of 500 to 700 r in 1 or 2 treatments is sufficient to eliminate hormonal function.

The contraindications to irradiation which we observe are listed below:

1. Any fibroid occurring in a woman under 40 should not be irradiated unless surgical treatment is contraindicated. The artificial menopause induced by irradiation should be avoided and can be avoided by conservation of ovarian tissue when surgery is done.

2. When the diagnosis is questionable, as, for example, when a fibroid cannot be differentiated with certainty from an ovarian tumor.

3. When the fibroid is larger than a 3½-months' pregnancy. Larger tumors are apt to produce pressure symptoms that are best relieved by surgery. They are also apt to contain areas of degeneration; hence they should be removed rather than irradiated.

4. When there is a complicating old or recent pelvic infection. Irradiation may light up the inflammatory processes. Salpingitis, complicating fibroids, usually causes pain, which is an indication for surgery.

5. When there is a complicating ovarian neoplasm.

6. When the fibroid is of the pedunculated submucous type. Irradiation of such a fibroid may cause necrosis with resulting serious infection. It will also fail to stop the bleeding.

7. When there is a large pedunculated subserous fibroid that is subject to possible degeneration and/or torsion.

8. When there is complicating malignancy of the cervix, the endometrium, or the ovary. Appropriate treatment of the malignancy naturally takes precedence over irradiation of the fibroid.

9. When there is a history of rapid growth before the menopause or, more particularly, when the history suggests postmenopausal growth. This is suggestive of malignant degeneration of the fibroid.

10. When there is abdominal pain, even though the pain is not explained on the basis of any of the above-mentioned complications.

11. When there is some other condition requiring surgical relief, such as symptomatic retroposition, prolapse, cystocele, relaxed vaginal outlet, or rectocele.

TOTAL VS. SUBTOTAL ABDOMINAL HYSTERECTOMY FOR BENIGN CONDITIONS OF THE UTERUS

From a review of recent gynecologic literature it is apparent that abdominal hysterectomy, both total and subtotal, has become a relatively safe operation in the hands of competent gynecologists. It is also apparent that there has been a great shift toward total hysterectomy in recent years In fact, in most clinics total hysterectomy has become the routine method of removal of the uterus. In our opinion, this trend toward total hysterectomy is justified, but we do not believe that it should be made an absolutely routine procedure.

In weighing the two procedures one should balance the advantages of removal of the cervix against the possibilities of an increased morbidity and mortality for the total operation. The advantages of removal of the cervix are that it is eliminated as a possible source of a troublesome discharge and also as a site where carcinoma may develop. The incidence of the development of carcinoma in the retained stump can only be estimated, since the true incidence cannot be determined except by following until their death a group of women who have been subjected to supravaginal hysterectomy. So far as we know, this never has been done, and the difficulties of such a study are obvious. The incidence of stump carcinomas, in relation to the total of cervical carcinomas, lies in the neighborhood of 3 per cent. This percentage has been quoted incorrectly at times as the incidence of the development of carcinoma in the retained stump; obviously, the true figure is much smaller. Scheffey made a follow-up study on 554 supravaginally hysterectomized women and found carcinoma in the cervical stump in 0.9 per cent of the cases. These were found from 6 to 21 years after the operation; hence, probably none was present at the time of operation. We have encountered personally only 2 cases of cervical carcinoma in women upon whom a supravaginal hysterectomy was done in our private practice, which does not represent an incidence of over 0.2 per cent. Wetterdal found malignancy in the cervical stump in 0.7 per cent of 288 women 10 years after a subtotal hysterectomy and contended that those who use total hysterectomy routinely have an exaggerated fear of cervical cancer. However, the retained cervix does constitute a possible source of leukorrhea and bleeding. Cariker and Dockerty studied 334 retained cervices of women who complained of symptoms referable to the cervix. Bleeding was the commonest complaint and was explained by both benign and malignant lesions. Twenty-three per cent of the bleeding cervices proved to have cancer, and they concluded that *total* removal of the uterus was desirable, a conclusion with which we would heartily agree. During the past several years we have studied thoroughly all cervices removed in performing total hysterectomy for supposed benign disease. In each instance the entire cervix was cut into blocks, and many, many sections were taken from each block. In the course of this thorough examination of 1,500 cervices very early but undoubted cancer was found in 0.6 per cent.

In attempting to judge the relative safety of the two operations one can prove that either procedure is safer, depending upon one's interpretation of figures found in gynecologic literature. Weir reports a mortality rate of 0.767 per cent in 1,436 total hysterectomies. The mortality rate in his series of 1,914 hysterectomies, of all types, was 1.2 per cent. Since this figure includes subtotal hysterectomies, obviously the mortality is higher in the subtotal group. Pearse reports on 1,243 supravaginal and 373 complete hysterectomies; the mortality rate of the series of the total operation was 2.9 per cent, while for the subtotal group it was 3.4 per cent. Danforth reports a mortality rate of 0.8 per cent for the subtotal operation and 3.66 per cent for the total. Masson reports a mortality of 1.3 per cent for the total operation and 1.8 for the subtotal. Most of these statistics are relatively old, and recent statistics from the better clinics show lower mortality for both groups of cases. For example, in 1,000 successive abdominal hysterectomies in our clinic Woodruff found only 2 deaths. Both of these were from pulmonary embolism. Also in 1,000 vaginal hysterectomies, many of which were done for small fibroids, the mortality was also 0.2 per cent. There was no mortality among the total abdominal hysterectomies. From the above figures one may justly conclude that either operation is relatively safe. However, to conclude that total hysterectomy is safer than subtotal would be to disregard the fact that the group of the subtotal operation usually includes the more difficult cases and the poorer operative risk. For example, in those clinics in which total hysterectomy is the rule, it is common for the operator to perform quickly a subtotal amputation when he encounters operative difficulties and/or is informed by the anesthetist that the patient's condition is critical. These cases are included in the subtotal group from which statistical data are compiled. Such data obviously cannot be used to prove the greater danger of subtotal hysterectomy, for the patient may be almost moribund when the decision for a subtotal hysterectomy is made.

As to morbidity, it is difficult to compare the two operations statistically. Danforth reports a morbidity of 28 per cent for the subtotal operation and 33 per cent for the total, but this slight difference, based on temperature elevation, is of little significance and does not tell the whole story. Today, in the better clinics, the incidence of ureteral and bladder injury is very small with either operation; however, the larger clinics are often called upon to repair damage done to ureters and bladders by less experienced operators. We have observed, as have also Norman Miller and Holden, an increased incidence of vesicovaginal fistulas resulting from total abdominal hysterectomies.

In view of the above considerations, what is the proper attitude in respect to total versus subtotal hysterectomy for benign uterine disease? On the gynecologic service at the Johns Hopkins Hospital we have done total hysterectomy in approximately 96 per cent of our cases in recent years. This percentage is lower than in some clinics and is lower than the percentage on the private service. It includes the operations done on colored patients in whom fibroids often are extremely large, and the complication of salpingitis is encountered more often than not. It is on these patients, particularly, that we occasionally perform the subtotal operation. We are inclined to attribute our very low mortality quoted above to the judgment which the staff exercised in selecting the proper operations in each case. It is sincerely hoped that our percentage of total hysterectomy never reaches 100. If it should, one would be inclined to believe that we had thrown clinical judgment to the wind. There are times in all surgery where discretion is the better part of valor.

In general, it is assumed on our service that a total hysterectomy will be done, and the cervix is left in only when, in the opinion of the operator, there is some good reason for doing so. Briefly stated, it may be said that when it is believed that the danger of removal of the cervix exceeds the danger of leaving it, the subtotal operation should be done.

Today, when total hysterectomy has become almost a routine procedure, the above discussion may seem antiquated to the young pelvic surgeon, but it is well for him to be familiar with the circumstances out of which our present practice has evolved.

OVARIAN MANAGEMENT AT HYSTERECTOMY FOR BENIGN DISEASE

Ovarian conservation versus ablation is considered here because the question of removal of normal or relatively normal ovaries occurs most often when hysterectomy is done for benign disease. The problem is an ancient one, and unfortunately the final answer is not yet forthcoming. Opinion in recent years has swung more to ovarian conservation. There are few active gynecologists today who follow the precept of Graves, who advocated the routine removal of ovaries in all women on whom hysterectomy was done, regardless of age. Among them are Grogan and Duncan, who in their writing state: "It was the considered opinion of the authors that the interest of the patient was best served by prophylactic castration (as opposed to ovarian salvage) and the institution of adequate hormonal substitution therapy which would serve to prevent postoperative occurrence of the menopause syndrome." At the other extreme are some gynecologists who practically never remove normal ovaries even though the patient is well past her menopause. Then there are many who routinely practice ovarian ablation after 45 when hysterectomy is done.

The question of the function of ovaries left in after hysterectomy has never been entirely settled. Grogan studied 30 residual ovaries that required removal. Sixty per cent contained either active corpora lutea or normally developing follicles. One of these ovaries was 16 years posthysterectomy. Wharton and Te Linde have studied the problem, using monkeys. They found no evidence that either subtotal or total hysterectomy had any effect on the remaining ovaries 2 years after the hysterectomy, as judged by the histology of the ovaries. Corpora lutea and follicles of all stages of development were found in the postoperative ovaries exactly as in ovaries with the uterus left in situ. It must be remembered that Grogan's study, showing 60 per cent of histologically normal ovaries, was made on ovaries which in his estimation required surgical removal. The percentage would undoubtedly be much higher if based on all residual ovaries.

The question of the effect of castration on atherosclerosis and/or osteoporosis is not yet settled. It is discussed fully in Chapter 6, Estrogen Replacement Therapy, to which the reader is referred.

From the above studies, together with

the clinical evidence which is observed daily in every gynecologist's office, it would seem that ovaries left in young women with good blood supply continue to function normally. We refer to the appearance of flushes and other menopausal symptoms appearing in the late forties and the early fifties in women who had a hysterectomy with ovarian conservation early in their menstrual life.

In recent years the question of ovarian function after the menopause has created considerable interest. Randall has been particularly interested in this phase of the subject. He attempted to estimate estrogen activity by vaginal smears in women after the cessation of their periods. He studied smears on women from 2 to more than 15 years after their last period and found a persistence of estrogen effect in 55.2 per cent. On comparing a group of women who had been castrated with a group of comparable ages who had had simple hysterectomy, there was evidence of estrogen deficiency in 30 per cent more of the castrated women than in the noncastrated. If these vaginal smear interpretations can be considered as really indicative of estrogen activity, it is apparent that many women receive estrogen from an extra-ovarian source. On the other hand, it is equally obvious that depriving a woman of her ovaries deprives her of her principal source of estrogen.

The question of the functions of the postmenopausal ovary has a bearing on the advisability of ovarian ablation. Current tissue incubation studies by Mattingly and Huang on the human menopausal and postmenopausal ovary, utilizing radioactive steriod precursors, demonstrate that the menopausal and postmenopausal ovarian stroma produce androgens primarily, while estrogens are synthesized in very limited amounts. Their study would support the position of removing both ovaries in women after the age of 45 to 50 who are undergoing pelvic surgery. They conclude that there is no valid data that supports the hormonal advantages of the postmenopausal ovary as an active endocrine organ.

Regardless of the correct answer on postmenopausal ovarian function, there can be no doubt of the undesirable effects of castration in the young. In addition to hot flushes, headaches, and general nervous instability, the local changes in the vagina are of great importance. The contracted vaginal outlet and the atrophic sensitive vaginal mucosa result in dyspareunia which may be very troublesome to the woman past 50 who has undergone her natural menopause; to the young woman it may constitute a major tragedy and even wreck her marriage. Although substitutional hormonal therapy is helpful in relieving the general and the local symptoms of castrations, it seldom equals the beneficial effect of the normally secreted estrogen.

Against the disagreeable symptoms of the menopause one must balance the possibility of malignancy developing in retained ovaries. Counseller has reported 65 such cases, but since the relation of these cases to the total number of hysterectomies is not available, the figure has no percentile meaning. Randall, on good statistical grounds, has estimated that the retained ovary at 40 has slightly less than a 1 per cent chance of becoming malignant. After 40 the percentage decreased. Benign tumors may also occur. After 50, Randall found 14 ovarian neoplasms per thousand women; 6 of these were benign, and 8 malignant.

It has been pointed out that if one subscribes to the view that all organs should be removed that are susceptible to cancer, there are organs with much greater neoplastic potential than the ovaries, notably the breasts.

From available evidence it would seem illogical to remove normal-appearing ovaries in women under 45, but what is the correct decision in the woman over 45 whose normal menopause is probably only a few years in the future?

The author considers the following factors:

1. *Temperament of the Patient.* We would be more inclined to spare at least 1 ovary in a woman whose temperament would indicate that the added psychic disturbance associated with the menopause would aggravate her already delicately balanced emotional status.

2. *Age of the Patient.* Within the limits of 45 and 52 or 53 we would be more in-

clined to perform oophorectomy toward the end of this period.

3. *Appearance of the Ovaries.* Often in this age group, there is a great variation in the appearance of the ovaries. In some individuals at 50 the ovaries appear to be quite youthful. There is no evidence of atrophy, and even a fresh corpus luteum may be present. Often there is quite a contrast between the 2 ovaries in the same individual. One or both ovaries might be spared on the basis of their youthful appearance. I would be especially inclined to spare such an ovary if the woman is youthful in appearance for her years, suggesting a persistence of good estrogen activity. The removal of 1 ovary, however, does not reduce the incidence of subsequent ovarian neoplasm by 50 per cent, because some ovarian tumors, benign and malignant, are bilateral from their incipiency.

TECHNIC: SUBTOTAL ABDOMINAL HYSTERECTOMY

Since the operation of subtotal abdominal hysterectomy is done most often for myomata, the great variation in size and shape of the uterus makes it necessary to deviate from any standard technic and, frequently, to improvise as one proceeds. Also, the complication of adnexal disease may prevent the carrying out of a uniform procedure. However, the surgeon should have some standard plan from which he can make any modifications that become necessary in the course of the operation. Such a standard technic is presented here:

One of the round ligaments is grasped with an Ochsner clamp near the uterine cornu and is ligated a short distance distal to the clamp with No. 0 chromic catgut. The ligament is cut between the clamp and the ligature. Thus the anterior leaf of the broad ligament is opened. The posterior leaf of the broad ligament is pushed forward through this opening with the surgeon's finger as shown in Figure 8-4 A. This portion of the broad ligament is quite avascular. It is incised with the scissors.

The next step depends upon whether the tube and the ovary are to be saved or removed. If they are to be saved, the tube and the ovarian ligament are triply clamped en masse as in Figure 8-4 B. The clamp in proximity to the uterus is to

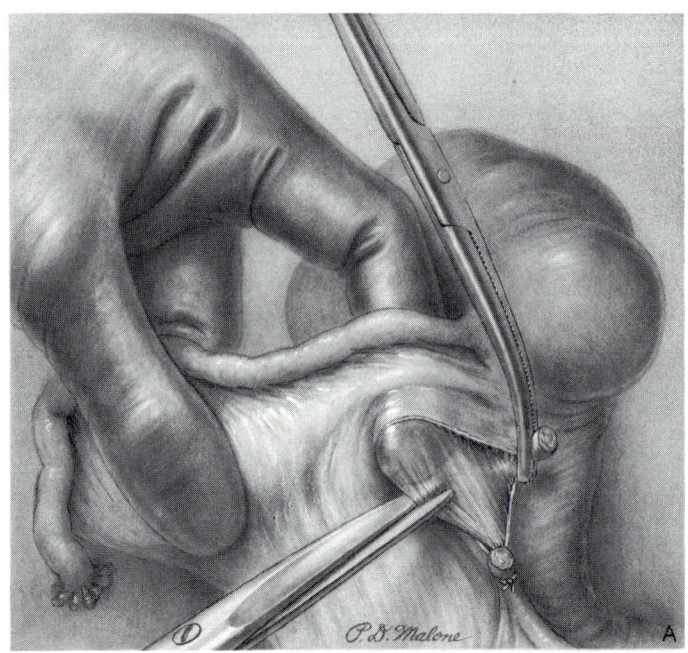

Fig. 8-4. Subtotal abdominal hysterectomy. (A) Round ligament has been ligated and cut, thus opening the anterior leaf of the broad ligament. Avascular area in the broad ligament is exposed and is being incised.

FIG. 8-4 (*Continued*). (B) The tube and the ovarian ligament are doubly clamped and cut as indicated by dotted line.

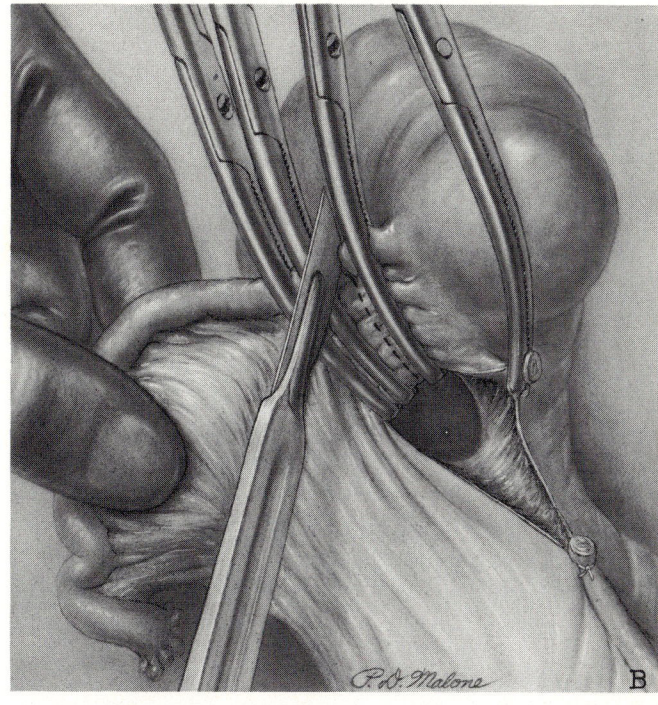

control back bleeding, and the incision is made between it and the next clamp. Thus the ovarian vessels are doubly clamped as they approach the anastomosis with the uterine. Double clamping of the ovarian vessels is our usual routine, and we believe that it is an excellent precaution. It prevents slipping and retraction of the cut vessels with the formation of a broad ligament hematoma. Furthermore, this ligation must be in the nature of a mass tie, and the crushing of the tissues by means of the second clamp affords a groove in which to tie the first suture ligature. The proximal clamp is removed as the suture ligature is tied, and the distal clamp is kept in place. Then the mass of tissue is transfixed with another suture of No. 0 chromic catgut distal to the first ligature as the distal clamp is removed.

There are instances in which the double-clamp technic cannot be used, but when it is feasible, we believe it to be a worthwhile precaution.

If the tube and the ovary are to be removed with the uterus, the infundibulopelvic portion of the broad ligament is clamped with 3 Ochsner clamps en masse as shown in Figure 8-4 C. The ligament is divided, and double ligation of the ovarian vessels by suture ligature of No. 0 chromic catgut is carried out. In general, it is good policy to ligate the clamped ovarian vessels as they are cut, rather than to leave all the clamps on until after the uterus is removed. By ligating them as one proceeds, the operative field is cleared of clamps, and if at any stage of the operation fast decisive action is necessary, there is less cluttering of the field by clamps which might have been disposed of earlier.

Clamping, cutting, and ligating of the round ligament, the uterine end of the tube, and the ovarian ligament or of the infundibulopelvic ligament are carried out in the same manner on the opposite side.

Next, the posterior leaf of the broad ligament on either side is cut parallel with the side of the uterus (Fig. 8-4 D). This step is not always done, although with large tumors cutting of the broad

158 Myomata Uteri

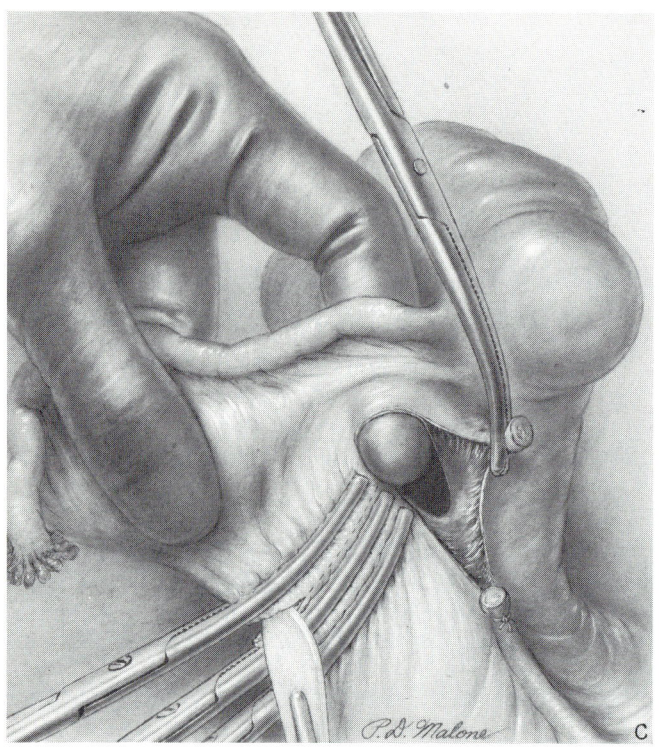

FIG. 8-4 (*Continued*). Subtotal abdominal hysterectomy. (C) When adnexa are to be removed, the infundibulopelvic ligament is doubly clamped and cut.

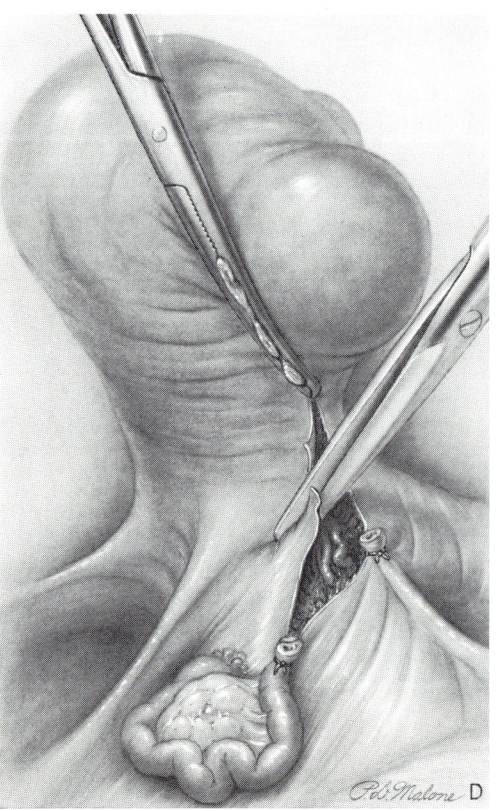

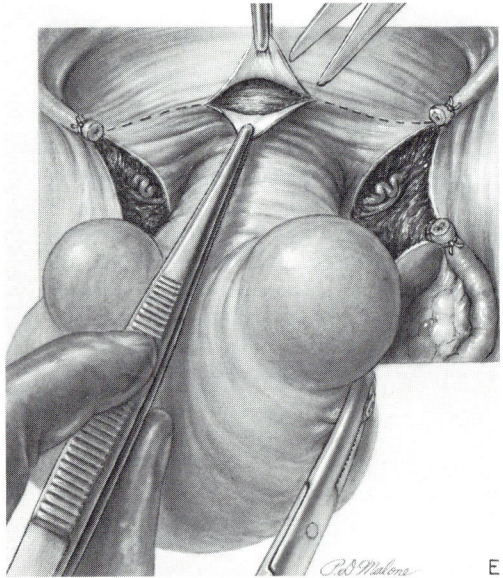

FIG. 8-4 (*Continued*). Subtotal abdominal hysterectomy. (D) The posterior leaf of the broad ligament is cut to secure better exposure of vessels for clamping. Often this step is not necessary. (E) Reflexion of the bladder peritoneum onto the uterus is cut, as indicated by dotted line joining the round ligaments.

ligament often better demonstrates the uterine vessels between the leaves of the broad ligament for clamping.

The reflexion of the bladder peritoneum onto the uterus is then picked up in about the midline, and it is cut as indicated in Figure 8-4 E. The incision through the peritoneum is carried laterally to the regions of the cut ends of the round ligaments. In cutting the peritoneum, care should be taken not to cut too deeply. If the cut is made just through the peritoneum a good line of cleavage is entered, but if the cut goes too deeply, bleeding will be encountered. With a sponge on a sponge holder, or with the finger, the bladder peritoneum usually can be dissected down easily by blunt dissection In the usual subtotal hysterectomy the bladder itself need be freed from the cervix little or none. Bleeding will be prevented by avoiding unnecessary dissection of the bladder from the cervix, but when a very low amputation of the cervix is desired, freeing of the bladder may be carried down to as low a point as necessary to carry out the amputation.

The uterine vessels that have been thus exposed are then triply clamped bilaterally with curved Ochsner clamps, as indicated in Figure 8-4 F. It is not necessary to dissect out these vessels for clear visualization; in fact, to do so may cause unnecessary bleeding. It is desirable to have these clamps that crush the loose tissue enveloping the uterine vessels bite into the edge of the cervix as shown in Figure 8-4 H. Of course, the upper clamp is intended to prevent back bleeding from the uterus, but the 2 lower clamps doubly clamp the uterine vessels. Then the corpus is amputated as indicated in the dotted line in Figure 8-4 F. The level of this amputation is variable, depending upon circumstances If it is desired to leave a little endometrium to permit a show of menstruation, the amputation may be done above the internal os. If, on the other hand, the endocervix is the source of leukorrhea, and for some reason a total hysterectomy is not thought

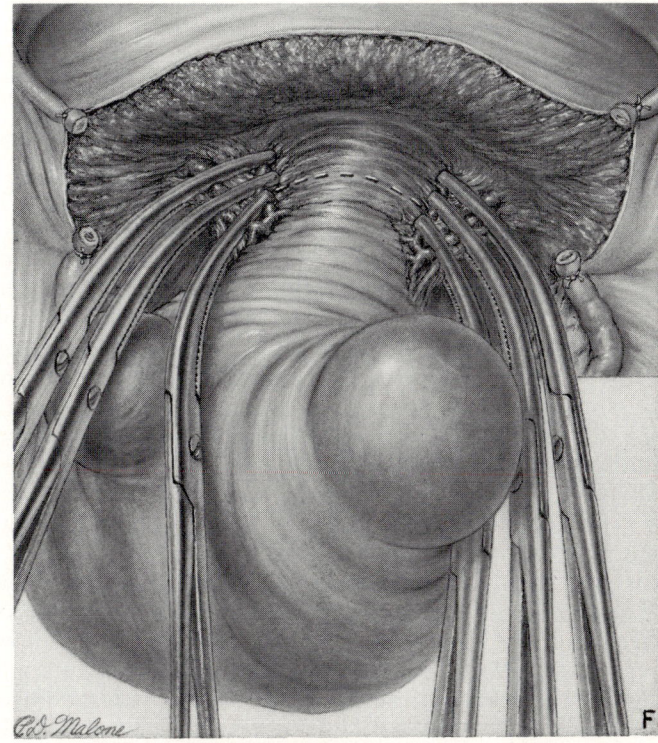

FIG. 8-4 (*Continued*). Subtotal abdominal hysterectomy. (F) Uterine vessels are doubly clamped, and clamps are also placed to control back bleeding. The line of amputation is indicated by a dotted line.

to be advisable, the amputation may be done very low, leaving almost no cervix. Regardless of the level of amputation, it is well to make a V-shaped cut as illustrated in Figure 8-4 G. This facilitates the closure of the stump.

The uterine vessels are doubly ligated with No. 0 chromic catgut, according to the preference of the operator. These sutures are placed into the substance of the cervix as indicated in Figure 8-4 H. As the first suture is tied, the lower clamp is removed, and if the bite of tissue is large, it may be well to loosen the upper clamp to permit the tissue to be compressed tightly by the ligature. As the second ligature is tied, the upper clamp is removed. Double clamping is of great value here, for if only one clamp is used and the tissue slips out of the ligature and retracts, the vessels must be caught again in the presence of bleeding. Attempts at clamping such retracted vessels in the basilar portion of the broad ligament may result in injury to the ureter.

The cervical stump is then closed, using figure-of-eight sutures of No. 0 chromic catgut on cutting needles (Fig. 8-4 H).

Next, the cervical stump is suspended by suturing the various ligaments to it. Figure 8-4 I shows this step when adnexa on both sides have been saved. The chromic catgut suture is first placed through the anterior surface of the cervix. It then picks up a bit of the round ligament. A bite or two is taken in the peritoneum between the round ligament and the tube. The tube to which the ovarian ligament has been tied is next included. One or two bites are taken in the posterior leaf of the broad ligament. In picking up the broad ligament one should be careful to include only the peritoneal edge under vision, because if bites are taken recklessly into the posterior leaf, it is possible to include the ureter in the suture. Finally, a bite is taken in the posterior surface of the cervix. An assistant grasps the ends of the round ligament and the tube as the suture is tied over them. This suture not only suspends the cervix but also partially peritonealizes the pelvis.

In case the adnexa have been removed, the suspension and the peritonealizing are done somewhat differently. In some cases the infundibulopelvic ligament is sufficiently mobile to be brought down to the cervix without tension, but often it is not. The leaves of the broad ligament are approximated with a continuous stitch of No. 000 chromic catgut, and the stump of the infundibulopelvic ligament is buried between the leaves of the ligament by a purse string.

The peritonization of the cervical stump is carried out by suturing the edge of the bladder peritoneum to the posterior surface of the cervix, using either interrupted or continuous No. 000 chromic catgut. To ensure covering over the cut ends of the ligaments and the tubes, it is often desirable to pick up these structures with the suture, as indicated in Figure 8-4 J, to cause them to invert beneath the serosa.

Due to the growth of the tumor and complicating adhesions, variations in the above-described technic of subtotal hysterectomy are common. For example, adhesions between the fibroid uterus and the anterior rectal wall often occur, and it may be impossible to sever them safely under vision from above downward. In such cases the corpus may often be amputated at the cervix and the adhesions cut safely from below upward. Figure 8-5 A shows such adhesions on sagittal view, and Figure 8-5 B shows them as they are visualized by the operator. Peritonization of the cervical stump in such cases is sometimes best done by lightly suturing the bladder peritoneum to the anterior rectal wall, which is still adherent to the cervical stump (Fig. 8-5 C).

One of the commoner surgical maneuvers performed in our clinic is the side-to-side amputation described by Kelly in 1898 in his *Operative Gynecology*. The difficulty in dissecting down to the uterine vessels on one side may be due to the development of a fibroid laterally to such an extent that no space between it and the pelvic wall can be developed to permit clamping of the uterine vessels. Often a large intraligamentary tumor serves as a barrier that cannot be circumvented. It

Technic: Subtotal Abdominal Hysterectomy

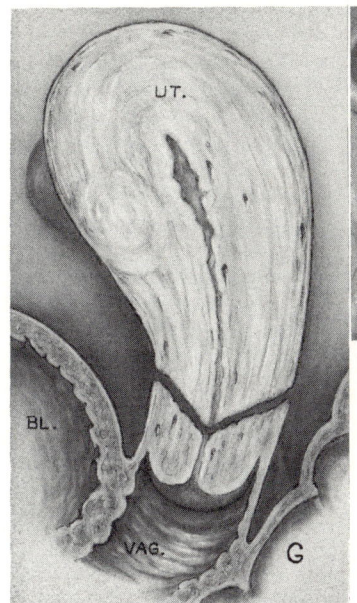
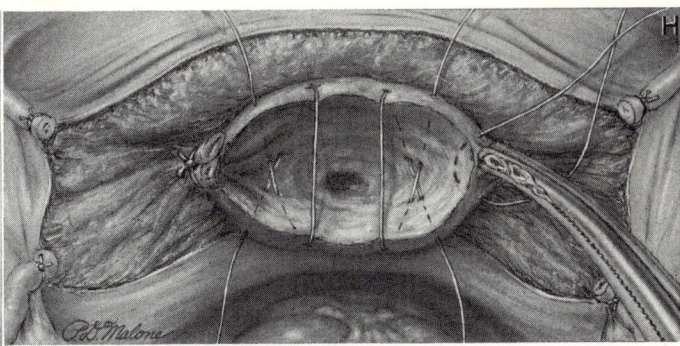
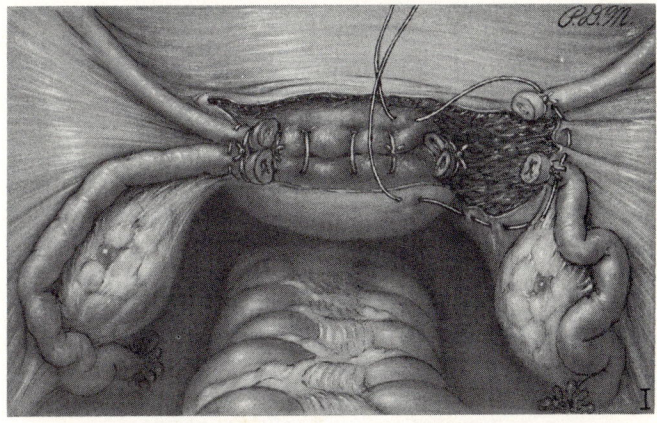
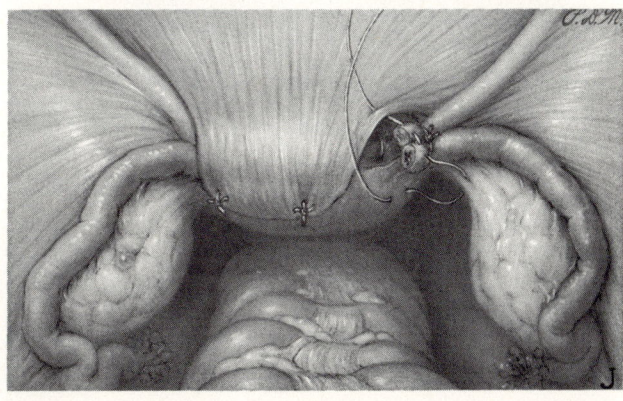

FIG. 8-4 (*Continued*). Subtotal abdominal hysterectomy. (G) Indicating method of coning out cervix to facilitate closing. (H) Indicating method of ligating the uterine vessels and suturing the cervix. (I) Demonstrating the method of suspending the cervix and partial peritonization. (J) Peritonization is completed by suturing the bladder peritoneum to the posterior surface of the cervix.

may also be due to a fixed, old adnexal inflammatory mass through which safe dissection is quite impossible. If, under such circumstances, the region of the uterine vessels can be reached on one side, they may be clamped, cut, and, if possible, ligated. The amputation is then made from that side to the opposite side, and the uterine vessels are clamped as they are approached (Fig. 8-6). If space permits, double clamping is desirable. Traction can best be made on the lower portion of the uterus with the volsellum, as shown in Figure 8-6. This controls back bleeding, and when there is bleeding from the uterine cavity, it is prevented from soiling the operative field.

As the amputation is done, an assistant grasps the cervical stump with a Jacobs tenaculum. By keeping traction on this, the danger of retraction of the cervix is prevented.

162 Myomata Uteri

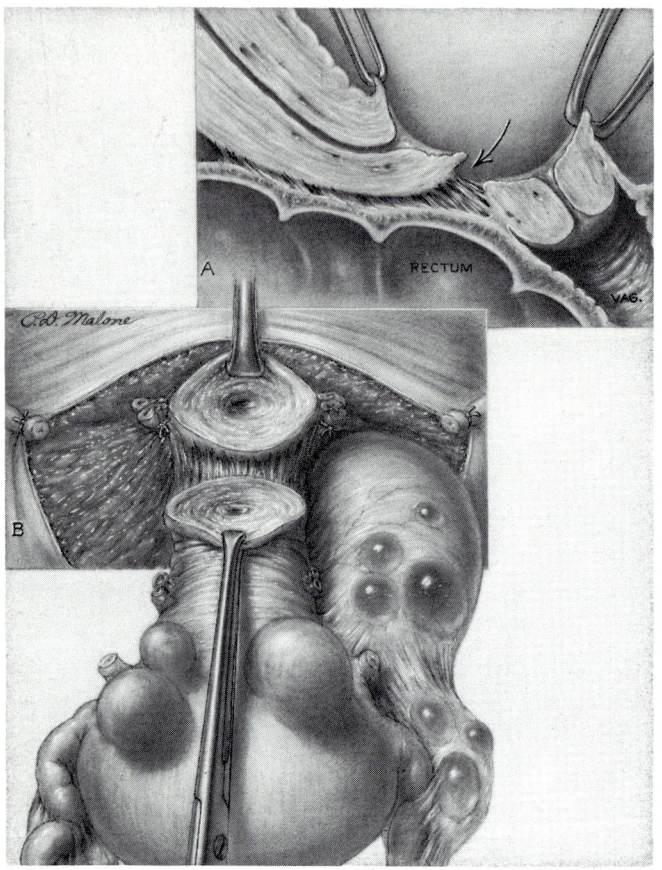

Fig. 8-5. Method of dissecting the uterus from the adherent rectal wall. (A) Dense adhesions between the rectum and the posterior surface of the uterus, which cannot be safely separated from above, are shown. (B) Uterine vessels are ligated, and the corpus is amputated from the cervix. Traction on the uterus upward exposes the adhesions which can usually be safely cut from below upward under direct vision. (C) Method of peritonization when the cul-de-sac is obliterated by adhesions or is raw due to freeing of the adherent mass from the cul-de-sac.

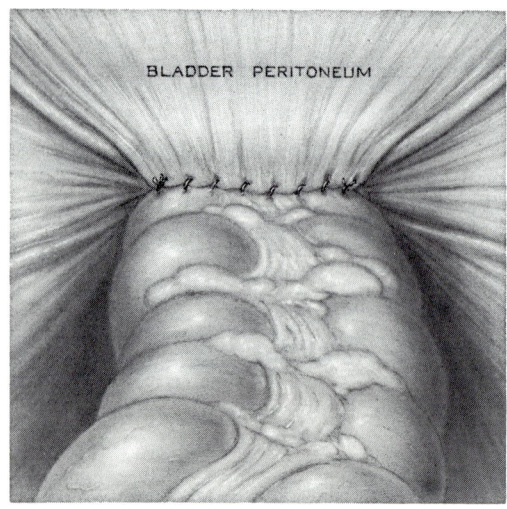

Total Abdominal Hysterectomy (Richardson's) for Benign Uterine Disease

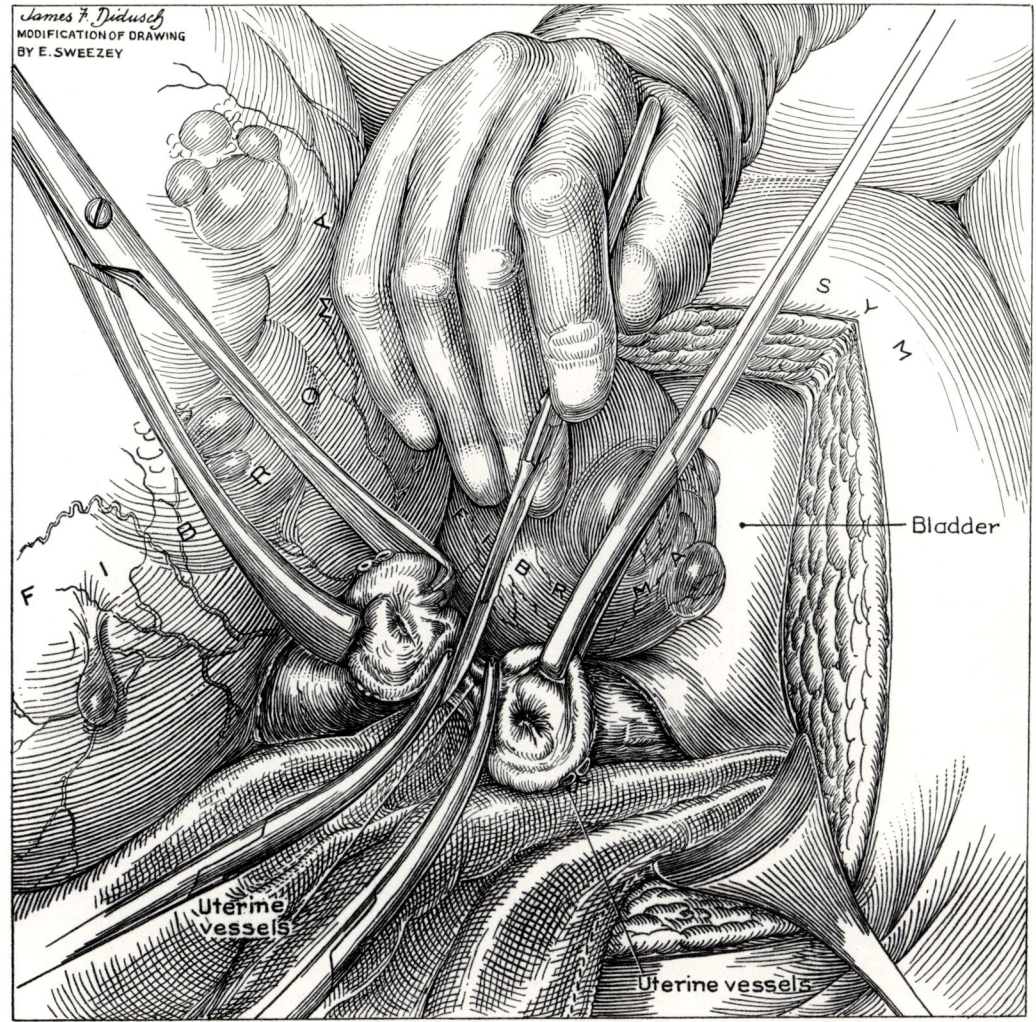

FIG. 8-6. Supravaginal amputation of a fibromatous uterus from right to left. The right uterine vessels have been clamped, cut, and tied. The left vessels are clamped as they are approached and are about to be cut.

After the base of the broad ligament is opened, dissection of the adnexal or fibroid mass from beneath usually can be done with less difficulty and greater safety. When there is an adherent adnexal mass, the infundibulopelvic ligament is often the last structure to be clamped, as it is isolated after the mass is freed from below upward.

TOTAL ABDOMINAL HYSTERECTOMY FOR BENIGN UTERINE DISEASE (RICHARDSON TECHNIC)

When in our judgment total abdominal hysterectomy is indicated for benign uterine disease, we remove the uterus, using the technic as described by E. H.

164 Myomata Uteri

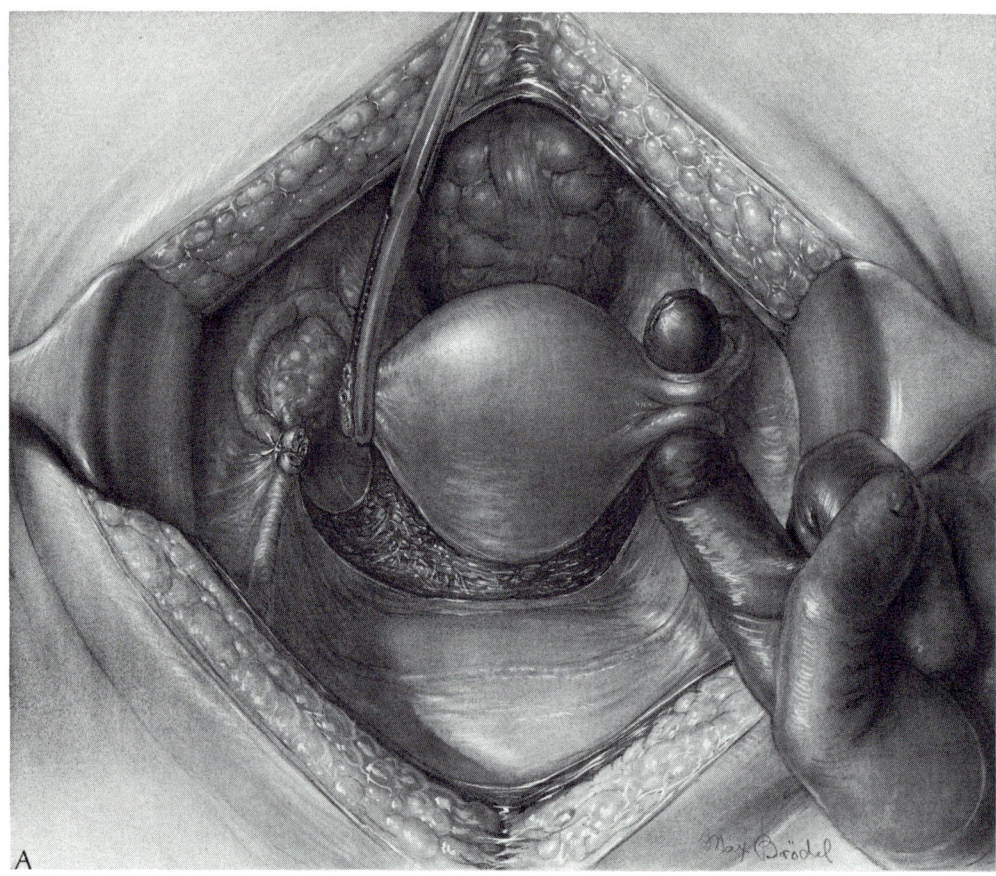

Fig. 8-7. Conservative total hysterectomy, Richardson technic. (A) The vesicouterine peritoneum has been incised transversely. The left round ligament, the fallopian tube and the utero-ovarian ligament are shown resting upon the index finger which has perforated the broad ligament. On the opposite side these structures have been divided and ligated. (Richardson, E. H.: A simplified technic for abdominal panhysterectomy. Surg. Gynec. Obstet., 48:252-256)

Richardson. We regard Richardson's contribution as a classic, and therefore his original article and illustrations are quoted here (Fig. 8-7 A to K). Certain modifications which we have used are discussed in the pages immediately after this description.

Technic of the Operation. 1. The bladder and the rectum should be empty. Preliminary, thorough surgical toilet of the vulva, vagina, and cervix is first carried out. In addition, the entire vagina, vaginal portion of the cervix, and, particularly, the external os and cervical canal are thoroughly treated with the official tincture of iodine, 20 per cent Mercurochrome or Scott's solution. The external os is then tightly closed by aseptic suture, and a dry sterile gauze pack is introduced into the vagina, one end of which is left outside, to which a clamp is attached, so that it can be readily withdrawn just before the vagina is opened above. The usual surgical toilet of the abdominal wall is then made, and the sterile draperies are properly arranged.

2. A lower midline incision is made from the symphysis pubix to the umbilicus.

3. Adequate exposure of the pelvis is secured through use of the Trendelenburg posture, together with the judicious use of wet gauze packs.

4. The body of the uterus is now grasped firmly with an appropriate instrument and lifted well up, provided only that its pathology is known to be benign in character.

Total Abdominal Hysterectomy (Richardson's) for Benign Uterine Disease

If, however, malignancy has been demonstrated or is suspected, the operation must be modified to include removal of both tubes and ovaries, and it is particulary stressed that no compression whatever should be applied to the uterus, either by instruments or by the surgeon's hands, until its extrinsic blood and lymphatic channels have been absolutely blocked by ligation and division of its four cardinal circulatory trunk systems, namely the two ovarian and the two uterine. This I believe to be a sound and effective precaution against the possible dissemination of malignant cells by squeezing them out into adjacent vascular currents.

5. A transverse, crescent-shaped incision is now made through the vesicouterine peritoneum at the upper margin of its loose attachment to the uterus and is carried laterally on each side to the uterine attachment of the round ligaments.

6. Into the angle of this incision on each side the index finger is introduced and burrowed bluntly through the loose areolar tissue of the upper portion of the broad ligament, perforating its posterior layer close to the uterus and below the level of attachment of the round ligament, the fallopian tube, and the utero-ovarian ligament.

7. This aperture is bluntly enlarged sufficiently to permit the approximation of these three structures to form a single pedicle, to which two stout clamps are applied, and amputation is done between them close to the uterus.

8. Transfixing ligatures replace the two clamps on the severed appendage stump, while the two applied to the cornua of the

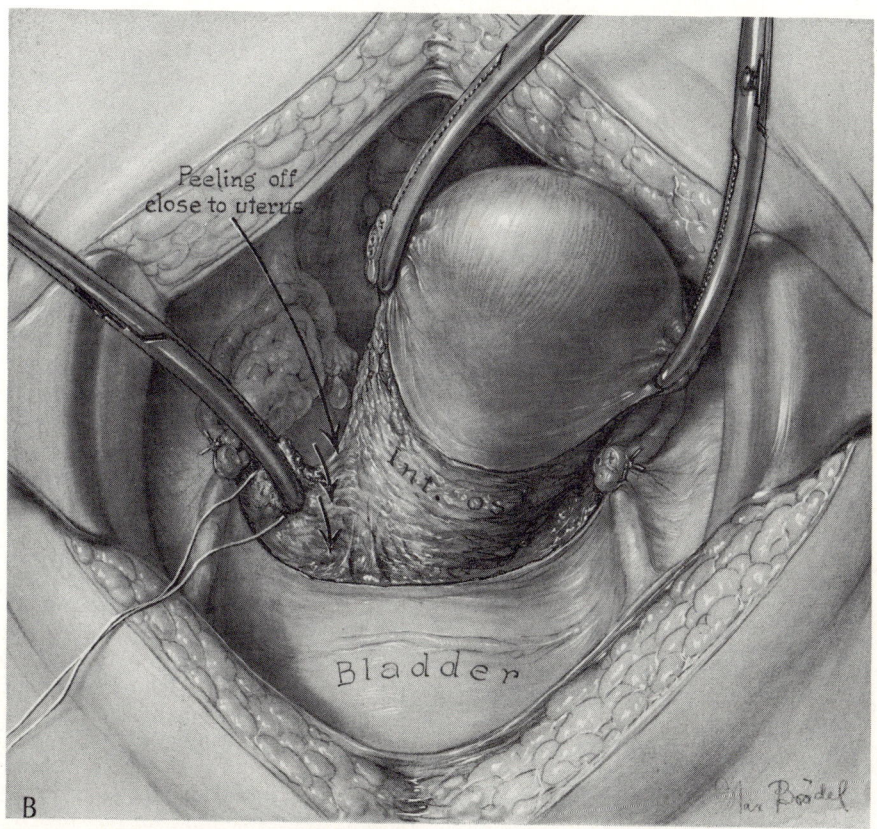

Fig. 8-7 (*Continued*). Conservative total hysterectomy, Richardson technic. (B) The right uterine vessels are shown clamped and divided with a ligature placed around them. The arrows indicate the line of dissection used to drop these vessels, together with the attached ureter, well away from the danger zone. (Richardson, E. H.: A simplified technic for abdominal panhysterectomy. Surg. Gynec. Obstet., *48*: 252-256)

166 Myomata Uteri

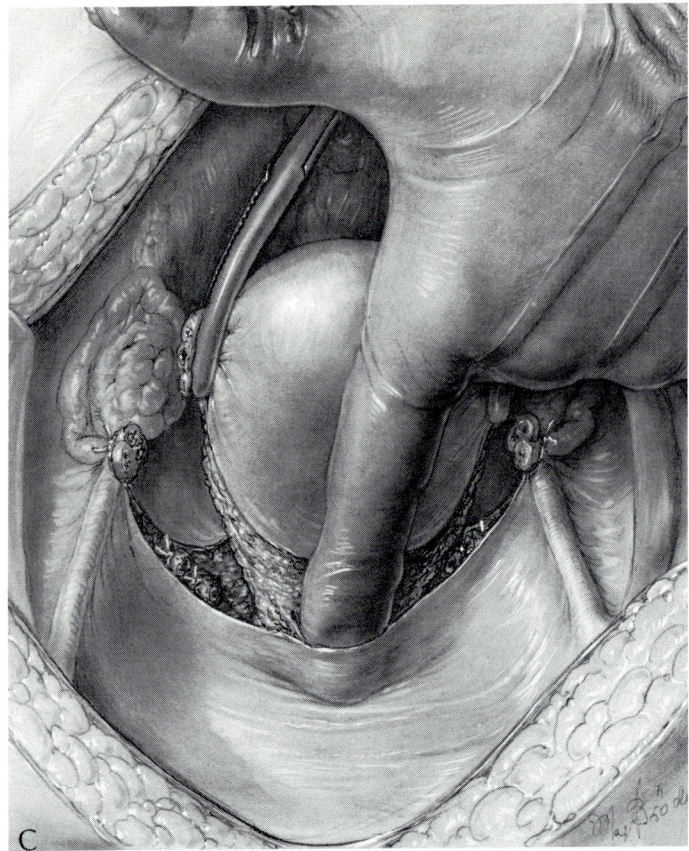

FIG. 8-7 (*Continued*). Conservative total hysterectomy, Richardson technic. (C) Here the bladder is being gently separated from the cervix by blunt dissection applied to its avascular central zone. Note that this dissection leaves the pubocervical (subvesical) fascia covering the cervix. To this structure the troublesome venous plexus is attached. Utilization of this anatomic fact to advantage is described in the operative technic. (Richardson, E. H.: A simplified technic for abdominal panhysterectomy. Surg. Gynec. Obstet., *48*:252-256)

uterus are henceforth used as tractors. The original instrument with which the body of the uterus was grasped for the purpose of elevating it is now removed.

9. Traction upward upon the uterus now brings clearly into view the skeletonized uterine vessels, which are clamped and divided on each side at the level of the internal os. Ligatures replace the clamps on these vessels, care being exercised not to include any cervical tissue in passing the needle.

10. The severed uterine vessels, with ease and safety, may now be bluntly dissected away from the cervix down to the point of their emergence above the thick basal segment of the broad ligament on each side.

11. The uterus is drawn strongly upward, and the bladder is easily separated by blunt dissection with the gauze-covered index finger first from the cervix and then from the anterior vaginal wall well down below the level of the external os. In most instances the line of cleavage along the course of least resistance here is between the bladder and the pubocervical (subvesical) layer of fascia, so that, after the bladder has been pushed well down, close inspection of the cervix anteriorly will disclose that it is covered with a thin but definite layer of fascia. It is in this fascia that the troublesome vascular plexus is contained. If now a T-shaped incision be made through the fascia with the transverse

cut a little below the level of the internal os and the vertical one over the middle of the cervix, the fascia layer together with the vessels may be easily freed from the cervix with the index finger and pushed laterally on each side, so that the vessels are nicely segregated adjacent to the basal segments of the broad ligaments.

Steps 10 and 11 serve further to drop the ureters well away from the cervix where damage to them is scarcely possible, if reasonable care is exercised in the subsequent application of clamps and sutures.

12. Strong traction upward and forward is exerted upon the uterus, and a transverse incision is made through its posterior peritoneal reflection 1 centimeter above the level of attachment of the two uterosacral ligaments. The lower peritoneal flap resulting is quite firmly attached to the posterior wall of the cervix, and sharp dissection vertically downward for at least 2 centimeters is necessary in order to free it sufficiently to permit introduction of the left index finger. Below this level the peritoneal and rectal attachment is quite loose, and blunt dissection is now utilized, first to free the peritoneum from the cervix, and then is continued downward to release the rectum from the vagina below the level of the external os. Bleeding does not occur in this step of the operation if care is exercised not to carry the dissection laterally on either side into the broad ligament zone.

13. If the uterus now be lifted well up, the two index fingers may readily be apposed below the level of the vaginal portion of the cervix by invagination of the anterior and posterior vaginal walls respectively, thus demonstrating that the bladder and rectum have been freed from the vagina sufficiently low down.

14. The two uterosacral ligaments are now clamped, divided, and ligated close to their cervical attachments.

15. The dense basal segment of the broad ligament on each side, together with the vascular plexus adjacent to it, which has been segregated through the earlier blunt dissection carried out over the central zone of the cervix in front and behind, may now be easily grasped close to the lateral border of the cervix, divided and securely ligated, the clamps being removed. If the cervix is elongated, this step has to be repeated at a lower level.

16. The vaginal vault now comes up into plain view on all sides, and the sterile gauze vaginal pack is withdrawn from below. Note

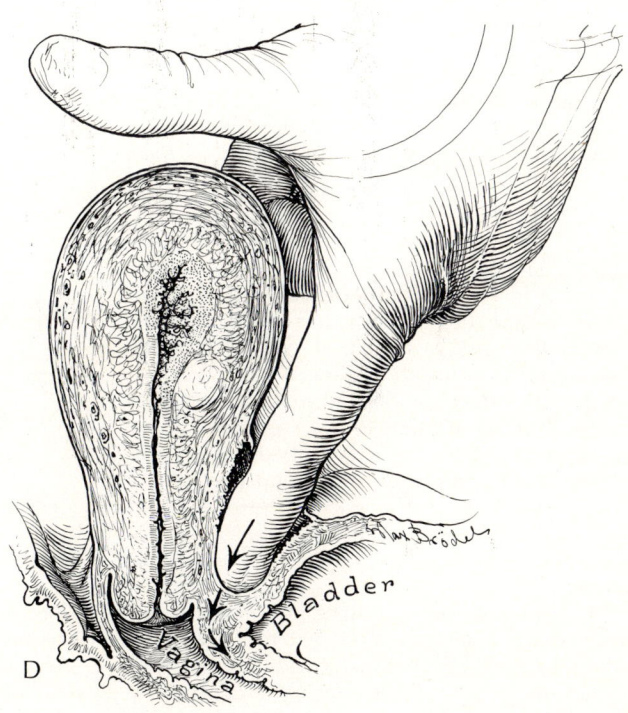

Fig. 8-7 (*Continued*). Conservative total hysterectomy, Richardson technic. (D) A sagittal view showing depth and direction of the vesicocervicovaginal dissection. This step serves to drop the ureters still farther away from the danger zone. (Richardson, E. H.: A simplified technic for abdominal panhysterectomy. Surg. Gynec. Obstet., 48:252-256)

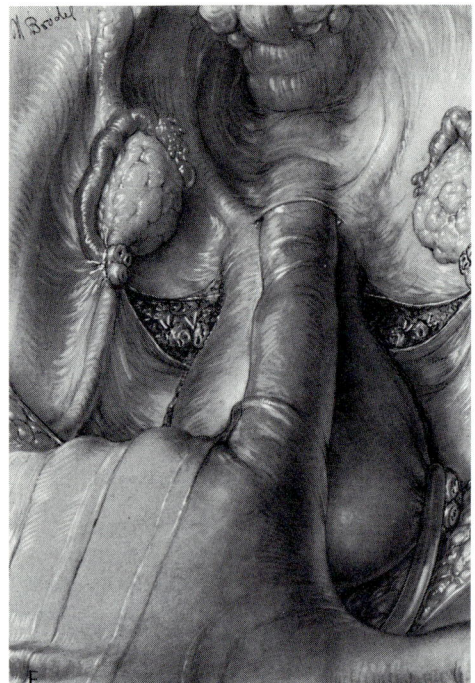

FIG. 8-7 (*Continued*). Conservative total hysterectomy, Richardson technic. (E) By means of the cornual traction clamps the uterus has been lifted strongly upward and forward over the pubis. A transverse peritoneal incision has been made 1 cm. above the attachment of the uterosacral ligaments. The method of applying blunt dissection to the avascular midsection of the cervix and the upper vagina is indicated. (Richardson, E. H.: A simplified technic for abdominal panhysterectomy. Surg. Gynec. Obstet, *48*:252-256)

mesial to the angle clamp; it now twice transfixes the stump of the basal portion of the broad ligament, forming within it a liberal mattress suture loop; from here the needle again enters the lumen of the vagina, piercing its posterior wall also 1 centimeter mesial to the angle clamp and, further, is made to transfix the stump of the uteroscaral ligament. When tied, this suture closes the lateral vaginal angle and snugly apposes to it for support both the strong basal segment of the broad ligament and the uterosacral ligament.

18. Further complete or partial apposition of the anterior to the posterior vaginal wall by suture, depending on whether or not drainage is to be employed, is now quickly executed.

19. A single mattress suture on each side now first engages the closed vaginal vault anteriorly and mesially to the angle suture, trans-

that even at this stage of the operation there are no clamps in the pelvis and that no troublesome hemorrhage has been encountered. The anterior vaginal wall is incised, the vagina promptly balloons, and the incision is extended around the cervix, four clamps being applied to the vaginal vault as it proceeds: one anteriorly in the midline, one laterally to each angle, and one posteriorly in the midline, as the entire uterus is lifted out of the pelvis, without the cervix at any time having come in contact with any intrapelvic tissue.

17. Special angle sutures now replace the two angle clamps as follows: the needle is first passed through the anterior vaginal wall into the lumen of the vagina 1 centimeter

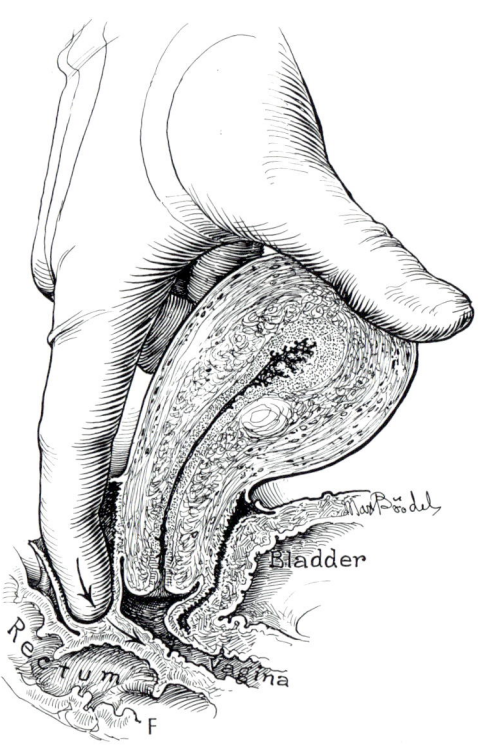

FIG. 8-7 (*Continued*). Conservative total hysterectomy, Richardson technic. (F) A sagittal view showing the bladder dissection completed and indicating depth and direction of the posterior dissection. (Richardson, E. H.: A simplified technic for abdominal panhysterectomy, Surg., Gynec. & Obst. *48*:252-256)

Total Abdominal Hysterectomy (Richardson's) for Benign Uterine Disease

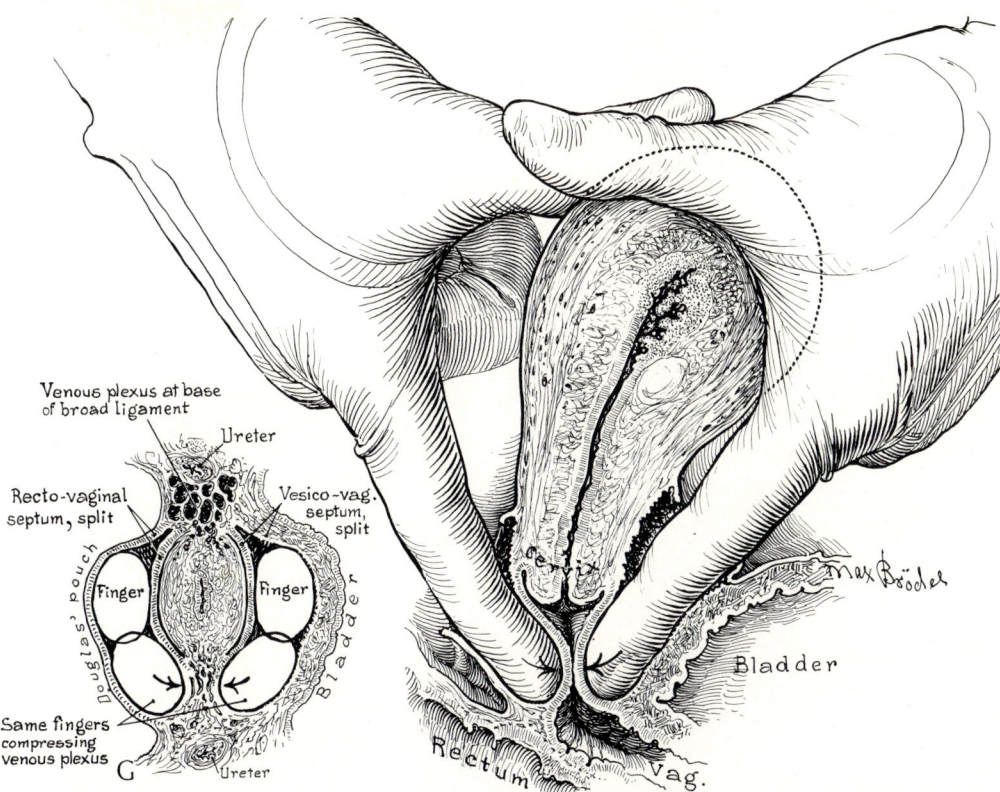

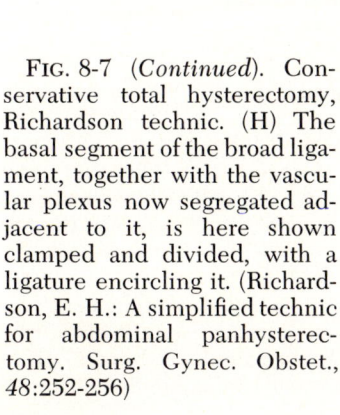

FIG. 8-7 (*Continued*). Conservative total hysterectomy, Richardson technic. (G) Testing the depth of the anterior and the posterior dissections. The inset shows the method of segregating the vascular plexus on each side into a narrow zone adjacent to the basal segment of the broad ligament. (Richardson, E. H.: A simplified technic for abdominal panhysterectomy. Surg. Gynec. Obstet., 48:252-256)

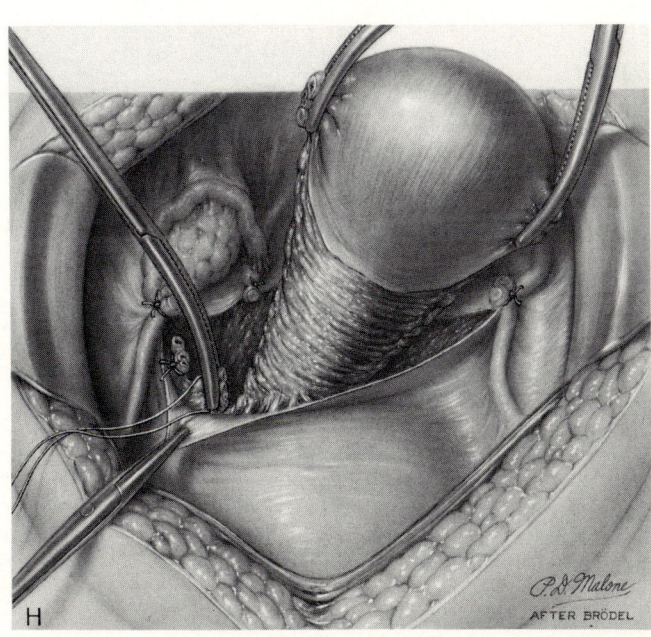

FIG. 8-7 (*Continued*). Conservative total hysterectomy, Richardson technic. (H) The basal segment of the broad ligament, together with the vascular plexus now segregated adjacent to it, is here shown clamped and divided, with a ligature encircling it. (Richardson, E. H.: A simplified technic for abdominal panhysterectomy. Surg. Gynec. Obstet., 48:252-256)

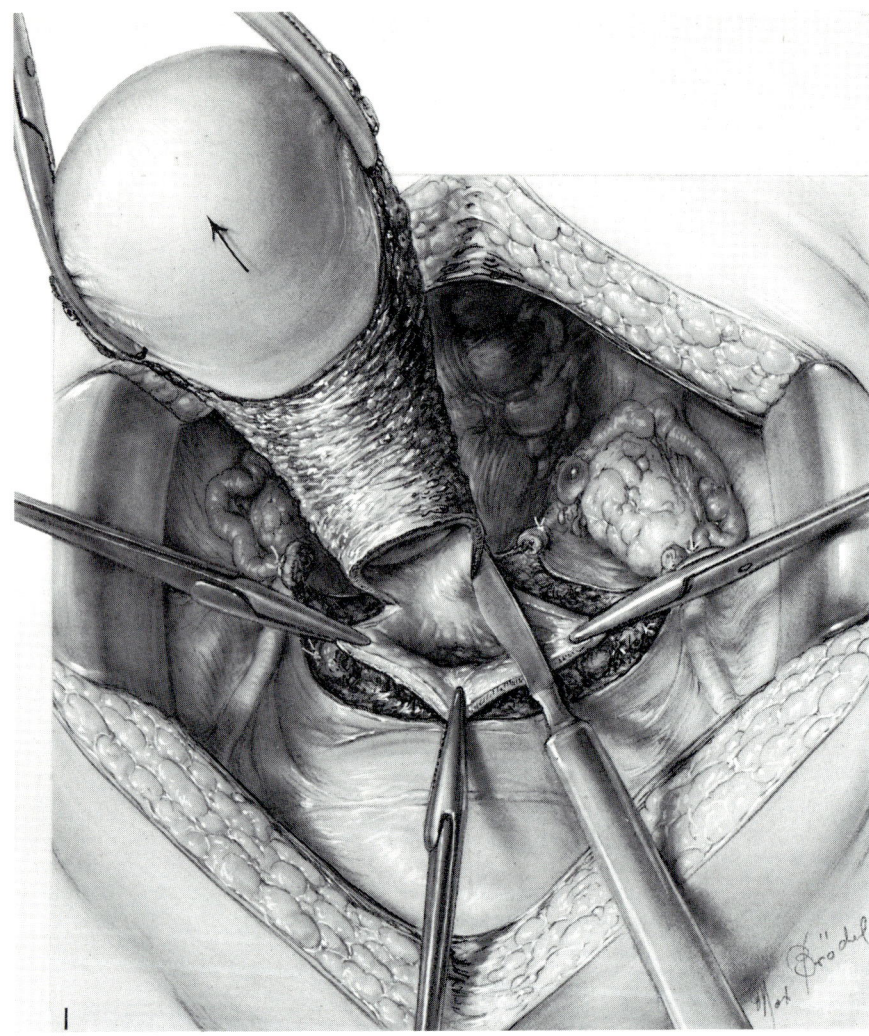

FIG. 8-7 (*Continued*). Conservative total hysterectomy, Richardson technic. (I) The dissection completed, the amputation across the vaginal vault is here shown. This should be done as closely as possible to the cervix in order to avoid shortening the vagina. Note that no instrument comes in contact with the cervix, nor does the latter touch the field of the operation at any time. (Richardson, E. H.: A simplified technic for abdominal panhysterectomy. Surg. Gynec. Obstet., 48:252-256)

fixes the stumps of the round and utero-ovarian ligaments, and passes back to engage the posterior vaginal wall opposite the point of entrance. When tied, this suture snugly apposes the round and utero-ovarian ligaments to the vaginal vault, thus affording additional support to the latter and at the same time neatly suspending the ovaries.

20. The cut margin of the vesicouterine peritoneum is now neatly sewed to the free edge of the posterior peritoneal flap, so that the pelvis is completely peritonealized with the vaginal vault and the ovaries strongly supported.

Modification A. If for any reason unilateral or bilateral salpingo-oophorectomy is indicated, the technic described becomes even simpler and is readily modified according to well-established procedure to meet this requirement.

Modification B. If exposure of the cervix for the lower dissection is rendered difficult by reason of a benign pathological condition in the corpus uteri, such as enlargement from a

Total Abdominal Hysterectomy (Richardson's) for Benign Uterine Disease

myomatous change, it is recommended that a subtotal hysterectomy at or above the level of the internal os first be done. The cervix may then be easily and speedily removed by means of the technic as described.

Summary

The perfected technic of this operation has been gradually developed during the past 4 years, in which period I have used it a number of times for various types of uterine disease. Thus far I have had no mortality and no postoperative complications, other than the minor ones uniformly associated with any major abdominal procedure. The operation is offered, not with the optimistic fancy that no untoward results will later be chargeable to it, but with the confident belief that it possesses the following distinct advantages.

1. Each step of the operation is anatomically and surgically sound in principle.
2. It is relatively simple, easy of execution, and consumes substantially less time than has been hitherto required by most operators for abdominal panhysterectomy.
3. There is complete freedom from hemorrhage or troublesome oozing throughout, which is accomplished by means of a carefully planned anatomic dissection that serves to segregate the vascular network surrounding the lower cervix, so that not more than four hemostatic clamps are required in the pelvis at any stage of the operation.
4. The danger of injury to the ureters is reduced to a negligible factor.

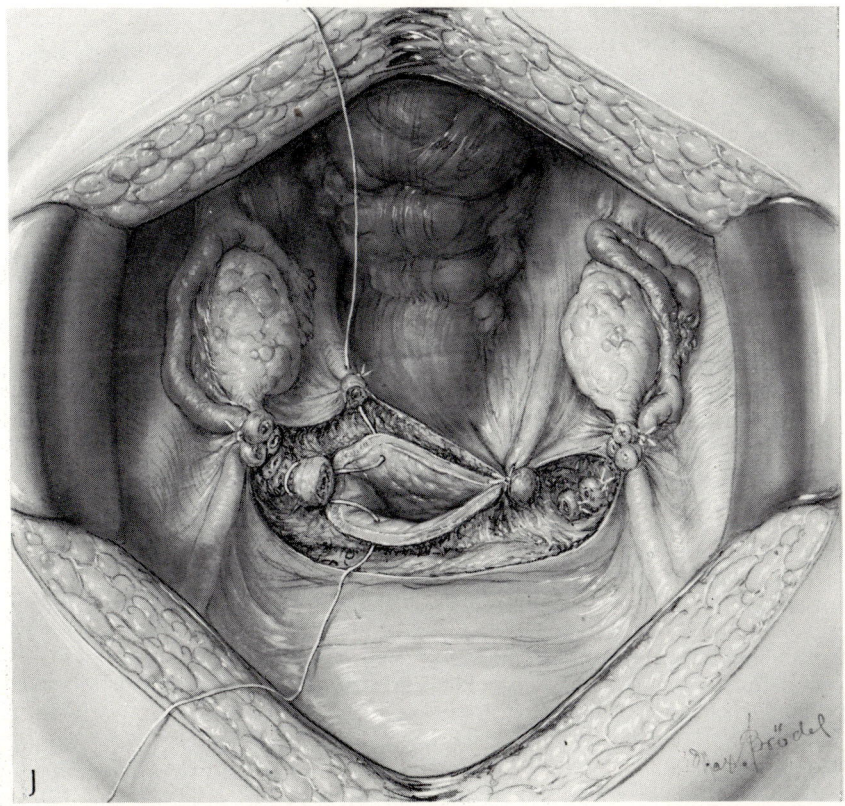

FIG. 8-7 (*Continued*). Conservative total hysterectomy, Richardson technic. (J) Illustrating the highly important angle stitch. Note that it first pierces the anterior vaginal wall 1 cm. from the lateral angle; it then twice transfixes the cardinal ligament to form a liberal mattress loop within this important structure; then it is passed through the posterior vaginal wall also 1 cm. from the angle and finally transfixes the stump of the uterosacral ligament. On the left side this suture has been tied, closing snugly the lateral angle of the vaginal vault and uniting with it the 2 strong supporting ligaments. (Richardson, E. H.: A simplified technic for abdominal panhysterectomy. Surg. Gynec. Obstet., 48:252-256)

172 Myomata Uteri

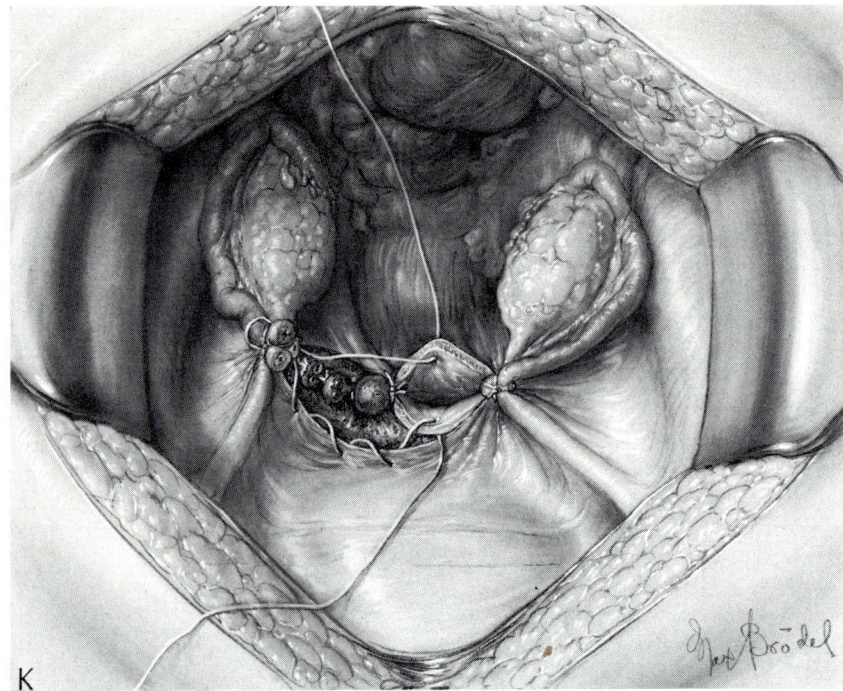

Fig. 8-7 (*Continued*). Conservative total hysterectomy, Richardson technic. (K) Left side of the pelvis has been peritonized. Right side is being peritonized in the same manner. (Richardson, E. H.: A simplified technic for abdominal panhysterectomy. Surg. Gynec. Obstet., 48:252-256)

5. The accurate identification and preservation of the substantial basal portions of the broad ligaments and of the uterosacral ligaments for later co-adaptation to the vaginal vault by a specially devised suture affords an efficient guarantee against later prolapse.

6. The possible contamination of the field of operation or of the peritoneal cavity from the cervix harboring virulent organisms is reduced to a minimum.

7. The special step recommended in the cases in which malignant disease is suspected (step 4) constitutes an additional protection against possible recurrence. This is a factor of unquestionable merit.

8. Finally, the factors which commonly produce shock and prompt exodus following panhysterectomy, such as excessive loss of blood, extensive mechanical insult to the tissues, and prolonged operative manipulations, are completely eliminated through this simplified technic.*

---

* Richardson, E. H.: A simplified technique for abdominal panhysterectomy. Surg. Gynec. Obstet., 48:252-256, 1929.

COMMENTS ON AND MODIFICATIONS OF RICHARDSON TECHNIC OF TOTAL ABDOMINAL HYSTERECTOMY

The technic of total abdominal hysterectomy above shown is, in the opinion of the authors, superior to any thus far described. It is logically planned to ensure complete hemostasis, to keep the pelvis free of interfering clamps at all times, and to utilize all ligamentous supports for the vagina. However, in adopting another surgeon's technic it is inevitable that each surgeon make a few modifications of the operation as originally described. This has been done without in any way changing the fundamental procedures, with the exception of the matter of drainage, which we have generally abandoned. Since our indications for abdominal panhysterectomy have been liberalized, many of the cervices removed are not badly infected. Although we carry out a careful preoperative vaginal toilet as suggested by Richardson, the final step of which is painting the cervix and the vagina with Scott's solution, we do not *routinely* suture the lips of the cervix. When the cervix is the source of a profuse discharge, when there is a pedunculated submucous fibroid peeking through the external os, or when there is reason to believe that the endometrial cavity is infected, we carry out the preliminary suturing of the external os. After painting the vagina and the cervix with Scott's solution we place a dry sponge against the cervix to absorb any secretions from the cervix or the corpus. This sponge is clamped and left protruding from the vagina so that it can be withdrawn by a nurse just before the vagina is opened.

The original Richardson technic calls for routine vaginal drainage. We have practiced tight closure of the vagina in a large series of cases and never have had occasion to regret it. On the basis of our experience, we now use drainage only in those cases in which the infection of the cervix or the endometrium is thought to be unusually severe. With the use of antibiotics our indications for drainage are becoming rarer and rarer. Within the past 15 years we cannot recall draining a single hysterectomy.

First, we wish to call attention again to the pubovesicocervical fascia, described by Richardson but not pictured in his original series of drawings. The fibers of this fascia extend from the level of the internal os of the cervix, beneath the mucosa of the anterior vaginal wall, to the symphysis. After the reflexion of the bladder peritoneum has been cut, and the bladder has been dissected downward this fascia is identified readily, and the fibers can be seen running parallel with the direction of the vagina and the cervix. The T-shaped incision in this fascia cut just below the level of the internal os is shown in Figure 8-8 A. As the edges of the fascia retract laterally, the light pink undersurface of the vaginal mucosa comes into view. The cut edges of the fascia usually bleed from the vessels within it. We wish to emphasize that this fascia layer is an important structure containing blood vessels that supply the upper vagina and the cervix. The proper disposition of this fascia is one of the most important points in carrying out panhysterectomy according to the Richardson technic. Since we have been closing the vagina almost routinely, we have modified the Richardson procedure slightly. We now carry out the cutting of the uterosacral ligaments and the freeing of the cervix and the vagina posteriorly, before making the T-shaped incision through the pubovesicocervical fascia. After completing the posterior steps of the operation, the cut edges of the fascia are clamped and sutured immediately after making the anterior fascial incision (Fig. 8-8 B). This ligation is done with No. 0 chromic catgut.

After the vagina and the cervix have been stripped of the fascia and freed from the basal portion of the broad ligament, only the vaginal mucosa is left, and it is usually thin enough so that the anterior and the posterior walls may be clamped together at either angle, as shown in Figure 8-8 C. For this purpose we have found the Heaney vaginal hysterectomy clamps exceedingly well adapted. Sometimes the vagina is so small that the clamps may be made to meet in the midline, thus keeping it completely closed when cut across. In most instances the closure is not complete, as in Figure 8-8 D, but only a small opening is left between the clamps. After the amputation, the center opening is closed immediately with a figure-of-eight suture of No. 0 chromic catgut, and then the lateral angles are closed, as indicated in Figure 8-8 D. Occasionally, the vaginal walls are so thick that the bilateral clamping is not feasible. In such instances it is better not to persist in the above-described technic but to abandon it in favor of the technic originally described by Richardson.

After the closure of the vagina, it is supported by suturing to it the pubovesicocervical fascia and the various ligaments utilized by Richardson. Since the vagina has been closed already, it is obvious that this must be done by a slightly different technic than that origi-

174 Myomata Uteri

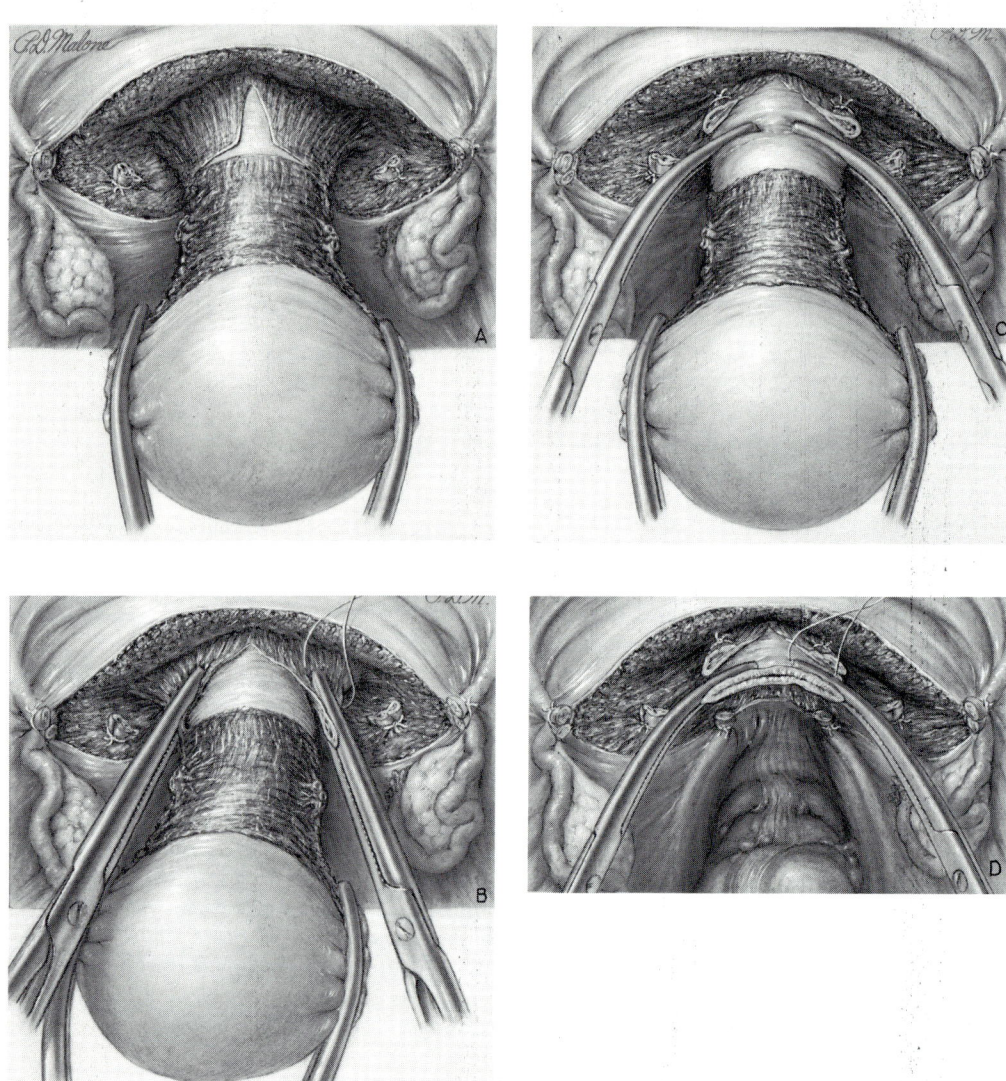

FIG. 8-8. Modification of Richardson's technic adapted to vaginal closure. (A) Demonstrating T-shaped incision into the pubocervical fascia as recommended by Richardson. (B) The fascial edges with contained blood vessels are clamped and sutured. (C) The vagina is closed as much as possible by placing 2 Ochsner clamps on it from each side just below the cervix. When the vagina is small, the ends of these 2 clamps may touch, thus completely closing it. Note that clamps include only the vagina, the fascia having been peeled off and clamped separately. (D) The central portion of the vagina is closed with a figure-of-eight suture of chromic catgut. The portion of the vagina held by the clamp is closed with a mattress stitch which perforates the vagina anteriorly at the nose of the clamp and posteriorly near the vaginal edge.

nally described by Richardson. Using No. 000 chromic catgut, the pelvis is finally peritonized completely.

The above method of dealing with the pubocervical fascia was described in the first edition of this book. We still use it as a routine procedure in most of our hysterectomies. However, there are instances in which it is not desirable to dissect the bladder free from the vagina sufficiently far to make the T-shaped incision. Adhesions or varicose veins between the bladder and the fascia may make it advisable to dissect the bladder free as little as possible. In such cases the fascia may be cut transversely at its insertion into the cervix, and the fascia may be dissected free from the vagina with the knife handle. In this manner it is impossible to injure the bladder, and the vessels lying between the bladder and the fascia are avoided. The vaginal clamps are inserted within the space beneath the fascia. These steps are shown in Figure 8-9.

Technic: Total Hysterectomy for Cervical Myoma

When total hysterectomy is done for a large cervical myoma, the danger lies in possible injury to the ureters, the bladder, or the rectum. Because of the enlargement of the cervix, any or all of these structures may be encroached upon and displaced.

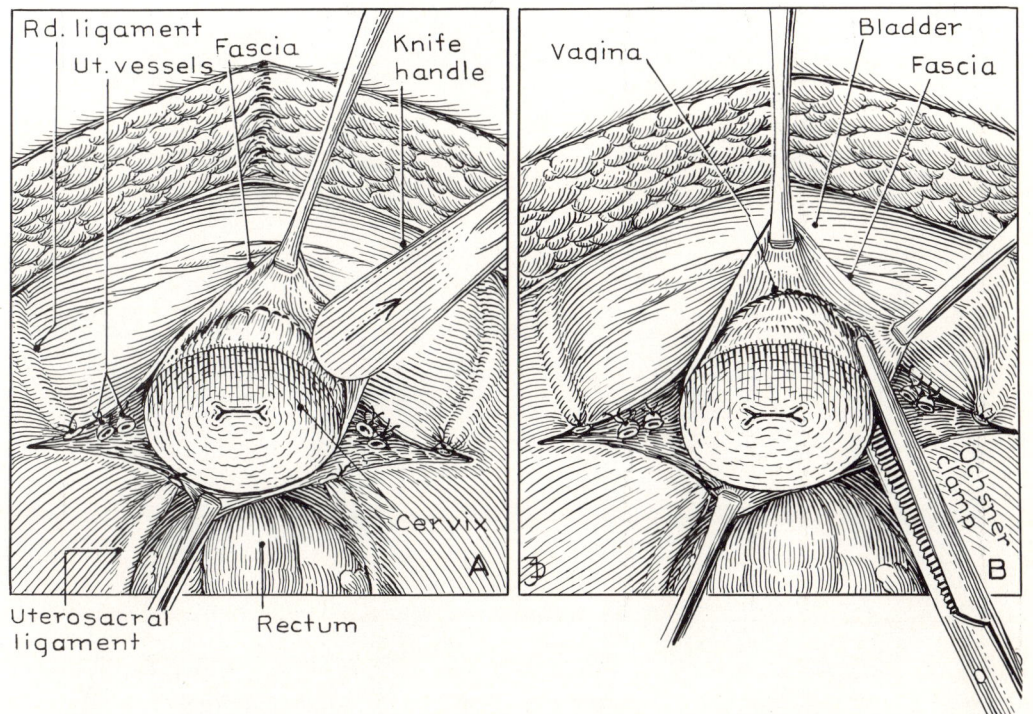

Fig. 8-9. Showing another method of performing total hysterectomy safely. The corpus uterus has been removed in order to demonstrate the technic more easily. (A) The fascial attachment to the cervix has been cut transversely, and the fascia is dissected free with the handle of the scalpel. (B) The paracervical tissues are clamped with the clamp inside of this fascial sheath. The lateral clamping can be carried down bilaterally to a point below the tip of the cervix. After this the cervix is amputated from the vagina.

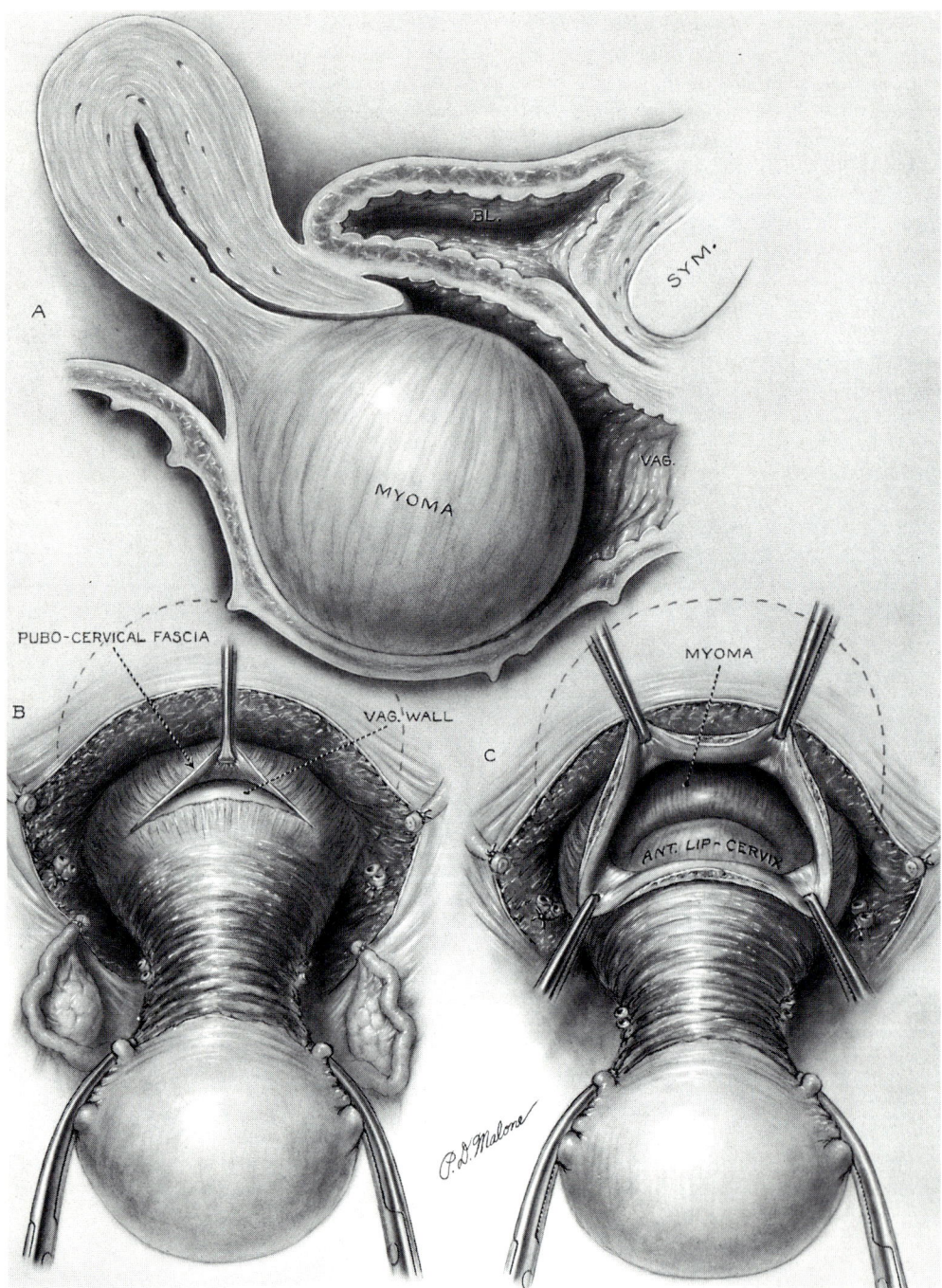

FIG. 8-10. Total hysterectomy for cervical myoma. (A) Sagittal section showing position of tumor. (B) A transverse incision is made through the pubocervical fascia, exposing the anterior vaginal wall. (C) The vagina has been entered through the anterior wall, exposing the tumor in the vagina. The excision is completed by trimming the tumor from its attachment to the vaginal wall posteriorly.

Figure 8-10 A illustrates a large myoma that has developed in the posterior lip of the cervix. Its removal from the vagina was quite impossible because it blocked the entire upper half of the vagina. Therefore, a total abdominal hysterectomy was required to remove this bleeding tumor.

The first part of the operation is exactly like the routine total hysterectomy However, special technic is required in excision of the cervix from the vagina. A transverse incision is made through the pubocervical fascia, just below its uppermost insertion into the cervix (Fig. 8-10 B). Then by blunt dissection this fascia is dissected downward from the vaginal wall. This maneuver absolutely safeguards injury to the ureters and the bladder, for if one cuts the vagina within this fascia, it is impossible to injure them.

The uterosacral ligaments are sutured and cut, and the peritoneum between these 2 ligaments is also cut. Using the index finger, the dissection is carried downward for a short distance in the midline posteriorly between the peritoneum and the vagina. It is assumed that the uterine vessels have been previously cut and sutured.

The vagina is then incised anteriorly where it has been bared of the pubocervical fascia. This exposes the anterior lip of the cervix and also the myoma arising from the posterior lip (Fig. 8-10 C). The wound is well protected with gauze because the remainder of the operation is not entirely clean, in spite of the most meticulous vaginal cleanup. A traction suture is placed in the myoma, and successive ones are used as the tumor is delivered through the vaginal opening. The vagina is trimmed from the tumor very closely as the tumor is pulled upward. The vaginal mucosa is clamped as necessary with Ochsner clamps. After the cervix has been completely cut from the vagina, the posterior surface is still attached to the anterior rectal wall by loose connective tissue. The cervix can now be dissected free from the rectal wall under vision, from below upward. The closure of the vagina and its suspension are done in a routine manner.

INJURY TO THE BLADDER

Injury to the urinary bladder can be avoided by performing the total hysterectomy within the pubocervical fascia. However, there are instances when, due to inflammation or neoplasm, this fascia is not easily dissected. Also, in doing the Wertheim or a modified Wertheim operation the fascia should not be dissected from the cervix or the vagina. When the bladder is injured accidentally at operation, this is not a serious catastrophy. Indeed, there are occasions when doing hysterectomy for malignancy it is desirable to remove a segment of the bladder with the uterus. Closure of the bladder with a double layer of No. 00 chromic catgut is all that is necessary. The first continuous suture should include the bladder musculature going to but not through the bladder mucosa (Fig. 8-11). It should be so taken as to invert the mucosa into the bladder. A second continuous suture should invert the first. A retention Foley catheter should be left in the bladder for 10 days postoperatively. In following this method of closure at the time of the primary operation there has never resulted a vesicovaginal fistula in our institution after abdominal hysterectomy.

POSTHYSTERECTOMY HEMORRHAGE

The most common serious posthysterectomy complication is bleeding. Fortunately, serious bleeding does not occur frequently. In a series of 1,000 consecutive hysterectomies reported by Gray there was bleeding sufficient to require resuturing in 0.8 per cent. Nevertheless, when profuse bleeding does occur, it may start suddenly and assume alarming proportions in a remarkably short time so that quick action is imperative and, indeed, may be lifesaving.

Bleeding noted directly after the operation is due to improper suturing of the vaginal cuff and should be attended to immediately by returning the patient to

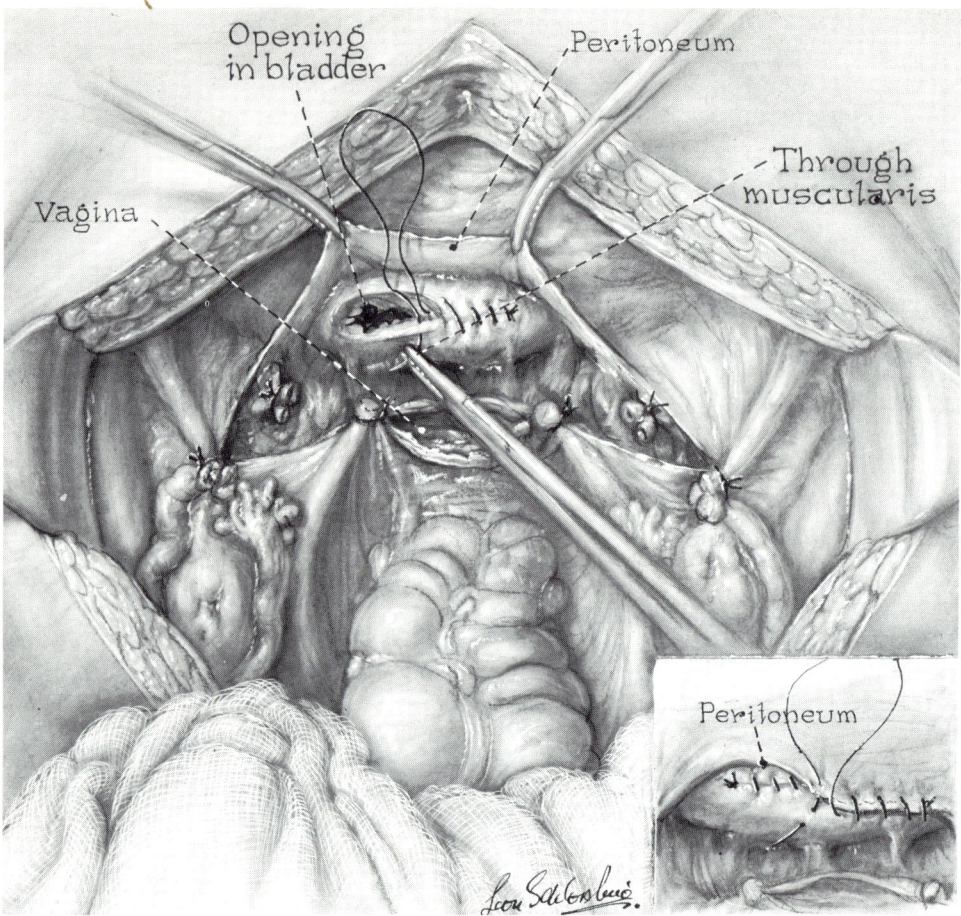

FIG. 8-11. Closure of accidental opening of bladder while performing total abdominal hysterectomy. The muscularis is closed with a continuous No. 00 catgut suture, inverting mucosa into bladder. The suture line is reinforced by bringing the peritoneum over the first layer of stitches and suturing it in place. This closure is anterior to the vaginal opening to make certain of no leakage into the vagina.

the operating room and suturing the cuff per vaginam. We have never had to reopen the abdomen for this rare complication. The more frequent posthysterectomy bleeding occurs from the end of the 1st to the end of the 2nd week. At this time the catgut becomes partially disintegrated, and the sutured vaginal mucosa edges slough and often separate. It is our belief that the rare occurrence of this type of bleeding is quite unavoidable and will occur regardless of the method of closure of the vaginal vault. In reviewing 1,000 cases of hysterectomy with 3 different methods of closure of the vaginal vault, Gray found no essential difference in the incidence of postoperative hemorrhage. A bit of bloody discharge is the rule at the 10th to the 14th day of convalescence. The patient should be reassured. She should not be permitted to take a douche, even though the rather foul-smelling discharge may be annoying to her. Reasonably brisk bleeding may often be controlled by vaginal packing, but one should not temporize too long. As soon as it becomes evident that the packing is not controlling the bleeding, the patient should be taken to the operating room, anesthetized, and placed in the lithotomy position for inspection of the vaginal vault and for suturing. We have always been able to control the bleeding by resuturing the edges of the vaginal incision with figure-of-eight sutures through the vaginal approach. Conceivably, opening of the abdomen might be necessary if the hemorrhage originates in the uterine vessels. Of course transfusions are used as necessary.

It is chiefly because of the possibility of late hemorrhage that we require abdominal and vaginal hysterectomized women to remain in the hospital for 14 days. We believe that this should be the rule whether or not early ambulation is practiced. This may be an annoying and expensive price for many women to pay for the small percentage of women who bleed. Nevertheless, we are convinced that a few women upon whom we have operated owe their lives to the prompt action of the hospital staff when the bleeding has been so sudden and profuse that transporting the patient to the hospital might have resulted in irreversible shock.

VAGINAL HYSTERECTOMY FOR THE MYOMATOUS UTERUS

Historically, the first reported vaginal hysterectomy was performed by Langenbeck of Göttingen in 1813 for suspected carcinoma of the cervix. Although this initial attempt to remove the uterus vaginally was complicated by profuse hemorrhage, the patient survived. Subsequent attempts were less successful, and the procedure was associated with a very high operative mortality due primarily to hemorrhage. The first documented vaginal hysterectomy in the United States was performed by Warren in 1829, a professor of anatomy at Harvard, and the indication again was for a malignant disease of the uterus. This patient also expired, and by the mid-19th century the vaginal hysterectomy had fallen into medical disfavor.

In the latter part of the 19th century interest in vaginal surgery was rekindled in the United States, and in 1879 Price of Philadelphia reported on 4,000 hysterectomies, of which 90 per cent were by the vaginal route. Later the technic for vaginal hysterectomy was refined by Heaney in this country, who reported on 565 vaginal hysterectomies for benign disease in 1934. Since that time, Kennedy and Campbell, Allen, Edwards, Aldrich, and the Mayo group have all championed the vaginal approach toward pelvic surgery.

The most frequent indication for vaginal hysterectomy is for removal of the small myomatous uterus. The authors' ideas on vaginal hysterectomy for uterine prolapse are discussed in Chapter 24, Malpositions of the Uterus, Cervical Stump, and Vagina. It is also a useful procedure when hysterectomy is required for definitive treatment of functional bleeding. In selected cases of carcinoma in situ it can be used to advantage. In this chapter, the pros and cons of vaginal hysterectomy will be concerned with the operation for the myomatous uterus.

For the small free myomatous uterus which can be delivered in toto, there can be little argument. Patients recuperate from the vaginal hysterectomy more rapidly than when the operation is done abdominally. Also, if vaginal plastic work is indicated, there is great advantage in being able to do all the surgery through one field. A parous outlet is usually an advantage in vaginal hysterectomy, but nulliparity by no means excludes this approach. As a matter of fact, the vaginal removal of the uterus in the nulliparous woman can on certain occasions be easier than on the parous woman. The lack of scarring in the vaginal vault and the cardinal ligament regions in the woman who has never borne children may more than compensate for the smaller vagina. Descensus of the uterus is not a requisite for vaginal hysterectomy, although a certain degree of it certainly facilitates the procedure. The presence of a low abdominal scar indicating previous pelvic surgery should make one evaluate the case very carefully before approaching the hysterectomy vaginally.

Previous cesarean sections are particularly apt to result in adhesions to the abdominal wall, and the operator should be especially careful in evaluating such cases before attempting vaginal removal. However, previous pelvic surgery does not absolutely exclude the vaginal approach. Ingram, Withers, and Wright have expressed optimism on vaginal hysterectomy following previous pelvic surgery, and it is their belief that the dangers of previous surgery have been overestimated. They report on 274 vaginal hysterectomies, of whom 26 per cent had undergone previous pelvic surgery. In only 2 instances was it necessary to complete the operation abdominally. A careful examination under anesthesia in order to estimate the mobility of the uterus is important in those who have had previous pelvic surgery. We have removed many myomatous uteri vaginally that have felt free in spite of previous surgery.

The size of the tumor should be considered carefully. It is true that often very large free fibroid uteri have been removed vaginally quite successfully, but the possibility of trouble increases with the size of the uterus. It is always well to have a laparotomy table set up in the operating room when vaginal hysterectomy is done. If the fibroid uterus is too large to be delivered through the vaginal incision relatively easily, it is far safer to resort to morcellation than to struggle to deliver a large tumor. Morcellation should not be attempted until after the uterine vessels are ligated. If it is impossible to expose the uterine artery area, the operator had best give up the vaginal approach. In most instances morcellation is most easily done anteriorly, but occasionally it can be accomplished more readily through the cul-de-sac. After drawing the uterus out as far as possible, orange-like slices are taken in the uterus until the uterus has been so reduced in size that it can be delivered readily. Then the hysterectomy is completed Often individual fibroids can be shelled out. The procedure of morcellation is usually surprisingly bloodless.

A history of abdominal pain is a relative contraindication to the removal of a fibroid uterus vaginally. Under such circumstances, exploration of the abdominal and pelvic cavities via a transabdominal route is preferable. Adnexal disease, especially salpingitis and endometriosis, contraindicates vaginal hysterectomy for fibroids. Occasionally, we have deliberately proceeded with vaginal hysterectomy in the known presence of a small, freely movable ovarian cyst, but in general adnexal disease is better approached abdominally.

Much has been written in recent years concerning pelvic cellulitis and cuff cellulitis. It is the opinion of the authors that this is chiefly due to inadequate hemostasis. The hematomas resulting from this often become infected and may require drainage, which is easily done per vaginum. Meticulous care in hemostasis will avoid most cases of cuff cellulitis.

A very rare complication of vaginal hysterectomy is injury to the sciatic nerve. It is thought to be due to either hyperextension of the lower extremities in the vertical position or excessive rotation of the thighs, with the knees and hip joints flexed.

The technic of vaginal hysterectomy is discussed in Chapter 24.

ABDOMINAL MYOMECTOMY

The earliest operation of myomectomy was done by Amussat in France in 1840. Howard A. Kelly, Charles P. Noble, and the Mayos wrote about myomectomy and practiced it extensively in this country during the early part of the 20th century. Victor Bonney, of London, and Isidor Rubin, of New York, were among the most enthusiastic myomectomists of the recent generation. For example, Bonney removed 225 tumors from one uterus.

This enthusiasm for the removal of multiple fibroids greatly exceeds that of the authors, although occasionally the performance of myomectomy for a large number of fibroids is indicated when the preservation of the uterus is of extreme importance to the patient.

A consideration of the indications, the contraindications, and the technic follows:

INDICATIONS AND CONTRAINDICATIONS

With few exceptions all indications and contraindications in medicine are relative, a fact that is especially true when one considers myomectomy versus hysteromyomectomy. It is difficult to lay down absolute criteria for the removal of, or the saving of, the uterus, but certain advantages and disadvantages of the two procedures will be discussed. It should be remembered that the only proved purpose of the uterus is childbearing, and while a few gynecologists have considered the endometrium to have an endocrine function, there is little real evidence to support such an idea; it has been abandoned by most gynecologists of today. The preservation of the function of menstruation is not important unless future childbearing is desired. Despite this, many women feel that the preservation of menstruation is essential to health, youth, and sexual life. A simple explanation will convince many of them of their error, but no explanation will suffice to satisfy others. The possibility of removal of the uterus should be discussed freely with the patient, for if the attitude of the patient is well understood by the surgeon, he will be greatly aided in making his decision at the operating table. Full permission from the patient to do whatever is necessary is essential, so that the gynecologist may be free to exercise his best surgical judgment. Because of technical reasons, discoverable only at operation, it is often difficult to be sure before operation that myomectomy is possible or wise. Should the removal of the uterus become necessary in the woman who is very desirous of retaining it, she will feel more kindly to the surgeon and will have less difficulty in becoming mentally adjusted to its loss if she has been told previously of the possibility of losing it.

The greatest reason for considering myomectomy is the patient's desire for future childbearing. In general, the younger the patient the greater the role this plays, but there are important exceptions to this rule. A woman who, for one reason or another, has had to defer marriage or childbearing until her middle thirties may feel a stronger desire for children than some girls in the early twenties; the wish of such an individual should be respected. The problem actually presents itself more often at this time of life, as fibroids more commonly give rise to symptoms in the 4th decade than they do in the 3rd. During the years of World War II the senior author performed more myomectomies than in the rest of his career. The reason was the great increase in sterility work. Many women who had practiced contraception for years were suddenly confronted with the possibility of a prolonged absence of their husbands. Many of these women were in their thirties. They decided to attempt a pregnancy, and when they failed to become pregnant, they consulted a gynecologist, only to find that they had fibroids; often the tumors were of considerable size. In many of such women the indications for myomectomy have been stretched in the hope of permitting future pregnancy. It is evident that Rubin's enthusiasm for myomectomy was probably based on the relative frequency of his discovery of fibroids in patients who consulted him, not for the usual symptoms of fibroids but because of sterility. It is obviously impossible, for technical reasons, to make a definite rule concerning myomectomy, but the more intense the desire of the women for children, the more one is justified in stretching the indications for myomectomy.

The twisting and/or the necrosis of a pedunculated fibroid during pregnancy is a special indication for myomectomy. Although such complications are rare, the performance of a successful myomectomy without interruption of the pregnancy is a surgical feat of supreme importance to the patient. Only when the patient experiences repeated attacks of acute pain, vomiting or fever should myomectomy be considered during pregnancy. Sedation should first be given an adequate trial. When myomectomy becomes a necessity, most authors believe that it should be done after the 90th day of pregnancy, when the uterus is less irritable and placental function is well established. However, the time of the onset of the symptoms may not give the gynecologist the choice of selecting the time for operation.

In women in the early or middle thirties who desire children, the performance of myomectomy can be an essential part of the treatment of sterility, or, in some instances, a desirable operation before permitting the patient to risk a pregnancy.

What are the chances of pregnancy following myomectomy? In Brown, Chamberlain and Te Linde's series there were 172 married women. All of these were followed for 2 or more years. Seventy-four, or 42.5 per cent, became pregnant, and 64 women delivered a total of 111 living children. Certainly, some of the myomectomized women practiced contraception, so it is probable that the 42.5 per cent is not a true index of the pregnancy potential. Occasionally, we have performed myomectomy primarily for the relief of sterility, and there were 21 patients in our series whose primary complaint was sterility, and myomectomy was the only treatment except for preoperative testing of tubal patency. Eleven of the 21 became pregnant. Nine went to term, and a total of 18 living children were born.

Bronnet et al. followed 95 patients from the Mayo Clinic for 5 to 20 years. Thirty-two per cent required subsequent hysterectomy.

In our series there were 8 patients whose primary complaint was repeated abortions, and no other abnormality was found to account for this. Then the operations were done for the relief of this, and all became pregnant following the surgery. However, only 4 went to term with living infants, the other 4 terminating in abortion, prematurity, or still birth.

There are a few absolute contraindications to myomectomy. Malignancy of any type in the uterus or the ovaries excludes myomectomy. If the tubes are closed with certainty, or if they have been removed previously, there is no justification for myomectomy. Under such circumstances the retained uterus is useless; also, it is often a source of future trouble. Diffuse adenomyosis of the uterine wall involving an appreciable part of the myometrium, being unencapsulated, is removed completely with great uncertainty, and an attempt at local excision should not be made.

Myomectomy at term, in conjunction with a cesarean section, is rarely justified. If there is a pedunculated subserous fibroid attached to the uterus with a small pedicle, cutting and suturing of the pedicle may be done easily. The removal of intramural fibroids from the uterus at term is not advisable.

Myomectomy is seldom justified in a woman over 35, and it is never a reasonable procedure when she is past 40. Only in those cases of late marriage in which childbearing is greatly desired should myomectomy be considered in the late thirties.

A uterus that is the site of a large number of fibroids had better be removed rather than subjected to multiple myomectomies. Rubin reports the removal of 33 myomas from one patient, and Victor Bonney has removed 225 fibroids from a single uterus. It is difficult for us to believe that the removal of such a large number of fibroids is ever justifiable; a uterus that is the site of many visible fibroids usually contains many invisible seed tumors that will eventually give trouble. Perhaps the possibility of an heir to a throne might justify a procedure such as that described above, but it would hardly seem good surgical judgment under ordinary circumstances. Furthermore, such a multiscarred uterus would be a poor receptacle in which to carry the fetus to term, and a still poorer organ to carry on the function of labor.

Race is an important factor in making the decision for myomectomy or hysterectomy. Because of the great tendency of the colored race to multiple fibroids we rarely practice myomectomy on the uterus of a colored woman. The possibility of future tumor formation is too great to justify the preservation of the uterus, although in rare instances, when the abdomen has been opened for other conditions, we remove small incidental myomata, thus preserving the uterus.

When myomectomy is considered, its technical difficulties and increased operative risk over hysterectomy always must be evaluated. In most cases myomectomy is a more difficult operation than hysterectomy except when the subserous tumor is pedunculated or the intramural fibroid is small. In recent years the mortality for the operation at the Mt. Sinai Hospital was 1.9 per cent. Although many series of hysteromyomectomies are reported with a mortality equal to this or even greater, hysterectomy is done in most of the better clinics today with a mortality of less than 1 per cent. Brown, Chamberlain and Te Linde had no mortality in 329 myomectomies on nonpregnant women and 1 death among 16 pregnant women. This woman had a gasbacillus peritonitis preoperatively with a twisted pedunculated fibroid, and the operation was undertaken as a desperate emergency measure. If a surgeon uses reasonable judgment in selecting his cases, it can be said that myomectomy carries no more mortality than a hysterectomy.

When considering myomectomy the patient wishes to know the possibility of further surgery, and it is well to have definite facts to give her. Brown, Chamberlain and Te Linde followed 234 myomectomy cases for 2 or more years. In 18.6 per cent myomas recurred, but in only 10.3 per cent was a hysterectomy required. Of course, the longer the cases are followed, the more recurrences there will be. Of the 176 cases followed for 5 or more years 31.3 per cent had recurrent fibroids, and hysterectomy became necessary for these fibroids in 16.5 per cent. Hysterectomy became necessary for other causes in an additional 4.3 per cent. Thus, over 20 per cent of the women on whom myomectomy was done required a later hysterectomy.

In a series of 95 patients upon whom myomectomy was done at the Mayo Clinic, 80 were married and 63 per cent of these became pregnant, 54 per cent being delivered of at least one living child.

There remains the problem of the method of delivery after myomectomy. We have never had a case of rupture of the uterus after a myomectomy at the Johns Hopkins. The same is true of the Mayo Clinic series.

It is our belief that the obstetricians are excessively cautious in not letting more of these women deliver vaginally. However in defense of their attitude one must remember that many of these women are elderly for childbirth, and that this may be their last chance at childbearing. In our series, 120 women were delivered vaginally, and 24 by cesarean section. The rule has been to perform cesarean section if the uterine cavity had been entered at the time of myomectomy, or if there was reason to believe by the postoperative course that the myomectomy wound was infected. Although this may be an excessively cautious attitude, it appears to be a safe one.

Technic:
Abdominal Myomectomy

Figure 8-12 illustrates a rather typical myomectomy for a large, single, intramural fibroid. An elliptical incision is made through the serosa over the tumor. This incision should represent an underestimate of the amount of serosa that is to be removed, for more can be trimmed off after the tumor is removed, whereas too radical excision of the serosa would be rather difficult of closure. The tumor is shelled out by a combination of sharp and dull dissection (Fig. 8-12 A). The knife handle is an excellent blunt dissector for this procedure. Often figure-of-eight traction sutures placed in the tumor afford convenient traction while enucleating the tumor. Often bleeding can be controlled to a large extent by pressure with the left hand (Fig. 8-12 B). Another excellent means of conserving blood loss is the suturing of the myometrium with interrupted or figure-of-eight sutures of No. 0 chromic catgut as the enucleation is done (Fig. 8-12 B). If the entire enucleation is done before suturing the myometrium and if the tumor is large, bleed-

184 Myomata Uteri

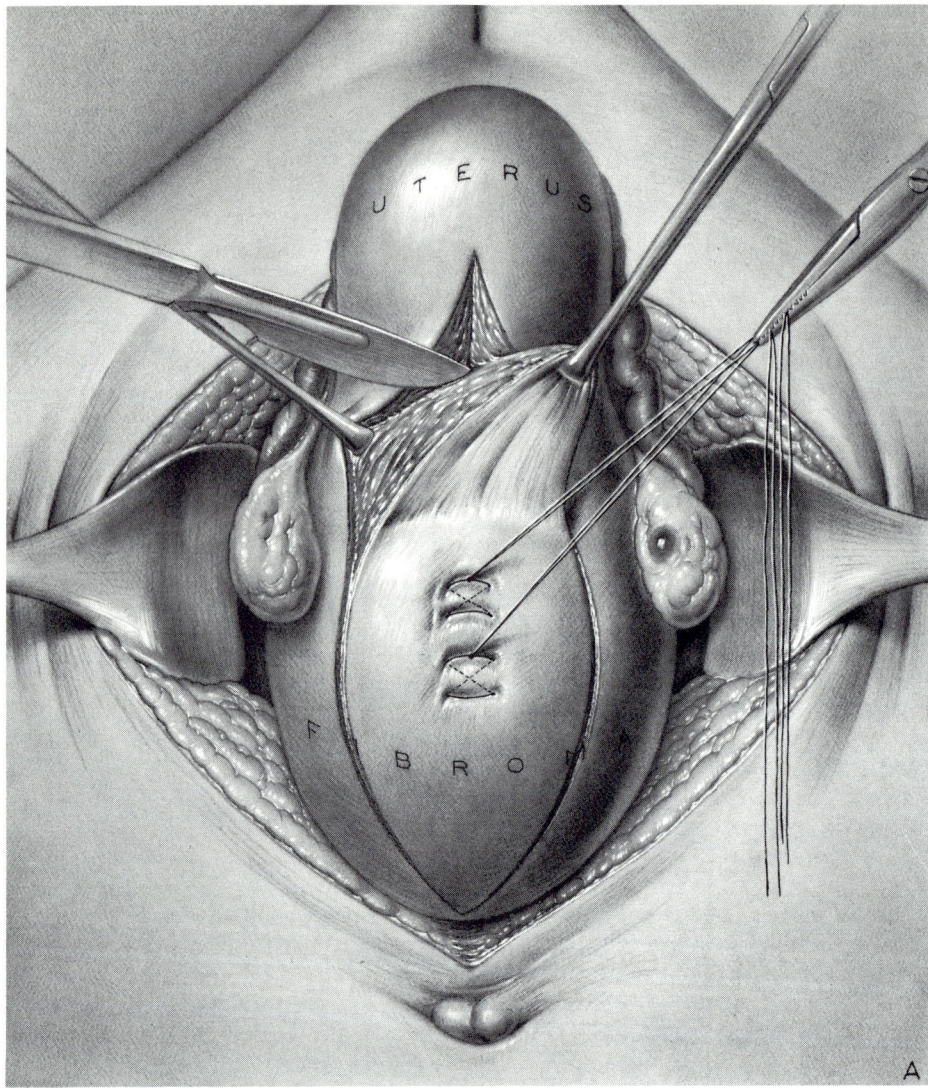

Fig. 8-12. Abdominal myomectomy for large intramural fibroid. (A) Figure-of-eight sutures of No. 2 chromic catgut have been placed through the tumor for traction. The tumor is being excised with sharp dissection.

ing may get out of control. The sutures in the myometrium, if left long, also serve as convenient traction sutures. After the myometrium has been approximated by one or more layers of sutures and the bleeding well controlled, the serosa is closed with a lock stitch of No. 0 chromic catgut (Fig. 8-12 C). A fine needle should be used for the serosal stitch; a nontraumatic needle is excellent.

When multiple myomectomy is necessary for fibroids in close proximity, frequently several tumors can be enucleated from one incision. In Figure 8-13 A two fibroids have already been enucleated, and the third is being shelled out with the knife handle. Figure 8-13 B shows a convenient method of holding a small subserous fibroid for enucleation. Figure 8-13 C shows traction suture in small fibroid used for this purpose. Figure 8-13 D represents the simplest form of myomectomy for a small subserous pedunculated tumor. One figure-of-eight

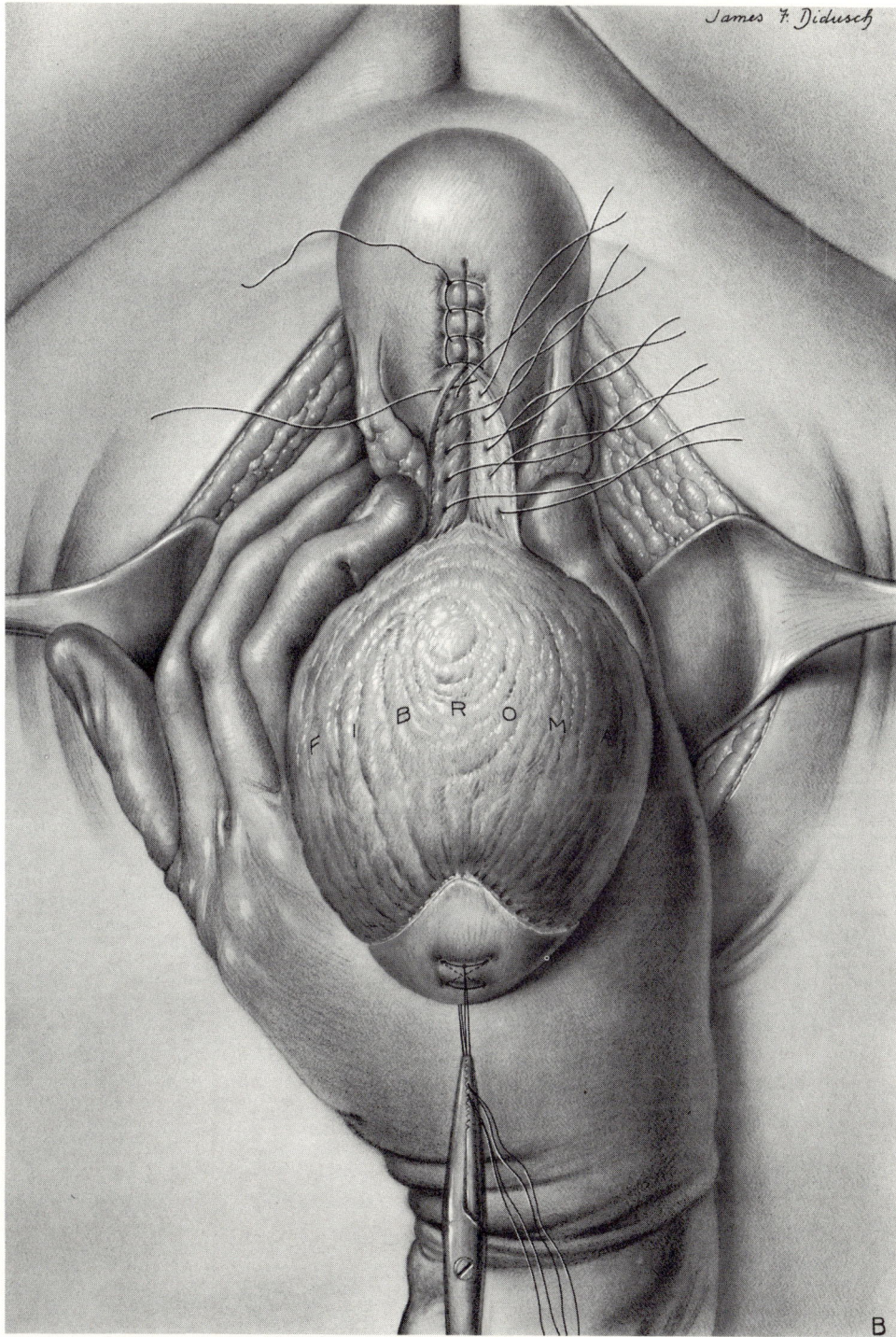

FIG. 8-12 (*Continued*). Abdominal myomectomy for large intramural fibroid. (B) Much blood loss is prevented by compressing the sides of the uterus. Excess of serosa has been excised, and myometrium is sutured with interrupted No. 0 chromic sutures as the tumor is excised.

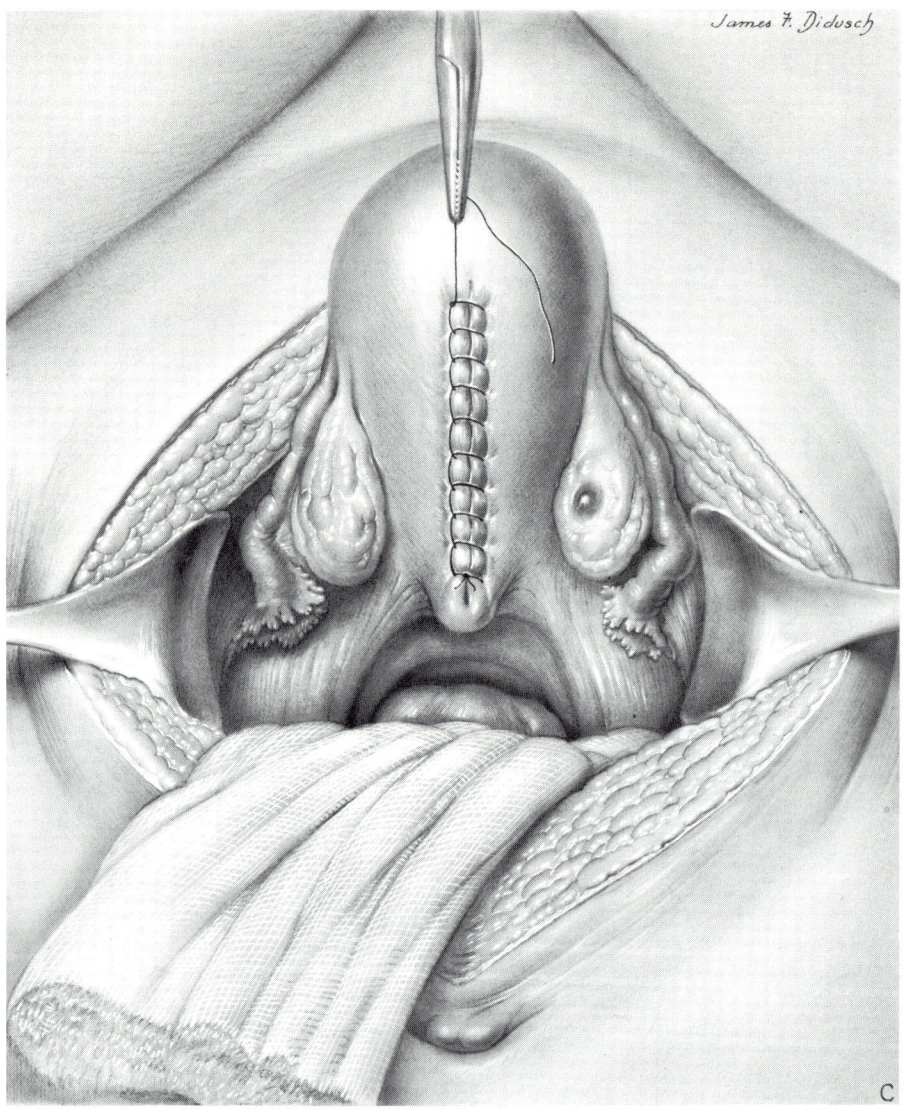

Fig. 8-12 (*Continued*). Abdominal myomectomy for a large intramural fibroid. (C) Approximation of serosa with continuous suture of No. 0 chromic catgut.

suture usually controls bleeding after such an excision.

When an extensive myomectomy for large fibroids is to be done, bleeding often can be reduced by the use of a tourniquet placed about the uterus just above the level where the uterine vessels approach the side of the uterus (Fig. 8-14) and rubber shod clamps on the ovarian vessels. Recently we have found the intramural injection of 20 to 30 cc. of a dilute solution of Neo-Synephrine (0.5 cc. of 1% solution in 100 cc. of saline) to be most effective in decreasing blood loss.

VAGINAL MYOMECTOMY

The removal of a pedunculated submucous fibroid that has worked its way down through the cervical canal and into the vagina is best accomplished by the vaginal route. Such fibroids are always infected, and, in general, the removal with the least manipulation is the best. When a submucous fibroid just "peeks" through the external os, the cervix can be closed over it by suture and a total abdominal hysterectomy done immediately.

When the myoma is not too large and sufficiently pedunculated, the pedicle is transfixed by a suture of chromic catgut at the highest possible point before cutting of the pedicle (Fig. 8-15). If the pedicle is so high in the cervical canal that it is impossible to transfix it, often it may be cut with the actual cautery at a low heat or with the electrosurgical knife with a combination cutting and coagulating current. We never have seen serious hemorrhage result from such cutting of the unligated pedicle. Frequently, the vessels in the pedicle are thrombosed. If bleeding should occur, it can be controlled easily by ligating the pedicle after removal of the tumor or, if this is impossible, by packing.

When the submucous myoma is very large and fills the vagina so completely

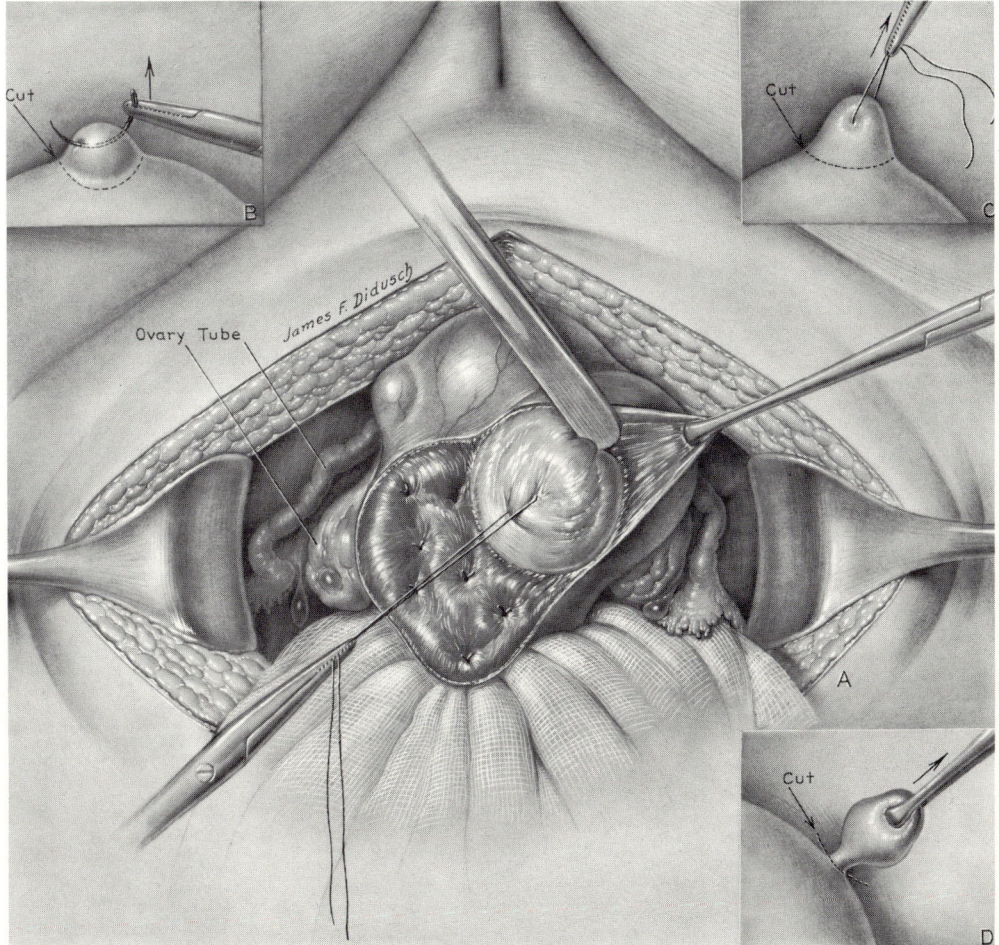

FIG. 8-13. Technical steps in myomectomy. (A) Multiple myomectomies through a single incision. Two myomas have already been enucleated, and dead space has been approximated with interrupted catgut sutures. A third is being enucleated. (B) An empty curved needle is a convenient instrument for grasping a small fibroid as it is enucleated. (C) A traction suture may serve equally well. (D) The simplest myomectomy for small pedunculated tumor.

188 Myomata Uteri

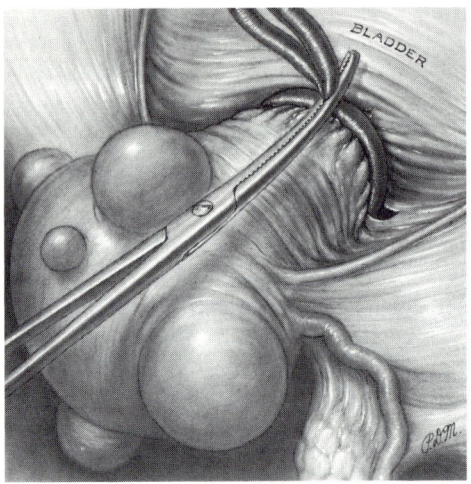

FIG. 8-14. A tourniquet has been placed around the cervix to reduce bleeding during myomectomy.

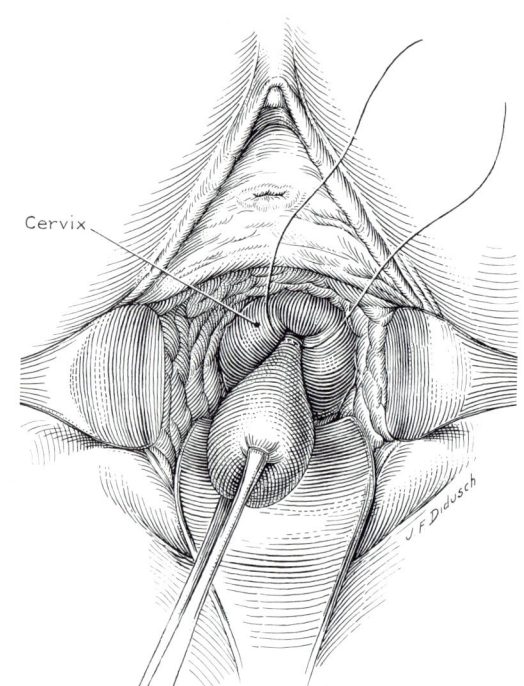

FIG. 8-15. Removal of small pedunculated submucous myoma. As traction is made on tumor, the pedicle is ligated as high as possible.

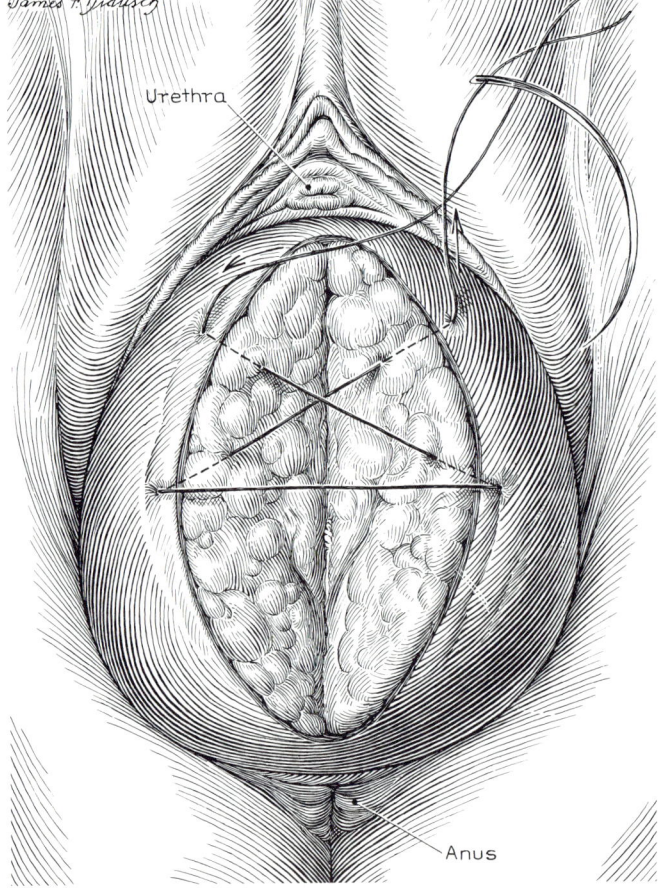

FIG. 8-16. Vaginal myomectomy by morcellation. A wedge-shaped piece of the myoma has been excised. A gross figure-of-eight suture is placed to control bleeding temporarily and to make traction.

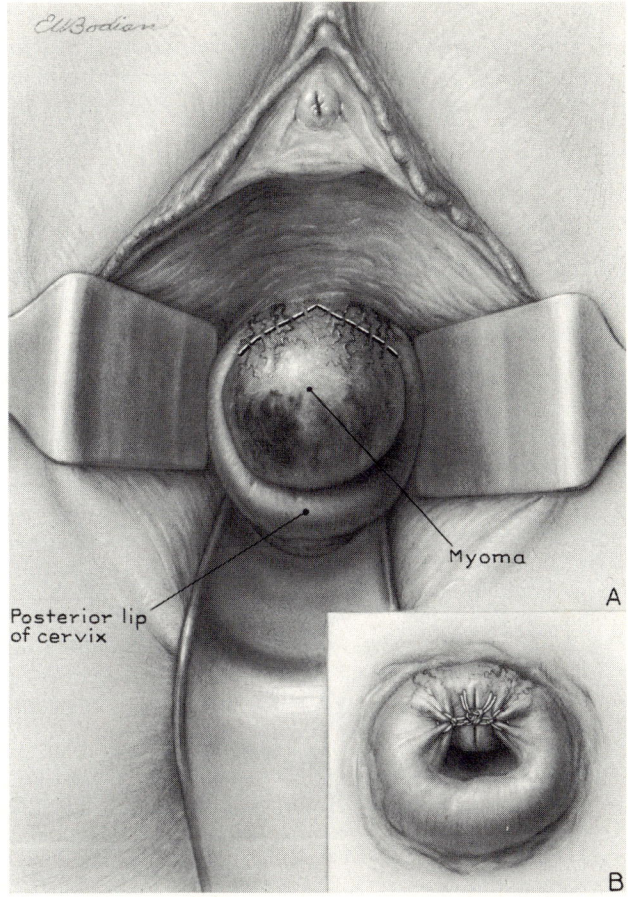

FIG. 8-17. Excision of cervical myoma. (A) Dotted line indicates incision. (B) The wound has been closed by tying together the two figure-of-eight sutures which were placed for hemostasis before the tumor was excised.

that the pedicle cannot be reached, it may have to be removed piecemeal. It is our practice to make wedge-shaped incisions in the tumor, reducing its size until sufficient room is afforded to permit access to the pedicle. Bleeding is controlled by grasping and compressing the remaining portions of the tumor or by temporarily suturing them (Fig. 8-16). Often there is surprisingly little bleeding when such tumors are cut into. Occasionally, one will discover a tremendous dilatation of the cervix with a huge tumor coming from it with no sign of a pedicle. Such tumors may be cut flush with the cervix, using the cautery or combination coagulating-and-cutting electrosurgical current. If this does not control bleeding satisfactorily, a tight vaginal packing with sulfanilamide-impregnated gauze may be used. Relieved of the pull of the portion of the tumor that has been removed, the remainder of the tumor often retracts up into the uterine cavity. At a later date the cervical lips may be sutured together and a total abdominal hysterectomy done. Before removing an infected submucous myoma the patient should be treated with penicillin and streptomycin, and these antibiotics should be continued for at least 2 days after the operation.

Vaginal Myomectomy for Cervical Myoma

Cervical myomata arising from the portio are generally discovered before they attain such size that hysterectomy is required, as described earlier in this chapter. Figure 8-17 shows a cervical myoma that has arisen from the anterior lip of the portio. Its abundant blood supply was easily visualized, as shown in the picture. Figure-of-eight sutures of No. 1 chromic catgut were first placed on either side of the anterior lip but were not tied until the tumor was excised with a wedge-shaped piece of cervical lip. Then the sutures were tied. This controlled bleeding satisfactorily. Next, the 2 suture ends were tied together; this neatly approximated the cut edges of the anterior lip.

BIBLIOGRAPHY

Amussat: Quoted by I. C. Rubin, Progress in myomectomy. Amer. J. Obstet. Gynec., 44: 197, 1942.

Bonney, V.: The technic and results of myomectomy. Lancet, 220:171, 1931.

Brown, A. B., Chamberlain, R., and Te Linde, R. W.: Myomectomy. Amer. J. Obstet. Gynec., 71:759, 1956.

Brown, J. M., Malkasian, G. D., Jr., and Symmonds, R. E.: Abdominal myomectomy. Amer. J. Obstet. Gynec., 99:126, 1964.

Copenhaver, E. H.: Hysterectomy: Vaginal vs. abdominal. Surg. Clin. N. Amer., 45:751, 1965.

———: Indications for hysterectomy. Lahey Clin. Bull., 15:29, 1966.

Cariker, M., and Dockerty, M.: The retained uterine cervix. Amer. J. Obstet. Gynec., 74: 379, 1957.

Corscaden, J. A., and Singh, B. P.: Leiomyosarcoma of the uterus. Amer. J. Obstet. Gynec., 75:149, 1958.

Counsellor, V. S., and Bedard, R. E.: Uterine myomectomy: Analysis of indications and results in 523 cases. J.A.M.A., 111:675, 1938.

Cullen, T. S.: Adenomyoma of the Uterus. Philadelphia, W. B. Saunders, 1908.

———: Successful removal of an eighty-pound cystic myoma intact. J.A.M.A., 48:1491, 1907.

Danforth, W. C.: Total hysterectomy, abdominal and vaginal. Amer. J. Obstet. Gynec., 42:587, 1941.

Evans, N.: Malignant myomata and related tumors of the uterus. Surg. Gynec. Obstet., 30:225, 1920.

Everett, H. S., and Scott, R. B.: The possible etiologic role of gynecologic lesions in the production of hypertension. Amer. J. Obstet. Gynec., 44:1010, 1942.

Everett, H. S., and Sturgis, W. J.: The effect of some common gynecological disorders upon the urinary tract. Urol. Cutan. Rev., 44:638, 1940.

Gray, L. A.: Indications, technics, and complications in vaginal hysterectomy. Obstet. Gynec., 28:714, 1966.

Grogan, R. H.: Reappraisal of residual ovaries. Amer. J. Obstet. Gynec., 97:124, 1967.

Grogan, R. H., and Duncan, C. J.: Ovarian salvage in routine abdominal hysterectomy. Amer. J. Obstet. Gynec., 70:1277, 1955.

Holden, F. C.: Partial colpocleisis as an approach to vesicovaginal fistula following total hysterectomy. Amer. J. Obstet. Gynec., 44:880, 1942.

Ingram, J., Withers, R., and Wright, H.: Vaginal hysterectomy after previous pelvic surgery. Amer. J. Obstet. Gynec., 74:1181, 1957.

Kelly, H. A.: Operative Gynecology. New York, Appleton, 1898.

Kelly, H. A., and Cullen, T. S.: Myomata of the Uterus. Philadelphia, W. B. Saunders, 1909.

Kimbrough, R. A., Jr.: Sarcoma of uterus. Amer. J. Obstet. Gynec., 28:723, 1934.

Masson, J. C.: Total versus subtotal abdominal hysterectomy. Amer. J. Obstet. Gynec., 14: 486, 1927.

Mattingly, R. F., and Huang, H. Y.: Steroidogenesis in the menopausal and postmenopausal ovary. Amer. J. Obstet. Gynec., 103:679, 1969.

Mayo, W. J.: Some observations on the operation of abdominal myomectomy for myomata of the uterus. Surg. Gynec. Obstet., 12:97, 1911.

Miller, N.: The surgical treatment and postoperative care of vesicovaginal fistula. Amer. J. Obstet. Gynec., 44:873, 1942.

Montague, A., Swartz, D. P., and Woodruff, J. D.: Sarcoma arising in leiomyoma of uterus: factors influencing prognosis. Amer. J. Obstet. Gynec., 92:421, 1965.

Noble, C. P.: Kelly and Noble, Gynecology and Abdominal Surgery. vol. 1. Philadelphia, W. B. Saunders, 1907.

Novak, E., and Anderson, D. F.: Sarcoma of the uterus: Factors influencing the results of treatment. Amer. J. Obstet. Gynec., 34: 740, 1937.

Novak, E. R., and Williams, T. J.: Autopsy comparison of cardiovascular changes in castrated and normal women. Amer. J. Obstet. Gynec. 80:863, 1960.

Pearse, R. L.: Supravaginal and total hysterectomy. Amer. J. Obstet. Gynec., 42:22, 1941.

Pratt, J. H., Lee, M. J., Jr., Hasskarl, W. F., and Brandes, R. W.: Morbidity after total abdominal hysterectomy. Amer. J. Obstet. Gynec., 61:407, 1951.

Randall, C. L., Birtch, P. K., and Harkins, J. L.: Ovarian function after the menopause. Amer. J. Obstet. Gynec., 74:719, 1957.

Randall, C. L., Hall, D. W., and Armenia, C. S.: Pathology in the preserved ovary after unilateral oophorectomy. Amer. J. Obstet. Gynec., 84:1233, 1962.

Randall, C. L., and Paloucek, F. P.: The frequency of oophorectomy at the time of hysterectomy Amer. J. Obstet. Gynec., 100:716, 1968.

Richardson, E. H.: A simplified technic for abdominal panhysterectomy. Surg. Gynec. Obstet., 48:248, 1929.

Rubin, I.: Progress in myomectomy: Surgical measures and diagnostic aids favoring lower morbidity and mortality Amer. J. Obstet. Gynec., 44:196, 1942.

Scheffey, L. C.: Carcinoma of the cervical stump J.A.M.A., 107:837, 1936.

Siddall, R. S., and Mack H. C.: Subtotal versus total hysterectomy. Surg. Gynec. Obstet., 60:102, 1935.

Te Linde, R. W., and Wharton, L. R., Jr.: Ovarian function following pelvic operations. Amer. J. Obstet. Gynec., 80:844, 1960.

Weir, W. C.: A statistical report of 1,914 cases of hysterectomy. Amer. J. Obstet. Gynec., 42:285, 1941.

Wetterdal, P.: Comparative study of total and subtotal hysterectomy in the treatment of uterine fibroids. Acta Obstet. Gynec. Scand., 33:350, 1954.

Woodruff, Donald: Personal communication.

Wuest, J. H., Dry, T. J., and Edwards, J. E.: Circulation, 7:801, 1953.

9

Endometriosis

LAWRENCE R. WHARTON, JR., M.D.[*]

Sampson has described endometriosis as the "presence of ectopic tissue which possesses the histological structure and function of the uterine mucosa. It also includes the abnormal conditions which may result not only from the invasion of organs and other structures by this tissue but also from its relation to menstruation."

In many respects it is an extremely fascinating condition. Though a benign process, it possesses the unique ability to invade tissues and to disseminate itself or metastasize by hematogenous or lymphatic routes or by implantation. These attributes are usually reserved for cancer alone. The solution of its etiology and treatment offers a stimulating challenge to gynecologists, and American gynecologists in particular have been responsible for most of the progress made in this disease.

Endometriosis is divided into two separate clinical and pathologic types; and, in fact, they appear to be essentially two different diseases. One is internal endometriosis, preferably called adenomyosis, which is the involvement of the myometrium by endometrium from within the uterine cavity. The other is external endometriosis, which is the involvement of tissues outside the uterus or the uterine serosa from without.

ADENOMYOSIS

Historically, adenomyosis was the first of these two diseases described, being first reported by Rokitansky in 1860. There was sporadic subsequent reports until 1896, when von Recklinghausen established it in his monograph as a definite pathologic entity. Cullen in 1897 reported his first case of "adenomyoma" of the uterus and in 1908 published the classic monograph on this disease, reporting 92 cases. He also recognized "diffuse adenomyoma of the uterus," now more properly known as adenomyosis.

Indeed, this disease does present itself in two distinct forms: (1) *diffuse adenomyosis*, which may involve either the anterior or posterior wall of the uterus or both to a varying degree (Fig. 9-1). It may be relatively localized but not encapsulated. The uterus is somewhat enlarged, rarely exceeding twice its normal size, and is more or less symmetrical. On sectioning the uterine wall, there is a coarse trabecular pattern of interlacing musculature and fibrous tissue, often with small dark hemorrhagic lacunae of endometrium; (2) *adenomyoma*, which is encapsulated as an ordinary intramural leiomyoma or may project into the uterine cavity, becoming a submucous adenomyoma (Fig. 9-2).

In regard to the origin of this process, von Recklinghausen contended that the intramural endometrium was derived from Wolffian tubular rests. Cullen, however, offered the most generally accepted

[*] Assistant Professor, Department of Gynecology and Obstetrics, School of Medicine, Johns Hopkins University.

theory, namely, that the tissue is of müllerian origin and is a direct downgrowth from the uterine cavity. In fact, he was able to show by serial sections in 55 of 56 cases of diffuse adenomyosis a direct continuity between the basalis of the endometrium and the edometrial islands within the areas of adenomyosis. These islands also usually have the histological appearance of the basalis, generally having a proliferative pattern or even one of cystic hyperplasia. Rarely do they show a full progestational effect but in pregnancy may have decidual reaction. This tissue, like that of the uterine endometrium is estrogen-dependent and becomes atrophic after the menopause.

The incidence of adenomyosis will vary widely from one laboratory to another since it is fundamentally a pathologic diagnosis. Its frequency will depend not only on the criteria for diagnosis but also on the thoroughness with which the removed uteri are studied. A reasonable criterion has been established by Benson and Sneeden, namely, that the area must extend at least 2 low-power fields into the myometrium. The incidence varies from 8 to 27 per cent and reaches its peak in the 5th decade. Most of these women are parous, frequently

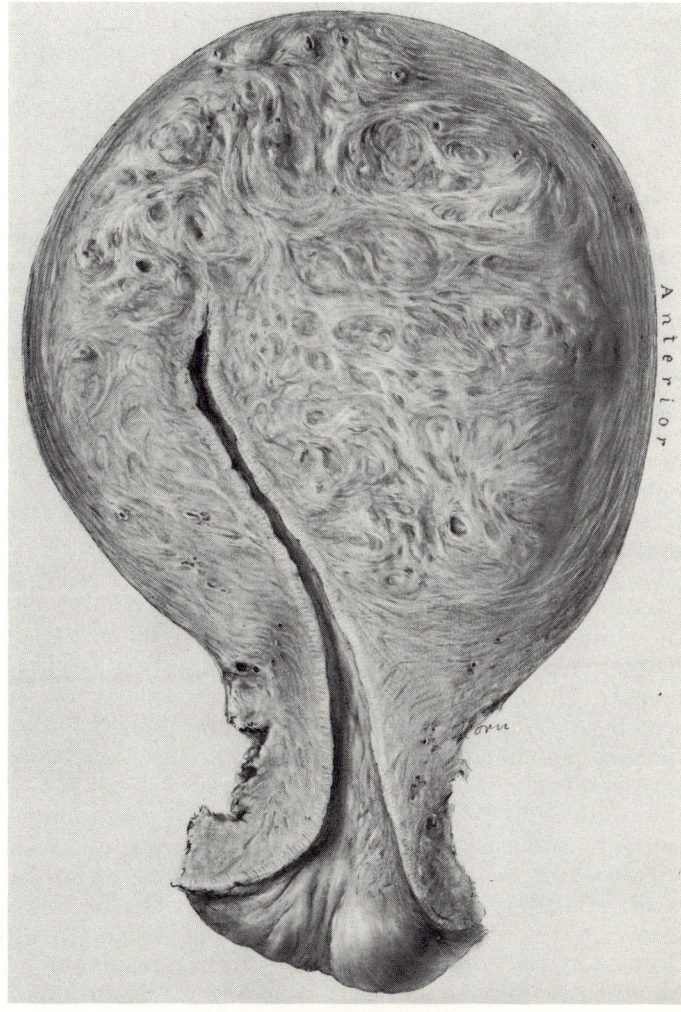

FIG. 9-1. Adenomyosis of uterus (after Cullen). A typical example with complete involvement of both anterior and posterior uterine walls. At the operating table such a uterus is moderately enlarged, usually symmetrically, and very firm to palpation.

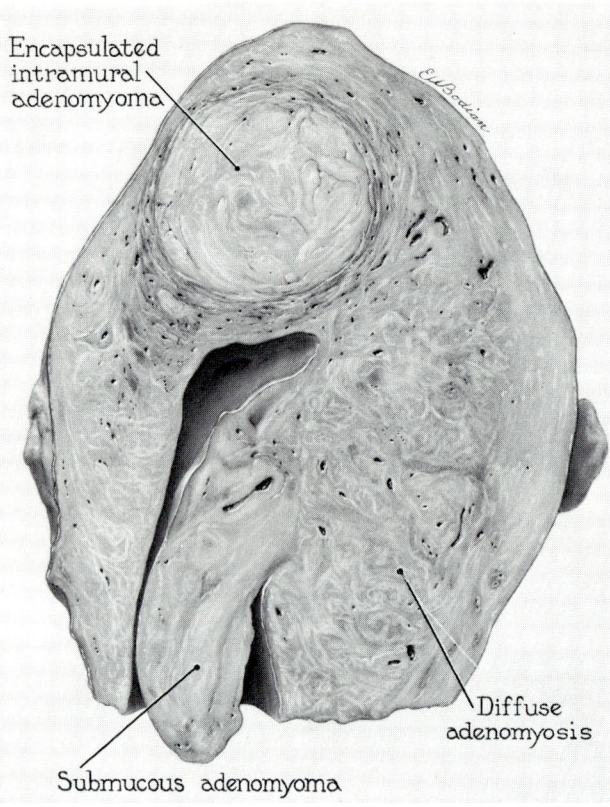

Fig. 9-2. Uterus showing 3 types of adenomyomatous growth: encapsulated intramural adenomyoma, submucous adenomyoma; and diffuse adenomyosis of both uterine walls.

multipara. About 12 per cent will have coexisting external endometriosis.

Symptoms

Adenomyosis is frequently an incidental pathologic finding and may be entirely asymptomatic, particularly when present to a minimal degree. When the myometrial involvement is more extensive, two symptoms are likely to occur, abnormal uterine bleeding and pain. The bleeding is usually in the form of menorrhagia. This may result from the increased endometrial surface area, from which bleeding may occur, or from submucous adenomyomas. The extensive involvement of the uterine wall also may interfere with the normal uterine contractility and cause excessive bleeding.

Pain when present is usually associated with menstruation and often is severe, grinding, or knife-like in nature. This dysmenorrhea probably results from bleeding within deep-lying islands of endometrium. Figure 9-3 shows the pathologic basis for these symptoms.

Pelvic Findings

The uterus may be firm and slightly enlarged. Usually it does not exceed twice its normal size. With the diffuse type of adenomyosis, the enlargement is usually symmetrical; hence the uterus is a rather globular organ. When an encapsulated adenomyoma is present, the uterus then may be irregular or asymmetrical. At times, particularly during menstruation, it is tender to palpation.

Differential Diagnosis

Adenomyosis should always be suspected in a woman with severe increasing dysmenorrhea and menorrhagia in the 4th or 5th decade. When the uterus is symmetrically enlarged and firm, the suspicion is likely to be confirmed. It is difficult to be certain of the diagnosis since functional uterine bleeding and a small symmetrical leiomyoma may present similar findings.

TREATMENT

Although the exact differential diagnosis is frequently difficult, it may be largely of academic interest. A curettage does not aid in establishing the diagnosis and is ineffectual as treatment. The same may be said of cyclic hormonal or progestagen therapy. The need for treatment, therefore, is based on continued menorrhagia and dysmenorrhea and not on whether the uterus is normal in size (functional bleeding), or whether it contains adenomyosis or a leiomyoma. The definitive treatment then is hysterectomy, either vaginal or abdominal, depending on the size of the uterus and the presence or absence of other pelvic abnormalities. At times in a younger patient who wishes to retain her reproductive capability, excision of an encapsulated adenomyoma should be considered in the same manner as one would consider myomectomy. This situation arises infrequently since most cases of adenomyosis occur in

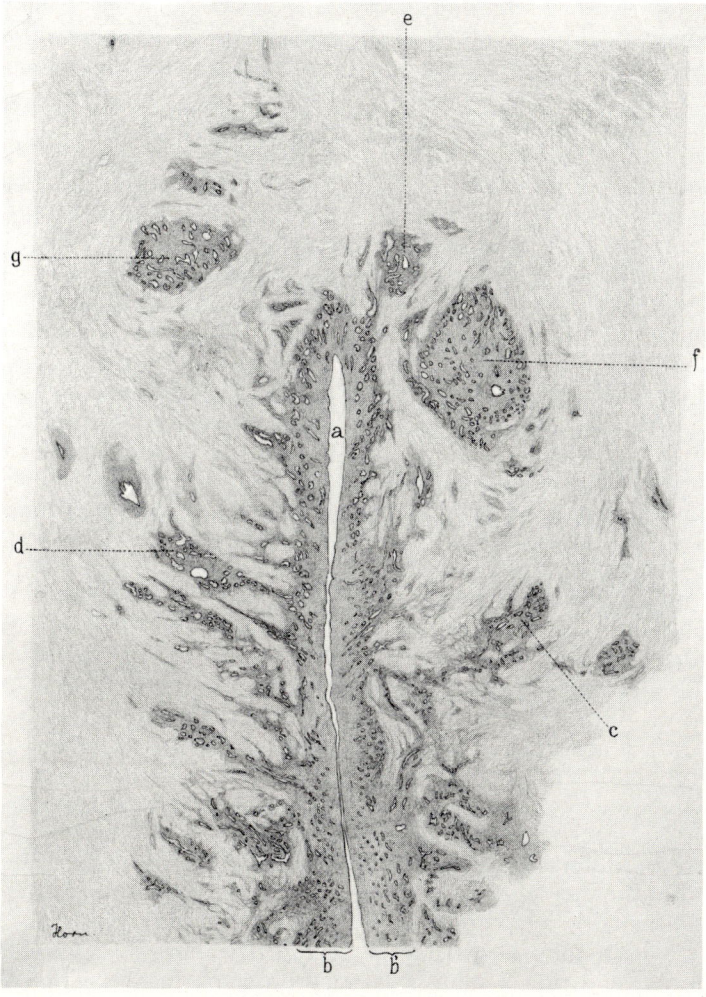

FIG. 9-3. Section through central portion of uterus with adenomyosis. (a) Uterine cavity. (b) The endometrium of the cavity. (c, d, e, f, g) Islands of displaced endometrium into which there is hemorrhage at the time of menstruation. The poor drainage of the menstrual blood with increased tension explains severe menstrual pain.

women no longer desirous of childbearing.

EXTERNAL ENDOMETRIOSIS

External endometriosis or ectopic endometrium growing elsewhere than in the uterine musculature from within is of clinical importance much more frequently than is adenomyosis. Although the two conditions have been found with about equal frequency histologically, many instances of adenomyosis show minimal invasion of the myometrium and are of no clinical significance, whereas in most cases of external endometriosis the ectopic endometrium is of clinical importance. Since 1897, when Pfannenstiel described the first case of adenomyoma of the rectovaginal septum, the condition has been recorded with increasing frequency. Endometriosis of the ovary was first described by Russell in 1899. This same case had a small endometrial nodule in the uterosacral ligament.

Although increased clinical awareness and better education in the field of gynecologic pathology without doubt have led to more frequent recognition of this disease, it is also probable that the disease is actually increasing in frequency. On the gynecologic service of the Johns Hopkins Hospital, endometriosis was found in 3.2 per cent of laparotomies in 1933 and 9 per cent in 1947. This increase was due to a greater incidence in private white patients in whom the incidence rose from 7.5 per cent in 1933 to 21.6 per cent in 1947. The incidence, therefore, of this disease is affected by the economic level of the patient, being much more common in private patients than in clinic patients. Several factors seem to affect this difference. Meigs believed that the greater age at which private patients married and, hence, the greater age at which they began childbearing made these women more susceptible to endometriosis. There seems to be little question, moreover, that pregnancy tends to decrease the incidence of endometriosis and confer some protection on the parous woman. Frequently 5 or more years may pass following a patient's last pregnancy before symptomatic endometriosis is discovered. Whether these benefits are the result of the hormones of pregnancy or the cervical dilatation at delivery is not certain.

The ectopic endometrium, wherever it may be, is dependent on the presence of ovarian hormones for its maintainence and is responsive in varying degrees to their stimuli. Scott and Wharton in studies on endometriosis in castrated rhesus monkeys showed that estrogen was important in maintaining active endometrial implants, and also that when estrogen-primed implants were subjected to progesterone-induced withdrawal bleeding, more active implants resulted. Each implant may then be considered a miniature uterus responding to these hormonal stimuli. Frequently the response to progesterone was found to be minimal, and in this respect the implants resemble the basalis of the uterine endometrium. In fact, this response is quite variable, and in the same patient some areas may show a good progestational response while others show none. The implants, however, are capable of exhibiting local withdrawal bleeding regardless of their histological pattern and degree of progestational response.

These implants in pregnancy or with progestagen therapy may show a marked decidual reaction. This response, too, is not entirely predictable. Because of the decidual reaction of the implants and the absence of menstruation, it has been a general impression that endometriosis improves during pregnancy. This concept has been questioned recently by McArthur and Ulfelder, who analyzed the reported cases of pregnancy and endometriosis and were unable to substantiate this.

The fact that endometriosis is dependent on ovarian hormones confines its clinical importance generally to the reproductive era of a woman's life. It has not been reported prior to the menarche, and the implants become atrophic after the menopause. Its peak incidence occurs in the 4th decade, with Scott and

Te Linde finding 49.5 per cent of their cases falling into this age group and 83.1 per cent occurring before the age of 40. Thus the so-called typical patient with endometriosis will be a nulliparous private patient in her thirties.

Distribution and Gross Pathology

Endometrial growths have been described in a great variety of places, chiefly within the pelvis, the ovary being the organ most frequently involved.

Figure 9-4 illustrates the distribution diagrammatically, and Table 9-1 shows the numerical incidence of the condition in the various pelvic structures.

In addition to these more common sites, some very unusual and rare locations have been reported. Navratil and Kramer described endometriosis in the extensor carpi radialis muscle and Mankin in the left thigh. There are at least a dozen cases of thoracic endometriosis reported (Bungeler and Fleury-Silveira, Laltes *et al.*, and Williams *et al.*). Some of these involve the pleura, producing pleuritic pain or pleural effusions, while others have involved the lung parenchyma, producing hemoptysis rather than the pleuritic symptoms.

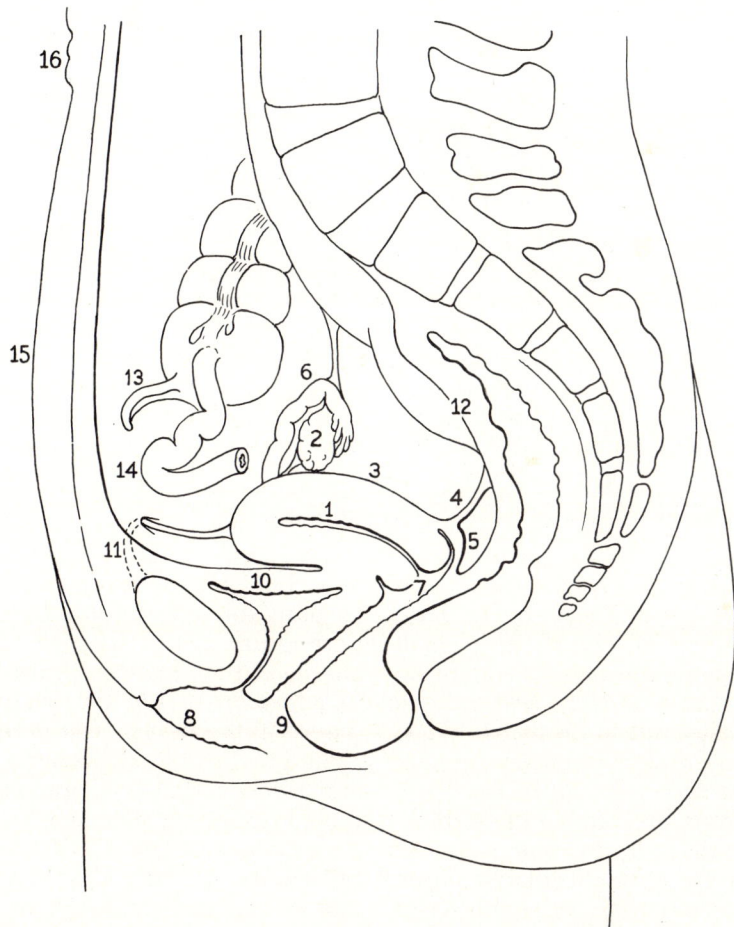

Fig. 9-4. Schematic drawing of sites of endometriosis. (1) Adenomyosis. (2) Ovary. (3) Serous surface of uterus. (4) Uterosacral ligament. (5) Cul-de-sac. (6) Tube. (7) Cervix. (8) Vulva. (9) Perineum. (10) Bladder. (11) Extraperitoneal portion of round ligament. (12) Rectosigmoid. (13) Appendix. (14) Ileum. (15) Abdominal scar. (16) Umbilicus.

TABLE 9-1. LOCATION OF EXTERNAL ENDOMETRIOSIS

TYPE	SITE	NUMBER	PER CENT
	Ovary—one	285	55.2
	Ovary—both	127	24.6
Superficial and small spots on serosa	Diffuse scattered pelvic	171	33.1
	Uterine surface	73	14.1
	Tubal surface	71	13.7
	Posterior cul-de-sac	24	4.7
	Uterosacral ligaments	19	3.7
	Anterior cul-de-sac	11	2.1
	Omentum	3	0.6
	Round ligaments	2	0.4
	Broad ligaments	1	0.2
	Small intestines	1	0.2
	Appendix	7	1.4
Intra-abdominal nodules	Rectovaginal septum	8	1.6
	Rectovaginal septum with rectosigmoid involvement	20	3.9
	Rectovaginal septum with vaginal extension	9	1.8
	Sigmoidal	4	0.8
	Anterior cul-de-sac	2	0.4
	Anterior cul-de-sac with bladder involvement	5	1.0
	Tube	8	1.6
	Broad ligament	4	0.8
	Round ligament	3	0.6
Extraperitoneal	Cervix	13	2.5
	Inguinal	4	0.8
	Umbilical	4	0.8
	Incisional-ventral	4	0.8
	Incisional-vulval	1	0.2

Total amounts to over 100 per cent because of multiple lesions.

The lesions of the ovary vary in size from small ones of pinhead size to those larger than a child's head. The small superficial lesions are more frequent on the convex ovarian surface and vary in color from dusky red to brownish black, depending on the state of preservation of the contained blood (Figs. 9-5 and 9-6). The larger cysts are often rather thick-walled and dull white in color, or in the thinner areas the dark chocolate-colored contents may darken the wall to brown or almost black (Fig. 9-7). The cysts, large and small, characteristically perforate when the pressure from intracystic hemorrhage becomes sufficiently great. The organization of the extruded blood seals over the defect in the cyst wall, and blood accumulates anew within the cavity until perforation again takes place. This discharge of blood with organization results in adhesions about the ovary and elsewhere in the pelvis. The peritoneum, irritated by this blood, becomes hyperemic and thickened. Upon opening the peritoneal cavity, the characteristic picture is a variable amount of old blood, free in the cavity. Usually this is very scanty, but in rare instances, where large cysts have ruptured, as much as 100 or 200 cc. may be present. When the cyst is dissected free, the point or points of previous perforations are inevitably broken into, and there is spilling of the cyst con-

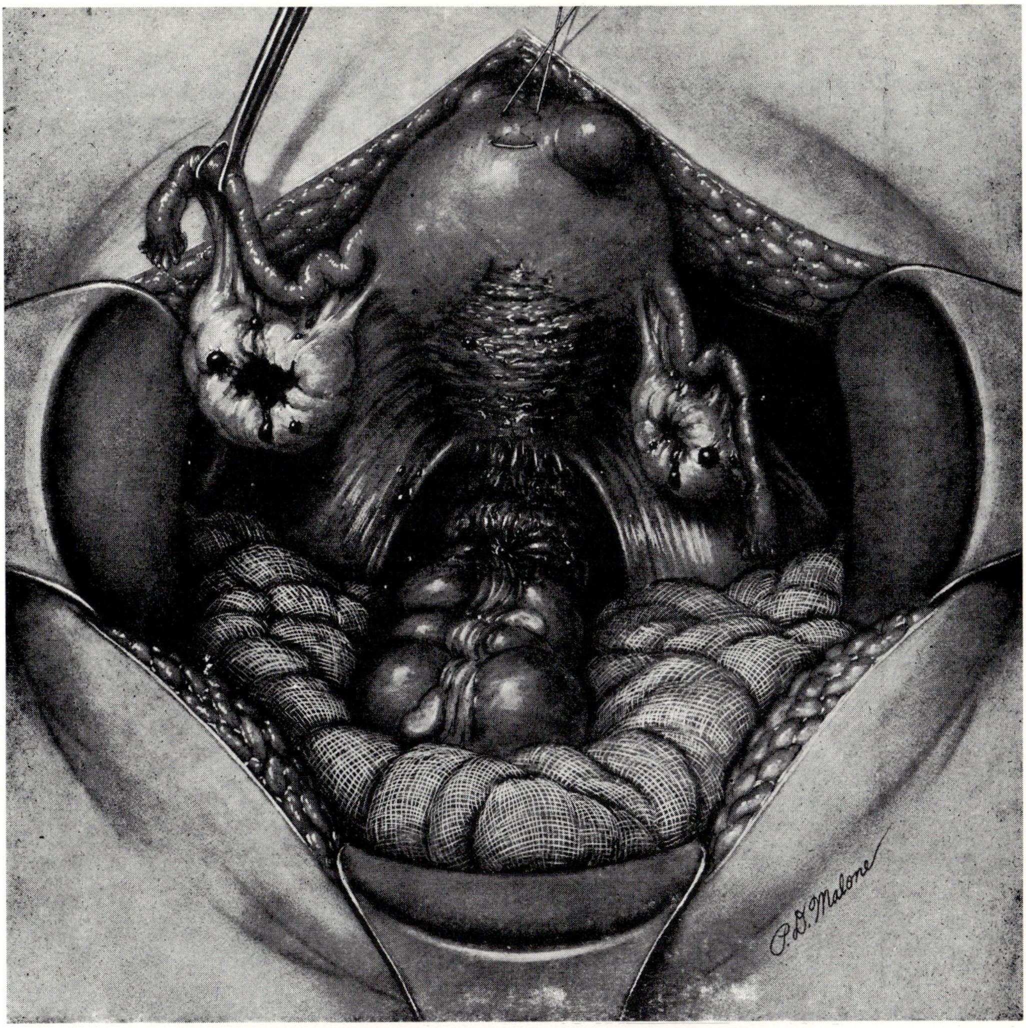

FIG. 9-5. Typical picture of pelvic endometriosis. Both ovaries, the uterosacral ligament, the posterior surface of the uterus and the rectal wall are involved.

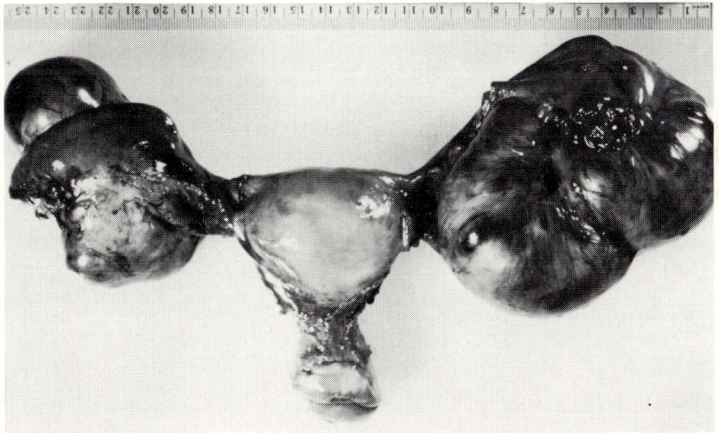

FIG. 9-6. The large endometrial cysts have almost completely destroyed the normal ovarian tissue.

200 Endometriosis

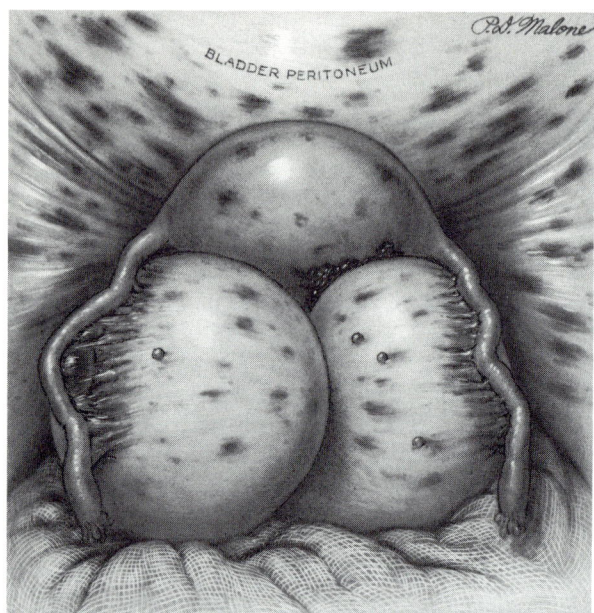

FIG. 9-7. Typical bilateral endometrial cysts of ovary. Old blood is disseminated on the pelvic peritoneum.

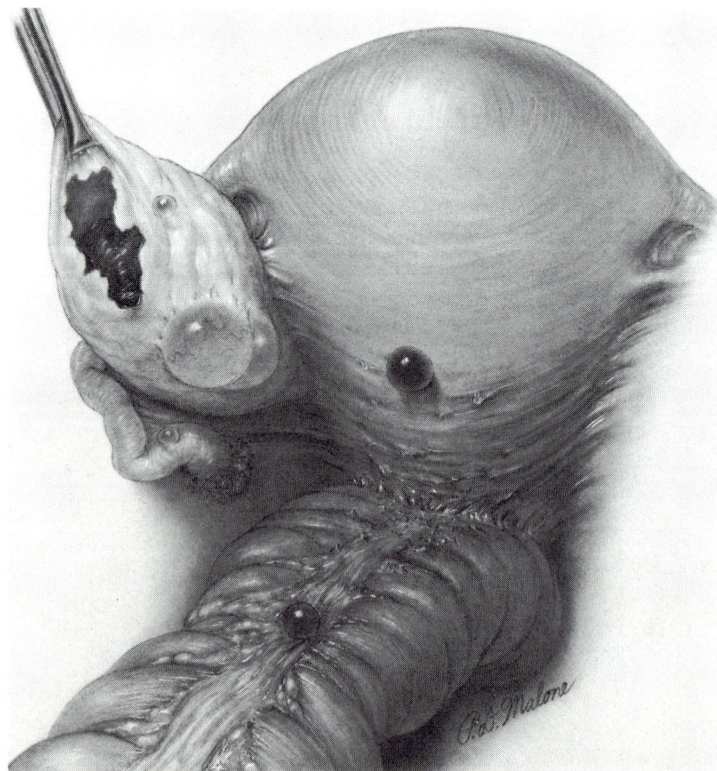

FIG. 9-8. Pelvic endometriosis with corpus luteum hematoma. A typical picture often seen at operation. The cul-de-sac is obliterated by dense adhesions. There is a large endometrial implant on the posterior surface of the uterus and the anterior surface of the rectum. The ovary contains a ruptured corpus luteum hematoma.

tents. Generally the contents are a thick brown fluid, from which the name of *chocolate cyst* has been derived; sometimes the contents are very thick, tenacious, and almost black in color. The Germans have called these *tar cysts*, and, indeed, the contents may resemble tar more than chocolate. The presumptive evidence is in favor of an endometrial cyst when, on dissecting free an adherent ovary or ovarian cyst, chocolate or tarry substance appears. This is not an invariable rule, since hemorrhage into corpora lutea and also into other types of ovarian cysts may give a similar picture (Fig. 9-8). However, the blood in a corpus luteum hematoma is much more apt to form a clot than to remain a thick fluid, as in an endometrial cyst. Hemorrhage into a serous cystadenoma may give a chocolate color to the contents; but the blood, being mixed with the serous contents, is not usually sufficient to alter the consistency of the fluid.

Next to the ovary the uterus is involved most frequently. The serous surface of this organ is often the site of many implants. They are usually very small, although occasionally they form dark vesicles as large as peas (Fig. 9-8). Wherever the endometrial lesion occurs on serosal surfaces there is apt to be a characteristic puckering of the serosa about the small dark lesion. Implants on the anterior surface of the uterus sometimes cause adhesions between it and the peritoneal surface of the bladder. Invasion of the bladder may extend through the entire thickness of the organ (Fig. 9-9). The lesions are more common on the posterior

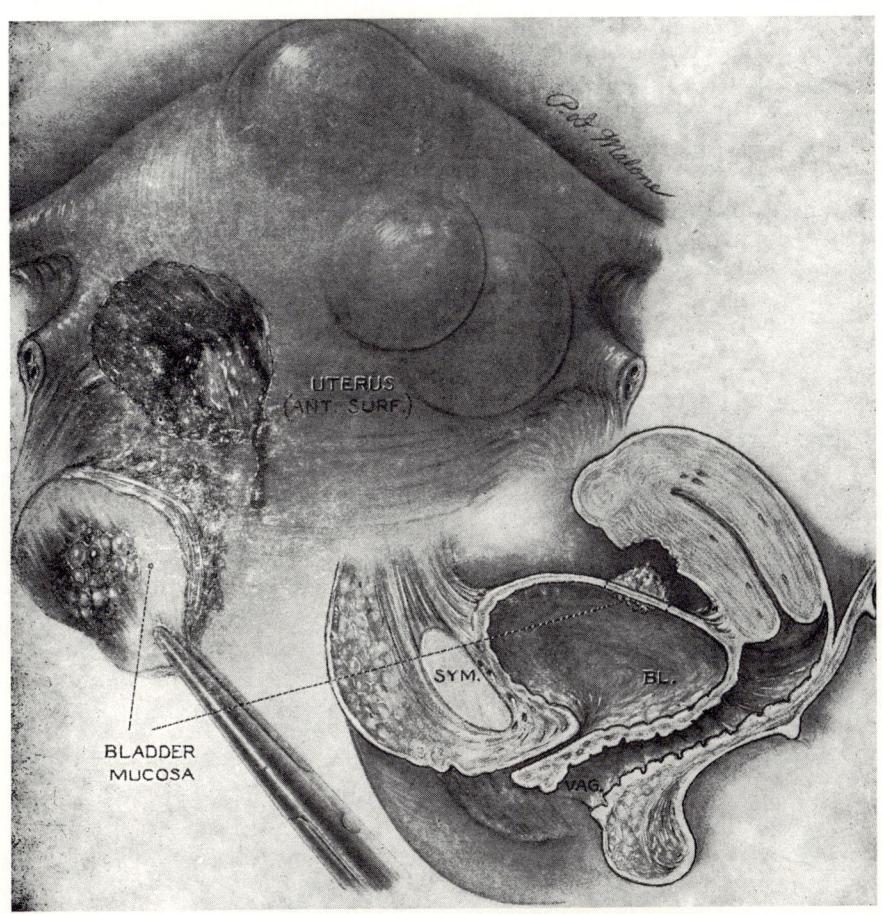

FIG. 9-9. Endometriosis, involving the bladder wall.

surface of the uterus and especially common on the lower portion. The cul-de-sac is a favorite place for endometrial "implants"; the posterior wall of the vagina and the cervix often become densely adherent to the anterior rectal wall, thus completely obliterating the cul-de-sac. The uterosacral ligaments on either side of the cul-de-sac are commonly involved in the endometrial growth and form small, puckered, shotty nodules along the course of the ligaments. An extension downward of the invasive endometrial process from the cul-de-sac and the uterosacral region brings it down into the rectovaginal septum, involving the anterior rectal wall and at times penetrating the mucosa of the posterior vaginal vault. This growth may be visible through a vaginal speculum as a dark nodular mass posterior to the cervix (Fig. 9-10).

Small endometrial implants may occur on the serosa of the round ligaments at any place within the peritoneal cavity, but a lesion of special interest is that described by Cullen in 1896, in which the extraperitoneal portion of the round ligament is involved in an adenomyosis process, forming a nodule in the region of the inguinal ring. Such a nodule may be from 1 to 3 cm. in diameter and is

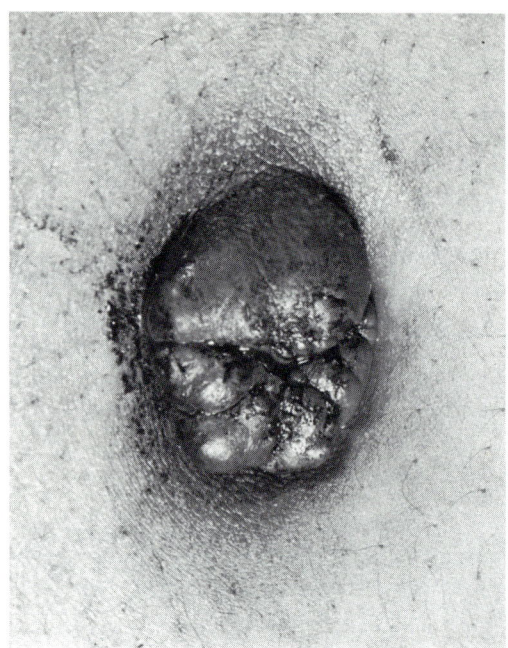

FIG. 9-11. Endometriosis of the umbilicus.

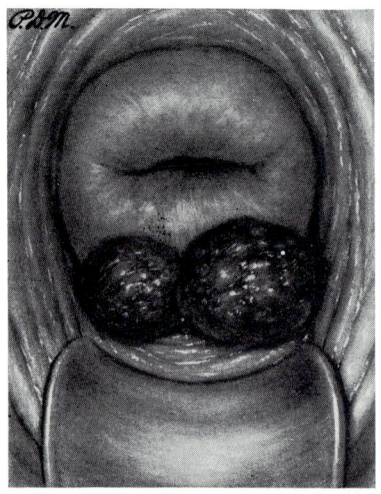

FIG. 9-10. Endometrial polyps growing in posterior vaginal fornix from cul-de-sac endometriosis.

usually blended diffusely with the surrounding adipose tissue. The round-ligament growths are composed of smooth muscle with islands of endometrium and dark areas that give evidence of hemorrhage. Many cases have been reported in the literature of endometriosis of the umbilicus. Here the endometrial tissue infiltrates the surrounding tissues and by hemorrhage forms bluish nodules, sometimes visible through the skin (Fig. 9-11).

Laparotomy scars from operations on the uterus and tubes occasionally are the site of endometrial growth; so also may be perineal, vaginal, or vulvar scars, particularly episiotomies, colporrhaphies, and Bartholin gland excisions. In such cases there frequently is a history of delayed wound healing. These growths appear as deep-lying or subcutaneous nodules infiltrating the fat, fascia, and muscle. Bleeding into the tissues at the time of menstruation causes cyclic local pain, tenderness, and discoloration of the tissues; but the nodule may lie too deep for one to detect the color change through the skin. If the nodule is superficial, there may be cyclic bleeding or ulceration with intermittent bleeding.

In addition to involvement of the anterior rectal wall with invasion of the rectovaginal septum, a prominent lesion in the upper rectum or sigmoid is not uncommon. Such a lesion causes a thickening and proliferation of the muscularis of the bowel, resulting in true adenomyosis. The degree of involvement may be sufficient to encroach on the bowel lumen and be responsible for partial or even complete obstruction. Usually, since the invasion is through the serosa and muscularis, the mucosa is not involved. This is an important diagnostic point in the differentiation by barium enema of endometriosis from carcinoma of the bowel since the latter arises from the mucosa. Endometriosis may involve the full thickness of the intestinal wall, even producing polypoid growths within the bowel lumen. Bleeding, often cyclic, then usually occurs, but also the diagnosis can be made by proctoscopy or sigmoidoscopy and a biopsy of the lesion. If these have not been done, at laparotomy it may be difficult to distinguish bowel endometriosis from carcinoma. The presence of endometriosis elsewhere in the pelvis generally gives a clue to the nature of the bowel lesion.

The appendix, cecum, and ileum are not infrequently involved in a process of endometriosis but rarely to the degree seen in the sigmoid and rectum. A loop of ileum may be caught in the pelvis, producing angulation and obstruction, either partial or complete. Biopsy of the lesion again is often necessary to establish the benign nature of the implant. Bowel resection or excision of the involved area should be done when obstruction is present, or when the size of the lumen is significantly compromised. Under such circumstances castration is not adequate treatment since subsequent fibrosis may further narrow the bowel lumen. Figure 9-12 illustrates an extensive growth of endometrium on an appendix.

The urinary tract is involved to a lesser degree than the bowel. As mentioned above, peritoneal implants on the bladder may infiltrate a part of the bladder wall or the entire bladder wall, causing symptoms of vesical irritability and occasionally hematuria. A more serious situation may arise when the ureter is compressed by an endometrial cyst or directly invaded by endometriosis in the pelvis. This in turn leads to ureteral obstruction and loss of renal function (Fig. 9-13).

There even have been a few cases of renal endometriosis reported. This may result from passage of fragments of endometrium up the ureter or by lymphatic or vascular metastasis along or in the ureteral wall.

Histology

Endometriosis in its various sites may present a variety of histologic pictures. In many instances, especially when located in the ovary, there are typical uterine glands and an abundance of typical endometrial stroma (Fig. 9-14). In the large chocolate cysts the epithelium lining the cavity is thinned out by pressure, sometimes to the point of being unrecognizable; indeed, in some areas the epithelium may be entirely lacking. Stroma, also, may be very scanty in some of the lesions, and one may be forced to search diligently for sufficient stroma to identify the tissue.

When the endometrium grows in a setting of smooth muscle, as in the round

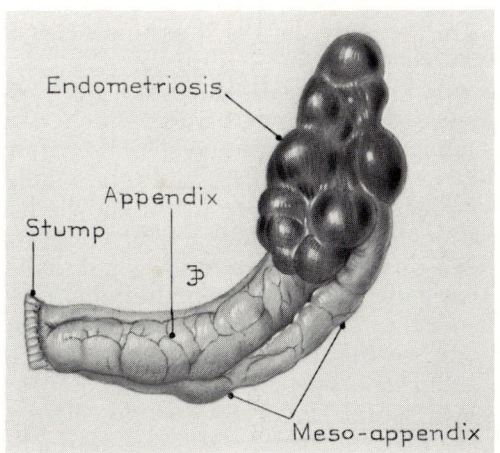

Fig. 9-12. Extensive endometriosis of the appendix.

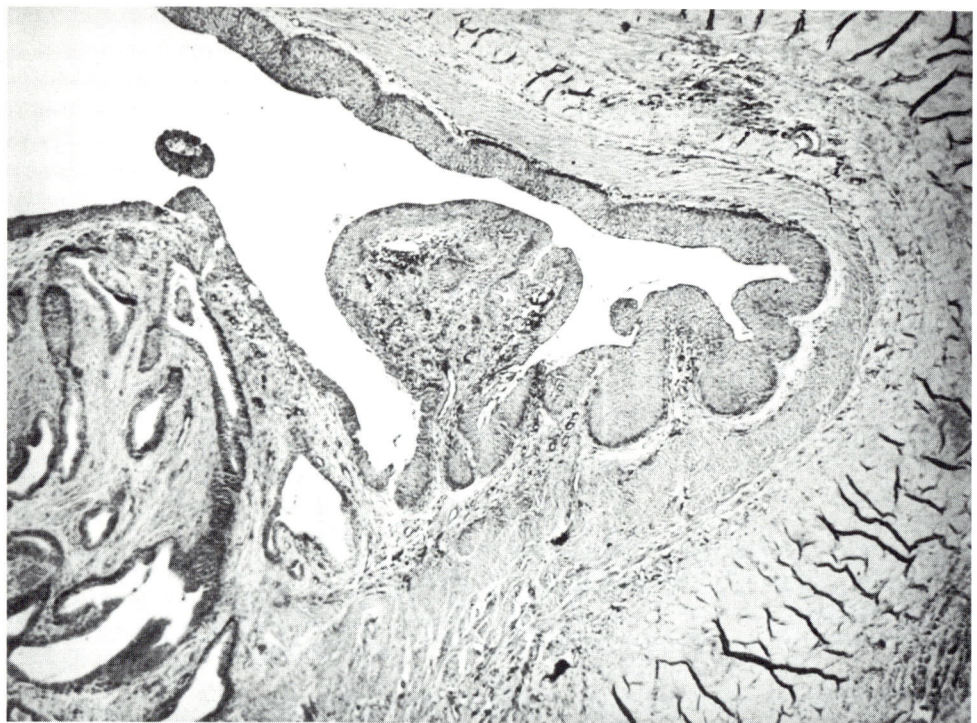

FIG. 9-13. Compression and invasion of the ureteral wall by endometriosis induced in experiments on monkeys.

or the uterosacral ligaments, or on the surface of the uterus, it often seems to stimulate the proliferation of the smooth muscle, which grows in whorls between the bits of endometrial tissue; thus histologically the growth may resemble that of internal adenomyosis.

In many instances the glands and the stroma go through the normal cyclic changes identical with those experienced by the endometrium in its normal site; during pregnancy a full decidual reaction is frequently noted (Fig. 9-15). However, the typical menstrual cyclic changes are not seen universally, and the endometrial pattern of the ectopic tissue may be purely proliferative, showing no progestational change; there are instances in which the typical Swiss-cheese pattern of hyperplasia is present.

In some of the cysts the epithelial lining resembles tubal epithelium, with ciliated and nonciliated cells. Sampson and Everet have described this, and the former has suggested the term *endosalpingiosis*. We have seen some cysts in which one part of the wall is lined by typical endometrium and another part by epithelium of the tubal type.

HISTOGENESIS

In the early days of reporting cases of endometrial lesions outside of the uterus, Cullen and Russell stated that they believed the ectopic tissue, which was histologically similar to that found within the uterus, was müllerian in origin. Subsequent developments in our knowledge of the physiology and the histology of reproduction have shown beyond doubt that these lesions are of müllerian origin, since they show all variations of response to the ovarian hormones characteristic of endometrium in its normal site. These early writers believed that the ectopic endometrial tissue was the result of misplaced embryonic müllerian rests but made no attempt to explain the mecha-

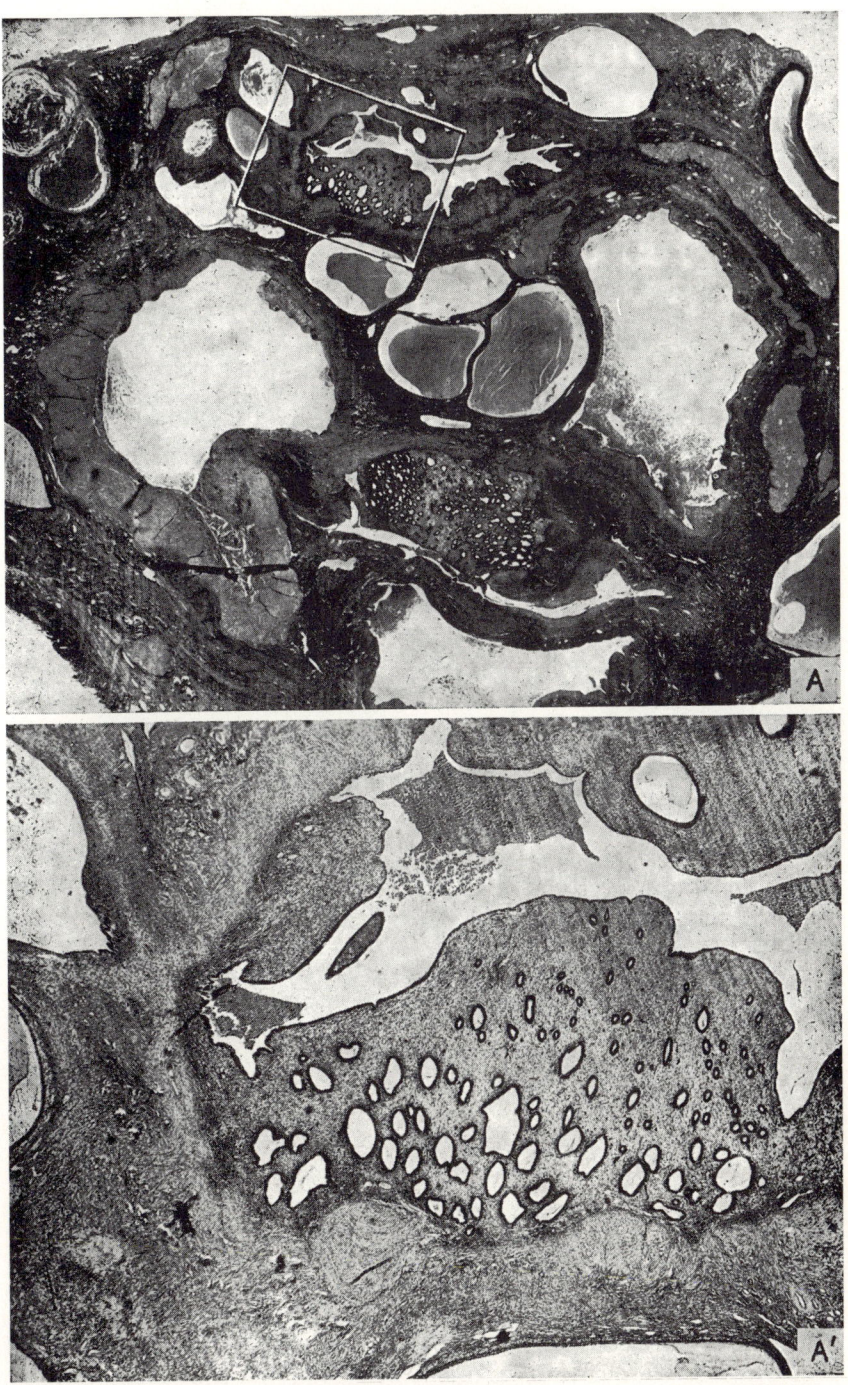

FIG. 9-14. Multiple endometrial cysts of ovary. (A) Lower-power section of most of ovary. (A') Higher-power section of one cyst wall.

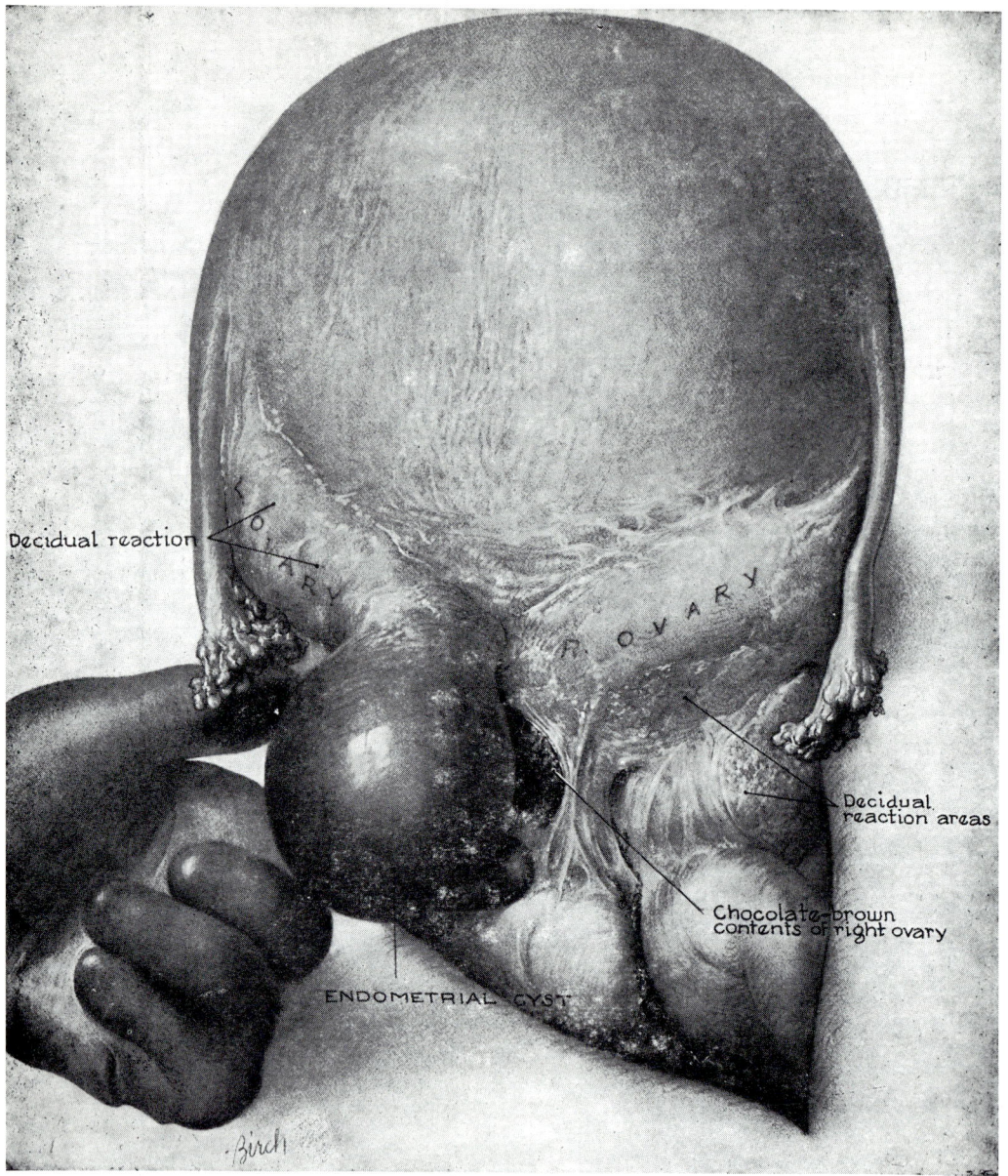

FIG. 9-15. Endometriosis associated with 36 weeks' pregnancy.

nism whereby the endometrial tissue was disseminated.

Not until Sampson's contributions, which first appeared in 1921, did gynecologists begin to bend seriously to the task of studying the histogenesis of this disease. At the outset it should be stated that the problem has not been solved completely. Sampson's contributions have been many, and he has given consideration to many speculations regarding the histogenesis of endometriosis. However, the theory which is generally considered as his most important contribution concerns itself with the question of whether or not the menstrual endometrium may flow in a retrograde manner out through the tubes, implant itself, and proliferate on the pelvic viscera.

Sampson has briefly stated his implantation theory as follows:

Ovarian and other forms of peritoneal endometriosis arise from the implantation of bits of müllerian mucosa, of either uterine or tubal origin, which, having been carried with menstrual blood escaping through patent tubes into the peritoneal cavity, have lodged on the surfaces of the various pelvic structures. The ectopic mucosa in these implants, regardless of their size or situation, may become additional foci for the spread of the endometriosis by direct extension and also by the implantation of bits of müllerian tissue which escape from them during their reaction to menstruation. This latter phenomenon is most spectacular in the ovary where ectopic endometrial cavities may attain a much larger size than elsewhere, forming the well-known endometrial cysts of that organ.

Sampson originally believed that the ovary acted as an incubator or hotbed for the development of implants on the peritoneum and might even impart greater virulence to the müllerian epithelium growing in it. He based this belief on the fact that in the cases studied by him up to 1922 the endometriosis was more extensive and more invasive in those cases that were associated with endometrial cysts of the ovary. However, the study of more material showed him that extensive pelvic endometriosis may occur without ovarian involvement; hence he considers unwarranted his earlier suggestion that the ovary imparts greater virulence to the müllerian epithelium.

Sampson has deliberately operated on many patients at the time of menstruation and has frequently observed blood coming from the ends of the tubes. This observation has been substantiated by many gynecologists, and it is generally believed that retroversion of the uterus augments this flow. Sampson has fixed and sectioned this blood and has demonstrated uterine mucosa in it, which he believed to be viable (Fig. 9-16).

Sampson's theory is undoubtedly the most widely accepted one offered in explanation of the phenomenon of pelvic endometriosis. Anyone who has repeatedly observed at the operating table

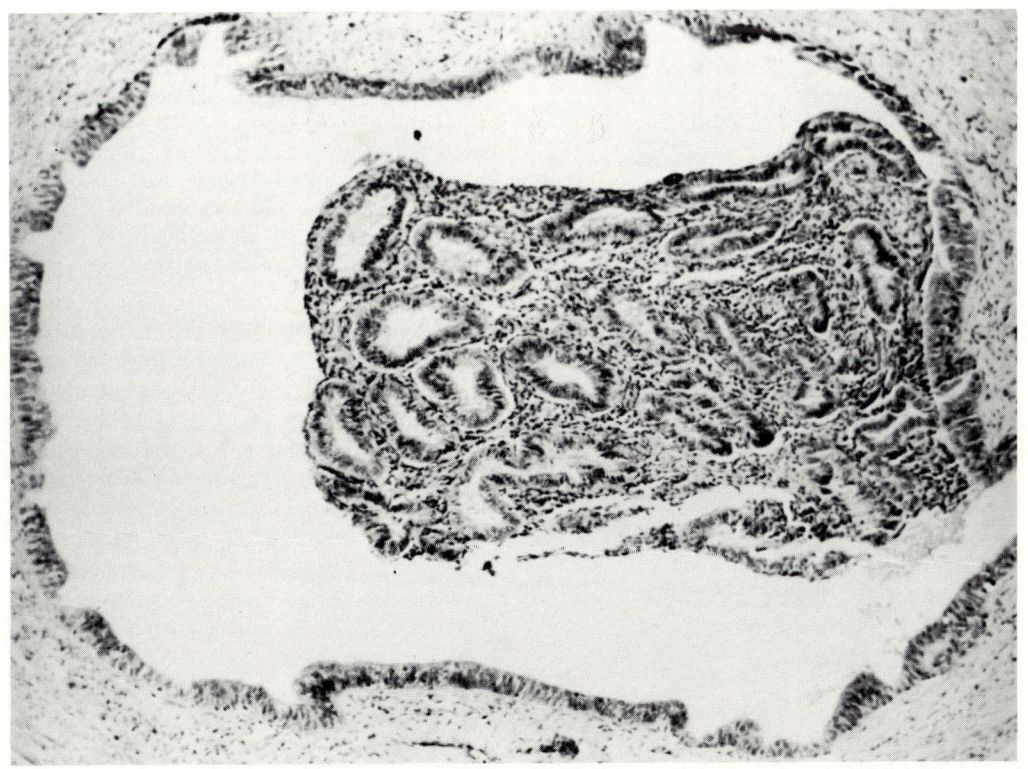

FIG. 9-16. A particle of endometrium in human tube.

endometrial cysts of the ovary associated with pelvic adhesions that are obviously the result of organizing old blood can scarcely doubt that these adhesions form from blood spilled from these cysts. If one couples this observation with the fact that many of these adhesions, when sectioned, show endometrial tissue, it is difficult to escape the conclusion that the peritoneal endometrial plaques are implants from the bloody contents of cysts. The question of whether or not the endometrial-lined cysts of the ovaries are the result of implantation of bits of cast-off menstrual endometrium via the tube would seem to be the crux of the problem.

There is no doubt from experimental studies that endometrium cut from the uterine lining and transplanted into the pelvic cavity or other areas will grow. Harbitz, Allen, Weinstein et al., Hobbs and Bortnick, and numerous other workers have successfully transplanted surgically removed pieces of endometrium in lower animals. Markee transplanted endometrium into the anterior chamber of the monkey's eye, where they grew through many menstrual cycles. Heim, Caffier, Traut, Hirsch and Jones, and others successfully cultured endometrium from surgically removed human uteri. The author repeatedly has seen endometriosis develop in the peritoneal cavity of rhesus monkeys following hysterotomy for recovery of fetuses (Fig. 9-17). Scott and Te Linde have transplanted bits of endometrial tissue removed by hysterotomy at various phases of the menstrual cycle and observed them by laparotomy to be growing up to 522 days.

Interesting as these observations are, until recently no unimpeachable experiments had been done to show whether or not the cast-off particles of menstrual endometrium are capable of implantation and growth. Therein lies the crux of the entire Sampson theory, for, as Sampson himself has said:

If bits of müllerian mucosa carried by menstrual blood escaping into the peritoneal cavity are always dead, the implantation theory, as presented by me, also is dead and should be buried and forgotten. If some of these bits are even occasionally alive, the implantation theory also is alive.*

Even the opponents of Sampson's theory have admitted that if it could be shown that cast-off menstrual endometrium is viable, Sampson's hypothesis would be strengthened greatly.

Novak has summarized the objections that have been raised to Sampson's theory:

(1) Retrograde menstruation, while it may occur, is a rarely observed phenomenon, as contrasted with the great frequency of endometriosis; (2) it is difficult to believe that

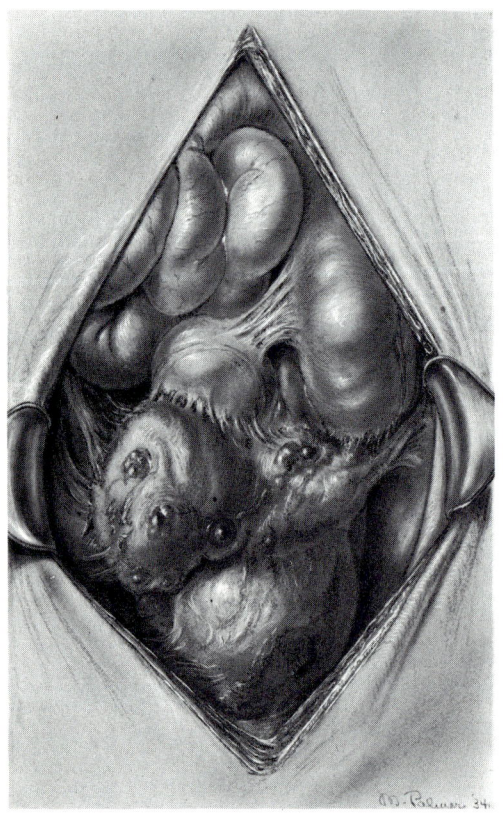

FIG. 9-17. Endometriosis involving intestines and lower abdomen of a monkey approximately 3 years of age following a hysterotomy to recover an early embryo.

---

* Sampson, J. A.: The development of the implantation theory for the origin of peritoneal endometriosis. Amer. J. Obstet. Gynec., 40:558, 1940.

endometrium thrown off in the uterus could enter the small uterine orifice of the tube, travel outward against the current and still be capable of implanting itself and growing upon the pelvic structures; (3) endometrium thrown off at menstruation is already degenerated or dead, so that it is not easy to conceive of its taking root in the peritoneum; (4) such experiments as those of Jacobson, showing that endometrium can grow in the peritoneum, have dealt with the normal, healthy endometrium of animals; (5) experiments such as those of Heim in monkeys, in which a utero-abdominal fistula was created, have all failed to show any development of endometrium in spite of the fact that the menstrual blood was emptied freely into the abdomen; (6) Sampson's theory could not explain endometriosis in certain locations, such as the umbilicus.*

Most of those who have been skeptical of accepting Sampson's theory have championed the theory of Ivanoff and of Meyer in one of its modifications. These two investigators independently advocated the idea that aberrant endometrium originates from abnormal differentiation of the coelomic epithelium, from which all the genital mucous membrane arises. This theory in its various modifications suggests that the pelvic peritoneum under certain stimuli, inflammatory or hormonal, may develop into endometrial-like tissue. We always have believed that the inflammatory stimulus to the pelvic peritoneum cannot be the answer, because in our colored wards, where pelvic inflammation is commonest, endometriosis is rarest. If the stimulus necessary to transform the pelvic peritoneum into endometrial tissue is hormonal, no one as yet has been able to explain just what abnormal hormonal stimulus is required to bring about the change.

Halban's theory of dissemination via the lymphatics appears to be relevant in only a few cases of endometriosis. The usual pelvic lesions of endometriosis do not follow the paths of the lymphatics. Endometrium has been found occasionally in the pelvic lymph nodes at operation, as reported by Javert, but this does not usually produce clinical endometriosis. This, however, appears to be the best explanation of endometriosis of the umbilicus, since Scott has shown in rhesus monkeys that lymphatics of the anterior wall may drain from the pelvis to the umbilicus.

By 1950 the discussion had become static. All of the arguments for and against the two major theories, retrograde menstruation and coelomic metaplasia, had been advanced, leaving perhaps the most fundamental question concerning the viability of cast-off menstrual endometrium unanswered. Scott and Te Linde then reported some experimental work which seems to have demonstrated the capability of growth of desquamated menstrual endometrium. The uterus of each of 10 rhesus monkeys (Fig. 9-18) was divided from its vaginal attachment and rotated on its ovarian axis to allow intraperitoneal menstruation to occur, spilling the menstrual flow in the cul-de-sac or upward toward the diaphragm. Six of the 10 animals developed typical areas of endometriosis within the peritoneal cavity (Figs. 9-19 and 9-20). Growing endometrium was found from 75 to 963 days after the reversal operation. The other 4 animals failed to survive.

The uterus of another monkey was rotated 90°, and the cervix was brought through the anterior abdominal wall, permitting menstruation to occur at this site (Fig. 9-21). The uterus subsequently retracted, leaving a sinus tract in the anterior abdominal wall. Endometriosis was found in this sinus tract (Fig. 9-22). In two additional animals the rotated cervix was implanted into the rectus muscle, permitting menstruation to occur in an area entirely free from the peritoneum or from tissue arising from the coelomic epithelium. Endometriosis was found adjacent to the reversed cervix in 12 and 19 months after the original operation.

It had been suggested that blood per se originating from the rupture of ovarian follicles or corpora lutea or escaping from the fimbria of fallopian tubes during

---

* Novak, E.: Gynecological and Obstetrical Pathology. Philadelphia, W. B. Saunders, 1940.

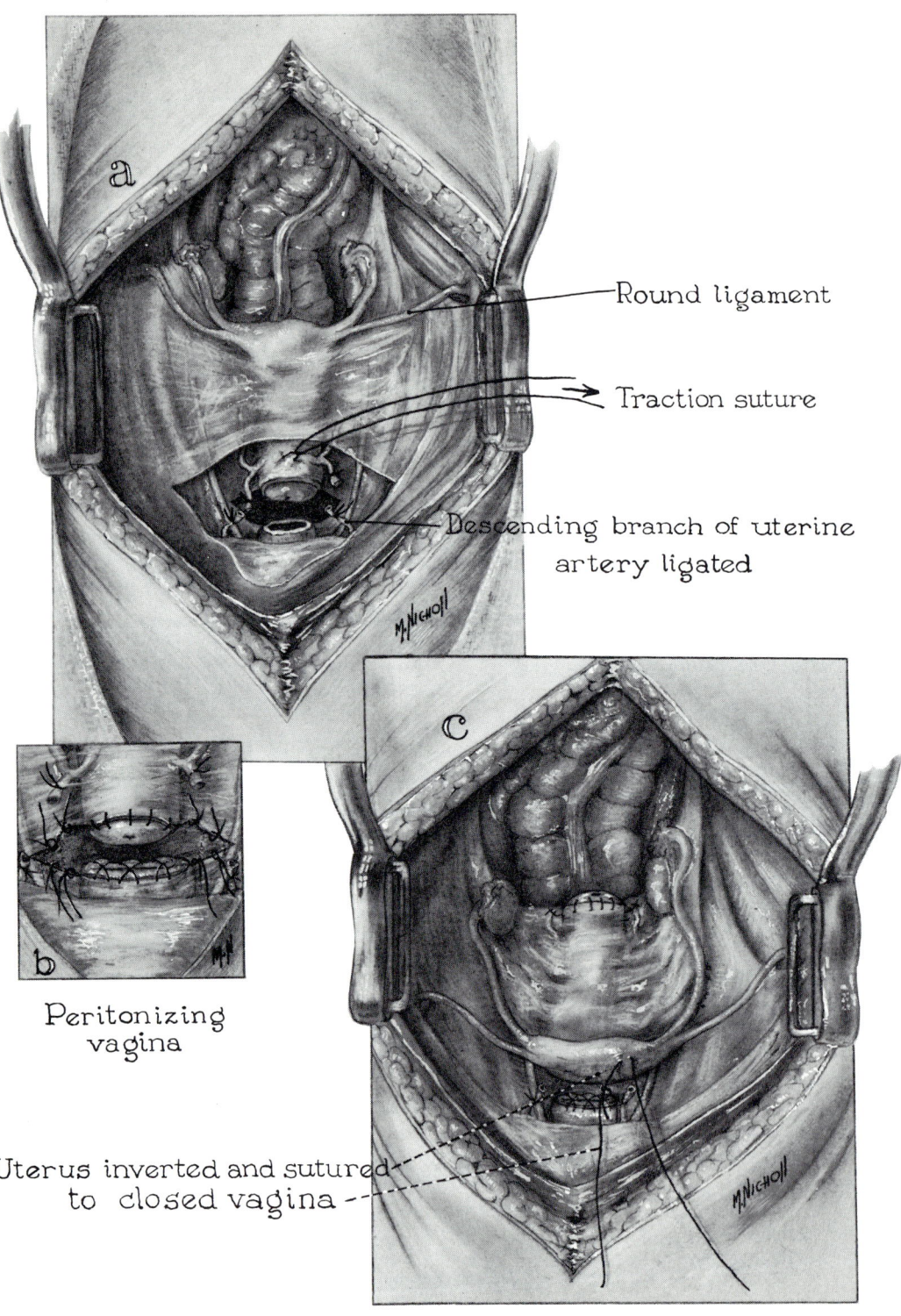

FIG. 9-18. The experimental surgical procedure on monkeys to allow intra-abdominal menstruation in which the entire uterus is separated from the vagina and turned through 180°.

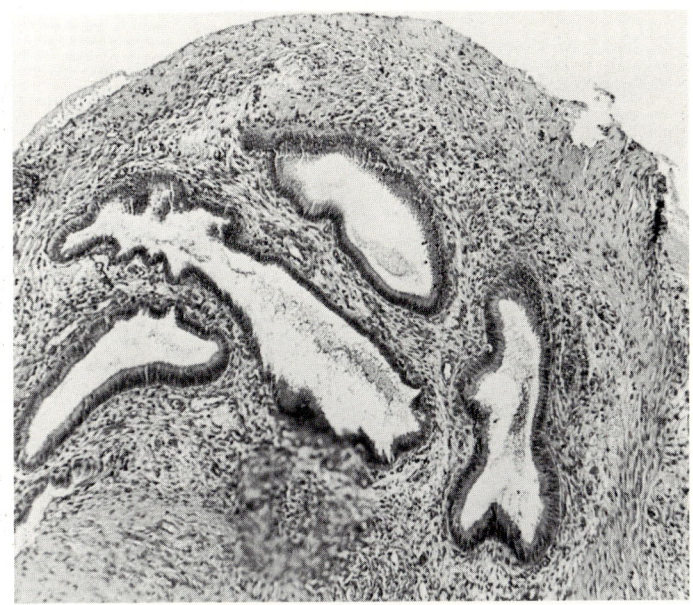

FIG. 9-19. Endometrial glands and stroma grossly appearing as a purplish area on the right lateral pelvic wall 404 days after turning the uterus through 180°. This was one of several such areas at some distance from the reversed cervix. (×100)

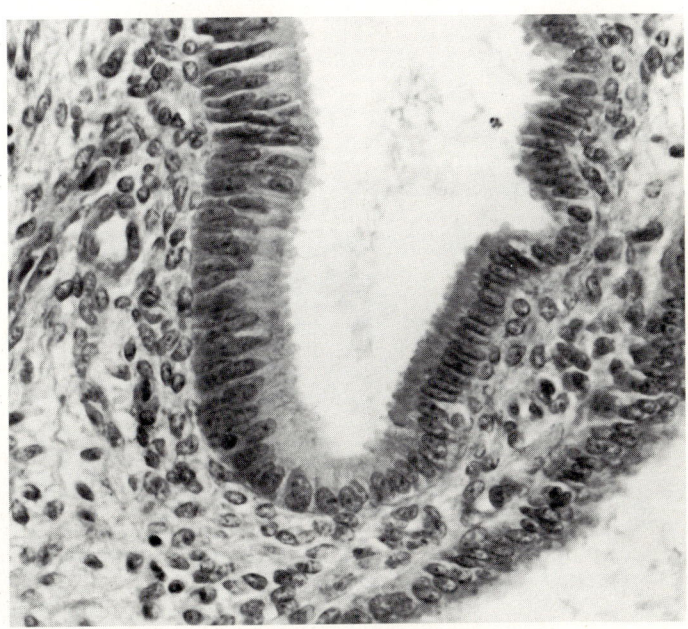

FIG. 9-20. High-power study of an area in Figure 9-19 to show the characteristic epithelium and stroma. (×500)

menstruation might incite metaplasia of the peritoneum and produce endometriosis. To test this theory, Scott, Te Linde, and Wharton injected venous blood obtained during 7 to 19 episodes of menstruation into the peritoneal cavity of 4 monkeys, and in no instance did endometriosis develop.

Ridley and Edwards finally in 1959 were able to transfer these findings from the experimental animal to humans. For 12 hours they caught the menstrual flow of 8 women through a cervical cannula. This material was centrifuged, and the sediment was injected into the rectus muscle of the same patient who was to

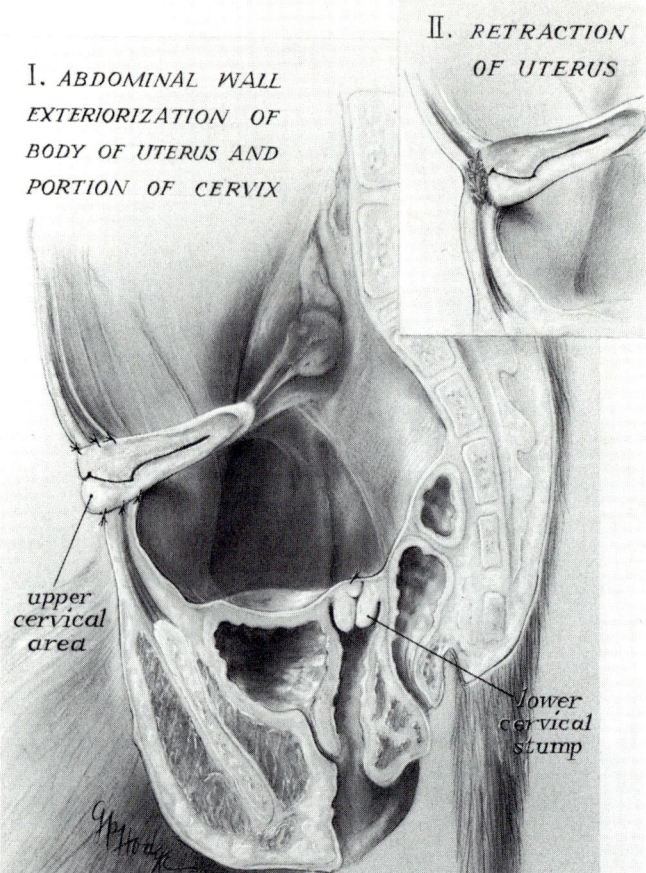

Fig. 9-21. The uterus, except for the distal portion of the cervix, was brought out through the anterior abdominal wall. The inset shows the retraction of the uterus and the scarring in the anterior abdominal wall.

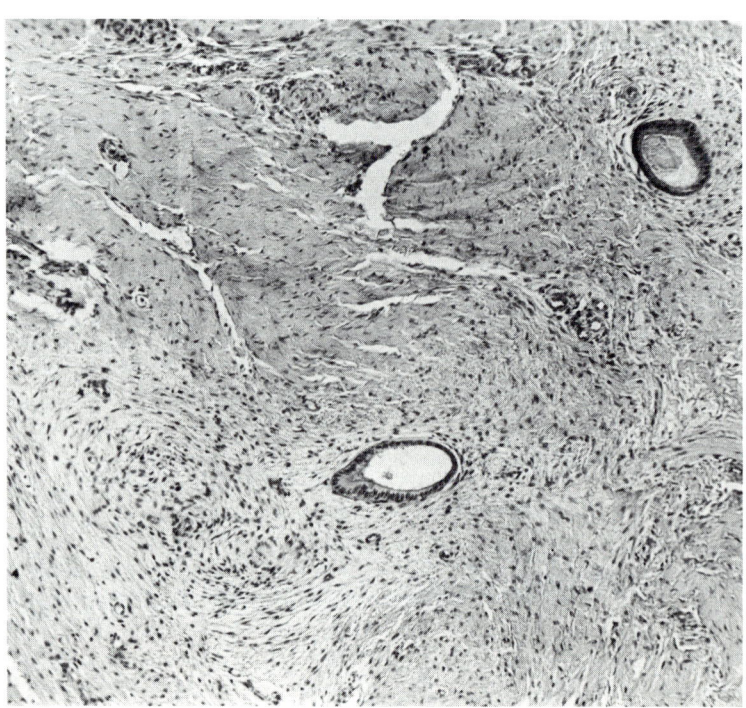

Fig. 9-22. Endometrial glands and stroma in the scar tissue along the line of uterine retraction 364 days after the surgical procedure in Figure 9-21. (×100)

have a laparotomy 90 to 180 days after the single injection. Six of these patients failed to show endometriosis in the injection site at laparotomy, but one had a definite area of endometriosis 175 days after injection, and the other patient had an area suggestive of endometriosis at 110 days.

Four women accidentally provided a clinical experiment. Three of these had a noncommunicating horn of a double uterus. In these women the only exit of the menstrual flow from the noncommunicating horn was through the fallopian tube, and each woman developed endometriosis in the ovary on the side of the rudimentary horn (Fig. 9-23). The 4th case was a maiden woman of 40 who developed dysmenorrhea and eventually amenorrhea, with recurring monthly pain. Examination showed the upper vagina to be obliterated completely by adhesions, and laparotomy showed endometriosis of the posterior surface of the uterus and cul-de-sac.

Desquamated human endometrium has been grown successfully on tissue culture by Keettel and Stein. The cultured cells had the appearance of fibroblasts and epithelial cells. In short, all these studies have given strong support to Sampson's theory of retrograde menstruation and implantation, showing that not only is menstruating endometrium viable but that it is also capable of growing and causing endometriosis.

The above experiments give no support to the theory of serosa metaplasia but give more or less conclusive support to Sampson's theory of retrograde menstruation. However, this theory fails to explain the occurrence of endometriosis

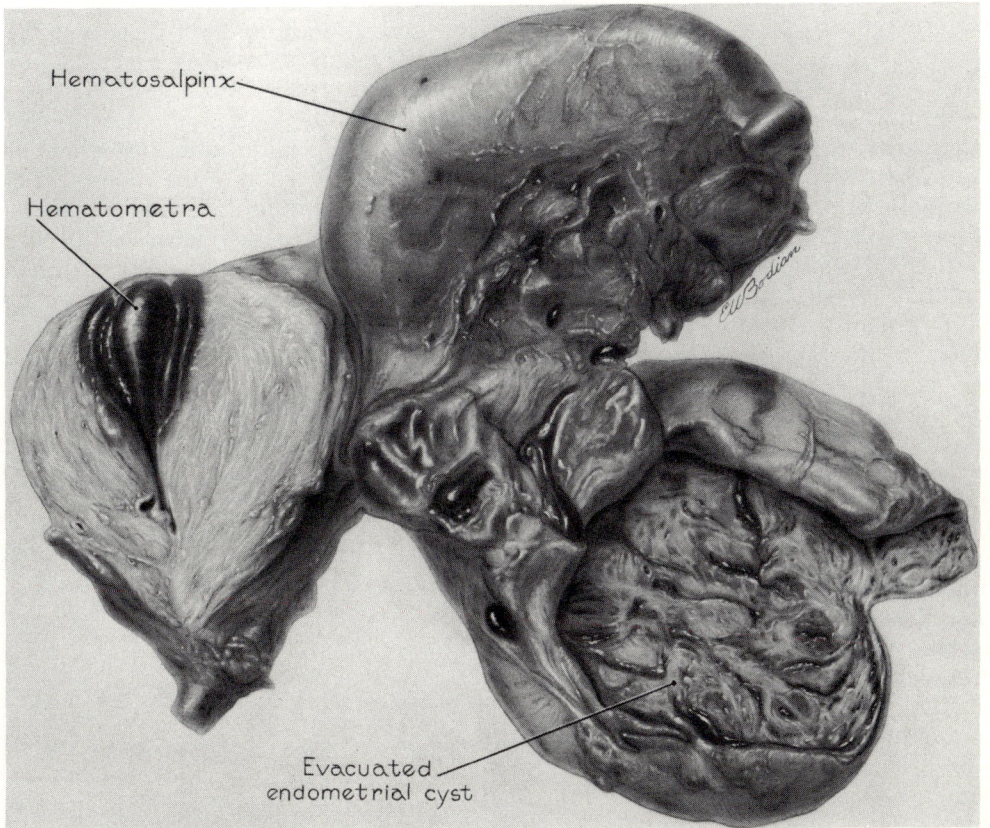

FIG. 9-23. Endometrial cyst occurring in a patient with a double uterus. The rudimentary horn did not communicate with the cervix; this resulted in hematometra, hematosalpinx, and an endometrial cyst in the respective ovary. (Mayo Clinic)

at the umbilicus. In view of the lymphatic drainage from the pelvic region to the umbilicus via the route of the urachus and obliterated hypogastric vessels, it would seem likely that endometrial particles are deposited in the umbilicus via the lymphatic channels. The possibility of this occurrence is borne out by one of Scott and Te Linde's experiments. A monkey developed extensive endometriosis of the pelvis with complete obstruction of one ureter. An autopsy revealed endometriosis in the nonfunctioning kidney, probably the result of deposits of endometrial particles from the pelvis via the periureteral lymphatics. The rare occurrence of endometriosis in the lung, forearm, and thigh is certainly not explained on Sampson's theory, and the only possible route would seem to be hematogenous. It is of historical interest that Sampson in the early days of his histological studies believed that endometrial particles could be disseminated via the bloodstream.

Symptoms

The most constant single symptom of endometriosis is **pain.** Exclusive of dysmenorrhea, Scott and Te Linde found pain to be present in 57.7 per cent of 243 cases operated upon primarily for endometriosis. Despite the great frequency of pain in these patients, we have repeatedly seen women with extensive endometriosis without the slightest discomfort. Conversely, some women with only a few small endometrial implants in the pelvis may have very severe pain. Since the lesions vary so much in size, number, and location, it is quite natural that the pain arising from them should vary in location and nature, but it is chiefly lower abdominal. It may be unilateral or bilateral, but is more often the latter; and it tends to be aggravated premenstrually or menstrually, leaving a postmenstrual residual pelvic soreness.

Endometrial cysts are inclined to rupture or leak varying amounts of their entrapped blood into the peritoneal cavity. This may occur suddenly and dramatically or intermittently. In either case the blood produces a chemical peritonitis of varying degrees with severe pain, rebound tenderness, and all other signs of peritoneal irritation.

Dysmenorrhea is also a frequent symptom of endometriosis. Although acquired dysmenorrhea is usually thought to be characteristic of this disease, an analysis of the cases of endometriosis fails to substantiate this pattern. In their study of 243 cases of endometriosis, Scott and Te Linde found that 51.4 per cent had had nonprogressive dysmenorrhea since their menarche, 19.3 per cent had progressive dysmenorrhea, and only 9.1 per cent acquired dysmenorrhea—probably coinciding with the development of endometriosis. Nevertheless, almost 80 per cent of the patients treated by surgery confirming the presence of endometriosis had dysmenorrhea, but it is still important to emphasize that extensive endometriosis can exist without any menstrual pain.

Involvement of the cul-de-sac of Douglas and the uterosacral ligaments frequently leads to **dyspareunia** and probably to low sacral backache. When the anterior rectal wall is involved, rectal pressure and painful defecation are common. With invasion of the mucosa of the sigmoid or rectum, bleeding per rectum at the time of menstruation can occur as well as diarrhea. With more extensive bowel infiltration, intestinal obstruction may result (Fig. 9-24).

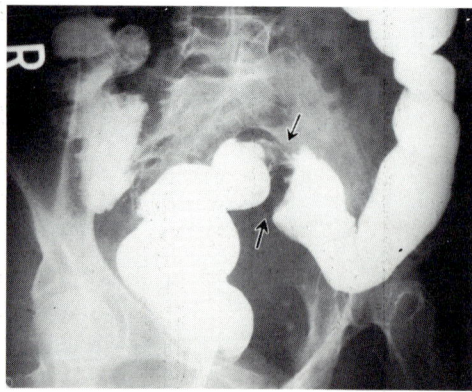

Fig. 9-24. Barium enema of patient with obstructive lesion due to endometriosis. This lesion was resected by a surgeon, who believed it to be carcinoma.

When endometriosis involves a scar in the abdominal wall, the umbilicus, inguinal region, or perineum, there usually is a nodule which undergoes painful swelling at intervals corresponding to menstruation. When these lesions are superficial, there may be a bluish discoloration from hemorrhage into the tissues and at times cyclic external bleeding when the skin is broken. Hematuria has been noted with vesical involvement.

The disparity between the extent of the endometriosis and the severity of the pain remains without adequate explanation. One sees many women in whom one makes with reasonable certainty the diagnosis of endometriosis on routine pelvic examination, and yet they may be completely asymptomatic. On the other hand, others with minimal findings on examination may have severe pain. Sturgis and Call have attempted to reconcile these observations by suggesting that superficial implants may expand more easily with hormonal stimulation, while the deeper islands of ectopic endometrium tend to be encased in fibrous tissue, making distention more difficult and more painful. This may be the case, but the supporting evidence is not yet convincing.

Abnormal uterine bleeding is often associated with endometriosis. It may be menorrhagia, metrorrhagia, or both. In the cases operated upon primarily for endometriosis, Scott and Te Linde encountered abnormal bleeding in 26.6 per cent. In further study of these cases, some associated lesions were found that obviously explained the bleeding. This reduced the incidence of abnormal bleeding with no cause other than endometriosis to 14.4 per cent. The menorrhagia and in some instances the metrorrhagia probably result from ovarian dysfunction due to ovarian involvement. At laparotomy one frequently finds old blood in the peritoneal cavity, and the intermenstrual spotting frequently appears to be due to the escape of the chocolate contents of the ovarian cysts into the abdomen and out through the uterus via the tubes.

Infertility is another common and important symptom. In all couples, it is generally estimated that the infertility rate is approximately 10 per cent. With endometriosis it is generally conceded that this rate is much higher. At the Johns Hopkins Hospital the absolute sterility rate was 33.3 per cent, and the relative sterility rate was 46 per cent; Counseller has reported rates of 32.1 per cent and 48.9 per cent. Haydon had reported a 53 per cent relative infertility rate. The cause of infertility may or may not be apparent. Tubal occlusion may occur, but most women with pelvic endometriosis have patent tubes unless peritubal adhesions have caused angulation and obstruction. Extensive destruction of ovarian tissue or replacement by endometrial cysts obviously can interfere with ovulation, while extensive periovarian adhesions can prevent the normal egress of the ovum. In addition, the numerous adhesions in the pelvis so typical of endometriosis, involving not only the ovaries, the pelvic peritoneum, but also the cul-de-sac, probably interfere with ovum transport, preventing the normal migration of the ovum from the ovary to the uterus via the tube. It is impossible of proof, but it would seem likely that the old peritoneal blood entering the tubal lumina would interfere with the action of the tubal epithelium cilia in propelling the ovum. Finally, dyspareunia has been known to limit sexual exposure. Despite these theories, there still are many instances in which minimal endometriosis appears to cause infertility without any apparent mechanical or endocrine abnormality. Conversely, the presence of endometriosis does not preclude pregnancy. Many women with endometriosis have had not only one pregnancy but several (Fig. 9-25).

Diagnosis

The symptoms discussed above always should suggest endometriosis, but any or most of them may be present with other pelvic conditions. There is no history sufficiently typical of endometriosis to justify the diagnosis on this basis alone; and if one operates without confirmatory pelvic findings, he will be disappointed often and find grossly normal pelvic

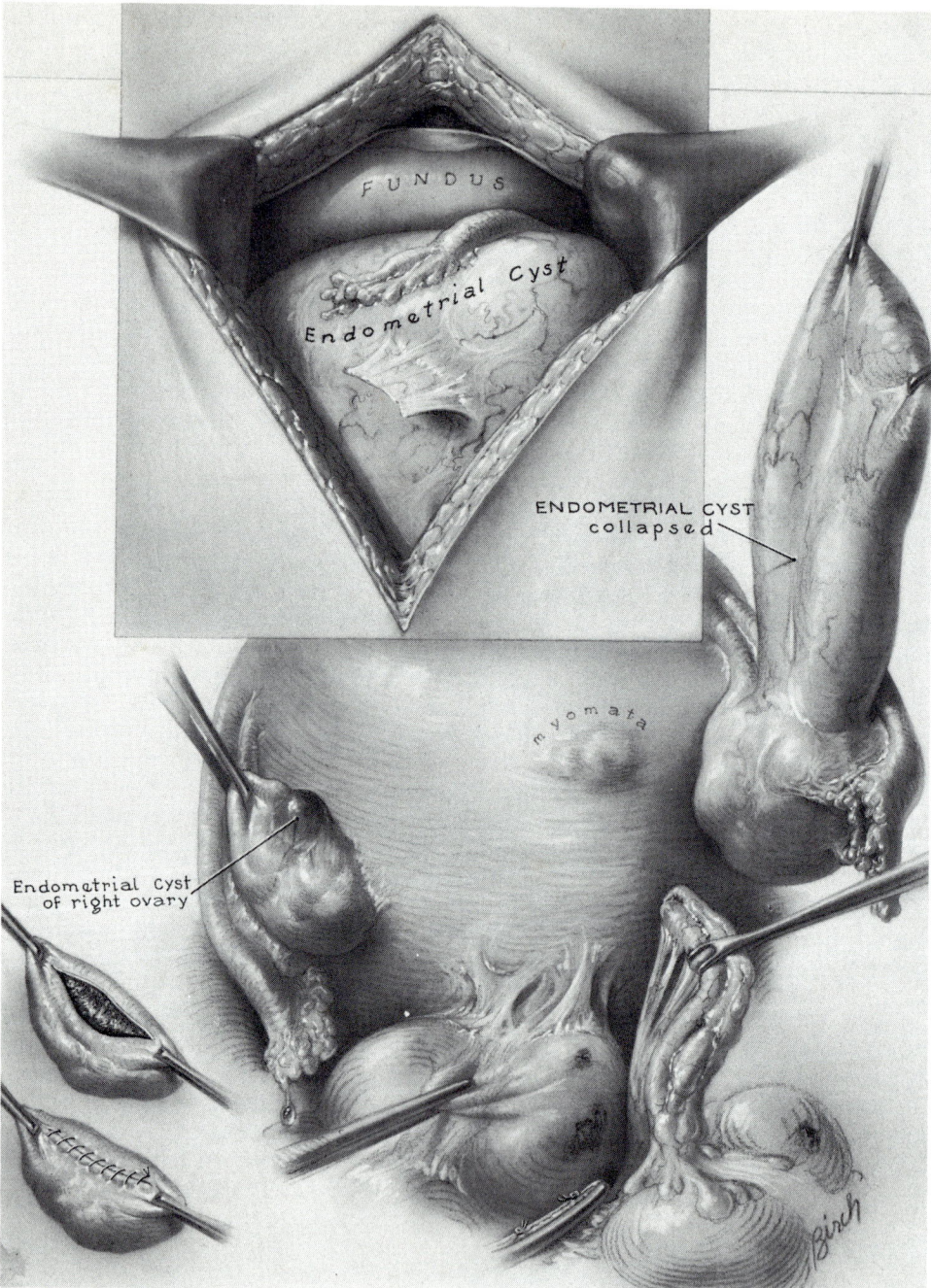

FIG. 9-25. Endometrial cyst of both ovaries associated with pregnancy of 12 weeks.

organs. In a disease with such a wide variation in distribution and character of the lesions, it is not surprising that the symptoms and signs are quite variable. If a cystic hemorrhagic nodule is visible at the umbilicus, in an abdominal scar, in the perineum, or in the vaginal vault, the diagnosis of endometriosis can be made with relative certainty. In the usual case of intra-abdominal endometriosis, the diagnosis must be made by bimanual examination. The finding of adherent adnexa in a woman in the menstrual years in whom gonococcal, tubercular, postabortal, or puerperal infection can be excluded with reasonable certainty should cause one to consider endometriosis. The presence of shotty induration in the cul-de-sac, in the uterosacral ligaments, or on the posterior surface of an adherent retroposed uterus is the most suggestive single pelvic finding of endometriosis. These nodular areas are frequently tender, particularly just prior to menstruation. When these findings are coupled with an enlarged ovary or an adherent ovarian cyst, the diagnosis is almost a certainty. Carcinoma of the ovary can reproduce most of these findings except that the nodules of metastatic carcinoma in the cul-de-sac usually are not as tender.

When the rectovaginal septum is involved, the pelvic and rectal findings may simulate carcinoma of the bowel or the induration and scarring of diverticulitis. Bluish cysts presenting in the posterior vaginal vault may be very helpful in deciding in favor of endometriosis. Moreover, they present a readily available biopsy site to confirm the diagnosis pathologically. On rectal palpation the mucosa is usually intact since endometriosis invades from outside the bowel wall. If the rectal mucosa is also involved, then proctoscopy and biopsy of the lesion will establish the diagnosis.

There still remains a group of women who have severe pelvic pain and other symptoms suggestive of endometriosis but lack definitive pelvic findings by examination. If the cul-de-sac is free from adhesions, culdoscopy is a very useful procedure. By this means women with minimal symptomatic endometriosis frequently can be distinguished from those whose symptoms are on a psychosomatic basis.

TREATMENT

Since endometriosis is usually a benign process becoming quiescent with the menopause, its presence does not necessarily constitute an indication for treatment. The need for treatment is dependent on the severity and type of symptoms, the palpable extent of the disease, the age and the general physical condition of the patient, the patient's desire for preservation of childbearing function, the psychological evaluation of the patient, and the presence or absence of other pathology in the reproductive tract. In the absence of palpable pelvic disease, exploratory laparotomy on the basis of symptoms alone is rarely indicated. Conversely, the presence of moderately extensive endometriosis may not require treatment when it is asymptomatic.

In considering the management of a case of endometriosis, the following four courses are available:

1. **Observation.** In the absence of significant symptoms and in the absence of an adnexal mass which might indicate an ovarian neoplasm, this certainly is the treatment of choice. Many cases of endometriosis can be managed in this way. Analgesics can be used frequently and satisfactorily to control dysmenorrhea and pelvic discomfort. If infertility is an important factor, active treatment is sometimes indicated.

2. **Hormonal Therapy.** Suppression of ovulation and menstruation either by pregnancy or artificially has been observed to cause an alleviation of symptoms and at times a clinical improvement of the disease process. Estrogens, progestogens, and androgens have been used.

3. **Surgery.** This may be considered as *conservative* when the reproductive potential is retained and hopefully increased, *semiconservative* when the reproductive ability is eliminated but ovarian function retained, and *radical* or *definitive* when ovarian function also is ablated.

4. **Irradiation.** Castration by external irradiation will treat endometriosis quite effectively. There are, however, very limited indications for this now rarely used method of treatment. Probably the only circumstance in which irradiation therapy may be applied would be in a woman with symptomatic endometriosis, recurrent after and proven by prior lapa-

rotomy when the patient is too poor a medical risk for definitive surgical treatment.

Hormonal therapy has been used rather extensively. Historically, estrogens were the first endocrine preparations used. Estrogens in sufficient doses can not only inhibit ovulation but also suppress menstruation. They do not induce a pseudopregnancy state, at least from the histologic aspect of the endometrium. If estrogens are used, diethylstilbestrol is the drug of choice. Karnaky has recommended starting at 0.5 mg. daily for 3 days and then increasing the dose rather rapidly to suppress breakthrough bleeding. Frequently, doses of 100 mg. daily will be reached, ultimately to produce a period of amenorrhea for a total time of 3 to 6 months. General experience has shown this method of treatment to be rather unsatisfactory. The diethylstilbestrol causes nausea and frequently rather severe bleeding. Furthermore, it appears to effect at best only temporary symptomatic relief and is not in any sense a cure. The areas of ectopic endometrium not only do not regress but frequently show areas of cystic hyperplasia, as one would expect. In general, this form of therapy is rarely used and has few advocates.

Androgens, usually oral methyltestosterone, may also be used to treat endometriosis. When doses of 10 mg. daily are used, ovulation and menstruation can be suppressed. Patients usually are not treated for more than 3 to 6 months because of the potential if not actual virilizing effects of this hormone. Another dosage schedule of 5 mg. daily for up to 6 months may also be used. At this level menstruation usually occurs and at times even ovulation. Pelvic pain has been relieved at least temporarily, and at times pregnancies follow such therapy. Histologically, the endometriosis appears to be unaffected, and the mechanism whereby this form of treatment achieves its results is not clear. Although androgens appear to achieve short-term palliation, one cannot use it for prolonged therapy, and hence this form of therapy has definite limitations.

The most popular form of hormonal treatment at this time is progestational agents. These are synthetic progesterone-like steroids which frequently are combined with an estrogen such as mestranol or ethinyl estradiol. Some are given parenterally (hydroxyprogesterone caproate and medroxyprogesterone acetate), but most are used orally, the most frequently used being norethynodrel and norethindrone. Kistner, one of the prime advocates of this form of therapy, has suggested the use of norethynodrel with mestranol (Enovid), beginning at 2.5 mg. daily for 1 week, then 5.0 mg. daily for 1 week, and 10 mg. daily for 2 weeks, followed by an indefinite maintenance dose of 20 mg. daily. This program has been used prior to and following conservative surgery for endometriosis as well as for primary treatment. In the case of the latter, the duration of treatment should be at least 12 months and may be continued for 2 to 3 years. This will not only produce anovulation and amenorrhea but also induce a pseudopregnancy state with a decidual reaction involving not only the uterine endometrium but also the ectopic endometrium. In 110 patients Kistner reports an improvement rate of 83 per cent, with remissions as long as 52 months and a 47 per cent pregnancy rate in those trying to conceive. Despite these impressive results, endometrial implants frequently become active after the cessation of the pseudopregnancy; and the patients to be treated by progestogens must be selected carefully and permanent cure not anticipated. The prime indication for this mode of treatment would appear to be in cases of symptomatic endometriosis recurrent after previous surgery.

Surgery finally remains the best form of therapy in most cases of symptomatic endometriosis. Definitive treatment consisting of abdominal hysterectomy and bilateral salpingo-oophorectomy is the preferred procedure in women with extensive endometriosis involving the pelvic structures and both ovaries, particularly if the patient is over 40. Unfortunately, there are younger women, a few in their twenties, whose ovaries have been so destroyed by endometriosis no functional ovarian tissue can be salvaged. These, too, must be subjected to the same procedure, as well as those patients who require a second laparotomy for recurrent endometriosis. The removal of all ovarian tissue is curative. We have not hesitated to use estrogens with care for menopausal symptoms after such procedures. There is the theoretical possibility that estrogens can reactivate endometriosis, but this must be a rare occurrence, as it has never been observed in the author's rather extensive experience.

On the other hand, many women with endometriosis are quite young and not only wish to retain their ability to reproduce but to enhance it, as in infertility. In the case of the latter, it is obvious that a thorough infertility study must be done to exclude other causes before the lack of pregnancy is attributed to endometriosis. When this has been done, or when there are other symptoms of endometriosis sufficient to require treatment, conservative surgery is advised. This consists of a laparotomy with the intent of destroying by resection or fulguration all areas of endometriosis possible. Large endometrial implants or endometrial cysts of the ovaries are best treated by resection. The smaller superficial implants are fulgurated, and the many adhesions so characteristic of endometriosis, involving the cul-de-sac, posterior surface of the uterus, and adnexa, are released. It is particularly important in problems of infertility to release any peritubal and periovarian adhesions which might interfere with ovum transport. To prevent the uterus from becoming adherent again in the cul-de-sac, a uterine suspension is performed, and frequently an ovarian suspension.

An important step in this procedure is a presacral neurectomy. This should be done in all cases in which dysmenorrhea is present and probably in cases of infertility as well, for should further endometriosis develop, this procedure is likely to prevent it from becoming symptomatic.

With conservative surgery there is always the chance of further problems with endometriosis. The risk, however, seems to be relatively small. Gray has noted a 4 per cent reoperation rate; Scott and Burt, a 2.7 per cent rate, whereas McCoy and Bradford reported a 21 per cent rate. In contrast, these authors reported pregnancy rates of 51 per cent, 64.1 per cent, and 63 per cent, respectively. These figures are considerably better than those with progestogen therapy. Surgery, since it is able to correct the mechanical problems caused by endometriosis as well as to remove it, remains the logical choice in the treatment of infertility.

There are women with symptomatic endometriosis that fall between those treated conservatively and those with the definitive procedure. These women, usually in their mid- to late thirties, have completed their childbearing careers and yet wish to avoid a premature menopause. In such instances removal of the uterus and other areas of pelvic endometriosis, but with preservation of some ovarian tissue, has much to recommend it. Such a procedure may seem illogical, since the retention of ovarian function might permit continued activity and symptoms from any residual endometriosis. This problem, however, arises infrequently, as shown by Scott and Te Linde, who found only 4.1 per cent of such patients subsequently required further surgery. Removal of the uterus eliminates dysmenorrhea and abnormal bleeding. In addition, it removes the main source of the ectopic endometrium. Endometrial implants probably can and do spread and cause daughter implants, but this may not occur very frequently. In monkeys with surgically created endometriosis in known locations, the fact that other implants have not been observed to arise from these areas suggests that secondary implantation is not a frequent occurrence.

When endometriosis causes ureteral or bowel obstruction, release of the obstruction is essential, particularly in the latter case, and a bowel resection is done. In ureteral obstruction with a nonfunctioning kidney, nephrectomy may be necessary; but if function can be preserved, a ureteroureteral or ureterovesical anastomosis should be considered. Other endometrial lesions involving the bladder wall, peritoneal surfaces, or rectovaginal septum may be removed and ovarian conservation practiced is justifiable. Endometrial lesions of the umbilicus, abdominal or other scars, vulva, and inguinal regions are infiltrating and should be excised by a wide margin so that endometrial remnants do not remain.

Finally, it should be stressed that surgery for endometriosis may be most difficult. The adhesions generally are extremely dense, often much more so than the usual inflammatory or postoperative type. Sharp dissection is often necessary, especially in freeing the uterus from the anterior rectal wall. Fortunately, the rectal wall is frequently thickened by fibrosis so that perforation of it is rare. Nevertheless, in making the dissection it is better to err in leaving a bit of cervical tissue on the rectum than vice versa. Another point to be stressed is that resection of part of an ovary is often a worthwhile procedure in young women. In general, in dealing with other ovarian pathology, a complete oophorectomy is preferable to resection if the opposite ovary is normal. This dictum does not apply too strictly in endometriosis, in which bilateral ovarian involvement occurs in about 25 per cent of the cases.

Kistner as well as others has employed progestogen therapy prior to proposed laparotomy for endometriosis and also following conservative surgery. Preoperatively it is thought to make the dissection easier and the implants more easily found as well as softer with the decidual reaction. Although we have not usually used this combined treatment preoperatively, it should be considered unless there is an ovarian mass present. Since there always is the possibility that the ovarian mass may not be an endometrial cyst but carcinoma, laparotomy should not be delayed by hormonal therapy. Generally we have not used hormonal therapy after conservative surgery, particularly in cases of infertility. Both the surgeon and the patient are usually anxious that she become pregnant as soon after surgery as is reasonable and practical, and we see no advantage in delaying this by progestogen-induced anovulation.

MALIGNANCY IN ENDOMETRIOSIS

It is natural that a woman in whom the diagnosis of endometriosis has been made should ask, "What relation does the disease have to cancer?" The correct answer to this question probably is that ectopic endometrium may become malignant in rare instances but has no more proclivity to do so than endometrium within the uterine cavity. Let us examine the evidence.

In 1925 Sampson, in reporting 7 cases of ovarian carcinoma of possible endometrial origin, outlined the criteria to establish such a diagnosis. They were: (1) there must be coexistence of benign and malignant tissues in the same ovary which have the same histologic relationship to each other as in carcinoma of the body of the uterus; (2) the carcinoma must actually be seen to arise in the benign tissue and not to invade it from some other source; (3) additional supportive evidence includes the presence of tissue resembling endometrial stroma about characteristic epithelial glands and the finding of old hemorrhage rather than fresh.

Among 516 cases of endometriosis reported by Scott and Te Linde, there were only 8 cases of ovarian malignancy. Three of these were papillary serous cystadenocarcinomas, two were epidermoid carcinomas arising in dermoid cysts, and one was a granulosa cell tumor. The remaining two cases were adenocarcinomas. In neither case could the transition from benign endometriosis to carcinoma be shown, but the histology of each tumor suggested that it might be of endometrial origin.

In 1957 Thompson collected 20 reported cases of ovarian malignancies arising in ovarian endometriosis. There have been other sporadic cases reported since that time. Aside from the fact that most of these malignant tumors are adenocarcinomas (there was 1 carcinosarcoma), 9 were adenoacanthomas, a tumor known to arise solely from endometrium. He also reported 17 cases of ovarian adenoacanthoma, 7 of which definitely arose from endometriosis.

In addition, there have been many reports of ovarian carcinomas having microscopic features of uterine endometrial carcinoma. These have been designated by the name *endometrioid carcinoma* and may or may not be associated with or originate from endometriosis. There also are very unusual instances of extraovarian malignancy arising in endometriosis in the rectovaginal septum. Lash and Rubenstone reported such a case in 1959, and Dockerty described 2 cases in 1954.

From this it would seem justifiable to conclude that endometriosis is capable of malignant change, but the incidence is extremely low and is of little importance in the clinical management of patients with this condition. Of greater clinical importance, however, is the rather common finding of a considerable enlargement of one or both ovaries in a case of obvious endometriosis. The much more common possibility of a coexisting ovarian malignancy unrelated to endometriosis must be considered, and exploratory laparotomy is then indicated even though the patient may have no symptoms.

BIBLIOGRAPHY

Allen, E.: Endometrial transplantation. Amer. J. Obstet. Gynec., 23:343, 1932.

Benson, R. C., and Sneeden, E. D.: Adenomyosis: A reappraisal of symptomatology. Amer. J. Obstet. Gynec., 76:1044, 1958.

Bungeler, W., and Fleury-Silveira, D.: Consideracoes sobre a patogenia endometriosis (a proposito de tres casos de endometriose externa). Arq. cir. clin. exper., 3:169, 1939.

Caffier, P.: Über Endometriumexplantation: Bisherige Ergebnisse, Wachstumsmechanik und Kritik. Z. Gynäk., 52:63, 1928.

Chinn, J., Horton, R. K., and Rusche, C.: Unilateral ureteral obstruction as sole manifestation of endometriosis. J. Urol., 77:144, 1957.

Counseller, V. S.: Endometriosis. Amer. J. Obstet. Gynec., 36:877, 1938.

———: The clinical significance of endometriosis. Amer. J. Obstet. Gynec., 37:788, 1939.

———: Surgical procedures involved in treatment of endometriosis. Surg. Gynec. Obstet., 89:322, 1949.

Cron, R. S., and Gey, G.: The viability of cast-off menstrual endometrium. Amer. J. Obstet. Gynec., 13:645, 1927.

Cullen, T. S.: Adenomyoma of the uterus. Bull. Johns Hopkins, 1896.

———: Adenomyoma uteri diffusum benignum. Johns Hopkins Hosp. Report, 6:133, 1897.

———: Adenomyoma of recto-vaginal septum. J.A.M.A., 62:835, 1914.

———: Adenomyoma of the uterus. Philadelphia, W. B. Saunders, 1908.

———: The distribution of adenomyomata containing uterine mucosa. Amer. J. Obstet. Gynec., 80:130, 1920.

Dockerty, M. B., Pratt, J. H., and Decker, D. G.: Primary adenocarcinoma of the rectovaginal septum probably arising from endometriosis. Cancer, 7:808, 1954.

Everett, H. S.: Probable tubal origin of endometriosis. Amer. J. Obstet. Gynec., 22:1, 1931.

Fallon, J., Bros, J. T., and Moran, W. G.: Endometriosis: 200 cases considered from viewpoint of practitioner. New Eng. J. Med., 235:669, 1946.

Gray, L. L., Keeler, J. E., and Nicolay, K. S.: Endometriosis in pregnancy, clinical observations. Amer. J. Obstet. Gynec., 63:511, 1952.

Goodall, J. R.: A Study of Endometriosis, Endosalpingiosis, Endocervicosis and Peritoneo-ovarian Sclerosis, A Clinical Pathologic Study. Philadelphia, Lippincott, 1943.

Graves, W. P.: Treatment of obstruc-

have been other sporadic cases reported since that time. Aside from the fact that most of these malignant tumors are adenocarcinomas (there was 1 carcinosarcoma), 9 were adenoacanthomas, a tumor known to arise solely from endometrium. He also reported 17 cases of ovarian adenoacanthoma, 7 of which definitely arose from endometriosis.

In addition, there have been many reports of ovarian carcinomas having microscopic features of uterine endometrial carcinoma. These have been designated by the name *endometrioid carcinoma* and may or may not be associated with or originate from endometriosis. There also are very unusual instances of extraovarian malignancy arising in endometriosis in the rectovaginal septum. Lash and Rubenstone reported such a case in 1939, and Dockerty described 2 cases in 1954.

From this it would seem justifiable to conclude that endometriosis is capable of malignant change, but the incidence is extremely low and is of little importance in the clinical management of patients with this condition. Of greater clinical importance, however, is the rather common finding of a considerable enlargement of one or both ovaries in a case of obvious endometriosis. The much more common possibility of a coexisting ovarian malignancy unrelated to endometriosis must be considered, and exploratory laparotomy is then indicated even though the patient may have no symptoms.

BIBLIOGRAPHY

Allen, E.: Endometrial transplantation. Amer. J. Obstet. Gynec., 23:343, 1932.

Benson, R. C., and Sneeden, E. D.: Adenomyosis: A reappraisal of symptomatology. Amer. J. Obstet. Gynec., 76:1044, 1958.

Bungeler, W., and Fleury-Silveira, D.: Consideracoes sobre a patogenia endometriosis (a proposito de tres casos de endometriose externa). Arq. cir. clin. exper., 3:169, 1939.

Caffier, P.: Über Endometriumexplantation: Bisherige Ergebnisse, Wachstumsmechanik und Kritik. Z. Gynäk, 52:63, 1928.

Chinn, J., Horton, R. K., and Rusche, C.: Unilateral ureteral obstruction as sole manifestation of endometriosis. J. Urol., 77:144, 1957.

Counseller, V. S.: Endometriosis. Amer. J. Obstet. Gynec., 36:877, 1938.

——: The clinical significance of endometriosis. Amer. J. Obstet. Gynec., 37:788, 1939.

——: Surgical procedures involved in treatment of endometriosis. Surg. Gynec. Obstet., 89:322, 1949.

Cron, R. S., and Gey, G.: The viability of the cast-off menstrual endometrium. Amer. J. Obstet. Gynec., 13:645, 1927.

Cullen, T. S.: Adenomyoma of the round ligament. Bull. Johns Hopkins Hosp., 7:112, 1896.

——: Adenomyoma uteri diffusum benignum. Johns Hopkins Hosp. Report, 6:133, 1897.

——: Adenomyoma of recto-vaginal septum. J.A.M.A., 62:835, 1914.

——: Adenomyoma of the uterus. Philadelphia, W. B. Saunders, 1908.

——: The distribution of adenomyomata containing uterine mucosa. Amer. J. Obstet. Gynec., 80:130, 1920.

Dockerty, M. B., Pratt, J. H., and Decker, D. G.: Primary adenocarcinoma of the rectovaginal septum probably arising from endometriosis. Cancer, 7:898, 1954.

Everett, H. S.: Probable tubal origin of endometriosis. Amer. J. Obstet. Gynec., 22:1, 1931.

Fallon, J., Brosnan, J. T., and Moran, W. G.: Endometriosis; 200 cases considered from viewpoint of practitioner. New Eng. J. Med., 235:669, 1946.

Gainey, H. L., Keeler, J. E., and Nicolay, K. S.: Endometriosis in pregnancy, clinical observations. Amer. J. Obstet. Gynec., 63:511, 1952.

Goodall, J. R.: A Study of Endometriosis, Endosalpingiosis, Endocervicosis and Peritoneo-ovarian Sclerosis, A Clinical and Pathologic Study. Philadelphia, J. B. Lippincott, 1943.

Graves, W. P.: Treatment of obstructing recto-

Gray, L. A.: The conservative operation for endometriosis—a report of 200 cases. J. Kentucky Med. Assoc. 56:1219, 1958.

——: The management of endometriosis involving the bowel. Clin. Obstet. Gynec. 9:309, 1966.

——: Surgical treatment of endometriosis. Clin. Obstet. Gynec. 3:472, 1960.

Halban, J.: Metastatic hysteroadenosis. Wein. Klin. Wchnschr. 37:1205, 1924.

——: Hysteroadenosis metastatica. Die lymphogene Genese der Sog. Adenofibromatosis heterotopica. Arch. Gynäk. 124:457, 1925.

Harbitz, H.: Clinical pathogenetic and experimental investigations of endometriosis especially regarding the localization in the abdominal wall (laparotomy scars) with a contribution to the study of experimental transplantation of endometrium. Acta Chir. Scand. 74(Suppl. 30):1, 1934.

Haydon, G. B.: A study of 569 cases of endometriosis. Amer. J. Obstet. Gynec. 43:704, 1942.

Heim, K.: Endometriosis. Ber. ges. Gynäk. Geburtsh. 17:641, 1930.

——: Lebens und Wachstumsbeobachtung an menschlichen Geweben und Geschwülsten im Explantationversuch und ihre Bedeutung für Klinische Fragen. Arch. Gynäk. 134:250, 1928.

Hirsch, E. F., and Jones, H. D.: The behavior of the epithelium in explants of human endometrium. Amer. J. Obstet. Gynec. 25:37, 1933.

Hobbs, J. E., and Bortnick, A. R.: Endometriosis of the lungs (an experimental and clinical study). Amer. J. Obstet. Gynec. 40:832, 1940.

Israel, S. M., and Woutersz, T. B.: Adenomyosis: a neglected diagnosis. Obstet. Gynec. 14:1068, 1959.

Ivanoff, N. S.: Drusigis Cystkaltiges Uterus-fibromyon complicert durch Sarcom und Carcinom (Adenofibromyoma cysticum sarcomatodes carcinomatorum). Monatsschr. Geburtsh. Gynäk. 7:295, 1898.

Jacobson, V. C.: The autotransplantation of endometrial tissue in the rabbit. Arch. Surg. 5:281, 1922.

Javert, C. T.: Observations on pathology and spread of endometriosis based on theory of benign metastasis. Amer. J. Obstet. Gynec. 62:477, 1951.

Karnaky, K. J.: The use of stilbestrol for endometriosis; preliminary report. Southern Med. J., 41:1109, 1948.

Keettel, W. C., and Stein, R. J.: The viability of the cast-off menstrual endometrium. Amer. J. Obstet. Gynec. 61:440, 1951.

Kerr, W. S.: Endometriosis involving the urinary tract. Clin. Obstet. Gynec. 9:331, 1966.

Kistner, R. W.: Current status of the hormonal treatment of endometriosis. Clin. Obstet. Gynec. 9:271, 1966.

Laites, R., Shepard, F., Tovell, H., and Wylie, R.: A clinical and pathologic study of endometriosis of the lung. Surg. Gynec. Obstet. 103:552, 1956.

Lash, S. R., and Rubenstone, A. I.: Adenocarcinoma of the rectovaginal septum probably arising from endometriosis. Amer. J. Obstet. Gynec. 78:299, 1959.

Long, M. E., and Taylor, H. C., Jr.: Endometrioid carcinoma of the ovary. Amer. J. Obstet. Gynec. 90:936, 1964.

Markin, Z. W.: Beiträge zur lehre von den endometrioden heterotopen. Arch. Klin. Chir. 175:314, 1933.

Markee, J. E.: Menstruation in intraocular endometrial transplants in the rhesus monkey. Contrib. Embryol. (Carnegie Inst. of Washington, Publ. No. 177), 28:223, 1940.

Maslow, L. A., and Learner, A.: Endometriosis of Kidney. J. Urol. 64:564, 1950.

McArthur, J. W., and Ulfelder, H.: The effect of pregnancy on endometriosis. Obstet. Gynec. Survey, 20:709, 1965.

McCoy, J. B., and Bradford, W. Z.: Surgical treatment of endometriosis with conservation of reproductive potential. Amer. J. Obstet. Gynec. 87:394, 1963.

Maurer, E. R., Schaal, J. A., and Mendez, F. L., Jr.: Chronic recurring spontaneous pneumothorax due to endometriosis of the diaphragm. J.A.M.A. 168:2013, 1958.

Meigs, J. V.: Endometriosis—its significance. Ann. Surg. 114:866, 1941.

——: Endometriosis. Ann. Surg. 127:795, 1948.

——: Endometriosis. Obstet. Gynec. 2:46, 1953.

Meyer, R.: Adenomatous proliferation of the serosa in an abdominal scar. Ztschr. Geburtsh. Gynäk. 49:32, 1903.

——: Über entzündliche heterotope Epithelwucherungen im weiblichen Genitalgebiete und über eine bis in die Wurzel des Mesocolon ausgedehnte benigne Wucherung des Darmepithels. Virchow's Arch. Path. Anat. 195:487, 1909.

Navratil, E., and Kramer, A.: Endometriose in

der Armmushkulatur. Klin. Wchnschr., *15*: 1765, 1936.
Novak, E.: Significance of uterine mucosa in fallopian tubes with discussion of origin of aberrant endometrium. Amer. J. Obstet. Gynec., *12*:484, 1926.
——: Pelvic endometriosis. Amer. J. Obstet. Gynec., *22*:826, 1931.
——: Gynecological and Obstetrical Pathology. Philadelphia, W. B. Saunders, 1940.
——: Adenoacanthoma of ovary arising from endometrial cyst. J. Mt. Sinai Hosp., *14*:529, 1947.
Preston, S. N., and Campbell, H. B.: Pelvic endometriosis: treatment with methyltestosterone. Obstet. Gynec., *2*:152, 1953.
Ridley, J. H., and Edwards, J. K.: Experimental endometriosis in the human. Amer. J. Obstet. Gynec., *76*:783, 1959,
Russell, W. W.: Aberrant portions of the mullerian duct found in an ovary. Bull. Johns Hopkins Hosp., *10*:8, 1899.
Sampson, J. A.: Perforating hemorrhagic (chocolate) cysts of the ovary. Their importance and especially their relation to pelvic adenomas of endometrial type ("adenomyoma" of the uterus, rectovaginal septum, sigmoid, etc.). Arch. Surg., *3*:245, 1921.
——: Intestinal adenomas of the endometrial type. Their importance and their relation to ovarian hematomas of endometrial type (perforating hemorrhagic cysts of the ovary). Arch. Surg., *5*:217, 1922.
——: The life history of ovarian hematomas (hemorrhagic cysts) of endometrial (mullerian) type. Amer. J. Obstet. Gynec., *4*:451, 1922.
——: Benign and malignant endometrial implants in peritoneal cavity and their relation to certain ovarian tumors. Surg. Gynec. Obstet., *38*:287, 1924.
——: Inguinal endometriosis. Amer. J. Obstet. Gynec., *19*:462, 1925.
——: Heterotopic or misplaced endometrial tissue. Amer. J. Obstet. Gynec., *10*:649, 1925.
——: Endometrial carcinomas of ovary arising in endometrial tissue of that organ. Arch. Surg., *10*:1, 1925.
——: Metastatic or embolic endometriosis, due to menstrual dissemination of endometrial tissue into venous circulation. Am. J. Path., *3*:93, 1927.
——: Peritoneal endometriosis, due to menstrual dissemination of endometrial tissue into peritoneal cavity. Amer. J. Obstet. Gynec., *14*:422, 1927.
——: Endometriosis following salpingectomy. Amer. J. Obstet. Gynec. *16*:461, 1928.
——: Pelvic endometriosis and tubal fimbriae. Amer. J. Obstet. Gynec., *24*:497, 1932.
——: The development of the implantation theory for the origin of peritoneal endometriosis. Amer. J. Obstet. Gynec., *40*:549, 1940.
Scott, R. B.: Endometriosis and pregnancy. Amer. J. Obstet. Gynec., *47*:608, 1944.
Scott, R. B., and Burt, J. H.: Clinical experimental endometriosis. Southern Med. J., *55*:129, 1962.
Scott, R. B., Nowak, R. J., and Tindale, R. M.: Umbilical endometriosis and the Cullen sign. Obstet. Gynec., *11*:556, 1958.
Scott, R. B., and Te Linde, R. W.: External endometriosis—the scourge of the private patient. Ann. Surg., *131*:697, 1950.
Scott, R. B., Te Linde, R. W., and Wharton, L. R., Jr.: Further studies on experimental endometriosis. Amer. J. Obstet. Gynec., *66*:1082, 1953.
Scott, R. B., and Wharton, L. R., Jr.: The effect of excessive doses of diethylstilbestrol on experimental endometriosis in monkeys. Amer. J. Obstet. Gynec., *69*:573, 1955.
——: The effect of estrone and progesterone on the growth of experimental endometriosis in rhesus monkeys. Amer. J. Obstet. Gynec., *74*:852, 1957.
——: The effect of testosterone on experimental endometriosis in rhesus monkeys. Amer. J. Obstet. Gynec., *78*:1020, 1959.
——: Effects of progesterone and norethindrone on experimental endometriosis in monkeys. Amer. J. Obstet. Gynec., *84*:867, 1962.
Stanley, K. E., Jr. Utz, D. C., and Dockerty, M. B.: Clinically significant endometriosis of the urinary tract. Surg. Gynec. Obstet., *120*:411, 1965.
Sturgis, S. H., and Call, B. J.: Endometriosis peritone—relationship of pain to functional activity. Amer. J. Obstet. Gynec., *68*:1421, 1954.
Te Linde, R. W., and Rutledge, F.: Culdoscopy, a useful gynecologic procedure. Amer. J. Obstet. Gynec., *55*:102, 1948.
Te Linde, R. W., and Scott, R. B.: Experimental endometriosis. Amer. J. Obstet. Gynec., *60*:1147, 1950.
Thomas, H. H.: Conservative treatment of endometriosis. Obstet. Gynec., *15*:498, 1960.
Thompson, J. D.: Primary ovarian adenocanthoma. Obstet. Gynec., *9*:403, 1957.
Trout, H. F.: Adult human endometrium in tissue culture. Surg. Gynec. Obstet., *47*:334, 1928.

Von Recklinghausen, F.: Die Adenomyome und Cystadenome der Uterus and Tubenwandung; ihre Abkunft von Resten des Wolff'schen Korpers. Berlin, August Hirschwald, 1896.

Weinstein, B. B., Weed, J. C., Collins, C. G., Lock, F. R., and Schlosser, J. V.: The effect of diethylstilbestrol dipropionate on endometrial transplants. Endocrinology, 27:903, 1940.

Williams, J. F., Williams, J. B., and Harper, J. W.: Thoracic endometriosis. Amer. J. Obstet. Gynec., 84:1512, 1962.

Wood, J. C., Geary, W. L., and Holland, J. B.: Adenomyosis of the uterus. Clin. Obstet. Gynec., 9:412, 1966.

Wryens, R. G., and Randall, L. M.: Endometriosis in postoperative scars. Proc. Staff Meet. Mayo Clinic, 16:817, 1941.

10

Presacral Neurectomy

GENERAL CONSIDERATIONS

The operation of presacral neurectomy has been described in the literature under a variety of names: presacral sympathectomy, presacral neurectomy, resection of the presacral nerve, and resection of the superior hypogastric plexus of Hovelacque. The operation was introduced by Jaboulay in 1898 but found little acceptance among gynecologists for many years. In 1925 Cotte began reporting on the operation and during succeeding years contributed many optimistic reports. In 1938 he reported 300 cases in which the operation had been done for primary dysmenorrhea, with success in all but 2. Since Cotte reports such a large series, it is obvious that his indications for the operation must be very liberal. The indications for presacral resection in this country, on the contrary, have been quite rigid for the most part; even from the larger clinics the number of cases reported is relatively small.

Our attitude toward the indications for the operation is a conservative one, but we have used it for both primary and secondary dysmenorrhea. Before considering this major operative therapy, complete medical therapy should be tried, such as nonhabit-forming sedatives, pain relievers, and, in most cases where medicine fails, cervical dilatation. Our attitude of almost complete pessimism about hormonal therapy has changed. The newer progestines are not infrequently successful in relieving primary dysmenorrhea; hence this operation is not indicated as often as formerly.

We have performed the operation more freely in connection with other procedures, such as suspensions, and conservative operations for endometriosis. In the endometriosis cases we believe that it should be done routinely whenever the uterus is not removed.

We have not used presacral resection for the relief of pelvic pain associated with inoperable pelvic carcinoma. It is our belief that the origin of such pain is apt to be too widespread to expect much relief from removal of the superior mesenteric plexus. In such cases we prefer to have the neurosurgeons either inject or sever the pain nerve fibers of the cord.

Some gynecologists, including Henriksen, have extended the use of presacral neurectomy for the cure of mittelschmerz, pruritus vulvae, and dyspareunia. We never have seen a case of mittelschmerz in which the pain was sufficiently severe to justify the operation. Perhaps it would be more nearly correct to say that in those cases of mittelschmerz in which the patients claimed very severe pain, we have concluded that the psyche played too great a role to make such patients good subjects for surgery. We have controlled pruritis by other methods. When dyspareunia is complained of, and no organic explanation is found, it generally should be concluded that the cause is psychic, and little can be expected from nerve resection.

In discussion an operation, the value of which is still not accepted universally, it is well to consider in some detail the operative results. Cotte claimed relief in all but 2 of 300 women on whom he operated for essential dysmenorrhea. In judging this report we cannot escape the conclusion that these excellent results, which are better than those reported from any other clinic, have been determined by a surgeon who is somewhat overenthusiastic about an operation of which he has been one of the chief promoters. In this country perhaps the most enthusiastic gynecologist is Greenhill, who states that "in severe dysmenorrhea, pelvic sympathectomy is almost 100 per cent successful." Ingersoll and Meigs report 81 per cent with complete relief, 4.5 per cent with partial relief, and 14.5 per cent with no relief when the operation was done for primary dysmenorrhea. In a group in which the operation was done for acquired dysmenorrhea, success was limited to 52.6 per cent. In a group of 68 patients with severe primary dysmenorrhea, Phaneuf reports satisfactory results in 58 per cent and considerable improvement in 28 per cent. Counseller and Craig of the Mayo Clinic, reporting on 14 cases of essential dysmenorrhea, obtained complete relief in 9 cases, 95 per cent relief in 2 cases, and 75 per cent relief in 3 cases. Henriksen, reporting on 42 cases of essential dysmenorrhea, obtained complete relief in 31 cases, some relief in 5 cases, and no relief in 6. Rutherford has reported on 23 cases followed for 2 years. In 13 he obtained 100 per cent relief; in 6 there was 75 per cent relief; and in 4 there was 50 per cent relief. Colcock from the Lahey Clinic followed 35 cases for at least 6 months; 70 per cent were followed over a year. Twenty-eight cases were completely relieved, 6 partially relieved, and there was 1 failure. The most recent results have been reported from Switzerland by Erb and Hauser, who report that the operation was done for severe dysmenorrhea in 118 patients, two thirds of whom had been unsuccessfully treated previously with hormones, physiotherapy, or both. Follow-up studies were available in 85. Freedom from symptoms or considerable improvement was achieved in 73 per cent, and slight improvement in 9 per cent, whereas the operation failed in 18 per cent.

Since the above statistics were published in the previous edition of this book, Black has made an excellent survey of the subject by reviewing the world literature, sending questionnaires to 800 obstetricians and gynecologists in the United States, and making a follow-up study of his own cases. Of the 2,516 cases of primary and secondary dysmenorrhea collected from the world literature between the years 1936 and 1963, satisfactory relief was reported in 79 per cent. Among the 7,378 cases reported by American gynecologists, there was satisfactory relief in 75 per cent. Of the author's own cases, there was satisfactory relief in 80 per cent.

These results from excellent clinics show, without doubt, that on the whole the results are satisfactory when the operation is used in selected cases of essential dysmenorrhea. All of the above-quoted American authors agree with us in our attitude of conservatism in performing the operation only on those cases in which other measures have failed.

It is more difficult to evaluate results when the nerve resection is performed in connection with other operative procedures which are also done for relief of pain. Those gynecologists who have expressed themselves on the subject hold the opinion that it is a worthwhile procedure, especially in connection with conservative operations for endometriosis in young women.

It is the universal opinion of the above-mentioned authors that the operation is quite harmless in its effect on the function of the bladder, the bowel, and the uterus; no effect has been noted on menstruation except to make it less painful. Many labors following this operation are virtually without pain except momentarily as the baby passes through the perineum.

artery, which is closely attached to the bony structures, usually escapes injury with the blunt dissection, but if it should be injured, usually bleeding can be stopped readily by making pressure directly against the subjacent bony structures. On a few occasions we have placed jelofoam in the retroperitoneal space to control oozing. After removal of the connective tissue and the nervous tissue, hemostasis is attended to, and the opening in the peritoneum is closed with a continuous suture of No. 0 plain catgut.

OVARIAN DENERVATION

Perhaps it would not be proper to conclude a chapter on the role of neurosurgery in dysmenorrhea without mentioning ovarian sympathectomy. Some gynecologists recognize the clinical entity of ovarian dysmenorrhea. The ovarian pain may be unilateral or bilateral and is said to be chiefly premenstrual but may be menstrual. Nausea is said to be an almost constant symptom. In our own experience a sharp differentiation between primary uterine and primary ovarian dysmenorrhea is not a simple matter and often is impossible. O'Donel Browne, of Dublin, makes such a differentiation and treats the severer cases of ovarian dysmenorrhea by ovarian denervation. His technic consists of division of both infundibulopelvic ligaments, their nerves and blood vessels, and simple ligature of the stumps with catgut. To avoid elongation of the divided ligaments with subsequent prolapse of the ovaries, the cut ends are sutured together. Of 21 ovarian denervations, he reports 14.2 per cent failures, 4.7 per cent partial successes, and 80.9 per cent successes. Our own experience with this operation is not sufficient to evaluate these results in the light of our own practice. The subject is discussed briefly here simply to call attention to a procedure which may or may not prove to be of value when tested by the gynecologic profession.

BIBLIOGRAPHY

Black, W. T., Jr.: Use of presacral sympathectomy in the treatment of dysmenorrhea. Amer. J. Obstet. Gynec., 89:16, 1964.

Browne, O'Donel: Survey of 113 cases of primary dysmenorrhea treated by neurectomy. Amer. J. Obstet. Gynec., 57:1053, 1949.

Colcock, Bentley: Presacral neurectomy for the relief of severe primary dysmenorrhea. Surg. Clin. N. Amer., 21:855, 1941.

Cotte, Gaston: La sympathectomie hypogastrique, A-t-elle sa place dans la thérapeutique gynécologique? Presse Méd., 33:98, 1925.

———: Die Resektion des Nervus praesacralis. Z. Gynäk., 57(I):77, 1933.

———: Resection of the presacral nerve in the treatment of obstinate dysmenorrhea. Amer. J. Obstet. Gynec., 33:1034, 1937.

Counseller, V. S., and Craig, W. McK.: The treatment of dysmenorrhea by resection of the presacral sympathetic nerves. Evaluation of the end results. Amer. J. Obstet. Gynec., 28:161, 1934.

Curtis, A. H., Anson, B. J., Ashley, F. L., and Jones, Tom: The anatomy of the pelvic autonomic nerves in relation to gynecology. Surg. Gynec. Obstet., 75:743, 1942.

Erb, H., and Hauser, G. A.: Results of Cotte's operation in dysmenorrhea. Gynecologia, 148:357, 1959.

Greenhill, J. P.: Sympathectomy for the relief of pelvic pain in women. J. Mt. Sinai Hosp., 14:363, 1947.

Henriksen, Erle: The role of the superior hypogastric plexus in gynecology. Western J. Surg., 49:1, 1941.

Ingersol, F. M., and Meigs, J. V.: Presacral neurectomy for dysmenorrhea. New Eng. J. Med., 238:357, 1948.

Keene, F. E.: The treatment of dysmenorrhea by presacral sympathectomy. Amer. J. Obstet. Gynec., 30:534, 1935.

Meigs, J. H.: Excision of the superior hypogastric plexus (presacral nerve) for primary dysmenorrhea. Surg. Gynec. Obstet., 68:723, 1939.

Pemberton, F. A.: Resection of the presacral nerve in gynecology. New Eng. J. Med., 213:710, 1935.

Phaneuf, L. E.: Presacral neurectomy in intractable dysmenorrhea. J. Mt. Sinai Hosp., 14:553, 1947.

Rutherford, R. N.: Presacral neurectomy. A gynecological and obstetrical follow-up. Western J. Surg., 50:597, 1942.

11

Pelvic Inflammatory Disease and Its Complications

GONORRHEA

Epidemiology

Gonorrhea and its clinical sequelae are rapidly becoming one of the top-ranking communicable disease problems in the United States and abroad. On a basis that only about 10 per cent of the new cases of gonorrhea are reported each year, it is currently estimated that 1.5 to 2 million new cases occur in the United States alone. The clinical problem was emphasized in 1967 by a reported 11.5 per cent national increase of gonorrhea cases over and above those of the fiscal year 1966. Not since the end of World War II has there been such an epidemic of this venereal disease, but even more tragic is the fact that gonorrhea among teenagers has reached a rate of 424.9 per 100,000, considerably more than twice the national rate of 178.6 for all age groups (USPH). In the calendar year 1966, the 15- to 24-year-old group, representing approximately 16 per cent of the total United States population, accounted for 46.1 per cent of all reported primary and secondary cases of syphilis and 57.5 per cent of all reported cases of gonorrhea. Similar statistics are evident in England, Wales, and other European countries. Utilizing a recently developed fluorescent antibody technic, Williams has found a 5.6 per cent incidence of gonorrhea in the initial prenatal clinic examination, while Kraus and Yen have demonstrated asymptomatic gonococcal infection in 5.73 per cent of antepartum patients during the 9th month of gestation. This basically asymptomatic nature of the disease in females is seldom realized. By examining known contacts, 90 per cent of females with proven gonorrhea are completely without symptoms and unaware that they are infected. This carrier state allows a large reservoir which perpetuates the survival of the organism. A similar asymptomatic state has also been shown to occur in a small percentage of males. On the international scene, the World Health Organization in 1963 officially estimated that 65 million new cases of gonorrhea occur each year. Griffiths has calculated that in some parts of Uruguay as many as half of the women have been sterilized by the age of 30 by gonorrhea. It is apparent that the problem of gonorrheal management is a major international health problem.

Several factors inherent in the natural course of gonorrhea contribute to the difficulty in management of the disease. The short incubation period allows rapid spread of the disease before epidemiologic methods can break the chain of spread. Since the gonococcus produces little immunity during its disease process, reinfection is common. Lucus et al. have demonstrated, following various treatment schedules, a 10 to 15 per cent reinfection rate in 1 month while these patients were under epidemiologic observation. In addition to the asymptomatic female carriers and the high reinfection rate in women, the gonococcus has developed an increasing tolerance to peni-

ANATOMY

It is obvious from reviewing the literature on the subject of presacral resection that the surgeons performing the operations have none too clear a conception of the nervous anatomy. Recognizing this fact, Curtis, Anson, Ashley, and Jones have made dissections on cadavers and have described and illustrated beautifully the anatomy of the pelvic autonomic nerves. The following is a direct quotation from their anatomic description:

The lumbar and lower thoracic sympathetic ganglia, and the superior, middle and inferior hypogastric plexuses constitute the sensory pathways from the pelvic viscera. A most important exception in gynecology is that the nerves from the ovaries, similar to their vascular supply, pass somewhat independently to the inferior mesenteric plexus, as do the sensory fibers from the lower bowel and fallopian tubes....

At the level of the bifurcation of the aorta the intermesenteric nerves join to form the superior hypogastric plexus, more commonly known as the "presacral nerve," which is the chief supply of the bladder, the rectum and the internal genitalia except the ovary and part of the fallopian tube. The location and relations of the superior hypogastric plexus are important because its removal is frequently resorted to for relief of intractable pelvic pain. It is usually a moderately wide plexus formed from two or three incompletely fused trunks of the intermesenteric nerves. In perhaps 20 per cent of the cases there is complete fusion, with resultant formation of a single nerve. The superior hypogastric plexus spreads out behind the peritoneum in a bed of loosely meshed areolar tissue which lies upon the bodies of the 4th and 5th lumbar vertebrae. In the midline the middle sacral artery is situated between the nerves and the anterior surface of the vertebral bodies. There is a bilateral communication between the "presacral nerve" and the lumbar sympathetic ganglia by means of fine nerve strands which pass from the ganglia to the nerves located behind the common iliac arteries.

The superior hypogastric plexus may or may not form a middle hypogastric plexus; when present the plexus is a flat expanse of neurofibrous tissue overlying the promontory and extending just below it; this plexus divides to form the bilateral inferior hypogastric plexuses, or hypogastric nerves. Each consists of two or three interlacing nerves, forming a low narrow plexus. The fibers of the inferior hypogastric plexus pass downward and lateralward near the sacral end of the uterosacral ligament, then forward over the lateral surface of the rectal ampulla to join the pelvic plexus, sometimes known as the uterovaginal plexus, the cervical ganglion, or the ganglion of Frankenhäuser, of which the hypogastric plexus furnishes the main sympathetic supply. The additional nerve supply to the pelvic plexus consists of fine fibers from the sacral sympathetic chain and parasympathetic branches (erigen or pelvic nerve) usually arising from the anterior roots of the sacral nerves....

The ovary derives its nerve supply mainly from the ovarian plexus, a meshwork of nerve fiber bundles which arise from the aortic and renal plexuses and accompany the ovarian artery throughout its course. The high source of the ovarian nerve supply is, as should be expected, with realization that the ovary is embryologically an abdominal organ. The ovarian plexus invests both the ovarian artery and the vein. It supplies fibers to the broad ligament and to the fallopian tube, as well as to the ovary, and communicates in the broad ligament with the pelvic plexus; through the latter plexus it supplies fibers to the uterus.*

Figure 10-1 demonstrates the above-described hypogastric plexuses as they appear in a typical dissected specimen.

TECHNIC: PRESACRAL NEURECTOMY

The operation is performed under general anesthesia through a midline incision beginning at the level of the umbilicus. Curtis advocates an incision extending well above the umbilicus. If the patient is obese, this may be necessary, but in thin individuals we have had no difficulty in getting adequate exposure with an infra-umbilical incision.

The bowel is packed well back, and the rectosigmoid is drawn to the left. A midline incision is made in the posterior parietal peritoneum, from a point above

---

* Curtis, A. H., Anson, B. J., Ashley, F. L., and Jones, Tom: The anatomy of the pelvic autonomic nerves in relation to gynecology. Surg. Gynec. Obstet., 75:743-745, 1942.

228 Presacral Neurectomy

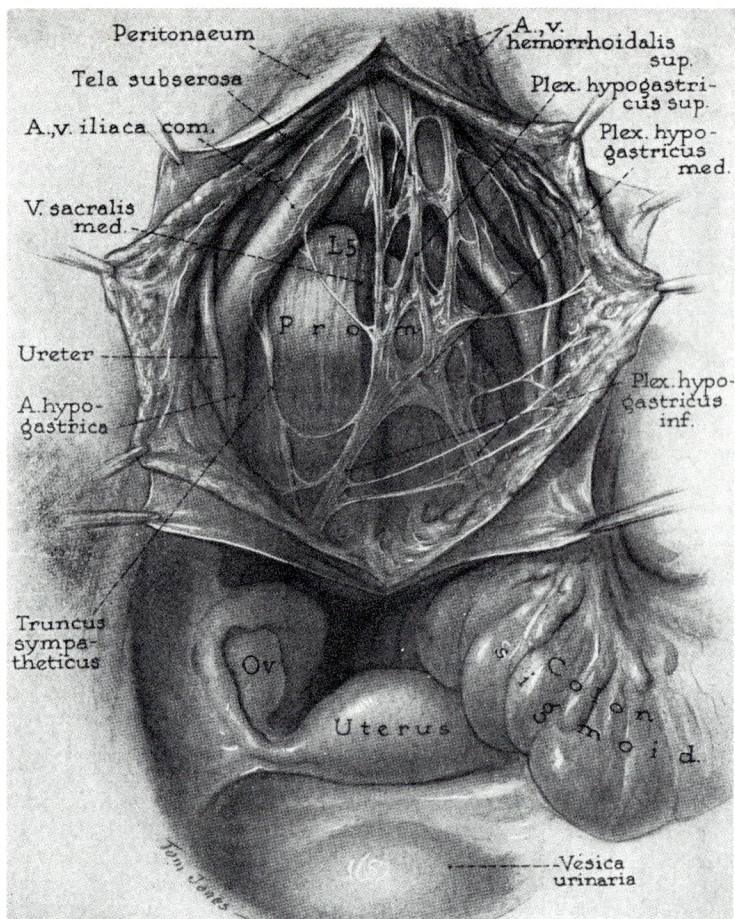

FIG. 10-1. Presacral nerves, in relation to peritoneal tissues. Anterior view of pelvis. Removal of the peritoneum and the retroperitoneal tissues, by strata, demonstrating the relation of the more prominent automatic elements to the heavy (deep) layer of retroperitoneal tissue. (Curtis, A. H.: A Textbook on Gynecology. Philadelphia, W. B. Saunders)

the bifurcation of the aorta to a point in the hollow of the sacrum opposite the 3rd or the 4th sacral vertebra. The retroperitoneal exposure is made by placing guy sutures on the edges of the peritoneum or by holding the edges apart with mucosa clips. Usually, exposure of the right ureter and the inferior mesenteric vessels is accomplished easily. Beginning on the right, all retroperitoneal connective tissue is dissected free between the right ureter and the inferior mesenteric vessels. A blunt dissector of some type is best for this dissection and minimizes bleeding. Two distinct layers of nerve-containing connective tissue are usually recognizable. The upper layer must be dissected free from the peritoneum. The deeper layer, which contains the main nerve trunks, is dissected from the vessels and the periosteum. Henriksen has suggested using an ordinary orangewood stick. The dissection is carried up to the origin of the inferior mesenteric artery, where the plexus is divided, and bleeding is controlled by fine catgut ties. The operator must avoid injury to the inferior mesenteric artery and its superior hemorrhoidal branch. All retroperitoneal nerve-containing tissue should be removed down to the level of the 2nd sacral nerve. The middle sacral

cillin. This relative resistance by the gonococcus to penicillin was little more than a laboratory curiosity a decade ago. While these resistant strains requiring 0.1 unit penicillin per mm. for in vitro inhibition were extremely rare in clinical practice, their commonplace occurrence now has necessitated the usage of higher doses of short-acting penicillin.

GONORRHEAL DISEASE OF THE LOWER TRACT

The natural history of this disease occurs in two stages. Initially, there is involvement in one or more structures of the lower genital tract 2 to 5 days after innoculation with the gonorrheal organism. The urethra, Skene's ducts, Bartholin's glands, cervix, or rectum may be involved. It is during this time that the disease remains asymptomatic and in the quiescent stage. The disease is most contagious during this latent, subclinical phase and can be disseminated widely if continued sexual contact occurs in the absence of adequate treatment. The upper genital tract, including the uterine cavity, tubes, and ovaries, may become secondarily involved from direct ascending infection, or this may occur at a later time, frequently associated with menses.

Although the difficulty in identification of *Neisseria gonorrhoeae* is well known, the culture method remains far superior to the Gram's smear procedure for identification of the organism. Improvement in the transport media for collection of the cervical swab and improvement in culture and incubation technics under anaerobic conditions have greatly improved the accuracy in identifying this organism.

METHODS OF CULTURE

The material from the urethral meatus, the cervix or the anal canal is collected on a cotton swab and immersed in a sterile test tube containing Stewart's transport medium (nonnutrient gelatin) specially buffered to prevent bacterial growth. This transport medium will preserve the gonococcus for 24 hours or longer but will not promote growth. Specimens are plated on Thayer-Martin V.C.N. chocolate medium, the inoculated plates are incubated at 37° C. under 5 to 10 per cent CO_2, and specimens are read at 24, 48, and 72 hours.

CLINICAL EVIDENCE OF INFECTION

Laboratory results should be interpreted carefully in the light of the history and the physical findings. Indeed, in some instances, particularly in the less acute cases, the diagnosis must be established or ruled out entirely on clinical grounds, since negative cultures and smears are not conclusive evidence of freedom from gonorrhea. Since the disease is almost invariably acquired by direct sexual contact, it is important to ascertain whether or not there has been recent activity. If examination indicates that the patient is not virginal, she should tactfully be given an opportunity to tell the true story. If vaginal discharge and/or burning and frequency of urination have developed following sexual exposure, and the laboratory examinations are negative, it is of the utmost importance to make contact with the male and have him examined for gonorrhea. Occasionally it is necessary to treat a woman who has been exposed to an infected male and has developed symptoms suggestive of gonorrhea on circumstantial evidence, when all laboratory tests are negative.

Examination of the recently infected woman may show a thick yellowish discharge coming from the vagina and/or the urethra. The urethral meatus may be edematous, and Skene's ducts may even be swollen by abscess formation. Bartholin's glands may be enlarged due to acute inflammation, and even large abscesses may develop in them. On the other hand, any or all of these signs are sometimes absent. As previously stated, 90 per cent of infected women are totally asymptomatic.

In searching for evidence, when chronic infection is suspected, one inspects and palpates Bartholin's and Skene's glands. The normal Skene's ducts are not palpable. After a neisserian infection, they may be thickened and even form chronic abscesses that discharge pus when compressed. Abscesses starting in Skene's ducts sometimes burrow between the urethra and the vaginal mucosa and form large abscesses. The infection occasionally is persistent in the urethra. Endoscopic examination may show small areas of granulation tissue along the course of the urethra. Normal Bartholin's glands are usually not palpable, or are palpable only as small structures about the size of kernels of wheat. When larger than this, there is a suspicion of infection, present or past. Bits of granulation tissue at the orifices of Bartholin's or Skene's ducts suggest old neisserian infection but are not pathognomonic of the disease.

Chronic neisserian infection of the cervix is not characteristic on inspection. It may appear exactly like any other chronically infected nulliparous or parous cervix. Infection is harbored deep in the cervical glands, most of which open into the cervical canal.

TREATMENT OF GONOCOCCAL INFECTION OF THE LOWER TRACT

Penicillin has become the principal agent of treatment of neisserian infections in the management of both asymptomatic and symptomatic *lower tract disease*. It is routine to give 4.8 million units of procaine penicillin G at one visit as the total therapy. In the past we have used long-acting penicillins such as benzathine penicillin G in the management of gonorrhea. It is apparent, however, that the prolonged low dosage of penicillin which persists after acute

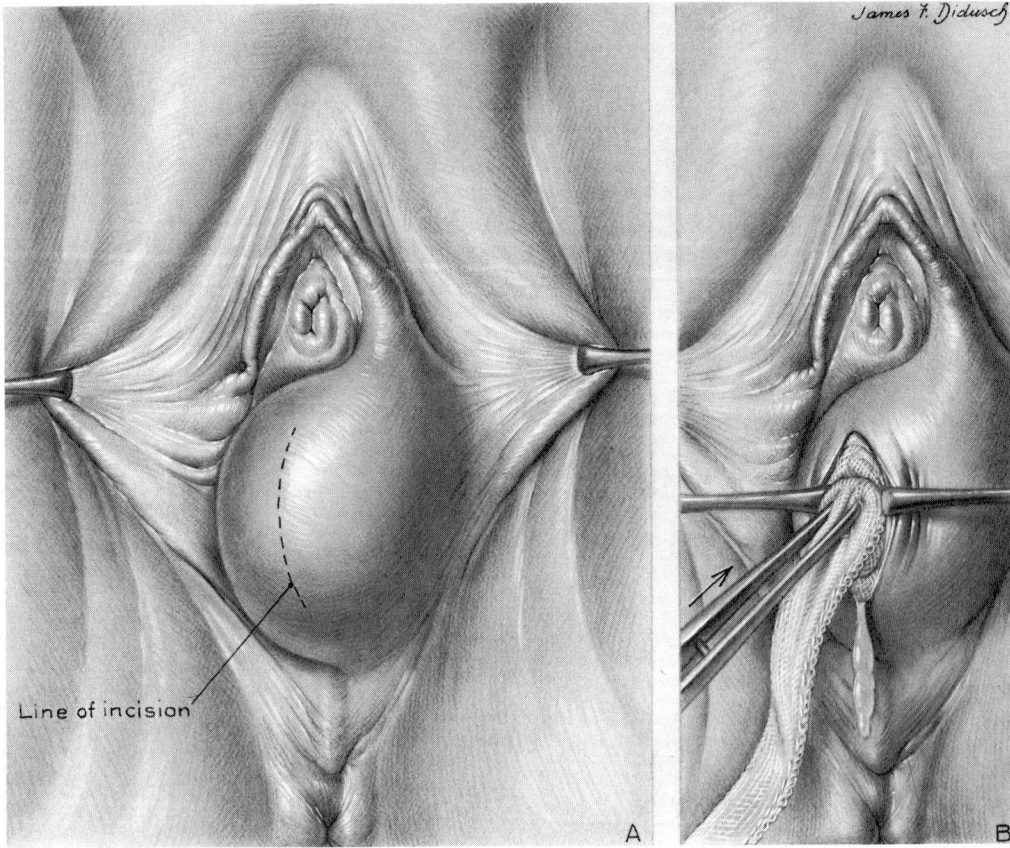

FIG. 11-1. Incision and drainage of Bartholin's gland abscess. (A) Dotted line indicates incision on mucosal surface. (B) Abscess cavity is packed with narrow gauze strip.

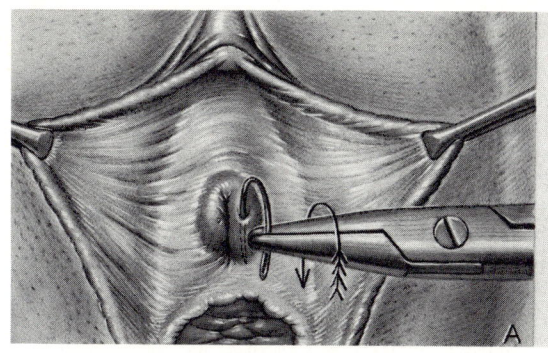 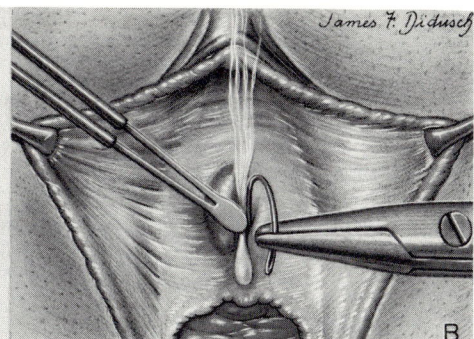

Fig. 11-2. Destruction of infected Skene's gland with cautery. (A) Curved needle is threaded into Skene's duct. (B) The gland is opened by cutting down to the needle. After the duct is opened, it is thoroughly destroyed with the cautery.

management is insufficient to prevent reinfection and may selectively allow more resistant forms to develop. Following this treatment, the patient is re-evaluated in 48 hours for symptomatic improvement. The cervix is cultured every week for 4 weeks before the woman is considered cured. For patients with penicillin sensitivity or resistance, 1 gm. of tetracycline is given orally as an initial dose, followed by 0.5 gm. of tetracycline 4 times a day for 3 days.

In cases of acute symptomatic gonococcal infection of the lower tract, rest in bed is desirable, but of less importance than in the treatment of upper tract infection. Avoidance of repeated unnecessary bimanual examinations is also desirable, and sexual continence is imperative. Warm douches keep the vagina and cervix clean, are conducive to the patient's comfort, and are thought to promote capillary dilatation and healing to the cervical and vaginal mucosa as a result of the temperature of the water.

Treatment of Residual Infections in the Lower Tract

From the previous discussion it is obvious that the treatment of gonorrhea has been completely revolutionized by penicillin therapy. Although the Bartholin gland and duct have been known to be a target of neisserian infection, as have other glandular structures of the lower genital tract, recently Reef has cultured the organism in 53.6 per cent of the cases of acute gonococcal infection by probing the normal-appearing Bartholin duct where there has been an absence of visible secretions from the gland. Bartholin's gland infection usually responds to penicillin therapy, coupled with local measures for symptomatic relief in the form of hot douches and sitz baths. In spite of this, some glands will go on to abscess formation and require incision and drainage (Fig. 11-1). Occasionally, chronic infection may persist in the glands, and cyst formation is common, even when all activity of the original infection has long since passed. Excision of the chronically infected gland and/or the cyst is indicated. For the technic of excision of Bartholin's gland cyst see Chapter 31.

Urethral infections are usually short-lived; this was true even before the use of chemotherapy. Since the advent of penicillin, residual infection in the urethra or Skene's glands and in the suburethral space is seen occasionally. When Skene's glands remain permanently infected, they may be destroyed by threading curved needles into the ducts and then destroying the ducts electrosurgically or with the actual cautery (Fig. 11-2). A suburethral diverticulum may arise from chronically infected paraurethral glands with resultant suburethral abscess formation and chronic urinary tract infection.

GONORRHEAL DISEASE OF THE UPPER GENITAL TRACT (ABOVE THE INTERNAL OS)

After the cervix has become infected, the course of the disease is variable. The disease in the cervix may persist as a chronic infection, or the infection may die out completely, even without treatment. In some instances, probably in a small minority of the cases, the infection proceeds above the internal os and infects the endometrium. This is particularly apt to occur during menstruation when the blood in the uterine cavity serves as an excellent culture medium for gonococci. Falk has studied the onset of gonorrheal salpingitis in Sweden and found that it occurred more often in the actual menstrual period and proliferative phase of the menstrual cycle than at any other time. Soon after the endometrium is infected, the salpinges become involved, probably by submucosal lymphatic spread. Not until the tubes are actually inflamed do symptoms appear which indicate that the infection has ascended above the cervix. Bilateral lower abdominal pain, distention, muscle spasm, fever, and leukocytosis are usually indicative of inflammation of the tubes and the pelvic peritoneum.

Differentiation of Acute Salpingitis from Appendicitis

One of the most frequent and most important differential diagnoses that the gynecologist is called upon to make is that between salpingitis and acute appendicitis. Hence the subject is worthy of special consideration. If the abdomen is opened for appendectomy in the presence of acute salpingitis, the patient is subjected to needless surgery, although as a rule no great harm results, provided that the operator resists the temptation to remove the acutely inflamed tubes. Failure to open the abdomen in the presence of an acutely inflamed appendix may result in rupture and even death. The decision is frequently difficult because all of the symptoms of salpingitis may be present in appendicitis, and vice versa.

Abdominal pain is usually the presenting symptom in both diseases. Characteristically, the pain due to appendicitis begins in the epigastrium and later localizes in the right lower quadrant. Characteristically, the pain due to salpingitis is low and bilateral. But often with appendicitis there are generalized abdominal cramps simulating the abdominal pain due to gonococcal peritonitis. Many times the disease of the two tubes is unequal; when the right adnexa are involved to a much greater degree than the left, the pain may be almost entirely right-sided, simulating that due to acute appendicitis.

Nausea and vomiting occur more frequently with acute appendicitis than with salpingitis, but they are by no means rare with the latter, especially in the more severe cases when considerable peritonitis is present. They may even be absent with an acutely inflamed appendix, and severe and persistent with acute salpingitis. In general, however, the absence of nausea and vomiting is a point in favor of salpingitis.

The degree of inflammation of the tubes is extremely variable, and, in a like manner, there is great variation in fever and leukocytosis. The same may be said of appendicitis. The average temperature in both conditions is between 100° and 101° F., but higher temperatures are commoner in salpingitis than in appendicitis, unless rupture has taken place, and peritonitis or abscess has developed. Although the average elevation of the leukocyte count in both conditions varies between 10,000 and 20,000, a continued rise in the white blood count or an increased number of immature forms during the acute phase of the disease is more commonly seen in appendicitis than salpingitis.

Intestinal distention is common in both conditions and is related to the degree of peritonitis present, regardless of the etiologic cause. Abdominal tenderness is apt to be more localized in the right lower quadrant in the unruptured appendix, and the maximum is usually at McBurney's point. With salpingitis the tenderness is usually bilateral, although it can be far more marked on one side than on the other. If the maximum tenderness happens to be on the right, it may simulate tenderness from appendicitis, but its lower position is usually helpful in pointing to tubal inflammation.

Muscle spasm is apt to be bilateral and low with salpingitis and limited to the right rectus region with appendicitis unless there is rupture with generalized peritonitis. Under these conditions the muscle spasm usually becomes generalized.

Psoas muscle tenderness from an inflamed appendix may be demonstrated by straight leg raising, which produces acute right lower quadrant symptoms when the muscle is placed on a stretch by such a maneuver. This clinical sign is typical of an acutely inflamed appendix.

The pelvic examination is the most important procedure in making the differentiation. An unruptured hymen almost certainly rules out gonococcal salpingitis. Evidence of acute Bartholin or Skene adenitis, urethritis, or cervicitis is strong evidence for salpingitis, particularly if the gonococcus is found in the smear from the cervix and/or the urethra. Tenderness on bimanual movement of the uterus and thickening in the adnexal region strongly suggest tubal infection, but it should not be overlooked that very early in the course of the tubal infection there may be no induration, and that tenderness may be the only abnormality noted on pelvic examination. If the symptoms have been existent for a week or more, the absence of adnexal induration is evidence against salpingitis. Occasionally, in appendicitis, induration can be felt high up on the right through the vagina due to inflammatory thickening of the cecum, the ileum, the meso-appendix on an abscess. Although usually situated higher than a tubo-ovarian abscess, an appendix abscess may be as low as the cul-de-sac. If bimanual palpation reveals normal nontender adnexa on the left, that is strong evidence against salpingitis, which is practically always bilateral.

If acute appendicitis cannot be ruled out with reasonable certainty, it is better to err on the side of operative intervention than to defer surgery. Under such circumstances, the gridiron-muscle-splitting incision is preferred. The appendix can be removed satisfactorily through this type of incision, and the right tube can be inspected satisfactorily. If an error in diagnosis is discovered at operation, the appendix should be removed, but the acutely inflamed tubes left undisturbed. The gridiron incision should be closed without drainage, even though very acute gonococcal peritonitis is present. Penicillin therapy should be started immediately.

TREATMENT OF ACUTE SALPINGITIS

The treatment of acute salpingitis in minimally symptomatic outpatients is essentially the same as that in lower tract disease. Unless there is marked improvement of symptoms in 24 to 48 hours, the patient is instructed to return for further therapy or hospitalization. Hospitalization is necessary, however, if the patient presents with fever, peritoneal or abdominal signs, or if there is question in the diagnosis. Intravenous aqueous penicillin, 1,000,000 units every 6 hours for 24 hours, is combined with 1,200,000 units of procaine penicillin given intramuscularly twice a day. Therapy is continued for 5 to 7 days, even though there is marked improvement in 24 hours in most cases. Wren demonstrated a 12 per cent penicillin-resistant form of gonococcus in hospitalized females who received 1,000,000 units of penicillin for 10 days. The organisms in these cases were shown to be resistant to blood levels of penicillin achieved by this treatment, but were susceptible to higher doses. Holmes *et al.* were able to study the response of gonorrhea in sailors in the United States Navy during long periods at sea, where the possibility of reinfection was virtually excluded. Of 63 such men, each of whom had a single intramuscular injection of 2,400,000 units of aqueous procaine penicillin G, the currently accepted dosage for men, 29 per cent failed to respond. By achieving higher dosage levels with the use of probenecid, there was only 1 failure. It is apparent that penicillin is the drug of choice in all cases of gonorrhea, but the early recognition of resistant form is imperative. If response to therapy is not prompt, 1 gm. streptomycin q.d. or 2 gm. of tetracycline q.d. is added to the management. In hospitalized patients the therapeutic level of penicillin is also considered effective against infectious syphilis. However, the therapy for these two diseases should not be combined routinely since the long-acting penicillin drugs may contribute to development of resistant gonococcal forms.

Douching with hot solutions, with the patient lying down, gives symptomatic relief, and it is our belief that the hyperemia caused by the heat promotes healing. Douches of plain hot water are probably of as much value as douches containing antiseptics. A douche powder that we find agreeable to the patient is as follows:

PULVIS MENTHAE COMPOSITAE

Oil of peppermint...... 4 cc.
Liquefied phenol ...... 8 cc.
Alum................. 30 cc.
Boric acid ....120 cc.
M. et Ft. Pulv. No. 1.
Sig: 2 teaspoonfuls to 2 quarts of warm water and use as a douche as directed.

Although this solution certainly has a minimum of antiseptic action, its pleasant "germicidal" odor and astringent effect seems to give the patient a sense of cleanliness that she desires. Sitz baths also give symptomatic relief.

Daily short-wave diathermy treatment is a more effective method of administering heat than by douching but is a little uncomfortable for the treatment of acute pelvic peritonitis. We find it of particular value in those cases that do not respond promptly to antibiotics, and in those cases in which marked pelvic induration or large masses persist. The degree of resolution of pelvic cellulitis that can be attained with regular, persistent diathermy over weeks and even months is truly remarkable. Often diathermy will quickly bring pelvic cellulitis to abscess formation in the cul-de-sac, and the cul-de-sac is easily drained by colpotomy (Fig. 11-3).

It is the considered opinion of the authors and of most American gynecologists that *laparotomy should be avoided while tubal inflammation is still active because:*

1. It is usually unnecessary, since the majority of patients can be made comfortable by conservative measures and never will require surgery. It is rare that laparotomy is required for the control of an acute salpingitis, although occasionally either a reinfection or an exacerbation of a tubo-ovarian inflammatory mass may produce intraperitoneal leakage requiring surgery, as discussed later in the chapter.

2. Pregnancy is quite possible in a large percentage of cases after acute infection of the tubes, if proper conservative therapy is carried out. The pregnancy rate is improved with intensive antibiotic therapy for acute infection of the tubes. In the study made in Sweden (Falk) there was an 84 per cent incidence of intra-uterine pregnancy after clinical recovery from gonorrheal salpingitis, a considerably higher incidence than that found in most statistics of previous years, in which only approximately 50 per cent fertility ensued. These improved results were ascribed to such factors as early diagnosis, early hospitalization, and adequate antibiotic therapy.

3. The patients operated on during the acute or subacute stage have a higher mortality and morbidity than those operated on for the inflammatory residue. Injuries to the bowel and the bladder are more common, and drainage, with its resultant adhesions, may be necessary; when operation is done on the residue, drainage is almost never necessary.

4. If surgery is undertaken during the acute or subacute stage, much more radical ovarian surgery is apt to be done. In spite of the best intentions for conservatism on the part of the operator, the appearance of the inflamed and often abscessed ovaries is such that he is more apt to remove both of them than he would be if he were operating after all active inflammation has subsided.

FIG. 11-3. Posterior colpotomy. (A) A transverse incision is made through the vaginal mucosa at the junction of the posterior vaginal fornix with the cervix. (B) A Kelly clamp is thrust through the abscess wall.

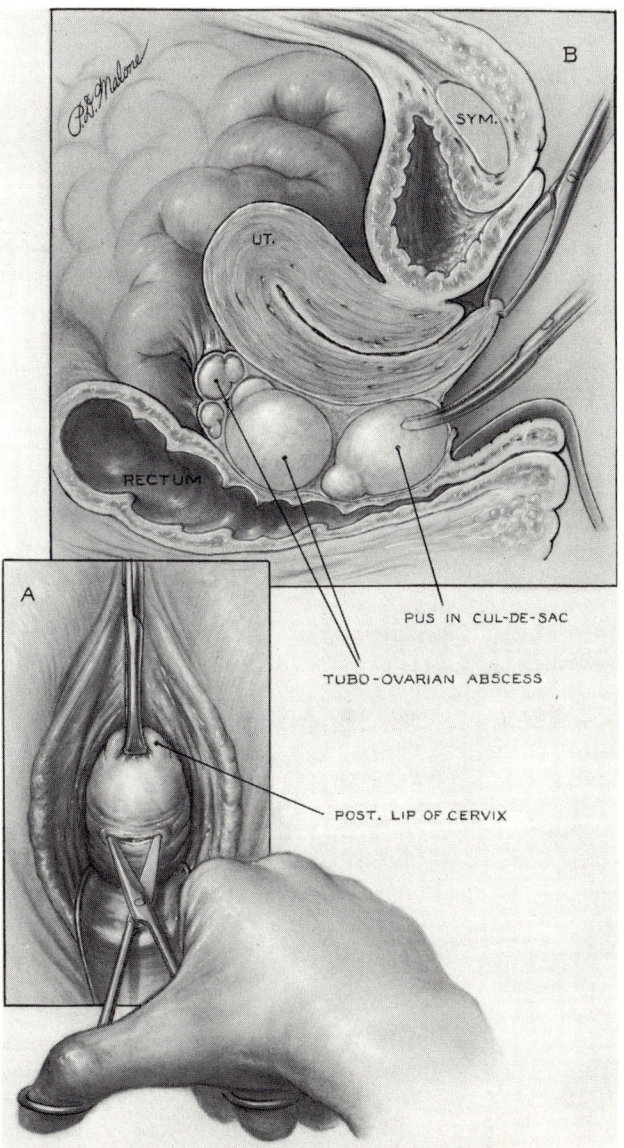

INDICATIONS FOR SURGERY DURING THE ACUTE STAGE OF SALPINGITIS

1. A fluctuant cul-de-sac abscess or a large tubo-ovarian abscess that does not respond to conservative treatment and is accessible to drainage through the posterior vaginal vault.
2. Rarely, the abdominal drainage of a large tubo-ovarian abscess is indicated when it fails to respond to conservative therapy and when it lies too high to be reached safely through the vagina. Such large thick-walled abscesses may fail to collapse and heal until drainage is established. It is our custom to open and drain them through gridiron incisions. This procedure is necessary only a few times a year on our service, in which pelvic inflammatory disease is common.
3. Rarely, a loop of small bowel may become adherent to an acute inflammatory mass, causing obstruction and requiring operative intervention.
4. As mentioned above, the removal of the appendix may be necessary for safety in cases in which the symptoms and the signs are too suggestive of appendicitis to justify a watchful waiting policy.

Technic: Posterior Colpotomy

Posterior colpotomy is done to evacuate pus and to establish drainage from a cul-de-sac abscess or a tubo-ovarian abscess. It is also done in a search for blood when tubal pregnancy is suspected.

Ideally, there are three requirements for colpotomy drainage of a pelvic abscess:

1. The abscess must be midline or nearly so.
2. It should dissect the rectovaginal septum to assure the surgeon that the drainage will be retroperitoneal. Occasionally, a cul-de-sac abscess may be successfully drained without dissecting the septum.
3. It should be cystic or fluctuant to assure adequate drainage.

The patient is placed on the table in the lithotomy position, and the posterior lip of the cervix is drawn downward and forward. It is essential that a thorough examination of the pelvis be made under anesthesia, so that the operator will have in mind the size and the position of the mass that is to be drained.

The vaginal mucosa is incised transversely with a scalpel, and the transverse incision is widened with a pair of long scissors at the reflexion of the vaginal mucosa onto the cervix (Fig. 11-3 A). With a long Kelly clamp the cul-de-sac is punctured (Fig. 11-3 B). As the abscess or hematoma wall is perforated, there is a definite sense of puncturing a cystic cavity; if blood or pus is present, some is soon seen in the upper vagina. The jaws of the clamp are spread, and the flow of liquid from the cul-de-sac is free. A culture is obtained from the purulent exudate and is sent to the bacteriology laboratory for appropriate culture and sensitivity. A direct smear is also made from the pus and examined for predominating organisms.

In puncturing an abscess, there is frequently more than one compartment, and it is desirable to insert a finger in the abscess cavity and explore. If another abscess wall is felt, often it may be punctured safely under the guidance of the finger. If pus is obtained, 2 cigarette drains are inserted into the abscess cavity.

If necessary to control bleeding of the vaginal wall, a catgut stitch or two are taken in the vaginal incision.

SURGERY FOR THE RESIDUE OF GONOCOCCAL TUBAL DISEASE

Although the gonococcus may be responsible for intitiating the acute salpingitis, the natural history of this organism as described by Lucas and coworkers is short-lived, while the residual chronic salpingitis is usually due to secondary invaders, notably coliform bacilli, which produce recurrent exacerbations and chronic symptoms. As a result of the initial infection or from subsequent secondary exacerbations, the fimbria are frequently occluded, and the tubes may be bound to the ovaries with adhesions. In addition, the bowel may become adherent to the broad ligament, and the fascia and loose connective tissue of the broad ligament may be converted to an indurated, brauny structure typical of "ligneous induration." If the chronic infection persists, serous secretion within the endosalpinx produces a hydrosalpinx which may ignite periodically with secondary infection and produce a pyosalpinx or chronic tubo-ovarian abscess. Rarely, there may be intra-abdominal rupture or leakage of an old tubo-ovarian abscess.

The symptoms of chronic pelvic inflammatory disease which most frequently require surgical treatment include (1) severe, persistent, and progressive pelvic pain, usually bilateral, although occasionally localized in one of the lower abdominal quadrants; (2) repeated exacerbations of pelvic inflammatory disease requiring multiple hospitalization and recurrent medical treatment; (3) the progressive enlargement of a tubo-ovarian inflammatory mass; (4) a history of previous colpotomy for drainage of pelvic abscess, and (5) severe dyspareunia related to the pelvic infection.

Selection of Operation

The decision having been made that operative intervention is necessary, the question of the proper operation has to be determined. The final decision is usually made with the abdomen opened. Consideration must be given not only to the pathologic lesions found at operation but also to the patient's age, parity, desire for children, and her previous history of pelvic disease. Because a knowledge of all these is essential to the best surgical judgment, it is desirable for the operator to be thoroughly familiar with the history.

Figure 11-4 illustrates the possible operative procedures for the residue of salpingitis. In addition to those pictured, there is the cornual tubal resection discussed and illustrated later in this chapter. The least surgery that can be done on a pelvic inflammatory residue is release of peritubal and periovarian adhesions. This is indicated occasionally in women in whom childbearing is desired, provided that the tubes can be demonstrated by retrograde tubal inflation with the abdomen open to be patent after the adhesions have been cut. It is uncommon to find both tubes in such a condition that their lumina can be restored so simply. More frequently, one tube is hopelessly closed, and the opposite one is patent after release of adhesions. Then unilateral salpingectomy may be indicated if preservation of the childbearing function is desirable. In a case in which the uterus is in retroposition and adherent, but the tubes patent, the adhesions should be released, and some type of suspension compatible with future pregnancy should be carried out.

In the majority of instances bilateral salpingectomy is necessary. Frequently one and occasionally both ovaries must also be removed. Since most operations for pelvic inflammatory disease are done on women under 35 years of age, the condition of the ovaries should be considered carefully before deciding upon bilateral oophorectomy. The decision to castrate should be made from the standpoint of the pelvic lesions and also after a consideration of the age and the emotional temperament of the patient. Our attitude toward bilateral ovarian removal is very conservative.

The senior author, in collaboration with Darner, followed a series of women on whom hysterectomy was done for fibroids, mostly complicated by salpingitis. The percentage of patients free from abdominal discomfort was slightly greater in those in whom ovarian ablation was done (88%) than in those in whom ovarian tissue was conserved (84.4%). This slightly poorer figure for the conservative group was more than compensated for by the absence of hot flushes and nervous symptoms that annoyed a great portion of the group upon whom total ablation had been done. If an ovary is to be preserved, as demonstrated in Figure 11-4 F, it is often preferable to leave the entire adnexa in place rather than to compromise the venous drainage to the ovary with resultant cystic change that may require an additional operative procedure. Once the continuity of the tubal lumen and uterine cavity is broken, the chronically inflamed tube does not produce subsequent symptoms, as shown by Falk in his series of cases with cornual tubal resection.

When all the adnexa are removed, it is our custom to perform a hysterectomy. When both tubes must be removed and ovarian tissue saved, we also remove the uterus unless there is a very good reason for conserving it. The pelvis is usually peritonized more easily after removing the uterus, which often is covered with shaggy adhesions. Furthermore, a possible source of leukorrhea and malignancy is thereby removed. We believe that there is usually little justification for the preservation of the uterus when a woman is to be sterilized by salpingectomy, if her condition permits the added surgery necessary to remove the uterus. In former years preservation of the uterus was a common practice in our clinic. The great number of myomata, functional bleeding uteri, and a small number of uterine carcinomata which we have observed in these sterile women have convinced us that there is little justification in most instances for preservation of the uterus. In all these women the cervix has been, or is, the site of infection; therefore total hysterectomy is the ideal operation. However, this procedure should not be

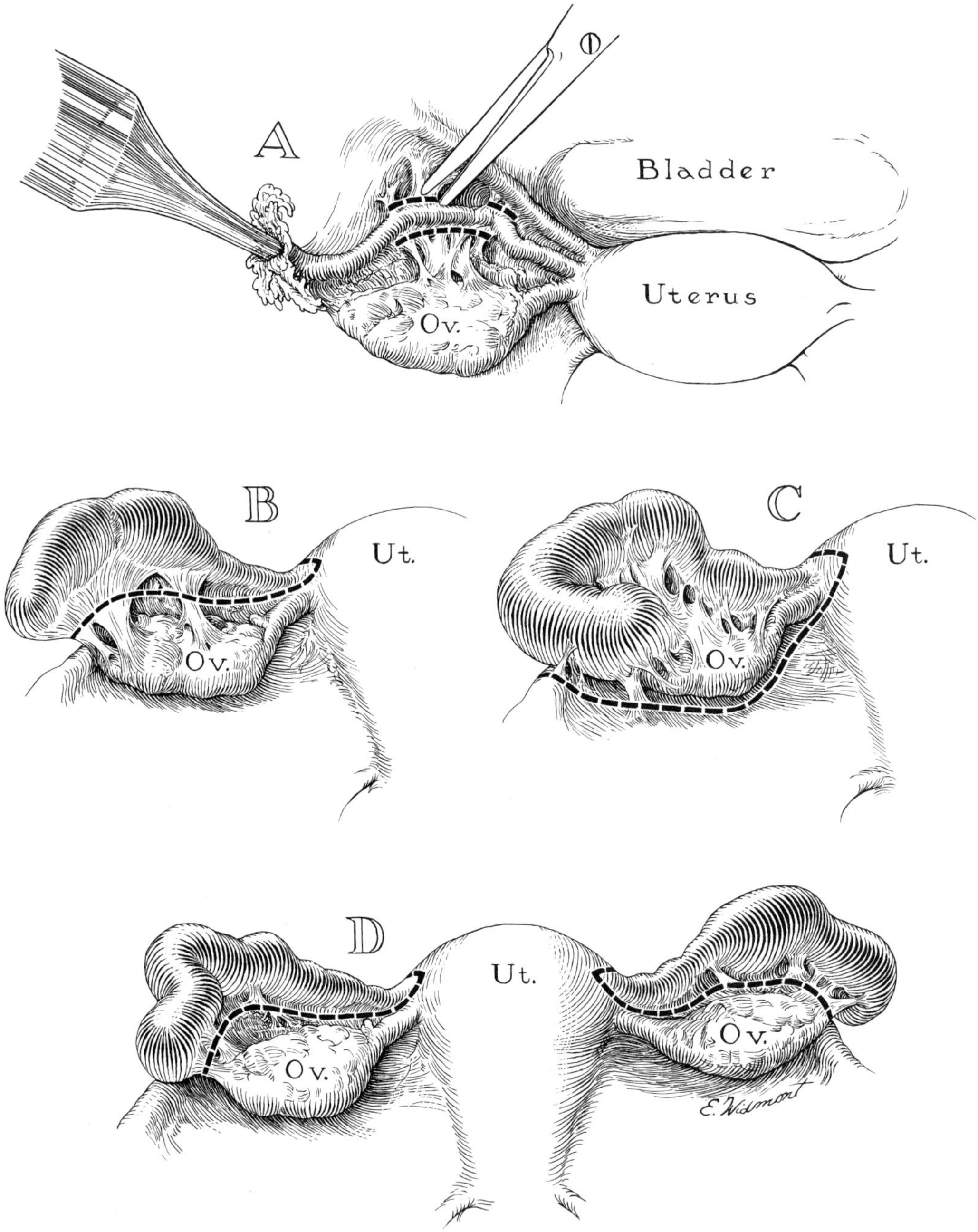

FIG. 11-4. Diagrammatic demonstration of possible operations for chronic salpingitis. (A) Release of peritubal adhesions. (B) Simple unilateral salpingectomy. (C) Unilateral salpingo-oophorectomy. (D) Bilateral salpingectomy.

an invariable rule. In many women with a severe pelvic inflammatory residue, the operation may be difficult, and discretion will dictate subtotal hysterectomy rather than the alternative of subjecting the patient to the further surgery necessary for removal of the cervix. This is particularly apt to be the case when the pelvic inflammatory residue is complicated by a large fibroid tumor.

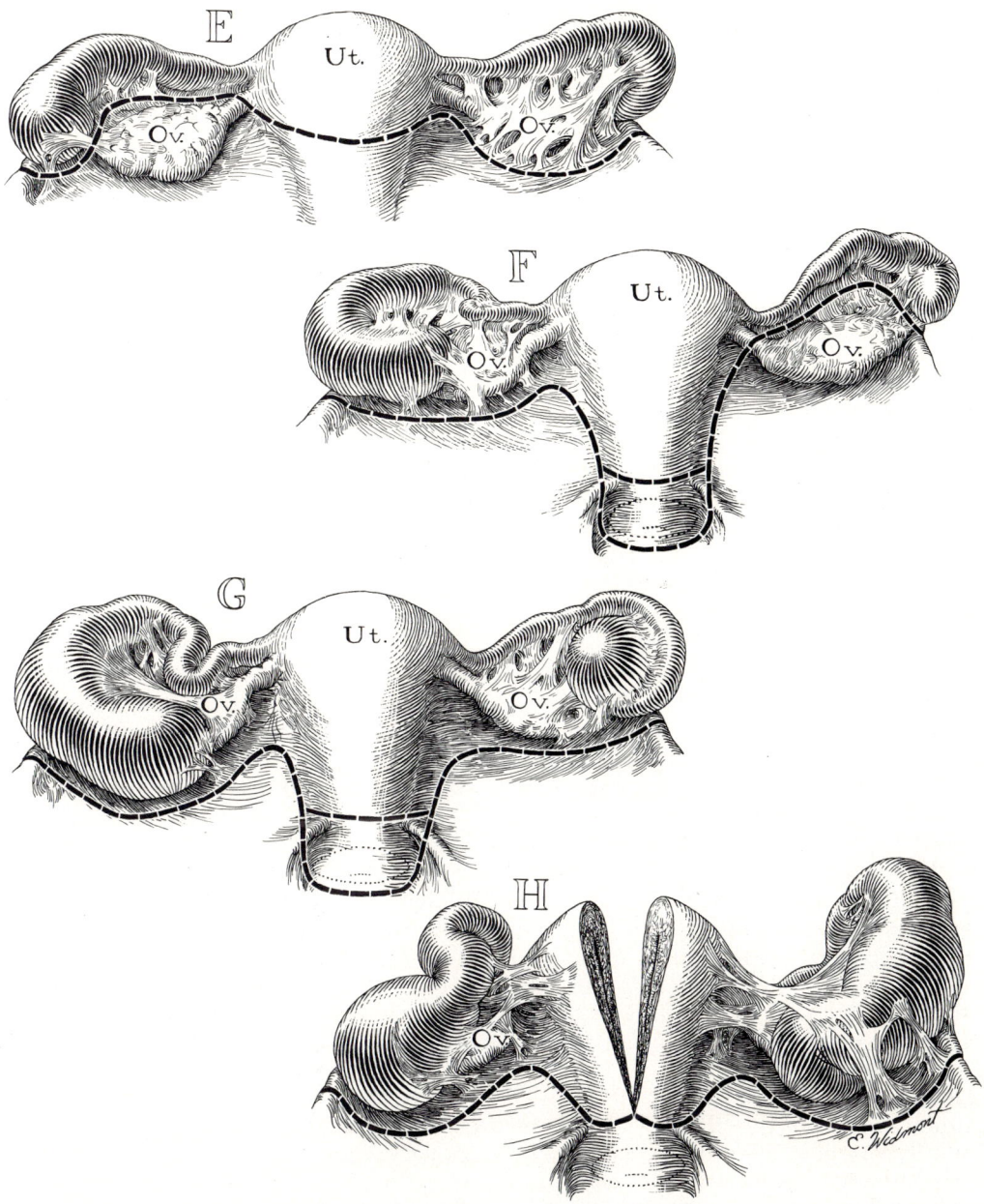

Fig. 11-4 (*Continued*). Diagrammatic demonstration of possible operations for chronic salpingitis. (E) Double salpingectomy, unilateral oophorectomy. (F) Double salpingectomy, unilateral oophorectomy and hysterectomy, total or subtotal. (G) Double salpingo-oophorectomy and hysterectomy, total or subtotal. (H) Bisection operation with complete adnexal ablation.

In spite of the very excellent reasons for hysterectomy with salpingectomy based on sound pathologic grounds, there is another factor that should enter into the decision. Before performing an operation for pelvic inflammatory residue, it is advisable to discuss the possibility of hysterectomy with the patient. A careful explanation to the sensible woman will usually cause her to consent to removal of the useless uterus, especially if dysmenorrhea or bleeding has been a prominent symptom. But unfortunately the emotions play a greater role than reason in many a woman's thoughts, and the idea of the absence of menstruation may suggest to her the loss of feminism and sex libido. Such ideas, unfounded as they may be, must be respected to prevent postoperative emotional upsets, and in such individuals preservation of the uterus is wise.

When the uterus is preserved, a proper suspension is essential to prevent its becoming adherent posteriorly. Usually, the modified Coffey procedure pictured on page 246 is sufficient, but occasionally, when there is a great tendency to retroversion, the modified Gilliam suspension may also be utilized to advantage.

Plastic operations for the restoration of tubal lumina for the cure of sterility are considered on pages 304 to 306.

Ruptured Tubo-ovarian Abscess

Of all the complications resulting from chronic pelvic inflammatory disease, the occurrence of intra-abdominal rupture of a tubo-ovarian abscess is the most infrequent but the most life-threatening sequela of this disease. For the 5-year period from 1959 to 1964 Mickal and coworkers reported an incidence of 14 per cent rupture of 661 tubo-ovarian abscesses admitted to the Charity Hospital in New Orleans. Pedowitz recently reported 29 cases of ruptured adnexal abscess at Kings County Hospital (15%) of 197 adnexal abscesses admitted from 1957–59. Although this is much higher than our own experience (5%), these statistics do reflect the seriousness of this complication. Such abscesses may rupture spontaneously or as the result of bimanual examination or accidental trauma. Bacteriologic study of the contents of the abscess is unrewarding in approximately 50 per cent of the cases in which no organism is isolated; in the remaining cases various aerobic and anaerobic organisms are found, of which the coliform group is more common. *E. coli* and *Aerobacter aerogenes* are the more frequently detected gram-negative coliform organisms. The gonococcus is rarely identified in such abscesses.

Diagnosis

The clinical symptoms are those of acute, progressive pelvic pain, which is usually so severe that the patient can accurately identify the time and place of its occurrence. Depending on the stoicism of the individual, the patient may seek medical advice immediately or delay consultation until generalized peritonitis and septic shock occur. Age is important in this group of cases. In our series the average age was 33 years, which is at least 10 years later in life than the average age of the primary attack of pelvic inflammatory disease of the colored female population on our service. Often there is a history of recurring attacks of pelvic inflammatory disease, and during the recent exacerbation there has been a sudden increase in the severity and the extent of abdominal pain. Examination usually reveals a temperature of over 101° F. and a pulse rate of over 110. There are signs of generalized peritonitis with a pelvic mass. Shifting dullness and diminished or absent bowel sounds may be noted. The leukocyte count is likely to be over 15,000. An abdominal film may reveal dilated loops of small bowel and free fluid in the abdomen. A culdocentesis is a valuable diagnostic aid and was positive for purulent material in 70 per cent of the New Orleans series. Shock may be present or may develop while the patient is under observation. The longer the delay in the operative treatment of this catastrophic disease, the higher is the primary mortality. In our own experience, death occurred less than 90 hours after the time of rupture in 88 per cent of the fatal cases, both operative and nonoperative.

Treatment

The treatment of these cases may be divided into three phases:

Preoperative Phase After Rupture. Operation should be undertaken after rapid but adequate preoperative preparation. The patient's blood should be grouped and cross-matched with 1,500 cc.

of blood. Monitoring of central venous pressure is essential for proper control of the hemodynamics of this condition. Blood transfusions should be started as soon as available. Emergency blood chemistry determinations are obtained, and intravenous fluids are started immediately including Ringer's lactate, normal saline or dextran 40. Vigorous antibiotic therapy should be undertaken. Penicillin, streptomycin, and intravenous chloramphenical are used at this stage because they are given parenterally. An indwelling Foley catheter is helpful in controlling fluid balance by monitoring the hourly urine output. Generally, it is advantageous to pass a Cantor or Miller-Abbott intestinal tube before operation. "Combat shock" is the watchword throughout treatment. The clinical features of this disease which warrant immediate laparotomy include a progressive increase in the pulse rate, a worsening of the abdominal signs of peritonitis, increase in abdominal distention, and a beginning drop in the blood pressure or central venous pressure.

Operative Phase. Blood transfusion should be started before surgery. The anesthetic of choice depends on the preference and experience of the anesthesiologist. (See Chapter 3, Anesthesia.)

The operation should be carried out as rapidly as possible. Although time is not a very important factor in some surgery, it is when dealing with these patients. The patient should not be put in Trendelenburg position until the abdomen is packed off, and no more Trendelenburg position than necessary should be used, to prevent the dissemination of pus into the upper abdomen. The operation of choice is the removal of the free pus, together with the abscess, the uterus, the tubes, and usually the ovaries. Rarely is it possible to leave some ovarian tissue. Even in the best surgical hands we believe that a subtotal hysterectomy is faster than a total and should be done in these critically ill patients. It is probable that the mortality would be increased if total hysterectomy were always done. Although we believe firmly in total hysterectomy, we do not believe in persisting in it when the danger of total hysterectomy exceeds the danger of leaving the cervix in.

As a rule, it is much easier to remove the corpus in these cases than to attempt a unilateral adnexectomy. Furthermore, the opposite adnexa is almost always involved, and subsequent operation may be necessary if conservation of one side is practiced, as was required in 35 per cent of Pedowitz's cases. If hemostasis is poor, or if considerable necrotic material is left behind, there may be some benefit from peritoneal drainage with cigarette drains through a stab wound or through the cul-de-sac. In any event, after closure of the peritoneum and the fascia, a small gutta-percha wick should be put in the subcutaneous fat. The pus from the abdomen should be cultured, and the organism tested for sensitivity to the various antibiotics.

Postoperative Phase. In the postoperative care, one should consider shock, infection, ileus, and fluid balance.

Septic shock should be combated with whole blood, Ringer's lactate or normal saline, and, if necessary, dextran 40 and norepinephrine intravenously. (See Septic Shock, this chapter.) Infection is usually controlled by penicillin, 30-60 million U./day; streptomycin, 1 gm./day, and intravenous chloramphenical 2-4 gm./day until the patient can take oral medication. The Fowler position may help prevent subdiaphragmatic abscess formation.

Constant intestinal suction by means of a Cantor or a Miller-Abbott tube is a very important feature of postoperative care. Adynamic ileus is often present and is best treated with the long tube.

Close attention to fluid balance and blood chemistry determinations is necessary. Not infrequently these patients have poor kidney function, and the fluid output and nonprotein nitrogen should be followed closely.

The results of the above therapeutic measures have been very gratifying. In earlier years medical treatment and simple drainage were the rule. Pedowitz and Felmus reported a mortality of 100 per cent in 1947 of the cases at Kings County treated by medical measures and occa-

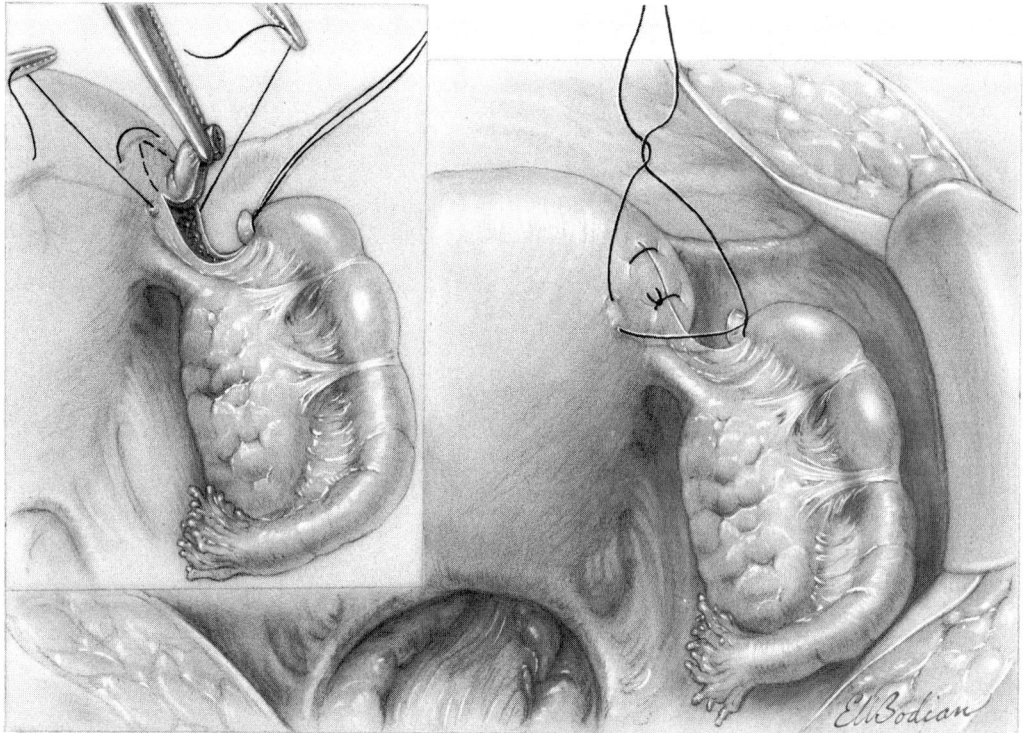

Fig. 11-5. Cornual excision of a diseased tube, according to Falk. Inset shows tube ligated and marks the line of excision. The picture proper shows that the cornual excision has been made and the wound closed with a figure-of-eight suture. The cornual end of the tube is being sutured to the anterior surface of the uterus.

sional incision and drainage, which was reduced to 3.1 per cent since that time by aggressive surgical management. Petroff reported 100 per cent mortality in the cases not operated upon and 66 per cent in the cases in which drainage only was carried out. He concluded that the treatment of choice was surgical. By intensifying their therapy since 1959, Mickal and coworkers have reduced their mortality to 5.12 per cent. On the Tulane unit at Charity Hospital, Johnson reports a reduction in the mortality rate to 10.7 per cent from 1962 through 1965. Vermeeren and Te Linde divided the cases in the Hopkins' clinic into 2 groups: those treated between 1925 and 1944 and those treated between 1945 and 1953. In the earlier group most of the cases were treated medically or by simple drainage. The mortality was 90 per cent. In the latter group, treated by the method outlined above, the mortality was reduced to 12 per cent. The deaths appeared to be due to septecemia and endotoxic shock with peritonitis and fluid imbalance. Our current mortality rate for this formerly lethal disease is 3.5 per cent.

Cornual Resection

In 1946 Falk introduced a conservative treatment of recurrent salpingitis by cornual resection (Fig. 11-5). This treatment was based on the fact that gonorrheal infection of the endocervix reaches the tube by direct mucosa-to-mucosa extension along the endometrium and the endosalpinx. Interruption of this glandular surface was considered a logical step in preventing reinfection. The major advantage of this procedure was the lack of interference of the blood supply of the ovary and preservation of the uterus in young women. Falk *et al.* reported a clinical cure rate of 85 per cent and an improvement in 14 per cent. At the present time, however, the use of antibiotics has essentially replaced the use of this operation. In the event that major symptoms from chronic pelvic inflammatory disease should develop, more definitive surgery as outlined is more commonly used today. Unfortunately, separation of the tubes from the uterus does not eliminate the chronic symptoms produced by pelvic pain from scar and enlarged hydrosalpinges.

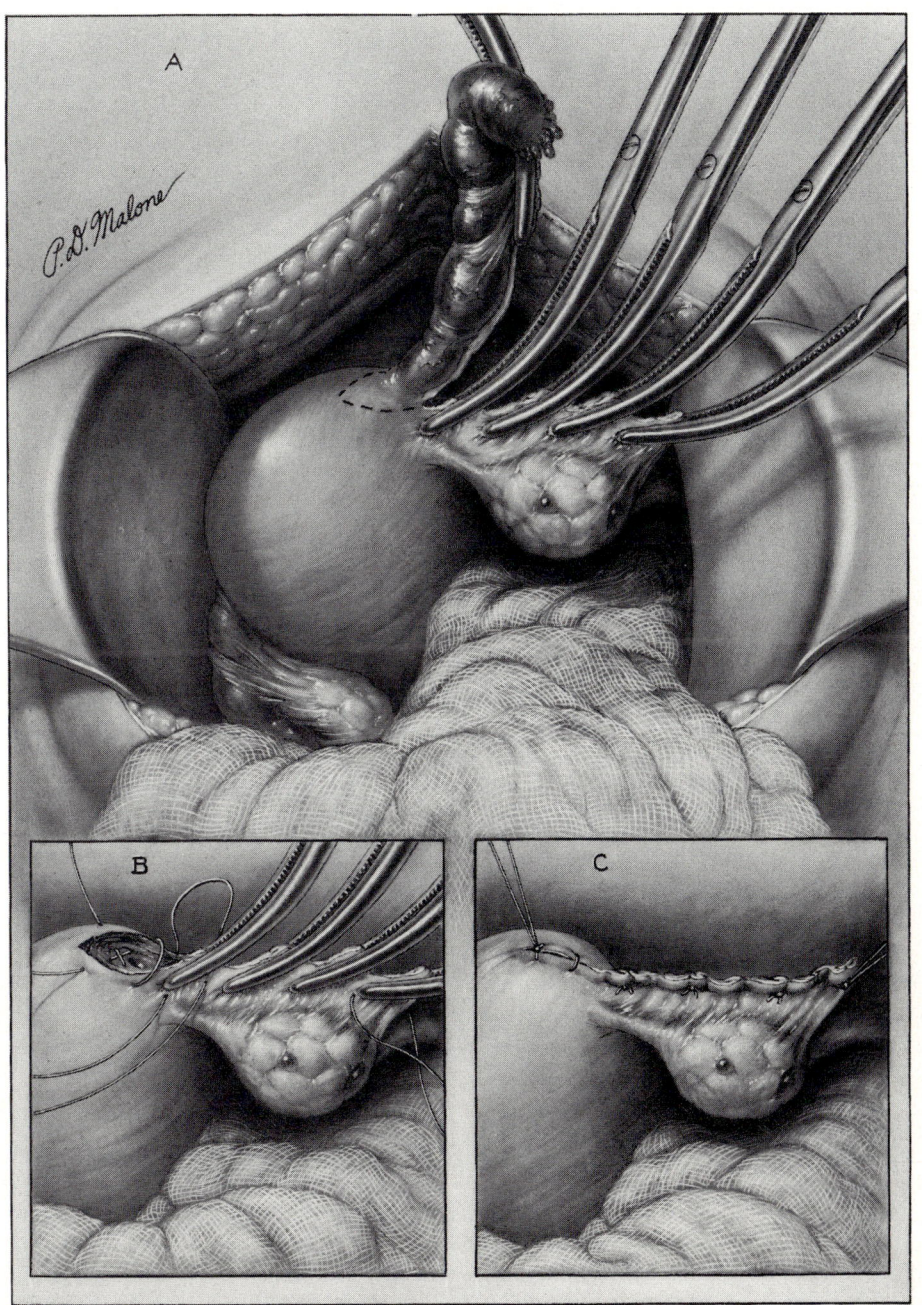

FIG. 11-6. Salpingectomy. (A) Mesosalpinx is clamped with multiple Kelly clamps and cut. Dotted line indicates cornual excision. (B) Cornual wound is closed with a figure-of-eight suture. (C) Mesosalpinx vessels are transfixed.

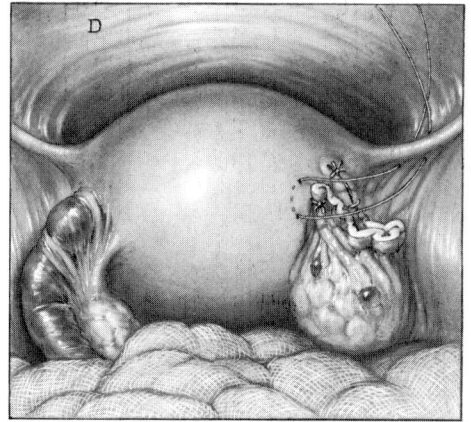
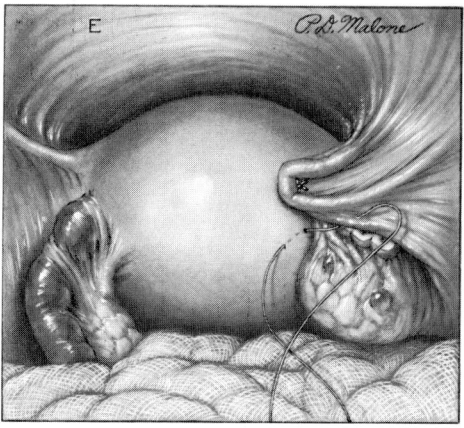
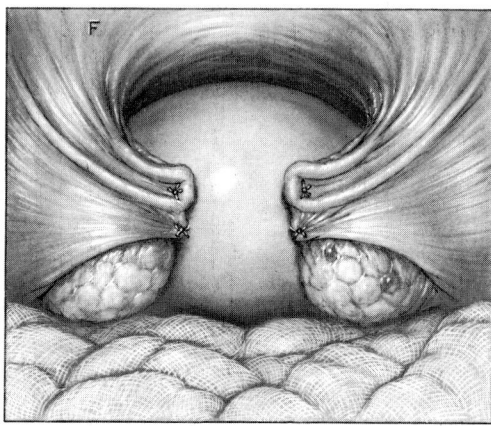

Fig. 11-6 (*Continued*). Salpingectomy. (D) Mesosalpinx has been turned back and sutured to cornu. Mattress suture is placed to cover operative area. (E) Round and broad ligaments cover cornual wound and mesosalpinx. (F) Modified Coffey suspension holds uterus forward and completely peritonizes operative area.

Technic: Salpingectomy

The adhesions binding the tube down are cut, and the tube is free. It is held up by a Kelly clamp placed on the mesosalpinx just beneath the fimbriated end. The mesosalpinx is then clamped and cut, taking a succession of small bites as close to the tube as possible (Fig. 11-6 A). By keeping the operative trauma as far as possible from the ovary that is to be retained, there is less danger of imperiling its blood supply. Experience has shown that the ovary whose tube has been removed is more apt to become cystic than the ovary whose tube has been undisturbed. Therefore it would seem logical to interfere as little as possible with the blood supply of the ovary by hugging the tube closely when excising it.

The tube is excised at the uterine cornu in a wedge-shaped manner as indicated by the dotted line in Figure 11-6 B. If there is palpable extension of the inflammation at the uterine cornu, the wedge may be rather large.

The wound at the uterine cornu is closed with one or more figure-of-eight sutures of No. 0 chromic catgut. The vessels in the mesosalpinx are ligated with mattress sutures of No. 0 chromic catgut. The mattress suture has the advantage that it will not slip off the tissue when tied as the clamp is withdrawn (Fig. 11-6 C).

If the broad ligament is sufficiently pliable, the distal end of the mesosalpinx is sutured to the cornu. This bunches up the cut edge of the mesosalpinx so that it can be covered easily with the broad ligament.

A mattress suture of No. 0 chromic catgut is taken to bring the broad and the round ligaments over the cornual wound

(Fig. 11-6 D). This suture passes just beneath the round ligament so that the ligament will not be strangulated when the suture is drawn tight. When this suture is tied, the cornual wound is covered with the broad ligament, and to some extent the uterus is suspended in a manner similar to that used in the Coffey suspension.

Usually a second mattress or interrupted suture is necessary to cover over the mesosalpinx completely, as shown in Figure 11-6 E.

At the conclusion of a bilateral salpingectomy the picture is as shown in Figure 11-6 F. The operative areas are completely covered with peritoneum. The uterus is held forward, and the ovaries are well suspended so that they cannot prolapse into the cul-de-sac.

Technic: Salpingo-oophorectomy for Chronic Salpingitis

The tubo-ovarian mass is first dissected free, and the infundibulopelvic ligament is identified. It is doubly clamped with

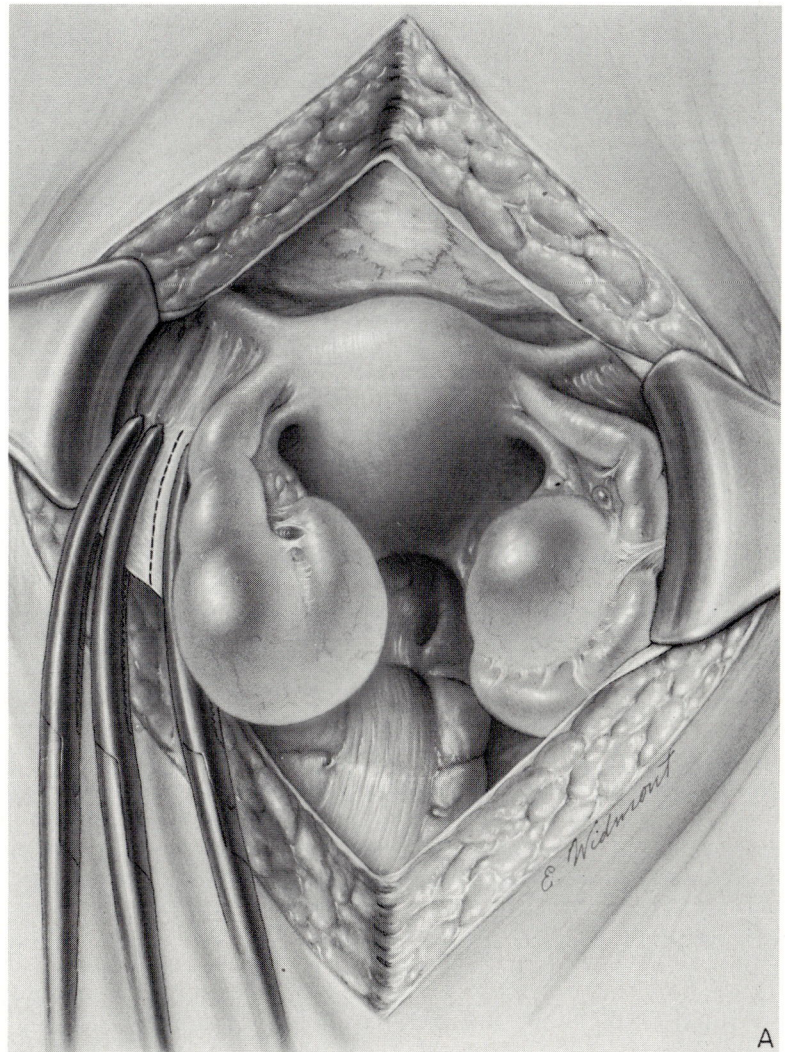

Fig. 11-7. Salpingo-oophorectomy. (A) The infundibulopelvic ligament is doubly clamped. Another clamp is placed to control back-bleeding. Dotted line indicates incision.

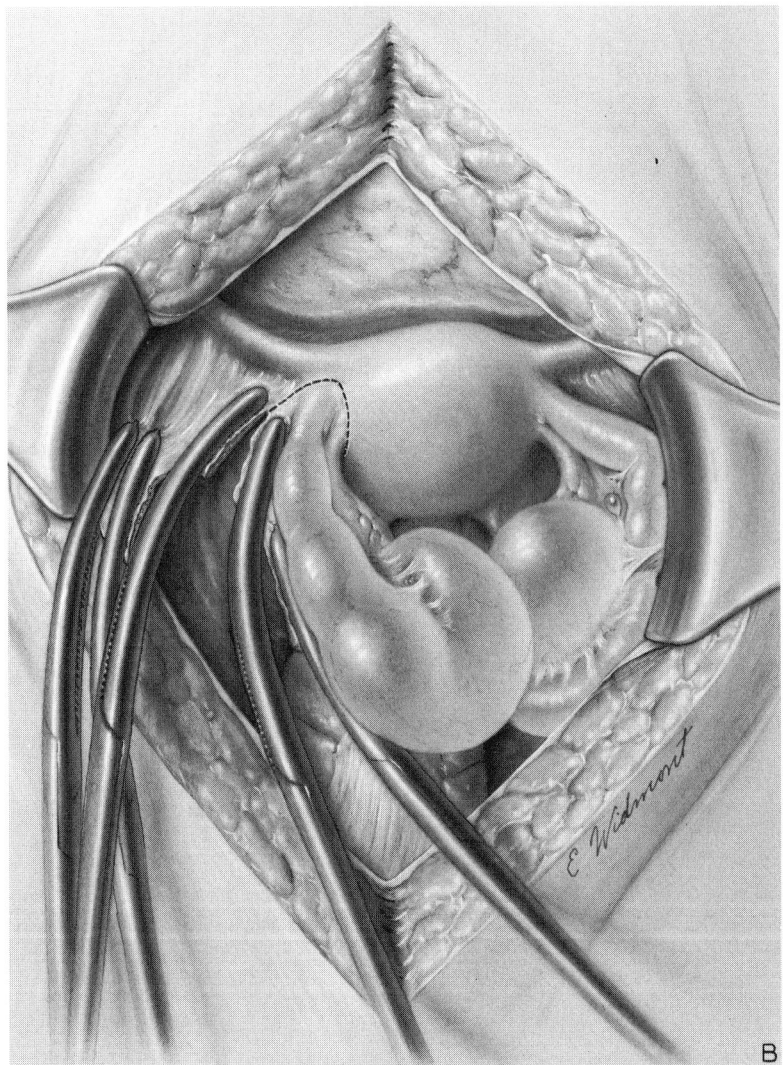

FIG. 11-7 (*Continued*). Salpingo-oophorectomy. (B) All of the mesosalpinx has been clamped and cut. Dotted line indicates wedge-shaped excision of tube and ovarian ligament at uterine cornu.

Ochsner clamps, and a third clamp is applied to control back-bleeding (Fig. 11-7 A).

The infundibulopelvic ligament is cut, and the remainder of the broad ligament attachment of the tube and the ovary is clamped and cut, as shown in Figure 11-7 B.

The uterine end of the tube and the ovarian ligament are excised from the uterus in a wedge-shaped manner as indicated by the dotted line in Figure 11-7 B.

The ascending uterine vessels are ligated just below the cornual wound, and the cornual incision is closed with a figure-of-eight suture of No. 0 chromic catgut (Fig. 11-7 C).

The infundibulopelvic ligament is doubly ligated, and the vessels in the broad ligament are ligated with No. 0 chromic catgut.

The cornual wound is peritonized, and the uterus is suspended to some degree by bringing the round and the broad ligaments over the uterine cornu with a

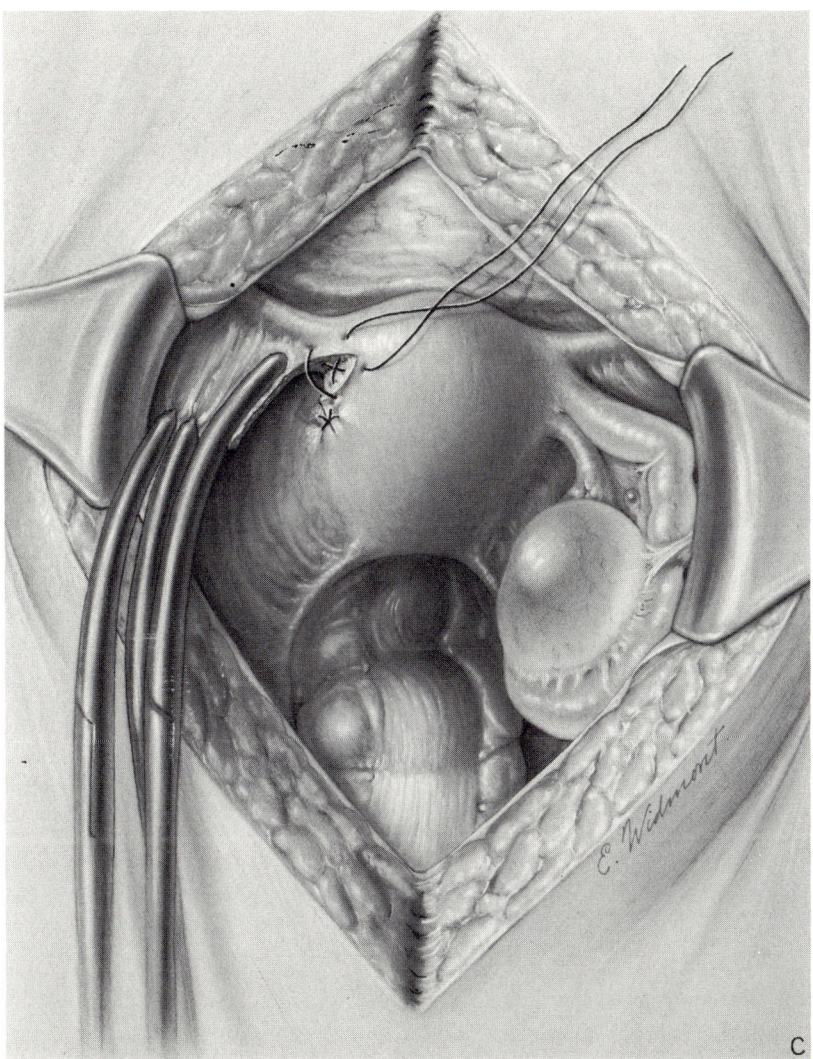

Fig. 11-7 (*Continued*). Salpingo-oophorectomy. (C) A suture has been placed so as to ligate the ascending uterine vessels just below cornual incision. The cornual incision is being closed with a figure-of-eight of No. 0 chromic catgut.

mattress suture of No. 0 chromic catgut, as shown in Figure 11-7 D.

Figure 11-7 E shows the completed unilateral salpingo-oophorectomy.

Technic: Bisection Operation

This operation is rarely indicated today but occasionally can be used to advantage in very severely inflamed pelves.

If possible, the reflexion of the bladder peritoneum is cut at the beginning of the operation, and the bladder is pushed down slightly with a sponge on a sponge stick. Because of the extensive pelvic inflammatory disease, it may be impossible to do this. In such instances care must be exercised in performing the bisection to avoid injury to the bladder, which may be adherent high up on the anterior surface of the uterus.

An incision is made down through the midline of the uterus until the level of supravaginal amputation is reached. Of necessity this may vary because of bladder adhesions. Bleeding from cut myometrium is controlled by grasping each

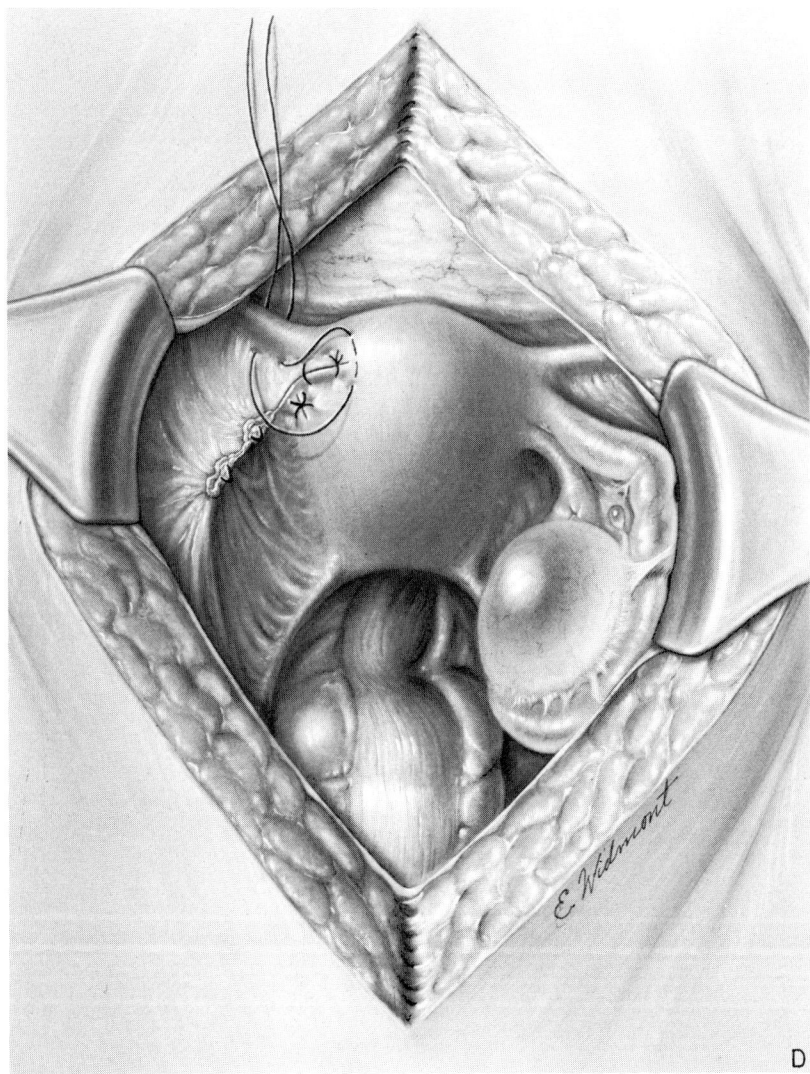

FIG. 11-7 (*Continued*). Salpingo-oophorectomy. (D) Infundibulopelvic ligament and rest of broad ligament vessels have been ligated. Cornual wound is being covered with the round and the broad ligament by use of a mattress suture of No. 0 chromic catgut.

half of the uterus with large vulsellum clamps. Then the incision is turned laterally to amputate half of the corpus uteri from the cervix. When the region of the uterine artery and veins is approached, the vessels are clamped with a curved Ochsner clamp (Fig. 11-8 A). After opening the broad ligament in this manner, the adnexal mass can usually be dissected free from its bed from below. The round ligament is isolated for clamping and cutting (Fig. 11-8 B). This operation is done only in the most severe cases of pelvic inflammatory disease when dissection of the adnexal mass cannot be done with safety from above. Therefore it is rarely done when adnexa are to be conserved; hence it is usually the infundibulopelvic ligament that is clamped, cut, and sutured.

The same procedure is carried out on the opposite side. Then the suspension of the cervix and peritonization are carried out as after the usual subtotal hys-

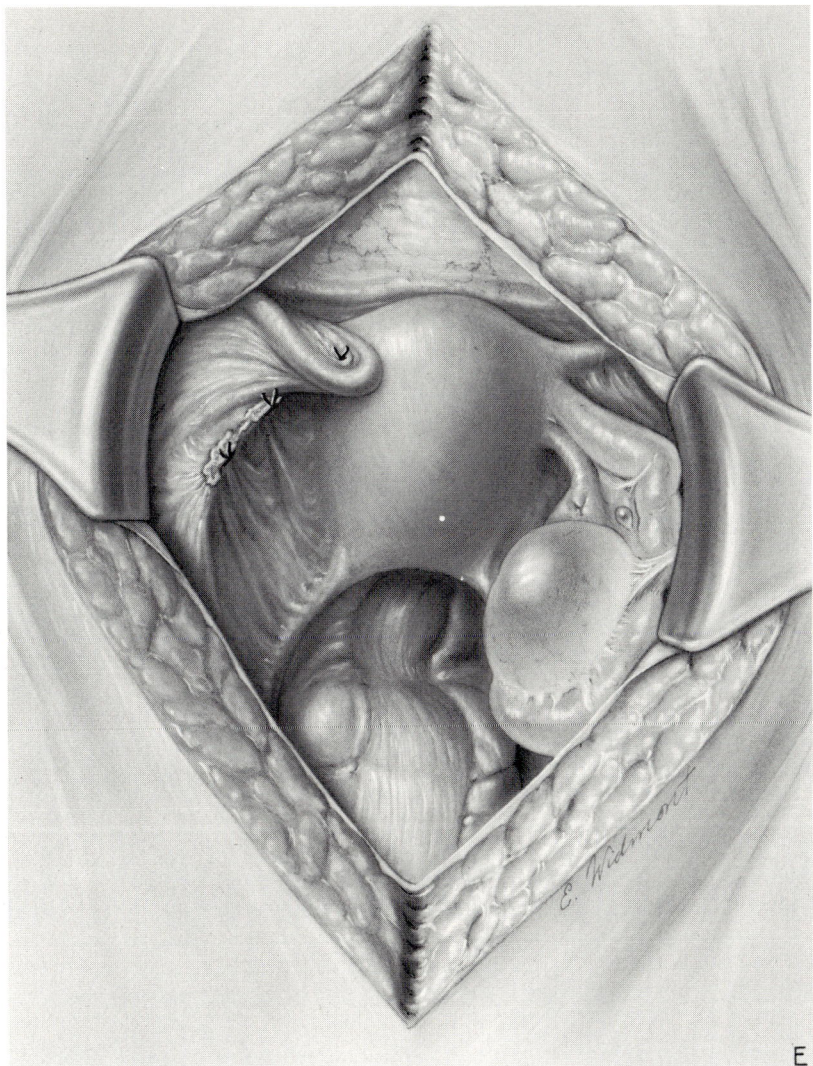

Fig. 11-7 (*Continued*). Salpingo-oophorectomy. (E) Shows operation completed on the left side.

terectomy. In this operation, as in the usual hysterectomy, the cardinal vessels are doubly ligated with No. 0 chromic catgut. Suture of the cervix is done with No. 0 or No. 1 chromic catgut, and peritonization is carried out with No. 000 chromic catgut.

Identification and Intubation of Ureter

Identification of the course of the ureter in the female pelvis where the pelvic anatomy has become obliterated as a result of chronic pelvic inflammatory disease is perhaps one of the most difficult and hazardous responsibilities of the gynecologist. In the surgical treatment of this disease, one frequently finds a tubo-ovarian inflammatory mass which is located between the leaves of the broad ligament and extends to the lateral pelvic wall. It is not uncommon for this "ligneous induration" of the thickened parietal peritoneum to obscure completely the location and course of the pelvic ureter so that dissection of the diseased adnexa produces a great surgical

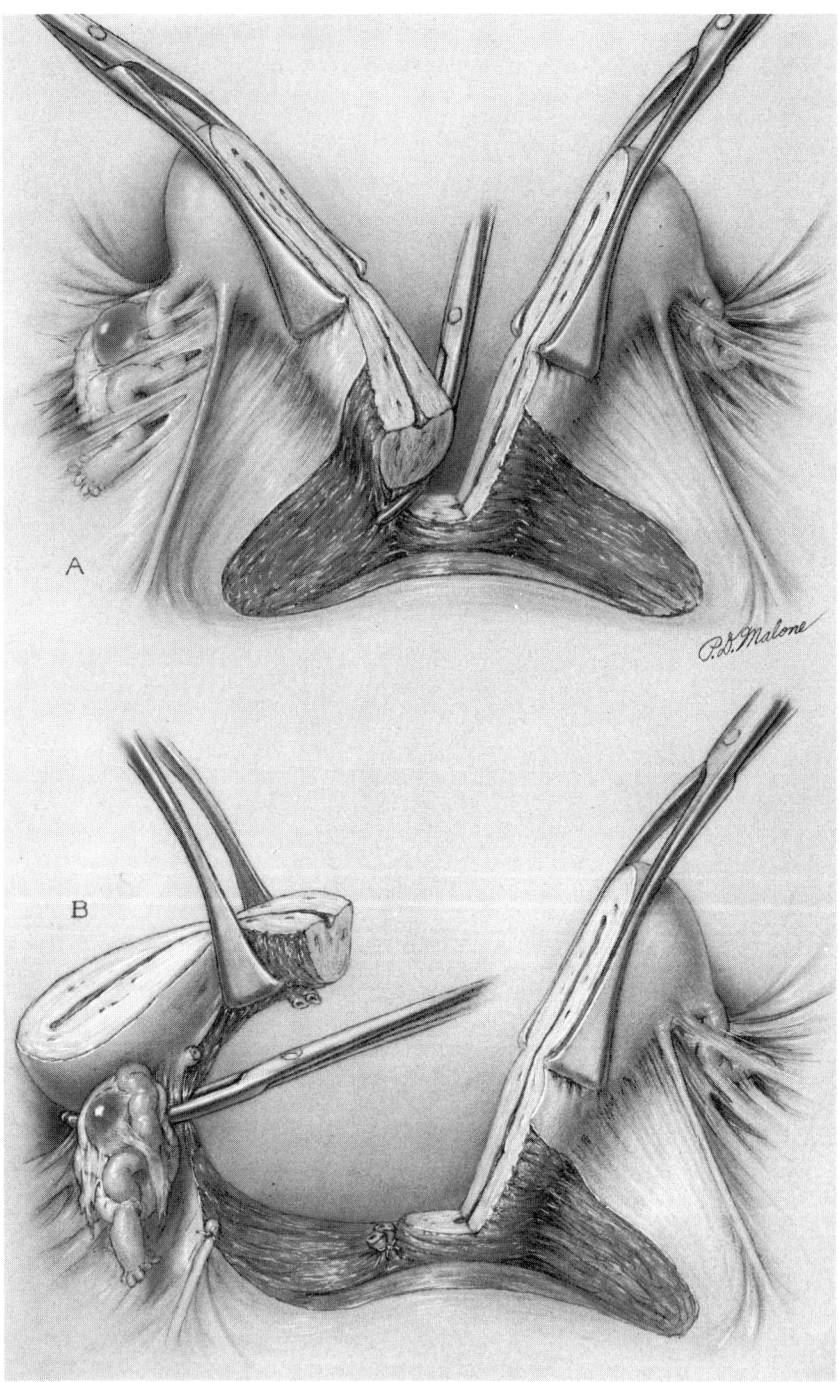

FIG. 11-8. Bisection operation. (A) The uterus has been bisected, and bleeding is controlled by grasping each half with vulsellum clamps. The right uterine vessel is being clamped. (B) Dissection has been carried laterally from below, and the infundibulopelvic ligament has been isolated and clamped.

risk to the urinary tract. Incorporation of the ureter into the posterior wall of an adnexal mass requires the pelvic surgeon to exercise great technical skill to avoid ureteral injury. Knowledge of the normal anatomic location of the pelvic ureters, as discussed in Chapter 12 (Operative Injury of the Ureters) is essential in order to identify accurately these vital structures *before* attempting to remove such adnexal masses blindly. Ideally, such patients should have the advantage of preoperative ureteral catheterization where there is clinical evidence of large, adherent adnexal masses, either benign or malignant. However, when the gynecologist finds himself confronted with such an anatomic problem at the time of laparotomy, we have no hesitancy in isolating, opening, and intubating the ureter as it crosses the pelvic brim near the bifurcation of the iliac artery.

Technic: Ureterostomy and Abdominal Catheterization of Ureter

The parietal peritoneum is opened lateral to the bifurcation of the iliac artery to avoid initial injury to the ureter, which is located medial to this landmark. Once identified, a small segment of the ureter is freed from the overlying peritoneum and stabilized by Allis clamps placed carefully on the periureteral fascia. A small 1-cm. longitudinal incision is made through the anterior wall of the ureter (Fig. 11-9). Particular care must be taken not to open the ureter transversally because of damage to the blood vessels which course the length of the ureter longitudinally. The posterior wall must not be traumatized because of the possibility of failure of healing and retroperitoneal fistula formation. A ureteral catheter, preferably No. 6 or No. 7, is then passed down the ureter, through the ureterovesical junction, and into the bladder (Fig. 11-9 A). A Silastic catheter is much more malleable and is preferable, in our hands, particularly in the case in which a splinting catheter is to be left in the ureter. In such instances the proximal end of the Silastic tube is threaded up the ureter to the kidney pelvis. The pelvic dissection is now performed with easy reference to the course of the ureter by gentle palpation of the indwelling catheter. At the completion of the procedure the catheter may either be removed or left in place and the small ureteral defect closed loosely with 2 or 3 interrupted sutures of No. 0000 chromic catgut which approximate serosa to serosa (Fig. 11-9 B). In such cases we have not found it necessary to drain the retroperitoneal space at the site of the ureterostomy unless there is some evidence of obstructive uropathy present which may influence healing and permit ureteral leakage.

Drainage at Laparotomy for Salpingitis

Views on drainage at laparotomy for pelvic inflammatory disease have changed markedly during the past several years. Whereas drainage was an everyday occurrence in gynecologic operating rooms of 3 decades ago, it is used only occasionally in our operating room today. Several factors are responsible for this change. Operations for acute and subacute pelvic inflammatory disease are avoided; hence pus is encountered less frequently. Even where small pockets of pus are encountered, experience has shown that the pus may be wiped away and the abdomen closed with impunity without drainage. Antibiotic therapy has also reduced the indications for drainage. The operator is justified in depending on antibiotics to be administered postoperatively to combat the infection.

Practically the only occasions when the authors use drainage in laparotomy for salpingitis, aside from drainage of ruptured tubo-ovarian abscesses, as discussed above, are those occasions when part of a necrotic abscess wall is, through necessity, left adherent in the pelvis, or when the bowel has been entered accidentally and its closure has not been entirely satisfactory. When an abscess is found densely adherent to the bowel wall or the region of the ureter, a thorough removal of all of the wall might result in damage to a viscus. In such cases small portions of necrotic abscess wall should be left in situ and a cigarette drain placed against the area. The ideal exit for such a

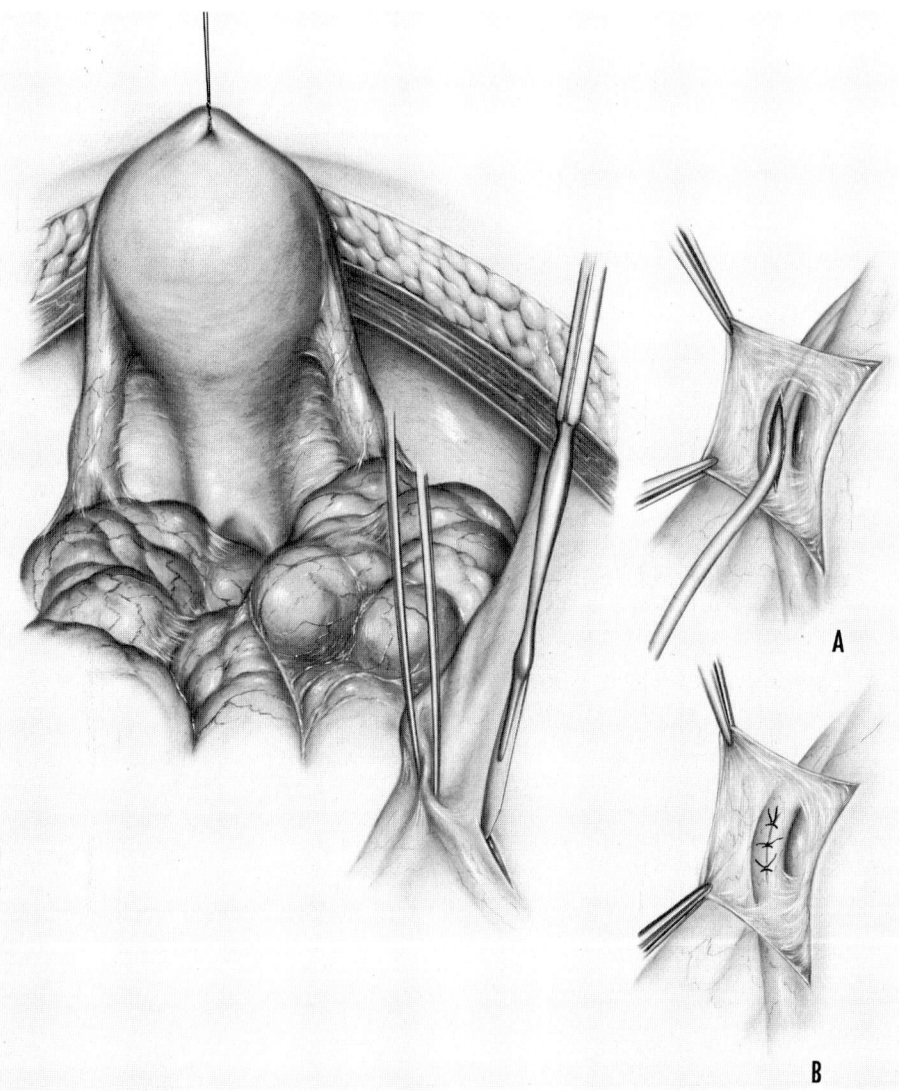

Fig. 11-9. Ureterostomy and temporary catheterization of pelvic ureter for identification. Ureter is identified as it enters the pelvis at the bifurcation of common iliac vessels. Peritoneum is incised on lateral side of ureter to preserve blood supply from medial side. (A) Shows small (1-cm.) incision through ureteral wall with insertion of Silastic tubing or ureteral catheter as splint. (B) Shows loose closure of ureteral incision with fine chromic sutures.

cigarette drain is through the cul-de-sac, as shown in Figure 11-10. Sometimes the cul-de-sac is completely obliterated by adhesions between the anterior rectal wall and the cervix. In such instances the use of the posterior vaginal vault for drainage is not feasible. When drainage is indicated under such circumstances, it should be done through a small stab wound in either lower quadrant which is most directly above the point to be drained (Fig. 11-11). We dislike drainage through midline incisions because of the danger of hernia formation and incisional infection, and only resort to it there when it is imperative and the condition of the patient is so precarious that the abdomen must be closed in the quickest possible

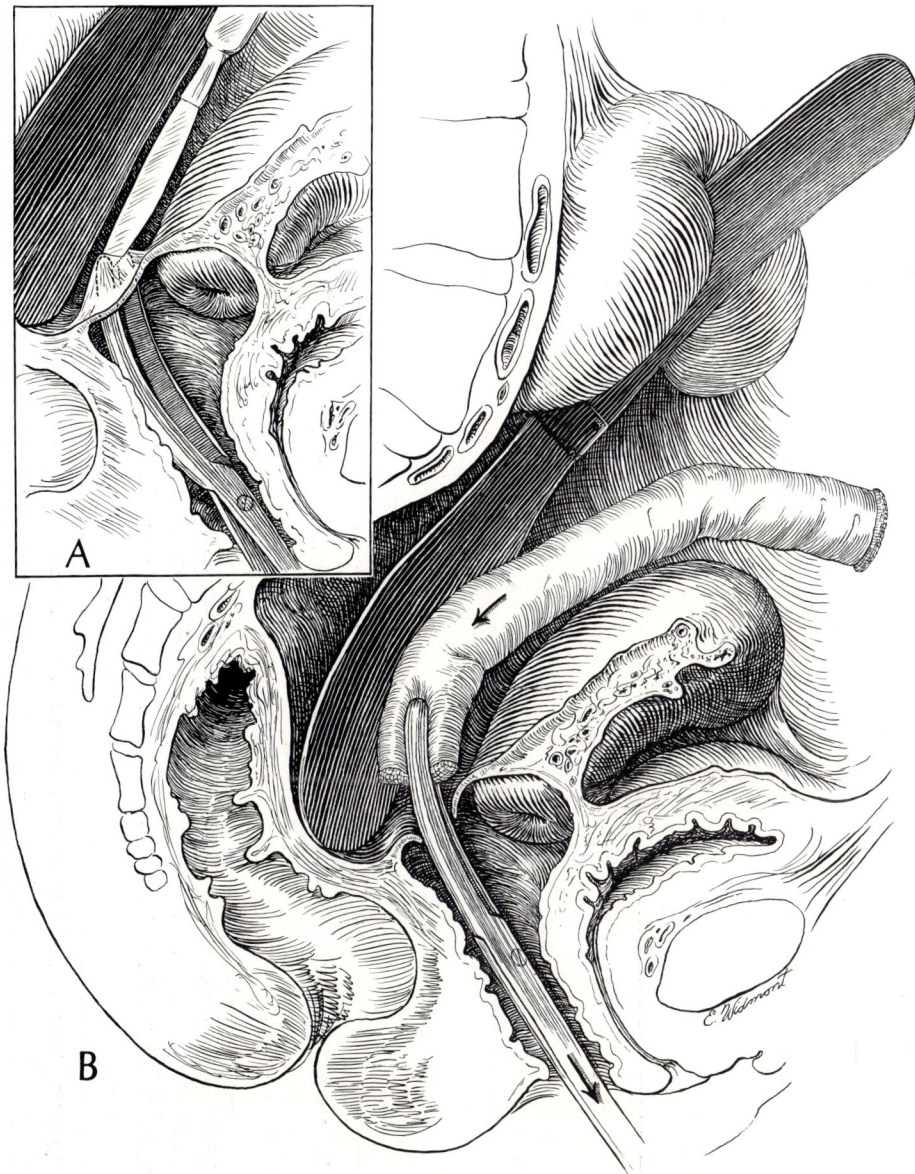

FIG. 11-10. Drainage of pelvis through cul-de-sac. (A) A long Kelly clamp is inserted into the vagina and opened slightly as the cul-de-sac is pushed upward. The scalpel incises between the jaws of the clamp. (B) Cigarette drain has been placed in the jaws of the clamp, and the clamp is withdrawn into vagina.

time. When the bowel has been entered accidentally and a perfectly satisfactory closure of healthy bowel wall effected, the abdomen is closed without drainage, and the patient is placed on streptomycin and penicillin. If the condition of the bowel wall is such that satisfactory closure cannot be done, a cigarette drain is placed down to the point of bowel injury and brought out through a stab wound.

An unruptured pelvic abscess that fails to present in the cul-de-sac may occasionally require abdominal drainage for control of a septic clinical course. Occasion-

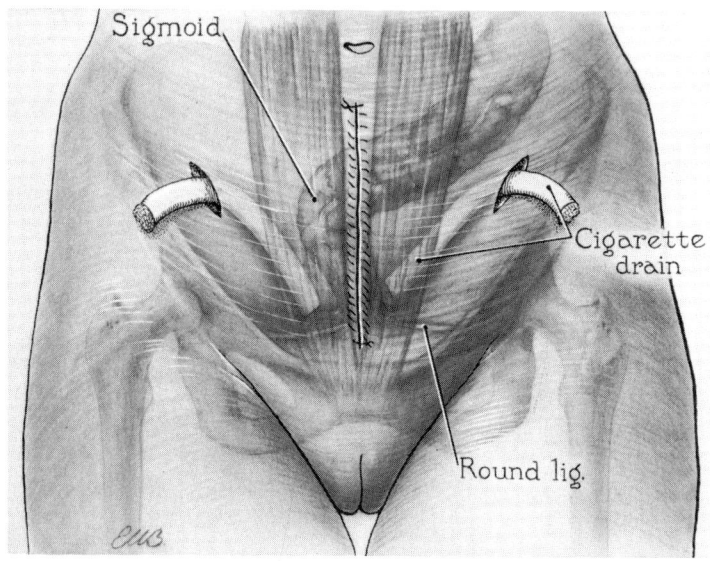

FIG. 11-11. Illustrating bilateral transabdominal drainage through stab wounds.

ally, puerperal infection may progress into a perimetritis and tubo-ovarian abscess which remains localized in the broad ligament region. A gridiron or stab wound incision in the lower quadrant of the abdomen provides an excellent retroperitoneal approach to the pelvic abscess. Care must be taken in directing a long Kelly clamp beneath the peritoneum into the pelvis to avoid trauma to the iliac vessels and the ureter, which cross the pelvic brim in this region. The cigarette drain is placed deep into the abscess cavity in order to avoid displacement by movement of the patient.

SEPTIC SHOCK

Historically, the rare occurrence of bacteremia and shock resulting from a severe infection of the female reproductive tract was usually lethal. During the past quarter of a century the effective control of gram-positive organisms with broad-spectrum antibiotics has accentuated the perplexing clinical problems of gram-negative bacteremia. Although the clinical entity of gram-negative bacteremia was first reported by Brill and Libman in 1899, the sporadic occurrence of shock associated with such infections was not clearly defined until 1951, when Waisbren pointed out the specific "shocklike picture" in patients with gram-negative bacteremia. The association of gram-negative shock with an endotoxin from the degenerating cell wall of gram-negative bacilli was first proposed by Borden and Hall in 1951 and confirmed by Braude and associates in 1953. While there is general acceptance of the view that endotoxin, a lipid polysaccharide, is the etiologic cause of neurogenic shock in gram-negative septicemia, the precise pathophysiologic changes resulting in irreversible shock are still unresolved.

In addition, a less frequent but more lethal type of septic shock results from an exotoxin, produced mainly by *Clostridium welchii* (*C. perfringens*), under anaerobic conditions. The histotoxic effect of this gram-positive, encapsulated bacillus produces not only profound vasomotor collapse with neurogenic shock but also massive intravascular hemolysis with secondary anemia, and a nephrotoxic effect resulting in acute tubular necrosis and aneuria. The tissue effect of gas gangrene is an anaerobic myositis, seen not only in the skeletal and smooth muscles but as a myocarditis as well. Such complications of an advanced stage of a *Clostridium* infection accounts for the high mortality rate, varying between 50 and 75 per cent.

Gram-Negative Endotoxic Shock

Septic abortion remains the most frequent clinical entity associated with endotoxic shock, which reportedly occurs in 2 to 6 per cent of such pelvic infections. While Deane and Russell report approximately 2 per cent incidence of septic shock of all abortion patients admitted to the Los Angeles County Hospital, endotoxic shock occurred in 18 per cent (Weil, 1964) of all obstetric patients admitted with bacteremia to this hospital. In general, when bacteremia from a gram-negative organism occurs, approximately 20 to 30 per cent of such patients will develop septic shock. In addition, septic shock is a recognized clinical complication of advanced pelvic neoplastic disease, ruptured tubo-ovarian abscess, chorioamnionitis and acute pyelonephritis. Except for the obstetric patient, the elderly patient is more susceptible to bacteremic shock, which is usually associated with some preciptiating event such as pelvic surgery, criminal induction of abortion, or instrumentation of the urinary tract. Patients with urinary tract infection, diabetes, and hepatic disease are more susceptible to bacteremic shock.

Pathophysiology of Endotoxic Shock

While numerous attempts have been made to identify the basic mechanisms underlying endotoxic shock, the current confusion results from reports on experimental animal studies that conflict with the clinical observations in the human. However, there have been few well-controlled studies in humans suffering from septic shock to provide a clear understanding of exact pathophysiology.

The essential features of endotoxic shock are characterized by sudden hypotension, decreased renal function, and peripheral pooling of blood, with resultant metabolic acidosis and cell death. The focal point of this septic event is the effect of endotoxin on the microcirculation of the peripheral capillary bed, producing increased peripheral vascular resistance involving particularly the vital organs and splanchnic circulation.

Clinical experience to date suggests that hypotension is caused initially by increased peripheral resistance and pooling of blood in the expansive capillary network, which includes more than 90 per cent of the vascular circulation. Recent evidence by Morris supports the view that the capillary bed of the lung may form part of this large peripheral reservoir. Similarities of the clinical and pathologic changes in septic shock with those seen in the generalized Shwartzman reaction, including disseminated intravascular coagulation, as described by McKay and others, suggests a hypersensitivity reaction as the etiologic factor. Clinical studies by Phillips and coworkers on patients with infected abortion confirm the findings of intravascular coagulation with renal cortical necrosis and activation of the fibrinolytic system with resultant hemorrhage. While intravascular coagulation is an attractive proposal for irreversible shock due to thrombotic plugging of the microcirculation, it is difficult to prove that these changes occur prior to the development of toxic shock rather than as a result of venous pooling. Treatment of septic shock with heparin could be useful only prior to the development of intravascular clotting and could be detrimental rather than beneficial if given after intravascular clotting had occurred.

The peripheral vascular effect of endotoxin, either directly or indirectly, is one of intense vasoconstriction resulting in structural injury to the vascular musculature and loss of vascular tone, with pooling of blood in the venules and veins. This neurotoxic effect of circulating endotoxin has been demonstrated by Fine by the absence of injury to the vascular musculature in areas that were denervated in advance of the injection of the endotoxin. Consequently, prevention of this vascular insult by the use of alpha-adrenergic blocking agents would be rational during the early stage of septic shock. Although Nickerson, Lillehei, and many others report the protective effects of phenoxybenzamine (Dibenzyline) in endotoxic shock, our own experience favors the use of isoproterenol (Isuprel), as explained below.

METABOLIC EFFECTS OF SEPTIC SHOCK

The most accurate method of monitoring the effects of anaerobic cellular metabolism from anoxia is by arterial pH and blood lactate levels. In one of the most elaborate clinical studies available in the human, MacLean and coworkers clearly demonstrate that the mortality in septic shock is related to two stages of the disease process. Early septic shock, in which patients are normovolemic before the onset of the bacteremia, is characterized by hyperventilation and respiratory alkalosis with an elevated blood pH, high central venous pressure, *low* peripheral resistance, elevated blood volume, hypotension, oliguria, and *warm*, dry extremities with elevated blood lactate levels. If recognized while the patient is still alkalotic, and if aggressive supportive measures are used to improve cardiac output by increasing blood volume to maximum levels and utilizing the inotropic effect of isoproterenol (Isuprel), the clinical result is quite successful when combined with appropriate surgery. In contrast, if the patient is hypovolemic at the onset of sepsis, the clinical picture is one of low central venous pressure, low cardiac output, *high* peripheral resistance, and *cold* cyanotic extremities. If septic shock is not detected until the patient is severely acidotic, as determined by a low arterial blood pH and a progressively rising blood lactate, cardiac output remains low despite all forms of treatment, and a high mortality rate results.

In 56 patients with septic shock studied by MacLean, only 6 of 38 patients died of shock when treatment was started before the onset of severe metabolic acidosis. Only 1 of 18 patients survived when treatment was started after the onset of metabolic acidosis. As demonstrated in their study, the requirement of 2 to 3 times the normal cardiac output is frequently necessary to provide adequate tissue blood flow. When septic shock is not recognized early and treated promptly by surgical drainage and hemodynamic support, these patients progress to an acidotic phase which is refractory to all present forms of therapy, and death is almost certain. Hyperbaric oxygen at 3 atmospheres of absolute pressure was not beneficial in MacLean's experience even though the arterial blood oxygen tension was elevated considerably. While the idea of delivering more oxygen to the tissue during shock is appealing, the value of hyperbaric oxygen remains to be established.

An additional prognostic feature of patients with septic shock is related to myocardial reserve. In the Montreal study by MacLean, patients who were unable to raise their cardiac index above 1 liter/minute/M^2 in response to treatment had a very poor survival rate.

BACTERIOLOGY

Gram-negative endotoxic shock may be produced by a variety of enteric bacilli, but the most common pathogen is *Escherichia coli,* which accounts for more than 50 per cent of the cases. In addition, *Klebsiella, Aerobacter aerogenes, Proteus, Pseudomonas,* and paracolon bacillus are known to produce clinical infection and shock. Frequently, two gram-negative species are cultured from the bloodstream, in which cases a much higher mortality rate is seen. In contrast, septic shock resulting from an exotoxin is produced primarily by *Clostridium welchii (C. perfringens)* although *C. novyi, septicum,* and *histolyticum* do produce similar histotoxic infections in man.

CLINICAL FEATURES

The earliest symptoms of septic shock are rarely recognized by either the clinician or the patient. These include mild anxiety, slight mental confusion, and disorientation. The earliest clinical signs are those of respiratory distress with hyperventilation, which is clinically misinterpreted as atelectasis, pneumonia, possible pulmonary embolism, or even myocardial infarction. If accurately detected at this early stage, hyperventilation is associated with a respiratory alkalosis, a normal or high central venous pressure, low peripheral resistance, hypotension, oliguria, elevated blood lactate, and warm, dry extremities. When the disease becomes clinically well established, shaking chills usually precede the onset of shock, and a spiking temperature, frequently above 104° F., is a common finding. Occasionally, patients will have a transient subnormal temperature, which may coincide with a low white blood count. When intense vasoconstriction has become well established with an increased peripheral resistance, the clinical picture is characterized by cold clammy skin, and shock. Nausea, vomiting, and diarrhea, occasionally bloody, are clinical manifestations of vasospasm involving the intestinal tract. Oliguria and subsequent anuria present clinical signs of advanced vasoconstriction and renal ischemia.

Treatment

In general, the same principles for the management of hemorrhagic shock apply equally to the patient with septic shock. For purposes of brevity, these will not be repeated in detail, but the reader is referred to Chapter 4 for a more detailed discussion. The practical approach to the control of septic shock is directed toward three parameters: (1) immediate replacement of a normal circulating blood volume with continuous monitoring of central venous pressure; (2) rapid bacteriostatic control of the gram-negative bacteremia with appropriate, effective antibiotics; (3) early surgical drainage and/or excision of the infected reproductive organ.

Due to the wide variety of clinical entities producing gram-negative shock, a therapeutic outline which would specifically relate to each clinical problem is beyond the scope of this presentation. However, a brief outline of our approach to the medical and surgical management of septic shock may be of interest:

1. Replacement of Intravascular Volume. A decrease in vasomotor tone produces peripheral vascular pooling and enlargement of the intravascular space. While whole blood is the most ideal agent for intravascular fluid replacement, due to its influence on oxygen transport to peripheral tissues, blood replacement should be limited to normal red cell mass as determined by blood volume studies. Admittedly, such radioisotope-labeled studies may not be completely accurate due to poor mixing of the blood and peripheral pooling, and yet it does serve as an additional guideline for whole blood replacement in the early stage of endotoxic shock. In order to replace the intravascular compartment adequately, it is essential to do so by central venous pressure monitoring, preferably by the subclavian or jugular route with the catheter placed in the superior vena cava for accurate recordings. The use of normal saline, low-molecular-weight dextran (mol. wt. 40,000) (dextran 40), and glucose are most effective in restoring the circulating blood volume to normal levels as measured by a central venous pressure of 15 cm. H_2O. Fluid requirements usually exceed clinical estimates of volume deficit when replaced by central venous monitoring. In fact, amounts of 8 to 12 liters of fluid are frequently required before adequate support of circulating blood volume is achieved. Accurate monitoring of the hourly urine output with measurement of specific gravity of the urine is one of the most sensitive clinical barometers available in determining adequate total blood volume.

In our experience the immediate results of fluid replacement depend more on the *amount* of fluid replaced than on the *type* of fluid used. Although advocated by some investigators, it is our feeling that lactate is undesirable as a volume replacement due to the presence of lactic acidosis as a consequence of shock.

Vigorous efforts should be made to correct severe acidosis with the use of bicarbonate, as it is our belief that myocardial contractility and vasomotor function of the pre- and postcapillary sphincters are adversely influenced by a high blood lactate level and a low pH. One must recognize, however, that acidosis will persist until adequate tissue oxygen replaces the anaerobic cell metabolism.

2. Antibiotics. While several blood cultures should be taken, preferably at the height of a febrile occurrence, it is important to initiate a broad-spectrum antibiotic coverage immediately in an effort to control the bacteremia rapidly. In addition, culture of the cervical canal or ruptured pelvic abscess and a direct smear for gram stain should be obtained prior to treatment for evaluation of the possible presence of gram-positive encapsulated rods *(Clostridium welchii)*. Chloromycetin is one of the most effective antibiotics against *E. coli* and other gram-negative bacilli. The combination of chloromycetin (1 gm. q.i.d.) and streptomycin (0.5 gm. b.i.d.) has produced the best clinical results in our hands. In addition, penicillin, although ineffective for gram-negative organisms in low doses, has recently been advocated in massive dose of 80 to 100 million units per day by Moore. In our own clinic, we give 30 to 60 million units of penicillin intravenously with I.V. chloromycetin and I.M. streptomycin daily. It is important to use the most sensitive antibiotic available since our experience corresponds with Weil's study, which revealed only 8.5 per cent survival when antibiotic treatment was administered to resistant organisms.

3. **Corticosteroids.** The addition of corticosteroids has been strongly advocated by Lillehei and others and has been shown to have a potentiating vasopressor effect when used concurrently with a vasopressor agent. When used in dosages of 50 mg./kg./day in the Los Angeles County Hospital study, Weil noted an improved survival (43%) when more than 300 mg. a day of hydrocortisone or its equivalent dosage of other corticoids was used. Where hydrocortisone of less than 300 mg. a day was used, there was a mortality of 85 per cent. One of the beneficial effects of pharmacologic doses of corticosteroids is the control of shock when large amounts of endotoxin are liberated into the bloodstream from sudden destruction and lysis of enteric bacteria. Though there is no evidence of adrenal insufficiency in such cases, the physiologic benefit of corticoids may be due to a positive inotropic (cardiac) effect and reduction of peripheral vascular resistance, thereby improving venous return. Dexamethasone (Decadron) is used in amounts of 40 mg. initially and 20 mg. every 4 to 6 hours. These drugs are discontinued when there is clinical evidence of cardiovascular stabilization and adequate peripheral circulation.

4. **Vasopressor Drugs.** The greatest area of controversy in the treatment of shock is related to the advisability of using vasopressor agents during acute hypotension. Based on the known pathophysiologic changes of intense vasoconstriction that occurs at the pre- and post-capillary bed with the production of venous pooling, further vasoconstriction would logically be considered detrimental. However, many studies have demonstrated the effect of agents such as metaraminol (Aramine) to be effective in mobilizing pooled blood with increased venous return. An additional pharmacologic advantage of metaraminol is its known inotropic effect of improving coronary perfusion and myocardial function. It has been shown in MacLean's experience that cardiac outputs of 2 or 3 times normal volumes may be required to provide adequate tissue blood flow. Therefore it is our opinion that any agent that would effectively improve myocardial contractility and cardiac output should be utilized during septic shock. Such inotropic effects can effectively counterbalance the potential adverse effects on the peripheral circulation.

However, the clinical responsiveness to vasopressor drugs must be the guideline in the continued and possibly inappropriate use of vasopressor agents. It is undesirable to raise the systemic pressure to normal preshock levels. An optimal systolic pressure level of 20 to 30 mm. Hg below the patient's normal arterial pressure should provide adequate tissue perfusion and peripheral circulation. In the absence of a clinical response, including improvement in arterial pressure, urinary output, central venous pressure, and peripheral circulation, continued use of vasopressor drugs in higher dosage is definitely contraindicated. Metaraminol is usually titrated by an intravenous drip of 200 mg. in 1,000 cc. of glucose or saline.

5. **Vasodilator Drugs.** The controversy regarding the potential benefit of antiadrenergic drugs (alpha-adrenergic blocking agents or beta-adrenergic stimulators) was initiated 20 years ago when Wiggers demonstrated the beneficial effect of an adrenergic blocking agent, dibenamine, on hemorrhagic shock in dogs. Continued interest in the pharmacologic principle of vasodilatation as an effective method of improving peripheral circulation in the treatment of shock has been championed by Nickerson, Lillehei, and others. Phenoxybenzamine (dibenzyline) in dosages of 1 mg. per kg. of body weight in 200 ml. of saline has shown definite improvement of patients in severe shock, as evidenced by a fall in central venous pressure, an increase in cardiac index, and a decrease in peripheral resistance with a positive diuretic effect. However, it has had only limited clinical use. The effect of chlorpromazine (Thorazine) has had wider clinical experience and is effective in producing splanchnic vasodilatation and improving urinary output. While we have also found this drug to be useful in improving peripheral circulation, its pharmacologic action is singular, and produces only alpha-adrenergic inhibition.

Our own preference, at the present writing, is the use of isoproterenol (Isuprel) because of its known pharmacologic effects of (1) beta-adrenergic stimulation, resulting in peripheral vasodilatation, (2) inotropic cardiac stimulation with improvement of coronary circulation and myocardial contractions, and (3) specific pulmonary vasodilatation. When given as a dilute infusion (2 mg. in 500 ml. of dextrose or saline) at the rate of .1 to .2 mg. per hour, this drug has been the most effective method of improving cardiac output in MacLean's experience. If the circulating blood volume is not completely replaced, isoproterenol will produce a transient drop in central venous pressure and can be used as a diagnostic tool for predicting adequate volume replacement.

6. **Other Medical Methods of Treatment.** Based on the recent reports of Hardaway, McKay, Phillips, and others on the demonstration of disseminated intravascular coagulation as a late stage of septic shock, there may be evidence of hypofibrinogenemia and release of circulating fibrinolysin with acute hemorrhage. This has stimulated the use of heparin in preventing intravascular coagulation, although the major clinical problem concerns the timing of this mode of therapy. When used after intravascular coagulation has already occurred, the added effects of heparin to that of a circulating fibrinolysin may alter the blood coagulation mechanism even further.

While hyperbaric oxygen has been advocated in the treatment of tissue hypoxia, limited experience with 3 atmospheres of absolute pressure by MacLean produced no effect on a rising arterial blood lactate and cellular hypoxia. Additional experience in this technic of increasing plasma oxygen is necessary.

Prophylactic antibiotics have not been useful in preventing septic shock, as was demonstrated by Weil, who reported the subsequent death of 16 of 18 patients who were being treated with the appropriate antibiotic prior to the bacteremic shock. Such use of prophylactic antibiotics is thought to develop drug-resistant strains of gram-negative bacteria and limit the effectiveness of antimicrobial agents when septic shock becomes clinically manifest.

7. **Removal of Focus of Infection.** Although it is an accepted clinical fact that the removal of the source of endotoxin-production is essential, the timing and extent of the surgical procedure remains in question. In the past decade the concept of management of septic abortion has changed gradually from the aggressive, immediate evacuation of all septic uteri by dilatation and curettage, to a more conservative view of delay in instrumentation of the uterus until the patient is afebrile for 12 to 24 hours, during which time metabolic and fluid balance is achieved. The question raised by Neuwirth and Friedman regarding the advisability of aggressive management of all patients with septic abortion, in view

of the fact that 95 per cent or more of such patients do not develop endotoxic shock, would seem to be legitimate.

Their experience in 173 cases of septic abortion at the Sloane Hospital for Women revealed an increased risk of postoperative fever and hypotension when curettage is undertaken while the patient is still febrile or within 12 hours of defervescence. While a conservative approach with antibiotics, oxytocics, fluids, electrolyte replacement, and curettage 24 hours after defervescence would seem advisable, Douglas and Beckman advise aggressive treatment with *early* evacuation of the uterus when hypotension is discovered. The use of primary hysterectomy is the most controversial aspect of the treatment and is rarely used except for (1) *Clostridium welchii* infections, (2) evidence of chemical infusion (soap, etc.), (3) uterine perforation, and (4) clinical deterioration or failure to improve by dilatation and curettage alone. In general, the successful evacuation of the intrauterine source of infection can be determined clinically by the clinical improvement in acidosis, as shown by MacLean and others. If a patient after dilatation and curettage shows a rising arterial blood lactate or develops shock after a favorable response, an additional surgical procedure is mandatory and usually requires hysterectomy.

While there may be legitimate debate regarding the conservative or aggressive treatment of septic abortion, clinical experience with ruptured tubo-ovarian abscess has been more clear-cut. Prior to 1950 the nonoperative management of this catastrophic event was associated with a mortality rate varying between 80 and 100 per cent. In our own experience at Johns Hopkins Hospital, prior to 1944, the mortality rate was 90 per cent when most of the cases were treated medically or by simple drainage. Between 1945 and 1953 the mortality was reduced to 12 per cent by immediate hysterectomy and bilateral salpingo-oophorectomy, and has been continually improved to the current rate of 3.5 per cent. At Charity Hospital in New Orleans, Michael and coworkers have reduced their mortality by the use of primary surgery to a rate of 8.6 per cent. Similar improvement in the mortality by such treatment for ruptured tubo-ovarian abscess with septic shock has been shown in practically every clinic in this country and abroad.

Summary

Since the successful treatment of gram-negative, septic shock is directly related to successful replacement of an adequate blood volume, re-establishment of peripheral circulation, and tissue oxygenation with reduction of anaerobic cellular metabolism and resultant acidosis, as well as elimination of the source of endotoxin-production, our approach to the management of this clinical entity can be summarized as follows:

1. Central venous pressure monitoring by the subclavian or jugular route.

2. Rapid replacement of blood volume, including blood, low-molecular-weight dextran, saline, and glucose until central venous pressure reaches its maximal normal level (15 cm. H_2O). Such efforts may require 8 to 12 liters of fluid replacement.

3. Repeated blood cultures and cervical canal cultures with gram stain of direct smear for determination of the bacterial agent and source of infection.

4. High-dose, intravenous, broad-spectrum antibiotic treatment using in combination chloromycetin (3-4 gm./day), streptomycin (1 gm./day) and penicillin (30 million units/day).

5. Intravenous hydrocortisone (or equivalent) in a minimum dosage of 50 mg./kg. per day with an initial loading dose of 1 gm. at the onset of treatment.

6. Vasopressor drugs, preferably metaraminol (Aramine), with cautious intravenous titration of vasopressor effect on central venous pressure, urinary output, and peripheral perfusion. Vasopressor is not used routinely but is recommended if urinary output remains low (less than 30 ml. per hour), and a low central venous pressure persists after adequate intravascular volume replacement.

7. Vasodilator agents are recommended when there has been no clinical response from modest doses of vasopressor drugs. Isoproterenol (Isuprel) given intrave-

nously (2 mg. in 500 ml. glucose or saline) .1 to .2 mg. per hour will usually demonstrate its pharmacologic effects by support of cardiac output, improvement in peripheral circulation, and pulmonary vasodilatation. Chlorpromazine (Thorazine) may be of equal benefit in dosages of $12\frac{1}{2}$ to 25 mg. q. 4 to 6 hours by improving peripheral circulation and increasing urinary output.

8. Early removal of the focus of infection is imperative. In cases of septic abortion, conservative medical management until the patient is afebrile for 24 hours, followed by dilatation and curettage, is our preferred treatment program. In cases of septic abortion with shock, early establishment of uterine drainage by D and C is imperative as soon as cardiovascular support can be achieved as outlined above. For cases of ruptured tubo-ovarian abscess, *Clostridium* infection, uterine rupture, or failure to respind to conservative therapy, it is important to achieve rapid cardiovascular stabilization, to be followed by immediate abdominal hysterectomy and adnexectomy for the control of circulating endotoxin or exotoxin.

MORTALITY

While the range of mortality in reported cases of septic shock varies between 20 and 80 per cent, the success of any therapeutic regime is dependent on the stage of the shock and the cardiovascular injury at the time treatment is initiated. Weil reports an overall mortality of 82 per cent from septic shock at Los Angeles County Hospital, whereas Douglas and Beckman have reduced their mortality to 22 per cent. The ability of the patient to respond to the intensive treatment as outlined will probably depend on the severity of the acidosis and the degree of cellular injury. The experience of MacLean suggests that if patients are not seen until they are profoundly acidotic, a low fixed cardiac output persists, and a high mortality results in spite of vigorous treatment. With newer technics currently under investigation for improvement of peripheral vascular circulation, it is anticipated that the next decade will show even greater success in the treatment of septic shock, which currently claims approximately 50 per cent of the lives of all patients treated in this country for this clinical entity.

TUBERCULOSIS OF THE FEMALE GENITAL TRACT

The first recorded case of tuberculosis of the female genital organs was described by Morgagni in 1761. It was found in the course of an autopsy on a young woman whose tubes and uterus were filled with caseous material. Since then there has been an enormous amount of literature on the subject. In the United States there has been a decline in the incidence of tuberculosis, and with this decline in the disease generally there has been a lessening of the incidence of genital tuberculosis. The reduced incidence noted in the United States has not been the case throughout many parts of the world. Halbrecht reported on Latent Female Genital Tuberculosis at an international symposium held in Basle in 1964. Reports from 15 European and Asian countries concerning the varied epidemiologic and pathologic aspects of female genital tuberculosis were in agreement that pelvic tuberculosis is still one of the major causes of primary and secondary infertility abroad. This documented fact is in marked contrast to the infrequent occurrence and clinical expression of this disease in the United States. Among the infertility patients at Johns Hopkins and Marquette, less than 1 per cent of the patients are found to have tuberculosis of the reproductive tract. Although it is frequently stated that tuberculosis is the etiologic factor in approximately 3 to 5 per cent of the cases of pelvic inflammatory disease in this country, it is evident from the recent literature that this disease has become much less frequent during the past decade. Involvement of the female genital organs is practically always secondary to a tuberculous focus elsewhere in the body and is considered to be transmitted by the bloodstream primarily from the lung or the urinary tract.

Clinical Features

Pelvic tuberculosis may occur at an early age, but the greatest frequency is between the ages of 20 to 40. In the series of cases from the Hopkins clinic, reported by Brown, Gilbert and Te Linde, the three most common symptoms included *menstrual disorder, pelvic pain*, and *decreased fertility*. In this study the following menstrual disturbances were noted:

	Per Cent
Menorrhagia	20.2
Amenorrhea	15.8
Oligomenorrhea	11.3
Dysmenorrhea	8.8
Polymenorrhea	6.3
Intermenstrual bleeding	10.1

Although amenorrhea is frequently stated to be a major symptom of pelvic tuberculosis, in our series excessive bleeding, including menorrhagia, polymenorrhea, and intermenstrual bleeding, accounted for 46.6 per cent of the menstrual abnormality. In contrast, amenorrhea and oligomenorrhea occurred in 27.1 per cent of the cases.

Abdominal pain, occurring in 69 per cent of the patients in our recent study, was more insidious in onset than the acute pattern associated with neisserian infection.

Fever is usually of a low-grade nature, varying between 99° and 100° F. but may on occasion produce a fulminating septic course, particularly when tuberculous peritonitis or abscess formation has occurred. A classic feature of this pattern of fever in pelvic tuberculosis is its failure to subside on high doses of broad-spectrum antibiotics. Such a clinical course should always alert the clinician to the possibility of a tuberculous infection.

Clinically, tuberculous peritonitis can be divided into three groups: First, in the "wet" type of peritonitis there is an outpouring of straw-colored fluid into the

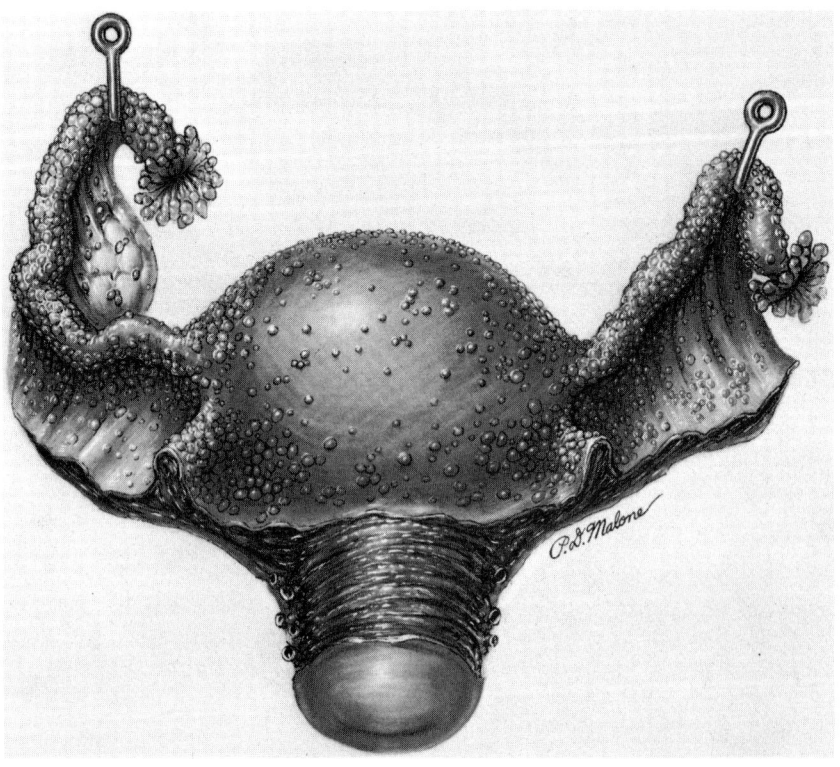

Fig. 11-12. Typical specimen of tuberculosis of generative organs as part of generalized tuberculous peritonitis.

peritoneal cavity, producing ascites. The peritoneum of the parietal wall and viscera is covered with innumerable small tubercles (Fig. 11-12). The tubes, in addition to being covered with miliary tubercles on the serosal surface, are usually slightly enlarged and distended with a patent fimbria, producing the characteristic "tobacco-pouch" appearance. Within the wall of the tube the histology is typical of tuberculosis, with tubercle formation, multinucleated giant cells and epithelioid reaction (Fig. 11-13). In advanced cases frank caseation is present. This pattern is more classically associated with hematogenous spread of the tuberculous organism to the peritoneal surfaces and the pelvic organs.

Another type of tuberculous peritonitis encountered in the female is the "dry" or adhesive type. Bowel adheres to bowel by innumerable dense adhesions that blend with the musculature. Indeed, the muscle of the bowel is often invaded to some degree by the tuberculous process. Separation of these adhesions is extremely difficult surgically, and accidental injury to the bowel is common. The pelvic organs show evidence of tuberculous salpingitis with enlargement of the tubes, and occasionally pyosalpinges and even tubo-ovarian abscess formation. This "dry" variety may represent the healed fibrotic end result of the "wet" ascitic pattern.

The third type of tuberculous peritonitis is of particular interest to the gynecologist. It represents an obvious direct extension of the tuberculous process from within the tubes to the surrounding peritoneum. On the serosa of the tubes and the uterus, on the sigmoid, and perhaps on the cecum, the appendix, or the lower ileum, there are scattered tubercles. It is possible that this localized peritoneal infection is in some instances the forerunner of the more extensive types of peritonitis discussed above. From a therapeutic viewpoint this form responds very satisfactorily to pelvic surgery.

Pathogenesis

The natural history of pelvic tuberculosis is best explained as a hematogenous disease from a primary infection in the lung, urinary tract, or other viscera. In the study of 132 patients in Toronto by Henderson and coworkers, approximately 60 per cent gave a history of tuberculosis or showed clinical evidence of it elsewhere in the body. The fallopian tubes are the most frequently involved pelvic organ, the reason for which is not fully understood but may be related to a dual blood supply. In general, the ovary is relatively resistant to tuberculous infection but may become involved in a tubo-ovarian inflammatory mass by direct spread of the disease. The endometrium is thought to be involved by direct extension of the lesion from the endosalpinx to the endometrial cavity. Between 70.9 per cent (Brown) and 61 per cent (Nogales) of the cases will show histologic evidence of tuberculous endometritis. The cervix and vagina are usually involved by either direct extension or vascular spread of the organism, but such lesions are infrequent and only rarely occur as primary sites of pelvic infection.

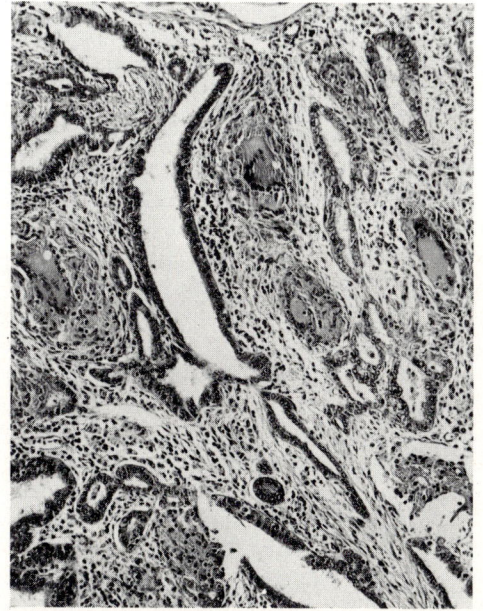

FIG. 11-13. Tuberculosis of the fallopian tube. Note the multinucleated giant cells.

Diagnosis

Although the clinical symptoms and signs of this disease should direct the clinician to the diagnosis of pelvic tuberculosis, the fact remains that over two thirds of the cases are diagnosed at the time of laparotomy performed for some other indication. A D and C or endometrial biopsy would be diagnostic in more than two thirds of the cases if such a procedure were performed in the evaluation of the patient. Acid-fast culture of menstrual blood is reportedly effective in detecting the organism in approximately 10 per cent of the cases, according to Overbeck. On pelvic examination, bilateral tenderness in the lower quadrants is the rule. The tenderness is usually less marked than with acute gonococcal or streptococcal infections. Occasionally, large tuberculous tubo-ovarian abscesses may be palpated through the abdominal wall. The classical "doughy" sensation to the broad ligament suggests a tuberculous inflammatory disease which is produced by a combination of thickening of the broad ligament, adherent bowel, and some ascitic fluid. The clinical detection of ascites is the strongest evidence obtainable in favor of pelvic tuberculosis. It was present in one fifth of the Hopkins' cases. However, other causes of ascites must be considered, including ovarian carcinoma and cirrhosis of the liver. In differentiating tuberculous salpingitis from neisserian infections, the finding of a virginal outlet in the presence of obvious tubal inflammation should lend strength to the diagnosis of pelvic tuberculosis.

In addition, failure of clinical response to broad-spectrum antibiotics is a clinical test which should strongly suggest tuberculosis.

Treatment

The currently accepted treatment of pelvic tuberculosis is long-term antituberculous chemotherapy. Of the various treatment regimes, a combination of streptomycin, 1 gm. daily for 2 months and then twice weekly; sodium paraamionsalicylic acid (PAS), 14 gm. daily, or PAS-C (a highly purified crystalline PAS acid), 6 gm. daily; and isoniazid (INH), 300 mg. daily in one dose before breakfast, is the accepted treatment of choice. Initially, such patients were treated for 1 year, but this has been extended to 18 to 24 months in most clinics. Such patients are followed closely for many years thereafter to observe them for the possibility of recurrence of the disease.

Surgery is reserved for specific indications, as outlined by Sutherland in his vast experience with this disease in Glasgow. In general, surgery is reserved for those patients who have failed to respond to an adequate trial of medical treatment, which usually consists of 6 months or more of antibiotic therapy. Our surgical indications for the treatment of pelvic tuberculosis include:

1. Persistence or enlargement of an adnexal mass after 3 to 6 months of antituberculous chemotherapy. The rare possibility of an ovarian tumor must always be considered even though pelvic tuberculosis is also present.

2. Persistence of pelvic pain or recurrence of pelvic infection while on medical therapy. Patients should be followed periodically with an endometrial biopsy for evaluation of recurrent infection.

3. Primary unresponsiveness of the tuberculous infection to chemotherapy as evidenced by persistent spiking temperature, leukocytosis, and elevated sedimentation rate. As is true of some abscesses of gonococcal or mixed bacterial infection with thick fibrotic abscess walls, adequate perfusion of the abscess cavity by high levels of antibiotics may be prevented. Such cases must be treated promptly by surgical measures.

The preferred surgical treatment includes a total abdominal hysterectomy and bilateral salpingo-oophrectomy. However, the very nature of this inflammatory disease may make such operative procedures technically difficult, with an increased risk of injury to bowel, bladder, or other viscera. Consequently, in the event of severe tuberculous pelvic infection and a "frozen" pelvis, it is occasionally necessary to perform only a subtotal hysterectomy. Because of the dense adhesions, there is frequently extensive blood loss from generalized venous oozing of the raw peritoneal surfaces, and identification of the pelvic ureter is occasionally troublesome in those cases in which the base of the broad ligament is involved in dense inflammatory change. In Sutherland's clinic, 5 per cent of his cases have required additional surgical treatment after failure of drug therapy. Approximately 10 per cent of Henderson's patients required surgical treatment in addition to the initial medical management.

RESULTS OF TREATMENT

Although pelvic tuberculosis can be cured with chemotherapeutic drugs, it is important to have close follow-up of the patient as recurrences do appear which require additional therapy. Kardos (Budapest) reports a cure rate of 89.9 per cent by chemotherapy in a personal series of 112 cases. In a collected series from the literature which included 1,474 cases, he found that the cure rate was only 82.8 per cent, varying from 65 to 95 per cent. In 168 cases in which Kardos removed the tubes following medical treatment for 10 months, tuberculosis was active in 35 per cent of the surgical specimens.

Of major importance is the occurrence of full-term pregnancy following treatment for genital tuberculosis. Shaffer's experience over the past 25 years is noteworthy in this respect. Of a total of 7,357 patients with genital tuberculosis collected from the literature, he found less than 100 of such patients had full-term pregnancies. Of this number, 64 case histories on study revealed that only 31 patients had genital tuberculosis proved by acceptable criteria. In addition, Sutherland noted that the incidence of tubal pregnancy was nearly double that of a normal full-term delivery following medical treatment for genital tuberculosis. According to Halbrecht, up to 20 per cent of all patients treated medically for genital tuberculosis sooner or later have ectopic pregnancies. This is an interesting observation, but the authors of this book have not had this experience.

It is evident, therefore, that the ultimate cure for pelvic tuberculosis must be achieved by irradication of dormant systemic tuberculosis through aggressive efforts in preventive medicine. The effectiveness of such public health measures are unequivocal, as evidenced by the decreasing rate of pelvic tuberculosis. The early treatment of asymptomatic patients with pulmonary tuberculosis whose disease is detected by routine screening procedures will undoubtedly continue to influence the declining frequency of this organism as an etiologic cause of pelvic inflammatory disease.

BIBLIOGRAPHY

Bircher, E.: Die chronische Bauchfelltuberkulose, ihre Behandlung mit Roentgenstrählen. Zbl. Gynäk., 32:31, 1908.

Brown, A. B., Gilbert, R. A., and Te Linde, R. W.: Pelvic tuberculosis. Obstet. Gynec., 2:476, 1953.

Brown, L., Brown, B. C., Walsh, M. J., and Pirkle, C. I.: Urethritis in males produced by Neisseria gonorrhoeae from asymptomatic females. J.A.M.A., 186:153, 1963.

Falk, H. C.: Interpretation of the pathogenesis of pelvic infection as determined by cornual resection. Amer. J. Obstet. Gynec., 52:66, 1946.

Falk, H. C., Mandelbaum, C., and Blinick, G.: Conservative treatment of salpingitis complicating myomata uteri. Ann. Surg., 132:247, 1950.

Falk, V.: Treatment of acute non-tuberculous salpingitis with antibiotics alone and in combination with glucocorticoids. Acta Obstet. Gynec. Scand., 44 (Suppl. 6):1, 1965.

Fiumara, N. J.: The treatment of gonorrhea. Tufts Folia Med., 9:12, 1963.

Freed, C. R., and Kimbrough, R. A.: Clinical evaluation of Falk's procedure. Amer. J. Obstet. Gynec., 60:416, 1950.

Gallanis, T. C., Dawson, F., and Harding, H. B.: Laboratory diagnosis of gonorrhea in premenarchal females and in adults. Obstet. Gynec., 29:401, 1967.

Greenberg, J. P.: A clinical study of tuberculous salpingitis, based on 200 cases. Bull. Johns Hopkins Hosp., *32*:52, 1921.

Griffiths, H. B.: Quoted by Trussell, R. R.: Pelvic inflammatory disease. Proc. Roy. Soc. Med., *61*:365, 1968.

Halbrecht, I.: Latent female genital tuberculosis. Int. J. Fert., *10*:157, 1965.

———: The relative value of culture and endometrial biopsy in the diagnosis of genital tuberculosis. Amer. J. Obstet. Gynec., *75*:899, 1958.

Henderson, D. N., Harkins, J. L., and Stitt, J. F.: Pelvic tuberculosis. Amer. J. Obstet. Gynec., *94*:630, 1966.

Henderson, D. N., Hopkins, J. L., and Stitt, J. F.: Pelvic tuberculosis. Amer. J. Obstet. Gynec., *80*:21, 1960.

Holmes, K. K., Johnson, D. W., and Floyd, T. M.: Studies of venereal disease. J.A.M.A., *202*:461, 1967.

Johnson, C. G.: Discussion of Kaplan, A. L., Jacobs, W. M., and Ehresman, J. B.: Aggressive management of pelvic abscess. Amer. J. Obstet. Gynec., *98*:482, 1967.

Kardos, F.: Late results in women with genital tuberculosis. Obstet. Gynec., *29*:247, 1967.

Koch, Marie: Personal communication.

Kraus, G. W., and Yen, S. S. C.: Gonorrhea during pregnancy. Obstet. Gynec., *31*:258, 1968.

Lachner, J. E., Schiller, W., and Tulsky, A. S.: Coincidence of tuberculosis of the endometrium with tuberculosis of the lung. Amer. J. Obstet. Gynec., *40*:429, 1940.

Lucas, J. B., Price, E. V., Thayer, J. D., and Schroeter, A.: Diagnosis and treatment of gonorrhea in the female. New Eng. J. Med., *276*:1454, 1967.

Medical News: Doubling the dosage of penicillin in treating gonorrhea recommended. J.A.M.A., *193* (8):23, 1965.

Malkani, P. K., and Rajani, C. K.: Pelvic tuberculosis. Obstet. Gynec., *14*:600, 1959.

Mickal, A., Sellmann, A. H., and Beebe, J. L.: Ruptured tubo-ovarian abscesses. Amer. J. Obstet. Gynec., *100*:432, 1968.

Nebel, W. A., and Lucas, W. E.: Management of tubo-ovarian abscess. Obstet. Gynec., *32*:382, 1968.

Nogales, F., Martinez, H., and Beato, M.: Erwägungen über die Pathogenese der Endometritis tuberculosa: 1011 Sälle mit Genital Tuberkulose. Arch. Gynäk., *203*:45, 1966.

Overbeck, L. Is tuberculosis of the female urogenital tract an entity? J. Obstet. Gynaec. Brit. Comm., *73*:624, 1966.

Pedowitz, P., and Bloomfield, R.: Ruptured adnexal abscess (tubo-ovarian) with generalized peritonitis. Amer. J. Obstet. Gynec., *88*:721, 1964.

Pedowitz, P., and Felmus, L. B.: Ruptured adnexal abscess with generalized peritonitis. Amer. J. Surg., *83*:507, 1952.

Reef, E.: Gonococcal bartholinitis. Brit. J. Vener. Dis., *43*:150, 1967.

Shaffer, C.: Tuberculosis of the genital tract. Amer. J. Obstet. Gynec., *91*:714, 1965.

Shapiro, L. H., and Lentz, J. W.: Clinical evaluation of treatment of gonorrhea in the female. Amer. J. Obstet. Gynec., *97*:968, 1967.

———: Final report on the effectiveness of oxytetracycline in the treatment of gonorrhea in females. Amer. J. Obstet. Gynec., *94*:536, 1966.

———: Large doses of penicillin for the treatment of gonorrhea in women. Obstet. Gynec., *30*:89, 1967.

Strauss, H., Horowitz, E. A., and Grunstein, I.: Cervical secretion in chronic gonorrhea in prostitutes. Amer. J. Obstet. Gynec., *45*:840, 1943.

Sutherland, A. M.: Latent Female Genital Tuberculosis. Basle, Karger, 1966.

———: The place of surgery in the treatment of genital tuberculosis in women. Acta Obstet. Gynec. Scand., *44*:163, 1965.

———: Treatment of genital TB in women. Bull. Sloane Hosp., Wom., *13*:127, 1967.

———: Tuberculosis of the endometrium. Obstet. Gynec., *11*:527, 1958.

Te Linde, R. W., and Darner, H. L.: End results in conservative and radical ovarian surgery. J.A.M.A., *90*:284, 1928.

Vermeeren, J., and Te Linde, R. W.: Intraabdominal rupture of pelvic abscesses. Amer. J. Obstet. Gynec., *68*:402, 1954.

Williams, W. J.: Incidence of asymptomatic gonorrhea in apparently healthy females using FA techniques. Public Health Lab., *22*:138, 1964.

Wren, B. G.: Gonorrhoea among prostitutes. Med. J. Australia, *1*:847, 1967.

SEPTIC SHOCK

Borden, G. W., and Hall, W. H.: Fatal transfusion reactions from massive bacterial contamination of blood. New Eng. J. Med., *245*:760, 1951.

Braude, A. I., Williams, D., Siemienski, J., and Murphy, R.: Shock-like state due to transfusion of blood contaminated with gram-negative bacilli. Arch. Intern. Med., *92*:75, 1953.

Braude, A. I., Siemienski, J., Williams, D.,

and Sanford, J.: Overwhelming bacteremic shock produced by gram-negative bacilli. A report of four cases with one recovery. Univ. Mich. Med. Bull., *19*:23, 1953.

Brill, N. E., and Libman, E.: Pyocyaneus bacillianemia. Amer. J. Med. Sci., *228*:153, 1899.

Cavanaugh, D., and McLeod, G. W.: Septic shock in obstetrics and gynecology: evaluation of metaraminol therapy. Amer. J. Obstet. Gynec., *96*:913, 1966.

Collins, V. J., Jaffee, R., and Zahony, I.: Shock, a different approach to therapy. Illinois Med. J., *122*:350, 1962.

Deane, R. M., and Russell, K. P.: Enterobacillary septicemia and bacterial shock in septic abortion. Amer. J. Obstet. Gynec., *79*:528, 1960.

Douglas, G. W., and Beckman, E. M.: Clinical management of septic abortion complicated by hypotension. Amer. J. Obstet. Gynec., *96*:633, 1966.

Fine, J.: Intestinal circulation in shock. Gastroenterology, *52*:454, 1967.

Hardaway, R. M.: Syndromes of Disseminated Intravascular Coagulation: With Special Reference to Shock and Hemorrhage. Springfield, Ill., Charles C Thomas, 1966.

Hardaway, R. M., James, P. M., Jr., Anderson, R. W., Brendenberg, C. E., and West, R. L.: Intensive study and treatment of shock in man. J.A.M.A., *199*:779, 1967.

Josey, W. E., Hock, W., Moon, E. C., and Thompson, J. D.: Analysis of 21 septic abortion deaths with special reference to the Shwartzman phenomenon. Obstet. Gynec., *28*:335, 1966.

Lillehei, R. C., Longerbeam, J. K., and Bloch, J. H.: Physiology in therapy of bacteremic shock. Experimental and clinical observations. Amer. J. Cardiol., *12*:593, 1963.

Lillehei, R. C., Longerbeam, J. K., Bloch, J. H., and Manax, W. G.: The modern treatment of shock based on physiologic principles. Clin. Pharmacol. Ther., *5*:63, 1964.

———: The nature of experimental irreversible shock with its clinical applications. *In* Hershey, S. G. (ed.): Shock, p. 193. Boston, Little, Brown & Co., 1964.

MacLean, L. D.: Blood volume vs. central venous pressure in shock. Surg. Gynec. Obstet., *118*:594, 1964.

MacLean, L. D., Mulligan, W. G., McLean, A. P. H., and Duff, J. H.: Patterns of septic shock in man, a detailed study of 56 patients. Ann. Surg., *166*:543, 1967.

McCally, M., and Vasicka, A.: Generalized Shwartzman reaction and hypofibrinogenemia in septic abortion. Obstet. Gynec., *19*:359, 1962.

McKay, D. G.: Disseminated Intravascular Coagulation. An Intermediary Mechanism of Disease. New York, Hoeber Med. Div., Harper and Row, 1965.

Michael, A., Sellman, A. H., and Beebe, J. L.: Ruptured tuboovarian abscess. Amer. J. Obstet. Gynec., *100*:432, 1968.

Moore, J. G.: Discussion of Douglas, G. W., and Beckman, E. M.: Clinical management of septic abortion complicated by hypotension. Amer. J. Obstet. Gynec., *96*:633, 1966.

Morris, J. A.: Bacteremic shock in obstetrics. *In* Marcus, S. L., and Marcus, C. C. (eds.): Advances in Obstetrics and Gynecology. p. 150. Baltimore, Williams & Wilkins, 1967.

Neuwirth, R. S., and Friedman, E. A.: Septic abortion. Changing concept of management. Amer. J. Obstet. Gynec., *85*:24, 1963.

Nickerson, M.: Drug therapy of shock. *In* Boch, K. D. (ed.): Shock, Pathogenesis and Therapy. p. 356. New York, Academic Press, 1962.

———: Sympathetic blockade in the therapy of shock. Amer. J. Cardiol., *12*:619, 1963.

Nickerson, M., and Carter, S. A.: Protection against acute trauma and traumatic shock by vasodilators. Canad. J. Biochem., *37*:1161, 1959.

Phillips, L. L., Skrodelis, V., and Quigley, H. J., Jr. An intravascular coagulation and fibrinolysis in septic abortion. Obstet. Gynec., *30*:350, 1967.

Spink, W. W.: The pathogenesis and management of shock due to infection. Arch. Intern. Med., *106*:433, 1960.

Waisbren, B. A.: Bacteremia due to gram-negative bacilli other than salmonella. A clinical and therapeutic study. Arch. Intern. Med., *88*:467, 1951.

Weil, M. H., Shubin, H., and Biddle, M.: Shock caused by gram-negative microorganisms; analysis of 169 cases. Ann. Intern. Med., *60*:384, 1964.

12

Operative Injury of the Ureters

CAUSES

Operative injury to the ureters occurs very rarely during pelvic surgery in the better clinics, but occasionlly even the best of surgeons may injure a ureter. The incidence of accidental ureteral ligation is difficult to determine with certainty, for there is no doubt that following a ureteral ligation at times the kidney may quietly cease to function; the patient or the surgeon never may become aware of the accident, but usually the outcome is not so happy. Ureteral injury occurs most often during hysterectomy—abdominal or vaginal—but it is about 6 times as frequent in the abdominal as in the vaginal. The accident may occur in other pelvic operations, such as the removal of a tubo-ovarian abscess or an adherent ovarian neoplasm. The Wertheim type of radical panhysterectomy for cervical carcinoma has contributed most heavily to ureteral injury. The dissection of the ureter required in this operation as originally done resulted in a high percentage of injury, even when performed by an expert; Wertheim himself reported an incidence of 10 per cent. Since the operation has been generally abandoned in this country in favor of radium therapy, ureteral injuries have decreased markedly. Recently, Meigs has revived interest in the Wertheim type of operation for cervical cancer; although he reported a series of 85 cases with no deaths, there still resulted an incidence of ureteral fistulae of 7.2 per cent. In our own clinic at Johns Hopkins Hospital there were 31 ureteral injuries occurring in 15,100 pelvic operations: 12,500 of these were abdominal procedures, and 3,600 vaginal operations, including 500 vaginal hysterectomies. The accident is a serious one with a relatively high mortality, as is evidenced by Bland in his report of 18.8 per cent for unilateral and 33.3 per cent for bilateral injuries.

Like all surgical accidents, prevention is better than cure; hence a consideration from this point of view deserves our attention. The injury usually occurs in one of four places: at the infundibulopelvic ligament, in the region of the uterine vessels, at any place between these two points where an inflammatory or neoplastic mass may be adherent to it, or where the ureter lies between the anterior vaginal wall and the base of the bladder (Fig. 12-1). The first of these places is the least frequent site of injury, but occasionally, when there is a short infundibulopelvic ligament due to distortion of the normal anatomy by a large ovarian or par-ovarian cyst or a large tubo-ovarian abscess, the clamp placed on the ovarian vessels may include the ureter. The second region, that of the uterine vessels, is the most common site of injury. If the uterine vessels are clamped carefully close to the uterus and tied with precision and care, the danger of ureteral injury is reduced markedly. The greatest danger of injury to the ureter is experienced in those cases in which the vessels slip from the clamps or the ligatures, and reclamping is attempted quickly and in the presence of profuse bleeding. Not infrequently, with large pelvic tumors, especially those that have developed between the leaves of the broad ligament, freeing of the tumor from the pelvic wall may endanger the ureter; identification and exposure of the ureter are necessary. When ureteral identification is desirable, it is well not to dissect it free from its bed for any greater distance than is necessary and also to leave as much periureteral tissue as possible attached to the ureter, for in this tissue lie important blood vessels that supply the ureter. Most of the fistulas that occur following the Wertheim panhysterectomy for carcinoma result from sloughing due to interference with blood supply rather than to direct injury of the ureter by the operator. It is well recognized that irradiation preceding the Wertheim operation greatly increases the danger of sloughing of the ureter. The irradiation, causing fibrosis of the nutrient vessels of the ureter, reduces the blood supply, and the surgical dissection often robs the ureter of the remainder. Also, in the radical total abdominal hysterectomy, as it is done in this clinic for microinvasive cervical cancer, identification of the ureter for some distance along its course is essential for safety. In such cases, preoperative catheterization of the ureters is advisable. Also, when an intraligamentary fibroid, an adherent ovarian cyst, or bad pelvic in-

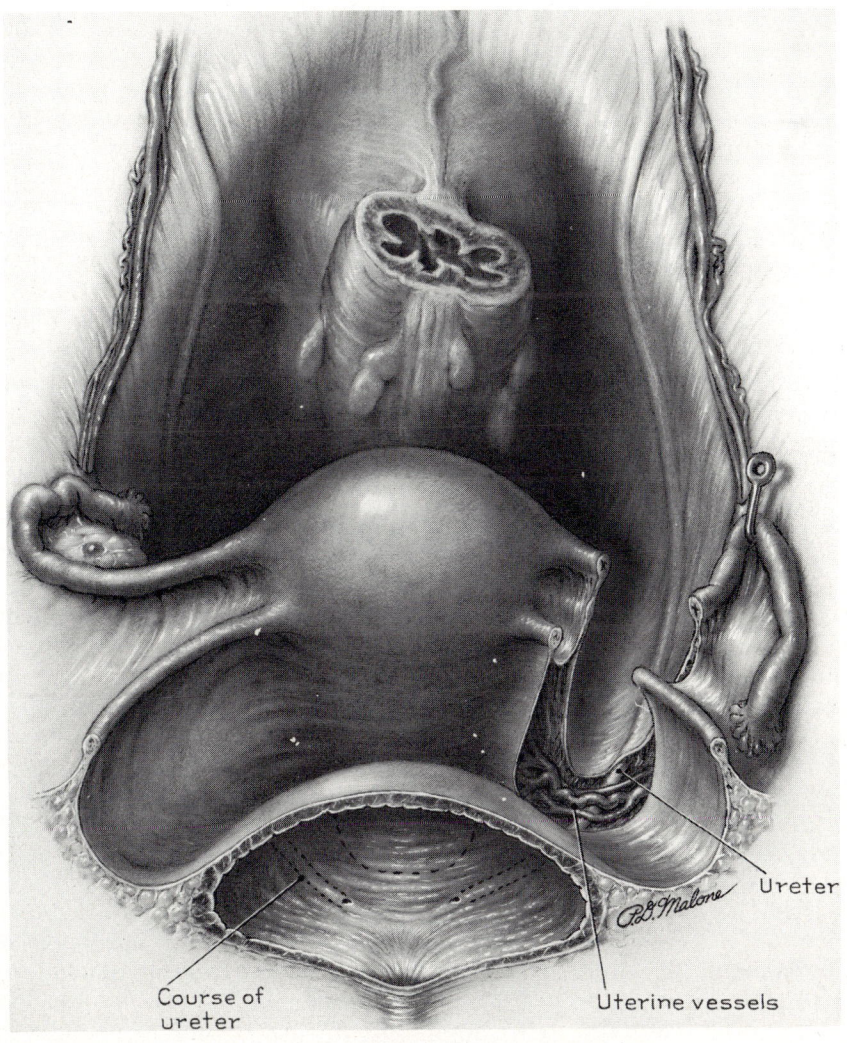

Fig. 12-1. Dissection showing relation of ureters to pelvic viscera.

flammatory disease suggests proximity or adherence to a ureter, preoperative catheterization is time-saving and a great safety factor. By this procedure not only can the ureter be identified more easily and speedily, but its course can be followed for as great a distance as is required without its complete dissection and without the attendant danger to its blood supply. Although the value of this safeguard is belittled by some surgeons who believe that they can locate the ureter at will, often we have seen experienced surgeons waste as much as a half hour in identifying the ureter. The saving of operating time in the course of a prolonged operation surely is well worth consideration. It is also the belief of some surgeons that ureteral catheterization increases the danger of ureteral fistulas, basing their claim upon their experience with the Wertheim operation for cervical cancer. It would appear to us that the stripping of the ureter for a long stretch and thus endangering the blood supply is the real factor concerned in the formation of these fistulas. In any event, we never have experienced a ureteral fistula following our wide panhysterectomy, without lymph node dissection, which we perform in this clinic for cervical cancer in situ. In performing less radical total abdominal hysterectomy for benign uterine disease avoidance of injury to the ureter anterior to the vagina can be accomplished by adhering to the Richardson technic, described elsewhere in this volume. Regardless of the particular technic used in total abdominal hysterectomy, care should be taken to dissect the bladder well down on the vaginal wall before the cervix is cut from the vagina and to note carefully what is included in each stitch as the vagina is sutured.

TREATMENT OF OPERATIVE URETERAL INJURIES

The treatment of ureteral injuries should be considered in the two groups into which they naturally fall: those recognized at the operating table and those discovered subsequently.

Injuries Recognized at the Operation. When a clamp or a ligature is discovered on a ureter *during the course of an operation*, it should be removed immediately, and the ureter should be inspected carefully. In many instances insufficient damage will have been done to prevent normal function of the ureter. If the damage is slight but the operator feels uneasy about its condition, a stab wound may be made and a cigarette drain placed extraperitoneally adjacent to the injury site as a safety valve. The peritoneum should be closed over this so that if there is leakage, it will be extraperitoneal. If the operator feels uneasy about simple drainage, a longitudinal slit may be made in the ureter above the injury and a polyethylene tube of suitable size threaded down the course of the ureter, left coiled in the bladder, and removed after 10 days. Obviously, there is room for judgment on the seriousness of the damage. If the ureter is discovered to be cut, or if there is damage that makes it appear incapable of spontaneous restoration, the operator has 3 choices. He may implant the severed ureter into the bladder, perform a ureteroureteral anastomosis, or he may simply ligate the upper segment of the ureter. The ideal repair should preserve normal kidney function and restore the function of the ureter. Implantation of the ureter into the bladder offers a closer approach to this ideal than ureteroureteral anastomosis. Hence, if the injury to the ureter is sufficiently low to permit it, implantation into the bladder is the preferred procedure. If the injury is too high for this, ureteroureteral anastomosis should be attempted. There are in our opinion only two occasions on which simple ligation of the injured ureter is justifiable: (1) when the operation has been of such magnitude that prolongation sufficient to perform an implantation or anastomosis would seriously risk the patient's life; (2) when a considerable section of the ureter has been removed, making impossible implantation or anastomosis. Before deliberate ligation is done, one should palpate the opposite kidney to determine its presence and, as far as possible, its normal condition. Experience has shown that ligation when the urine is uninfected usually results in an asymptomatic, afunctional kidney. Ligation of the ureter under these circumstances should be done with a strong nonabsorbable material. If palpation reveals absence of the opposite kidney or any evidence of abnormality, the proximal end of the ureter should be brought out to the skin and permitted to drain until the condition of the opposite kidney can be determined.

Bilateral cutting or severe damage of the ureters is rare, and still more rare is its discovery at the operating table. When one is confronted with such a serious accident at the operation, bilateral anastomosis or implantation must be done. In case the patient's condition does not permit repair on both sides, one must be repaired and the opposite ureter brought out to the skin to permit functioning of that kidney until it can be determined that the repaired ureter is working satisfactorily.

Injuries Undiscovered at the Operation. *Bilateral ligation* soon becomes apparent as anuria results. For the first 48 hours this is usually the only symptom, but soon thereafter the blood urea nitrogen of the blood begins to rise, and the patient shows signs of uremia. If the obstructions are unrelieved, death usually results within 7 to 10 days. If no evidence of serious kidney disease was discovered in the preoperative urinalysis, one can be quite certain that anuria for 48 hours postoperatively signifies bilateral ureteral injury. Before resorting to surgery it is our custom to attempt passing ureteral catheters to demonstrate definitely the ureteral obstructions or, as is rarely possible, to overcome one or both of the obstructions. When one is certain that the condition exists, the sooner treatment is instituted, the better. We feel strongly that bilateral nephrostomy is preferable to attemtping deligation. In attempting transabdominal deligation one is subjecting a patient who has had a laparotomy a few days previous to a second one, and the mortality is high.

The technical difficulties of working in the ureteral regions, which so recently were subjected to operative trauma, are great, and the deligations may be unsuccessful. In contrast with this, bilateral nephrostomy is done quickly, the patient soon begins to pour forth quantities of urine, and the blood urea nitrogen drops rapidly. Urinary secretion is immediately stimulated postoperatively by intravenous injections of glucose and saline solution. Occasionlly, the ureteral lumina will re-establish themselves spontaneously after nephrostomy or pyelostomy. If they do not, an attempt may be made to open the ureters by ureteral catheterization, although such attempts often fail. If ureteral catheterization fails to overcome the obstruction, a laparotomy should be performed 6 weeks after the nephrostomies, and the necessary ureteral plastic work should be done. The condition of the patient will then be sufficiently good to permit the meticulous painstaking work which is necessary to give permanent normal ureteral function.

Unilateral ureteral injury which is unrecognized at the operation may become apparent later by (1) symptoms of pyelitis, (2) evidence of ureterovaginal or ureterocervicovaginal fistula, and (3) the appearance of a mass in the kidney region due to hydronephrosis. As previously stated, complete and permanent occlusion of one ureter in the absence of infection sometimes leads to renal atrophy without symptoms, local or constitutional. The appearance of chills and fever, postoperatively, may indicate a simple acute postoperative pyelitis, but when these symptoms persist under the usual medical therapy, the possibility of ureteral injury should be considered. Ureteral catheterization will determine whether or not the ureter has been occluded. It is possible, but not likely, that the obstruction can be overcome with the ureteral catheter. If one is fortunate enough to overcome the obstruction, the catheter should be left in the ureter for 10 to 14 days to permit drainage of the kidney and healing of the injured ureter. If the obstruction cannot be overcome and the symptoms of pyelonephritis are present, a nephrostomy should be done at once to permit drainage of the infected urine and preserve the kidney substance until 6 weeks or more have passed, when the patient's local and general condition are such as to ensure success in the necessary work on the injured ureter.

At times, the appearance of urine in the vagina gives the first intimation of ureteral injury. If there has been cutting of the ureter without ligation, the urine may appear almost immediately postoperatively. Since most ureters which are cut at operation are also ligated, several days may elapse before the ligature sloughs off and permits drainage. Since most ureteral damage today is the result of stripping the ureter of its blood supply, as in the Wertheim operation, several days elapse before sloughing has progressed to the point of permitting urinary drainage. In our experience the vaginal drainage usually becomes evident in such cases from the 10th to the 21st postoperative day. After total hysterectomy this enters the vagina directly via a fistulous tract from the ureter. Following subtotal hysterectomy, the urine usually enters the vagina via the cervical canal. In other cases the appearance of the fistula may be preceded by an attack of pyelitis; then the drainage afforded by the fistula may result in subsidence of the temperature. In other cases the evidence of pyelitis may appear after the evidence of fistula formation, for there is a tendency for all fistulous openings to contract; this leads to ureteral obstruction and pyelitis. Occasionally, the fistula may close spontaneously with re-establishment of the ureteral lumen, and because of this a reasonable period of expectant treatment is permissible. If the policy of watchful waiting is pursued for several weeks, intravenous urograms should be done repeatedly to note the effect on the kidney (Fig. 12-2). If hydronephrosis is observed to be developing, nephrostomy or the plastic work on the ureter should be done without delay. The choice of these two procedures depends upon the local condition and also the general condition of the patient. The spontaneous cessation of drainage through

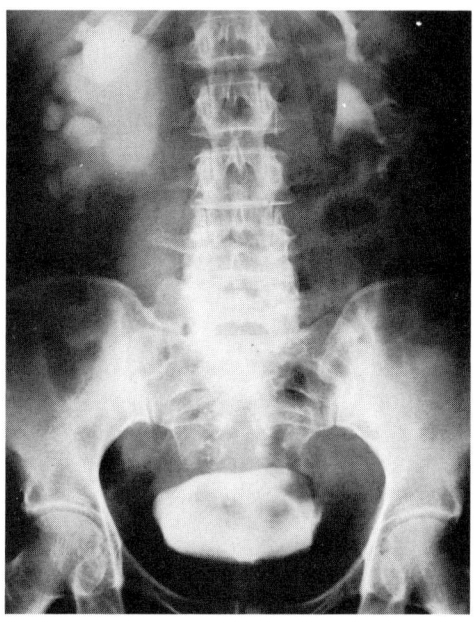

FIG. 12-2. Urogram showing effect of ureteral injury at Wertheim operation. After 3 weeks the kidney still shows considerable function but has developed a marked hydronephrosis.

the vagina may mean infrequently a diversion of the urine elsewhere, as into the peritoneal cavity; this has been reported by Hunner and Everett.

As the hydronephrosis develops, judgment is required on when to take the next step. If there is spiking fever, nephrostomy or pyelostomy should not be delayed. If the hydronephrotic kidney is uninfected, usually one may wait as long as 6 weeks before attempting surgery on the ureter, but one may vary this time, depending on the extent of the previous surgery in the region of the ureter and on the rapidity with which the hydronephrosis appears to be developing.

One of the first studies indicated after the appearance of urine in the vagina should be an attempt to prove whether the urinary fistula communicates with the bladder or the ureter. A convenient way to do this is to fill the bladder with a weak solution of methylene blue and place a gauze sponge in the vagina; if the vaginal sponge remains free of methylene blue, the evidence points to the ureteral fistula. Inspection of the vaginal vault gives no information as to the side on which the ureter is damaged. Usually, the fistula can be located exactly by the passage of a ureteral catheter on the suspected side. As a rule, it is impossible to force the catheter past the point of injury because of scarring and stricture formation. If by good fortune the catheter is made to pass the injured point in the ureter, it should be left in for 10 to 14 days, during which time the fistula usually will heal. Before undertaking the operation for repair or implantation of the ureter, a differential phthalein test should be done with the opposite ureter catheterized to determine beyond question the function of the kidney on the uninjured side. The output from the fistula may be caught in a bedpan. A knowledge of the function of the opposite kidney is invaluable to the surgeon when making his decisions while attempting to repair or reimplant the injured ureter.

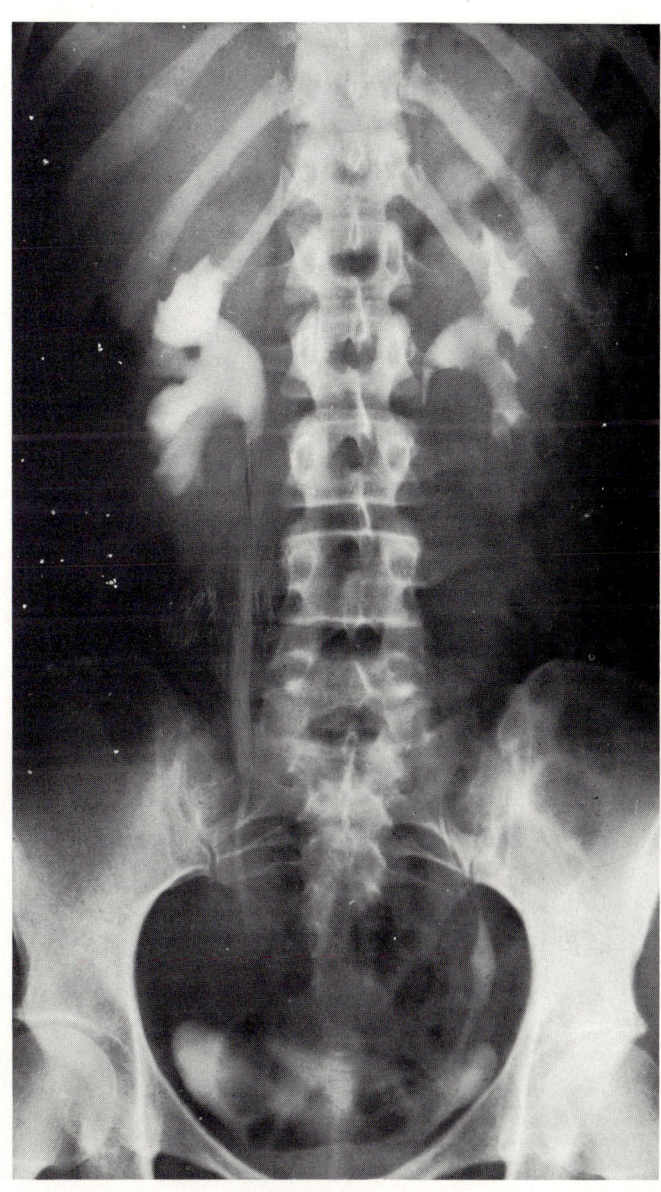

FIG. 12-3. Intravenous urogram taken several months after bilateral plastic operation on ureters, following bilateral ligation.

Only when the final operation is undertaken can one decide on the exact procedure, and that must be done after investigating the local conditions from within the abdomen.

We have been able, on one occasion, to re-establish the ureteral lumen by simply opening the ureter longitudinally above the acquired stricture, tunneling through the occluded segment and allowing the catheter to stay in place for 14 days. Retrograde pyelograms done on this patient a year afterward showed that little permanent damage had been done to the kidneys (Fig. 12-3). Kidney function was normal on both sides. If the injury is at the level of the uterine vessels or below, vesical implantation is usually preferable to anastomosis. In some instances when the shortened ureter will not quite reach the bladder, the bladder may be elongated by rolling up a flap. The blood supply of the bladder is so abundant that generally this can be accomplished without fear of sloughing.

When a hydronephrotic kidney mass makes its appearance several months or years after the operation, and ureteral catheterization indicates a complete ureteral obstruction, a nephrectomy may be necessary, but if the hydronephrotic sac is asymptomatic, it may be left undisturbed.

Technic: Ureteroureteral Anastomosis

The anastomosis may be done at the time of injury at the original operation or subsequently. If done at the time of injury, a ureteral catheter, preferably a No. 7 or No. 8, is threaded up the upper segment and down the lower segment into the bladder, where it is permitted to curl up as shown in Figure 12-4. More recently we have used silicone tubing (Silastic), 0.078 cm. in diameter, for the ureteral splint as it is less traumatic to the ureter and bladder, is quite inert, and can be left in the ureter for longer periods of time without obstructing it. If the anastomosis is done at some time subsequent to the original injury, the patient is first cystoscoped, and a catheter is passed up the ureter until it meets the obstruction. This enables the operator to identify the lower segment of the ureter easily. In view of the relatively recent operation, postoperative edema and changes in the tissues may make the identification of the ureter difficult without the aid of the catheter. The ureter is opened at the site of injury, and silicone (Silastic) tubing is passed up to the kidney pelvis. The other end of the Silastic tube is tied onto the tip of the catheter, and the catheter is withdrawn from the urethra by our assistant. Formerly, we used ureteral catheters, but the lumen of the Silastic tubing is much larger in proportion to the total diameter of the tube; we now prefer this silicone tubing.

The ureter having been thus splinted by the Silastic tubing, the two ends are drawn together and united by 3 to 4 interrupted sutures of No. 000 chromic catgut, placed through the outer coats of the ureter (Fig. 12-4). Before the abdomen is closed, drainage is established extraperitoneally by the use of a cigarette drain through a small stab wound. This drain is easily placed, under direct vision, to a point near the site of anastomosis. Then the peritoneum is closed over the ureter. If, during the postoperative course, there is any reason to believe that drainage from the ureter is not going well, the end of the tubing can be brought out through the urethra and irrigated.

The above-described technic is suitable in the usual case, but there is a special precaution which may be taken when, due to the condition of the ureter, it is feared that the anastomosis is not as satisfactory as one might desire. In such a case, urinary leakage at the anastomosis might seem likely, and it might be desirable to leave the indwelling ureteral tubing in place for more than the usual 10 days. The urine may be diverted by making a short longitudinal slit in the ureter a short distance above the anastomosis and a Silastic tube threaded up toward the kidney pelvis, bringing the other end out through the incision. This has the added advantage of permitting irrigation and being certain of drainage without bringing the end of the indwelling catheter out through the urethra.

This is demonstrated in the diagram shown in Figure 12-4.

TECHNIC: IMPLANTATION OF THE URETER INTO THE BLADDER

The ureter is dissected free from its bed for a sufficient distance to permit its implantation into the bladder without tension. Since most ureteral injuries follow hysterectomy, the uterus is out of the way, and usually the bladder can be brought up to the shortened ureter if the ureter cannot be brought down to the bladder in its usual position. There is no advantage in performing the implantation retroperitoneally; hence the implantation is usually done in the vertex of the bladder. The ureteral injury for which the implantation here pictured was done followed an anterior colpotomy for drainage of an abscess; hence the presence of the uterus makes the implantation somewhat more difficult. The shortest route to the bladder was through an opening made in the broad ligament.

The lower end of the ureter is split for about 5 mm., and a substantial bite is taken into each part of the divided end by

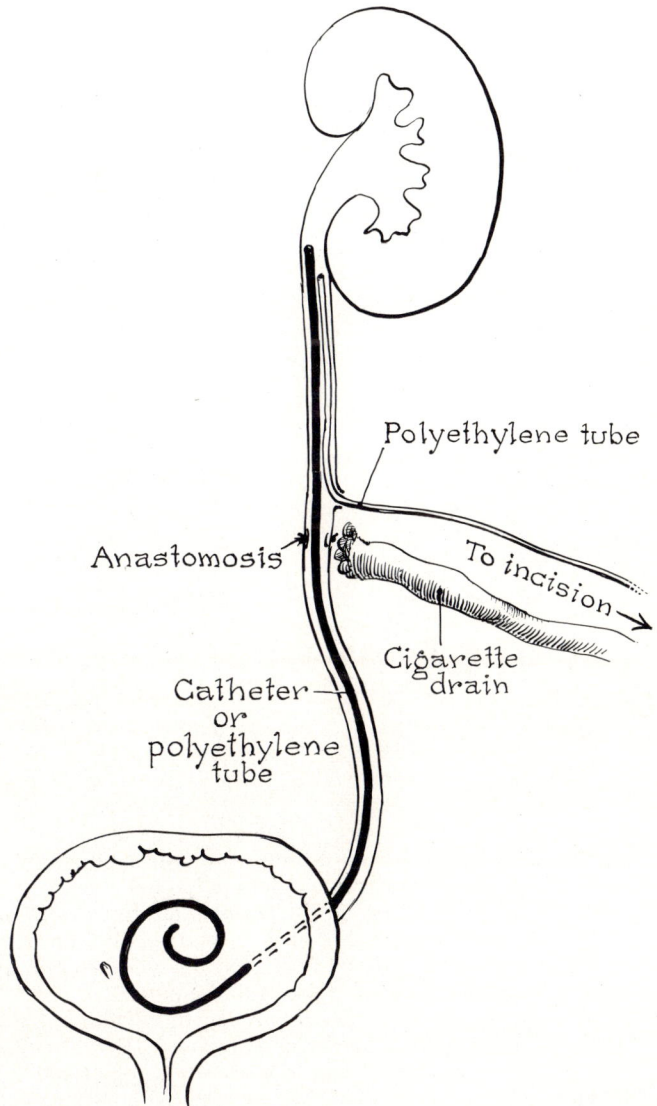

FIG. 12-4. Diagram showing anastomosed ureter. A catheter of polyethylene tube has been threaded up to the kidney pelvis and down into the bladder. A smaller polyethylene tube is inserted into the upper segment of the ureter through a slit-like incision about 1 cm. above the anastomosis. One cigarette drain is placed down to the site of the anastomosis.

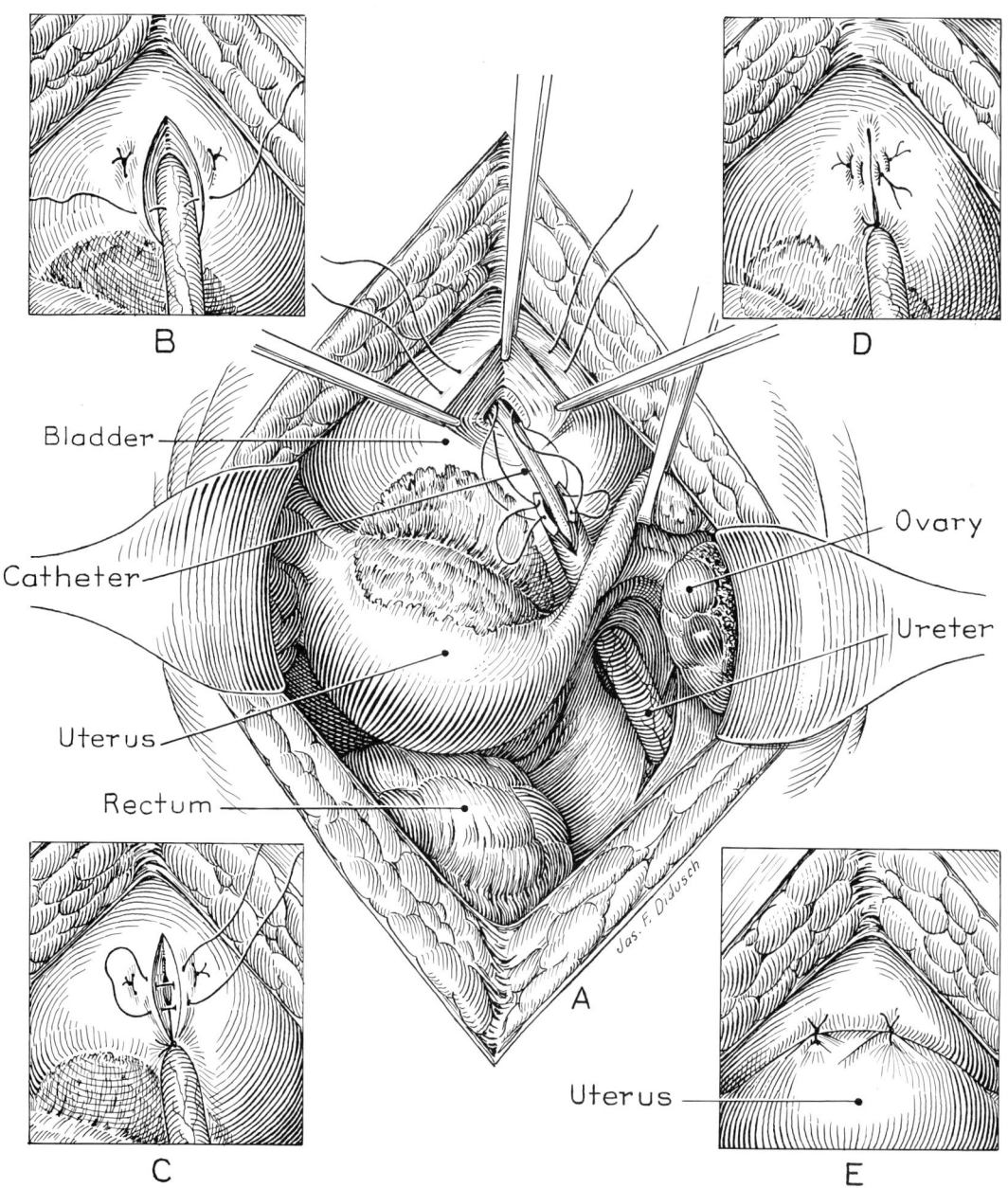

FIG. 12-5. Implantation of the ureter into the bladder. (A) The ureter has been dissected free and cut across. An opening has been made through the broad ligament into the bladder, and the end of the catheter has been introduced into it. Mattress sutures have been placed in the end of the ureter, passed into the bladder and out through the wall of the bladder. (B) Mattress sutures have been tied, and a fixation suture has been placed through the bladder wall and the muscular coat of the ureter. (C) The bladder-wall incision is approximated with a mattress stitch. (D) This mattress stitch has been tied, and implantation has been completed. (E) The uterus and the serosal surface of the bladder are sutured together to relieve any tension that might develop at anastomosis.

the use of No. 00 chromic catgut. A Silastic tube is threaded up the ureter for several centimeters. An opening is made into the bladder at the point selected for the implantation. The edges of the opening are held with mucosa clips, and the end of the catheter is introduced into the bladder. The 2 sutures that were previously placed in the lower end of the ureter are then rethreaded, and, with a fairly large round needle, they are introduced into the bladder and carried out through the wall, as shown in Figure 12-5 A. The sutures are carried out on opposite sides of the incision so as to hold apart the slit ends of the ureter (Fig. 12-5 A). These sutures are tied, as shown in Figure 12-5 B, thus drawing the ureter into the bladder. A third stitch is taken to fix the ureter to the bladder wall. This stitch passes through the edges of the incision in the bladder wall and picks up the wall of the ureter (Fig. 12-5 B). A mattress suture is used to complete the closure of the bladder wall (Fig. 12-5 C and D). Finally, in this particular case the uterus is sutured to the bladder to cover over the raw area caused by separation of the bladder from the uterus, to which it had been adherent. Pulling the bladder toward the uterus by these stitches also relieves tension on the anastomosis and fixes the structures in position for healing (Fig. 12-6).

Preceding a planned anastomosis, it is well to insert a ureteral catheter through the urethra and leave it coiled in the bladder. The Silastic tubing used for splinting the anastomosis is threaded onto the tip of this catheter and tied tightly

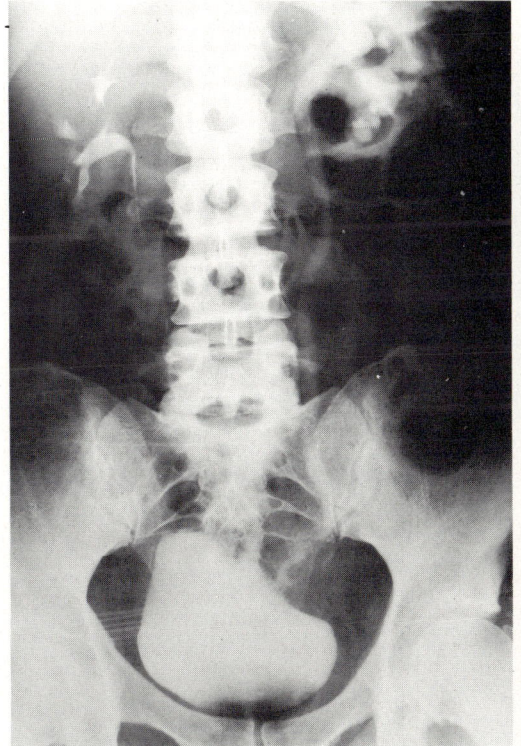
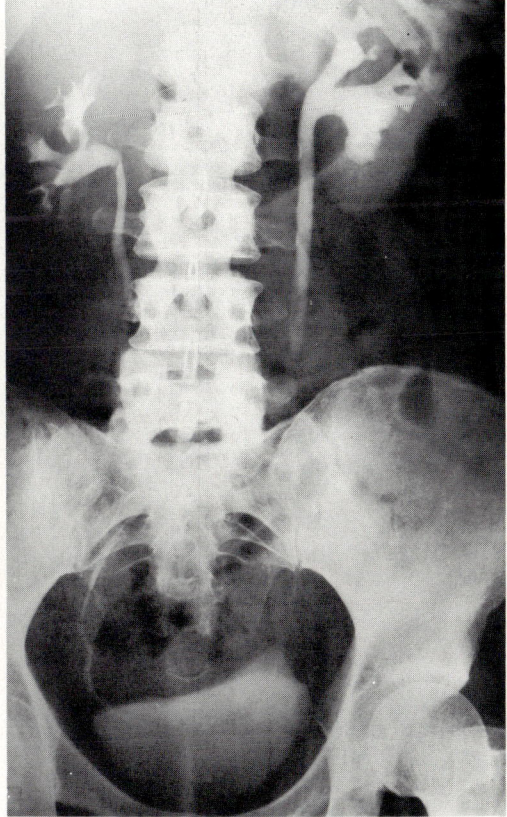

FIG. 12-6. (*Left*) Urogram taken 2 weeks after operative injury to left ureter. Hydronephrosis is developing, but the patient is still draining urine from the vagina. Ureter was reimplanted 6 weeks after injury. (*Right*) Urogram taken 5 weeks after implantation of injured left ureter into bladder, showing ultimate result. Note how the bladder was pulled up to meet the shortened ureter.

with silk suture, and the catheter is withdrawn from the urethra. The tubing is strapped to a Foley catheter, and the Foley is strapped to the patient's thigh. The tube is removed in 10 days, and the Foley is left in the bladder for another day or two. During the 10 days the tubing is irrigated only if it fails to drain freely, and then only a few cc. of 1 per cent neomycin solution is used.

BIBLIOGRAPHY

Bergman, H. (ed.): The Ureter. New York, Paul B. Hoeber, 1967.

Bland, P. B.: Surgical injuries of ureter. Med. J. & Rec., *121*:389, 1925.

Curtis, A. H.: Management of ureteral injuries with discussion of surgical indications in patients who require ureteral transplantation. Surg. Gynec. Obstet., *48*:320, 1929.

Everett, H. S.: Gynecological and Obstetrical Urology. Baltimore, Williams & Wilkins, 1944.

Everett, H. S., and Mattingly, R.: Urinary tract injuries resulting from pelvic surgery. Amer. J. Obstet. Gynec., *71*:502, 1956.

Hunner, G. L., and Everett, H. S.: Ureteroperitoneal fistula with urinary ascites and chronic peritonitis. J.A.M.A., 95:327, 1930.

——: Ureteroperitoneal fistula with urinary ascites—a second case. J. Urol., 28:333, 1932.

Meigs, J. V.: The Wertheim operation for carcinoma of the cervix. Amer. J. Obstet. Gynec., *49*:542, 1945.

Wertheim, E.: Zur Frage der Radikaloperation beim Uteruskrebs. Arch. Gynäk., *61*: 627, 1900.

——: Die erweiterte abdominale Operation bei Carcinoma colli uteri. Berlin, Urban and Schwarzenberg, 1911.

13

Surgery of the Double Uterus

INDICATIONS FOR SURGERY

Surgery upon the double uterus (Fig. 13-1) may be required for a variety of symptoms or complications resulting from the congenital abnormality. Undoubtedly, the operation was done in the past on many occasions without proper indications. Ruge, in 1882, first reported the excision of a uterine septum in a woman who had had 2 abortions. She subsequently carried to term. The strongest advocate of the plastic operation was Paul Strassmann, of Berlin, who first unified a bicornate uterus through the anterior cul-de-sac in 1907. He subsequently performed 17 unifications. His son, Erwin Strassmann, has continued

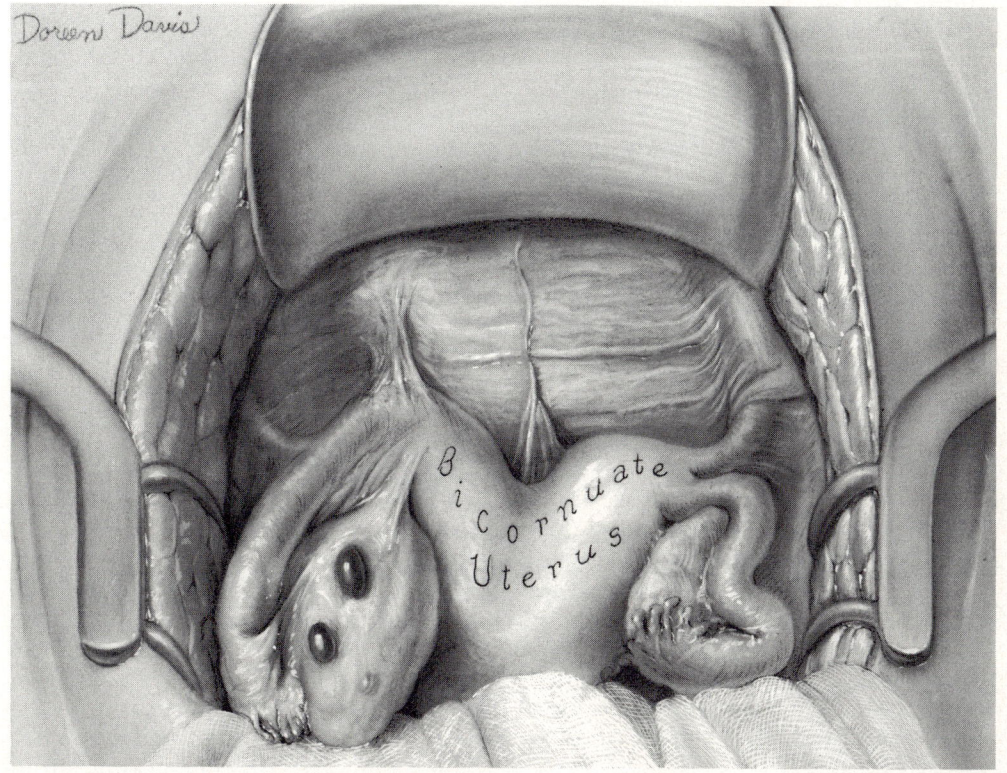

FIG. 13-1. Typical bicornuate uterus.

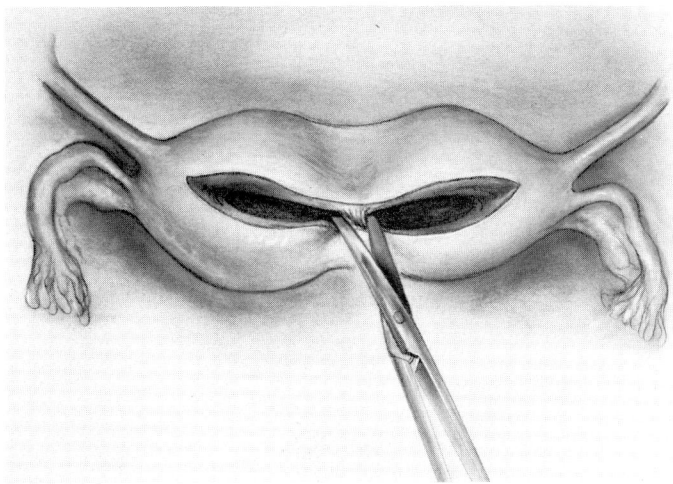

Fig. 13-2. Strassmann operation, showing incision of septum. This is now only of historical interest.

interest in the operation and has collected 123 such operations carried out over the past 70 years. The indications for which these operations were done were habitual abortion, dysmenorrhea, menometrorrhagia, sterility, dyspareunia, and premature delivery. It is obvious that many of these conditions would not be considered proper indication for the operation today. The surgical procedures used for the unification described here differ in an important detail from the Strassmann procedure. In the latter, the uterine incision is transverse from cornu to cornu across the uterine fundus with the final suture line in the anteroposterior midplane of the uterus. Such a procedure incises rather than excises the septum. (Fig. 13-2).

The operation herein reported attempts to excise the muscular septum by a triangular incision, resulting in a final vertical midline incision. This has the additional advantage of avoiding injury to the cornua.

Although there are perhaps other indications, we have found the following indications requiring surgery on the double uterus:

1. Hematometra occurring in a rudimentary horn or in a completely septate uterus in which one uterine cavity does not communicate with the other cavity or the cervical canal.
2. Pyometra occurring in one or both horns, resulting from infection in the cavity from which drainage is inadequate.
3. Habitual abortions, occurring as a result of the congenital abnormality, *after excluding endocrine or metabolic disturbances which might account for the abortions.*

SURGERY FOR HEMATOMETRA

Operation for hematometra for a noncommunicating rudimentary uterus consists of excision of the rudimentary uterus and adnexa. Figure 9-23, shown in Chapter 9, Endometriosis, shows such a case encountered at the Mayo Clinic. The retention of menstrual blood resulted in hematometra, hematosalpinx, and unilateral pelvic endometriosis. The rudimentary uterus and the unilateral adnexa were excised by Counseller, and subsequently the patient was delivered of a full-term child.

A rarer condition is the one shown in Figure 13-3, in which a bicornate uterus was associated with a complete septum. One cavity failed to communicate with the other uterine cavity or the cervical canal. The patient complained of incapacitating dysmenorrhea, which lasted for 5 days, and a tense cystic mass was palpable in the right half of the pelvis.

Operation consisted of making an incision through the anterior wall of the

Surgery for Pyometra

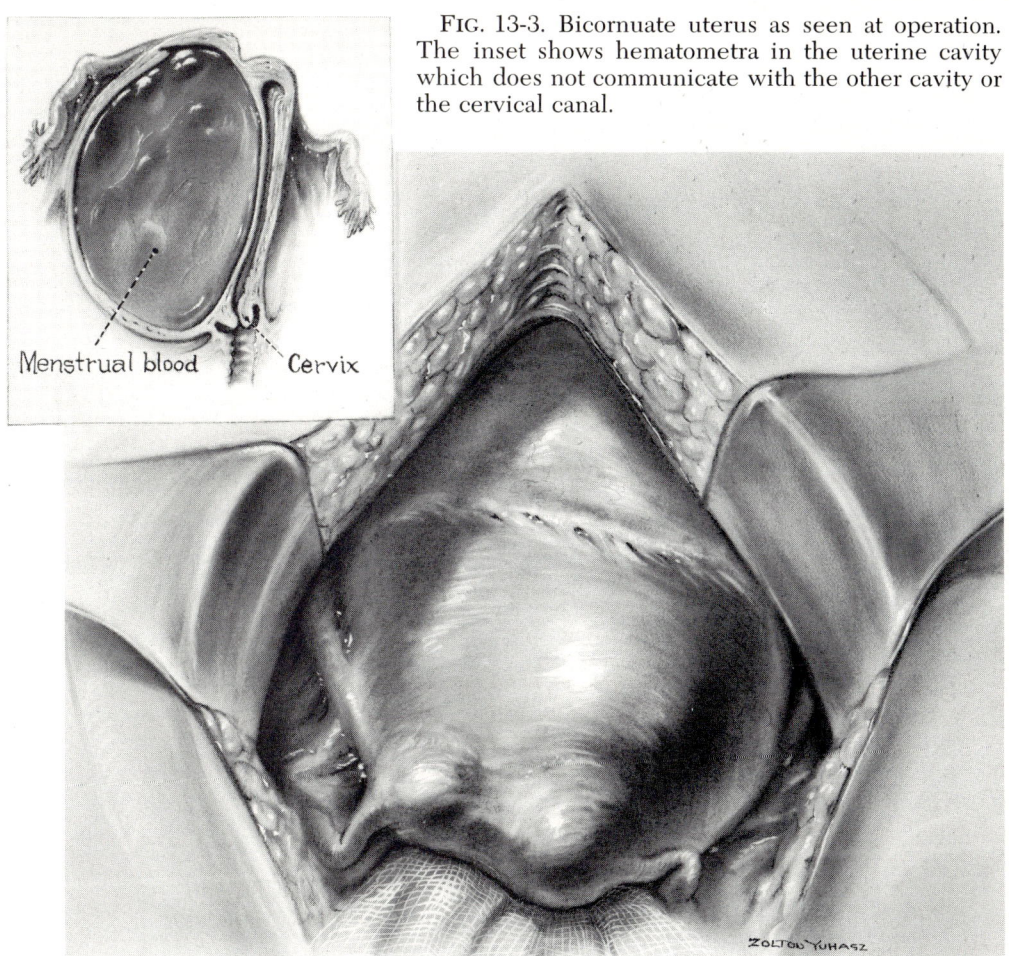

Fig. 13-3. Bicornuate uterus as seen at operation. The inset shows hematometra in the uterine cavity which does not communicate with the other cavity or the cervical canal.

cystic right portion of the uterus. It was found to contain old menstrual blood. The entire septum was excised, and the uterus was reconstructed by anastomosis of the two cavities. A continuous lock stitch joining endometrium to endometrium was reinforced by interrupted myometrial sutures (Fig. 13-4 A). The plastic reconstruction of the uterus was completed by a third layer of interrupted sutures, uniting myometrium and serosa (Fig. 13-4 B).

A hysterogram taken 15 months after the operative procedure showed a rather large but symmetrical uterine cavity. Two years after the operation the patient reported that she was menstruating painlessly every 2 to 3 months. She was only 16 years old at this time and was not married.

SURGERY FOR PYOMETRA

Faulty drainage of one or both horns of a double uterus may make infection more serious than in the normal uterus. Pyometra and/or pyosalpinx may result and eventually may require major surgery. Figure 13-5 is the uterus of a women whose left uterine horn was infected by artificial, intra-uterine insemination. The infection reached the peritoneal cavity, and a pelvic abscess resulted. This was drained by culpotomy, and the patient was in relatively good health for 4 years.

284 Surgery of the Double Uterus

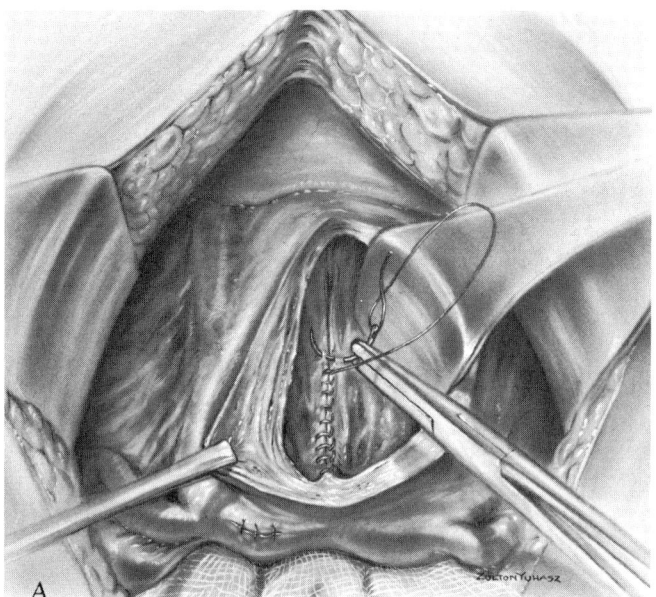

Fig. 13-4 A. The septum of the bicornuate uterus seen in Figure 13-3 has been excised, and anastomosis is being made, uniting the two cavities.

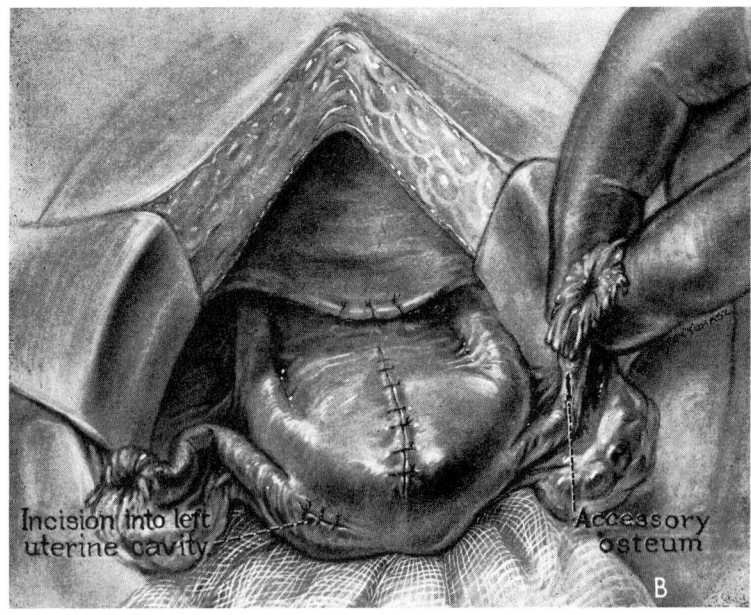

Fig. 13-4 B. Anastomosis is completed. The small incision in the left uterine cavity was made before the septum was removed for the purpose of orientation.

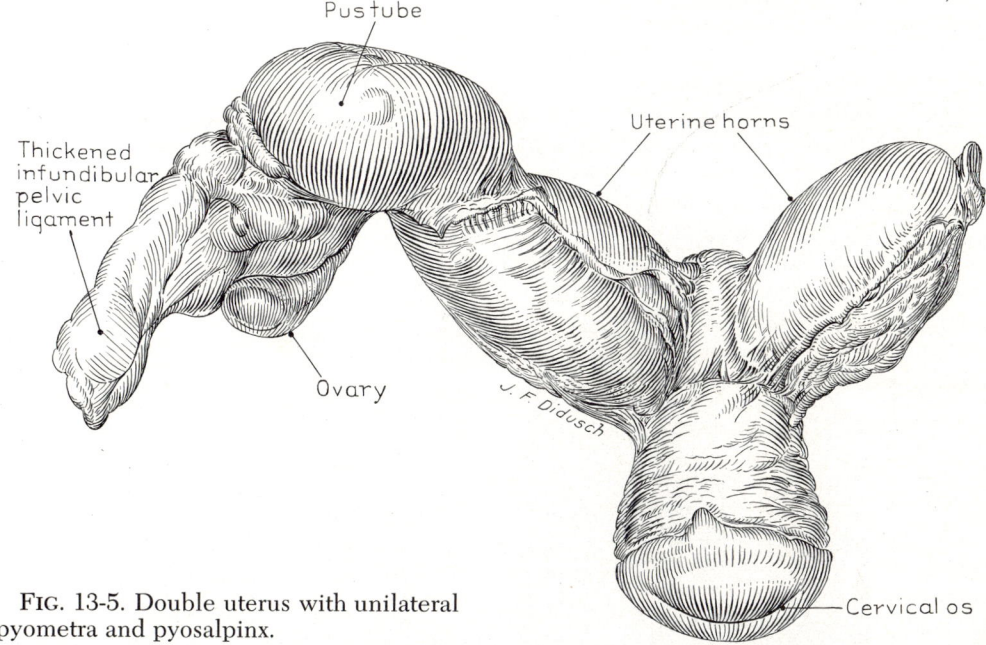

FIG. 13-5. Double uterus with unilateral pyometra and pyosalpinx.

Then she developed severe abdominal pain, and on one occasion there was a sudden gush of a large quantity of pus from the vagina. In spite of this spontaneous emptying of the pyometra, the patient continued to have pain, and surgery became necessary. The unilateral pyometra and pyosalpinx shown in Figure 13-5 were found. Because the patient had been married and sterile for 10 years, the entire double uterus and left adnexa were removed. The right adnexa, being normal, were saved. The patient has remained well since the operation.

SURGERY FOR HISTORY OF HABITUAL ABORTION

Probably the most important indication for surgery on the double uterus is for the cure of habitual abortion. There is no doubt that pregnancies occurring in the double uterus abort more frequently than when occurring in the normal uterus. Miller collected 67 pregnancies in didelphic uteri with an abortion rate of 28.3 per cent. Smith in an analysis of 35 such patients noted an overall abortion incidence of 23.5 per cent. Schauffler reported on 11 patients with 32 pregnancies and 17 abortions, an incidence of 53 per cent. Hoyt C. Taylor reported 11 patients, 8 of whom were exposed to pregnancy. There were 12 pregnancies with 4 abortions, or 33 per cent. Jones and Jones, in reviewing 52 pregnancies in 21 women at the Johns Hopkins Hospital, found an incidence of abortions of 27 per cent. All of the above figures are substantially higher than the 10 to 15 per cent usually quoted as the overall population abortion incidence.

The incidence of abortions is higher in those patients in whom there is a septate uterus (Fig. 13-6) than in those patients having completely double uteri (Fig. 13-7). This indicates that if two definite corpora can be felt on bimanual examination, the prognosis for completion of pregnancy is better than when the uterus feels normal or slightly notched, and the septum is demonstrable only on hysterography. Hence, all patients with a history of habitual abortion should have a hysterosalpingogram.

In spite of the recognized increased incidence of abortions in women with duplication of the uterus, it does not hold

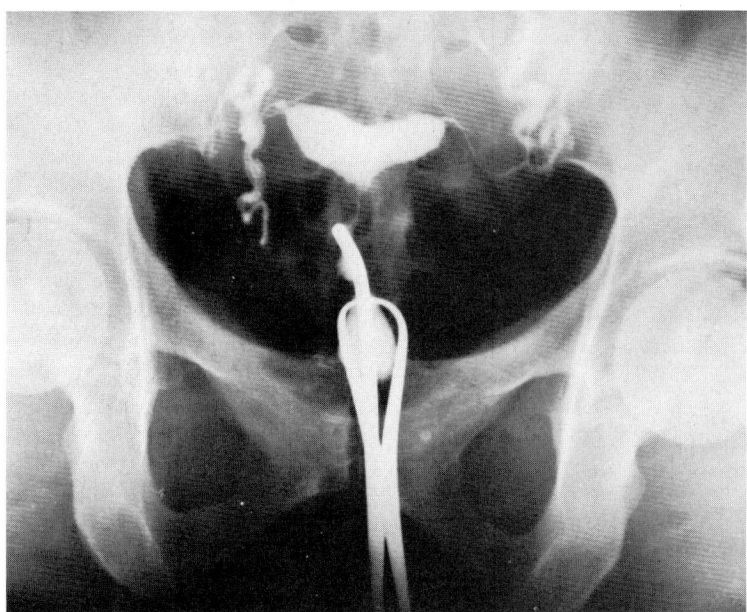

FIG. 13-6. Hysterogram of bicornuate uterus with thick septum.

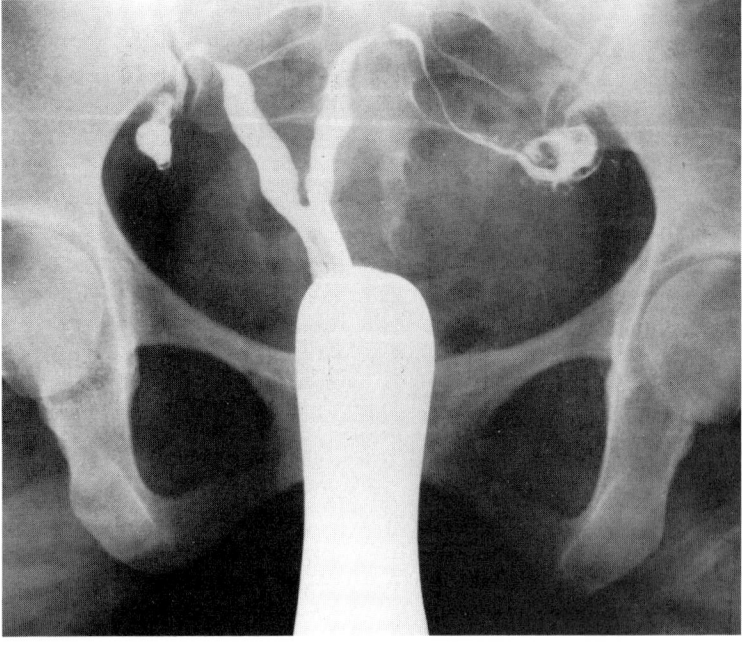

FIG. 13-7. Hysterogram of two completely separate corpora with a single cervix.

that the double uterus in a woman with a history of habitual abortion necessarily accounts for the abortions.

In the last edition of this book a case was reported of a women with a double uterus who had been married for 5 years and had had 4 miscarriages. Complete endocrinologic and metabolic studies showed a serious inadequacy of luteal function, with evidence of thyroid and adrenal disturbance. Therapy for these abnormalities resulted in a living child without surgical correction of the double uterus. Since that time, Jones and Jones have had greater experience with this condition and suggest a complete endocrinologic investigation before deciding on surgery. A premenstrual endometrial biopsy for evaluation of the luteal phase is particularly important. A review of the status of the other endocrine glands should be made as well as an evaluation of the nutritional status and possible stress evaluation. An estimation of the normalcy of any pregnancy which occurs while the patient is under investigation is carried out by serial quantitative determinations of serum chorionic gonadotropin, as well as urinary pregnanediol when necessary.

When an endocrine abnormality is discovered, it should be corrected before considering surgery. Jones and Jones found that among 98 women with some degree of uterine duplication, there had been 321 pregnancies with an abortion or premature rate of 43 per cent. Among 31 of these patients in whom some endocrine abnormality or abnormalities were found, there had been 72 pregnancies, only 8 of which had gone to term. After proper therapy correcting the endocrine abnormality there were 58 pregnancies, 44 of which went to term. There were only 8 premature babies and 6 abortions. Most of the premature babies lived, so that there was a total of 51 living children.

Treatment was directed chiefly toward the luteal-phase defect, which most of these patients exhibited, by direct supplementation of the luteal phase preconceptionally by 12.5 mg. of progesterone, or its equivalent, daily, shifting to 17-hydroxyprogesterone caproate after pregnancy occurred, and administering this in amounts from 250 to 500 mg. per week, depending upon the pregnanediol values. Background factors such as nutritional defects, excess smoking and drinking, and stressful situations were eliminated insofar as possible. Furthermore, treatment directed at thyroid abnormalities and adrenal disorders was carried out as indicated.

After those cases with an endocrine disorder have been excluded, there remains a substantial percentage of patients in whom the duplication of the uterus plays a role in the high rate of abortions or premature deliveries. Jones and Wheeless report on 22 such patients. There had been 86 pregnancies in this group, 82 of which had terminated in abortion and 4 in premature delivery. There were only 2 living children. After a unifying operation there were at the time of their report 37 pregnancies, 25 of which had gone to term. Nine aborted, and there were 3 premature deliveries.

Technic

The method of unifying a double uterus varies, depending on the degree of duplication. With a septate uterus such as that shown in Figure 13-8, a longitudinal incison is made in the anterior and the posterior uterine wall. The septum is excised, and the two portions of the uterus are sutured together with 3 layers of interrupted catgut sutures. In the case pictured in Figure 13-8, pregnancy occurred within a year after such a unification. Figure 13-9 shows the same uterus at full term as the baby was delivered by cesarean section.

When there is a more complete duplication, such as that shown in Figure 13-10, a different technic is used. In addition to the duplication of the corpus uteri, there was a small septum at the external os. This was first excised from below. Then a laparotomy was done. The medial walls of both uteri were excised. A male rubber catheter was then pushed down through the cervix, and the two halves were sutured together in 3 layers as shown in Figure 13-11 and 13-12. After completion of the operation the catheter was withdrawn.

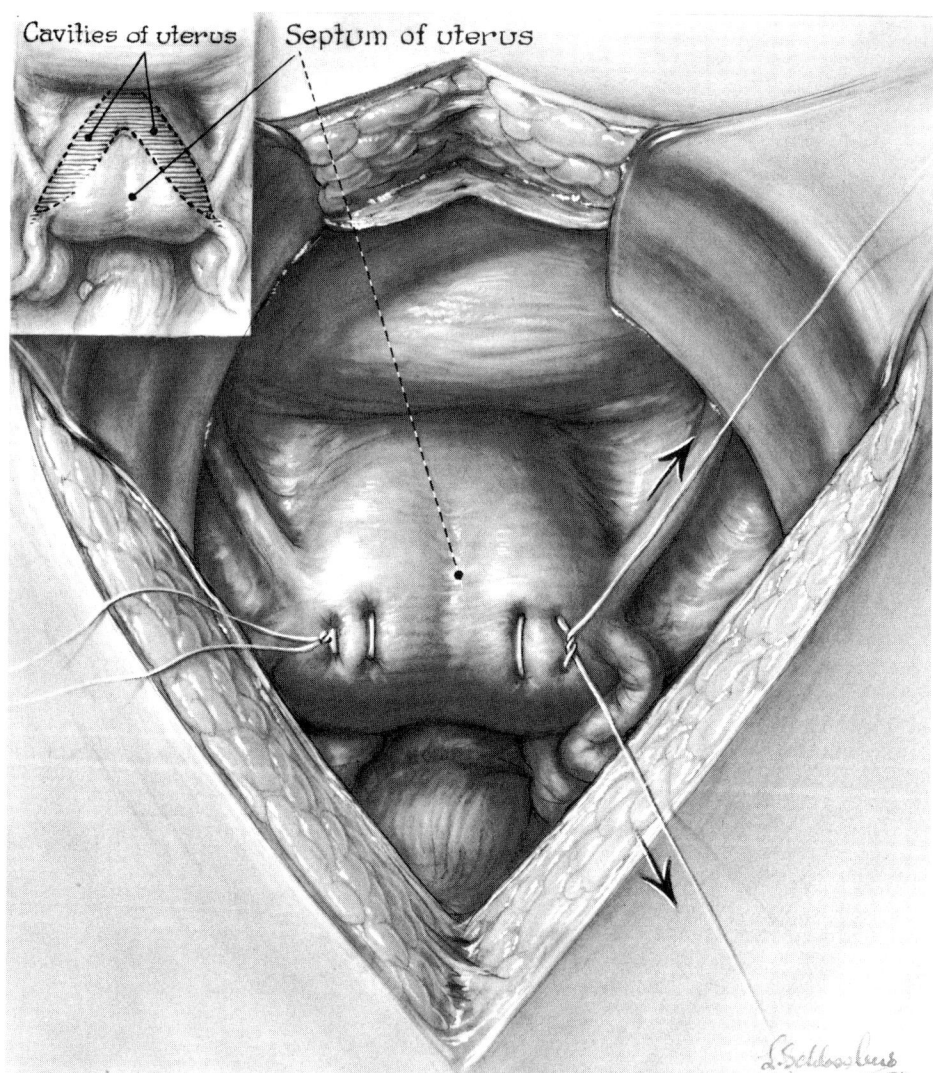

Fig. 13-8. Appearance of the uterus at operation. The inset shows the cavities as found after opening the uterus.

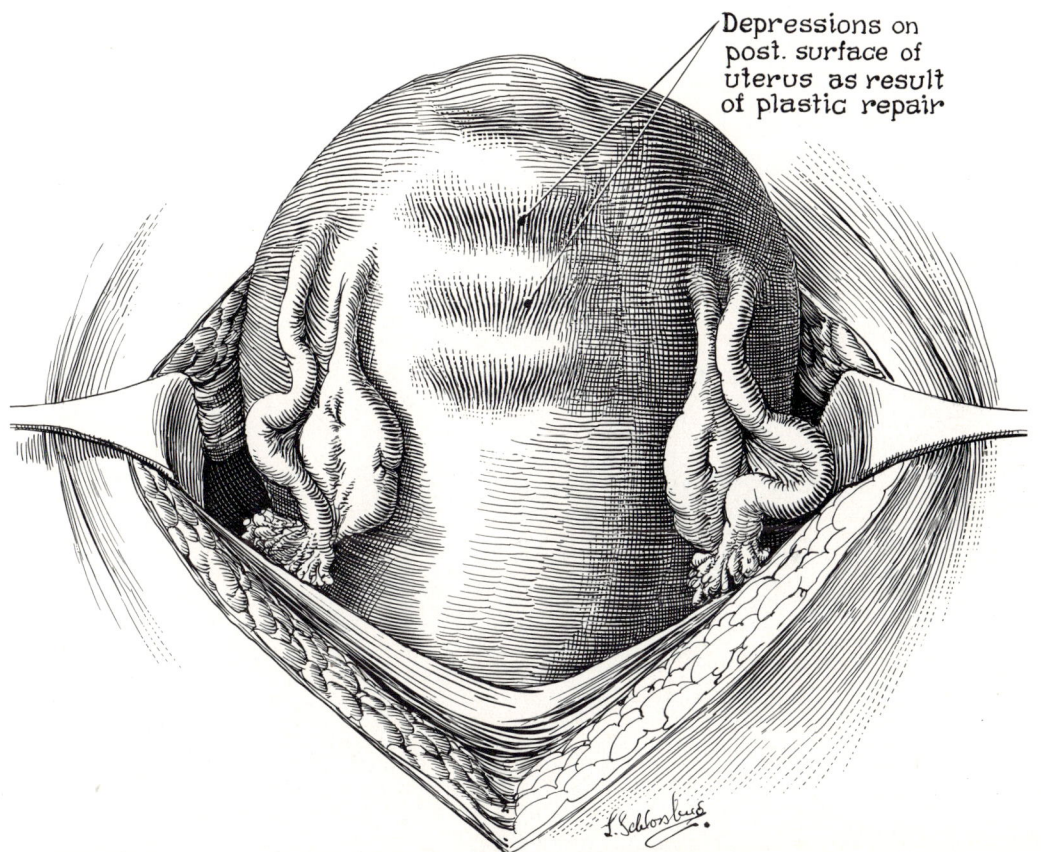

FIG. 13-9. Posterior surface of term uterus, showing scarring from plastic repair.

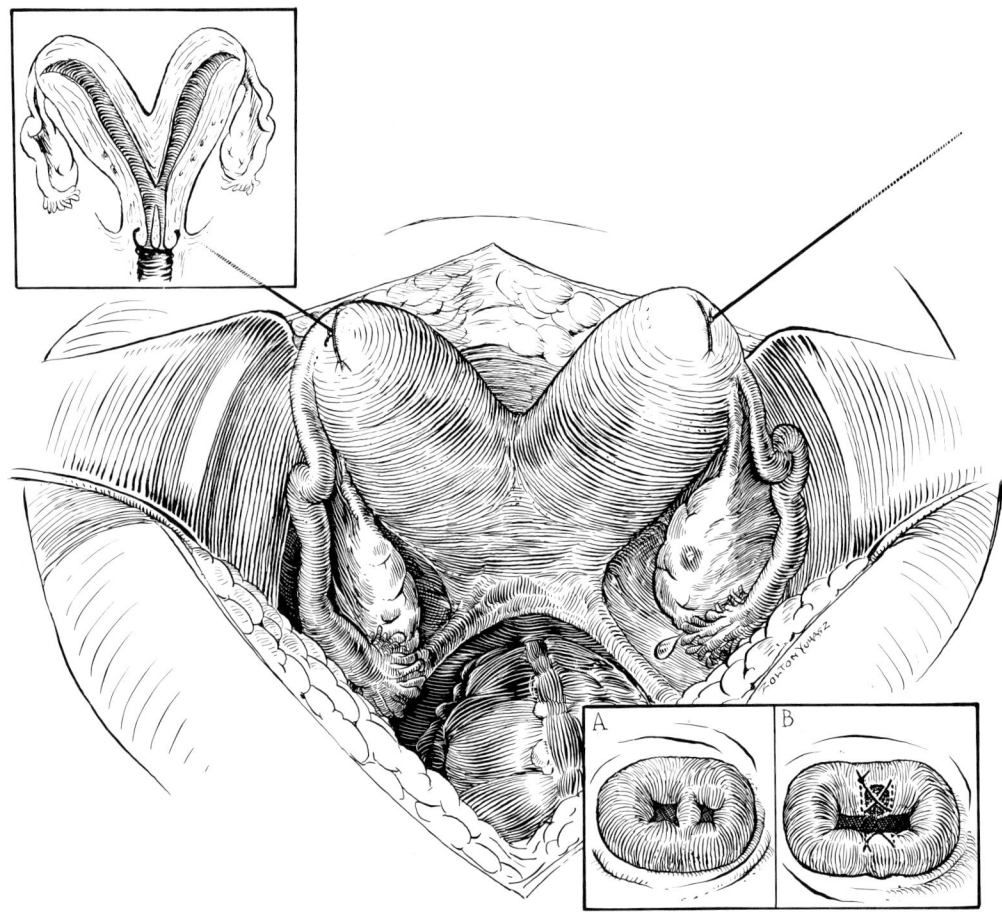

Fig. 13-10. Double uterus with double external os divided by septum but with single cervical canal higher up. Septum at external os was first excised from below, as shown in Figure 13-11.

Surgery for History of Habitual Abortion 291

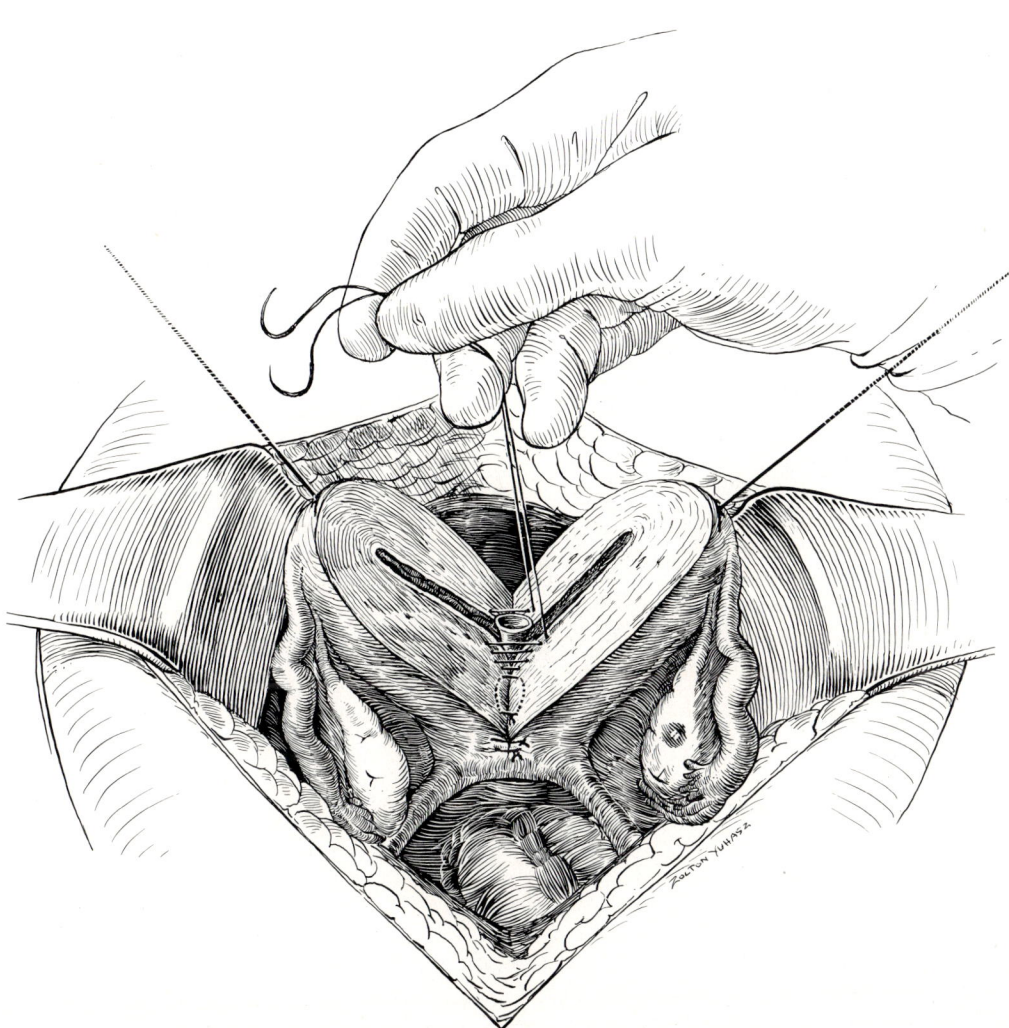

FIG. 13-11. The medial portions of both uteri have been excised. A catheter has been inserted downward through the cervix. Suturing is done around the cathether in the uterine cavity. The 3 layers of closure of the myometrium and the serosa are indicated in this sketch.

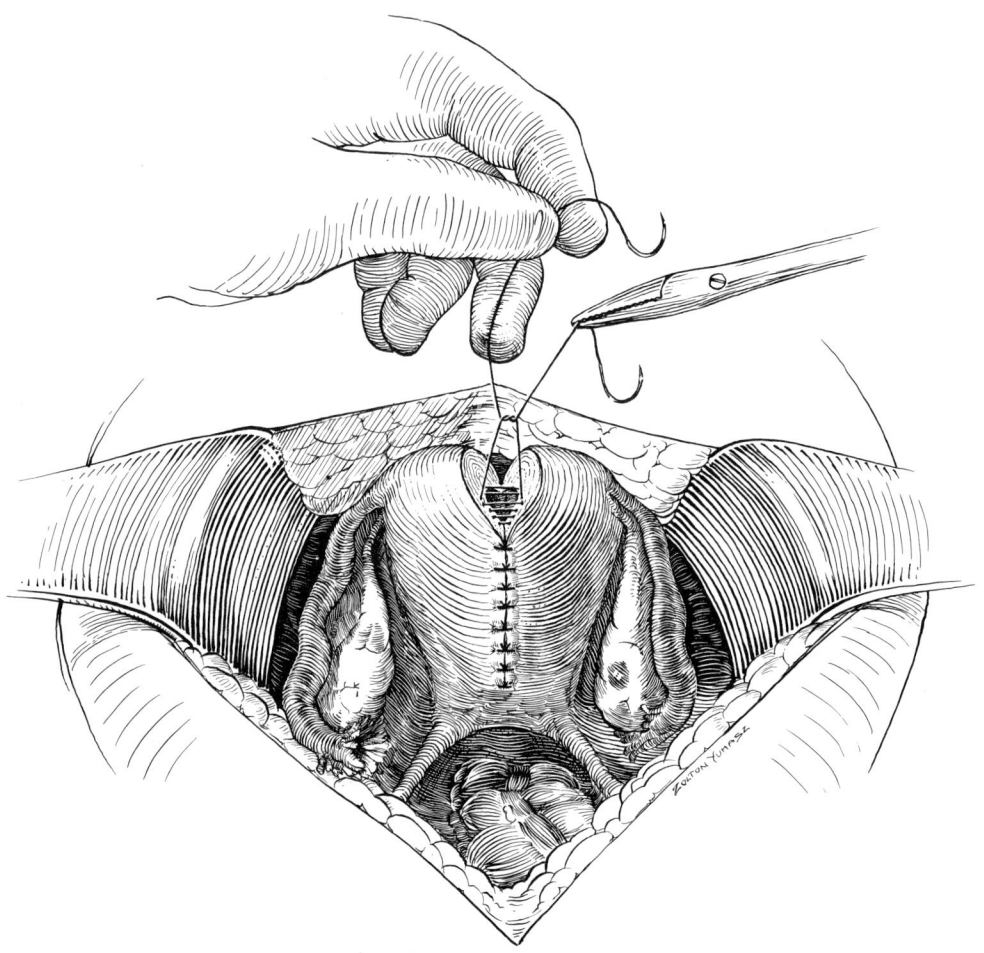

Fig. 13-12. The closure is almost complete, and the resulting single uterus appears to be almost normal.

BIBLIOGRAPHY

Jones, H. W., Jr., and Jones, G. S.: Double uterus as an etiological factor in repeated abortion: indications for surgical repair. Amer. J. Obstet. Gynec., 65:325, 1953.

Jones, H. W., and Wheeless, C. R.: Salvage of the reproductive potential of women with anomalous development of the müllerian ducts: 1868-1968-2068. Amer. J. Obstet. Gynec., 104:348, 1969.

Miller, N. F.: Uterus didelphys. Amer. J. Obstet. Gynec., 4:398, 1922.

Ruge, P.: Fall von Schwangerschaft bei Uterus septus. Z. Geburtschilfe Gynäk., 10:141, 1884.

Schauffler, G.: Double uterus with pregnancy. J.A.M.A., 117:1516, 1941.

Smith, F. R.: Significance of incomplete fusion of müllerian ducts in pregnancy and parturition with report on 35 cases. Amer. J. Obstet. Gynec., 22:714, 1931.

Strassmann, E. O.: Plastic unification of double uterus. Amer. J. Obstet. Gynec., 64:25, 1952.

Strassmann, P.: Die operative Vereinigung eines doppelten Uterus; nebst Bemerkungen über die Korrektur der sogenannten Verdoppelung des Genital-Kanales. Zbl. Gynäk. Leipz., 31:1322, 1907.

Taylor, H. C.: Pregnancy and the double uterus. Amer. J. Obstet. Gynec., 46:388, 1943.

14

Infertility

GENERAL CONSIDERATIONS

For purposes of clarity, the term *infertility* should be considered separately from the more ominous classification of *sterility* and the broader topic of *reproductive failure*. In brief, infertility relates to those factors in married couples that temporarily interfere with conception. This may be either *primary*, in which conception has not occurred previously, or *secondary*, in which there has been a previous pregnancy with transient difficulty in conceiving again. In contrast, sterility is concerned with more serious reproductive problems in which the etiologic factors preclude the possibility of future pregnancy. It is obvious that the infertility status of an individual may change from one category to another, depending on the success or failure of treatment of the underlying factors.

The frequency of this clinical problem varies between countries, but in the United States it includes 12 to 15 per cent of all married couples in whom fertility is either temporary or permanently impaired. According to Southam, 60 per cent of normal married couples will achieve pregnancy within 6 months of marriage, and 75 per cent will become pregnant within the first year. After 2 years of marriage, 82 per cent of such normal couples will achieve a pregnancy. In contrast, after 1 year of involuntary infertility, 30 per cent of such couples ultimately are proven to be sterile, while after 2 years there is a sterility rate of 54 per cent. The fertility rate of a married couple is also related to age. According to Southam, there is an infertility rate of 31.3 per cent of couples over the age of 35 and a 70 per cent infertility rate over the age of 40. In comparison, there is only a 4.5 per cent infertility rate between the ages of 16 to 20.

Advances in reproductive physiology during the past quarter century have interrelated many problems of infertility with the field of endocrinology. Many etiologic factors must be thoroughly evaluated in order to initiate proper treatment. These include (1) anovulation, (2) luteal phase defects, (3) cervical factors, (4) tubal factors, (5) male factors, and (6) immunologic factors.

Since it is impractical to attempt to discuss the accumulated literature relating to each factor influencing infertility, a practical approach to the investigation of this entity is presented below.

DIAGNOSTIC EVALUATION

1. Detection of Ovulation. An accurate history of regular menstrual periods is perhaps one of the most useful clinical methods of predicting ovulation. In fact, some investigators state that menses cannot occur in a perfectly regular fashion for any length of time without cyclic ovulation. This fact is easily documented by a written record of the dates of each menstrual period as well as by an accurate basal body temperature chart (BBT) demonstrating a biphasic thermogenic temperature curve. A persistent rise of the basal temperature of at least 0.5° F. following ovulation should persist for approximately 14 days. Although the oral temperature is usually satisfactory to demonstrate this thermal change, in cases of an erratic temperature pattern, rectal temperatures may be taken before rising each morning for more accurate monitoring of the basal temperature. Ovulation may also be confirmed by an endometrial biopsy, which demonstrates secretory endometrium, as shown in Figure 14-1. A daily vaginal smear for evaluation of the maturation index will show a midzone shift following ovulation, but this study is difficult to obtain due to the limits of patient cooperation.

There are many factors which may interfere with cyclic ovulatory function, including the central nervous system, endocrine factors, and dysfunction of the ovary, to mention only a few. These require specific treatment before ovulatory cycles will resume. In some instances, such as premature ovarian failure, ovulation will not recur.

There has been one endocrinologic breakthrough, however, since the last edition of this text concerning the treatment of hypothalamic dysfunction with clomiphene citrate, 50 mg./day $\times$ 5 days each month. This compound presumably acts as an antiestrogen and enhances the activation of FSH and LH releasing factors from the hypothalamus, which initiates ovulation. The drugs must be used repeatedly each month until normal hypothalamic function returns.

2. **Luteal Phase Defects.** Even though ovulation has been documented, there may be insufficient progesterone support of the endometrium due to inadequate maintenance or function of the corpus

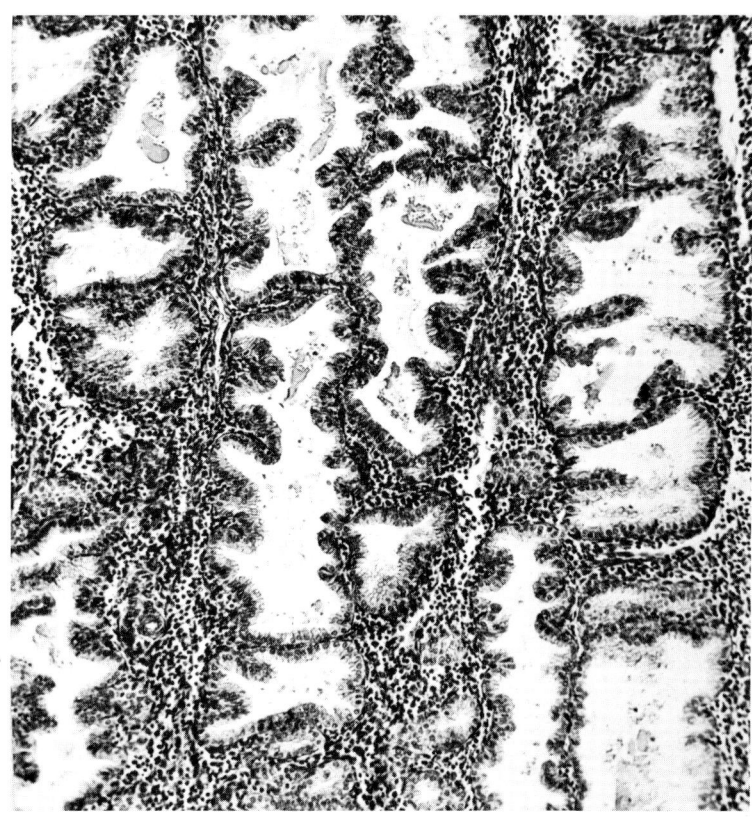

FIG. 14-1. Premenstrual secretory endometrium.

luteum, which may be related to gonadotropin stimulation, primarily LH. This is a difficult diagnosis to establish as it requires accurate histologic dating of the endometrium, which has been described by Noyes, Hertig, and Rock. A premenstrual endometrial biopsy taken on day 25 of the menstrual cycle should not vary histologically more than 48 hours from the day of the cycle. Daily 24-hour urine determinations of pregnanediol following ovulation will further document an inadequate luteal phase. In a normal menstrual cycle, progesterone is excreted in the urine as pregnanediol at day 21 in approximately 6-10 mg./24 hrs. A pregnanediol excretion of 2.5 mg. or less per day at this time suggests a luteal phase deficiency. In addition, a deficiency of progesterone excretion is demonstrated by either a slow BBT rise or a premature fall of the temperature after ovulation has occurred. After 2 or more cycles in which there is failure of such correlation, this diagnosis may be made, and the luteal phase should be supplemented with small daily doses of progestins. We have used 10 mg. of oral medroxyprogesterone acetate (Provera) with good success in such cases, given for 10 days after BBT evidence of ovulation. This defect, which is usually central in origin, is reportedly present in 5 to 10 per cent of infertile patients and may be responsible for either failure of implantation of the blastocyst following fertilization or early spontaneous abortions.

3. **Cervical Factors.** Changes in the cervical mucus have been studied by many investigators, including Lamar, Shettles, and Delfs (1940), Pommerenke (1946), and more recently by Marcus and Marcus (1963). Cervical mucus is most receptive to sperm penetration and migration at midcycle during a high estrogen peak, at which time the mucus is copious, watery, and is reduced in viscosity (spinnbarkeit of 5 cm. or longer). Normal cervical mucus is increased in amount at midcycle due to estrogen stimulation of the endocervical glands and is clear and relatively acellular. Crystallization of the mucus upon air drying on a glass slide is a term called *ferning*. Such a ferning pattern is due to precipitation of sodium and potassium salts in the cervical mucus in the presence of high estrogen levels, which does not occur following ovulation in the presence of progesterone. Improvement in the quality (decreased viscosity) and quantity of cervical mucus may be obtained by giving small daily doses of oral estrogen, such as 0.1 mg. of stilbestrol.

Chronic cervicitis, producing a tenacious, mucopurulent discharge, may provide a "hostile" environment for sperm penetration and migration through the cervical canal and should be treated by clearing the infection with cauterization, vaginal suppositories, douches, and, if necessary, systemic antibiotics. The endocervical glands may be infected, as evidenced by WBC's in the cervical mucus on microscopic examination. In the presence of unexplained infertility, such a finding should be treated adequately with 7 days of broad-spectrum antibiotics. On the other hand, it is remarkable that some women conceive despite profuse cervical leukorrhea.

Cervical stenosis may play a major role in infertility. This may result from a congenital anatomic defect, or may occur following severe endocervicitis, radical cauterization, or cervical conization. It is important always to sound the cervical canal and uterine cavity for demonstration of patency of the cervical canal. There is no doubt clinically that women often become pregnant following cervical dilatation after a long period of infertility.

4. **Tubal Factors.** Perhaps the most serious, as well as most frequent factor influencing infertility is related to anatomic and physiologic alterations of the fallopian tube. Tubal peristalsis and the ciliary action of the fimbriae are responsible for ova pickup from the ovarian cortex or peritoneal cavity prior to fertilization of the gametes in the outer third of the fallopian tube.

The most common disease which produces anatomic deformity of the tube is gonococcal endosalpingitis. Unless treated early, this infection will produce tubal occlusion at various locations from the uterine cornu to the fimbriae, with resultant tubal obstruction, hydrosalpinx, or tubo-ovarian inflammatory masses. (See Chapter 11, Pelvic Inflammatory Disease and Its Complications.) The initial infection is usually the most damaging to the tubal mucosa and motility since the gonococcus frequently is followed by secondary infections of staphylococcus, streptococcus, or coliform organisms, resulting in chronic and irreversible tubal damage. Even though complete obstruction of the fallopian tube may not occur with such infections, fusion of the fimbriated appendages or impairment of ciliary activity may produce infertility by interference with ovum pickup and transport. Peritubal scarring resulting from pelvic endometriosis or from other causes of extrapelvic infection (appendicitis, diverticulitis, etc.) may produce similar interference in tubal motility. Impaired tubal motility explains an infertility rate of approximately 30 per cent of patients with endometriosis even though there is demonstrable evidence of tubal patency.

Because of the increased frequency of tubal factors as a major cause of infertility, tubal function studies should be carried out early in the investigation of the infertile couple. The remainder of the infertility evaluation should also be completed due to the fact that in approximately 15 per cent of such cases there are two or more factors involved. Basically, there are three currently available methods of observing tubal function, namely, (1) tubal insufflation (Rubin's test), (2) hysterosalpingography, and (3) culdoscopy and laparoscopy. These methods are discussed further in this chapter under Special Diagnostic Studies.

5. **Male Factors.** The infertile couple must be evaluated as a biologic unit since approximately 30 per cent of barren marriages are due to male factors. Although a normal sperm count includes 60 million sperm/ml. of ejaculate, the lower limits of normal should include at least 20 million/ml., according to MacLeod. Recent evidence from Baeyertz in New Zealand reaffirms our clinical impression that the quality and viability of the sperm are as important as the quantity. At least 40 per cent of the cells must show excellent motility, and no more than 40 per cent of the total sperm population should demonstrate anatomical abnormalities. In the New Zealand study (Baeyertz), 10 per cent of 158 patients studied with full sperm counts had counts below 10 million/ml., and of these 37 per cent conceived. In the Hopkins clinic, Jones reports a 25 per cent pregnancy rate in couples where the count was below 20 million/ml. Hotchkiss found semen counts as low as 2.25 million/ml. in husbands whose wives were pregnant. However, it is generally believed that the lower the sperm count, the lower is the fertility rate.

The initial assessment of the adequacy of male sperm is obtained by postcoital examination (Sims-Huhner test). This test is performed at midcycle, approximately 8 to 12 hours following intercourse. The patient is instructed not to douche following coitus, and the cervical mucus is obtained from the endocervical canal by a fine glass pipette. The finding of less than 5-10 motile sperm/hpf would suggest a male factor and requires a complete semen analysis and a urological examination of the male. Such factors as hypospadias and retrograde ejaculation as well as the "virgin wife" are coital factors that require investigation.

An important factor in male infertility has been confirmed in recent years following the initial report by Tulloch in 1952 on the relationship between varicocele of the spermatic vein and infertility. Since that time, numerous reports have confirmed the high incidence of infertility with varicocele of the left testis. The entrance of the left internal spermatic vein at right angles to the renal vein in contrast to the oblique entry of the right internal spermatic vein into the vena cava is considered to be a possible anatomic cause of either poor venous drainage on the left side or retrograde blood flow into the left spermatic vein from the kidney (Fig. 14-2). Although the exact mechanism of interference with spermatogenesis is unclear, a temperature change in the scrotum is thought to be a major factor in the normal production of the male gamete. MacLeod reports im-

FIG. 14-2. Varicocele of left testis demonstrating entrance of spermatic vein at right angles to the renal vein with potential reversal of venous drainage of left kidney and testis, which may produce venous dilatation and varicocele formation.

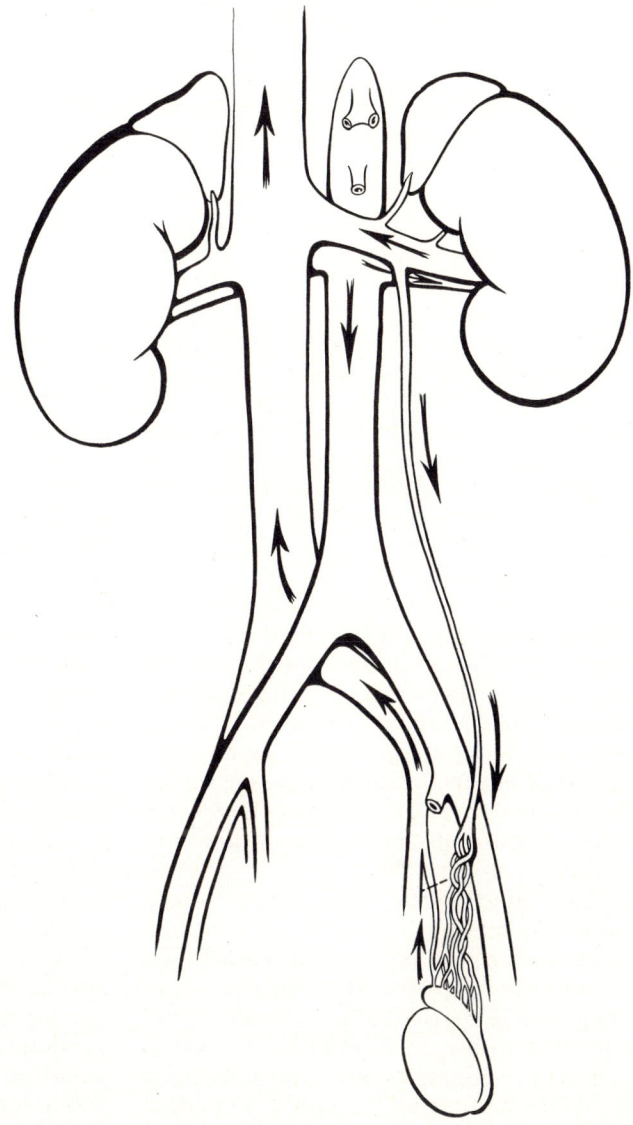

provement in the semen quality following ligation of the varicocele in 185 patients with oligospermia, poor motility, and increased abnormal forms. The most consistent improvement was found in sperm motility and morphology, which resulted in a significant conception rate of 40 per cent. Many pregnancies occurred with very low sperm count levels (under 20 million/ml.).

One additional subtle etiologic factor should be searched for in the infertile male, namely, the adrenogenital syndrome, in which there is a congenital enzymatic deficiency of the adrenal gland in cortisol synthesis. Although such cases are infrequent, the only clinical expression of this entity in the adult male is short stature and azospermia or oligospermia. Due to the increased adrenal secretion of androgens, pituitary gonadotropins are suppressed through the hypothalamus, with resultant decreased spermatogenesis. Such androgenicity is undetectable in the male except by an elevated 17-ketosteroid (above 20 mg./24 hr.) and pregnanetriol determinations. The 17-ketosteroids are easily suppressed by a cortisone suppression test. Although much less frequent, this syndrome is similar to the female variety, which produces primary amenorrhea, and it must be treated with continuous cortisone replacement each day. Under such therapy, the gonadotropin-releasing factors from the hypothalamus are increased, with release of pituitary gonadotropins and improvement in the male in spermatogenesis.

In general, most other causes of azospermia are relatively refractory to medical therapy. Although the rebound phenomena is frequently attempted with the temporary use of methyltestosterone, the clinical results of this method of stimulating gonadotropin release are quite poor.

6. **Immunologic Factors.** These have recently been implicated in an antigen-antibody reaction by Franklin and Dukes, resulting from an antigen on the surface of sperm, which gradually produces a specific antibody in the serum of the female. This antibody reacts as an antigen-antibody isoagglutinin when sperm enters the female reproductive tract. Such sperm agglutination and/or immobilization has been demonstrated in normal infertile couples by immunologic tests on samples of male semen and serum from the spouse. Such an immunologic response is reportedly improved by either coital abstinence or the use of a sheath for 6 months or longer, following which sperm migration is markedly improved through the cervical canal, uterine cavity, and fallopian tube.

Behrman has also initiated pioneer investigative work on other immunologic factors which may play an active role in infertility where there is no obvious explanation. The demonstration of auto-immune antibodies in the male serum which produce agglutination of his own sperm in his seminal fluid is an intriguing and complicated problem in infertility. Similarly, ABO (H) incompatibility between husband and wife is considered to be another immune mechanism whereby blood group antigens on the surface of the semen are agglutinated or immobilized by circulating antibodies in the female. In such cases, artificial insemination with sperm from a donor with blood group compatibility has been a successful method of treatment.

SPECIAL DIAGNOSTIC STUDIES

TUBAL INSUFFLATION

Tubal insufflation was first described by Rubin in 1920, and although there have been modifications of the original technic, this test rightfully bears his name, the Rubin's test. The procedure includes an endocervical cannula connected by rubber tubing to a mercury manometer and a source of carbon dioxide. Gas is gradually increased in rate of flow through the system to approximately 30-60 ml./min. The vagina is filled with sterile water to submerge the cervical os in order to detect any leakage of gas from the cervical canal. Tubal patency may be determined by a direct-writing recording device for a permanent record or by oscultation of the lower abdomen for the sound of gas passing from the tubes into the peritoneal cavity. Although normal fallopian tubes will demonstrate patency at pressures below 100 mm. Hg, the test is still considered to be in the normal range if patency is demonstrated below 180 mm. Hg. At higher pressures, however, there is a higher incidence of partial tubal obstruction. At pressures of 200 without demonstrable patency, the test is considered to be negative, and the tubes are either in spasm at the cornu or are pathologically obstructed. However, this test is considered only one of several methods of evaluating tubal patency, and a negative Rubin's test cannot be interpreted conclusively as evidence of tubal obstruction. A recent study by Sweeney and Gepfert from the New York Hospital documents this fact by reporting a 50 per cent pregnancy rate ultimately in patients whose tubal insufflation tests have recorded pressures of greater than 180 mm. Hg. The Rubin's test can only be interpreted, therefore, as a study of gross tubal function and must be either repeated or combined with other studies for final evaluation of tubal patency.

In general, it is preferable to perform the tubal insufflation prior to midcycle, about the 10th day, to avoid the objection of possibly transporting particles of endometrium through the tube if performed during the late secretory phase. We have not had this experience, having used the tubal insufflation test premenstrually as an opportunity to evaluate the histology of the endometrium at the same time. However, we do recognize the infrequent case in which gas has failed to pass through the tubes premenstrually, or in which tubal patency has been demonstrated subsequently during the first half of the cycle.

It is our preference to combine the tubal insufflation test with an adequate examination of the pelvic organs under anesthesia and a dilatation and curettage. A pelvic examination under anesthesia provides immeasurable clinical information which may not be available by an examination while the patient is awake. Thickening of the adnexal region of even a minimal degree should make one suspicious of old tubal disease, and an adequate examination of the ovaries for size and mobility provides much information on the pathology of the reproductive tract. Although it must be remembered that there may be complete occlusion of the tubes from salpingitis without the slightest palpable evidence of adnexal disease, thorough evaluation of the pelvis with the patient anesthetized and relaxed may frequently demonstrate evidence of other disease, such as nodularity of the cul-de-sac or uterosacral ligaments from endometriosis that would be difficult or impossible to detect otherwise.

Hysterosalpingography

Hysterosalpingography is a permanent, visual record of the presence or absence of tubal patency and was first described by both Carey and Rubin in 1914. This test is usually reserved for patients demonstrating a negative tubal insufflation study or as a confirmatory tubal examination. This study should not be performed in the latter part of the cycle due to the increased incidence of oil emboli in pelvic venogram or lymphangiogram when the vascularity of the endometrium and uterus is increased. Lipiodol, which made its appearance in 1922, was later abandoned by Rubin because of the occurrence of oil granuloma and lipoid salpingitis. Rubin noticed some persistence of oily media after hysterosalpingography in two thirds of the cases of one series he conducted. However, less than half of the cases of lipoid salpingitis recently reported by Elliott *et al.* could be attributed to oily contrast media, while the remainder were thought to be due to the piston action of solid instruments, with the dissemination of lubricant jelly, mineral oil used to lubricate cervical dilators, starch powder, and the like. More recently a water-soluble, opaque media (Salpix) has been used in our clinic to avoid such complications. Although the rapid absorption and egress of this dye eliminate the use of the delayed 24-hour film, we have not found this to be a disadvantage with this procedure.

As is true of the tubal insufflation study, interpretation of the hystersalpingogram must be done with some reservation. Sweeney and Gepfert recently reviewed the results of hysterosalpingography at New York Hospital and found 107 cases of tubal pathology in a group of 510 patients studied. Thirteen of the 107 patients with tubal pathology (12%) became pregnant, although most of these occurred in patients in whom the tubal obstruction was described as unilateral. Only 1 patient conceived of those patients in whom there was x-ray evidence of bilateral tubal occlusion.

Altemus *et al.* are convinced that the complications and shortcomings resulting from conventional hysterography can be overcome by supplementing the study with fluoroscopic visualization of the uterus and tubes, employing image intensification. The 30-second fluoroscopic exposure is equivalent in irradiation to one conventional radiographic exposure and can avoid the necessity for multiple films when there is inadequate uterine or tubal filling. This technic also avoids excessive venous or lymphatic injection when the dye is visualized in the myometrium. Although fluoroscopy has not been a part of the technic of hysterosalpingography at Hopkins, it has been found useful at Marquette.

Technic

The optimum time for performing hysterosalpingography is about a week after the cessation of the previous menstrual period. The patient is placed in the lithotomy position on an x-ray table that is equipped with a Bucky diaphragm. It is assumed that a previous careful bimanual pelvic examination has been made recently so that the operator is familiar with the size and the position of the uterus and the condition of the adnexa. A bivalve speculum is placed in the vagina, and the cervix is exposed. The anterior lip of the cervix is grasped with a 2-prong tenaculum, and the cervix is swabbed with cotton swabs soaked in Zephiran. The last swab is inserted into the cervical canal and is rotated. A uterine sound is inserted to determine the direction and the length of the uterine cavity. Then the cannula is introduced in the same direction, but not to the full depth of the cavity. Grasping the tenaculum and the cannula in one hand, the operator manipulates the syringe with the other. At present we are using Salpix, which we have found to be very satisfactory for visualization. There has been no evidence that it causes irritation. About 2 cc. of the dye is injected, and the exposure is made. In some clinics, fluoroscopy is performed prior to taking the x-ray.

This film is developed and inspected. If fluoroscopy and the film indicate the media is entering the uterine cavity, 3 or 4 cc. more is injected, and the film is developed. If inspection of that film indicates incomplete filling of the uterine cavity, more dye is injected, fractionally, (a few cc. at a time) until a filled cavity is visualized. The dye is injected under low pressure; in case resistance is encountered, the injection is discontinued, and an x-ray is taken, developed, and inspected.

When visualization of the tubes is desired, more dye is usually necessary, but in most cases about 6 cc. will suffice. If more is needed, it may be injected, provided that fluoroscopy or the first film shows the dye within the uterine cavity. Since the aqueous dyes are absorbed quickly, there is no object in taking a 24-hour film, as was previously often done when Lipiodol was used.

Figures 14-3 to 14-5A show the results of hysterosalpingogram studies concerned with tubal patency.

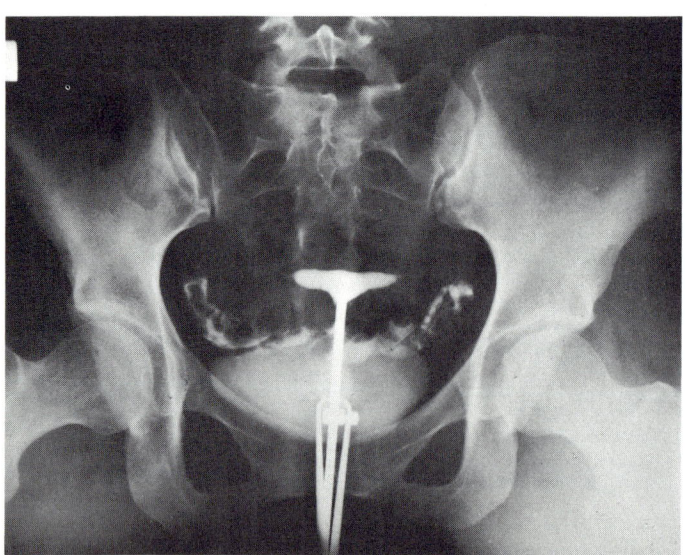

Fig. 14-3. A normal hysterosalpingogram. The dye has spilled into the peritoneal cavity. The bladder is also outlined by a cystogram.

FIG. 14-4. Bilateral hydrosalpinges with the dye.

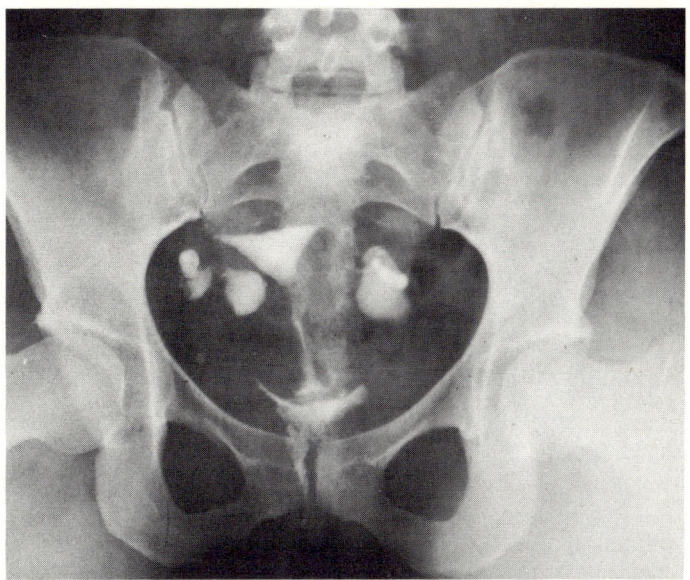

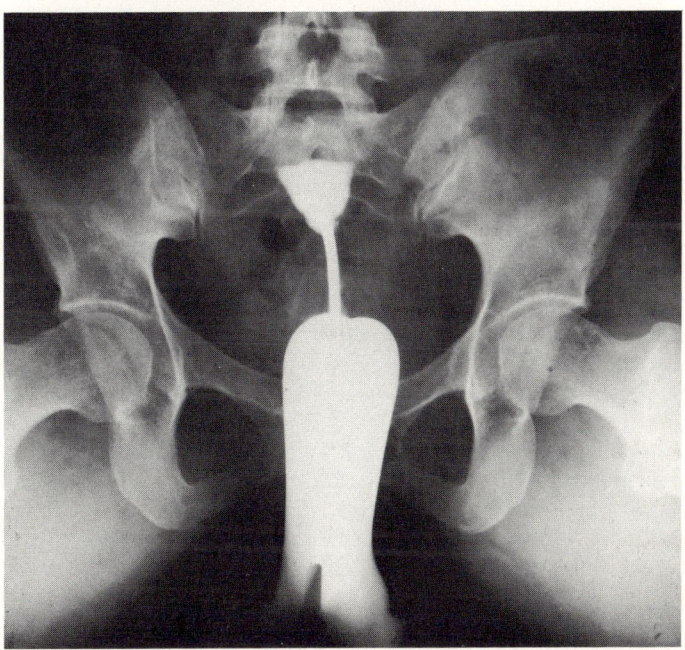

FIG. 14-5. Normal uterine cavity with tubes occluded at cornua.

Culdoscopy; Laparoscopy

Culdoscopy, although discussed in detail in Chapter 15, requires emphasizing at this time because of its importance in the assessment of the fallopian tubes in cases of prolonged infertility. It is particularly useful when there is a discrepancy between the tubal insufflation study and the hysterosalpingogram.

Peretz and Sharf demonstrated that approximately 30 per cent of patients with tubal occlusion diagnosed by tubal insufflation and hysterosalpingography failed to reveal occlusion at the time of culdoscopy. The main information provided by these two studies concerns tubal patency or obstruction, whereas direct inspection of the adnexa with the culdo-

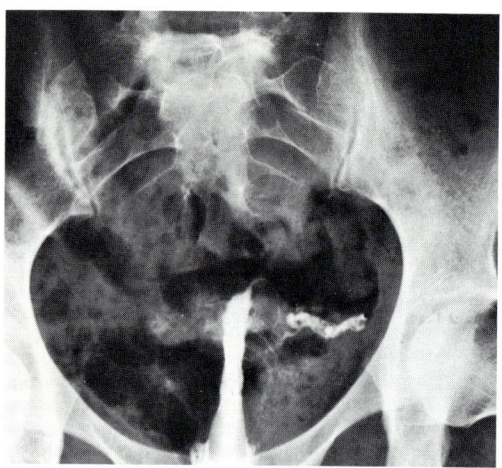

Fig. 14-5 A. Endometrial sclerosis (Asherman's disease) with partial obliteration of uterine cavity and obstruction of cornual portion of right tube.

scope provides an excellent opportunity for evaluation of tubal patency and motility, peritubal adhesions, and other pelvic disease such as possible endometriosis or unsuspected ovarian pathology. By inserting a No. 14 Foley catheter with a 5-cc. bag into the cervical canal and inflating the bag with 2 cc. of sterile water, indigo carmine may be instilled into the uterine cavity with direct visualization of the presence or absence of dye from the fimbriated end of the tube. While culdoscopy is the most difficult of all the tubal function studies to perform, it is perhaps the most informative. It is our policy to evaluate the pelvis by culdoscopy prior to considering definitive surgery for correction of tubal disease.

The recent introduction of a malleable intraperitoneal probe through a second puncture site enables the operator to manipulate the pelvic organ and greatly to improve visualization. Marshall terms this technic "dynamic culdoscopy." A superb improvement in the light source by means of fiber optic glass bundles has greatly enhanced the visibility of this procedure.

Laparoscopy, a renewed innovation, provides the same information of tubal function as culdoscopy except that the approach is through the abdominal wall rather than the cul-de-sac. It does have the advantage of making possible the observation of the fallopian tubes from the anterior surface of the broad ligament and consequently may provide a more direct view of the fimbriae than when they are observed through the cul-de-sac. Sufficient time has not elapsed as yet to evaluate critically its advantages over culdoscopy. However, the same information can be obtained with the laparoscope as with the culdoscope.

OPERATIVE TREATMENT

Treatments To Be Considered Prior to Major Surgery

Before turning to the various operative procedures which are sometimes indicated in sterility, the therapeutic aspects of uterotubal insufflation should be considered. It is the authors' belief that this procedure may be as effective in relieving tubal obstruction as any of the other major operative procedures. The most important therapeutic effect of insufflation is its effect on the tubes. Mild intratubal agglutinations may be separated, mucous plugs in the tubes may be dislodged, and adhesions at the fimbriated ends may be broken.

The therapeutic effect of repeated Rubin's tests was evaluated by Rubin in 118 cases of strictured tubes. Of these cases, 31 per cent eventually became pregnant as against 26 per cent of the cases with normally patent tubes. The time of pregnancy in relation to insufflation gives some idea of the benefit of Rubin's test. Within 2 months of the test 38 per cent of the successful women were gravid; 64 per cent of the pregnancies occurred within 6 months, and 18 per cent more of the pregnancies occurred in the following 6 months. Rutherford reports a 63 per cent pregnancy rate following repeated Lipiodol insufflations. Vesell reported a pregnancy rate in 29 per cent of 100 patients who had an initial tubal function study which suggested occlusion. With repeated insufflations monthly from 6 to 28 months, 29 of these patients ultimately became pregnant.

Considering the above results, one certainly should exhaust the possibilities of insufflation therapy before considering major surgery for relief of infertility.

The following procedures, major and minor, are at times indicated in the treatment of sterility:

Dilatation and curettage is done routinely in connection with Rubin's test. It is our belief that cervical dilatation is of value in some cases.

Cervical cauterization is done to clear up tenacious mucopurulent discharge in cases of sterility, and the results are often gratifying. The technic of this operation and the postoperative care are described in Chapter 20, Nonmalignant Cervical Lesions and Their Treatment.

Pelvic laparotomy is performed after at least three negative tubal function studies confirm a definite tubal factor. Tubal plastic surgery may also be performed in conjunction with a pelvic operation, performed primarily for relief of other symptoms. Many procedures have been described, but most of them may be included among the following procedures.

SALPINGOLYSIS

Peritubal adhesions may result from postabortal or puerperal infection, previous appendicitis, or pelvic endometriosis. The simple release of adhesions about the tube or the fimbriated extremity may reveal a patent tube when tested with syringe or indigo carmine inserted through the fimbriae or a Foley catheter inserted in the cervical canal. If there has been no damage to the fimbriated end of the tube, this procedure has the highest pregnancy rate of all tubal procedures, approximately 35 to 40 per cent.

CORNUAL IMPLANTATION

Preservation of function of the fimbriated end of the tube with cornual implantation has been considered to be one of the most successful methods of tuboplasty, but the end results of many series, including our own at Johns Hopkins, have been disappointing. Although the pregnancy rate varies between 10 and 35 per cent, the number of live births in many reported series rarely exceeds 10 per cent. Unfortunately, there is a high rate of tubal pregnancy and abortion in this group of patients. One of the better reports of this procedure comes from the recent experience at the Mayo Clinic in 75 cases of tubal reconstructive surgery in which there were 10 live births (45%) of 22 cornual implantations. This was the best experience in the entire series at the Mayo Clinic since there were only 2 other live births in the 75 cases, for a live birth rate of 16.0 per cent. Shirodkar has the largest series of cases in which tubal implantations have been done. He reports a 35 per cent pregnancy rate for 140 women who had uterotubal implantations. Shirodkar attributes his success to the use of a polyethylene intrauterine loop (Fig. 14-6) which splints the tubal anastomoses and remains in the dome of the uterus. The polyethylene loop remains in place for 4 months and is then removed through the cervix by hooking the loop in the uterus through the cervical canal.

TECHNIC: REIMPLANTATION OF DISTAL PORTION OF TUBE INTO UTERUS

The obstructed proximal end of the tube is excised. The remaining distal portion is tested for patency with a Chetwood syringe containing sterile saline. A small wedge-shaped piece of tissue is excised at the cornu, sufficient to permit the insertion of the tube into the uterine cavity. The uterine end of the shortened tube is split longitudinally for about a centimeter or slightly less. With No. 000 chromic catgut, a bite is taken into each half of the split end. Each end of both sutures is then threaded on a curved needle. The needle is inserted through the cornual opening and carried out through the myometrium. After the four ends of the two sutures have been brought out through the uterine wall, the two ends attached to each flap are tied together. Thus the end of the tube is drawn into the uterine cavity, and since it is split, the lumen is more apt to be kept open at the point of implantation (Fig. 14-7). In recent years we have used

304 Infertility

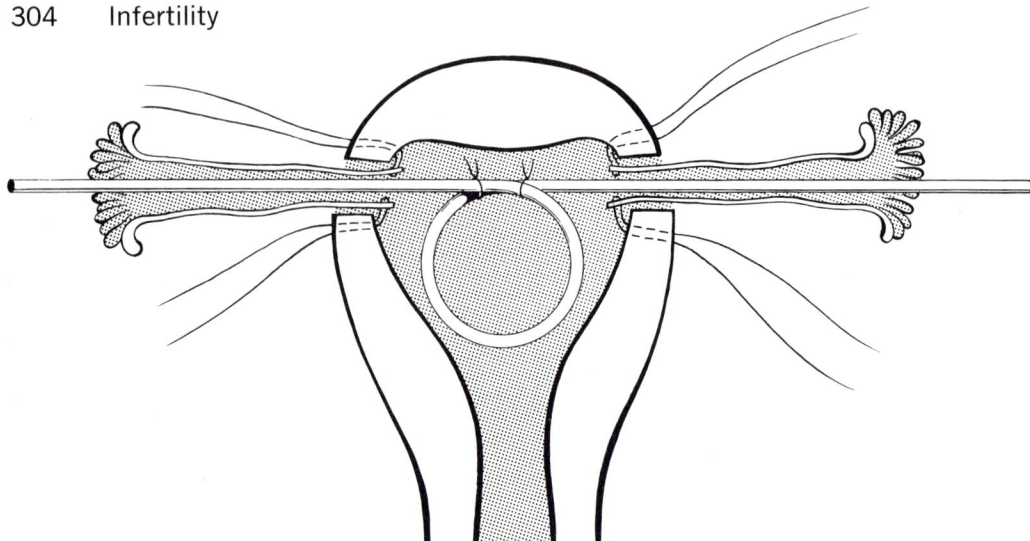

FIG. 14-6. Intra-uterine polyethylene loop (Shirodkar) showing method of splinting tubal anastomosis of cornual implantation. Note that indwelling tube avoids bacterial contamination of vagina and abdominal wall.

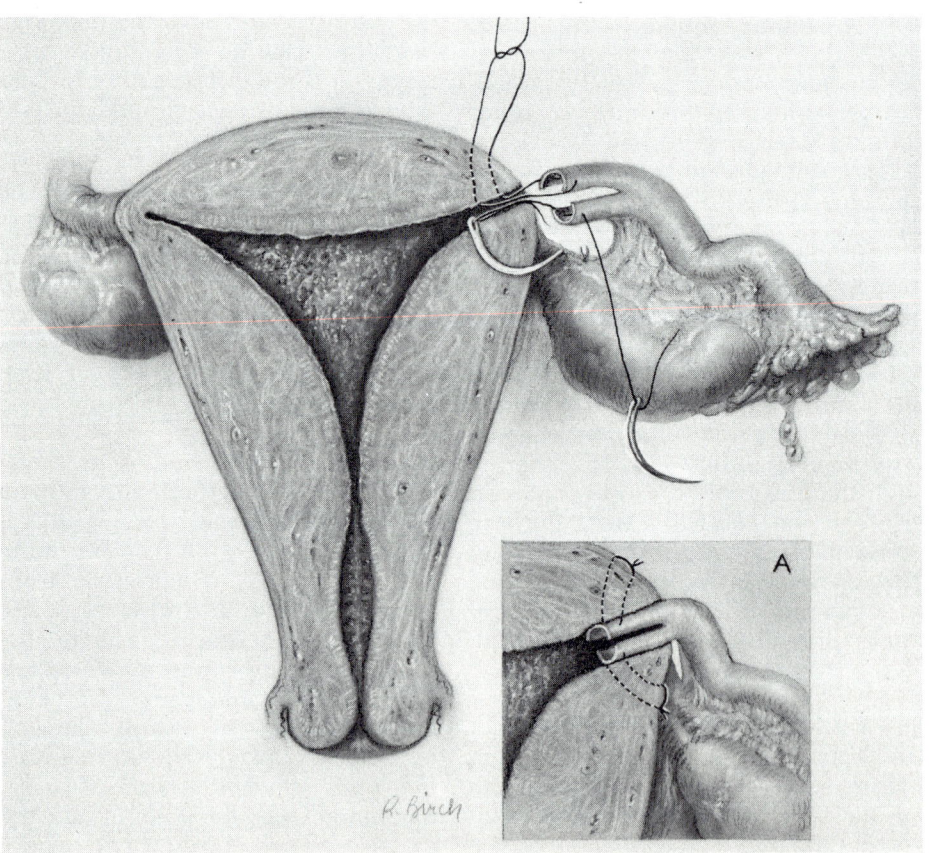

FIG. 14-7. Implantation of a shortened tube into the uterus. The split tube is drawn into the uterine cavity through an opening at the cornu. Inset A shows tube sutured in the cornu.

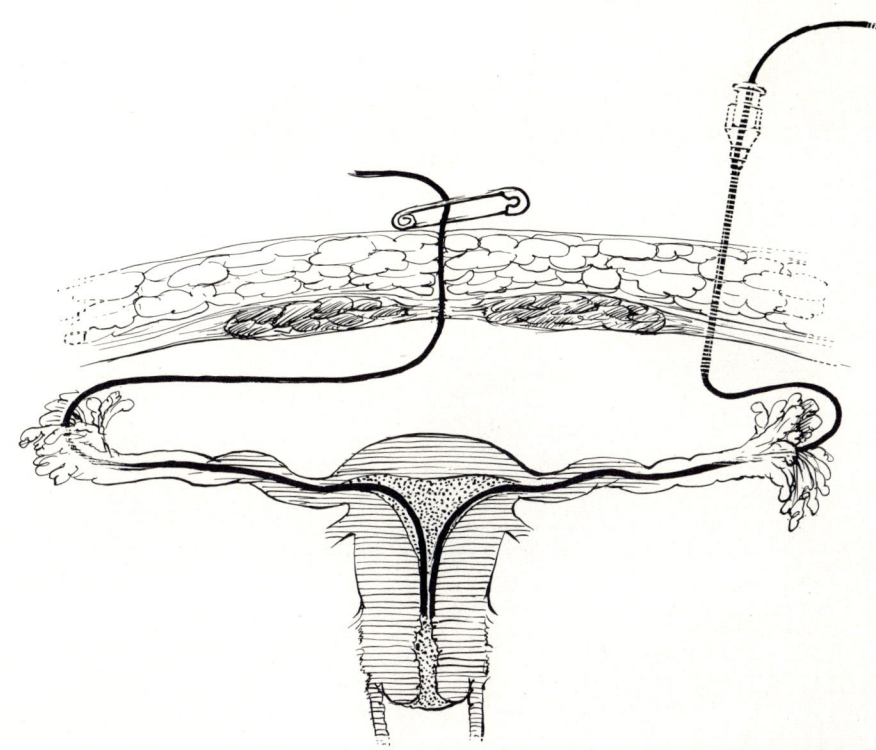

Fig. 14-8. Showing method of bringing tubing out through midline incision or laterally through needle which is then withdrawn.

a small polyethylene tube placed within the fallopian tube and extending into the uterine cavity. The distal end of the polyethylene tube is brought out of the abdomen through the incision and is withdrawn after 2 to 4 weeks.

Overstreet has suggested bringing the tubing out laterally to the incision and threading it through a needle which perforates the abdominal wall, as shown in Figure 14-8.

Currently we are using Shirodkar's polyethylene loop, which does not require exteriorization and can be left in place for 3 to 4 months (Fig. 14-6). Polyethylene tubing has been shown to be completely inert in its effect on the tissues of laboratory animals, and the frequency with which we have found the tubes to be patent following its use in plastic tubal operations indicates that it is equally innocuous in the human tube. Tubal insufflation should be done within 48 hours after removal of the polyethylene tubing and again after 6 weeks to test the patency of the implanted tube. The use of hydropertubation of a solution consisting of physiologic saline (40 ml.), 50 mg. hydrocortisone, and 2,000 U. penicillin through the cervical canal postoperatively remains of questionable value at the present time. Swolin from Sweden begins this treatment on the 9th postoperative day while the patient is still hospitalized and obtains good surgical results.

SALPINGOSTOMY

Salpingostomy has the lowest yield of pregnancies and live births of all the tubal plastic procedures. Although Sovak reported the cuff salpingostomy in 1932 as a means of maintaining patency of the reconstructed distal fallopian tube, subsequent pregnancy even in patent tubes has been infrequent due to inflammatory change in the wall of the tube and impairment of ciliary function. In our own clinic, Woodruff and co-workers have re-

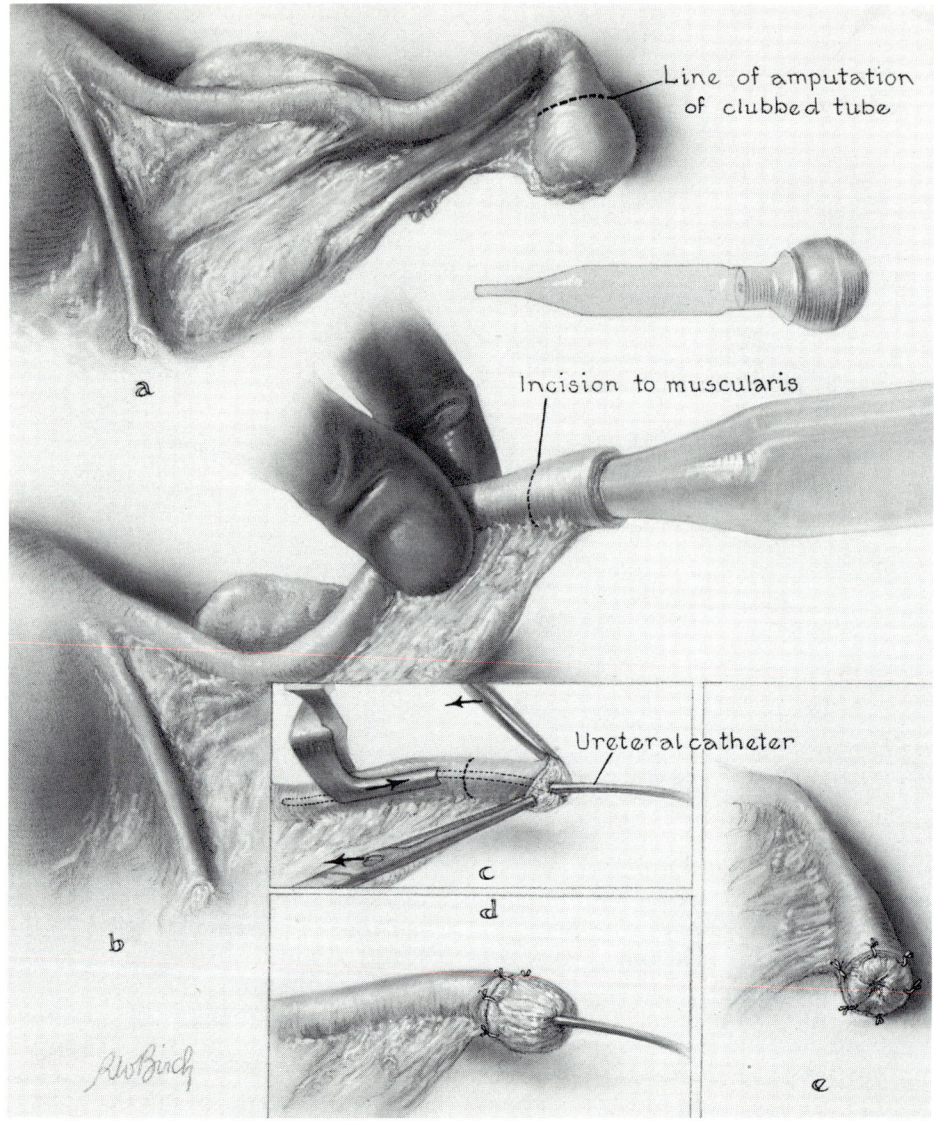

Fig. 14-9. Cuff salpingostomy (Sovak Method). (a) Line of amputation of clubbed tube. (b) Circular incision into muscularis. (c) Cuff is reflected. (d) Cuff is sutured to serosa. (e) Newly formed end of tube.

cently reported 96 cases with only 3 patients achieving a live infant in the 34 having salpingostomy procedures. In 32 such cases reported from the Mayo Clinic, there were 6 pregnancies, although 5 resulted in abortion or were ectopic, with only 1 live birth. Only recently has there been an improvement in this method as reported by Mulligan at Harvard, where his most recent series between 1955–59 included 45 cases with the use of a silicone rubber (Silastic) hood. Although he achieved a tubal patency in 87 per cent of the cases, he reported only 21 per cent had term deliveries, with 8 per cent of the pregnancies being ectopic. While the use of this prosthesis has improved the pregnancy rate in the Boston clinic, it has the disadvantage of requiring a second laparotomy after approximately 3 months.

Technic: Cuff Salpingostomy (Sovak's Method)

The tube is carefully freed from its adherent bed, and no instruments are used in handling it to avoid injury to its delicate tissue. The distal portion of the tube is excised proximal to the point of obstruction (Fig. 14-9 a). The patency of the tube is then tested with a Chetwood syringe or uterine insufflation with indigo carmine by means of an intracervical catheter. If the tube is open, a gurgling sound can be heard as the air enters the uterine cavity, or dye can be seen flowing from the fimbriated end of the tube. If the remaining portion of the tube is found to be patent, the Chetwood syringe is inserted again, and a circular cut is made through the musculature of the tube about 1.5 cm. from the end (Fig. 14-9 b). A French urethral catheter or small polyethylene tube is then passed into the tubal lumen for about 3 cm. A Bonney clamp is placed over the tube containing the catheter or polyethylene tube so that the tip of the clamp is just within the circular incision. Two Allis clamps are used to grasp gently the ends of the tube. The tube is pulled backward, and at the same time the Bonney clamp is pushed forward (Fig. 14-9 c). Thus a cuff is formed at the end of the shortened tube. The cuff is held in place by a few delicately placed sutures of No. 000 chromic catgut (Fig. 14-9 d and e). The fine polyethylene tubing is passed into the uterine cavity, and the distal end of the polyethylene tubing is brought out through the abdominal incision. It is desirable to suspend the tube to the side of the pelvic wall to prevent the end from becoming adherent in the cul-de-sac. The polyethylene tube is removed after 6 weeks, and an insufflation is done to test the patency of the tube.

Estes Procedure

Attempts to restore fertility after salpingectomy, by means of implanting the pedicled ovary into the uterine cavity, were first made by Tuffier of Paris. He implanted the whole ovary through a midline incision in the posterior wall of the uterus. The few pregnancies resulting from this procedure almost always ended in abortion, and in some instances the uterus gave birth to the implanted ovary. This operation has been almost universally abandoned. One recent report from Ghosal in India reports a case of utero-ovarian implantation. Apparently the patient menstruated normally following the operation and reportedly had 5 pregnancies during the subsequent 10 years. However, when implantation is done today, the majority of operators follow the technic described by Estes, or some modification of it.

Estes recommends excision of the convex surface of the ovary and implantation of the remainder into the uterine cornu in an opening made in the myometrium, communicating with the cavity (Fig. 14-10). It seems illogical to us to excise the cortex of the ovary, since this portion contains most of the follicles. In the few instances in which we have performed this operation, we have implanted the unexcised ovary into the cornu.

Estes has reported 50 cases in which he has performed this operation, and in which he has complete case records. Four of the 50, or 8 per cent, became pregnant; 2 of these went to term, giving a 4 per cent success rate. Von Graff collected 41 cases from the literature in which the ovary was transplanted into the uterine cavity. There were 3 pregnancies, an incidence of 7.5 per cent. One of the 3 went to term, making the incidence of live births 2.5 per cent. Reiprich collected 200 cases of ovarian transplants of all types, 2.5 per cent of which became pregnant. Although operations of the Estes type result in a low percentage of successes, it must be said in its defense that in many instances the operation is incidental to a salpingectomy, and that the abdomen is opened primarily for relief of pain. The necessity of another laparotomy for removal of a cystic ovary, implanted at the uterine cornu, probably occurs no more frequently than after salpingectomy in general. Presentation of this data is primarily for historic purposes since there has been no favorable recent ex-

308   Infertility

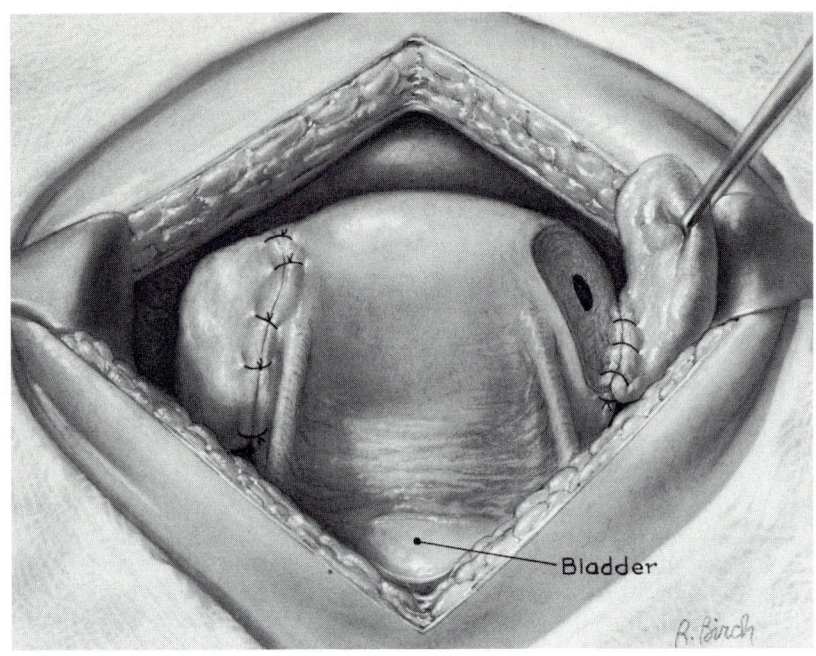

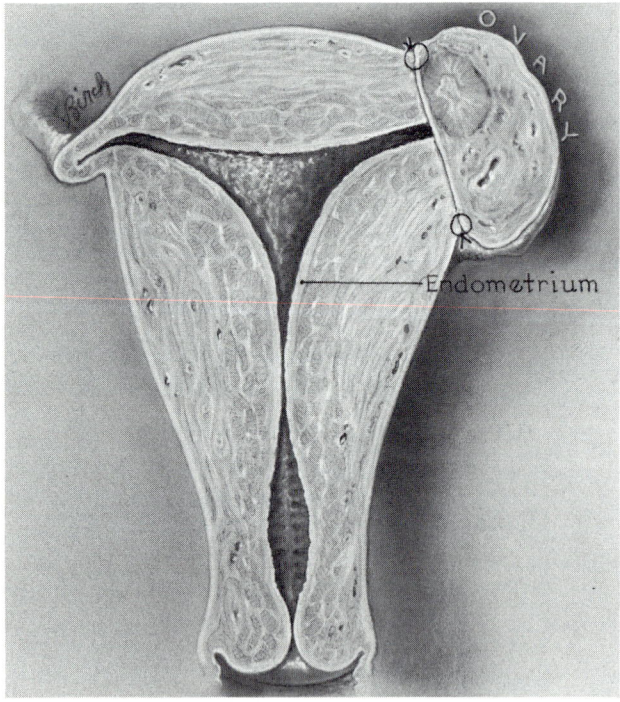

Fig. 14-10. Estes operation for sterility after salpingectomy. (*Top*) Excision of myometrium at the cornua opens the uterine cavity. The right ovary has been sutured to the cornu. The left is being sutured in place. (*Left*) Section of the uterus showing how ovulation into the uterine cavity is possible.

perience with this procedure in most clinics performing tubal surgery.

Summation of Experience

From the above discussion and statistics, it is obvious that the chances for full-term pregnancy following various plastic procedures are in the neighborhood of 10 to 15 per cent. Our most recent experience from the Hopkins clinic was reported by Crane and Woodruff and included 96 operations performed during a 25-year period, 1940-65. Although the corrected pregnancy rate was 22.2 per cent, the term-pregnancy success rate was only 10 per cent. Greenhill surveyed a group of clinics in this country and accumulated data on 2,113 tuboplastic procedures, with a full-term pregnancy rate of 15 per cent. In a recent review of the literature by Llusia from Madrid, of 7,416 patients who were treated surgically, 17.2 per cent became pregnant, and 4.2 per cent had ectopic pregnancies, for a full-term rate of 13 per cent. In contrast, of 1,034 infertile patients treated medically, 15.9 per cent became pregnant, and 2.2 per cent had ectopic pregnancies, for a term-pregnancy rate of 13.7 per cent. Since only about 1 per cent of gynecologic surgery in the major clinics in the United States is performed for reconstructive tubal surgery, it is probable that there is inadequate experience by the occasional operator to achieve excellence in this field. Buxton, in discussing the poor outcome in term pregnancy (9%) resulting from 23 cases undergoing similar bilateral tubal surgery, an experience which is similar to our own, states:

It is our feeling that significant improvement in the results of tubal surgery will not come from further refinements in technique. Improvements must come from increased knowledge of tubal function and physiology so that more rational selection of cases for surgery can be made.

BIBLIOGRAPHY

Altemus, R., Charles, D., and Yoder, V. E.: Conventional hystero-salpingography used in the evaluation of sterility problems. Fertil. Steril., *18*:713, 1967.

Baeyertz, J. D.: A review of 307 cases of infertility. Aust. New Zeal. J. Obstet. Gynaec., 7:204, 1967.

Behrman, S. J., Beuttner-Janusch, J., Hellgar, R., Gershewitz, H., and Tew, W. L.: ABO(H) blood incompatibility as a cause for infertility: A new concept. Amer. J. Obstet. Gynec., 79:847, 1960.

Cary, W. H.: Note on determination of patency of the fallopian tubes by the use of collargol and x-ray shadow. Amer. J. Obstet. Gynec., 69:426, 1914.

Crane, M., and Woodruff, J. D.: Factors influencing the success of tuboplastic procedures. Fertil. Steril., *19*:810, 1968.

Cullen, T. S.: A normal pregnancy following insertion of the outer half of a fallopian tube into the uterine cornu. Bull. Johns Hopkins Hosp., *33*:344, 1922.

Elliott, G. B., Brody, H., and Elliott, K. A.: Implications of "lipoid salpingitis." Fertil. Steril., *16*:541, 1965.

Estes, W. L., Sr.: A method of implanting ovarian tissue in order to maintain ovarian function. Penn. Med. J., *13*:610, 1909.

Estes, W. L., Jr.: Ovarian implantation. Surg. Gynec. Obstet., 38:394, 1924.

Estes, W. L. Jr., and Heitmeyer, P. L.: Pregnancy following ovarian implantation. Amer. J. Surg., 24:563, 1934.

Franklin, R. R., and Dukes, C. D.: Antispermatozoal antibody and unexplained infertility. Amer. J. Obstet. Gynec., 89:6, 1964.

Ghosal, K. K.: Ovarian function after Estes' operation. J. Obstet. Gynec. of India, *16*:540, 1966.

Glass, R. H., and Buxton, C. L.: Tubal plastic surgery. Fertil. Steril., *18*:80, 1967.

Greenhill, J. P.: Present status of plastic operations on the fallopian tubes. Amer. J. Obstet. Gynec., 72:516, 1956.

Hanton, E. M., Pratt, J. H., and Banner, E. A.: Tubal plastic surgery at the Mayo Clinic. Amer. J. Obstet. Gynec., 89:934, 1964.

Holden, F. C., and Sovak, F. W.: Reconstruction of the oviducts; an improved technic with report of cases. Amer. J. Obstet. Gynec., 24:684, 1932.

Hotchkiss, R. S.: Methods in sperm analyses and evaluation of therapeutic procedures. J.A.M.A., *107*:1849, 1936.

Huhner, M.: The diagnosis of sterility in the male and female. Amer. J. Obstet. Gynec., 8:63, 1924.

Jones, G. E. S. (Disciple of Baeyertz, J. D.): A review of 307 cases of infertility. Obstet. Gynaec. Survey, 23:691, 1968.

Katsh, S.: Immunology, fertility and infertility: A historical survey. Amer. J. Obstet. Gynec., 77:946, 1959.

Lamar, J. K., Shettles, L. B., and Delfs, E.: Cyclic penetrability of human cervical mucous to spermatozoa in vitro. Amer. J. Physiol., *129*:234, 1940.

Llusia, J. D.: Results of treatment of tubal obstruction. Acta Ginec. (Madrid), *17*:241, 1966.

MacLeod, J.: Male infertility. Advances Obstet. Gynec., *1*:432, 1967.

———: Further experiences on the role of varicocele in human infertility. Fertil. Steril., *20*:545, 1969.

Marcus, C. C., and Marcus, S. L.: The cervical factor in infertility. Clin. Obstet. Gynec., 8:15, 1965.

Marcus, S. L., and Marcus, C. C.: Cervical mucus and its relation to infertility. Obstet. Gynec. Survey, 18:749, 1963.

Marshall, J. R.: The intraperitoneal probe and dynamic culdoscopy. Obstet. Gynec., 27:733, 1966.

Moszkowski, E., Woodruff, J. D., and Jones, G. E. S.: The inadequate luteal phase. Amer. J. Obstet. Gynec., 83:363, 1962.

Mroueh, A., Glass, R. H., and Buxton, C. L.: Tubal plastic surgery. Fertil. Steril., 18:80, 1967.

Mulligan, W. J.: Results of salpingostomy. Int. J. Fertil., 11:424, 1966.

Noyes, R. W., Hertig, A. T., and Rock, J.: Dating the endometrial biopsy. Fertil. Steril., 1:3, 1950.

Parmer, V. T.: Tuboplasty in the treatment of sterility. J. Obstet. Gynaec. of India, 17:302, 1967.

Peretz, A., and Sharf, M.: Culdoscopy in gynecologic diagnosis: A review of 404 cases of endoscopic examination. Amer. J. Obstet. Gynec., 82:582, 1961.

Pommerenke, W. T.: Cyclic changes in the physiological and chemical properties of cervical mucus. Amer. J. Obstet. Gynec., 52:1023, 1946.

Reiprich, W.: Die operative Behandlung der Tubensterilität und experimentelle Studien über die Erfolgsaussichten der freien Eileiterverpflanzung. Z. Geburtsh. Gynäk., 104:1, 1933.

Riva, H. L., Andreson, P. S., DesRosiers, J. L., and Breen, J. L.: Further experience with culdoscopy. J.A.M.A., 178:873, 1961.

Rubin, I. C.: Non-operative determination of patency of fallopian tubes in sterility: Intrauterine inflation with oxygen and production of a subphrenic pneumoperitoneum. Preliminary report. J.A.M.A., 74:1017, 1920.

——: Retention of Lipiodol in fallopian tubes with special reference to occlusive effect in cases of permeable strictures. New York J. Med., 36:1089, 1936.

——: Röntgendiagnostik der Uterus tumoren mit Hilfe von intrauterinen Collargolinjektionen. Vorläufige Mitteilung. Zbl. Gynaek., 38:658, 1914.

——: Therapeutic aspects of uterotubal insufflation in sterility. Amer. J. Obstet. Gynec., 50:621, 1945.

——: Uterotubal insufflation with special reference to technic. Amer. J. Surg., 50:614, 1940.

Rutherford, R. N.: The therapeutic value of repetitive lipiodol tubal insufflations. Western J. Surg., 54:145, 1948.

Schwimmer, W. B., Ustay, K. A., and Behrman, S. J.: An evaluation of immunologic factors of infertility. Fertil. Steril., 18:167, 1967.

Shirodkar, V. N.: Contributions to Obstetrics and Gynecology. Edinburgh, E. & S. Livingston, 1960.

——: Further experience in tuboplasty. Aust. New Zeal. Obstet. Gynec., 5:1, 1965.

Siegler, A. M., and Hellman, L. M.: The tubal plastic operations: A critical analysis of 43 cases. Fertil. Steril., 14:300, 1963.

Southam, A. L.: What to do with the "normal" infertile couple. Fertil. Steril., 11:543, 1960.

Sovak, F. W.: Operative treatment of sterility. Amer. J. Surg., 33:406, 1936.

Steptoe, P. C.: Gynecological endoscopy-laparoscopy and culdoscopy. J. Obstet. Gynec. Brit. Comm., 72:535, 1965.

Sweeney, W. J., III: Hysterography—accuracy of preoperative hysterosalpingography. Obstet. Gynec., 11:640, 1958.

Sweeney, W. J., III, and Gepfert, R.: The fallopian tube. Clin. Obstet. Gynec., 8:32, 1965.

Swolin, K.: 50 Fertilitätsoperationen: Literatur und methodik. Acta Obstet. Gynec. Scand., 46:234, 1967.

Thomas, H. H., and Dunn, D.: Salpix as a medium in hysterosalpingography. Fertil. Steril., 7:155, 1956.

Tuffier, T.: Conservation et transposition dans l'uterus d'un fragment d'ovaire, après salpingectomie pour suppuration. Grossesse consecutive dans un cas. Bull. et mém. Soc. chir. Paris, 48:1051, 1922.

Tuffier, T., and Letulle, M.: Transposition de l'ovaire avec son pédicule vasculair dans cavité l'uterus après ablation des trompes uterine pour annexites. Bull Acad. de Méd., Paris, 3 s., 91:362, 1924.

Tulloch, W. S.: Consideration of sterility. Subfertility in the male. Trans. Edinburgh Obstetrics Society, 54:29, 1951; Edinburgh Med. J., 29, March 1952.

Vesell, M.: Multiple utero-tubal insufflations in cases of sterility due to tubal occlusion. Amer. J. Obstet. Gynaec., 68:810, 1954.

Von Graff, E.: Operative treatment of female sterility. J. Iowa Med. Soc., 26:31, 1936.

15

Culdoscopy

Since 1901, when Kelling of Dresden demonstrated inspection of the peritoneal cavity of a dog by means of the Nitze cystoscope, peritoneoscopy in one form or another has been used sporadically by a few surgeons both in Europe and in America. The work at the Johns Hopkins Hospital was developed by Shackelford of the general surgical service, who stimulated our interest in it in relation to gynecology. In many instances we found peritoneoscopy to be a very useful procedure. Nevertheless, it often left something to be desired. Previous abdominal surgery, resulting in adhesions, often prevented the passage of the peritoneoscope through the peritoneal cavity into the pelvis. Also, if there was a possibility of the pelvic lesion's being of an acute inflammatory nature, peritoneoscopy was contraindicated, for there was danger of disseminating the infection through the peritoneal cavity.

The culdoscope was introduced by Decker and Cherry in 1944 and has been in use in our department since 1946. In 1957 Josey, Thompson, and Te Linde reported on our experience with 594 cases, and we have continued to use it regularly since. With increased experience we have come to regard it as a useful procedure and consider it a necessary part of the armamentarium of every modern gynecologic operating room.

INSTRUMENT

The apparatus is pictured in Figure 15-1. There is a special trochar with a guard on the sheath about 3 cm. from the tip to prevent introducing the trochar too far. A valve is attached near the head of the sheath through which CO_2 gas can

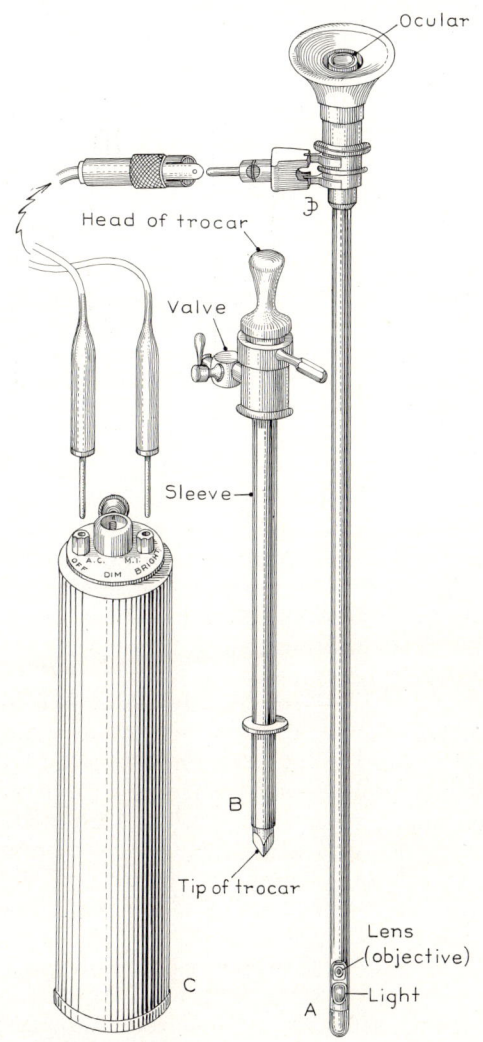

FIG. 15-1 (A) Culdoscope. (B) Trocar. (C) Battery.

311

be introduced into the peritoneal cavity. We never have made use of this, since the results with air have been quite satisfactory. The trocar proper can be fixed in the sheath by means of a special locking device at the head of the sheath. The culdoscope proper consists of a longer metal tube with ocular and objective lenses with a prism to deflect the light so as to make the abdominal contents visible through the ocular. Just distal to the objective lens is a small electric bulb which is illuminated by means of a dry-cell battery. The one pictured in Figure 15-1 is supplied by the manufacturers, but we have made a larger one which gives better illumination.

In 1963 Clyman described a new set of instruments, the panculdoscope, with fiber optic light source, through which a biopsy can be taken.

PROCEDURE

Properly administered, any anesthesia can be used successfully, the type depending in a great measure on individual preference. In our series the anesthesia used in about 90 per cent of the cases was intravenous Pentothal Sodium, usually supplemented by nitrous oxide and oxygen. Cyclopropane, ether, caudal and spinal anesthesia were used occasionally. In many clinics local anesthesia is apparently used much more frequently than in ours, and quite successfully. Pentothal Sodium has been so satisfactory in our hands that we rarely use local today. We have had no anesthetic deaths, but it should be emphasized that the patient should be *routinely* intubated before putting her in the knee-chest position. She is held in the knee-chest posture by two assistants, each grasping a thigh as he stands beside the patient facing the operator. Various apparatuses have been devised for holding the patient in the knee-chest posture, but if assistants are available, we prefer them.

The patient is draped with an ordinary fenestrated sterile sheet. A posterior vaginal retractor is inserted into the vagina, and the posterior lip of the cervix is grasped with a tenaculum. By making gentle traction on it the posterior fornix is put on a stretch and punctured with the trocar. The fornix is punctured about an inch behind the cervix (Fig. 15-2). It is very thin at this point, being formed of only vaginal mucosa and peritoneum, held together by a bit of areolar tissue. The trocar thus enters the pelvis between the two uterosacral ligaments. The novice is apt to make the puncture too close to the cervix in his desire to avoid injury to the rectum. This error will result in stripping up of the peritoneum from the posterior surface of the uterus, and the cul-de-sac will not be entered. There is a flange on the sheath of the trocar which automatically prevents its introduction too far. As the trocar is withdrawn from the sheath there is an audible inrush of air. The sterile culdoscope is then inserted through the sheath (Fig. 15-3). Thus the culdoscope never touches the vaginal mucous mem-

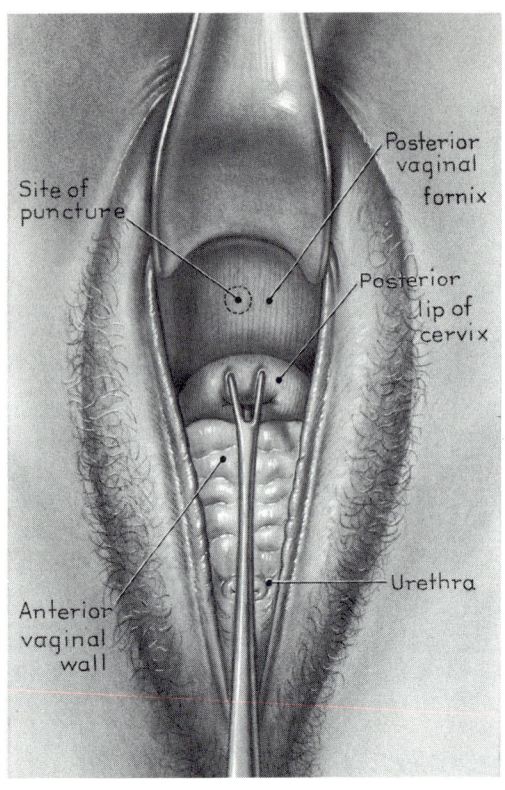

Fig. 15-2. View of vagina with patient in the knee-chest position, showing site of puncture.

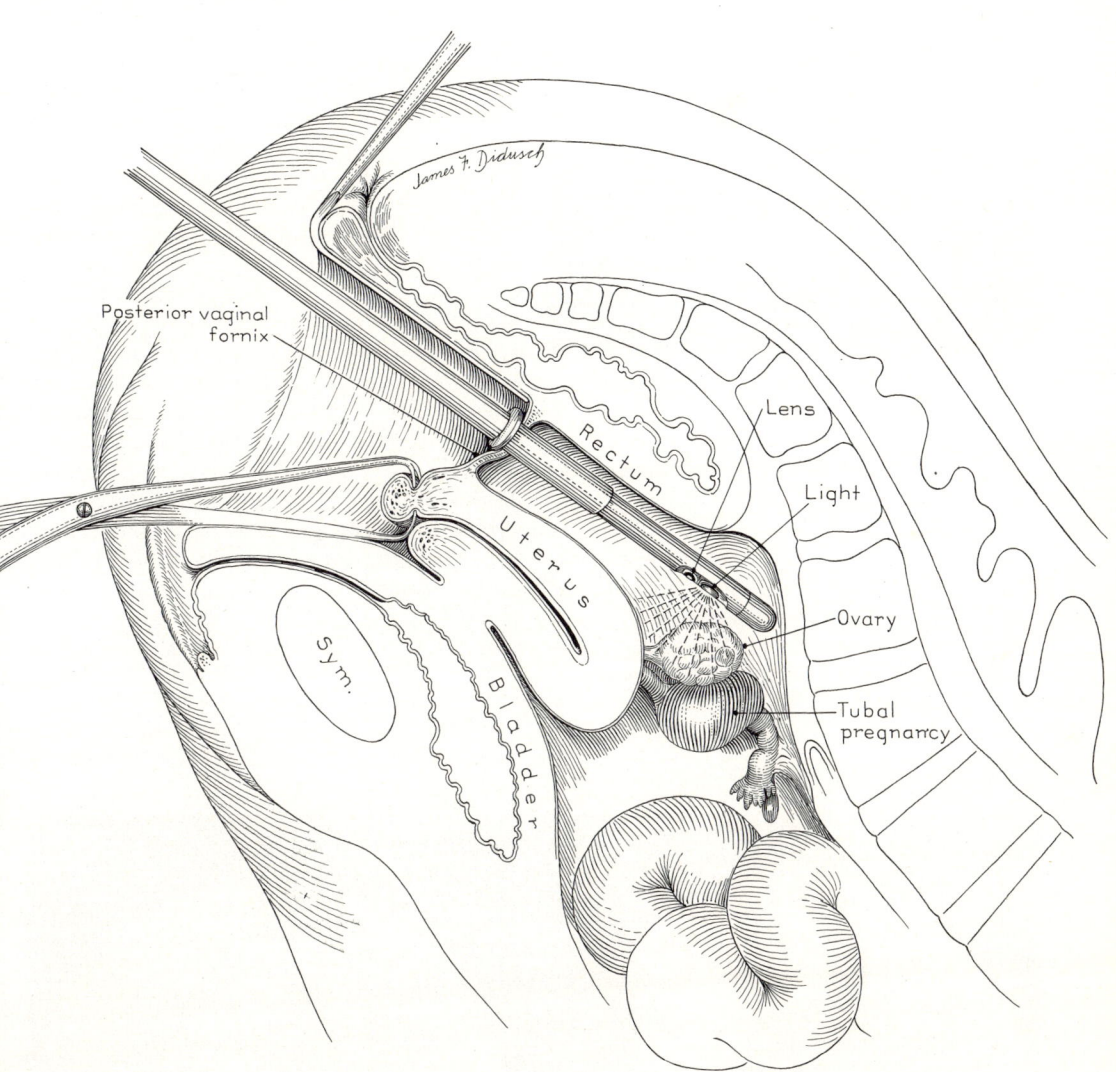

FIG. 15-3. Sagittal section, showing culdoscope viewing pelvic viscera.

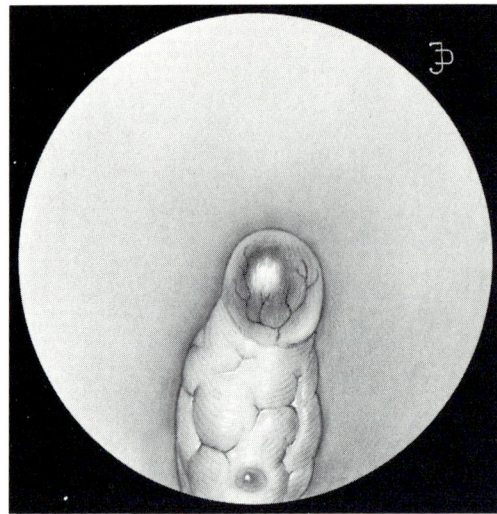

Fig. 15-4. Normal ovary with corpus luteum.

can be visualized. Figures 15-4 to 15-6 show an artist's view of several normal or nearly normal viscera. The culdoscope may be moved from side to side and rotated as necessary. The direction of vision is indicated by a marker on the eyepiece. The pelvic viscera may be moved so as to be brought into view by manipulation with the tip of the culdoscope, by movement of the cervix with the tenaculum, or by having an assistant make pressure at various points in the suprapubic region. Occasionally, the lens, if introduced cold, may become foggy due to body heat. Therefore it is well to dip the tip of the culdoscope in warm water and then wipe dry just before inserting the culdoscope. The lens magnifies structures to some degree, depending on the distance from the object. As the tip of the culdoscope is drawn away from the object, a larger field is visualized. If the object of the culdoscopy is the inspection of the tubes in connection with an investigation of sterility, a self-retaining screw-tip cervical cannula is introduced in the cervical canal. This is connected by means of a small rubber or

brane, and the possibility of infection is reduced to a minimum.

The uterus, the tubes, the broad ligaments, the uterosacral ligaments, the infundibulopelvic ligaments, the rectal wall, the sigmoid, the small intestines, and often the cecum and the appendix

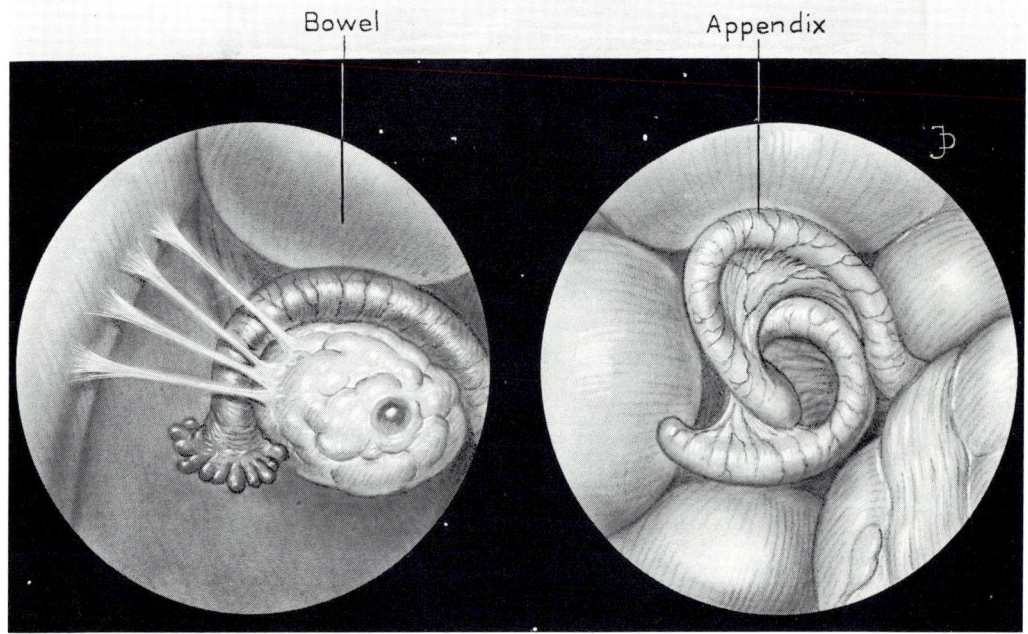

Fig. 15-5. (*Left*) Ovary with a few adhesions. (*Right*) Appendix.

Procedure 315

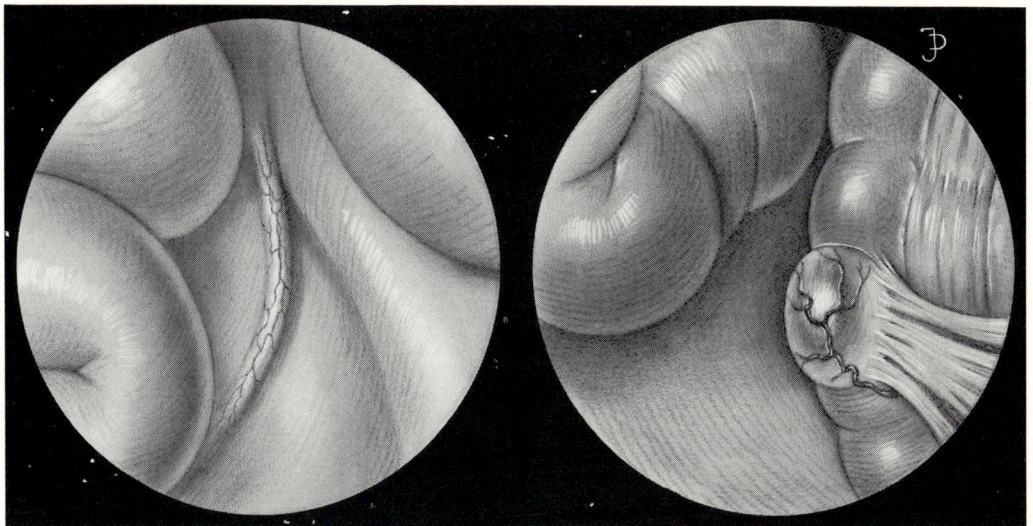

Fig. 15-6. (*Left*) View of ureter occasionally seen. (*Right*) Small bowel and sigmoid with serosal bleb and adhesions.

plastic tubing to a syringe filled with methylene blue. As the fluid is forced in, distention can be seen proximal to the point of obstruction. If the tube is patent, methylene blue solution can be seen dripping from the fimbriated end.

Figures 15-4 to 15-14 illustrate views of the various pelvic organs and diseases as seen through the culdoscope.

On completion of the examination the

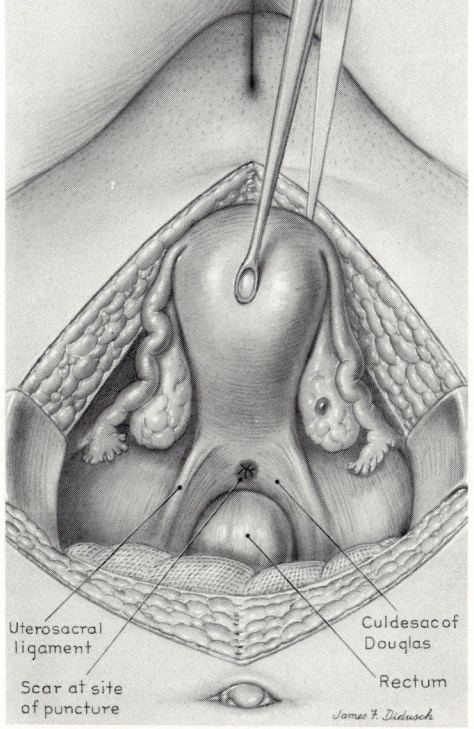

Fig. 15-7. View of culdoscopic wound 2 days after culdoscopy.

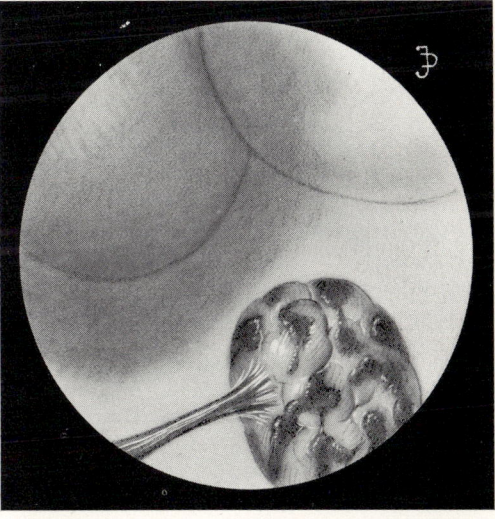

Fig. 15-8. Small blood clots adherent to an ovary. The dark area above is a large blood clot which is out of focus at the moment. Seen with ruptured tubal pregnancy.

culdoscope is withdrawn, but the sheath is left in place as the patient is placed on her side. Pressure is made upon the abdomen to force the air out of the peritoneal cavity. Failure to do this adds greatly to the postoperative discomfort. The vaginal wound is not sutured, and we have had no appreciable hemorrhage from it. Figure 15-7 shows the wound from within the abdomen 2 days after culdoscopy.

INDICATIONS

The culdoscope was used in our series of 594 cases for the following reasons:*

TABLE 15-1. INDICATIONS FOR CULDOSCOPY

	NO. OF CASES
1. To rule out or establish the diagnosis of ectopic pregnancy	356
2. To rule out or establish the diagnosis of endometriosis	51
3. As part of endocrinologic investigation	43
4. To search for a cause of unexplained abdominal or pelvic pain	45
5. As part of the investigation for sterility	37
6. To determine the nature of pelvic masses	31
7. Suspected pelvic tuberculosis	21
8. Miscellaneous	10
Total	594

The reasons for using the culdoscope in our series of patients are listed in the above table. It was possible to place all but 10 of the cases in one of 7 major categories. These 10 patients, representing only 1.8 per cent of the total, had culdoscopy for such rare indications as congenital absence of the uterus, precocious puberty, postmenopausal bleeding and dysmenorrhea. Since there is some overlapping of the indications, it was necessary to assign arbitrarily certain cases to the category that, from a careful study of the records, appeared

---

* Josey, W. E., Thompson, J. D., and Te Linde, R. W.: Southern Med. J., 50:713, 1957. Matter to the end of the chapter, except for material in regular text type, is from this source.

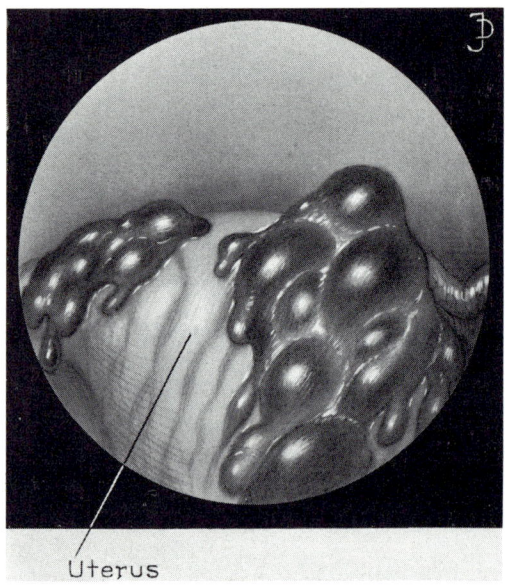

FIG. 15-9. Blood clot seen on fundus of the uterus in case of ruptured tubal pregnancy.

to be the predominating one. For example, several patients who were sterile were suspected of having endometriosis, as were some of those in the group classified as having "unexplained abdominal pain."

Ectopic Pregnancy. The most frequent indication for culdoscopy was that of ruling out or establishing the presence of ectopic pregnancy. This was the reason for the procedure in 356, or well over half of our cases. An impression of ectopic pregnancy by culdoscopy led to laparotomy in 81 patients. The diagnosis was confirmed in 57 of these. The discrepancy between the large number of suspects and the relatively few verified cases is explained by the great many Negro women in our outpatient department who eventually are proven to have pelvic inflammatory disease, but in whom the clinical picture closely mimics that of ectopic pregnancy.

The 24 cases in which the diagnosis was not confirmed at operation constitute the false positives and represent approximately 7 per cent of the culdoscopic operations done for suspected ectopic pregnancy. In exactly half of the falsely positive group the diagnosis at laparotomy was corpus luteum hematoma, of which 8 had ruptured, resulting in hematoperitoneum. Surgical intervention must be regarded as justifiable in the cases in which there was significant bleeding from a corpus

Indications 317

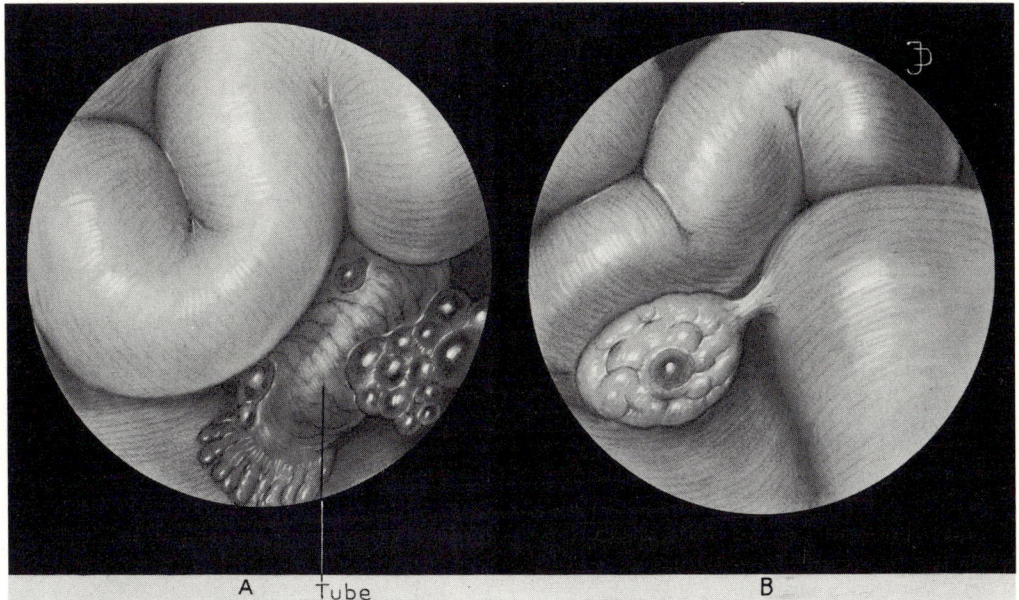

FIG. 15-10. (A) View of tubal abortion. (B) View of the opposite side on which previous salpingectomy had been done for tubal pregnancy.

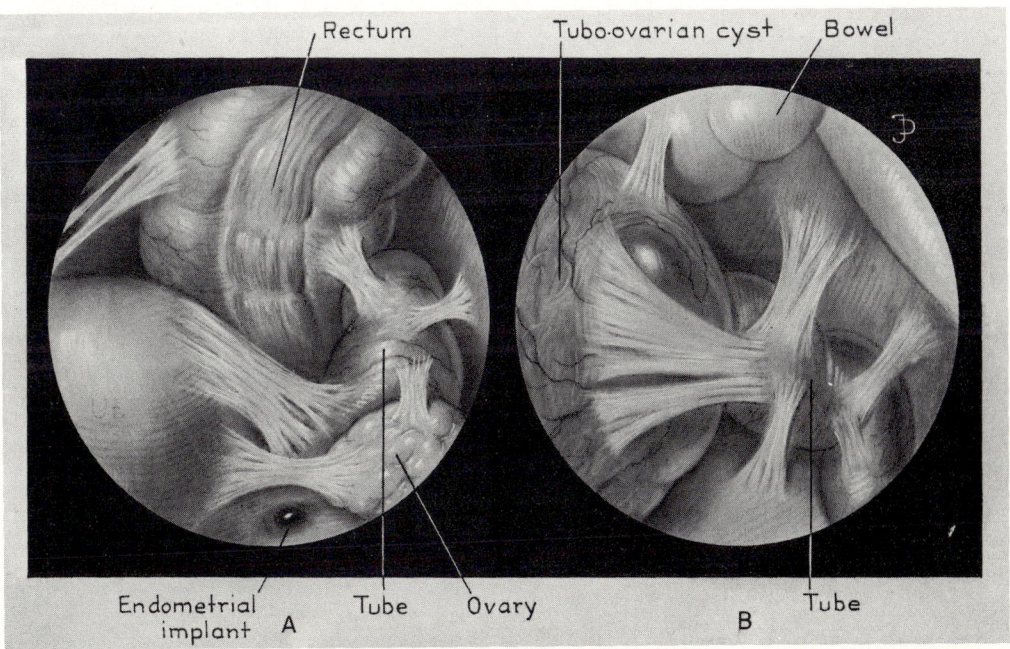

FIG. 15-11. (A) Endometrial implant and adnexal adhesions. (B) Tubo-ovarian inflammatory cyst and adnexal adhesions.

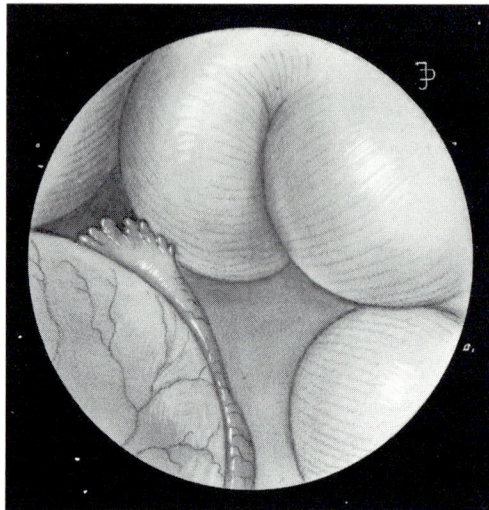

Fig. 15-12. Culdoscopic view of portion of an ovarian cyst and tube.

luteum hematoma. Furthermore, since surgery is not infrequently indicated to relieve pain caused by a corpus luteum hematoma, it cannot be said that these patients had unnecessary operations.

With the culdoscope it is sometimes impossible to distinguish between the bluish, cystic mass of a corpus luteum or follicle hematoma and that of a tubal pregnancy. However, one is often able to make this differentiation by using the culdoscope, in which case surgical intervention may be averted. This is revealed by our study which shows that a culdoscopic diagnosis of corpus luteum or follicle hematoma was made 13 times in the total series, but in only 3 of these patients was the hemorrhage sufficient to necessitate operation.

If those who were found to have corpus luteum hematomas are disregarded, there remain 12 patients who were operated upon either unnecessarily or with questionable justification. They include 6 cases of pelvic inflammatory disease, 2 of intra-uterine pregnancy, 1 patient with the finding of a cystic ovary and 1 with small myomata uteri. Only 2 patients had perfectly normal pelvic organs.

There were two false negative examinations for ectopic pregnancy. In one of these there was a divergence of opinion between two observers regarding the culdoscopic findings.

Occasionally, one encounters serious pelvic disease other than ectopic pregnancy when culdoscopy is done to rule out or establish that diagnosis. Eight patients were operated upon for other conditions revealed preoperatively by the culdoscope, such as dermoid cyst, ruptured pyosalpinx and, of course, ruptured corpus luteum hematoma.

It should not be inferred that culdoscopy is the usual method of establishing the diagnosis of ectopic pregnancy in our clinic. On the contrary, during the period of study a total of 415 ectopic pregnancies were treated on the gynecologic service and in only 13.7 per cent was the diagnosis made using the culdoscope. If a patient presents herself with the clinical manifestations of hemorrhagic shock and the history and pelvic findings point toward the presence of a ruptured ectopic pregnancy, immediate laparotomy is indicated. Furthermore, in less dramatic cases the diagnosis can often be made with reasonable certainty by other means. Frequently, however, the findings may be quite suggestive but the usual methods of examination fail to settle the question. Some of these patients will eventually be found to have an ectopic pregnancy, and for this reason they must be carefully observed if expectant management is elected. In such cases culdoscopy is of great value, for if ectopic pregnancy can be ruled out, the patient may be spared the expense of prolonged hospitalization, and both she and the surgeon relieved of the anxiety engendered by uncertainty.

On the positive side we believe that culdos-

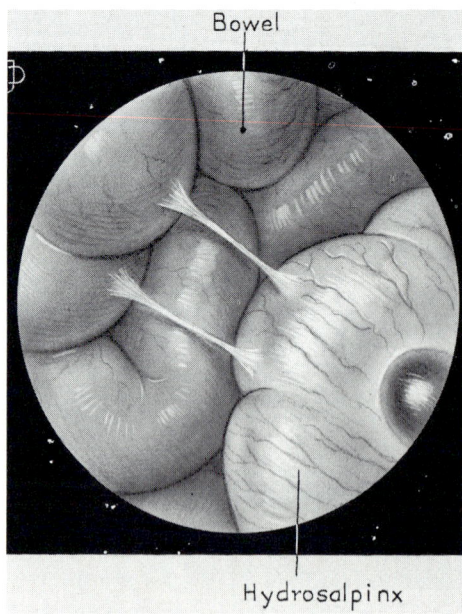

Fig. 15-13. Hydrosalpinx which was differentiated from ovarian cyst by culdoscopy.

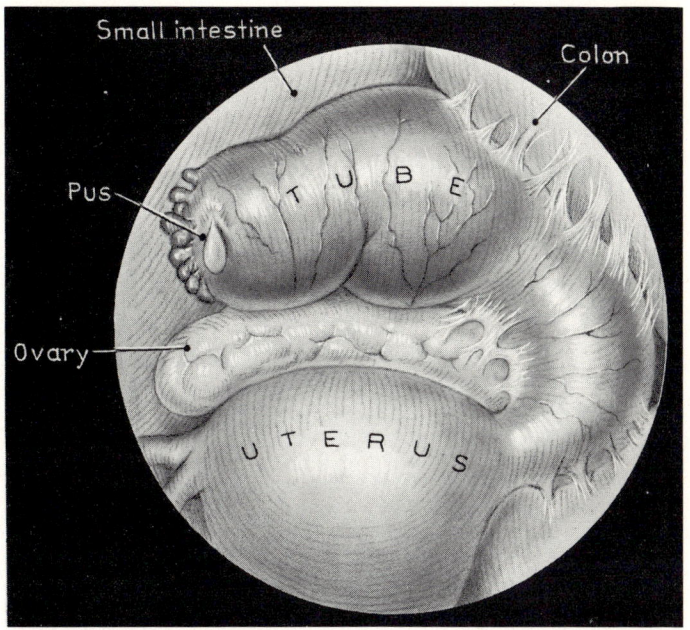

FIG. 15-14. Pus tube as viewed through the culdoscope.

copy can be relied upon to pick up many early cases prior to rupture or tubal abortion. If there is little or no blood in the pelvis, culdocentesis is without value. The same is true of colpotomy unless the incision is large enough and pelvic conditions are suitable to permit tubal visualization. Of the 57 ectopic pregnancies diagnosed by culdoscopy, the fallopian tube was found to be completely intact in 15 cases. In many of the others only a few small clots were present, so that puncture of the cul-de-sac probably would have failed to produce blood.

Endometriosis. Suspected endometriosis was the indication for culdoscopy in 51 patients. The lesions were demonstrated in 10, and in 3 patients the diagnosis was later confirmed by laparotomy. Endometriosis was diagnosed 14 times when culdoscopy was done for other reasons. It is our opinion that many pelves are explored unnecessarily for suspected endometriosis, simply on the basis of a history of severe dysmenorrhea. Without palpable evidence of this disease, such explorations frequently result in negative findings. Culdoscopy will often prevent such unnecessary surgery.

On the other hand, endometrial blebs and scarring can at times be seen with the culdoscope even though the pelvis is normal to palpation. Nevertheless, failure to identify the lesions culdoscopically does not entirely rule out the presence of endometriosis. Often one is unable to visualize all surfaces of the ovaries. Similarly, one is rarely able to see the vesico-uterine fold and although the uterosacral ligaments may be seen, their attachments to the uterus are very difficult to visualize.

A number of patients in this group were found to have pelvic inflammatory disease rather than endometriosis. This differentiation is easily made with the culdoscope, and the exact diagnosis thus made is valuable in planning further therapy.

Endocrine Investigation. Forty-three patients had culdoscopy as part of an investigation for the cause of endocrine disorders. The majority of them were amenorrheic, but 3 had abnormal uterine bleeding. Eleven patients with unexplained amenorrhea had positive findings, including hypoplasia of the ovaries and ovarian agenesis.

Whenever there is a question of ovarian disease that cannot be established by pelvic examination, we regard culdoscopy as a very useful procedure. At least portions of the ovaries can usually be visualized even when the tubes are obscured by adhesions or loops of bowel.

The appearance of the ovaries in patients with the Stein-Leventhal syndrome is quite characteristic. Culdoscopies were done in 16 patients suspected of having this syndrome;

in 7 of these the diagnosis confirmed by visualizing the typical large, pale, multicystic ovarian surfaces.

Marshall and Hammond, working at the National Institute of Health with the newer culdoscope of Clyman, which can take biopsies, have had a rather extensive experience. They have concluded that its greatest usefulness is for the evaluation of nonmalignant disease states, of endocrinologic or genetic conditions such as oligomenorrhea, secondary and primary amenorrhea, the Stein-Leventhal syndrome, hirsutism, Turner's syndrome, and other types of dysgenesis or agenesis.

Unexplained Abdominal Pain. The search for a cause of obscure abdominal or pelvic pain can be time consuming, expensive for the patient, and frequently unrewarding for the physician. Many of these patients undoubtedly have pain on a psychosomatic basis. Occasionally, however, a cause has been found at culdoscopy and later corrected. If on the other hand no disease can be demonstrated, one may then more confidently assure the patient that no organic lesion is present or refer her for psychiatric evaluation if this seems indicated.

In this group of 45 patients, about one third had pathologic findings which might have accounted for their symptoms. Five of them were subsequently operated upon for the lesions demonstrated.

An interesting observation has been made by Polishuk and Sharf, who performed culdoscopy on 35 patients during menstruation, seeking an explanation for dysmenorrhea. In 15 women in whom severe pain began before the onset of menstruation, menstrual blood was found in the peritoneal cavity. In 12 women in whom pain began after the onset of bleeding, in only 2 was menstrual blood seen in the peritoneal cavity. In 8 control cases without dysmenorrhea, no blood was found. These findings would seem to offer a rational basis for therapeutic clinical dilation in selected dysmenorrhagic women.

Sterility. The use of the culdoscope as an adjunct to the investigation of infertility is perhaps the most controversial. Its diagnostic and prognostic value undoubtedly depends on the experience of the operator. Unfortunately, its value in selecting patients for tubal plastic or other corrective operations is to some degree nullified by the notoriously poor results in this type of surgery. On the other hand, if the tubes are patent and no abnormalities can be visualized, one may then assure the patient that there is nothing that can be done surgically to aid conception.

Possible etiologic factors that have been demonstrated in our cases of sterility include pelvic adhesions, endometriosis, pelvic inflammatory disease, tubal occlusion as shown by injection of methylene blue, ovarian cysts, and absence of evidence of corpus luteum formation.

Pelvic Masses. When there was uncertainty as to the nature of a pelvic mass, culdoscopy revealed the correct diagnosis in a remarkably high percentage of our cases. Four of the 31 culdoscopies in this group were regarded as unsatisfactory. In every one of the others it was possible to visualize the mass in question. The most frequent findings were pedunculated myomata, hydrosalpinges, and simple ovarian cysts. Dermoid cyst was diagnosed twice and confirmed by laparotomy in each instance. In two other patients the diagnosis of ovarian endometriosis was made.

If an encapsulated ovarian tumor or ovarian cyst is seen which might be malignant, biopsy is contraindicated. If there is disseminated growth suggestive of malignancy, there is no contraindication to taking a biopsy of a nodule, and the microscopic diagnosis of the specimen may be useful in planning definitive treatment.

Pelvic Tuberculosis. The culdoscope was used 21 times to look for evidence of pelvic tuberculosis. Definite tuberculous lesions were discovered in two patients. In one of these the pelvic organs appeared normal but a number of tubercles were seen on a loop of small bowel. In the other patient the pelvic peritoneum was seen to be studded with tubercles. It is noteworthy that both curettage and culture of ascitic fluid had failed to establish the diagnosis. This case clearly demonstrates that culdoscopy can be a valuable aid in the diagnosis of pelvic tuberculosis.

FAILURES

The examination was regarded as unsatisfactory in 45 cases, or in 7.6 per cent of patients so studied. In view of the inexperience of the operator in many of our cases, this would appear to be a relatively low failure rate. Inability to enter the peritoneal cavity accounted for 15 failures. This is occasionally true because the puncture is made too close to the cervix and the peritoneum is merely stripped off the posterior surface of the uterus. In this event it is sometimes feasible to open into the peritoneal cavity with a Kelly clamp and insert the telescope directly into the cul-de-sac.

It is not always possible to visualize completely the adnexa following successful passage of the culdoscope. In many patients, however, it is not essential that both tubes and ovaries be seen in order to arrive at a diagnosis. For this reason we have followed the policy of designating an examination as "unsatisfactory" only if no useful diagnostic information was gained. In such cases the commonest reasons for failure were dense pelvic adhesions, fixed masses in the cul-de-sac, and inability to visualize the adnexa in question due to their fixation in an anterior position or to adherent loops of bowel.

COMPLICATIONS AND MORBIDITY

Usually there is no appreciable bleeding from the site of puncture following culdoscopy. In only 8 cases was it deemed necessary to suture the posterior vaginal fornix. Extra-peritoneal perforation of the rectum occurred three times; no untoward results ensued. Two patients are known to have developed retroperitoneal emphysema due to entry of the trocar into the areolar tissue behind the cervix (Fig. 15-15 A). The air was spontaneously absorbed in a few days. In one instance it was necessary to readmit a patient for drainage of an infected hematoma in the cul-de-sac. Another patient complained of a severe backache following culdoscopy under spinal anesthesia. It was felt by the orthopedic consultant that the cause was back strain due to the prolonged maintenance of the knee-chest position. Postoperative abdominal and shoulder pain are occasionally troublesome, but nearly always are due to a failure to express all the air possible from the abdomen at the conclusion of the procedure.

Marshall and Hammond saw mild venous bleeding at the biopsy site in two instances among their 25 cases. In each instance the bleeding was controlled by coagulation.

A few patients have been allowed to return home within 6 to 8 hours after culdoscopy. In general, however, they are kept in the hospital for 1 to 2 days. Most instances of significant postoperative fever have been due to a flare-

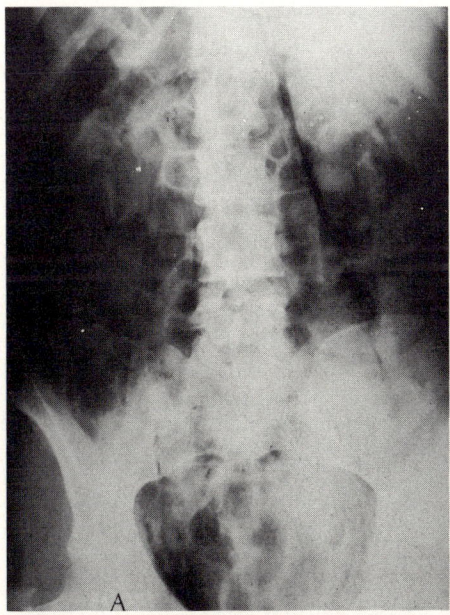 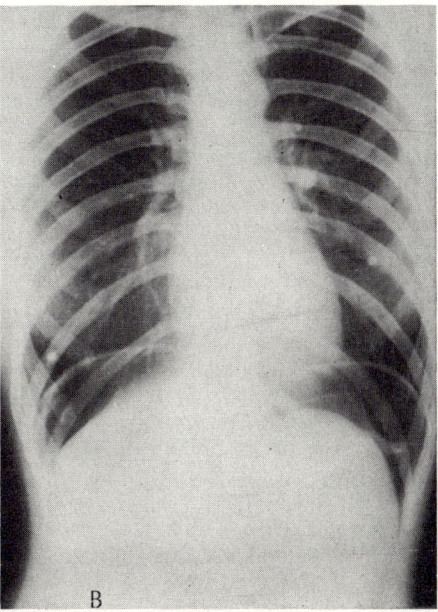

FIG. 15-15. (A, *left*) Retroperitoneal air, resulting from the trocar's failing to enter the peritoneal cavity. (B, *right*) Air under diaphragm, resulting from failure to press on abdomen to evacuate air following culdoscopy.

up of pelvic inflammatory disease. Only 15 patients who had a culdoscopy, but were not subjected to laparotomy, developed fever above 100.8°. Because of the prevalence of pelvic inflammatory disease on our ward service, antibiotics have been administered liberally. We do not consider this necessary in the majority of cases.

OUTCOME OF CONCURRENT INTRA-UTERINE PREGNANCY

Early intra-uterine pregnancy was found at the time of culdoscopy in 45 patients. In a few others an incomplete abortion was completed concomitantly by curettage. Follow-up studies were available on 28 pregnant patients. Of these, 23 delivered uneventfully. Four of the 5 women who subsequently aborted had uterine bleeding and cramplike pain on admission to the hospital, suggesting that abortion was threatening prior to culdoscopy.

EVALUATION OF CULDOSCOPY AND CONTRAINDICATIONS

Although we are convinced that many patients have been spared a laparotomy by the use of culdoscopy, to support this belief objectively we felt it would be necessary to have a comparable series of patients in whom culdoscopy was not done. A strictly comparable series must be made up of cases in which the same diagnostic problems present themselves. Such a series is to be found in the group of patients who were culdoscopic failures, since they may be regarded as not having had culdoscopy at all. There were 45 patients in this group, and in 42.2 per cent laparotomy was done, whereas only 21.1 per cent of the larger group who had successful culdoscopic examinations were subjected to laparotomy. These data add statistical support to our clinical impression that culdoscopy, if used successfully, will substantially reduce the number of patients requiring laparotomy.

Although the most significant contribution of culdoscopy is that of enabling the gynecologist to avoid unnecessary pelvic surgery, the experience of our clinic upholds the broader viewpoint that culdoscopy is a valuable adjunct to the more usual diagnostic methods. It is a relatively safe procedure in the hands of experienced culdoscopists and closely supervised trainees.

The chief contraindications are the presence of a fixed mass or dense adhesions in the cul-de-sac, and inability of the patient to assume the knee-chest position due to debilitation, arthritis, cardiac disease and the like.

BIBLIOGRAPHY

Angell, J. H., and Te Linde, R. W.: Further experiences in culdoscopy. Ann. Surg., *135*: 690, 1952.

Beling, C. A.: Selection of cases for peritoneoscopy. Arch. Surg., *42*:872, 1941.

Clyman, M. J.: A new panculdoscope—diagnostic, photographic, and operative aspects. Obstet. Gynec., *21*:348, 1963.

———: Importance of culdoscopy in fertility studies. New York J. Med., *66*:1867, 1966.

Decker, A.: Simple technic to test tubal patency. Amer. J. Obstet. Gynec., *50*:227, 1945.

———: Artificial pneumoperitoneum by cul-de-sac puncture; new technic for pelvic pneumograms. New York State Med., *46*:314, 1946.

———: Pelvic culdoscopy. *In* Progress in Gynecology. p. 95. New York, Grune & Stratton, 1946.

———: Culdoscopy. Philadelphia, F. A. Davis, 1967.

Decker, A., and Cherry, T. H.: Culdoscopy; new method in diagnosis of pelvic disease—preliminary report. Amer. J. Surg., *64*:40, 1944.

Hall, R. B.: Culdoscopy in infertility investigation. Fertil. Steril., *4*:486, 1967.

Josey, W. E., Thompson, J. D., and Te Linde, R. W.: Ten years experience with culdoscopy: an analysis of 594 cases. Southern Med. J., *50*:713, 1957.

Lamb, E. J., Guderian, A. M., and Cruz, A. L.: Culdoscopy in infertility. Obstet. Gynec., *33*:822, 1969.

Marshall, J. R., and Hammond, C. B.: Ovarian biopsy performed under culdoscopic visualization. Amer. J. Obstet. Gynec., *96*:1022, 1966.

Polishuk, W. Z., and Sharf, M.: Culdoscopic findings in primary dysmenorrhea. Obstet. Gynec., *26*:746, 1965.

Riva, H. L., Hatch, R. P., and Breen, J. L.: Culdoscopy, an analysis of 1500 consecutive cases. Obstet. Gynec., *12*:610, 1958.

Te Linde, R. W., and Rutledge, F. N.: Culdoscopy: a useful gynecological procedure. Amer. J. Obstet. Gynec., *55*:102, 1948.

16

Ectopic Pregnancy

The term *ectopic pregnancy* includes any gestation located outside the uterine cavity. Although the fallopian tube is the most common site of this entity, accounting for more than 95 per cent of such gestations, other sites of extra-uterine implantation include: (1) the broad ligament, (2) the peritoneal cavity, and (3) the ovary. The frequency of ectopic pregnancy varies considerably among clinics throughout the world, ranging between 0.3 and 2.2 per cent of all pregnancies. In 1953 Anderson restudied the ratio of ectopic pregnancies in Baltimore during the 5-year period of 1949–53 and found 1 ectopic gestation in 223 white births and 1:115 in Negro women for a combined incidence of 0.56 per cent (1:178).

A more recent report by Timonen and Niemien from Finland reveals a higher ectopic pregnancy rate of 1.4 per cent during the years 1954–65, an incidence nearly 3 times greater than that of the Baltimore experience. While the frequency of this disease seems to have increased over the past 2 to 3 decades, the mortality rate has been greatly reduced. During the past decade, deaths in the United States from ectopic pregnancy have decreased from 7.2 per cent of total maternal mortality in 1957 to the most recent report of 5.9 per cent in 1965, as reported in the Vital Statistics of the United States. In general, the overall mortality from ectopic pregnancy in a well-staffed hospital should be less than 0.5 per cent. This figure varies significantly in relation to maternal mortality statistics among racial groups. The death rate from ectopic pregnancies in the city of Baltimore is reportedly 15 times greater for Negro than for white women. The common denominator in such deaths is delay in establishing the diagnosis and in initiating surgical treatment of the disease.

Considering the incidence of tubal pregnancy, it should be pointed out that there is an increased frequency of this condition following the initial ectopic pregnancy. In general, approximately 10 per cent of subsequent gestations will result in a repeat ectopic pregnancy. Expressed in a different way, once a woman has a tubal pregnancy, her chance of having another is approximately 20 times greater than that of women in the general population.

ETIOLOGY

Mechanical Obstruction. Pre-existent pelvic inflammatory disease is considered to play the most important role in the pathogenesis of ectopic pregnancy. Kleiner and Roberts recently conducted a prospective study on the factors causing tubal pregnancy and demonstrated histologic evidence of chronic salpingitis in 53 per cent of their cases. However, none of the tubes that were cultured revealed any bacterial growth. It has been postulated that the current treatment of acute salpingitis with antibiotics may be responsible for the reported increase in the incidence of ectopic pregnancies. Prior to the antibiotic era, the acutely inflamed tube usually became totally occluded, so that permanent sterility resulted. While intensive antibiotic therapy administered early in the course of the disease may hasten tubal healing prior to complete tubal obstruction from fibrosis (see Chapter 14, Infertility), agglutination of the cilia and synechial bands within the tubal lumen may occur and result in partial tubal obstruction. The clinicopathologic study of Kleiner and Roberts would support this thesis, as chronic follicular salpingitis was the most common single finding in their study of tubal pregnancy.

Peritubal adhesions resulting from peritonitis from puerperal or postabortal pelvic infection may also partially obstruct the fallopian tube. In the above study of ectopic pregnancies, 37 per cent of the tubes with normal endosalpinx had moderate or extensive peritubal adhesions at the time of laparotomy.

Other factors related to impairment of tubal transport of the fertilized ovum include previous tubal plastic procedures; in patients with such a history, the subsequent ectopic pregnancy rate varies between 10 and 20 per cent. While congenital abnormalities of the tube, such as diverticula and accessory ora, were formerly though to play an etiologic role in ectopic pregnancy, such findings are difficult to document at the time of surgery, particularly after tubal rupture or abortion has occurred.

Other Factors. As reviewed by Pauerstein and coauthors, the oviduct is an organ of multiple functions and not merely a conduit for ova and sperm. There is recent evidence to suggest that the ampullar and isthmic portions of the tube behave differently, both in spontaneous contractility and in response to various pharmacologic agents. A partial block occurs normally in the region of the ampullar-isthmic junction and may be directly responsible for impairment of ova transport as a result of altered tubal physiology. The influence of estrogen and progesterone on tubal mobility has received conflicting reports from animal experiments. However, in analyzing our personal data on ectopic pregnancies during the past 5 years, we were impressed with the observation that 12 per cent of 162 such patients in Milwaukee were taking "birth-control" pills of varying estrogen and progesterone combinations. This finding is difficult to evaluate and must be considered in relation to the percentage of the population taking such pills.

Transperitoneal migration of the ovum has been postulated as an additional factor and is supported by the finding of the corpus luteum of pregnancy in the opposite ovary from the side of the gestation in approximately 15 per cent of the reported cases.

PATHOPHYSIOLOGY

When the fertilized zygote is impaired in its transport from the outer third of the fallopian tube, the lytic properties of the developing trophoblast cause erosion of the tubal mucosa and small blood vessels, with the development of a miniature placental site. There is poor development of the decidua of the tubal mucosa, and a protective Nitabuch layer is absent. The rapid growth and invasive properties of the trophoblast are uncontrolled, which may result in one of three complications:

1. Continued invasion and digestion of the musculature of the tube may occur, with rupture into the peritoneal cavity, which usually results in extensive intraperitoneal hemorrhage. More infrequently, trophoblastic penetration of the tubal wall may occur between the peritoneal reflection of the broad ligament on the tube, with intraligamentary rupture. This rare event can result in secondary implantation and a broad-ligament pregnancy, which has a reported occurrence of approximately 1 in every 245 ectopic pregnancies, according to Ziel and co-workers.

2. Tubal abortion is the most common result of tubal pregnancy and is associated with an insufficient blood supply and nutrition for the developing pregnancy. In such cases necrosis and dis-

lodgment of the anchoring trophoblastic villi accompany retrovillus hemorrhage. Bleeding continues, which results in abortion and hemorrhage from the fimbriated end of the tube. The intraperitoneal hemorrhage from *tubal abortion* is less serious than that associated with *tubal rupture.*

3. On rare occasions the gestational process may undergo spontaneous regression and gradual phagocytic absorption of the necrotic tissue or may become calcified in the tube as a lithopedion. The number of tubal pregnancies that are never diagnosed but treated conservatively as salpingitis is unknown, but this clinical error must occur more often at the present time than prior to the availability of broad-spectrum antibiotics.

While these changes are taking place in the tube, the endometrium undergoes a true decidual reaction and may become quite thick. The myometrium also hypertrophies, becomes softened, and will produce slight uterine enlargement. Frequently it is difficult to identify such anatomic changes in the earliest stages of an extra-uterine pregnancy.

When tubal abortion or rupture occurs, the fetus usually dies promptly, unless the trophoblastic villi remain partially attached to the tubal wall while developing a parasitic blood supply in the peritoneal cavity. With fetal death there is regression of the corpus luteum due to a decrease in the secretion of chorionic gonadotropin from the degenerating trophoblast. A concomitant decrease in the blood estrogen and progesterone levels takes place, which produces shedding of the decidua, either as a complete cast of the uterine cavity or, more frequently, in small fragments mixed with blood. Occasionally, uterine bleeding may occur prior to death of the fetus, which probably represents fluctuations in circulating blood steroid levels.

SYMPTOMS

The symptoms of tubal pregnancy are protean, depending chiefly on whether the pregnancy is intact, aborted into the peritoneal cavity, or ruptured through the tubal wall. The amount of associated hemorrhage is one of the most important factors in the occurrence of clinical symptoms. The cardinal symptoms include the triad of pain, bleeding, and menstrual irregularity.

Pain. Although pain is the most common manifestation of this entity, it may vary in severity. Acute, severe, unilateral pain is usually associated with the acute episode of tubal abortion or rupture with hemorrhage into the peritoneal cavity. The pain may be persistent and become generalized over the lower abdomen or may be spasmodic and crampy in nature. It usually becomes localized to one of the lower abdominal quadrants. If sufficient intraperitoneal bleeding occurs, blood will collect in the cul-de-sac and produce rectal pressure and tenesmus. In addition, subdiaphragmatic collection of blood will produce reflex shoulder pain in approximately 15 to 20 per cent of the cases. When there is minimal tubal leakage of blood into the peritoneal cavity, the symptoms are more chronic and insidious. Such cases are much more difficult to differentiate from such conflicting conditions as pelvic inflammatory disease, appendicitis, and a leaking corpus luteum hematoma.

Bleeding. Vaginal bleeding or spotting may precede, present simultaneously, or follow the occurrence of pain. In many cases the blood is mixed with cervical mucus and may simulate a chocolate discharge. Occasionally a decidual cast is passed spontaneously, but more frequently decidua is shed in small pieces and mixed with blood, which may persist for weeks. Such symptoms make the diagnosis difficult to differentiate from threatened or incomplete abortion.

Menstrual Irregularity. In most cases there is a history of one or more missed periods, but this symptom is perhaps one of the most difficult to document accurately. Due to the fact that bleeding can occur at any stage of the extra-uterine gestation, depending on the fluctuations of the blood progesterone level, it must be recognized that any form of menstrual irregularity is compatible with the diagnosis of ectopic pregnancy. In our experience, more than 50 per cent of the cases have periods of amenorrhea of 6 to 12 weeks' duration.

CLINICAL FINDINGS

Shock. It is evident that patients seek medical attention earlier today than in previous decades, as shown by our finding of profound shock with systolic blood pressure below 70 mm. Hg in only 20 per cent of ectopic pregnancies at Milwaukee County Hospital. Others have reported shock as frequently as in 32 per cent of such cases. With significant intraperitoneal hemorrhage there is extreme pallor, with calmminess of the skin, sweating, and rapid pulse. Intraperitoneal hemorrhage produces irritability of the stomach and small bowel, which may cause nausea and vomiting even though the patient is in a semicomatose state.

Pelvic Mass. A unilateral adnexal mass, clearly separable from the ovary and bowel, in conjunction with such symptoms and signs is a conclusive finding in establishing the diagnosis of an ectopic pregnancy. Unfortunately, it has been our experience that only 35 per cent of such patients have a clearly defined, unilateral adnexal mass. Caution must be exercised in repeated examinations of the adnexa to avoid excessive pressure on the tube, which might produce rupture or abortion with resultant hemorrhage. It is best therefore that only 1 or 2 experienced examiners perform a pelvic examination in the patient who is thought to have an unruptured ectopic pregnancy.

Cullen's sign — or the "blue navel" of ectopic pregnancy — is seen only rarely, but when present, it is a significant finding that indicates extensive intra-abdominal hemorrhage. Although this phenomenon was first described by Hofstätter (1909), its classic description by Cullen in 1918 stimulated clinicians throughout the world to look for this sign, which gradually inherited his name. Discoloration of the peritoneum signifies intraperitoneal blood and is best seen through the thinnest area of the abdominal wall at the umbilicus. This finding can occur in other pathologic states than ectopic pregnancy, including acute pancreatitis and hemorrhage from the intestinal tract or from other intra-abdominal sites. Abdominal wall discoloration can also occur in other areas from such causes as hernias and incisional scars and is thought to represent intra-abdominal fluid which accumulates between fascial planes after traversing the peritoneal membrane. In cases of ruptured ectopic pregnancy, this condition is rarely seen unless accompanied by massive intra-abdominal bleeding, with significant distention of the peritoneal surface, which produces the translucent effect in the umbilicus.

DIAGNOSTIC PROCEDURES

Culdocentesis. In recent years the use of culdocentesis has increased in this country and abroad and has resulted in an earlier diagnosis of hematoperitoneum. This technic of placing a needle in the cul-de-sac has now experienced wide usage with no significant complications. The advantage of this diagnostic procedure includes the opportunity to evaluate the peritoneal cavity immediately whenever the examiner suspects intraperitoneal bleeding by the sensation of cul-de-sac bulging or crepitus. A No. 18 gauge spinal needle is inserted through the posterior fornix between the uterosacral ligaments at the site of the maximum bulge after infiltration of the vagina and septum with approximately 5 cc. of 1 per cent Xylocaine (Fig. 16-1). In many instances the local anesthetic is not used as the discomfort of entering the peritoneal cavity is very brief. The needle is attached to a 20 cc. Luer-Lok syringe, and the needle is directed horizontally to avoid posterior displacement into the rectum or sigmoid. Even if the bowel is accidentally punctured, we have seen no difficulty resulting from this procedure. The detection of nonclotting blood in the peritoneal cavity is most useful in establishing a clinical diagnosis, particularly when other signs and symptoms of intraperitoneal hemorrhage are inconclusive.

FIG. 16-1. Culdocentesis.

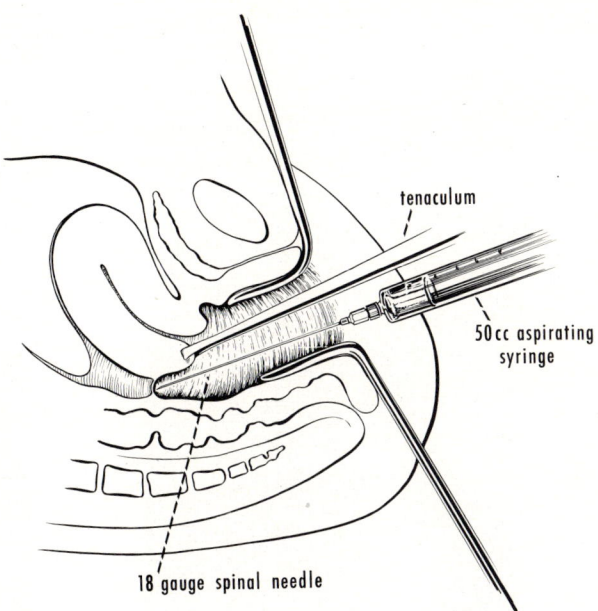

Once this finding is established, immediate exploratory laparotomy should be undertaken after stabilization of the vital signs. Significant hematoperitoneum is always a surgical emergency, and consequently this procedure is helpful in the early treatment of such acute conditions.

Examination under anesthesia is one of the most accurate methods of evaluating the pelvic organs and may give confirming evidence of a unilateral adnexal mass clearly separate from the adjacent ovary. However, in early gestations, either intrauterine or extra-uterine, the pelvic examination may not reveal the location of the pregnancy. The absence of a mass on pelvic examination under anesthesia therefore does not definitely rule out a tubal pregnancy. It will, however, assist in differentiating a symptomatic ovarian cyst, such as a corpus luteum hematoma or a twisted physiologic cyst, as well as bilateral pelvic inflammatory disease, from the list of possible diagnoses.

Dilatation and Curettage. A curettage is of assistance in differentiating the patient with an incomplete abortion from the patient with chronic symptoms of an ectopic pregnancy if villi are found in the curettings. However, a dilatation and curettage should not be performed unless the patient is bleeding, to avoid interrupting a threatened abortion. The presence of decidua with no trace of chorionic villi is helpful, but not absolute evidence, of tubal pregnancy (Fig. 16-2). A spontaneous complete abortion may have only residual decidua as evidence of a previous pregnancy. In general, decidua is found in the endometrium unless the fetus has been dead for a significant period of time, or there has been sufficient uterine bleeding to permit complete shedding of all the decidua.

The experience of Romney, Hertig, and Reid in their study of the endometrium in 115 cases of ectopic pregnancy reaffirms this fact, as over 75 per cent of these cases showed endometrium with no specific decidual change. Our own experience confirms their findings and is a constant reminder that the absence of decidua does not rule out an existing ectopic pregnancy (Fig. 16-3).

ARIAS-STELLA REACTION. There has been recent emphasis on the Arias-Stella reaction of the endometrial glands in association with pregnancy. This endometrial picture was first described by Polak and Wolfe in 1924 in a case of tubal pregnancy. It was not until 1954, however, that Arias-Stella re-emphasized the atypical endometrial features found

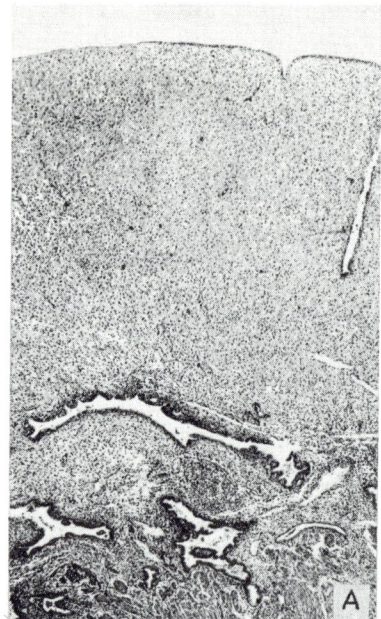 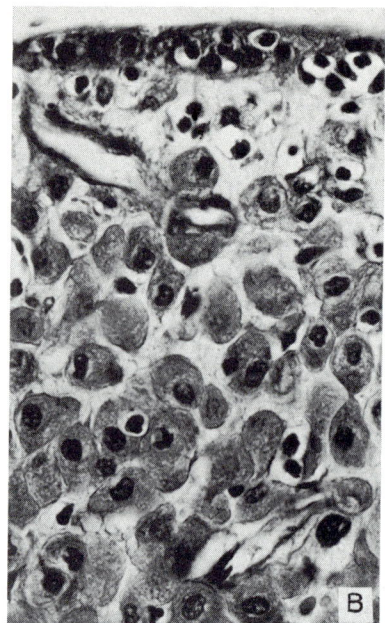

FIG. 16-2. (A) Low-power magnification of endometrium, showing very heavy compacta layer. Glands show secretory change. (B) High-power magnification of section taken near the surface showing very marked decidual-like changes of the stroma cells.

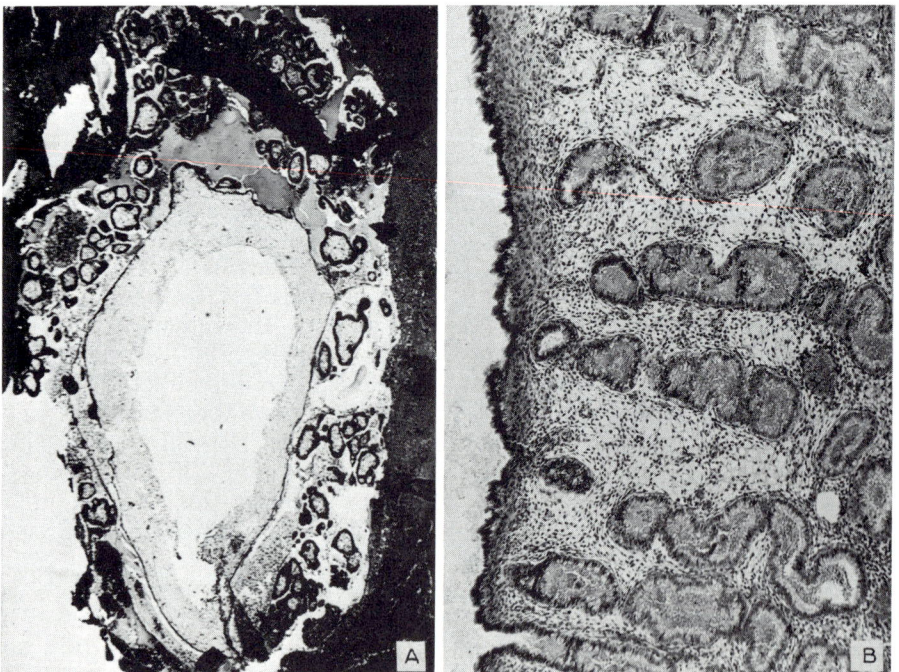

FIG. 16-3. (A) Early embryo found in tube. (B) Endometrium from same case, showing late interval secretory glands and absolutely no decidual change in the stroma.

in association with abortions, syncytial endometritis, hydatidiform mole, and choriocarcinoma. In addition, only one case of ectopic pregnancy was included in his initial study, in which he concluded that this histologic endometrial pattern "may be of value in making a presumptive diagnosis of the presence of active chorial tissue in which the chorial tissue is not in a position accessible to the curette." Lloyd and Fienberg have defined the A-S reaction in glandular epithelial cells as follows:

1. Nucleus—increase in size associated with hyperchromasia or pyknosis; often folding of nuclear membrane.
2. Cytoplasm—abundant vacuolated cytoplasm, usually eosinophilic staining.
3. Desquamation of such cells into lumen of glands.

Their experience, as well as that of others, reveals that the presence of this endometrial reaction (Fig. 16-4) cannot be related to the exact site of pregnancy. While it may raise the clinical suspicion of extra-uterine pregnancy, it is considered to be an involutional, regressive phenomena of the endometrium, which occurs after fetal death and cessation of hormonal stimulation.

Culdoscopy; Laparoscopy. We have found culdoscopy to be a most useful procedure in the unruptured ectopic pregnancy in which the diagnosis is not confirmed by either history or pelvic findings. Suspected tubal pregnancy remains our greatest indication for culdoscopy. For example, of 186 culdoscopic examinations performed at Johns Hopkins Hospitals during a 3-year period, 86 were done because of suspected tubal pregnancy. We have found this procedure most useful in attempting to differentiate a tubal pregnancy from pelvic inflammatory disease or a symptomatic ovarian cyst. Direct observation of the tube, adnexa, and pelvis provides accurate information on the pelvic pathology. The greatest benefit of this procedure has been to avoid a needless laparotomy in the absence of significant pelvic pathology.

More recently, laparoscopy has been used for the same indications and may

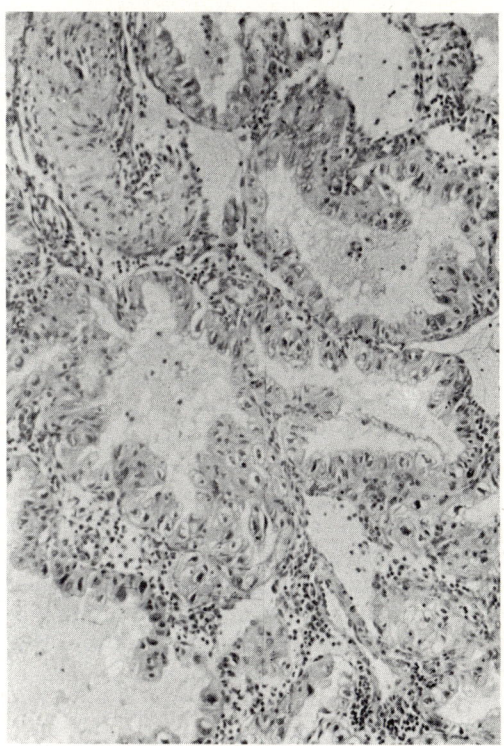

FIG. 16-4. Arias-Stella reaction in endometrial cells associated with ectopic pregnancy, showing nuclear enlargement, irregularity, and hyperchromasia with cytoplasmic vacuolation.

prove to have more widespread acceptance because of the positional advantage for the patient and the wider range of visibility of the entire peritoneal cavity.

Colpotomy. This procedure is useful for diagnosis of an adnexal mass suggestive of an ectopic pregnancy when the lesion is accessible in the cul-de-sac. In general, we have reserved this procedure in ectopic pregnancies for cases in which tubal rupture or abortion is suspected. It is important that the adnexa be free and mobile, to permit adequate inspection through the vagina. In general, it is not our preference to remove a tubal pregnancy through a colpotomy incision, due to the difficulty of obtaining adequate hemostasis which is associated with the complication of a pelvic hematoma. However, a tubal pregnancy which is in direct view of the colpotomy incision may be easily excised by the experienced gynecologist without difficulty. In such cases the patient's postoperative course is usually much more rapid, and the duration of hospitalization is decreased as compared to that following the use of laparotomy.

Other Diagnostic Procedures. Blood counts should be done, but in the acute cases these are of little value in accurately assessing circulating blood volume. Falling hematocrit levels in a well-hydrated patient will provide more accurate clinical evidence of intraperitoneal bleeding. The white blood count usually is only mildly elevated, but we have seen marked leukocytosis. Frequently there is an increased number of juvenile forms due to the presence of blood in the peritoneal cavity as well as the tubal pathology. Pregnancy tests, in general, may be of some diagnostic assistance when positive, provided that the report is accurate, but this will give only biologic evidence of a gestation and does not define its location. However, the rapid, immunologic pregnancy tests, including the precipitation test and hemoagglutin-inhibition test, have a high false negative rate in view of the low serum level of circulating human chorionic gonadotrophin (HCG). Consequently, a negative value is of no assistance whatsoever in assuring the clinician of the absence of a gestational process.

TREATMENT

General Considerations

The diagnosis of tubal pregnancy with intraperitoneal bleeding constitutes one of the few surgical emergencies in gynecology. The major cause of maternal death from this condition is directly related to the delay in establishing a diagnosis and initiating surgical treatment. Irreversible shock secondary to uncontrolled intraperitoneal hemorrhage is the common denominator in most deaths from ectopic pregnancy today. Even an unruptured tubal pregnancy that is diagnosed by culdoscopy, laparoscopy, or colpotomy requires immediate surgical treatment to avoid the risk of subsequent intra-abdominal hemorrhage and shock.

Although the treatment for this condition is surgical, the operative procedure of choice depends on several factors, including the age and parity of the patient, her desire for future childbearing, the condition of the opposite oviduct, the surgical risk of the patient, and the anatomic location of the pregnancy, as well as other pelvic pathology. In general, such cases fall into one of two surgical methods of treatment, either *radical treatment*, including salpingectomy, salpingo-oophorectomy or hysterectomy, or *conservative treatment*, with preservation or reconstruction of the damaged tube if possible.

The primary treatment of tubal pregnancy in this country must be defined as *radical* with less than 5 per cent of the reported cases managed by *conservative* surgical technics. This therapeutic approach is contradictory to our knowledge of the high incidence of infertility and nulliparity among such patients, approximately 30 to 35 per cent, as well as the known fact that subsequent term pregnancies occur in only 25 to 30 per cent. Since the severity of the hemorrhage dictates the extent of surgery that is indicated, the patient with an unruptured tubal pregnancy serves as the ideal candidate for a conservative operative procedure.

In considering the urgency of pelvic laparotomy in the operative treatment of tubal pregnancy, the cases fall into three groups.

In the first group, with obvious symptoms and signs of tubal rupture and shock from internal hemorrhage, the immediate treatment is replacement of intravascular volume with whole blood, low molecular weight dextran, or balanced salt solution (Ringer's lactate). In such cases central venous pressure monitoring is helpful in avoiding excessive blood volume replacement, with resultant pulmonary edema. Hematocrit values are rarely accurate at this point due to the contracted blood volume and hemoconcentration. Blood volume studies are unfortunately time-consuming and of no practical value in such conditions. The operation should be undertaken at the first possible moment that the patient's cardiovascular system can be adequately supported for a general anesthetic. Careful monitoring of the urinary output is essential in such acute cases, as discussed in another section of this text under Hemorrhagic Shock. Since operative speed and skill is essential in the surgical control of such hemorrhage, it is important that the surgeon be an experienced operator with surgical judgment and dexterity.

In the second group the diagnosis is reasonably certain, but there is no evidence of acute hemorrhage, and the patient is in good condition. In many of these cases early rupture or tubal abortion has taken place, but the amount of intraperitoneal bleeding is minimal and consequently does not constitute an acute surgical emergency. Ideally, such patients should be operated on immediately, but in the event that surgery is temporarily delayed, they should be kept under close observation with frequent observations of blood pressure, pulse, and respiration, or an increase in abdominal distention, which would be evidence of continued intra-abdominal bleeding.

In the third group the history or physical findings are quite atypical. Various diagnostic procedures are desirable and often necessary to establish the diagnosis with some degree of certainty before undertaking laparotomy. Into this group fall some unruptured cases, some old long-standing ruptured or aborted cases, and some recently aborted or ruptured cases in which the history and/or physical findings deviate greatly from the typical. It is in this third group that the diagnostic procedures discussed above are of the greatest value. Usually it is quite safe in any well-regulated hospital to await the outcome of these tests while the patient is under careful observation. On the whole, patients will fare better if this group is studied carefully than if operation is quickly begun without complete investigation.

Extent of Operative Procedure

Speed is seldom of prime importance in gynecologic surgery. However, when dealing with a ruptured tubal pregnancy with massive abdominal hemorrhage, it may prove to be the difference between complete recovery and the rare case of irreversible shock, acute tubular nephrosis, and ultimate death of the patient. If hemorrhage has been great, rapid removal of the tube and control of the source of bleeding in the mesosalpinx is all that should be done. Occasionally it is necessary to remove the ovary with the tube by clamping the infundibulo-pelvic ligament when the ovary has become inseparable from the gestational process. Every effort should be made, however, to preserve the ovary, if possible.

If bleeding has been slight and the patient's condition is quite satisfactory, time should be taken to inspect the opposite tube carefully and to evaluate its potential function. If necessary, methylene blue solution should be instilled into the uterine cavity with a syringe and needle to demonstrate patency of the remaining tube. In cases of sterility in which the contralateral tube is destroyed or surgically absent, a conservative operative procedure should be considered, depending on the patient's interest in future child-bearing.

Rarely, when the blood loss has been slight and the patient's condition is perfectly satisfactory, a hysterectomy is indicated when fibroids are present and/or the contralateral tube is surgically absent. Although such cases are infrequent, a patient with a recurrent ectopic pregnancy in whom the remaining pregnant tube is irreparably damaged, would constitute an indication for hysterectomy in preference to the alternative of leaving a barren uterus for future menstrual dysfunction. However, it is important that a discussion of the various alternatives be held preoperatively, so that the full understanding and agreement of the patient may be secured, and her wishes on continuing to menstruate may be clearly known by the surgeon. In general, the closer to the menopause this condition occurs, the greater the indication for such a procedure. In the younger patient the primary effort would be to perform either a conservative operation on the remaining fallopian tube or to preserve the uterus solely for psychological purposes.

332 Ectopic Pregnancy

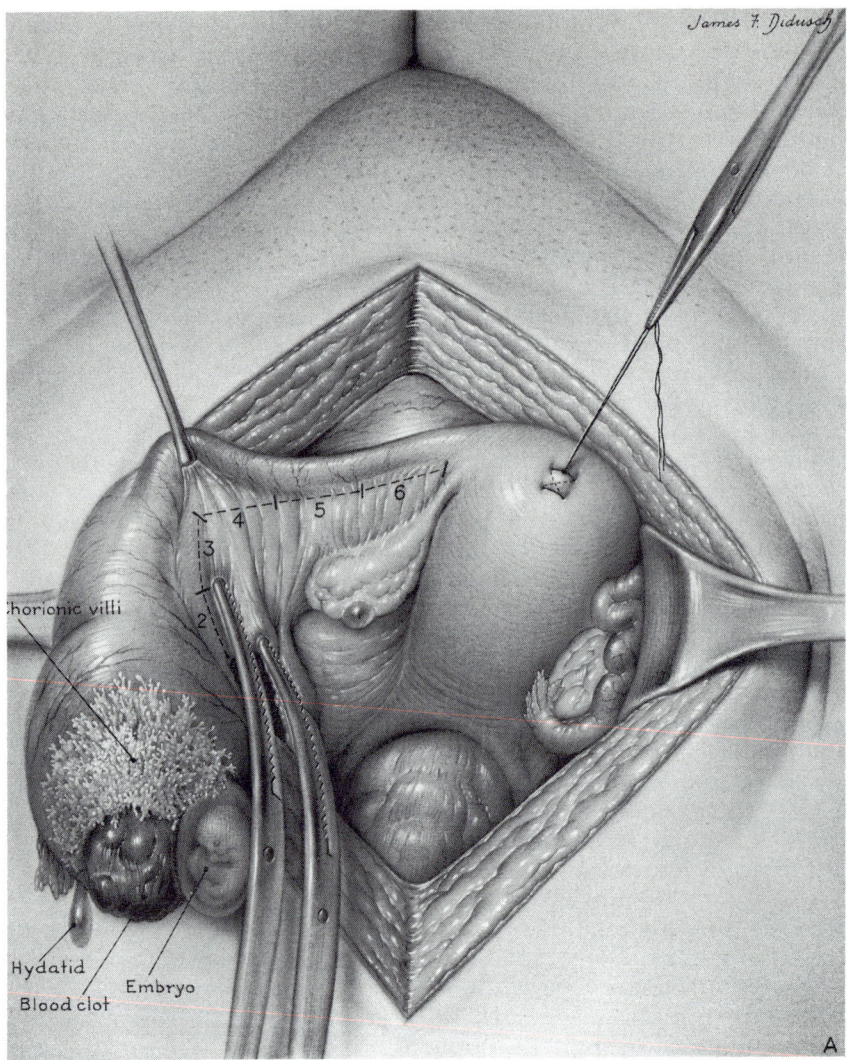

Fig. 16-5. Salpingectomy for tubal pregnancy. (A) The tube has been delivered, and the mesosalpinx is being clamped and cut, using a succession of Kelly clamps.

When the patient's condition is satisfactory, there is no objection to removal of the appendix. The argument sometimes used against appendectomy, that there is an increased morbidity from the presence of intra-abdominal blood with such a procedure, is not valid in accordance with current statistics.

In spite of there being some difference of opinion on the disposition of intra-abdominal blood, it is our preference to irrigate the peritoneal cavity thoroughly to remove all of the remaining blood and clot in an effort to reduce the development of pelvic adhesions, which may impair subsequent fertility.

Technic: Simple Salpingectomy for Tubal Pregnancy

The distended tube is lifted out of the pelvis, and the mesosalpinx is clamped with a succession of Kelly clamps as close to the tube as conveniently possible (Fig. 16-5 A). The tube is excised with a small wedge at the uterine cornu (Fig. 16-5 B). The peritoneum of the meso-

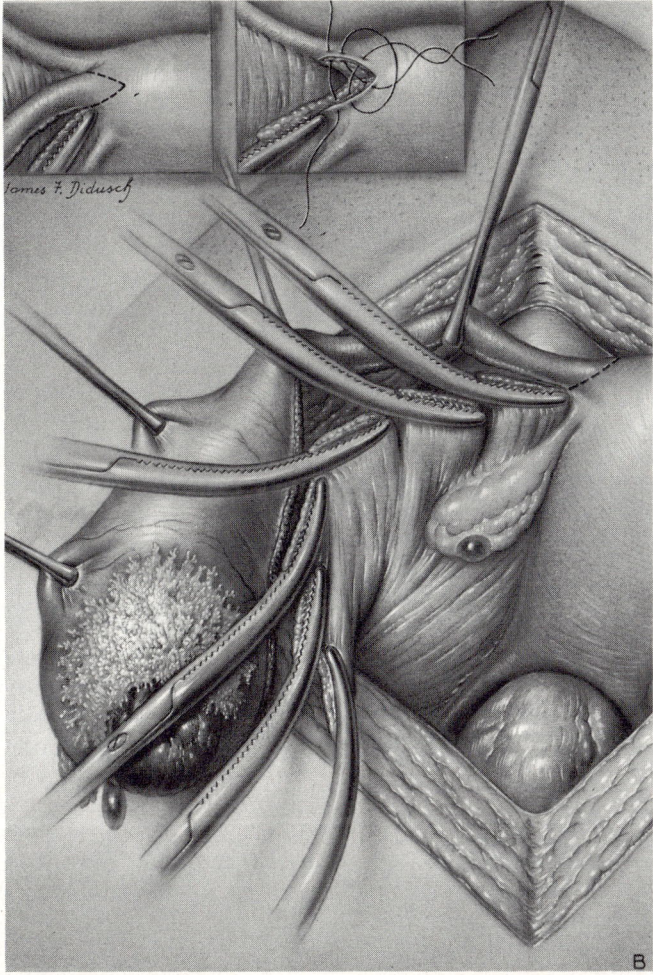

FIG. 16-5 (*Continued*). Salpingectomy for tubal pregnancy. (B) The mesosalpinx has been completely clamped and cut. The dotted line indicates the line of excision of the tube at the cornu. Inset shows suture of the excised cornu.

salpinx is usually in relatively good condition, permitting its closure and control of hemorrhage by a continuous lock stitch of No. 0 chromic catgut. This suture may be started at the uterine end, closing the incision in the uterus first and continuing laterally, or, if more convenient, the closure may be made from the outer end inward (Fig. 16-5 C^1).

The two ends of the suture are then tied together, forming a loop of the mesosalpinx, which is very convenient for peritonization (Fig. 16-5 C^2).

Peritonization is effected, and the fundus is held forward, by suturing the round and the broad ligaments over the uterine cornu (Fig. 16-5 C^3). The method of placing the peritonization suture should be noted in Figure 16-5 C^3. The needle with No. 0 plain catgut first penetrates the broad ligament from its anterior surface, just below the round ligaments, 1 or 2 cm. from the cornu. The next bite is taken in the fundus of the uterus a little medial to the uterine wound. This bite is taken from the anterior surface, posteriorly. The suture is then placed through the broad ligament from behind, about 1 cm. lateral to the point where the suture was begun. When this suture is tied, the

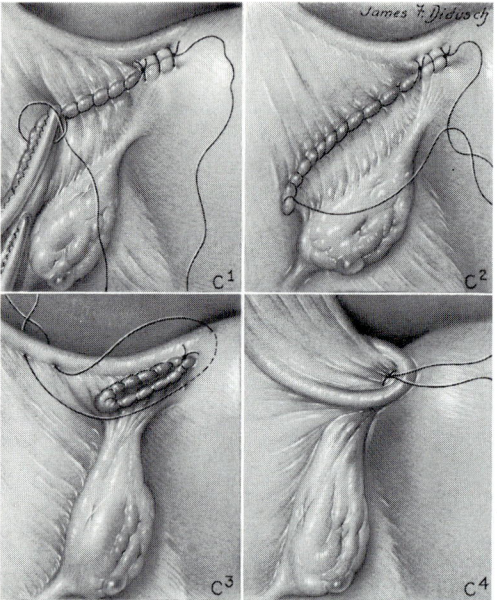

FIG. 16-5 (*Continued*). Salpingectomy for tubal pregnancy. (C^1) Showing method of suturing the mesosalpinx by using a lock stitch for hemostasis. (C^2) The mesosalpinx has been completely sutured. The end of the suture has been left long for tying to suture at the cornu. (C^3) The mesosalpinx is thus folded back on itself so that it may be peritonized easily. The method of placing of mattress suture for peritonization is also shown. (C^4) Peritonization is completed by tying mattress suture, which brings the broad and the round ligaments over the uterine cornu.

cornual wound and the mesosalpinx are nicely peritonized (Fig 16-5 C^4).

Conservative Procedures in Tubal Pregnancy

The extent of pelvic surgery for the treatment of a tubal pregnancy must be individualized at the time of operation. Conservation of the fallopian tube in the past has been reserved primarily for young patients with a recurrent tubal pregnancy or for those in whom the contralateral tube is destroyed or surgically absent. Consideration of conservative surgery has been advocated recently even when the opposite tube appears normal, in view of the apparent sterility of more than 50 per cent of such cases.

The early experience of Rubin in 1934 demonstrated that the contralateral, apparently healthy oviduct was patent in only 12.3 per cent of the cases following removal of a tubal pregnancy. He found complete occlusion of the remaining uterine tube in 44.4 per cent and partial occlusion in 43.2 per cent. Only those patients who present no surgical risk for a slightly longer operative procedure should be considered as candidates for a conservative operative procedure. Ideally, patients with an unruptured tubal pregnancy or tubal abortion have the best opportunity for successful conservation of such a fallopian tube. The recent experience of Timonen and Nieminen from Finland in the use of conservative tubal surgery is most encouraging. Of a total of 1,067 patients with tubal pregnancy during the years 1954–65, 22.5 per cent were given conservative treatment, including longitudinal section of the tube, manual expression of the ovum, tubal resection, and, rarely, tubal reimplantation. Resection was mostly performed in cases of tubal rupture, whereas longitudinal tubal section was performed most frequently in cases with an unruptured tubal pregnancy. A transabdominal polyethylene catheter was left in place for 6 weeks, with postoperative irrigation with a penicillin (200,000 units)-hydracortisone (50 mg.) solution injected daily (4 cc.) during the 1st week. Subsequent full-term pregnancies were more frequent in the cases treated by longitudinal tubal section, with a rate of 36.1 per cent. This figure should not be construed as an indication that the ovum passed through the repaired tube. Most of these patients were left with a tube on the opposite side, and it seems more than likely that the ovum passed through the uninvolved tube. Manual expression and squeezing of the ovum from the ampulla of the tube produced the highest complication rate, with a 24 per cent incidence of recurrent extra-uterine pregnancy, suggesting inadequate evacuation of the gestational contents. This conservative method of treating tubal pregnancies is not recommended. While the rate of recurrent ectopic pregnancy utilizing such conservative treatment is 12.5 per cent, this correlates well with the ectopic pregnancy rate following tuboplastic procedures in the nonpregnant state.

The conservative management of tubal pregnancy will undoubtedly play only a minor role in the surgical treatment of this condition. It is included in the revision of this text for the occasional patient who would meet such criteria.

INTERSTITIAL PREGNANCY

Interstitial pregnancy occurs in that portion of the tube that lies within the wall of the uterus. It is a rare condition, but the consequences of mismanagement are so disastrous that some space should be devoted to its consideration. Before 1893 the only available reports were from autopsies. Since then the literature presents more than 200 cases that will stand critical analysis. Rare as the condition is, accounting for 3 to 4 per cent of all tubal pregnancies, it occurs more commonly than primary ovarian or primary abdominal pregnancy.

The etiologic factors concerned in interstitial pregnancy are the same as those responsible for tubal pregnancy of the ordinary variety, the most important of which are pelvic inflammatory disease, congenital abnormalities, operative trauma, and tumors. Of particular interest are those occurring in the tubal stump after salpingectomies. Kalchman and Meltzer have reviewed the literature on the subject and report 73 cases of interstitial pregnancy following total salpingectomy, with two additional cases of their own, and an additional 24 following partial salpingectomy. Ectopic pregnancy accounted for 60 per cent of the indications for salpingectomy. Too vigorous a cornual resection was considered to be one of the major factors in subsequent interstitial pregnancy. The problem for speculation in such cases is whether the ovum entered the interstitial portion of the tube from the abdominal or the uterine end. Attempts have been made to classify interstitial pregnancies based on the position of the ovum in the interstitial part of the tube, but most cases are seen in a stage too far advanced to permit accurate classification, or they have ruptured, and therefore are still more difficult to classify.

The gestational sac is better protected in the interstitial portion of the tube than in the remainder of the tube, and as a result, such pregnancies usually are somewhat further advanced when they rupture. Eventually, the chorionic villi erode into the blood vessels at the uterine cornu, and hemorrhage results. This hemorrhage is apt to be much greater than that associated with the ordinary tubal pregnancy, since the anastomosis of the uterine and the ovarian vessels makes it one of the most vascular areas in the female pelvis. The severe hemorrhage associated with rupture usually throws the patient into serious shock with great suddenness. The abdomen becomes rigid and tender, due to the presence of the intraperitoneal blood. Frequently, before rupture the patient has some discomfort and a sense that all is not well with the pregnancy. After 2 or 3 months of amenorrhea, vaginal spotting begins. Asymmetry of the uterus of a patient who has missed her period suggests the possibility of a pregnant bicornuate uterus, a pregnancy in a fibroid uterus, or an interstitial pregnancy. Previous knowledge of the shape of the uterus may confirm or exclude the possibility of a bicornuate uterus. The firmness of the protrusion on the uterus suggests a fibroid. A soft, tender, asymmetric enlargement at one cornu suggests an interstitial pregnancy. Because of the fact that rupture often occurs late when the cornual enlargement is palpably enlarged, a fairly large percentage of interstitial pregnancies are diagnosed before rupture. While earlier reports included a very high maternal mortality rate from interstitial pregnancy, the series reported by Kalchman and Meltzer includes a mortality rate reduced to 2.7 per cent.

TREATMENT

The surgical procedure for the treatment of interstitial pregnancy in Kalchman and Meltzer's report of 75 cases includes the following:

TABLE 16-1*

Procedure	No.	%
Cornual resection	26	34.7
Hysterectomy	26	34.7
Simple repair	22	29.3
Unknown	1	1.3
	75	100.0

* Kalchman, G. G., and Meltzer, R. M.: Amer. J. Obstet. Gynec., 96:1142, 1966.

Contrary to previous experience, cornual resection and simple repair of the cornual defect comprised 64 per cent of the procedures, whereas hysterctomy was performed in only 34.7 per cent. As reported by the authors, this more conservative approach probably reflects the interest in preservation of childbearing function of this highly infertile group. Fortunately, the more conservative management of this condition can be accomplished effectively today without jeopardizing the patient's life, even though such cases are known to produce massive hemorrhage due to frequent involvement of the adjacent uterine artery. The availability of rapid blood replacement and more accurate physiologic monitoring and control of such acutely ill patients has greatly improved the surgical risk of patients with this pregnancy complication. However, hysterectomy remains the treatment of choice in those patients in whom the pregnancy has advanced to such a stage that repair of the cornua would be technically difficult and time-consuming. In such instances it is far preferable and safer to perform a hysterectomy. In performing cornual resection, one must accept the infrequent but serious risk of uterine rupture in any subsequent pregnancy.

Figure 16-6 illustrates excision of an interstitial pregnancy by cornual resection with removal of the adjacent ovary and tube. The tube should be removed rather than implanted, for the reimplanted tube offers an excellent opportunity for another tubal pregnancy as well as a site for uterine rupture in the event of a future pregnancy. The ovary can usually be preserved with this procedure.

Technic: Excision of Interstitial Pregnancy With Salpingo-Oophorectomy

Figure 16-6 A illustrates the ruptured interstitial pregnancy, and the dotted line shows the line of excision.

The salpingo-oophorectomy is done in the usual manner. As the ascending uterine vessels are approached near the cornu, a suture ligature is placed about the vessels (Fig 16-6 B). The interstitial pregnancy is excised in a V-shaped manner, and the myometrium is approximated with figure-of-eight sutures of No. 1 chromic catgut. In doing this, it is found necessary to cut the round ligament. The round ligament is resutured to the cornu, and the uterine serosa is approximated with a continuous lock stitch (Fig. 16-6 C). The round and the broad ligaments are brought over the cornual wound with a few mattress sutures of No. 1 chromic catgut (Fig. 16-6 D).

Figure 16-7 shows a method of excision of interstitial pregnancy in which a layer of mattress sutures is laid and tied before the pregnancy is removed. After the sac is removed, the superficial musculature and serosa are approximated by a second layer of sutures. This technic may save considerable blood loss.

ABDOMINAL PREGNANCY

The occurrence of an abdominal pregnancy is perhaps one of the most rare, as well as most serious types of extra-uterine gestation. The frequency of this entity is quite variable, ranging between 1 per 3,371 total deliveries (Beacham) to 1 in 20,000 full-term deliveries in Finland. Perhaps the largest reported experience with this entity to date has been that of Beacham and co-workers, who have treated 65 cases at the Charity Hospital in New Orleans from 1937 through 1961. Their review of 553 cases in the literature

Abdominal Pregnancy

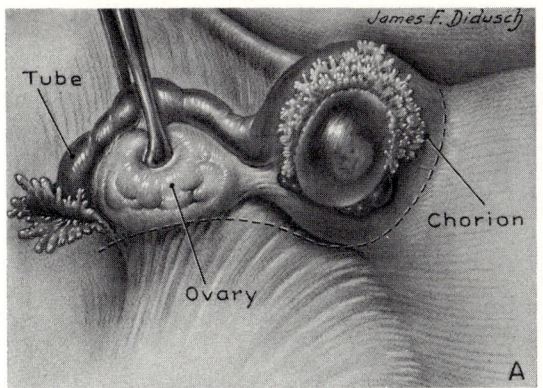
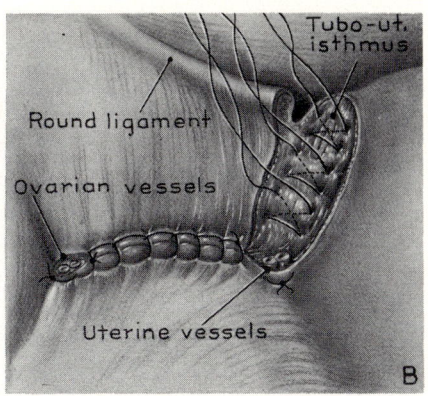
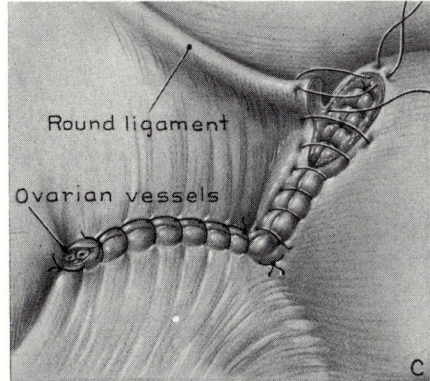
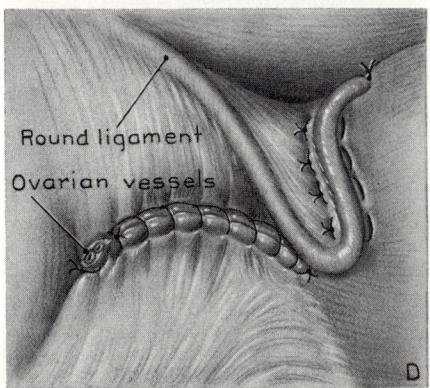

Fig. 16-6. Cornual resection of interstitial pregnancy. (A) Dotted line denotes line of excision. (B) Tube, ovary, and cornual pregnancy have been excised. Myometrium is being approximated with figure-of-eight sutures of No. 1 chromic catgut. Note that the uterine vessels have been ligated. (C) The round ligament, which was cut, is being resutured to the cornu. The ovarian vessels have been ligated, and the broad ligament has been closed with a continuous lock stitch. Serosa of the uterine wound is closed with a simple continuous stitch. (D) The cornual wound is covered over with the round and the broad ligaments.

revealed a racial incidence of approximately 60 per cent Negro. In the Charity Hospital experience, however, 95 per cent of their cases were found in the Negro population. This reflects not only the predominant racial distribution of patients at the New Orleans Charity Hospital but also the high incidence of tubal inflammatory disease associated with this group of patients.

Abdominal pregnancies are classified as either *primary* or *secondary*. Most of the reported cases result from early tubal abortion or rupture with secondary implantation of the pregnancy into the peritoneal cavity. The authenticity of primary abdominal implantation of a fertilized ovum has been difficult to prove. However, isolated cases have been reported in the recent literature following Studderford's description of the criteria of this entity in 1942, which include the following: (1) the normal condition of both tubes and ovaries, with no evidence of recent or remote injury, (2) absence of any evidence of uteroperitoneal fistula, and (3) the presence of a pregnancy related exclusively to the peritoneal surface and young enough to eliminate the possibility of secondary implantation following primary nidation in the tube.

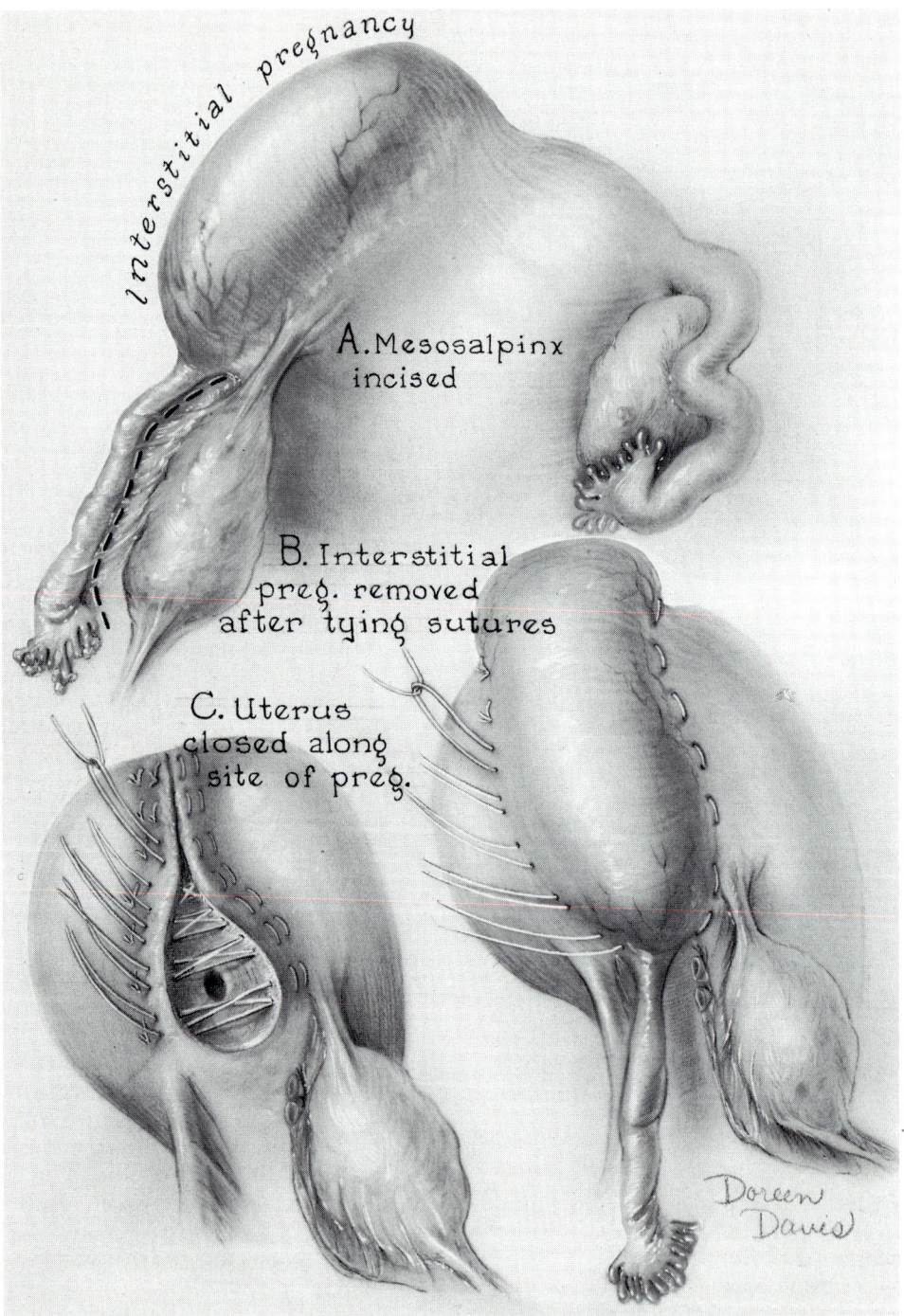

Fig. 16-7. Demonstrates a method of reducing hemorrhage by laying a row of mattress sutures which are tied before opening the sac for removal of pregnancy. Musculature and serosa are then closed by a more superficial line of sutures.

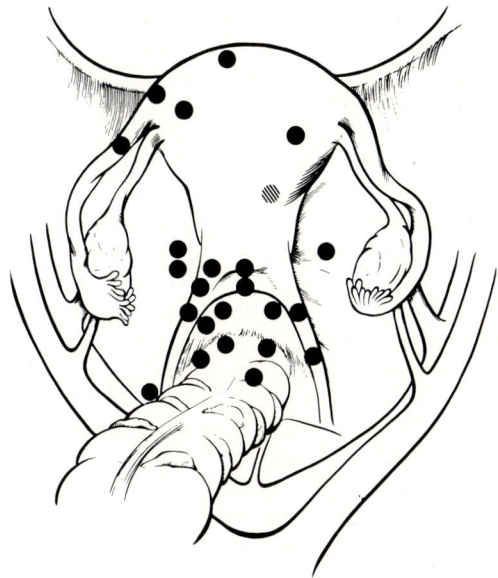

Fig. 16-8. Sites of previously reported primary pelvic pregnancies. (Friedrich, E. G., and Rankin, C. A.: Primary pelvic peritoneal pregnancy. Obstet. Gynec., *31*: 649, 1968)

Friedrich has recently collected 24 cases from the literature in which the gestation was less than 12 weeks in duration, and the implantation was limited solely to the pelvis. In addition to his own case, which was located on the anterior leaf of the broad ligament, there are undoubtedly other isolated experiences that have not been reported. The sites of previously reported primary peritoneal pelvic pregnancies are shown in Figure 16-8. Such findings suggest that the cul-de-sac may function as a receptacle for ova and sperm in the process of human fertilization. Explanation of such a primary peritoneal implantation would suggest failure of the fallopian tube to engulf the fertilized zygote for transportation into the uterine cavity. If this theory is correct, however, one wonders why this condition is not seen more frequently than presently recorded.

It is well recognized that secondary abdominal pregnancy is far more common than primary implantation. This condition results from a tubal gestation which attaches itself to the other viscera as the enlarging placenta spreads either through the wall of the tube or is aborted out through the fimbriated end. There is some doubt whether the placenta can be completely detached from its tubal implantation, extruded from the tube, and reimplanted on the pelvic viscera. It is probable that the placenta retains some tubal attachment which supplies blood to the fetus as the remainder of the placenta gains a foothold on its new peritoneal site. Rare types of secondary abdominal pregnancies have been reported following spontaneous separation of an old cesarean scar, uterine perforation during clinical abortions, and after subtotal hysterectomy.

The diagnosis of an abdominal pregnancy is quite difficult and yet very important to establish at an early stage of pregnancy to avoid the possibility of catastrophic hemorrhage from separation of the placenta. The patient's history is usually documented with symptoms of abdominal discomfort, fetal movement beneath the abdominal wall, and the presence of the fetal movements high in the upper abdomen. Confirmation of the diagnosis requires demonstration of the fetus outside the uterine cavity. If the uterus can be palpated separately from the fetal parts, the abdominal pregnancy can be confirmed either by hysterosalpingogram or failure of oxytocin induction of labor. The most effective method of diagnosing an abdominal pregnancy is by x-ray, including AP and lateral films. Radiologic features suggestive of this entity include malposition of the fetus, with the most common attitude of the fetus found in the transverse lie. Often there is the pose of the characteristic "swimming attitude," with the fetus in a transverse position, the spine cephalad and the limbs caudad, as though swimming in the abdominal cavity. Frequently, gas in the maternal small bowel can be seen overlying the fetus. The classic finding of fetal small parts overlying the maternal spine in the lateral position was first noted by Weinberg and Sherwin in 1956 and, when present, is a fairly reliable sign. However, this can also occur with sacculation of the uterus, with a fetus in transverse lie within the uterus. In addition, the fetus stands out clearly on an x-ray film with sharp details of fat lines and epiphysial centers.

Experience varies in the accuracy of the diagnosis but this is rarely greater than 50 per cent prior to operation. Once the diagnosis is established, it is our opinion that surgery should not be delayed because of the high perinatal mortality rate as well as maternal risk if intra-abdominal placental separation should occur. While maternal deaths are rare from this condition, Clark and Guy report an extremely high fetal wastage, with an overall fetal salvage of only 11 per cent in 26 pregnancies. One of the major factors in fetal survival is related to intact fetal membranes. When the membranes are ruptured, the fetus usually dies in the peritoneal cavity or from respiratory distress in the immediate neonatal period. There is also a very high incidence of fetal anomalies, which are thought to be related to the extra-uterine environment of the fetus.

Management of the placenta remains a controversial issue but probably is best treated by clamping the cord and closing the abdomen without drainage. The placenta can be removed secondarily after complete cessation of function as determined by quantitative chorionic gonadotropin titers, at which time it can be assumed that the circulation has undergone fibrosis. Thompson reports leaving a placenta in the peritoneal cavity for a period of 13 years without evidence of physical harm to the patient. We have recently treated such a case by the use of methotrexate to hasten trophoblastic degeneration as determined by serial HCG titers. Repeated 5-day courses of this antimetabolite drug were given, using 10 mg. daily by mouth, which is approximately half the usual dose for patients with trophoblastic tumors. However, other authors feel the placenta should be removed at the time of laparotomy if accessible and if its removal can be accomplished without excessive blood loss. When in doubt, however, it is best to leave the placenta in place and await sclerosis of its blood supply.

OVARIAN PREGNANCY

Although this condition was first reported in 1862 by Saint Maurice from France, it was not until 1878, following Spiegelberg's well-preserved criteria for the diagnosis of ovarian pregnancy, that this entity became accepted. These criteria require:

1. That the tube, including the fimbria ovarica, be intact and the former clearly separate from the ovary.
2. That the gestation sac definitely occupy the normal position of the ovary.
3. That the sac be connected with the uterus by the utero-ovarian ligament.
4. That unquestionable ovarian tissue be demonstrated in the walls of the sac.

Because of the difficulty in fulfilling all of these criteria, Hertig has estimated that this entity occurs once in every 25,000 to 40,000 pregnancies. Although there have been many reports in the English literature in the past half century, the exact number of cases is uncertain. Boronow and co-workers collected 62 cases from the literature from 1950 through January 1963, and estimated that there were at least 150 cases of ovarian pregnancies documented in the English literature. There have been several additional reports since that time.

Most of the cases of ovarian pregnancy are extrafollicular in origin, while approximately 15 per cent of such gestations are reportedly intrafollicular. The latter classification requires a well-identified corpus luteum in the wall of the gestational sac in addition to the other criteria. Several theories are presented for mechanisms of ovarian pregnancy and include (1) obstructed ovulation, (2) inadequate tubal peristalic function, (3) favorable surface implantation site of decidua or endometriosis, (4) parthenogenesis, and (5) chance.

The diagnosis is usually made by both symptoms and signs similar to other forms of ectopic pregnancy, including unilateral adnexal pain, vaginal bleeding, and amenorrhea. Occasionally ovarian pregnancies persist for a longer period of time than other forms of ectopic pregnancies. The diagnostic procedures are similar to those described previously, but because of the ovarian location of the gestation, it is more frequently misdiagnosed as an ovarian cyst.

The treatment depends on the extent of the ovarian pregnancy and the amount of intraperitoneal hemorrhage at the time of diagnosis. If detected early enough, an ovarian resection of the gestation is possible, with conservation of the ovary. Unfortunately, this is usually not possible, and more frequently than not, an oophorectomy is required. If the adjacent fallopian tube is adherent, it may be necessary to remove the oviduct as well. Occasionally an ovarian pregnancy is combined with an intra-uterine pregnancy, as recently reported by Ashley.

OTHER FORMS OF ECTOPIC PREGNANCY

Combined Pregnancy. Coexistent intra-uterine and extra-uterine pregnancies were first described by Duverney in 1708. Over 500 cases of such heterotopic pregnancy have been recorded to date. Approximately 50 per cent of the cases are associated with death of the intra-uterine twin. Although there was some original thought given to the possibility of multiple ovulation at 1-month intervals, the current explanation suggests simultaneous multiple ovulations, with each ovum subjected to an equal risk of an ectopic implantation. Various combinations of pregnancies may occur, including abdominal, ovarian, and tubal along with the intra-uterine implantation. The most frequent combination is the tubal-intra-uterine pregnancy.

The diagnosis is usually suspected when a slight increase in the size of the uterus is noted at the time of removal of the ectopic pregnancy. However, due to the fact that uterine size varies greatly, depending on the duration of the extra-uterine gestation, this clinical sign is frequently overlooked. It is usually not until the patient fails to menstruate in subsequent months after removal of the ectopic gestation that clinical suspicion of an additional gestation is aroused. Continued enlargement of the uterus and positive pregnancy tests confirm the diagnosis. Although there is little information to evaluate the condition of the children who survive the neonatal period, there is concern that such cases associated with shock from the extra-uterine pregnancy may produce permanent brain damage, as suggested by recent pathologic examinations of the central nervous system in the report by Jolly and Norman.

If the combined pregnancy is suspected at the time of laparotomy for the ectopic gestation, it is advisable to continue the patient on supplemental progesterone postoperatively until the pregnancy test confirms or denies the presence of an additional gestation.

Cervical Pregnancy. The cervix is a rare but hazardous site for placental implantation because of the complication of hemorrhage associated with penetration of the cervical wall and with involvement of the uterine blood supply. This freak location for trophoblastic implantation is more commonly associated with placentation in the lower uterine segment, with secondary extension into the cervical canal. Bleeding is frequently late due to the excellent blood supply in this region and occurs only when the gestational process begins to enlarge the cervical canal with progressive growth.

This diagnosis is frequently confused with a neoplastic process because of its marked vascularity and friable appearance. Unfortunately, excessive bleeding may occur if the placenta is mistaken for a tumor and biopsied. In such cases it may be necessary to evacuate the gestation by dilatation and curettage for control of the bleeding. Occasionally this is unsuccessful, and with continued bleeding a hysterectomy is necessary. A true cervical pregnancy is incompatible with a viable fetus and will usually produce symptoms within the first trimester of pregnancy.

BIBLIOGRAPHY

Arias-Stella, J.: Atypical endometrial changes associated with the presence of chorionic tissue. A.M.A. Arch. Path., 58:112, 1954.

Ashley, D. J. B., and Lloyd, M. I.: Coexisting ovarian and uterine pregnancy. J. Obstet. Gynaec. Brit. Comm., 73:152, 1966.

Barnes, A. B., Grover, J. W., and Sudduth, S. S.: Simultaneous intra- and extra-uterine pregnancy: Report of a case. Obstet. Gynec., 31:50, 1968.

Beacham, W. D., Hernquist, W. C., Beacham, D. W., and Webster, H. D.: Abdominal pregnancy at Charity Hospital in New Orleans. Amer. J. Obstet. Gynec., 84:1257, 1962.

Boronow, R. C., McElin, T. W., West, R. H., and Buckingham, J. C.: Ovarian pregnancy: A report of 4 cases and a 13-year survey of the English literature. Amer. J. Obstet. Gynec., 91:1095, 1965.

Clark, J. F. J., and Guy, R. S.: Abdominal Pregnancy. Amer. J. Obstet. Gynec., 96: 511, 1966.

Cullen, T. S.: New sign in ruptured extrauterine pregnancy. Amer. J. Obstet. Gynec., 78:457, 1918.

Dougherty, R. E., and Diddle, A. W.: Intrafollicular ovarian pregnancy: Management with ovarian conservation. Obstet. Gynec., 33:20, 1969.

Fallon, J., and Manning, J. J.: A variant of the Hofstäter-Cullen sign in intra-abdominal hemorrhage from ectopic pregnancies with a note on the mechanism of its production. New Eng. J. Med., 240:747, 1949.

Fontanilla, J., and Anderson, G. W.: Further studies on the racial incidence and mortality of ectopic pregnancy. Amer. J. Obstet. Gynec., 70:312, 1955.

Foster, H. W., and Moore, D. T.: Abdominal pregnancy. Report of 12 cases. Obstet. Gynec., 30:249, 1967.

Friedrich, E. G., and Rankin, C. A.: Primary pelvic peritoneal pregnancy. Obstet. Gynec., 31:649, 1968.

Grech, P., and D'Sa, A. L. M.: Radiological diagnosis of advanced extrauterine pregnancy. Brit. J. Radiol., 38:848, 1965.

Hofstätter, R.: Über einen Fall von durch Tubargravidität komplizierter akkreter Nabelherniae. Wien. Klin. Wschr., 22:524, 1909.

Hreshchyshyn, M. M., Naples, J. D., Jr., and Randall, C. L.: Amethopterin in abdominal pregnancy. Amer. J. Obstet. Gynec., 93: 286, 1965.

Jolly, G. F., and Norman, R. M.: Co-existing intra- and extrauterine pregnancy associated with cerebral malformation in the surviving twin. J. Obstet. Gynaec. Brit. Comm., 72:125, 1965.

Kalchman, G. G., and Meltzer, R. M.: Interstitial pregnancy following homolateral salpingectomy: Report of 2 cases and review of literature. Amer. J. Obstet. Gynec., 96:1139, 1966.

Kleiner, G. J., and Roberts, T. W.: Current factors in causation of tubal pregnancy: A prospective clinicopathologic study. Amer. J. Obstet. Gynec., 99:21, 1967.

Lloyd, H. E. D., and Fienberg, R.: The Arias-Stella reaction: A nonspecific involutional phenomenon in intra- as well as extrauterine pregnancy. Amer. J. Clin. Path., 43:428, 1965.

McElin, T. W., and LaPata, R.: Angular pregnancy. Report of a case. Obstet. Gynec., 31:849, 1968.

Pauerstein, C. J., Woodruff, J. D., and Zachary, A. S.: Factors influencing physiologic activities in the fallopian tube: The anatomy, physiology, and pharmacology of tubal transport. Obstet. Gynec. Survey, 23:215 1968.

Polak, J. O., and Wolfe, S. A.: A further study of the origin of uterine bleeding in tubal pregnancy. Amer. J. Obstet. Gynec., 8:730, 1924.

Reid, D. W. J., and Vant, J. R.: Ovarian pregnancy. Obstet. Gynec., 21:450, 1963.

Riva, H. L., Kammeraad, L. A., and Anderson, P. S.: Ectopic pregnancy: Report of 132 cases and comments on the role of the culdoscope in diagnosis. Obstet. Gynec., 20:189, 1962.

Robb, H.: Ectopic gestation with special reference to the treatment of tubal rupture. Amer. J. Obstet. Gynec., 56:6, 1907.

Romney, S. L., Hertig, A. T., and Reid, D. E.: Endometria associated with ectopic pregnancy: Study of 115 cases. Surg. Gynec. Obstet., 91:605, 1950.

Rubin, I. C.: The status of residual tube following ectopic pregnancy in relation to sterility and further pregnancy. Amer. J. Obstet. Gynec., 28:698, 1934.

Sherrin, D. A.: Ectopic pregnancy: A review of 113 selected cases. Canad. Med. Assoc. J., 95:535, 1966.

Siddall, R. S.: The occurrence and significance of decidual changes of the endometrium in extrauterine pregnancy. Amer. J. Obstet. Gynec., 31:420, 1936.

Skulj, V., Pavlic, Z., Stoiljkovic, C., Bacic, G.,

and Drazancic, A.: Conservative operative treatment of tubal pregnancy. Fertil. Steril., 15:634, 1964.

Spiegelberg, O.: Zur Casuistik den ovarialschwangenschaft. Arch. Gynaek., 13:73, 1878.

Stromme, W. B., McKelvey, J. L., and Adkins, C. D.: Conservative surgery for ectopic pregnancy. Obstet. Gynec., 12:294, 1962.

Studderford, W. E.: Primary peritoneal pregnancy. Amer. J. Obstet. Gynec., 44:487, 1942.

Tan, K. K., and Yeo, O. H.: Primary ovarian pregnancy. Amer. J. Obstet. Gynec., 100:240, 1968.

Thompson, L. R.: Abdominal pregnancy at term with late removal of the placenta. Amer. J. Surg., 111:272, 1966.

Timonen, S., and Niemien, U.: Tubal pregnancy, choice of operative method of treatment. Acta Obstet. Scand., 46:327, 1967.

Turunen, A.: Acht Fälle von Ausgetragener, Extrauterin-Schwangerschaft. Ann. Chir. Gynaec Fenn., 55:85, 1966.

Vital Statistics of the United States. Vol. 2 (Mortality), Part A, pp. 1-40. Washington, D.C., Govt. Print. Off., U.S. Census Bureau, 1967.

Webster, A., and Price, J. J.: Cervical pregnancy. Amer. J. Obstet. Gynec., 99:134, 1967.

Webster, H. D., Jr., Barclay, D. L., and Fischer, C. K.: Ectopic pregnancy: A 17 year review. Amer. J. Obstet. Gynec., 92:23, 1965.

Weinberg, A., and Sherwin, A. S.: A new sign in roentgen diagnosis of advanced ectopic pregnancy. Obstet. Gynec., 7:99, 1956.

Ziel, H. K., Miyazaki, F. S., Baker, T. H., and White, J. D.: Advanced intraligamentary pregnancy. Obstet. Gynec., 31:643, 1968.

17

The Intestinal Tract in Relation to Gynecology

LARRY C. CAREY, M.D.[*]

The gynecologist is likely to encounter disease of the gastrointestinal tract in four ways. First, primary gynecologic disorders may involve the gastrointestinal tract. An example of such involvement would be intestinal obstruction from tubo-ovarian abscess, endometriosis, or pelvic cancer. Second, primary gastrointestinal disease may be found during the course of pelvic surgery; such disease might be occult colon cancer, regional enteritis, or colon diverticulitis. Third, primary gastrointestinal disease may mimic pelvic disease. Acute intraabdominal or intrapelvic disorders may be quite difficult to assess accurately preoperatively; colon diverticulitis, Meckel's diverticulitis, acute small bowel obstruction, volvulus, or other processes may mimic acute gynecologic disorders. Fourth, the postoperative complications of gynecologic surgery frequently involve the gastrointestinal tract. Fistula formation, adynamic ileus, and intestinal obstruction may be imposing problems after major gynecologic surgery. The following discussion is intended to outline the diagnosis and treatment of the more common gastrointestinal diseases which the gynecologic surgeon is likely to encounter.

INTESTINAL OBSTRUCTION

Small Bowel Obstruction. Etiologically, hernias and adhesions account for the vast majority of cases of small intestinal obstruction. Other causes, such as metastatic carcinoma, primary tumor, intraabdominal abscess, volvulus, intussusception, gallstone ileus, and congenital disorders, occur in varying frequency. Recent review shows small bowel obstruction from adhesions to be increasing and that from hernias to be decreasing. Undoubtedly the increasing enthusiasm for hernia repair is in part responsible for this changing trend. The type of surgery preceding intestinal obstruction caused by adhesions is most often gynecologic. This observation is related to the fact that gynecologic surgery is very common, and the mechanical problem is enhanced by the dependence and narrowness of the pelvic space.

Pathophysiology. Intestinal obstruction is an area of surgical illness where great improvement in survival rate has occurred with increased understanding of the pathophysiology of the disorder. Forty years ago mortality of 40 to 60 per cent was not uncommon. Presently mortality is between 10 and 20 per cent for all patients with obstruction of the small intestine. If a single factor could be altered which would most greatly affect mortality, it would be lessening the delay between onset of symptoms and surgical intervention. There are few diseases not involving overt hemorrhage in which delay in treatment adversely influences outcome as it does in obstruction of the small intestine. The difference between simply dividing an adhesive band to relieve an early obstruction and resecting

---

[*] Associate Professor of Surgery, University of Pittsburgh School of Medicine.

two feet of black, gangrenous perforated ileum in the presence of extensive peritonitis and gram-negative shock may be as little as 12 hours in time.

How does this small difference in time create such a greatly different problem? Obstruction of the small intestine causes distention. The distention occurs as a result of fluid collection proximal to the obstruction, but of much greater importance is swallowed air. Well over 70 per cent of the air in the gastrointestinal tract is swallowed. In his classic experiments, Wangensteen showed that animals could survive for long periods with complete small bowel obstruction if the esophagus was simultaneously ligated to prevent air swallowing. The tension on the surface of a cylinder increases as a function of the diameter and intraluminal pressure ($T = \pi DP$). Since the veins and arteries enter the intestinal wall tangentially, the tension on them increases rapidly with distention. The veins having the lower pressure of the two show the effect of the increase in tension first. As they are stretched, resistance in them increases, and flow slows. Arterial vessels with their higher pressure are not affected as soon. Fluid rich in protein and salt begins to exude from the capillaries. Edema is the result. Intraluminal fluid accumulation increases both from decreased absorption and weeping of edema fluid. Blood cells begin to escape from the capillaries, venous flow finally stops, arterial flow continues, blood accumulates in the wall and then the lumen of the bowel, gangrene occurs, intestinal integrity is lost, and peritonitis quickly follows.

Older patients have a greater tendency to tolerate the discomfort of intestinal obstruction without seeking medical advice until late in the disease. The need for prompt action on the part of any physician dealing with intestinal obstruction is clear. If inordinate delay has occurred prior to seeing the patient, the need for haste is even greater. The adage that states, "One never goes to bed on intestinal obstruction," is well conceived.

Diagnosis. The clinical story of intestinal obstruction is usually one of sudden onset of crampy abdominal pain. Reflex vomiting may be associated with the first symptoms and then stop, only to start again as the obstruction persists. The pain is periodic with the pain-free intervals longer than the periods of pain. The pain is classically periumbilical.

Inspection of the abdomen initially may show little change. As obstruction persists, distention will occur. In the very thin, loops of intestine will become visible beneath the abdominal wall, and peristalsis may be seen.

The bowel sounds of obstruction are characteristic. The high-pitched, tinkling metallic sounds may occasionally be heard without a stethoscope. The sounds suggest the presence of the air-fluid interface which exists.

Palpation in the early stage of the disease may disclose no tenderness. As distention progresses, it is usual to find tenderness over the point of obstruction. One must remember that distended loops of bowel are painful when disturbed, and so vigorous examination may produce misleading signs. Any evidence of peritoneal irritation should sound the alarm to consider strangulation, and plans for operative intervention should begin.

Laboratory tests of help will be those suggesting hypovolemia and specifically plasma volume loss. Increase in hematocrit, with high urine osmolarity and normal serum osmolarity, may be helpful. The presence of leukocytosis is distressing, and levels of over 15,000 after hydration should suggest strangulation.

The x-ray findings of small bowel obstruction must be interpreted in light of the clinical evidence. If the clinical evidence points toward intestinal obstruction and x-rays show distended bowel with air-fluid levels, the diagnosis is confirmed. Early in the course of the disease x-rays may show very little. Late in intestinal obstruction, as the bowel becomes filled with fluid, air-fluid levels may be very small or even absent. The importance of an upright or lateral decubitus film cannot be overstressed. Flat films of the abdomen may be of no benefit and, indeed, may be misleading. Contrast material may be helpful in separating adynamic ileus from obstruction. Recent reports have supported the use of thin barium suspensions rather than the more irritating water-soluble media. If the contrast material has not reached the cecum within 6 hours, small bowel obstruction rather than ileus is likely.

Preoperative Preparation. The keystone of preoperative preparation for surgery for small bowel obstruction is the correction of existing hypovolemia. It has been shown that nearly 50 per cent of the plasma volume and 30 per cent of the blood volume may be sequestered in intestinal obstruction. Blood pressure, pulse rate, clinical appearance, central venous pressure, hematocrit, urinary output, and urine and plasma osmolarity are all helpful in evaluation of the degree of hypovolemia. Central venous pressure and hematocrit, along with pulse and urinary output, should be monitored as fluid replacement is accomplished with balanced salt solution and whole blood. If a specific electrolyte disturbance exists, such as hypochloremic alkalosis of high intestinal obstruction, it should be corrected. Usually, the loss of extracellular fluid with normal electrolyte concentration results in no apparent electrolyte disturbance. As soon as central venous pressure, pulse, and urinary output indicate volume to be replaced, surgery should be undertaken. Preoperative antibiotics are useful, especially when strangulated obstruction is suspected. Choice of a drug effective against colon organisms is important.

Operative Procedure. The choice of incision should be one which allows exploration of the entire abdomen. If possible, the incision should not be over a previous one. The obstructing adhesion may be directly under a previous incision, and injury to the bowel may be difficult to avoid.

After opening the peritoneum, a loop of collapsed bowel should be located and followed backward until the point of obstruction is found. The nondistended bowel is much easier to handle and less susceptible to injury. The point of obstruction is more easily identified in this manner. Unless the patient's condition is grave, all adhesions should be taken down and the loops of bowel returned to the peritoneal cavity. During the course of taking down the adhesions, great care should be used. Handling of the intestine with sponges or pads should be avoided, and only the gloved hand should be used. Sharp dissection is the only safe method of dispensing with adhesions. The ease with which distended bowel can be torn may come as a disastrous surprise to the neophyte. If the bowel is injured, it should be repaired with interrupted 4-0 silk sutures. There is no need to repair tears unless the mucosa is injured. Rents in the serosa are not dangerous.

Identification of viable bowel may be extremely difficult. A variety of methods have been tried involving electrical impedance and dye injection. None has become popular. All bowel obviously necrotic should be resected. If areas of questionable viability remain, re-exploration after 24 hours may be necessary to assure that no necrotic intestine has been overlooked. Such factors as color, peristalsis, serosal appearance, and consistency are not reliable. Brisk bleeding from the cut end of the bowel may be helpful.

Nonoperative Treatment. In general, there are three instances in which nonoperative treatment for intestinal obstruction should be considered. Patients with known widespread intra-abdominal cancer may be sometimes successfully treated by using intestinal intubation. The occasional patient who has had multiple operative procedures for intestinal obstruction, and who is known to have dense intra-abdominal adhesions, may also do well with nonoperative treatment. Last, those occasional patients who develop obstructions in the early postoperative period are candidates for nonsurgical treatment.

If nonoperative treatment is used, one of the long small intestinal tubes should be used. Our preference is the Miller-Abbott tube with the balloon containing 2 cc. of mercury. A nasogastric tube is passed simultaneously and connected to intermittent suction to avoid continued distention. The long tube is not connected to suction since this will often interfere with its passage. The patient should be placed in the lateral position with the right side dependent. Frequent x-rays will demonstrate the progress of the tube through the pylorus. After passing the ligament of Treitz, it may be attached to intermittent suction and the nasogastric tube removed.

Careful surveillance must be maintained for the previously described signs of strangulation. If they occur, operative intervention must be immediate.

REGIONAL ENTERITIS

Regional enteritis is a granulomatous inflammatory process involving usually the small intestine in its distal portion. It may be encountered by the gynecologic surgeon occasionally and usually unexpectedly. Clinically, the disease usually causes diarrhea, weight loss, and abdominal pain. The usual factors which make surgery necessary are either acute exacerbation of the inflammatory process or intestinal obstruction from edema and cicatrix. Fistula formation is common and in females may involve the bladder and/or vagina. When encountered unexpectedly, unless obstruction is present, no surgery should be performed since medical treatment may be quite successful.

The extent of the disease should be thoroughly documented since "skip-areas" are common.

Definitive surgery should, where possible, be directed at resection of the diseased bowel. Usually, removal of the terminal ileum and right colon and performance of an ileotransverse colostomy are needed. Bypass procedure has been recommended but seems less satisfactory than resection in most cases since it is attended by a higher recurrence rate.

MECKEL'S DIVERTICULUM

Meckel's diverticulum is a congenital malformation of the small bowel and is a remnant of the vitelline duct. The diverticulum occurs in the terminal 24 to 48 inches of ileum. Occasionally, gastric mucosa is found in the sac, and perforation or hemorrhage may result from ulceration. These diverticula should be resected if they have caused difficulty or have narrow necks. The technic is simply that of clamping the base and excising the pouch. Closure of the resulting defect is best accomplished with interrupted 3-0 Lembert sutures. Care need be taken to avoid narrowing the bowel lumen.

INTESTINAL FISTULA

Fistula formation is one of the more annoying and difficult problems associated with intra-abdominal surgery. It is often associated with technical error in intestinal anastomosis, para-anastomotic abscess, or an anastomosis performed in diseased bowel. Broadening of the scope of gynecologic surgery to include radical pelvic dissection has greatly increased the frequency with which the gynecologist encounters fistulas of the intestinal tract. This is in the main attributable to previous irradiation damage to the intestine.

The great variation in the severity of physiologic disturbance resulting from an intestinal fistula depends on the location of the fistula. Fistulas of the stomach, duodenum, or high jejunum may be devastating. The volume of electrolyte-rich fluids lost from such a fistula may cause life-threatening imbalance in a very short time. Distal ileal or colonic fistulas may be very well tolerated and cause no greater disturbance than an ileostomy or colostomy.

There are occasions when the diagnosis of a fistula may be very difficult. If the intestinal opening is small, drainage may be intermittent. At times, a wound infected with enteric organisms will drain material resembling intestinal contents. In these instances the oral administration of a dye, such as powdered charcoal or carmen red, may readily establish the diagnosis. Contrast material may be injected into the cutaneous opening to determine whether a fistula exists.

radiographic appearance should establish the correct diagnosis. Occasionally, in the mental-defective the colon may be huge and full of stool, and the characteristic x-ray picture is not present. The surgical treatment consists of simply untwisting the loop of bowel, but colostomy may be necessary occasionally. Primary resection is not indicated unless gangrene has occurred, and primary anastomosis is never justified.

Volvulus of the cecum is quite rare. It occurs usually in the very elderly and is managed by simple derotation.

If elective surgery is planned which may involve colotomy, the question of bowel preparation is raised. There is little controversy over the mechanical preparation. Clear liquid diet for 24 hours preoperatively combined with saline cathartic, such as Fleet's Phospho-soda, and saline enemas the evening prior to surgery are very effective measures.

There is considerable controversy over the use of nonabsorbable antibiotics. Many surgeons feel that the increased risk from altering colonic flora is greater than the benefit derived from bowel preparation. Still others feel strongly that systemic antibiotics are important. The controversy is not resolved. The administration of a large dose of tincture of opium the evening prior to colon surgery makes the bowel much easier to manage technically. Thirty ml. of paregoric is quite effective.

Technic

Open End-to-End Anastomosis (Fig. 17-1). This operation follows intestinal resection. Crushing clamps are placed obliquely on the intestine, with the apex on the mesenteric side. This gives some advantage in providing a large lumen at the anastomotic site. With fine needles (french eye are excellent), a row of 3-0 silk mattress sutures is used to approximate the serosal surfaces. The crushing clamps are then removed and a mucosal layer of 4-0 silk Lembert sutures placed. At the angles, the sutures become interrupted Connell sutures, with the knots on the luminal aspect. The serosal suture line is then completed with mattress or Lembert sutures. Using continuous absorbable suture on the mucosal layer is quite acceptable. When the lumen is small, however, continuous sutures are more likely to narrow the anastomotic stoma. After completing the anastomosis, the mesenteric rent is repaired with fine sutures. Care must be taken not to injure the blood supply to the suture line.

Closed Anastomosis (Fig. 17-2). This method is particularly useful in ileocolostomy construction with unprepared bowel. Four crushing clamps, such as Allen clamps, are placed across the unopened bowel to isolate the segment to be removed. As with all anastomoses, moist pads are used to isolate carefully the gut from the peritoneal cavity. The mesentery of the segment to be resected is divided in a wedge.

Careful placement of hemostats on the mesenteric vessels is critical. Suture ligation of these vessels is much safer than simple ligation. If a vessel is lost and retracts into the mesentery, attempts to find and control it may result in further vascular damage, necessitating a greater bowel resection. The time spent carefully isolating and ligating these vessels will be well rewarded.

After the bowel to be resected has been removed, the clamps on the cut ends are approximated, and 4-0 silk Lembert sutures are placed through the bowel wall to include the mucosa about 3 mm. apart around the entire circumference. The clamps are then removed, and the cut, crushed ends of bowel separated to ensure that no suture has been placed across the lumen. The sutures are then tied. As they are tied, any needed additional ones are placed. Patency of the lumen is assured and the mesenteric defect repaired. This anastomosis carefully performed is quick, safe, and assures maximum patency. For the surgeon who only occasionally performs an anastomosis, it is an excellent method. The area of greatest difficulty is at the site of mesenteric attachment to the bowel wall; by carefully dissecting the mesentery off the bowel for 5 mm., trouble can be avoided. If this is not done, the bowel wall may be missed and the sutures

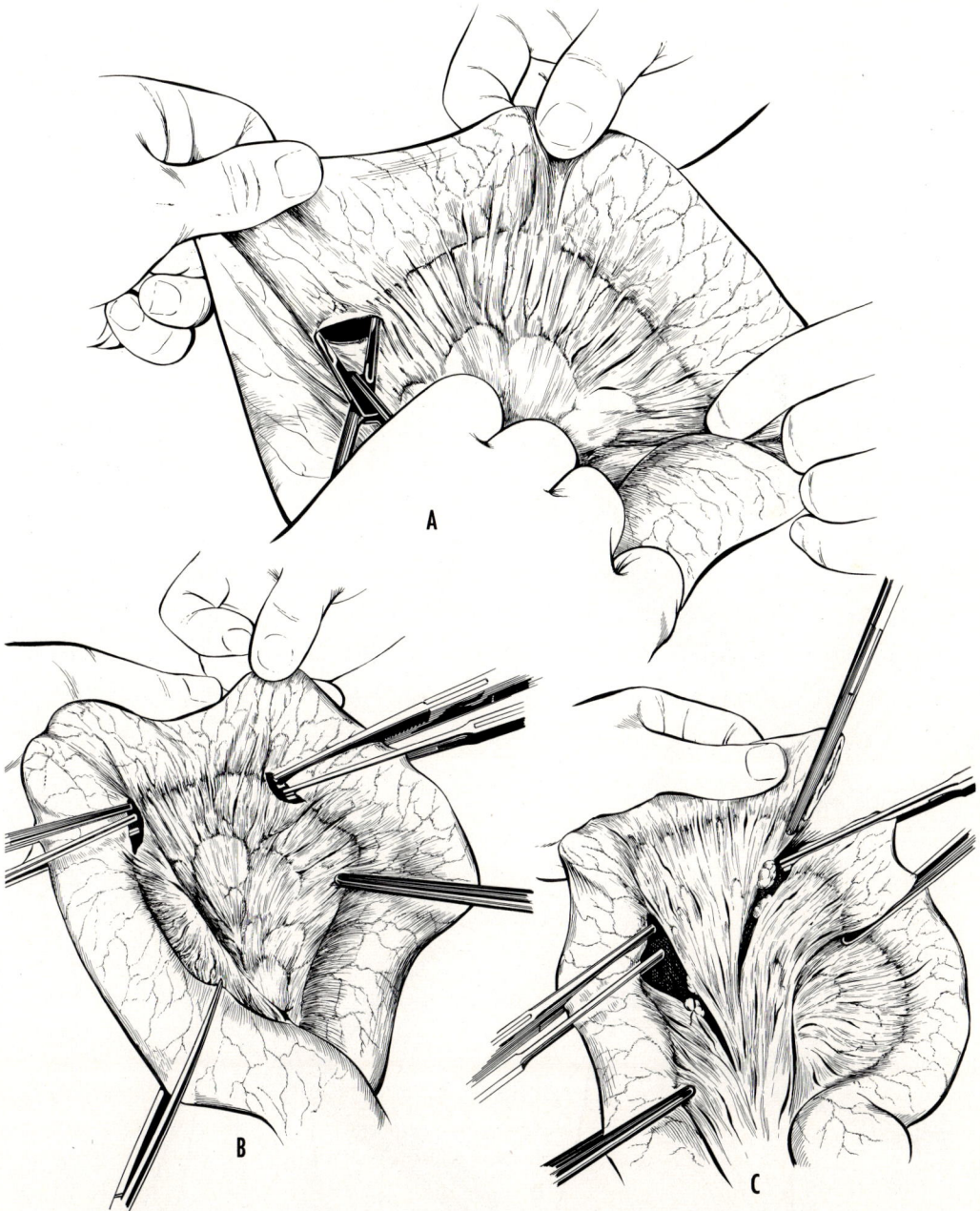

Fig. 17-1. Open end-to-end anastomosis. (A) The mesentery is carefully dissected from the intestine. (B) The resected segment is defined by clamps. Note the noncrushing clamps proximally placed to control spill. (C) Note the individual ligatures on the mesentery. Suture ligation of these vessels is important.

placed in the mesenteric fat, with disastrous results.

Side-to-Side Anastomosis (Fig. 17-3). This method of anastomosis is less popular than end-to-end. It may be quite useful in excluding a segment of the intestinal tract as in regional enteritis. The two segments of bowel to be anastomosed are approximated with stay sutures. A distance of about 4 inches between these

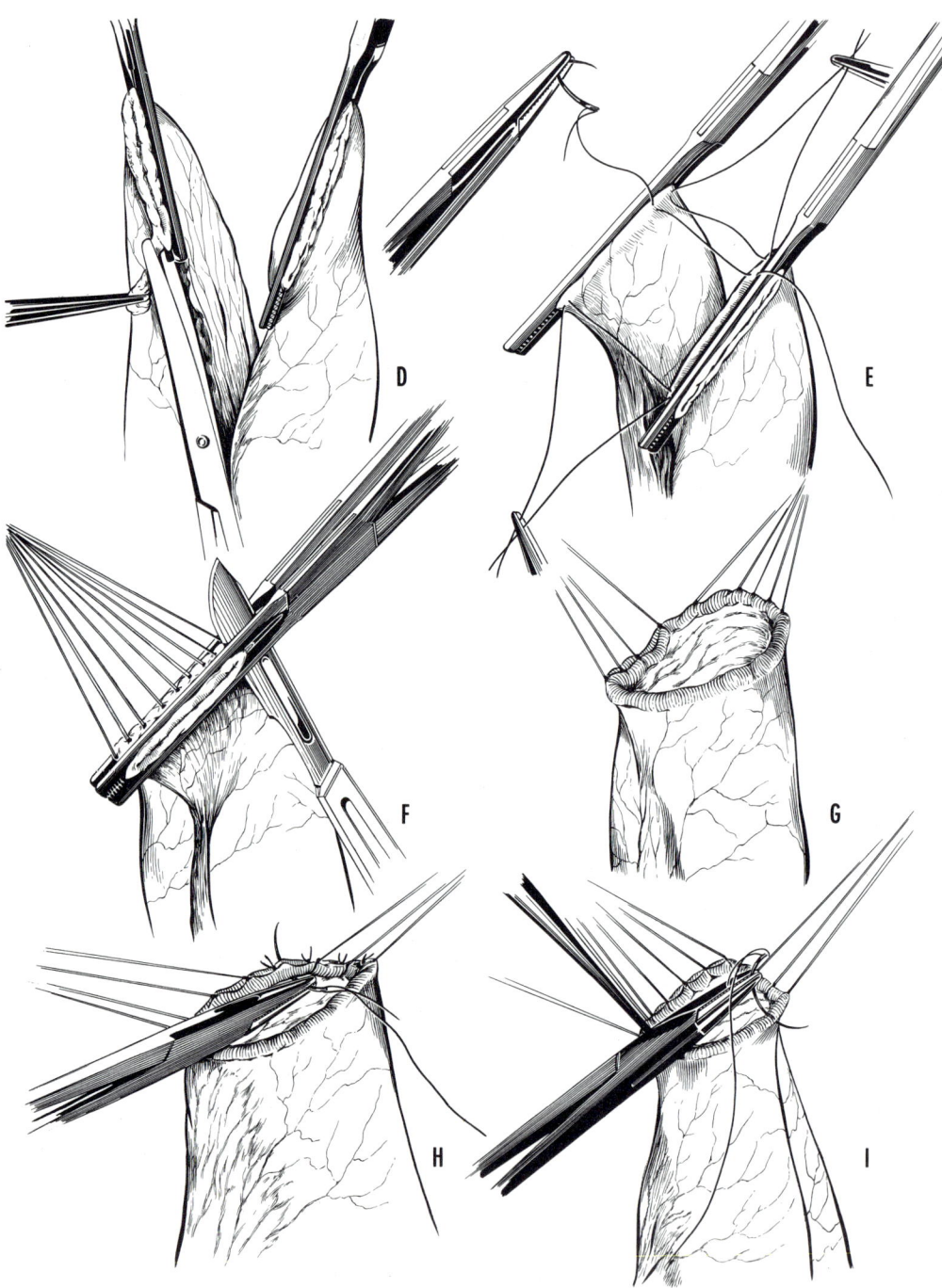

FIG. 17-1 (*Continued*). Open end-to-end anastomosis. (D) Emphasizing the importance of careful dissection of the mesentery from the intestine. (E) Posterior interrupted sutures about 5 mm. apart. (F) Trimming away the crushed end of the bowel. (G, H) Note that the posterior serosal sutures are not cut until the first mucosal suture has been placed. (I) Beginning to "turn the corner."

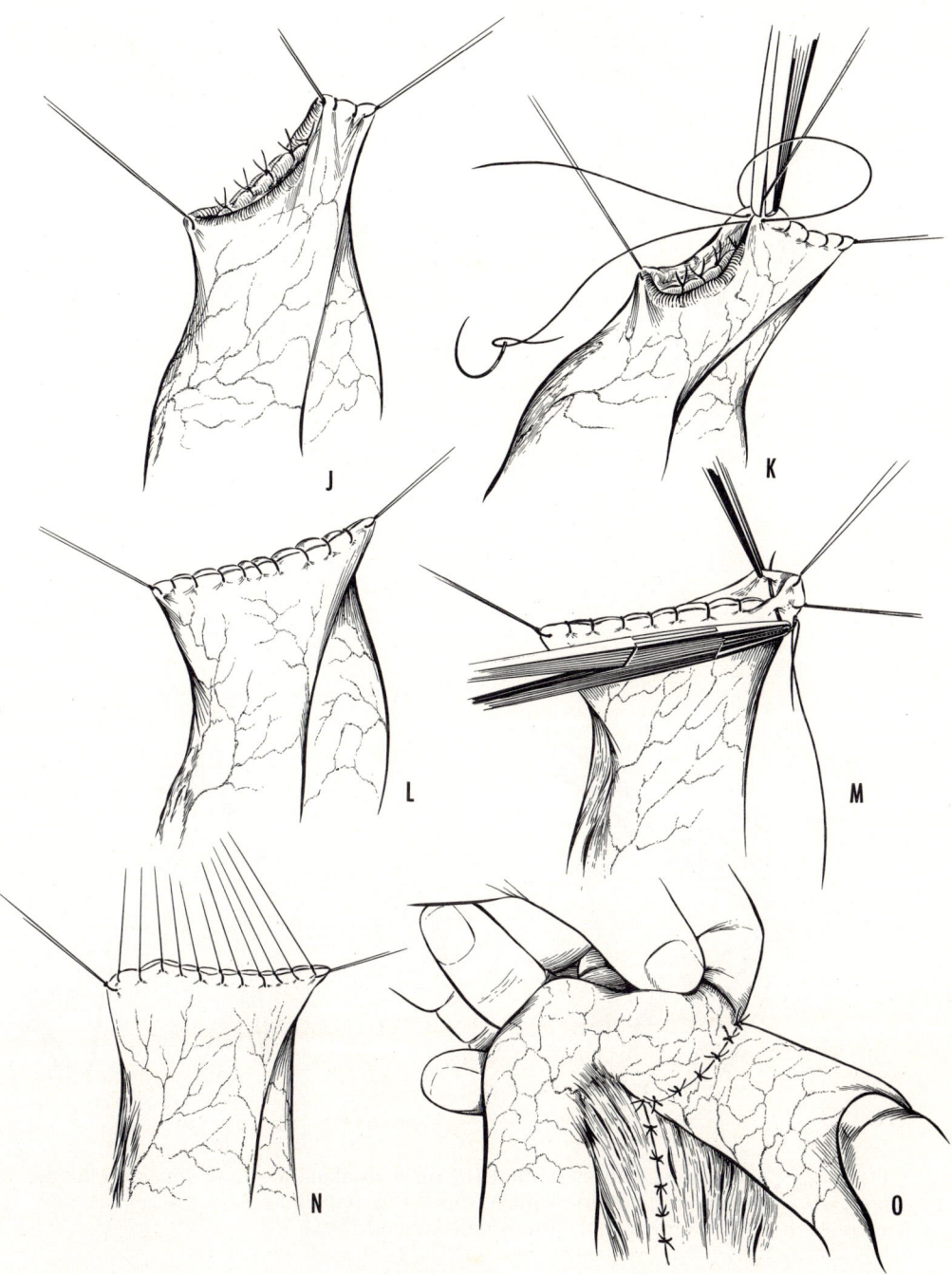

Fig. 17-1 (*Continued*). Open end-to-end anastomosis. (J) The inverting suture is continued anteriorly. (K) Note the placement of each suture before cutting the previous one. (L, M) Completion of the anterior mucosal suture line and beginning the anterior serosal one. (N, O) The anastomosis is complete and the mesenteric defect closed.

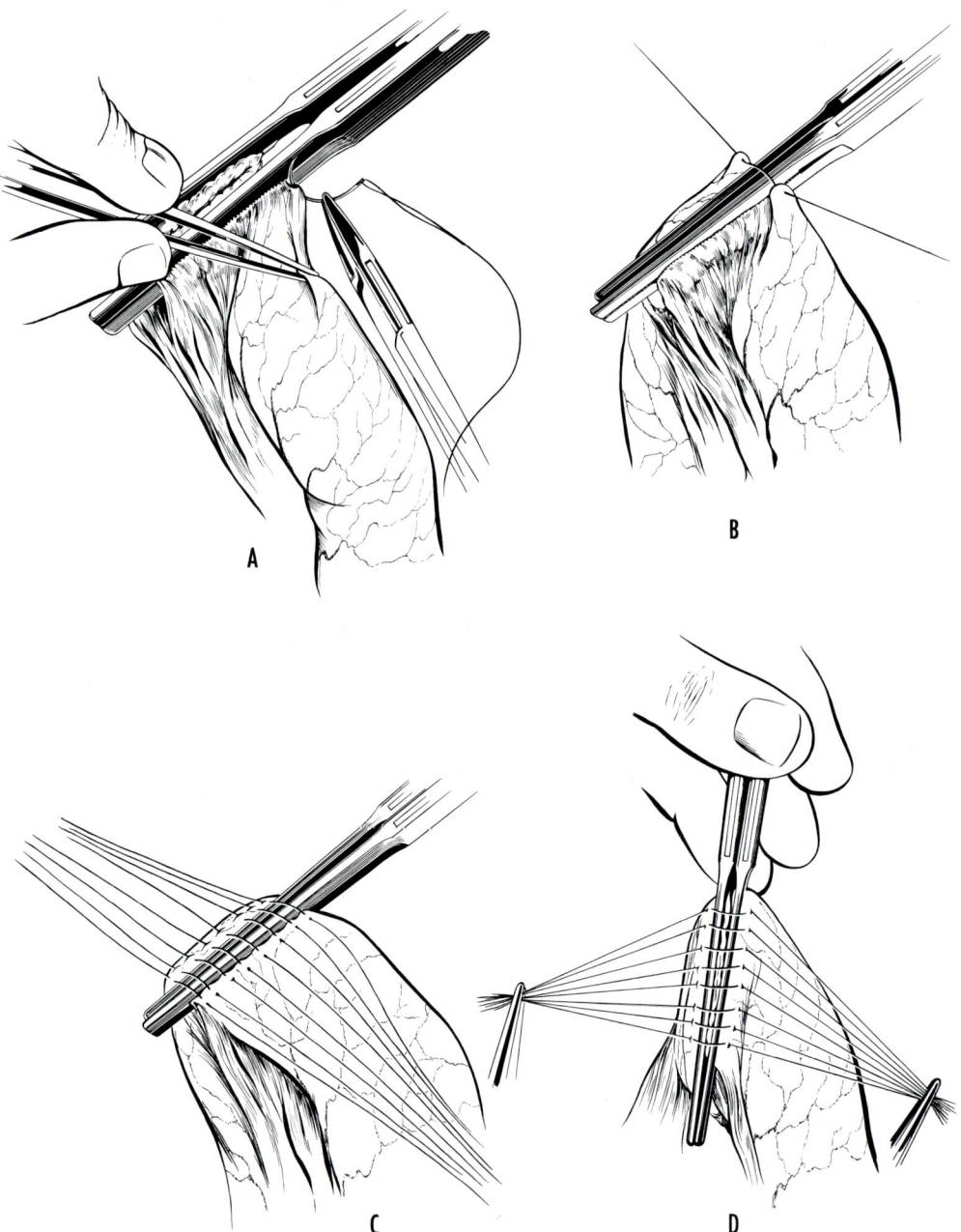

FIG. 17-2. Closed anastomosis. (A) Note the placement of the suture very close to the clamp. (B) Demonstrates the first suture completed. (C) The row of sutures has now been placed. (D) The clamp on the intestine is rotated 180°.

sutures is ideal. Serosal mattress sutures of 3-0 silk are placed. With noncrushing clamps, the segments to be connected are isolated. This aids in controlling bleeding and also in avoiding contamination. Both segments of bowel are then opened with parallel incisions about 3 mm. from the suture line. Mucosal sutures may be either continuous or interrupted. The larger lumen in this method makes continuous suture less hazardous. The serosal suture line is then completed.

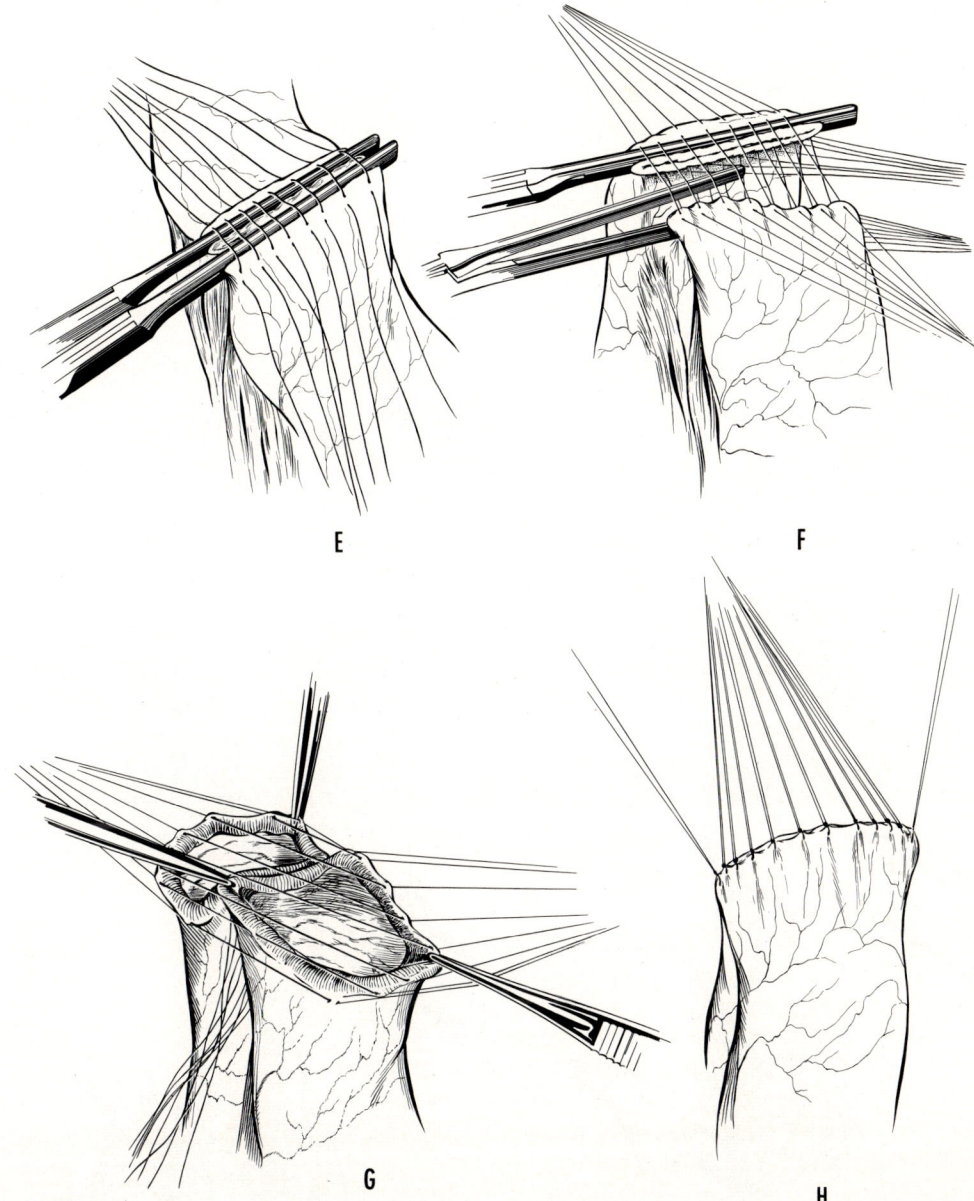

FIG. 17-2 (*Continued*). Closed anastomosis. (E) Following rotation of the clamp, the suturing is completed. (F) Clamps being removed prior to tieing the sutures. (G) The lumen is inspected to assure that no sutures have been placed across the lumen. (H) Sutures tied. One layer is adequate. The mesenteric defect is closed as in Figure 17-1 (N and O).

An important aspect of this technic is to place the initial suture line in a perfectly straight line. Angulation may interfere with stomal function.

Enterostomy. The safest method for the performance of an enterostomy is shown in Figure 17-4. Two concentric purse-string sutures of 3-0 silk are placed in the bowel wall. A stab wound is made and a catheter inserted. The sutures are tied and the bowel is sutured to the anterior abdominal wall. Omentum may be pulled up to the catheter to assist in controlling any possible leakage.

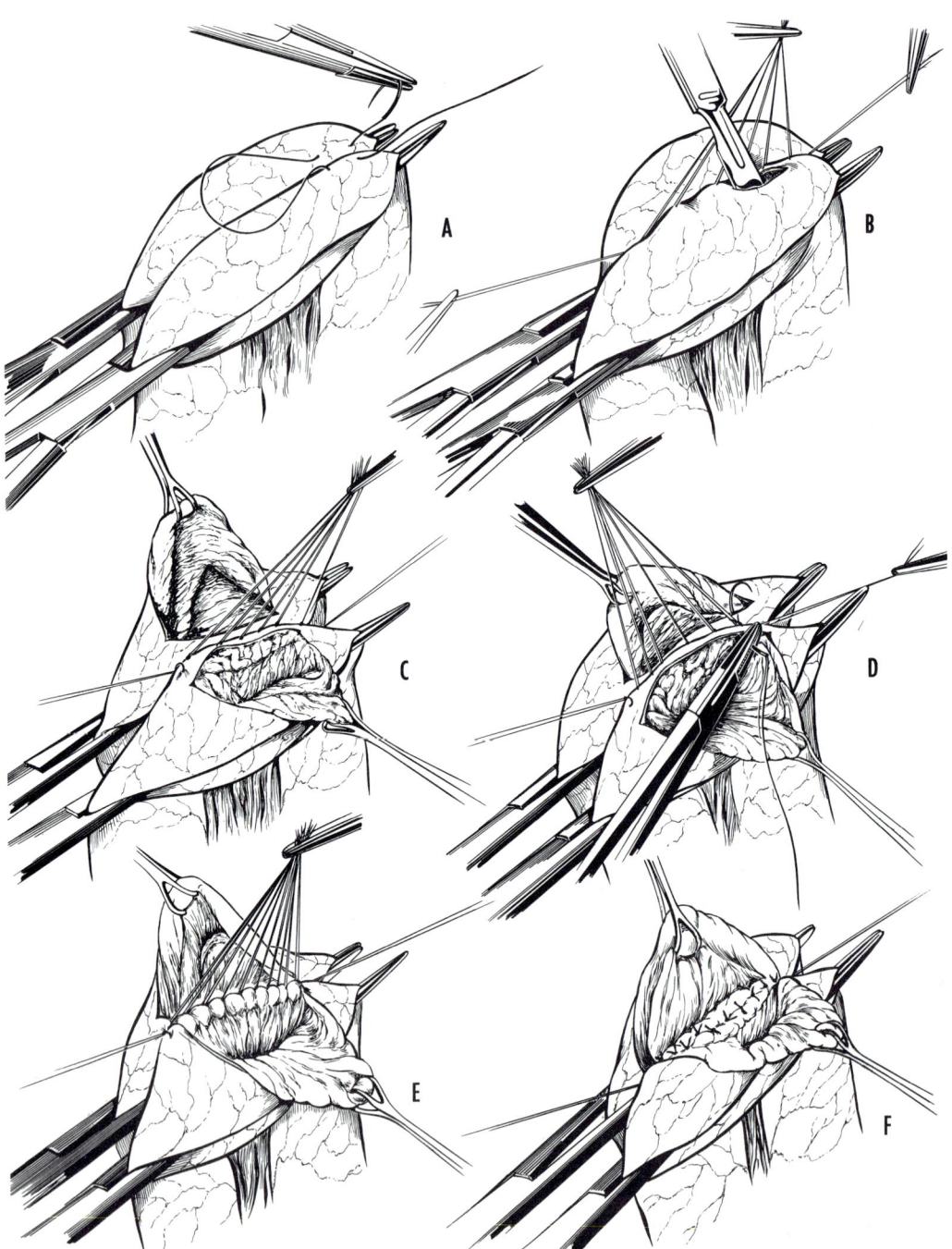

FIG. 17-3. Side-to-side anastomosis. (A) Horizontal mattress sutures are used on the posterior row. (B) The noncrushing clamps avoid spill as the bowel is opened. (C, D) The posterior serosal suture line is completed and the first mucosal suture placed before cutting the serosal ones. (E, F) Completion of the posterior mucosal sutures.

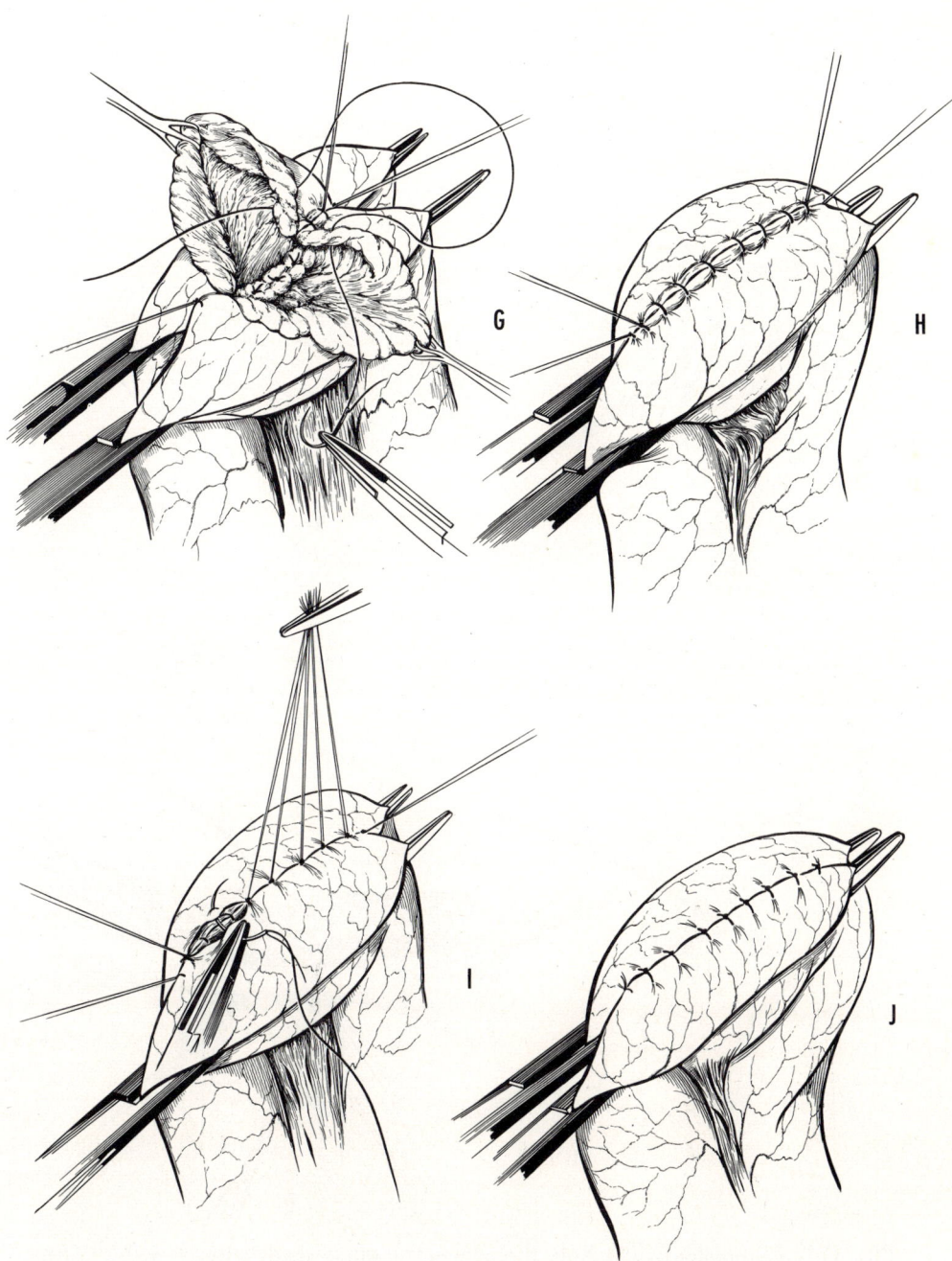

Fig. 17-3 (*Continued*). Side-to-side anastomosis. (G, H) Completion of the anterior mucosal suture line. Continuous suture can be used more safely in side-to-side than in end-to-end anastomosis. (I, J) Completion of the anterior serosal suture line.

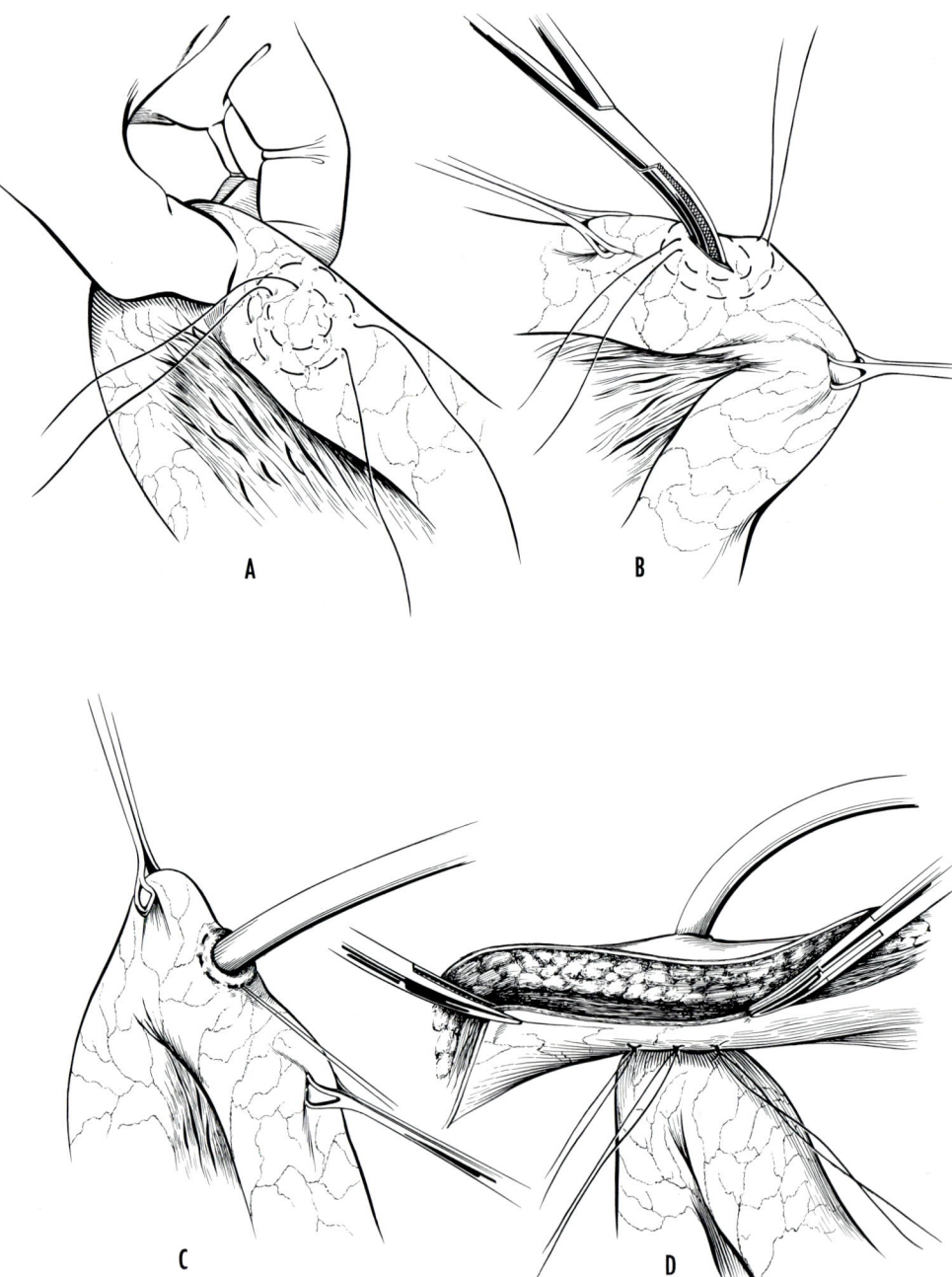

Fig. 17-4. Enterostomy. (A) Note the concentric purse-string sutures with the free ends opposite each other. (B) After a stab wound with scalpel, the patency of the mucosal wound is established with a clamp. (C) After introducing the tube the purse-string sutures are both tied. (D) The intestine is tacked to the peritoneum.

SURGERY OF THE ANUS AND RECTUM

There is no occasion for the gynecologic surgeon to perform major rectal surgery electively; however, on many occasions when doing vaginal plastic operations, gynecologists can very conveniently remove a symptomatic hemorrhoid with great satisfaction to the patient. That being the case, this segment of the text will deal primarily with the nonoperative management of rectal disorders.

Hemorrhoids. Man has paid several rather dear premiums for having assumed upright posture; not the least of these is hemorrhoids. Few human afflictions cause more discomfort without posing any threat to life.

The story of the pathophysiology of hemorrhoids is quite simple. Increased pressure in the perianal and rectal veins causes distention with dilatation of the veins (Fig. 17-5). It is assumed that as the vein walls are chronically distended, varices develop. Internal hemorrhoids are covered with mucous membrane and protrude into the rectal lumen (Fig. 17-6). They are quite painless, and the prime symptom is bleeding, which may occasionally be severe enough to require transfusion. As the hemorrhoids enlarge, they may protrude through the anal opening. When this occurs, the mucocutaneous junction becomes exposed, and itching and burning may be severe. Occasionally, as a hemorrhoid prolapses through the anal opening, the external sphincter goes into spasm, and the hemorrhoid may be strangulated, with resulting gangrene. This is an excruciatingly painful process. Rupture of a hemorrhoid, with hemorrhage into the perianal subcutaneous tissue, is also quite painful and is identified clinically as a thrombosed hemorrhoid.

One of the more common associated conditions with hemorrhoids in the female is pregnancy. Several theories have

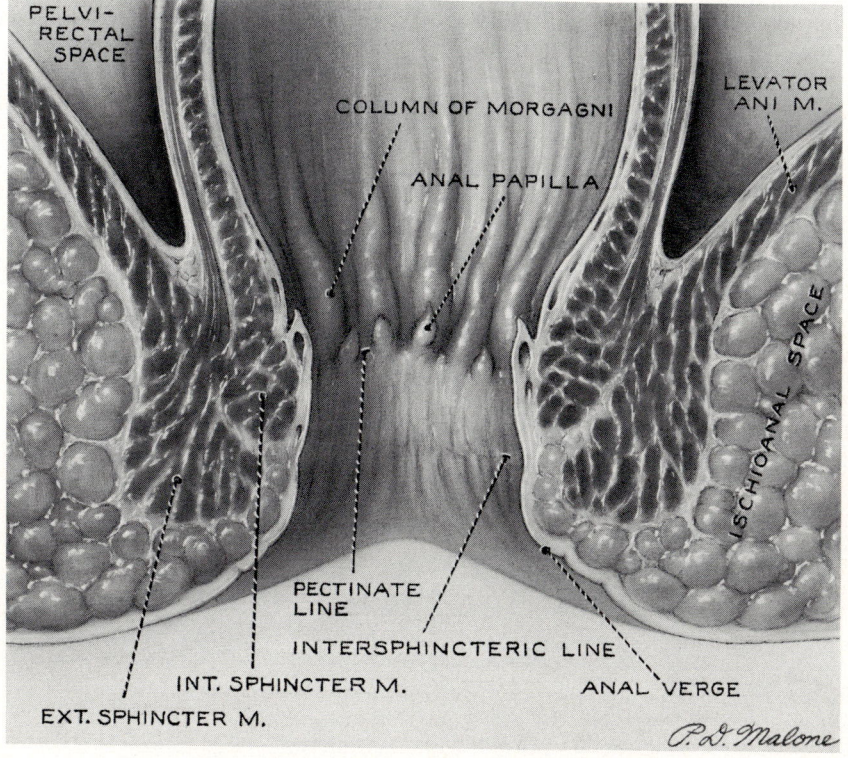

FIG. 17-5. Normal anatomy of anus and lower rectum.

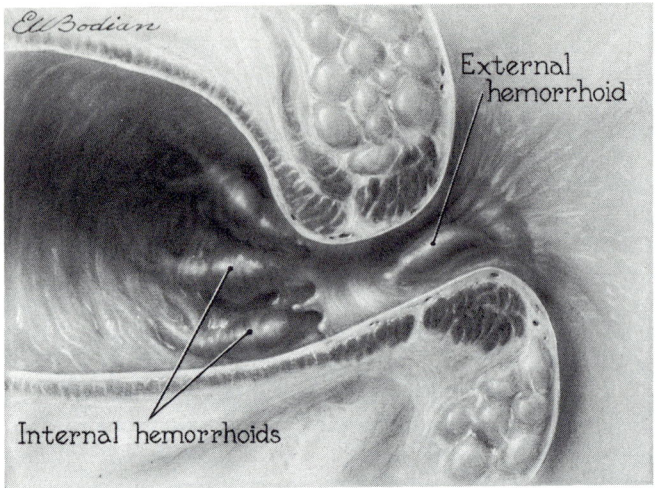

FIG. 17-6. Showing position of external and internal hemorrhoids.

been proposed. Possibly the increased blood volume, plus pelvic venous congestion, is a factor; arteriovenous fistulas may be of importance. If symptoms can be managed until parturition, surgery may not be necessary.

Local treatment is often quite beneficial. Relief of constipation by the administration of an emollient is important. Sitz baths, 2 to 4 times a day, are helpful. Suppositories with local anesthetic agents may be of benefit. In the case of prolapse or acute thrombosis, cold compresses of saturated magnesium sulfate solution may bring great relief. Perianal injections of local anesthetic agents may be required to relieve sphincter spasm.

Occasionally symptomatic protruding hemorrhoids are excised at the time of vaginal surgery by the radial technic, as shown in Figure 17-7. This avoids an extra operative procedure and has caused no increased morbidity in my experience. At the end of a week a digital examination is made gently. This is painful but prevents adhesions formation and con-

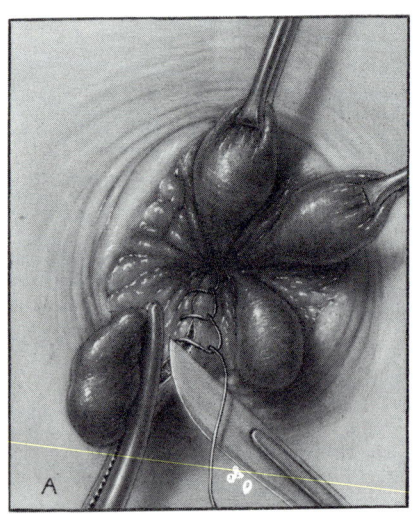
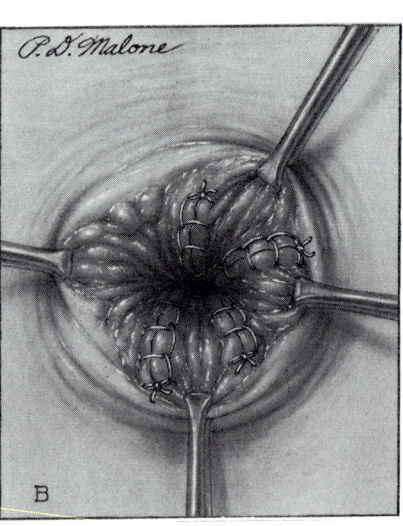

FIG. 17-7. Typical radial operation for internal hemorrhoid. (A) Groups of hemorrhoids are retracted with mucosa clips, and one mass of hemorrhoids is being excised. (B) The wounds have been sutured with continuous lock stitch of No. 0 chromic catgut.

striction. It is advisable to have the patient return to the office about 2 weeks after leaving the hospital for another digital examination. If there is any tendency to stricture formation, the patient should return at weekly intervals as long as necessary. This prophylactic attention often prevents the formation of a troublesome stricture later.

Anal Fissure. This is a condition that rarely needs surgical treatment unless the fissure becomes chronic with scar formation. The problem is usually created by hard stool tearing the mucous membrane in passing. Once the tear occurs, sphincter spasm follows. Each subsequent bowel movement aggravates the problem.

Management is not different from that for hemorrhoids. Constipation must be alleviated and sphincter spasm relieved.

Fistula in Ano. Fistula in ano most often makes its presence known by the development of a perirectal abscess. The fistula usually begins in the anal crypt (Fig. 17-8). It is preceded by an inflammatory process in the crypt, which then extends through the rectal wall to contaminate the fat-containing perirectal spaces. The poor blood supply of this space makes it extremely vulnerable to infection. Fistula development is complete when the abscess drains spontaneously or is drained surgically. In the acute stage, management is aimed at the control of sepsis. Basic to the control of sepsis is the provision of adequate drainage. Systemic antibiotics should be given if evidence of systemic reaction, such as leukocytosis, fever, or tachycardia, is present. Special attention needs to be given the very elderly, the debilitated, and those with associated illness such as diabetes.

The external opening of a fistula in ano often gives a clue as to where the internal opening can be found. The principle is called Goodsell's law of the fistula. It is illustrated in Figure 17-9. Knowledge of this principle can be of assistance

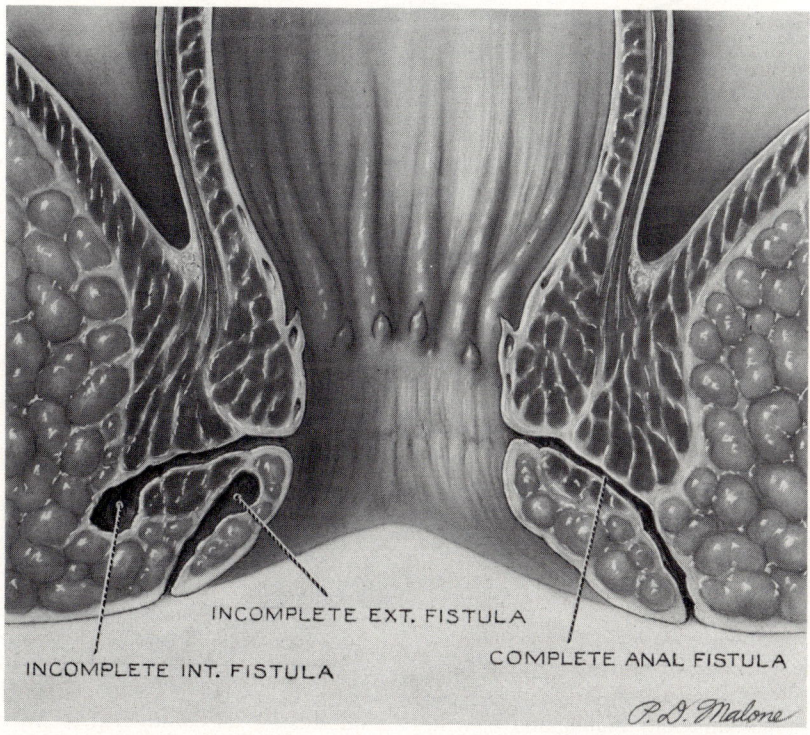

Fig. 17-8. Schematic illustration demonstrating three types of fistulas.

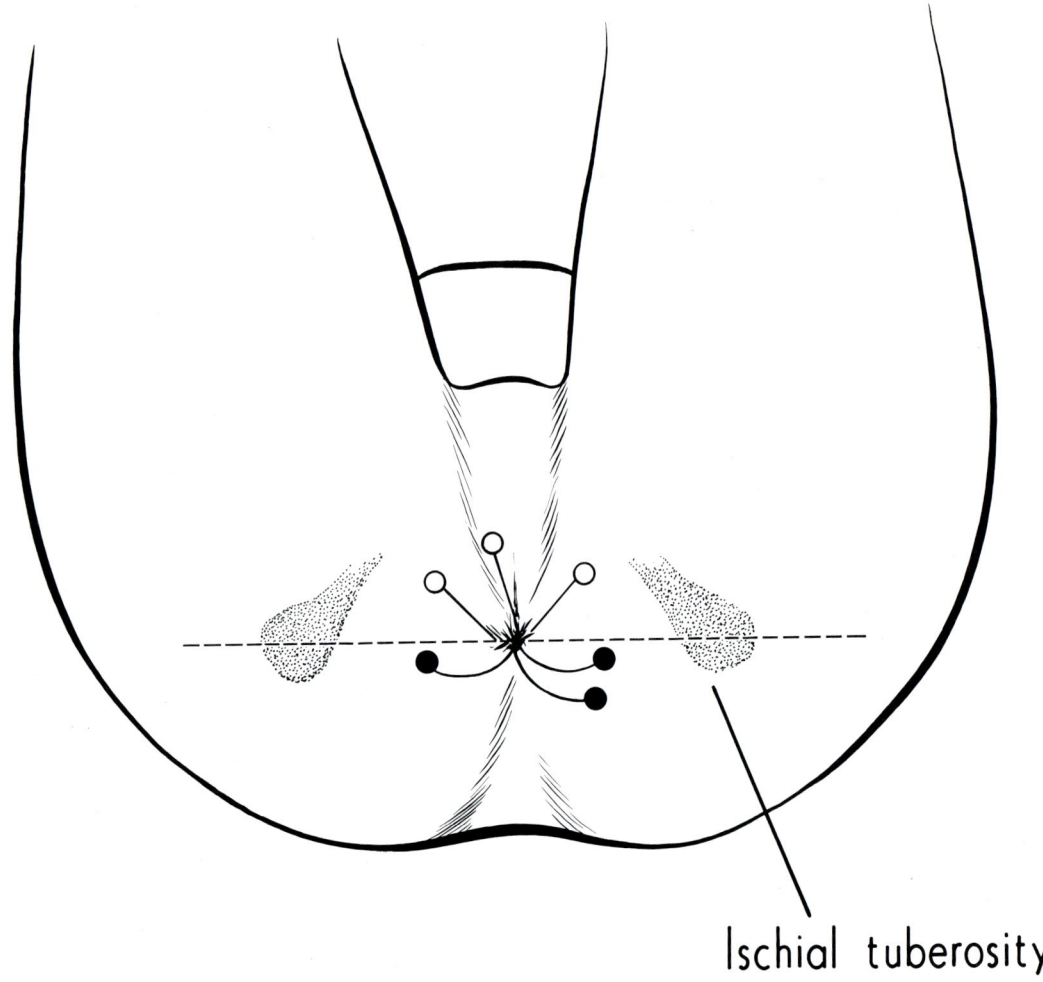

FIG. 17-9. Goodsell's law of the fistula. This rule is not absolute but generally will give a clue to the site of the internal opening of a fistula-in-ano. External openings posterior to the line between ischial tubero sites enter in the midline. Those anterior tend to have a radial course.

in probing a fistula, seeking the internal opening. There is little need for the gynecologic surgeon to perform definitive surgery for a chronic fistula in ano. The need is to drain or improve spontaneous drainage of a perirectal abscess.

BIBLIOGRAPHY

Adrwitz, A., Smith, D. F., and Rosensweig, J.: The acutely obstructed colon. Amer. J. Surg., *104*:474, 1962.

Barnett, W.: Experimental strangulated intestinal obstruction—a review. Gastroenterology, *39*:34, 1960.

Barnett, W. O., Truett, G., Williams, R., and Crowell, J.: Shock in strangulation obstruction: mechanisms and management. Ann. Surg., *157*:747, 1963.

Becker, W. F.: Acute adhesive ileus; study of 412 cases with particular reference to abuse of tube decompression in treatment. Surg. Gynec. Obstet., 95:472, 1952.

Berry, R. E.: Obstruction of the small bowel: an evaluation of pathology and treatment. Ann. Surg., *154* (Suppl.):102, 1961.

Brown, D. B., and Toomey, W. F.: Diverticular disease of colon. Brit. J. Surg., *47*:485, 1960.

Burns, F. J.: Bleeding after hemorrhoidectomy. Dis. Colon Rectum, 5:281, 1962.
Drapanas, T., and Stewart, J. D.: Acute sigmoid volvulus. Amer. J. Surg., *101*:70, 1961.
Edmunds, L. H., Jr., Williams, G. M., and Welch, C. E.: External fistulas arising from the gastrointestinal tract. Ann. Surg., *152*: 445, 1960.
Eisenhammer, S.: The anorectal and anovulval fistulous abscesses. Surg. Gynec. Obstet., *113*:519, 1961.
Harbison, S. P.: The principle of complete exclusion in fistulas of the small intestine. Surgery, *28*:384, 1950.
Lo, A. M., Evans, W. E., and Carey, L. C.: Review of small bowel obstruction at Milwaukee County General Hospital. Amer. J. Surg., *111*:884, 1966.
McKittrick, L. S., and Sarris, S. P.: Acute mechanical obstruction of small bowel; diagnosis and treatment. New Eng. J. Med., *222*:611, 1940.
Mikal, S. J.: Fluid and electrolyte abnormalities in small bowel obstruction. Amer. J. Proctol., *13*:243, 1962.
Miller, T. G., and Abbott, W. O.: Intestinal intubation: practical technique. Amer. J. Med. Sci., *187*:595, 1934.
Nelson, S. W., Christoforidis, A. J., and Roenigk, W. J.: Dangers and fallibilities of iodinated radiopaque media in obstruction of the small bowel. Amer. J. Surg., *109*: 546, 1965.
Quan, S. H., and Stearns, M. W., Jr.: East postoperative intestinal obstruction and postoperative intestinal ileus. Dis. Colon Rectum, *4*:307, 1961.
Romsdahl, M. M., and Cole, W. H.: Diverticulitis of the colon. Arch. Surg., *86*:751, 1963.
Saitzstein, E. C., Marshall, W. J., and Freemark, R. J.: Gangrenous intestinal obstruction. Surg. Gynec. Obstet., *114*:695, 1962.
Schier, J., Symmonds, R. E., and Dahlin, D. C.: Clinicopathologic aspects of actinic enteritis. Surg. Gynec. Obstet., *119*:1019, 1964.
Shamblin, J. R., Symmonds, R. E., Sauer, W. G., and Childs, D. S., Jr.: Bowel obstruction after pelvic and abdominal radiation therapy: factitial enteritis or recurrent malignancy? Ann. Surg., *160*:81, 1964.
Silen, W. M., Hein, M. F., and Goldman, L.: Strangulation obstruction of the small intestine. Arch. Surg., *85*:121, 1962.
Smith, G. A., Perry, J. F., Jr., and Yonehiro, E. G.: Mechanical intestinal obstructions; study of 1,252 cases. Surg. Gynec. Obstet., *100*:651, 1955.
Snyder, E. N., and McCranie, D.: Closed loop obstruction of the small bowel. Amer. J. Surg., *111*:398, 1966.
Wangensteen, O. H., and Rea, C. E.: The distention factor in simple intestinal obstruction: an experimental study with exclusion of swallowed air by cervical esophagostomy. Surgery, 5:327, 1939.
West, J. P., Ring, E. M., Miller, R. E., *et al.*: A study of causes and treatment of external postoperative intestinal fistulas. Surg. Gynec. Obstet., *113*:490, 1961.
Williams, L. F., Hughes, C. W., and Bowens, W. F.: Obstruction of the small bowel. Amer. J. Surg., *104*:376, 1962.

18

The Vermiform Appendix in Relation to Gynecology

The appendix, lying in close proximity to the pelvic viscera, plays an important, although often undiscerned role in gynecology. Acute inflammation of the appendix commonly extends to the right adnexa and less frequently involves the left. Nather and Ochsher have reported 9 abscesses resulting from appendicitis on the left side of the lower abdomen. Faulkner and Weir have reported 3 cases of young women with inflammatory masses in the left side of the pelvix, all directly traceable to previous attacks of appendicitis. In all 3 the major pelvic lesion occurred on the left side with minor involvement of the right adnexa. The history and the intact hymen left no doubt that inflammation of the appendix, rather than primary salpingitis, was responsible for the lesion in each case. When appendiceal rupture takes place, bilateral tubal involvement is common, and complete or partial tubal closure may ultimately result. Accordingly, sterility or tubal pregnancy may be the final sequela. However, it should be remembered that the inflammation is peritubal, and in many cases, even when a large appendiceal abscess forms in the pelvis, the tubal lumina may be left intact.

The differential diagnosis between acute appendicitis and acute salpingitis is one of the most frequent that the gynecologist is called upon to make. It is also a serious one, and a mistake may be fatal to the patient. For a discussion of the differential diagnostic points, the reader is referred to the section on acute salpingitis. However, in passing we should like to say that we have found culdoscopy of considerable value in making a differential diagnosis; on several occasions it has prevented laparotomy.

In spite of the best surgical judgment there will be occasions in which the differentiation is doubtful. In such cases it is better to remove the appendix when there is serious suspicion of its involvement. It is our custom to do this through a muscle-splitting, gridiron incision. A low midline incision will provide a better opportunity for intra-abdominal and pelvic exploration when there is serious doubt regarding the exact origin of the clinical findings. If the case proves to be one of salpingitis, the operator may remove the appendix without any untoward effect upon the course of the salpingitis.

According to Loeffler and Stearn, the first recorded incidental appendectomy was carried out in in 1734 by Amyard in London at the time of a hernia repair. Although more than two and one third centuries have passed since this event, there is still debate among gynecologists and obstetricians on the advisability of incidental appendectomy at the time of pelvic surgery. An excellent review of this controversy has been published by Loeffler and Stearn from England, who have found no adverse complications from routine appendectomy. Since the establishment of the Hopkins clinic, appendectomy has been a routine incidental procedure in all pelvic laparotomies, except in those cases in which it would be inadvisable to prolong the operation. For many years Curtis voiced opposition to this on the basis of "increased morbidity, some increased mortality in relatively serious cases and a rather too frequent incidence of chronic postoperative discomfort in the region of the appendectomy."

In 1957 McCall and Bolton disagreed with the routine removal of the appendix during gynecologic laparotomies. The British view is similar, as voiced by Howkins, who sent a questionnaire to 31 British surgeons, among whom only 5 removed the appendix routinely. MacLeod and Howkins have maintained the view of the late Victor Bonney that "the appendix should be removed only where preoperative symptoms indicate it or when the appendix is found to be diseased."

Our own experience has not brought us into agreement with this point of view. If judgment is exercised in omitting appendectomy in the seriously ill patients, we have noted no untoward effects, except perhaps for a slightly increased postoperative right lower quadrant discomfort.

Powell *et al.* and, more recently, Loeffler and Stearn have compared series of patients, with and without appendectomy. In both reports incidental appendectomy was not found to influence the morbidity, mortality, or hospital stay even when done with the presence of blood in the peritoneal cavity. Pratt reports no increase in febrile morbidity in 373 patients undergoing abdominal hysterectomy, of whom approximately one half had prophylactic appendectomy.

In view of these facts, our own opinion concerning incidental appendectomy is that this procedure may avoid subsequent laparotomy for symptoms referable to the appendix. Boyd and Hofmeister cite 17 cases in which appendectomy was performed during a 12-year interval on female patients who had previous pelvic surgery. The differential diagnosis of acute appendicitis could have been eliminated and such cases may have been altered if the appendix had been previously removed. A report by Lee on data from National Health Service hospitals in England and Wales reveals that from 7,000 to 8,000 women have unnecessary, nonincidental appendectomies each year. It is thought that routine appendectomy at the time of pelvic surgery would help to lower this incidence of unnecessary and erroneous surgery. It is important also to inform the patient during her convalescence whether or not her appendix was removed.

TREATMENT OF ACUTE APPENDICITIS

There is general agreement among surgeons that the treatment of acute appendicitis in the nonperforated stage is immediate appendectomy. Clinical experience and innumerable reports on mortality clearly show the advantage of early operation. Numerous recent reports, including those from Egdahl, as well as Ashley and Morris, and Cantrell and Stafford, document the decreasing mortality of appendicitis without perforation (approximately .08%) while even following perforation of acute appendicitis the overall mortality has been reduced to approximately 5.0 per cent. Obviously the influence of antibiotics and earlier surgical intervention have played a role in these improved statistics.

Thus there is no controversy concerning the treatment of the appendicitis per se, but there is considerable difference of opinion concerning the treatment of the two principal complications, namely, peritonitis and abscess. It has been the rule on both the general surgical and the gynecologic services at the Johns Hopkins Hospital and Milwaukee County Hospital to perform immediate operation when the diagnosis is made, regardless of the stage of the disease. At the present time we still believe in this as a general policy.

However, it is only fair to consider the views of those who advocate expectant treatment in those cases in which rupture is diagnosed. In the first place, it becomes obvious that there is no perfect unanimity of opinion among this group. Some would operate immediately when evidence of rupture exists, provided that the peritoneal infection is limited to the region of the appendix. They would not operate when they find evidence of diffuse peritonitis. Others would not operate when there is evidence of localized peritonitis but would when generalized peritonitis has developed. Some of the conservative group would not operate on palpable, well-walled-off appendiceal abscesses. Others, who would not operate when there is generalized peritonitis, would operate on these abscesses with or without removal of the appendix. If the abscess is drained without removal of the appendix, most surgeons are agreed that the appendix should be removed later.

Harvey Stone has challenged the plan of waiting in acute ruptured appendicitis. His objection seems to be a logical one, namely, the impossibility of recognizing exactly the extent of the lesion from clinical signs. How frequently an unruptured, partially gangrenous appendix is removed when the clinical and laboratory data strongly suggested rupture! To permit such an appendix to remain in the abdomen would greatly jeopardize the patient's chances of recovery. Such a mistake in judging the extent of the lesion is possible by the best of surgeons, and as long as that possibility exists, there is danger in the "waiting" treatment of appendicitis.

Our general rule is to operate immediately through a McBurney incision in all cases of acute appendicitis, regardless of the stage of the disease. There is only one rare exception to this rule. Occasionally, one encounters a well-walled-off abscess that is palpable abdominally in a patient whose history suggests strongly that she is improving. It is apparent from her history that she is not as ill as she was previously, and that the walled-off abscess is subsiding. Such a patient should be kept under close observation with frequent white blood counts, differential counts, and repeated radiological evaluation of the dilated bowel pattern for documented evidence of clinical improvement. Operation should be deferred as long as improvement continues. During the period of being watched the patient should have the advantage of intensive antibiotic therapy. If there is evidence of spread of infection, or if the patient's general condition becomes worse, surgical intervention is carried out immediately. Our reason for making this exception to the rule of immediate operation is the experience of the authors in observing a few cases that fell into this category; in those instances the patients were operated upon and died of obstruction and/or peritonitis with septic shock. In retrospect, it appears that such patients probably would have continued to improve if surgical intervention had been omitted at that stage.

When appendiceal abscesses are operated upon, it is our custom to make a gridiron incision directly over the abscess. The abscess cavity is entered with the greatest of care to prevent breaking up of the adhesions that are responsible for the walling-off of the abscess. If the appendix can be removed readily without danger of injury to the bowel wall or of dissemination of the infection, appendectomy is done; if appendectomy is not feasible, the abscess is simply drained. Intensive antibiotic therapy is begun. When the abscess localizes in the cul-de-sac, it is drained by colpotomy; two cigarette drains are placed in the cavity. Generally, we get the patient back in the hospital and perform an appendectomy 6 or 8 weeks after the abscess has ceased to drain.

Perhaps the term "immediate operation" should be defined. In the usual case of unruptured appendicitis the operation is done as soon as the operating room can be made ready. On the other hand, very ill patients with abscess or generalized peritonitis are often dehydrated, the serum electrolytes may be abnormal, gastric and intestinal distention is marked, and there may be circulatory collapse from gram-negative shock. Often conservative treatment for a few hours will greatly improve the patient's condition and enhance her chances of recovery after operation. Such patients are admitted to the hospital and placed in the Fowler's position. A Levin or Kantor tube is passed, and suction is started. High-dose, intravenous antibiotics are initiated to include 30 to 60 million units of penicillin and 4 gr. of Chloromycetin per day, in an effort to produce rapid blood levels and tissue perfusion of the antibiotics.

Postoperatively, supportive treatment is continued in the ill patients. All food and fluids by mouth are forbidden. Suction is continued until distention has disappeared, and there is evidence of intestinal activity. Intensive antibiotic therapy is continued until the patient is well on her way to recovery.

APPENDICITIS IN PREGNANCY

Acute appendicitis occurring during pregnancy is a serious condition from the standpoint of the mother and the fetus. Brant, in a recent review from the Hammersmith Hospital in London, found 12 cases of acute appendicitis in 42,936 deliveries between the period 1945-64 for an incidence of appendicitis of 1 in 1,789 cases (0.06%). This was of the same order as the percentage in earlier reports by Baer, Reis, and Arens (0.17%), by Cosgrove at the Margaret Hague Maternity Center (0.07%), and by Randall and Baetz (0.1%). In most clinics acute appendicitis is noted primarily in the first 2 trimesters of pregnancy. Black, however, has noted equal incidence in all 3 trimesters, and Child and Douglas suggest that the disease may be more common in late pregnancy than is diagnosed, but that many cases may be attributed to other complications of pregnancy, such as pyeltis, degeneration of a fibroid, or a small area of concealed placental separation. The difficulty in diagnosing appendicitis in the last trimester of pregnancy may also explain the greater severity of the disease during this period, with the high incidence of premature labor. Labor and delivery of a patient with a ruptured appendix are two of the most serious, yet frequent, complications of this disease. Not only is prematurity of the newborn a common problem, but the condition of the patient worsens rapidly. Prior to delivery the pregnant uterus served as a partial barrier of the abscess from the peritoneal cavity. Uterine contractions, which may be initiated by the adjacent inflammatory process, will disrupt this anatomic barrier, and generalized peritonitis follows delivery and involution of the uterus.

Although there has been marked improvement in the mortality of acute appendicitis in pregnancy during the past 2 decades, it is still much higher than that in the nonpregnant state. Brant has summarized the reports appearing from 1950 until 1965, which include 5 maternal deaths in 256 cases of acute appendicitis in pregnancy for a mortality rate of 2 per cent. As is true in the nonpregnant patient, the higher mortality is associated with ruptured appendicitis and abscess formation.

Differential Diagnosis

The classic symptoms of abdominal pain, nausea, vomiting, and constipation are common to both pregnancy and appendicitis. Abdominal discomfort is frequently attributed to round ligament stretching since only 50 per cent of the patients have peritoneal irritation with rebound tenderness. The change in position of the appendix during pregnancy makes the interpretation of abdominal pain and tenderness more difficult than in the nonpregnant woman. One can interpret pain and tenderness much more intelligently if one bears in mind these changes. Baer, Reis, and Arens studied 70 women with normal appendices roentgenologically at regular intervals throughout pregnancy and the puerperium. They showed that the base of the appendix undergoes upward and outward displacement after the 3rd month caused by the enlarging uterus, reaching the level of the iliac crest at the end of the 6th month. After the 7th month of pregnancy, in 88 per cent of their cases, the appendix was found above the crest of the ileum (Fig. 18-1). However, in interpreting these findings in relation to abdominal pain and tenderness, one must remember

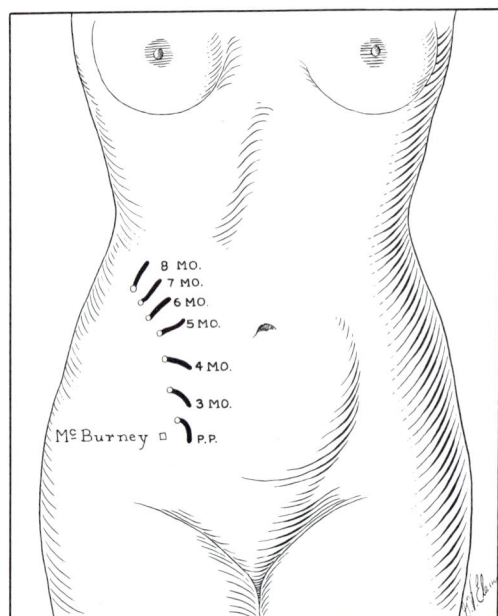

Fig. 18-1. Showing change of position of appendix during pregnancy. (After Baer, Reis, and Arens)

that in dealing with the abnormal appendix, in which previous attacks of appendicitis are frequent, there may be adhesions that fix it in a low position and do not permit its upward displacement. Due to the fact that the appendix is embryologically a midline structure, the afferent sensory fibers to this vestigial organ registers pain more frequently in the periumbilical region, as well as on both sides of the abdomen. Once local peritonitis occurs, however, the maximum tenderness is usually located in the position of the appendix.

The most frequent organ of confusion with appendicitis in pregnancy is the kidney, in which an acute urinary tract infection is frequently misdiagnosed. Due to the fact that urinary tract symptoms occur in more than 50 per cent of the cases of appendicitis in pregnancy, the patient is frequently treated initially for pyelitis of the right kidney. It is not uncommon for white cells to appear in the urine from an overlying peritoneal infection from appendicitis, which further confuses the clinical picture. This complication is more frequently seen in late pregnancy, when the appendix rises higher in the peritoneal cavity in the region of the renal pelvis and upper ureter. Acute torsion of an ovarian cyst will also mimic the clinical signs of appendicitis in pregnancy, but in general there are fewer intestinal symptoms with this entity, and the onset is more abrupt. Torsion of an ovarian cyst can be traced frequently to strenuous physical activity, namely, dancing, swimming, coitus, etc.

Although a mild leukocytosis is common in pregnancy, one should observe the white count frequently for a gradual or rapid increase and particularly for the change in polymorphonuclear leukocytes. A white count above 16,000/cu. mm. and a differential count of more than 80 per cent polymorphs suggest an acute inflammatory process but are not specific for appendicitis. One must always be aware of the occasional case in which the white count remains normal throughout the acute phase of the disease.

All of the above factors tend to make the diagnosis of appendicitis more difficult in pregnancy; hence a tendency to delay operation is common. The important thing for the clinician to bear in mind is a *possibility* of appendicitis, remembering that the symptoms of acute appendicitis are the same in a pregnant as in a nonpregnant patient. The clinician should have no concern about the possibility of removing a normal appendix during pregnancy but should bear in mind the fact that this additional operation is a small price to pay for the increased risk to the life of the mother and fetus of a delay in the diagnosis of this disease.

PERINATAL MORTALITY

There has been considerable improvement in the combined fetal and neonatal (perinatal) mortality from the earlier reports of 34 per cent by Meiling and 36 per cent as reported by Black in his collected series. The experience of Hoffman and Suzuki, which was 11 per cent fetal mortality when the infection was limited to the appendix but 35 per cent fetal mortality when the infection had spread beyond the appendix, is a testimony to the fact that stimulation of labor is a direct result of the severity of the infection rather than the stage of the gestation when appendicitis occurs.

TREATMENT

Immediate operation is the treatment for acute appendicitis in pregnancy, regardless of the duration of pregnancy or the stage of the disease. Antibiotic therapy should be initiated as soon as the patient comes under observation.

If the pregnancy is 3 months or less in duration, the appendix may be removed through the usual gridiron incision. The further advanced the pregnancy, the higher should be the incision (Fig. 18-1). Bronstein and Freidman stress the importance of centering the incision over the point of maximum tenderness, which usually means a high lateral oblique muscle-splitting incision. Anderson suggests turning the patient on her left side to minimize displacement and handling of the uterus, while Parker has advocated the use of the transverse muscle-cutting-incision at the level of the umbilicus for better access than the paramedian incision. Although there has been much debate over the years on the advisability of cesarean section combined with appendectomy, it is our conviction that the appendectomy should be done alone as quickly and atraumatically as possible, and that the patient should be given intensive antibiotic therapy and the supportive addition of 200 to 400 mg. of progesterone I.M. daily to decrease uterine irritability until the acute inflammatory process has subsided. In case of rupture and frank abscess formation, the patient should be treated immediately, the same as in the nonpregnant state, with the understanding that a much higher incidence of premature labor will occur with delay in surgical treatment, during which time the infection may be disseminated and the risk of fetal and maternal mortality increased.

INCIDENTAL APPENDECTOMY FOLLOWING CESAREAN SECTION

Until recently, the removal of the appendix incidentally at cesarean section was considered to be ill-advised. Larsson was one of the first to advocate it in 1954, and since that time additional proponents of this procedure include Israel and Roitman, Powell *et al.*, Speirs *et al.*, and Champion and Doolittle. In 1959, Sweeney of Cornell undertook a study to compare the results of 230 patients with cesarean section on whom appendectomy was done with 230 cesarean-section patients without appendectomy. Except for a 16.8-minute increase in operative time for those with appendectomy, there was no increase in operative risk, no difference in postoperative febrile morbidity, and no increase in the duration or hospitalization in the two groups. However, a careful critic would admit a slight increase in postoperative ileus and wound infection in those cases with appendectomy. Upon histologic study of the appendices, 2 were found to be acutely inflamed and 2 contained carcinoid. This rare, low-grade malignant appendiceal tumor has such a low incidence of occurrence (less than 0.3%) that prophylactic appendectomy is not indicated on this basis alone. Greenwald and Fenton, however, reported a case of an ovarian abscess secondary to appendectomy at the time of cesarean section and felt that "the risk inherent in the dual operation must be greater than cesarean section alone. What remains to be proven is whether this risk is small enough, compared to the hazards of acute appendicitis, to warrant appendectomy at abdominal delivery." At the present time the majority of clinical experience would answer this question in favor of routine appendectomy in the uncomplicated cesarean section in order to avoid future confusion and complications from this organ.

TECHNIC OF APPENDECTOMY

The appendix and the cecum are delivered. Usually this is a simple matter, but in some instances an immobile cecum, adhesions, or retrocecal position of the appendix may make this difficult. Often the retrocecal appendix can be

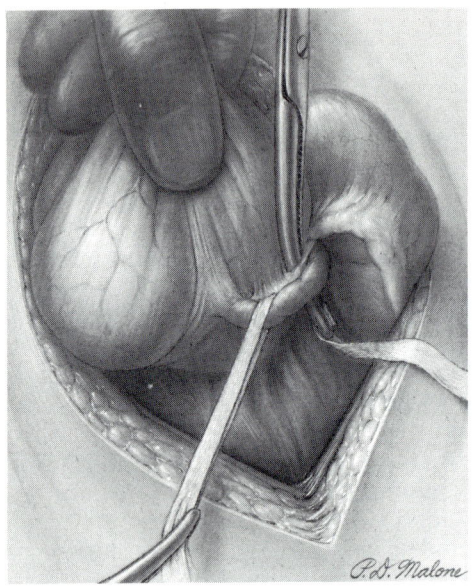

FIG. 18-2. Technic of appendectomy. Showing method of delivering retrocecal appendix, using successive pieces of tape in a hand-over-hand manner.

delivered by using pieces of tape in a hand-over-hand manner, beginning at the base (Fig. 18-2). When the appendix is mobile, the mesoappendix may be conveniently grasped near the tip of the appendix with a Kelly clamp and the appendix supported with a Babcock clamp (Fig. 18-3).

The mesoappendix can then be ligated en masse with No. 0 chromic catgut, if it is sufficiently mobile (Fig. 18-3 A). The ligation by a single suture is advantageous when possible in that the cut mesoappendix is then very easily peritonized. Often ligation of the mesoappendix en masse is not feasible, and if this is the case, it is clamped with Kelly clamps in a succession of small bites; each bite is ligated individually.

A purse-string suture of medium silk is placed about the base of the appendix (Fig. 18-3 B). The circumference of the

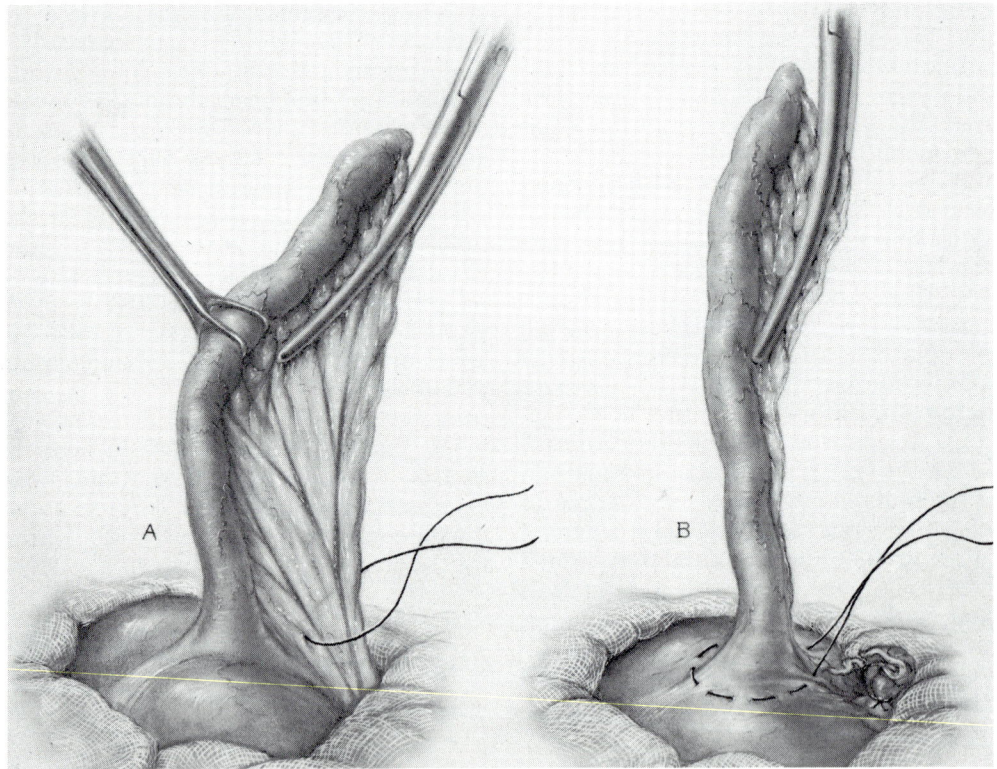

FIG. 18-3. Technic of appendectomy. (A) Appendix is delivered and supported with Kelly and Babcock clamps as the mesoappendix is ligated. Often this can be done with a single ligature as illustrated. (B) A purse string of medium silk has been placed about the base of the appendix.

Technic of Appendectomy

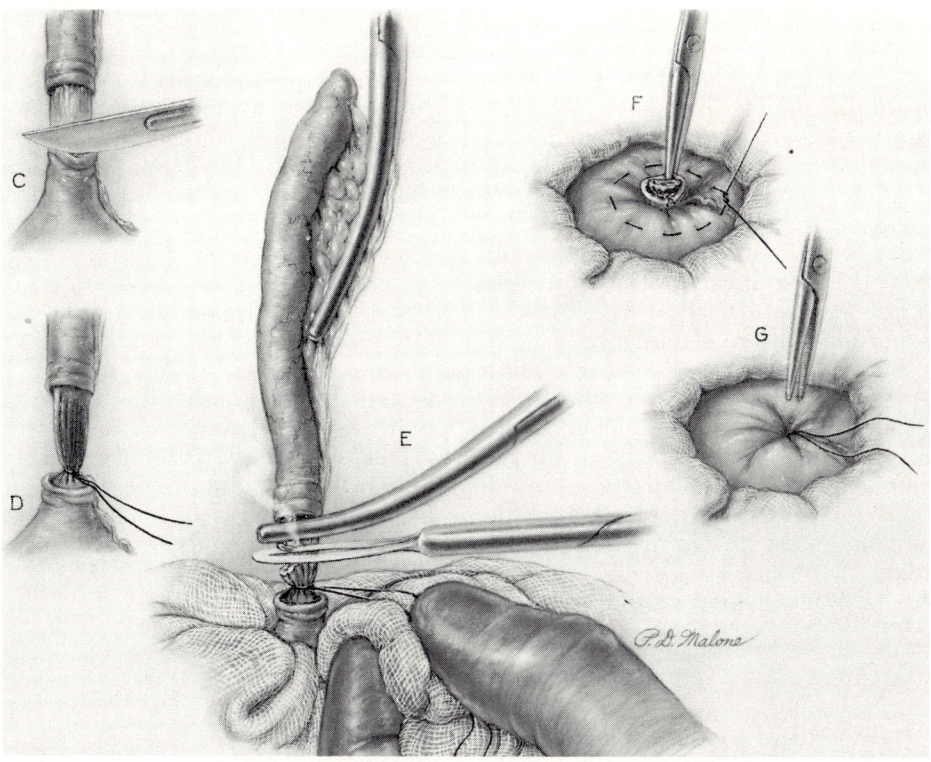

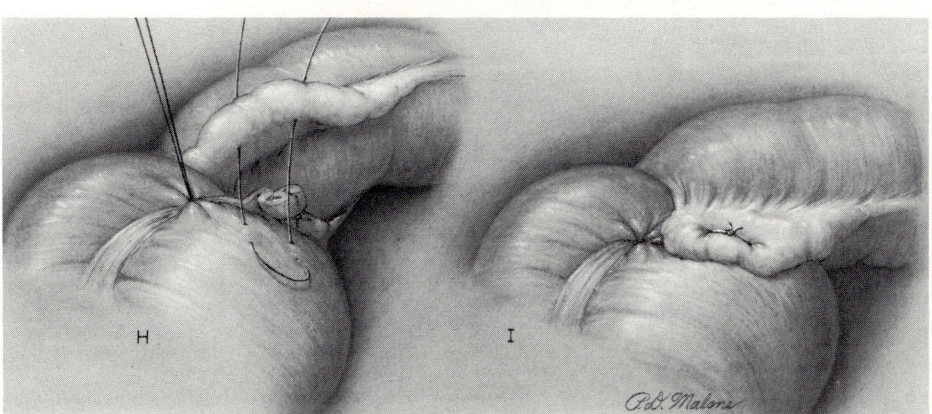

Fig. 18-3 (*Continued*). Technic of appendectomy. (C) An incision through the serosa is made about the appendix near its base, and the serosa is pushed down. (D) The appendix has been crushed at the point where it has been freed of serosa and ligated with catgut. (E) A Kelly clamp is placed on the appendix just distal to the point of amputation, and the appendix is amputated with the cautery. (F) The stump is inverted as the purse string is drawn tight. (G) The mosquito clamp is withdrawn as the purse-string suture is tied. (H) Showing simple method of peritonizing the mesoappendix stump. Fine silk is used for this. (I) Completed appendectomy.

purse string should be great enough to permit easy inversion of the stump. A half-knot is placed in the silk.

A cuff of peritoneum is turned back after making a circular incision about the base of the appendix (Fig. 18-3 C).

The appendix is crushed at the point of denudation with a Kelly or Halsted clamp and tied with No. 2 plain catgut (Fig. 18-3 D).

A Kelly clamp is placed on the appendix a short distance distal to the ligature, leaving sufficient space between the ligature and the clamp to permit the passage of the cautery without burning of the ligature.

The appendix is amputated with the cautery (Fig. 18-3 E). Amputation with the knife and cauterization with carbolic acid and alcohol are equally good technics, but the latter involves a few more steps than the simple use of cautery. The appendix and the attached clamps are dropped into a small basin kept on the operating table for receiving the appendix and for the instruments that might be contaminated in doing the appendectomy.

The peritoneal edge of the appendix stump is grasped by the assistant with a mosquito clamp, and the ligature about the base of the appendix is cut short. The sponge, with which the operator protected his finger while holding the ligature, is placed in the "appendix basin."

The stump is inverted, and the purse string is drawn tight (Fig. 18-3 F and G). The mosquito clamp is dropped into the "appendix basin," and the basin is passed from the operating table.

If the appendix is entirely retrocecal, the mesoappendix need not be peritonized, but generally the cut mesoappendix is peritonized with interrupted sutures of fine silk. Often there is a convenient flap of fat at the terminal portion of the ileum that may be used to cover over the mesoappendix by inserting 1 or 2 mattress sutures of fine silk (Fig. 18-3 H and I).

BIBLIOGRAPHY

Anderson, R. E., Pontius, G. V., and Witkowski, L. J.: A modified technique for the removal of the appendix during pregnancy. Amer. J. Surg., 93:117, 1957.

Ashley, J. S. A., and Morris, J. N.: Deaths from appendicitis. Lancet, *1*:217, 1967.

Baer, J. L., Reis, R. A., and Arens, R. A.: Appendicitis in pregnancy, with changes in position and axis of normal appendix in pregnancy. J.A.M.A., 98:1359, 1932.

Bierman, H. R.: Human appendix and neoplasia. Cancer, *21*:109, 1968.

Black, P.: Acute appendicitis in pregnancy. Brit. Med. J., *1*:1938, 1960.

Boyd, A., and Hofmeister, F. J.: Caesarean section and associated surgery. Obstet. Gynec., *24*:533, 1964.

Brant, H. A.: Acute appendicitis in pregnancy. Obstet. Gynec., *29*:130, 1967.

Bronstein, E. S., and Freidman, M.: Acute appendicitis in pregnancy. Amer. J. Obstet. Gynec., *86*:515, 1963.

Burwell, J. C., and Brooks, J. B.: Acute appendicitis in pregnancy. Amer. J. Obstet. Gynec., *78*:772, 1959.

Cantrell, J. R., and Stafford, E. S.: The diminishing mortality from appendicitis. Ann. Surg., *141*:749, 1955.

Champion, P. K., and Doolittle, J. E.: Appendectomy at caesarean section. Obstet. Gynec., *18*:200, 1961.

Cosgrove, S. A.: Surgical complications of pregnancy. Amer. J. Obstet. Gynec., *34*: 469, 1937.

Curtis, A. H.: A Textbook of Gynecology. ed. 1. Philadelphia, W. B. Saunders, 1930.

Egdahl, R. H.: Current mortality in appendicitis. Amer. J. Surg., *107*:757, 1964.

Faulkner, R. L., and Weir, W. C.: Left-sided pelvic lesions subsequent to appendicitis. Amer. J. Obstet. Gynec., *45*:874, 1943.

Greenwald, J. C., and Fenton, A. N.: Ovarian abscess secondary to incidental appendectomy at caesarean section. Obstet. Gynec., *14*:593, 1959.

Hoffman, E. S., and Suzuki, M.: Appendicitis in pregnancy. Obstet. Gynec., *67*:1338, 1954.

Howkins, J.: Appendectomy during gynecological operations. Lancet, *1*:1016, 1956.

Israel, S. L., and Roitman, H. B.: Caesarean section and prophylactic appendectomy: The passing of a prejudice. Obstet. Gynec., *10*:102, 1957.

Kocsard-Varo, G.: Physiologic role of tonsils, adenoids and the appendix in immunity. Med. J. Australia, *2*:873, 1964.

Larsson, E.: Elective appendectomy at time of cesarean section. J.A.M.A., *154*:549, 1954.

Lee, J. A. H.: "Appendicitis" in young women. An opportunity for colloborative clinical research in the National Health Service. Lancet, *2*:815, 1961.

Loeffler, F., and Stearn, R.: Abdominal hysterectomy with appendectomy. Acta Obstet. Gynec. Scand., 46:435, 1967.

MacLeod, D., and Howkins, J.: Bonney's Gynaecological Surgery. ed 7, p. 547. London, Hoeber Med. Div., Harper & Row, 1964.

McCall, M. L., and Bolton, K. A.: Martius Gynecological Operations. ed. 7. Boston, Little, Brown & Co., 1957.

McVay, J. R., Jr.: The appendix in relation to neoplastic disease. Cancer, 17:929, 1964.

Meiling, R. L.: Appendicitis complicating pregnancy, labor and puerperium. Surg. Gynec. Obstet., 40:495, 1947.

Nather, K., and Ochsner, A.: Abscess on left side with appendicitis. Deutsche Z. Chir., 188:144, 1924, abstracted in Surg. Gynec. Obstet., 40:495, 1925.

Parker, R. D.: Acute appendicitis in late pregnancy. Lancet, 1:1252, 1954.

Powell, D. V., Holmes, D. E., Beath, D. H., Yard, G. H., and Noel, P. J.: Incidental appendectomy in obstetrics and gynecology. Obstet. Gynec., 12:727, 1958.

Pratt, J. H., Lee, M. H., Hasskarl, W. F., and Brandes, R. W.: Morbidity after total abdominal hysterectomy. Amer. J. Obstet. Gynec., 61:407, 1951.

Randall, C. L., and Baetz, R. W.: Surgery during pregnancy. Obstet. Gynec., 3:100, 1954.

Speirs, R. E., Baum, A. H., Williams, E. R., and Boles, R. D.: Elective appendectomy at the time of Cesarean section. Amer. Surg., 25:558, 1959.

Stone, H. B.: The management of acute appendicitis—arguments and controversies. W. Virginia Med. J., 36:505, 1940.

Sweeney, W. J.: Incidental appendectomy at cesarean section. Obstet. Gynec., 14:588, 1959.

19

Sterilization

ELEANOR DELFS, M.D.*

GENERAL CONSIDERATIONS

Sterilization has a permanent place in surgery, although there are and always will be differences of opinion on the medical, the eugenic, the religious, and the legal aspects of the subject. In the hands of responsible medical men it can be a force for great good in relieving physical and mental distress. In the hands of the unscrupulous, it has potentialities for evil that are equally great. The gynecologist is generally called upon to perform the sterilization, and therefore he carries the major medical and legal responsibility. Though he may depend considerably on the opinions of the internist or psychiatrist in their fields, he needs familiarity with all aspects of the problems to reach a sound judgment in each case.

The legal status of sterilization is not uniform throughout the United States. Twenty-eight states have passed eugenic laws of some type. In general, these may be divided into two groups:

1. Those that make sterilization mandatory under certain conditions without the consent of the patient or those responsible for her.

2. Those that require consent of the patient and/or those responsible for her.

The validity of the Virginia law was tested in the Supreme Court of the United States, and the now famous decision was written by Justice Oliver Wendell Holmes:

It is better for all the world if, instead of waiting to execute degenerate offspring for crime or to let them starve for their imbecility, society can prevent those who are manifestly unfit from continuing their kind. The principle that sustains compulsory vaccination is broad enough to cover cutting the fallopian tubes.

However, in several other instances the enacted state laws have been declared unconstitutional.

Myerson has drawn attention to the fact that even though in some states laws have permitted eugenic sterilization for many years, relatively few of the patients who should or could have been sterilized under those laws have actually been sterilized. He attributes this to the fact that laws cannot be ahead of public opinion and cannot be enforced successfully if public sentiment does not favor them. Gampbell has reviewed the state laws and concluded that therapeutic sterilization is permissible in all states, and that, except in 3 states which expressly forbid it (Connecticut, Kansas, and Utah), purely contraceptive, permissive sterilization carries no greater criminal or civil liability than that associated with any other medical procedure. Since in some states there is no law regarding sterilization, it becomes the duty of the medical profession to act in the matter according to its best judgment and to be well informed on the subject.

---

* Professor, Department of Gynecology and Obstetrics, Marquette School of Medicine.

Ideas regarding sterilization vary greatly in different hospitals. In Catholic hospitals surgical sterilization is absolutely prohibited unless it occurs incidentally in connection with an operation done primarily for the removal of diseased organs. Other hospitals are quite liberal in their indications. In order to obtain the combined judgment of the more responsible members of the staff and to protect the doctor doing the sterilization, some hospitals have committees to act on recommendations for sterilization.

For the physician's protection it has been our practice for many years to require the signatures of both husband and wife to a letter requesting sterilization. The letter is written in simple nonmedical language so that there can be no doubt of the ability of the signers to understand its contents. In case of sterilization for psychiatric reasons, it is well to obtain, if possible, the signature of the patient as well as the responsible member or members of her family. A few sterilizations done for psychiatric conditions are performed on underage children of extremely low mental status. In such instances the signatures of the mother and the father are required.

The majority of sterilizations done in the United States at present are on a voluntary basis for medical indications or for multiparity and socioeconomic reasons, the procedure being requested by the woman and her husband. The incidence of puerperal sterilization was found to be 3.2 per cent of live births by Starr and Kosasky and 1.7 per cent by Moore and Russell. Campbell estimated from a survey that about 200,000 operations preventing pregnancy are done yearly in the United States in women between 18 and 39 years, over one half being solely for sterilization.

INDICATIONS

A study of indications for sterilization was made by Guttmacher at the Mt. Sinai Hospital in New York. The study is of particular interest because he divided the patients into private and public ward groups. It is apparent that the indications in the two groups vary considerably. On the private service there were 119 cases with the following indications:

	CASES
Multiparity	26
Repeated cesarean sections	65
Heart disease	4
Hypertensive disease	3
Previous vaginal plastic operations	5
Varicosities	4
Eugenic reasons	2
Diabetes, psychiatric disorders, poor obstetric history, asthma, previous nephrectomy, brain tumor, epilepsy, chronic back pain, 3rd degree uterine prolapse, and obstructing pelvic tumor	1 each

On the ward service there were 425 cases with the following indications:

	CASES
Multiparity	340
Repeated cesarean sections	51
Heart disease	9
Hypertensive disease	6
Diabetes	6
Psychiatric disorders	5
Poor obstetrical history	2
Varicosities, eugenic reasons, asthma, obstructive jaundice, carcinoma of the cervix, and Hodgkin's disease	1 each

Sterilization was offered for socioeconomic reasons to women at the birth of the 6th child regardless of the mother's age, to mothers between 30 and 35 years after the 5th child, and to mothers over the age of 35 after the 4th child. These views seem to be reasonably conservative. Sterilization is entirely voluntary on the part of the patient and her husband, and the carrying out of such a program undoubtedly spares many mothers mental and some physical suffering.

In general, the indications for sterilization can be divided into four groups: (1) psychiatric, (2) medical, obstetric, and gynecologic, (3) socioeconomic, and (4) potential fetal defect.

Psychiatric Indications. Psychiatric problems may be an indication for sterilization on either a mandatory or a voluntary basis. Several potential risks may present: the possibility of transmission of deficiency or susceptibility to mental illness to the child, the provision of a poor and damaging environment for children, and the exacerbation of maternal psychiatric illness by the stress of increasing responsibilities. Myerson, in summarizing the report of an investigation by a committee of the American Neurological Association, points out that though there are possibly some hereditary bases for schizophrenia, manic-depressive psychoses, some epilepsy, and feeblemindedness, heredity is by no means the whole picture. Such hereditary risk alone is often not definite enough to constitute strong indication for sterilization. Other factors are more evident and measurable, and certain practical considerations will indicate a reasonable course in most cases.

Young girls who are minors and childless should not be sterilized except under extreme circumstances. With psychological testing showing mental age under 6 years in individuals who are adolescent or older, few would oppose sterilization, as such persons cannot care for themselves or any children they might produce. Mildly retarded individuals usually should not be sterilized until they have a couple of children. They may manage a small family satisfactorily but usually welcome sterilization to avoid being overwhelmed by more than they can handle.

Women who are seriously psychiatrically ill on a chronic or recurrent basis may be candidates for sterilization, particularly if they are multiparous. Sterilization is preventive in that it reduces the number of children at risk and minimizes the deterioration of environment which larger numbers may produce. Since most women with psychiatric problems do not want large families, their voluntary sterilization does not deny essential human rights; in actual fact, it often extends their right of choice.

Medical, Gynecologic, and Obstetric Indications. Indications for therapeutic abortion in various medical conditions given in Chapter 22 are, with few exceptions, indications for sterilization as well. In most cases serious enough to require therapeutic abortion, sterilization is mandatory regardless of the parity. How and when it is accomplished will vary with the type of termination procedure and condition of the patient. Sterilization may be done with propriety more liberally than therapeutic abortion. Multiparous women with chronic hypertensive vascular disease, heart disease, chronic renal or pulmonary disease, diabetes, etc., not severe enough to demand abortion may often be well advised not to invite additional risks of future pregnancies.

Gynecologic plastic operations for extensive relaxations, prolapse, and the like are most often done in women of considerable parity when the family is complete, and sterilization is usually indicated to protect the repair. This indication is decreasing because of the wider use of vaginal hysterectomy in such situations.

The major obstetric indication is the presence of cesarean section scars. The danger of scar rupture is small (0.5 to 2.0%, depending on the type of scar) but is ever present. Repeated sections have additive risks of anesthesia and laparotomy as well. It is our practice to offer sterilization with the 3rd section and strongly recommend it with the 4th; in a woman of parity over 4 who requires primary cesarean section, it is justifiable to accompany it with sterilization if the patient desires to avoid risks.

Great multiparity has been widely considered an indication for sterilization, as supported by Eastman's demonstration in 1940 that the maternal mortality was 3 times as high in women of parity over 8 as in women of lesser parity. In 1955 he pointed out that improved obstetric management had reduced maternal mortality so that the risk of pregnancy did not significantly exceed the operative risk for sterilization. Mortality is not the only consideration, however, as the woman of great parity may suffer various complications, anemia, fatigue, and overwork, which adversely affect her life and that of her family. Sterilization is still justified for many, particularly if they cannot use contraception successfully.

Socioeconomic Indications. Distress from socioeconomic factors is a major indication for sterilization in some areas but is controversial to many. It is closely bound to multiparity. Parents with limited resources, personal or economic, may manage a few children, but the burden may become more than they can cope with if they have no means of limiting their families. The plight of the children is more desperate than the parents', as the children may lack adequate nutrition and essential care. Financial aid frequently has failed to stabilize the family or improve the status of unwanted children. The availability of more effective contraceptives may be expected to decrease the need for sterilization on socioeconomic indications.

Potential Fetal Defect. Severe iso-immunization is an acquired condition which may be an indication for sterilization in carefully selected cases. Congenital malformations and deficiencies may or may not be hereditary; therefore, careful consideration of the family history and the genetic nature of the particular condition is necessary before sterilization is considered. Sterilization of childless individuals should be undertaken usually only in conditions of seriously handicapping nature and high probability of manifestation and with urgent request of the woman. Parous women who carry a hereditary trait or have already given birth to affected children are more evident candidates. An example is the study of congenital anomaly of the central nervous system by Labrum and Wood, who found that women who had delivered an infant with such an anomaly had a 12 per cent incidence of repeat central nervous system anomaly in the next pregnancy. After 2 anomalies the expectation of a normal term pregnancy decreased to only 13 per cent. Moloshak has summarized the mode of transmission and empiric risk of many anatomical anomalies, coagulation defects, errors of metabolism, and other genetic aberrations as a guide to clinical counseling.

OPTIMUM TIME FOR STERILIZATION

Sterilization accompanying cesarean section is a common and convenient time to do the procedure when section is needed. However, the sterilization should not be used as an indication for cesarean section. Section carries considerably greater risks of hemorrhage, shock, and postoperative complications than does vaginal delivery followed by puerperal tubal ligation. Samuels found in vaginal delivery with tubal ligation a morbidity of 3 per cent and other complications of 4.8 per cent but in cesarean section and tubal ligation a morbidity of 8.9 per cent and other complications of 8.9 per cent.

Puerperal sterilization is best done in the first 24 to 36 hours after delivery. We prefer to wait at least 6 hours to reduce the likelihood of bleeding and permit rest after labor. It is not done later than 48 hours postpartum as bacteria are present in the uterus by this time, and the postoperative course is more likely to be febrile. If there has been premature rupture of membranes, intrapartum fever, manual removal of the placenta, or any factor predisposing to infection and postoperative complications, the procedure should be deferred until involution is completed. The advantages of early puerperal sterilization are the easy access to the uterus, which may be approached by a small incision over the fundus a short distance below the umbilicus, and the convenience of combining postpartum and postoperative convalescence with minimal additional hospitalization.

Interval sterilization may be done 6 weeks after delivery or at any later period in the nonpregnant individual. Women with cardiac disease, marked hypertension, renal disease, or acute toxemia should not be subjected to sterilization in the labile early puerperium but should have an interval procedure when they are well stabilized.

Sterilization may be done in conjunction with vaginal plastic repairs and is strongly indicated when extensive operations are done. Vaginal hysterectomy and the Spalding-Richardson composite operation automatically sterilize.

METHODS AND EFFICACY

A large number of procedures have been devised to accomplish sterilization, but most of them have had limited use. Overstreet has made a critical review of commonly used methods, their strong and weak points, and their failure rates (see Table 19-1). Garb's review is also an extensive material source. Only those methods which we use frequently or which meet a special purpose will be discussed here.

Irradiation sterilization is used very infrequently and only in women over 40 years of age who are bad surgical risks. As it is effective only if it suppresses ovarian function, the resulting menopause may be disturbing to younger women. External radiation of 1,500 to 2,000 r is given to each ovary over a 3-week period, the larger dose being used for younger women.

Surgical sterilization can be done by either vaginal or abdominal route. Boysen and McRae recommended the vaginal operation by choice and reported 0.6 per cent failures in nonpregnant women. Failures were 16.6 per cent when done in conjunction with therapeutic abortion, which would seem to invalidate the method in the puerperal woman. We use the vaginal route only when sterilization accompanies a vaginal plastic procedure. The Pomeroy method is most easily done in this situation.

The Pomeroy technic (Figs 19-1 and 19-2) is the most widely used and simplest of all methods. The failure rate is relatively low (1 in 340) except when accompanying cesarean sections, when the rate increases to 1 in 50, according to Prystowsky and Eastman. We use this procedure in puerperal or interval sterilizations if there are technical reasons for doing so, such as marked vascularity of the mesosalpinx making mobilization of the tube difficult, lessened mobility at times with use of local anesthesia, or need to shorten operating time because of poor condition of the patient. Occasionally, it is used with cesarean section for technical reasons but is not the procedure of choice.

The Irving sterilization has a very high success rate and is our procedure of choice accompanying cesarean section particularly, even though it may be asso-

TABLE 19-1. FAILURE RATES OF STERILIZATION METHODS*

STERILIZATION METHOD	APPROXIMATE FAILURE RATE	
	At Cesarean Section	Noncesarean
Tubal methods		
Cornual resection	Unknown	1 in 35
Madlener	1 in 50	1 in 70
Cooke	Unknown	1 in 250
Pomeroy	1 in 50	1 in 300
Irving	Extremely low— less than 1 in 1,000	
Uchida	No reported failures in nearly 5,000	

* Adapted from Overstreet, E. W.: Clin. Obstet. Gynec., 7:109, 1964.

ciated with somewhat more bleeding. It is preferred in puerperal and interval ligations as well unless there is some obstacle to its ready accomplishment.

The Uchida sterilization likewise has a reported high efficacy. It is somewhat similar to the Irving method except that the mesosalpinx is ballooned by saline injection, a pocket formed, and the proximal end of the cut and ligated tube buried in the mesosalpinx rather than in the uterine wall.

Vaginal hysterectomy has been used as an alternative to tubal ligation in some areas in recent years. When there is any pelvic pathology such as chronic cervical dysplasia, menorrhagia, pelvic relaxations, or uterine descensus, vaginal hysterectomy and repair may solve the whole problem well, particularly in the multiparous women beyond 30 years of age. Operation should be deferred 4 to 6 months after pregnancy to permit regression of vascularity. The use of hysterectomy for the sole purpose of sterilization may be questioned as it is a more extensive procedure with potential for more operative complications than tubal ligation. Under optimal conditions with an experienced operator, the risks are small, but this is not the case in all circumstances in which sterilization may be contemplated. Some women (or their husbands) are psychologically disturbed by the loss of the uterus and menstrual function, and attitudes should be explored before elective choice of hysterectomy.

Total hysterectomy following cesarean section has been advocated as a method of sterilization, and a considerable literature has accumulated on this subject in the last decade or so. Several sizable series without mortality have been published, but the operation is not without hazard. Pritchard *et al.* documented average blood loss in cesarean section hysterectomy at 1,400 cc. Pletsch forthrightly reported 4 per cent of cases of operative hemorrhage and shock and several of postoperative hemorrhage and hematomas requiring secondary operation.

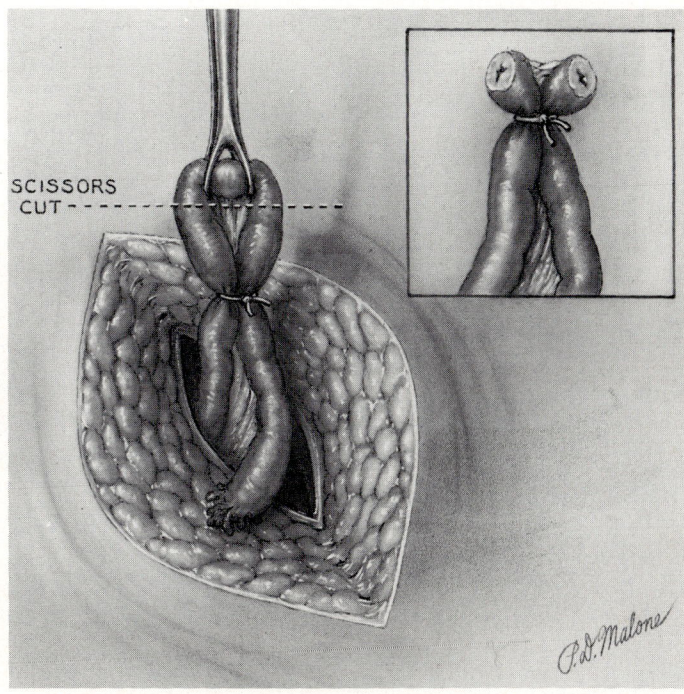

FIG. 19-1. Pomeroy tubal sterilization. The tube has been withdrawn through a short midline incision, and a knuckle has been ligated. Inset shows knuckle excised with divergent ends.

380 Sterilization

Ward and Smith also reported 2.5 per cent requiring surgery for postoperative bleeding, and 80 per cent of their patients were transfused. Most series report transfusion required by 50 to 80 per cent of patients. Bladder injuries are a hazard, O'Leary and Steer reporting 1.8 per cent and Pletsch 6.5 per cent. Postoperative morbidity varies from 8 to 30 per cent. O'Leary and Steer found 30 per cent morbidity, which was twice as high as that in their series of cesarean section with tubal ligation. In general, our practice has been to limit cesarean-section hysterectomy to patients with pathology requiring hysterectomy and to carry out tubal ligation in the remainder.

Technic: Pomeroy Operation for Tubal Sterilization

A short midline incision is made at approximately the level of the fundus of the postpartum uterus. One tube is delivered with a Babcock clamp which grasps the tube at about the middle. As the loop of the tube is held up, it is ligated with No. 1 plain catgut (Fig. 19-1). The loop is then cut off with the scissors, as shown in the dotted line. At the completion of the operation the two severed

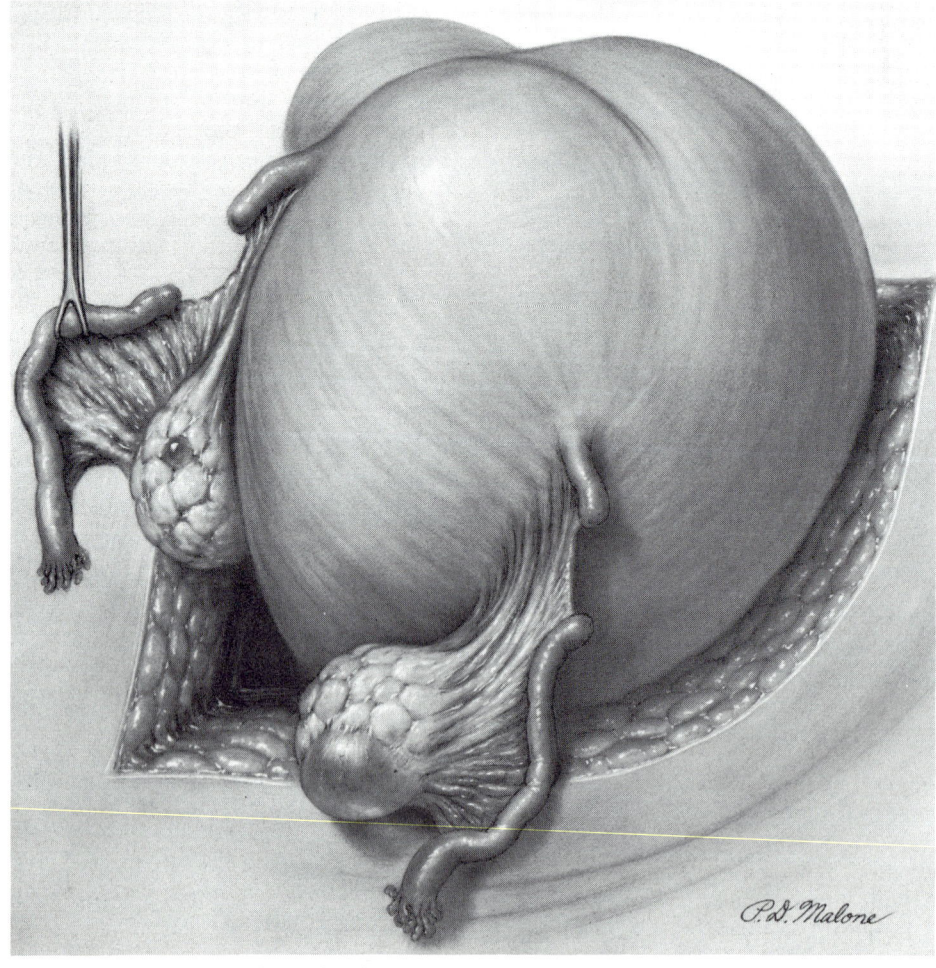

Fig. 19-2. End result of Pomeroy sterilization done 3 years before.

ends of the tube have a tendency to diverge from one another, as shown in the inset. This process is repeated on the opposite side, and the midline incision is closed.

Figure 19-2 shows the tubes as they appeared at laparotomy some years after Pomeroy sterilization. The healed-over tubal ends are widely separated.

Technic: Modified Irving Sterilization

The tube is doubly ligated with No. 0 chromic catgut about 1 inch from the uterine cornu and then severed. The sutures on the proximal end of the tube are left long (Fig. 19-3 A). This tubal stump is then mobilized by dissecting it free from the mesosalpinx. A very small nick is made in the serosa on the posterior surface of the uterus near the cornu in as avascular an area as possible, and the musculature is penetrated with a mosquito clamp for about ½ inch, spreading the clamp sufficiently to admit the tube (Fig. 19-3 A). One of the ligatures attached to the tubal stump is threaded with a round needle. The

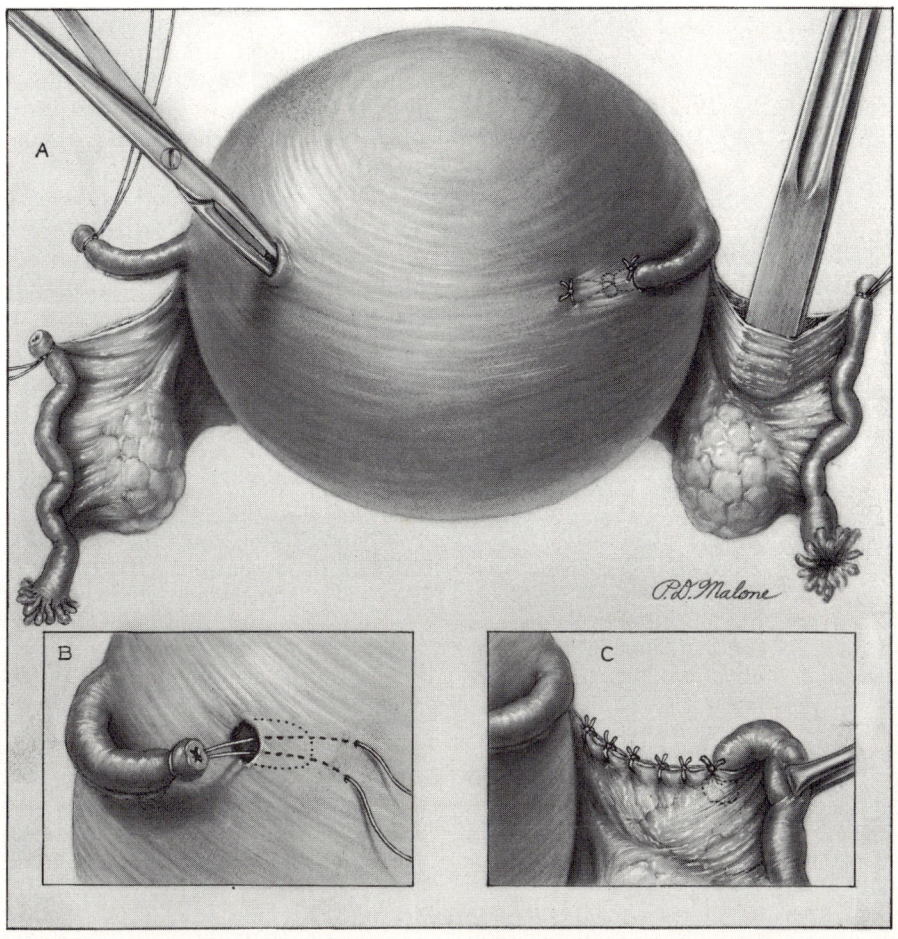

FIG. 19-3. Modified Irving sterilization. (A) Tubes have been cut and are being buried in musculature of posterior uterine wall. (B) Showing method of burying proximal tubal end. (C) Broad ligament is closed, and distal end of tube is buried.

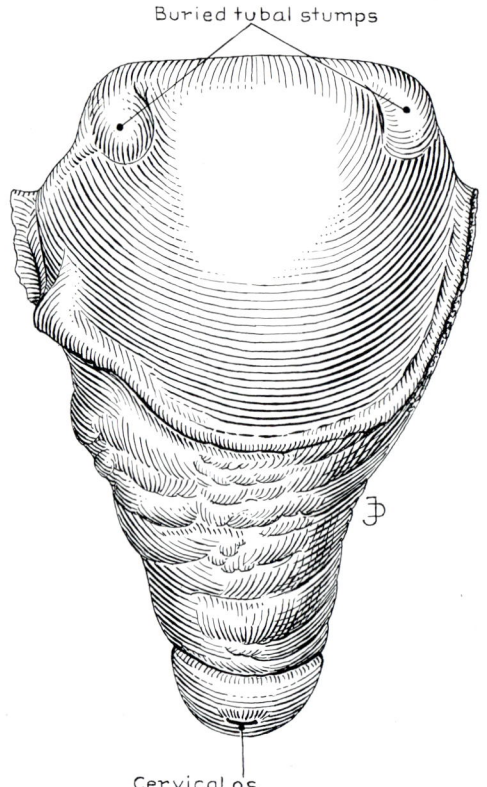

FIG. 19-4. Demonstrating late result of tubal sterilization by the Irving technic.

needle is thrust to the bottom of the pocket guided by a grooved director and carried out to the uterine surface. The other suture attached to the tubal stump is treated in a similar manner, bringing it to the surface of the uterus about ½ inch from the first suture (Fig. 19-3 B). Traction is made on the sutures, and thus the tubal stump is buried in the uterine musculature. Then the sutures are tied together. A stitch of fine catgut or a silk purse string is used to close the edges of the pocket more tightly about the tube.

According to Irving's original description of the operation, the ligated end of the distal portion of the tube is buried between the leaves of the broad ligament (Fig. 19-3 C). This makes a very neat appearance but adds nothing to the effectiveness of the sterilization. Occasionally, a blood vessel may be nicked during this step, and this accident is annoying. The burying of this end of the tube is optional with the operator.

Recently, we removed a uterus several years after an Irving sterilization and had an opportunity to view the end result of the operation. Figure 19-4 illustrates the findings.

BIBLIOGRAPHY

Aldridge, A. H.: Temporary surgical sterilization with subsequent pregnancy. Amer. J. Obstet. Gynec., 27:741, 1934.

Boysen, H., and McRae, L. A.: Tubal sterilization through the vagina. Amer. J. Obstet. Gynec., 58:488, 1949.

Campbell, A. A.: The incidence of operations that prevent conception. Amer. J. Obstet. Gynec., 89:694, 1964.

Committee of the American Neurological Association for the Investigation of Eugenic Sterilization: Eugenical Sterilization. New York, Macmillan, 1936.

Eastman, N. J.: Hazards of pregnancy and labor in the "grand multipara." New York J. Med., 40:1708, 1940.

Gampbell, R. J.: Legal status of therapeutic abortion and sterilization in the United States. Clin. Obstet. Gynec., 7:22, 1964.

Garb, A. E.: A review of tubal sterilization failures. Obstet. Gynec. Survey, 12:291, 1957.

Guttmacher, A.: Puerperal sterilization on the private and ward services of a large metropolitan hospital. Fertil. Steril., 8:591, 1957.

Hallat, J. G., and Hirsch, H.: Total hysterectomy for sterilization following cesarean section. Amer. J. Obstet. Gynec., 75:396, 1958.

Irving, F. C.: A new method of insuring sterility following cesarean section. Amer. J. Obstet. Gynec., 8:335, 1924.

Labrum, T., and Wood, C.: Congenital nervous system anomalies. Obstet. Gynec., 18:430, 1961.

Moloshak, R. E.: Fetal considerations for therapeutic abortion and sterilization. Clin. Obstet. Gynec., 7:82, 1964.

Moore, J. G., and Russell, K. P.: Maternal medical indications for female sterilization. Clin. Obstet. Gynec., 7:54, 1964.

Myerson, A.: Certain medical and legal phases of eugenic sterilization. Ann. Intern. Med., 18:580, 1943.

O'Leary, J. A., and Steer, C. M.: A 10-year review of cesarean hysterectomy. Amer. J. Obstet. Gynec., 90:227, 1964.

Overstreet, E. W.: Techniques of sterilization. Clin. Obstet. Gynec., 7:109, 1964.

Pletsch, T. O.: Cesarean hysterectomy for sterilization. Amer. J. Obstet. Gynec., 85:254, 1963.

Pritchard, J. A., Baldwin, R. M., Dicky, J. C., and Wiggins, K. M.: Blood volume changes in pregnancy and puerperium. Amer. J. Obstet. Gynec., 84:1271, 1962.

Prystowsky, H., and Eastman, N. J.: Puerperal tubal sterilization. J.A.M.A., 158:463, 1955.

Samuels, B.: Puerperal sterilizations: A ten-year survey at Touro Infirmary. Obstet. Gynec., 18:454, 1961.

Starr, S. H., and Kosasky, H. J.: Puerperal sterilization. Amer. J. Obstet. Gynec., 88:944, 1964.

Uchida, H.: Uchida's abdominal sterilization technique. Proc. Third World Congress Obstet. Gynec., 1:26, 1961.

Ward, S. V., and Smith, A. H.: Cesarean hysterectomy: Combined section and sterilization. Obstet. Gynec., 26:858, 1965.

PART THREE

Vaginal Operations for Benign Disease

20

Nonmalignant Cervical Lesions and Their Treatment

Nowhere in gynecology is there such confusion as in the terminology and the exact understanding of benign cervical lesions. Before discussing operative measures for dealing with these lesions, some clarification of the pathology and definition of terms as accepted and used by the authors are necessary.

CONGENITAL PSEUDO-EROSION

This term, as used here, refers to a reddened zone about the external cervical os found in a considerable percentage of nulliparous women (Fig. 20-1). It does not appear to be the result of inflammation, although such cervices are probably more susceptible to infection than others. The reddened zone is due to the fact that the columnar epithelium, which in the normal average cervix ends at the external os, in some cases meets the stratified squamous epithelium at a variable distance outside of the os. Tissue biopsied from such a zone is found to be covered with a single layer of columnar epithelium; because of this the subjacent blood vessels color the area deep red, in contrast with the dull pink of the rest of the portio, which is covered with stratified epithelium of several cell layers in thickness. Because of the frequent occurrence of this condition in young virginal women without any abnormal cervical discharge, we believe it to be of congenital origin. Therefore we prefer the term *pseudo-erosion*. Norman Miller has suggested the term *ectoplasia*. This term undoubtedly is more descriptive of the condition than any other thus far suggested but has not been accepted generally. Curtis takes exeption to our point of view and that of Miller and states that in a large percentage of cases there is actual ulceration. He believes that the destruction of the cervical epithelium is the result of maceration of the epithelial

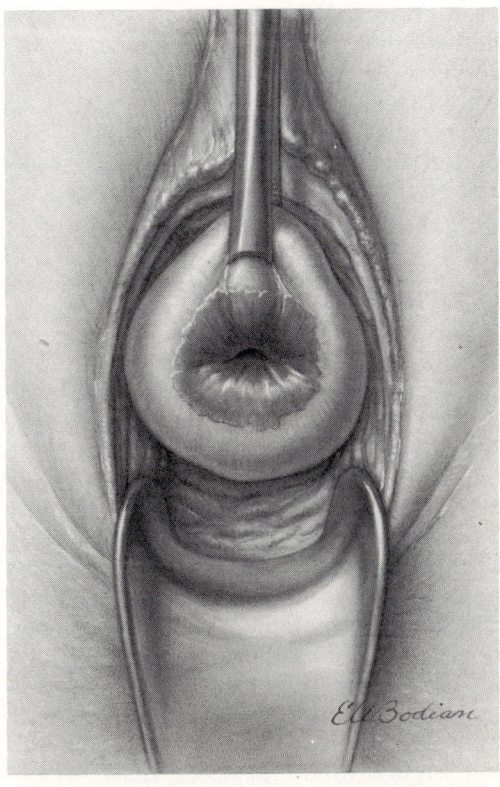

Fig. 20-1. Pseudo-erosion or ectoplasia of nulliparous cervix.

covering by cervical discharge. Therefore, he clings to the term *erosion*. Because in many of the cases there is no discharge and an intact epithelial covering, we cannot subscribe to this point of view. On the other hand, it must be admitted that a cervix with a pseudo-erosion is more susceptible to nonspecific infection than a cervix whose portio is covered entirely by the thicker stratified epithelium. This infection may result in real, but superficial ulceration. We believe that the term *erosion* should be reserved for those cases in which there are infection and actual loss of surface epithelium. It seems important to distinguish between these two lesions, because the pseudo-erosion, per se, requires no treatment, but when there are infection and an annoying discharge, the cervicitis should be treated. In the past, many of the pseudo-erosions have been treated unnecessarily by applications of medications and by the cautery. After destroying the columnar surface epithelium, usually it is replaced by stratified epithelium; the appearance of the cervix changes, but nothing else is accomplished. Such treatment, which is the result of lack of understanding of the underlying pathology, is meddlesome and should be avoided.

CERVICAL LACERATIONS

Lacerations of the cervix of sufficient degree to be a source of future trouble result almost exclusively from childbirth or abortions. Lacerations of the cervix incurred by cervical dilatation in performing a diagnostic curettage may give rise to acute hemorrhage at the time but seldom give future trouble. Childbirth tears are usually bilateral but may be unilateral or may radiate out from the external os into the anterior or the posterior lip. At the time of the laceration, infection is permitted to enter the cervical tissues and may lay the foundation of a persistent chronic cervicitis and a resulting vaginal discharge. As a result of bilateral laceration and infection, scar tissue forms, and as it contracts, the endocervical canal is turned outward. This eversion or ectropion (Fig. 20-2) exposes the deep-red endocervix to view through a speculum. Infection is the rule in this type of cervix, and small abrasions may occur on the everted surface. When rubbed with a cotton applicator, slight bleeding usually is easily induced. Profuse mucopurulent leukorrhea is common from such a cervix. The treatment of cervical lacerations is discussed later in this chapter in considering cervicitis and the various operative procedures.

CERVICITIS

Acute cervicitis is usually the result of gonococcal infection, and consideration is given to it in the chapter on gonorrhea. As a result of delivery or abortion, the cervix frequently becomes lacerated, and the bacterial flora of the vagina enters the cervical stroma and infects it. The acute phase of this infection is transient, but the organisms frequently persist in the tissues, and chronic cervicitis results.

Chronic cervicitis is one of the commonest of gynecologic lesions; in fact, if one were to consider the condition from a strictly histologic point of view, one would be forced to the conclusion that the majority of cervices are to some degree infected, for it is unusual to examine a section of a cervix histologically without seeing some evidence of infiltra-

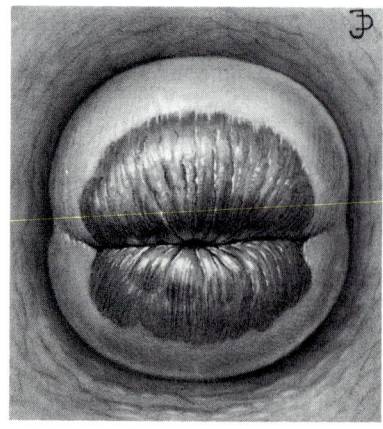

FIG. 20-2. Lacerated cervix with everted endocervix.

tion by inflammatory cells. The usual microscopic picture of the chronically inflamed cervix is that of infiltration with round cells and to some degree with plasma cells and polymorphonuclear leukocytes. Even in the lesser degrees of inflammation the infiltration is well down into the depths of the cervical tissue, concentrating especially about the glands to their full depth. These compound mucus-secreting glands extend down into the cervical interstitial tissue for as much as a centimeter. It is important to recognize this deep penetration of the infection if one is to treat the condition intelligently; the futility of applying medication to the surface of the cervix in attempting to eradicate the infection is obvious. From histologic examination of innumerable cervices we conclude that the term *endocervicitis* should be abolished. Even though there is no visible evidence of inflammation of the portio, the infection extends deep into the cervical tissue from the endocervix, and the term *cervicitis* describes the condition much more accurately. As a result of the deep infection of the glands, they are stimulated to hypersecretion of mucopurulent secretion, which is the source of the troublesome leukorrhea.

The appearance of the chronically infected cervix is extremely variable. It may appear quite normal through the speculum, even when a profuse discharge is pouring from the external os. When there is an old laceration, the appearance varies greatly, depending upon the amount of ectropion. The everted endocervix is deep red even when normal; when inflamed, it appears angry and often granular. This everted mucosa is exposed to the vaginal flora, and, if not originally infected, such a cervix is apt to become so. Small abrasions are common on the everted tissue, and rubbing the tissue with a cotton applicator frequently causes bleeding. The infection often results in sealing together the lumina of the cervical glands, and retention cysts result. These nabothian follicles may be numerous and range in size from a few millimeters to a centimeter. On palpation, such cysts are often felt elevated above the surface of the cervix as shotty nodules; the sensation is quite different from that encountered from friable, carcinomatous tissue. Upon opening the glands, they pour forth glary fluid, which may be quite clear or mixed with pus.

As a part of the routine gynecologic examination, the cervix should be inspected under good illumination. One of the dividends that has resulted from cytology is that it has made doctors "cervical inspection conscious." The appearance of the inflamed cervix, and especially the everted lacerated cervix, frequently makes biopsy of a suspicious area necessary to differentiate it from cancer. The microscopic criteria necessary to a diagnosis of early carcinoma are discussed at length in the chapter on cervical cancer in situ. There are certain benign lesions of the cervix that simulate malignancy, and a familiarity with these lesions is necessary to prevent serious errors in the histologic interpretation of biopsy specimens. Mistakes are commonly made in the interpretation of these lesions; hence many uteri are sacrificed unnecessarily. The lesion most often confused with early cervical cancer is *epidermidization* or *squamous metaplasia*. These two terms are applied to the condition because of a difference in the theories of its origin. Robert Meyer believes that during the healing process of cervicitis the stratified squamous epithelium creeps along the basement membrane beneath the columnar epithelium, lifting up and destroying the latter. The microscopic picture frequently seen would seem to support this theory. The term *epidermidization* would seem to be a suitable one for this process. The term *metaplasia* has arisen from the belief of some histologists that there is an actual metaplasia of the columnar cells into cells of the stratified squamous type. Novak doubted this theory but felt that some theory other than that of Meyer is necessary to explain the islands of stratified epithelium lying deep in the cervical glands, far removed from the stratified squamous surface epithelium, and having no continuity with it. He suggests the possibility that these squamous epithelial islands may arise from indifferent cells, beneath the cylindrical cells, possessing differentiation potentialities which permit them to develop into squamous epithelium. Regardless of the origin of this abnormal epithelium, the fact is that it may form patterns that simulate early cancer. This resemblance is most apparent under low power (Fig. 20-3). Under high power the cells look distinctly less active than those of early cancer (Fig. 20-4). Mitotic figures are absent or rare, hyperchromatosis is lacking, and the cells are uniform in size and staining qualities. To the inexperienced the low-power microscopic picture may strongly suggest cancer, but to the experienced gynecologic pathologist the picture is so familiar that it can be recognized at a glance. Nevertheless, in every case a careful high-power examination should be made for confirmatory evidence. The final answer to the malignant potentialities of these lesions can be determined only by a careful follow-up study of a series of women from whom such biopsy specimens were obtained. The senior author has made such a follow-up study, following the cases for several years. In no instance was it found that cervical cancer developed on the basis of pre-existing epidermidization or squamous metaplasia.

The treatment of chronic cervicitis should be considered from the point of view of its ability to produce an annoying discharge, to act as a focus of infection, to prevent conception, and to predispose to cancer. There is no doubt about the desirability of eradicating the source of the disagreeable discharge, and for this reason cervicitis is most frequently treated. There is one necessary word or warning. One should make certain before treating the cervix that it is the origin of the discharge, and that the discharge does not arise from the inflamed vagina. The question of treating cervicitis for the eradication of an infection that might be acting as a focus for some distant disease is not easily answered scientifically with certainty. Among good gynecologists and internists one encounters wide variation in opinion. There is no doubt that the cervix may harbor virulent streptococci, but the proof that they are responsible for the disease elsewhere is lacking.

The clearing up of a thick mucopurulent discharge is desirable as an aid to fertility, and we have seen pregnancies occur after doing so. On the other hand, how frequently does pregnancy take place in spite of a severe cervicitis with a profuse thick mucilaginous leukorrhea!

Finally, cervices which are the site of rather marked infection should be treated as prophylaxis against the development of cancer. There is definite clinical evidence that cervicitis in some measure predisposes to subsequent cervical malignancy. The subject is discussed in full in the chapter on cervical carcinoma, to which the reader is referred.

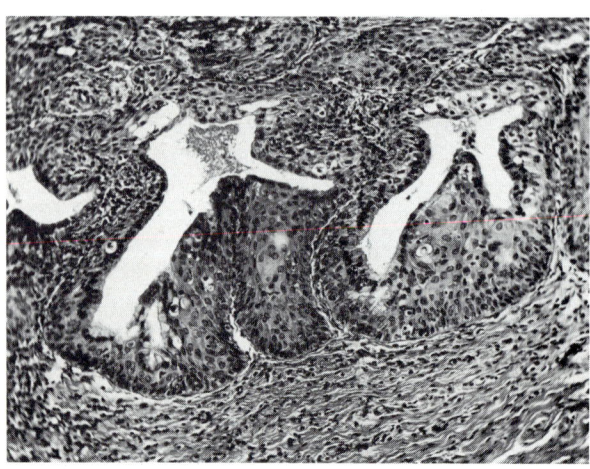

Fig. 20-3. Epidermidization or squamous metaplasia in cervical glands.

FIG. 20-4. Marked epidermidization in cervical polyp. (A) Low power, showing many epithelial pearls. (B) High power, showing benign nature of epithelial cells.

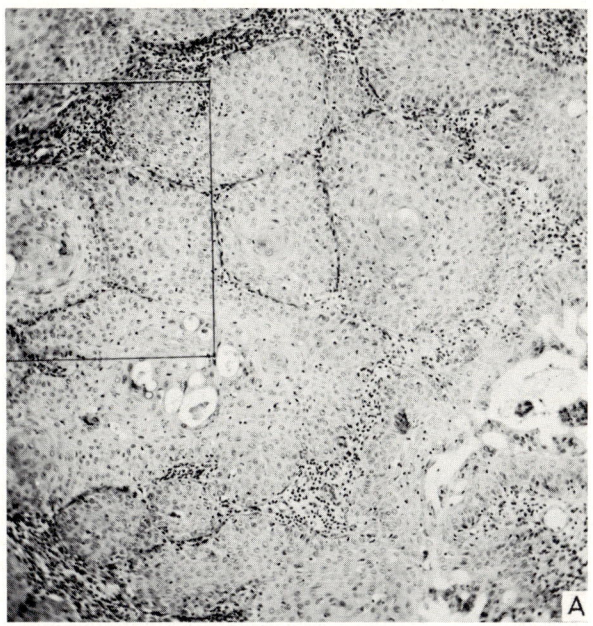

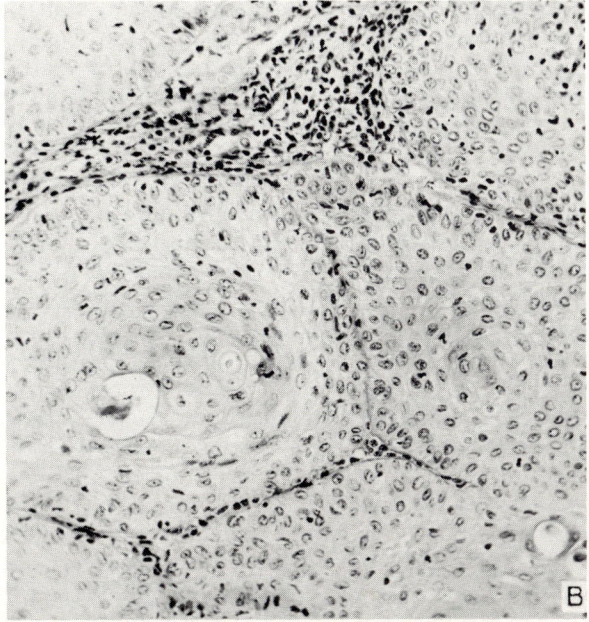

At the outset we should like to condemn the practice of total hysterectomy as a method of treating chronic cervicitis. It is done all too frequently when a lesser procedure will clear up the discharge. If the operator attempts to justify the major surgery on the grounds that the cervix is suspicious of malignancy, he is at fault. If the cervix is malignant, an ordinary total hysterectomy is not adequate treatment. If it is not malignant, the treatment has been excessive. Smear and proper biopsying of the cervix will definitely establish or rule out malignancy, and these procedures should be done before definitive treatment is undertaken.

The various procedures for the treatment of chronic cervicitis are considered later in this chapter. The operative procedures of cauterization, conization, Sturmdorf tracheloplasty, amputation, and trachelorrhaphy are evaluated in the light of our present experience.

STRICTURE OF THE CERVIX

Acquired stricture of the cervix is a common lesion, and its consequences may be serious. The most common etiologic factors in the formation of cervical stricture are the various therapeutic operative procedures directed at the cure of cervicitis. If these are performed improperly, or if the cervix is not taken care of adequately during the period of convalescence, complete or partial occlusion of the cervix, either at the external os or within the canal, may result. Conization of the cervix is more apt to result in stricture than cauterization. The circular scar, resulting from certain types of cervical amputation or radium applied for either benign or malignant uterine disease, may cause the cervical canal to contract and form occluding adhesions within its lumen. Likewise the normal menopause may so shrink the upper vagina and/or the cervix as to obstruct drainage completely. In addition to these etiologic factors, which are generally recognized as being responsible for cervical stricture, Curtis believed that any instrumentation of the cervical canal, such as curettage or instrumental abortion, may result in occlusion of the canal by adhesions. He also believed that gonorrheal disease is perhaps the commonest of all the causes of cervical stenosis. Our clinical experience has not brought us to agree with him, but we do admit the finding of cervical stenosis occasionally when nothing in the history gives a clue to its etiology. Our experience on the wards, where gonorrhea is very prevalent, and our laboratory examination of the uteri from patients operated upon for the residue of gonococcal disease have not led us to conclude that it plays an appreciable role in the subsequent development of cervical stricture.

Acquired cervical stenosis, occurring before the menopause, gives rise to severe dysmenorrhea and, if the occlusion is complete, hematometra, hematosalpinx, and hematoperitoneum result with severe lower abdominal pain and signs of peritoneal irritation. Brownish discharge during the month is common, as the retained uterine blood eventually finds its way through the cervical canal. The possible relationship of this condition to pelvic endometriosis is worthy of consideration but has not been proved. Adhesions in the cervical canal may cause pocketing of infectious material and be responsible for persistent purulent discharge.

After the menopause pyometra often, although not always, results from cervical occlusion (Fig. 20-5). Lower abdominal pain, fever, and a history of intermittent purulent discharge are common. On the other hand, we have noted on several occasions complete occlusion of the cervical canal in elderly women on whom operation for prolapse was being performed without pyrometra.

The treatment of cervical stenosis is thorough dilatation. Considerable searching and probing with the uterine sound or fine probe may be necessary to locate the external os or to find the passage into the uterine cavity. This is especially true in elderly women. When the occlusion is due simply to sealing together of the cervical lips externally, the membrane may be punctured and the external os easily dilated without anesthesia. This condition obtains not uncommonly after cervical cauterization and also spontaneously after the menopause. When there is stenosis higher in the canal, anesthesia must be resorted to in order to secure adequate dilatation. One must be governed in the degree of dilatation by the condition of the cervix. When the cervix is large and strong, as in the premenopausal woman, dilatation may be more vigorous than in the atrophic postmeno-

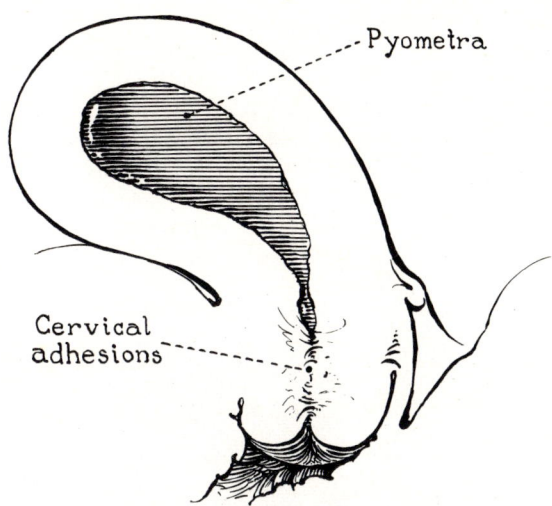

FIG. 20-5. Pyometra, resulting from benign cervical stricture due to postmenopausal cervical adhesions.

pausal cervix that may be torn easily. When pyometra is present, the least instrumentation necessary to secure drainage is the wisest. Even after simple cervical dilatation, there may be a flare-up of temperature. Endometrial or endocervical carcinoma is justly suspected in all cases of postmenopausal pyometra and particularly when the discharge is blood-tinged. However, curettage never should be done at the time of dilatation, but the patient should be given antibiotic therapy and return for curettage a month after the drainage has been established.

CERVICAL POLYPS

Cervical polyps are among the commonest lesions encountered in gynecology. They may be single, but multiple polyps are not uncommon. Cervical polyps may appear at any time after puberty, but they develop more frequently in the latter half of menstrual life and after the menopause. Etiologically, they are considered by most gynecologists to be dependent upon cervicitis, but this generally accepted view is difficult to prove, and we confess to some skepticism. Cervical polyps are commonly encountered in virginal women with no history of leukorrhea to cause one to suspect pre-existing cervicitis. Furthermore, chronic cervicitis is such a common lesion that the occurrence of polyps with it may well be coincidental. It is probably more nearly in keeping with scientific facts to admit that the cause of polyp formation on the cervix is as much unknown as the cause of other benign neoplasms.

The term *polyp* is strictly a morphologic one, and there is considerable variation in the histologic composition of different polyps. Most of them are pedunculated and connected to the cervix with a slender pedicle, but fibrous and fleshy elevations that are sessile probably represent polyps in the process of growth. Most polyps arise from the endocervix; hence they are covered with a single layer of columnar epithelial cells. Like the endocervix, such polyps are deep red in color (Fig. 20-6) and bleed easily on contact. Histologically, they are tree-like structures, rich in glands with connective tissue cores that are composed of loose connective tissue with many blood vessels (Fig. 20-7). Much less commonly, polyps arise from the vaginal surface of the portio. These are grossly different in appearance as well as histologically. They are light pink in color due to the fact that they are covered with thick squamous epithelium. The pedicle connecting a polyp of this type with the cervix is apt to be thicker than that of the endocervical polyp, and the whole structure is firm and fibrous (Fig. 20-8). Glands do

394 Nonmalignant Cervical Lesions and Their Treatment

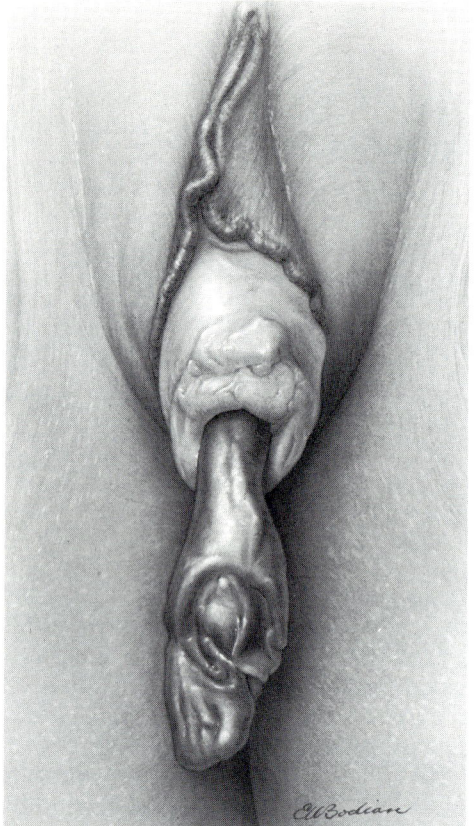

FIG. 20-6. Large cervical polyp arising from endocervix associated with prolapse of the uterus.

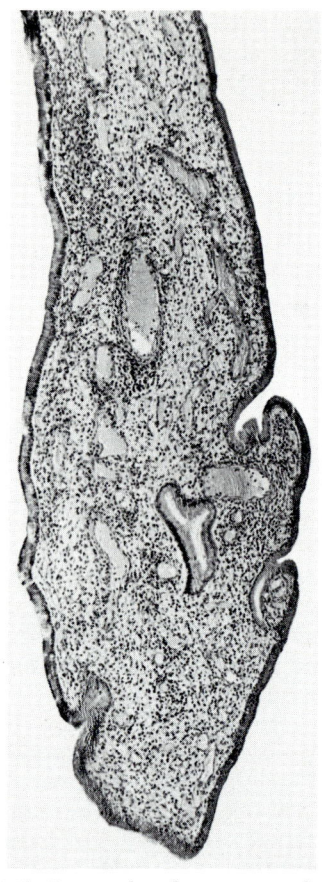

FIG. 20-7. Cervical polyp arising from endocervix.

occur in polyps of this type, but usually they are much sparser than in the endocervical polyp.

The relation of cervical polyps to malignancy deserves special consideration, for errors in the interpretation of the histologic patterns are not uncommon. The incidence of carcinomatous change in originally benign cervical polyps is very small, but such change does occur, making it desirable to examine histologically each cervical polyp that is removed. Also, on rare occasions an endocervical malignancy may protrude from the external os as a polypoid structure, resembling the ordinary benign polyp. Special consideration should be given to epidermidization or squamous metaplasia in relation to cervical polyps, for the condition is extremely common in polyps, and not infrequently it is erroneously diagnosed as malignant. Figure 20-4 shows extreme squamous metaplasia with pearl formation that occurred in a benign polyp. The patient from whom this polyp was removed was followed for over 10 years and remained free from symptoms. The rules for distinguishing between malignancy and benignancy in cervical polyps are the same as those for elsewhere in the cervix, and because of the great incidence of cancer-like benign changes in polyps, it is important always to bear them in mind.

Cervical polyps are often entirely asymptomatic and are incidental findings in the course of routine pelvic examinations. Freedom from symptoms is much

Fig. 20-8. Removal of large polyp with heavy pedicle by cautery. Dotted line indicates line of excision.

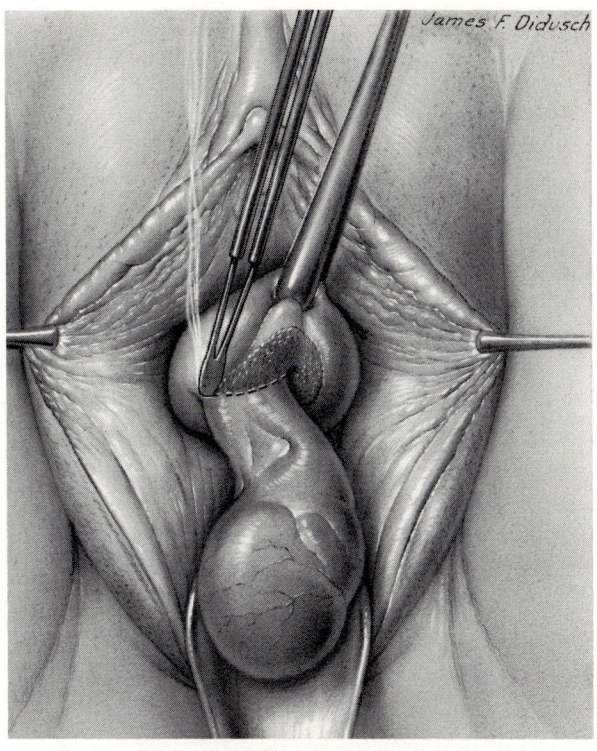

more apt to be the case when polyps arise from the surface of the cervix than from the endocervix. Endocervical polyps are much more liable to ulceration and infection; hence mucopurulent discharge results that is often blood-tinged. A common history is one of spotting a few days before and after the menstrual periods or after coitus.

The finding of a cervical polyp, symptomatic or asymptomatic, is indication for its removal and microscopic section. A small polyp is easily twisted off with a Kelly clamp in the office or the outpatient department (Fig. 20-9). If a cervix is found to have a tendency to the re-formation of polyps, the patient should be anesthetized and the cervix well dilated, so that the canal can be thoroughly curetted and the site of polyp formation touched with the cautery. Often a radial cauterization is necessary to clear up the accompanying cervicitis. Large polyps with broad fibrous pedicles arising from the portio may be best removed by the cautery (Fig. 20-8).

LEUKOPLAKIA OF THE CERVIX

Leukoplakia of the cervix (Fig. 20-10) has been much discussed in recent years as a possible precancerous lesion. There is little unanimity of opinion on the microscopic picture as well as the interpretation of leukoplakia in its relation to cancer. In the opinion of the authors the term *leukoplakia* should be considered only as a descriptive clinical term, indicating a white area on the cervix, without attempting to infer the presence of a particular microscopic picture. Biopsied leukoplakic tissue may show a variety of histologic pictures. In some specimens we have detected little, if any, change from the normal; in others there is simple hyperkeratosis with slight basal cell overactivity; in a very few we have found undoubted carcinoma in situ. It must be emphasized that most leukoplakic areas are not malignant, and Meyer believes that there is little or no justification for the belief that cancer develops on leukoplakic areas any more than on cervical

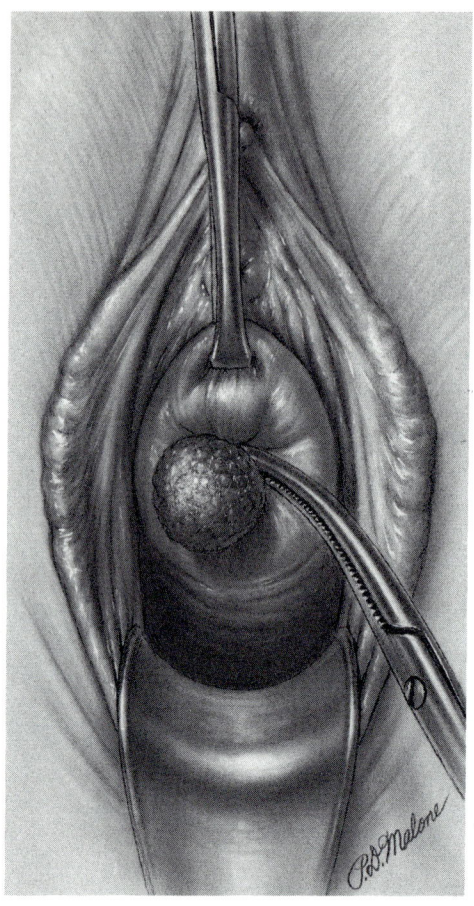

FIG. 20-9. Polyp attached to endocervix. Pedicle grasped with Kelly clamp and about to be twisted off.

to page 152. When benign disease of the cervix alone is the cause for operation, the following procedures are useful, provided that the indications and the contraindications discussed with each procedure are observed.

CAUTERIZATION OF THE CERVIX

In 1906 there appeared in the *Journal of the American Medical Association* an article on "The Treatment of Leucorrhea with the Actual Cautery" by Guy L. Hunner. This article was destined to initiate the general use of the actual cautery in modern gynecology for the treatment of chronic cervicitis. Although many other procedures have been proposed and used from time to time, cervical cauterization still remains the most generally useful method at our disposal, while some of the other procedures have been discarded or have continued to be used on special indication. Hunner's method was "cauterization by deep radial incisions," and this *method* has made cauterization popular by virtue of its excellent results. At the time of his original publication in 1906, Hunner was not aware that the actual cautery had been used upon the human cervix. Later he became interested in ascertain-

polyps. From a practical point of view the question boils down to the advisability of biopsying all leukoplakic areas. We believe that this should be done, just as we biopsy cervical polyps, and in a very small percentage early cancer will be found.

OPERATIVE PROCEDURES

The various operative procedures for the eradication of benign cervical disease are discussed in the following pages. It is understood, of course, that the complete elimination of the cervix by total hysterectomy is desirable *when hysterectomy is otherwise indicated.* For a consideration of this the reader is referred

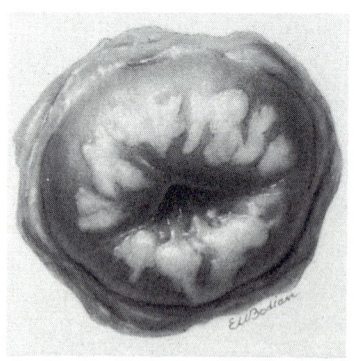

FIG. 20-10. Leukoplakia of the cervix. All of the leukoplakic areas in this case proved to be intra-epithelial carcinoma, but real invasive carcinoma was found on cutting up the whole cervix.

ing whether or not anyone had preceded him with this idea. In 1935 he published "A Historical Summary" on the subject.

The following quotation from Hunner's historical sketch indicates that the use of the cautery is hardly a modern innovation, but that it had been used extensively and abandoned at a much earlier period because of generally unsatisfactory results:

According to the English gynecologist, James Henry Bennet, Celsus used the actual cautery for treating ulcers of the prolapsed uterus. About the middle of the last century Jobert de Lamballe, the talented Paris surgeon, used the actual cautery in treating the ulcerated cervix as well as in cases of severe inflammatory hypertrophy. Bennet says that Jobert always used the conical ivory speculum to protect the vaginal walls from the radiated heat, but this "is not, however, indispensable. One or two olive-shaped cauteries, heated to whiteness, may then lie extinguished on the part of the cervix which has to be cauterized. An eschar, more or less deep, is thus formed, as by cauterization with *potassa fusa*. It is necessary that the cautery should be brought to a white heat, or otherwise it adheres to the tissues on being withdrawn. But little pain is experienced by the patient, either at the time or subsequently, the eschar falling off from the sixth to the tenth day, according to the depth of the cauterization. When the actual cautery is used to remove inflammatory hypertrophy, two or more cauterizations may be necessary to restore the neck of the uterus to its natural size."

It appears from Bennet's discussion of the relative merits of the actual cautery and the Vienna paste (which Bennet preferred) that both methods involved the entire circumference of the cervical canal, and unless used with discretion, serious stenosis resulted. It is probable that the preponderance of bad results in the hands of the profession at large finally led to the practical abandonment of these methods so successfully practised by a few discreet surgeons as far back at 1840.[*]

Hunner's contribution is the introduction of a *method* of cauterization by which the disadvantages, which led to the abandonment of the use of the cautery on the cervix, were overcome. His method consists of making deep radial strokes for the destruction of the deep cervical glands with the surrounding areas, leaving enough healthy stroma between the cautery strokes to ensure against future stenosis and dystocia. The necessity of fairly deep strokes becomes obvious if one is familiar with the histology of the cervix. The bases of the racemose glands lie as much as a centimeter deep in the cervical stroma, and superficial cauterization destroys only the mouths of the glands and leaves the bases untouched.

Hunner first used the Paquelin cautery with quite satisfactory results, but later with the improvement in thermocauteries, he displaced the Paquelin cautery with a more modern type. Figure 20-11 shows the cautery that the senior author has found admirably adapted to cervical cauterization. It is inexpensive and rarely gets out of order. The small light bulb gives adequate illumination to visualize the cervix well, and the blades are sufficiently heavy to burn widely and deeply enough to destroy the glands. It is less clumsy than the larger cauteries in general use in operating rooms. Because of the ease with which it can be handled, it is admirably suited for office use without anesthesia.

Hunner originally advocated office cauterization without anesthesia. To the inexperienced, this might appear unnecessarily cruel, but there is a complete absence of heat-conducting nerve fibers in the cervix, and if one is careful to keep the cautery away from the vagina, there is no sensation of burning. The slight discomfort in the abdomen that some patients experience with it is due to the insertion of the cautery blade into the cervical canal. The same sensation can be reproduced by the insertion of a cold applicator. The absence of anesthesia is naturally an advantage, and we have practiced it extensively with satisfactory results. When the vagina is large and parous and the cervix large, lacerated, and patulous, the operation can be carried out with the greatest of ease. Also, in

---

[*] Hunner, Guy L.: The cautery treatment of cervicitis: a historical summary. Journal-Lancet, 55:59, 1935.

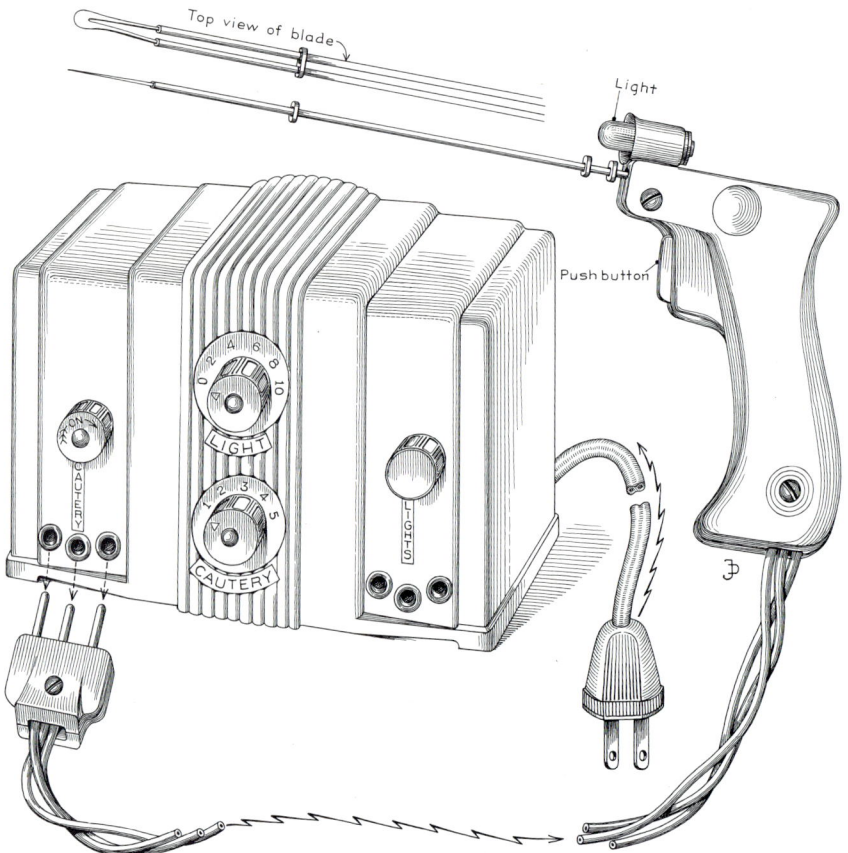

Fig. 20-11. Small cautery well adapted for cervical cauterization.

many nulliparous women it can be done quite satisfactorily, but when the cervical canal is of very small caliber, considerable dilatation may be a prerequisite to satisfactory cauterization, and this cannot be done adequately on the unanesthetized patient. The disadvantages of anesthesia were greater in the era in which Hunner published his views than they are today. Nitrous oxide and ether anesthesia are not pleasant to take, and even less pleasant on recovery. Intravenous Pentothal Sodium is pleasant both on administration and on recovery, and after cervical cauterization the patient may return to her home on the same day. When done under anesthesia, the cauterization is usually more thorough than when done on the unanesthetized patient, and in almost all instances only one cauterization is required. The ultimate result is usually as good when cauterization is done piecemeal on the unanesthetized woman, but since a period of sloughing of a few weeks follows each cauterization, the prolonged period in which there is a foul discharge is objectionable. However, in many instances the cauterization can be completed at once quite satisfactorily without anesthesia.

Following the cauterization there is an increase in vaginal discharge, and it is well to warn the patient of this. Within a day or two a watery discharge usually appears. As the burned tissues become necrotic and infected, the discharge increases and becomes foul-smelling. At about the 10th or the 12th day it is not unusual for the discharge to become tinged with blood, and in some instances there is real bleeding. Very rarely, alarming hemorrhage occurs which must be controlled by a tight vaginal pack. Douching, using some douche powder containing a deodorant, is advised, beginning 2 days after the cauterization. The patient should be warned not to insert the nozzle too high in the vagina in order to lessen the chance of initiating bleeding. When the discharge becomes very profuse and foul, 2 douches a day may be desirable. In approximately 3 weeks the sloughing is complete, and the discharge gradually is reduced as healing takes place. Complete healing usually requires about 5 weeks. Even though the cauterization is done by the proper radial method, precaution should be taken against resulting cervical stenosis. As prophylaxis against this, the patient is instructed to return a month after the cervix has healed completely. The patency of the cervical canal is then tested with a sterile uterine sound. If evidence of stenosis exists, dilatation is done. For this purpose the author uses a small pointed dilator (Fig. 20-12). Dilatation may be done quickly with this but not painlessly; however, the pain is momentary.

The value of cervical cauterization as prophylaxis against cancer is suggested by Scheffey, who states:

For many years I have made it a point never to leave a cervix uncauterized when performing supravaginal hysterectomy and in no instance, that I know of or learned later, did cancer develop in these cauterized cervices. In furthering this plan I treated all cervices alike, whether intact or attended by the trauma of childbirth, infection or congenital maldevelopment.*

Such a statement representing almost the entire lifetime experience of one who was in charge of an active gynecologic clinic is of great importance as evidence for infection as an etiologic factor in cervical malignancy. However, today, when total hysterectomy has become an

---

* Sheffey, L. C.: Definitive methods for the prompt diagnosis and management of pelvic malignancy—a prophylactic approach. First Asiatic Congress of Obstetrics and Gynecology, Tokyo, Japan, 1957.

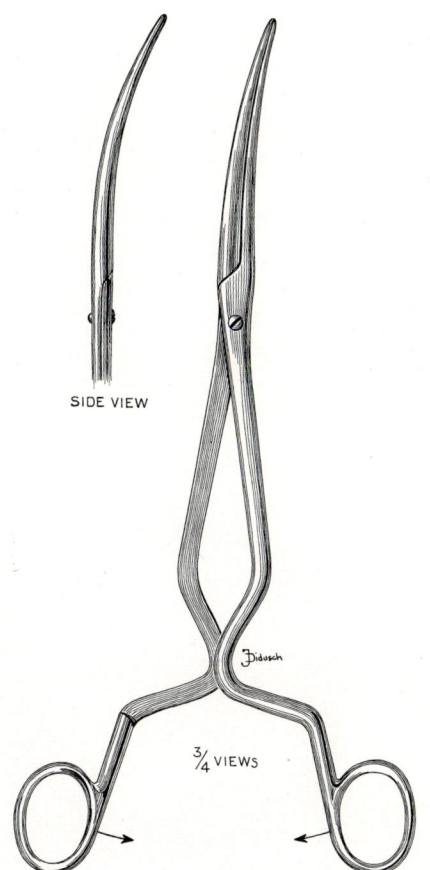

FIG. 20-12. Special pointed dilator, used to prevent cervical stenosis following cauterization.

almost routine procedure, it has less practical application.

TECHNIC:
CERVICAL CAUTERIZATION

If the cauterization is done under anesthesia, the cervical canal is thoroughly dilated; if done on the unanesthetized patient, little or no dilatation can be done. Deep radial strokes are taken with the very hot cautery blade (Fig. 20-13 B). These strokes are carried well up into the cervical canal. If there is considerable eversion of a lacerated cervix, the radial strokes are carried well out on the everted surface. After the radial cauterization, individual nabothian cysts may be destroyed as shown in Figure 20-13 C. The final result is usually a remarkably

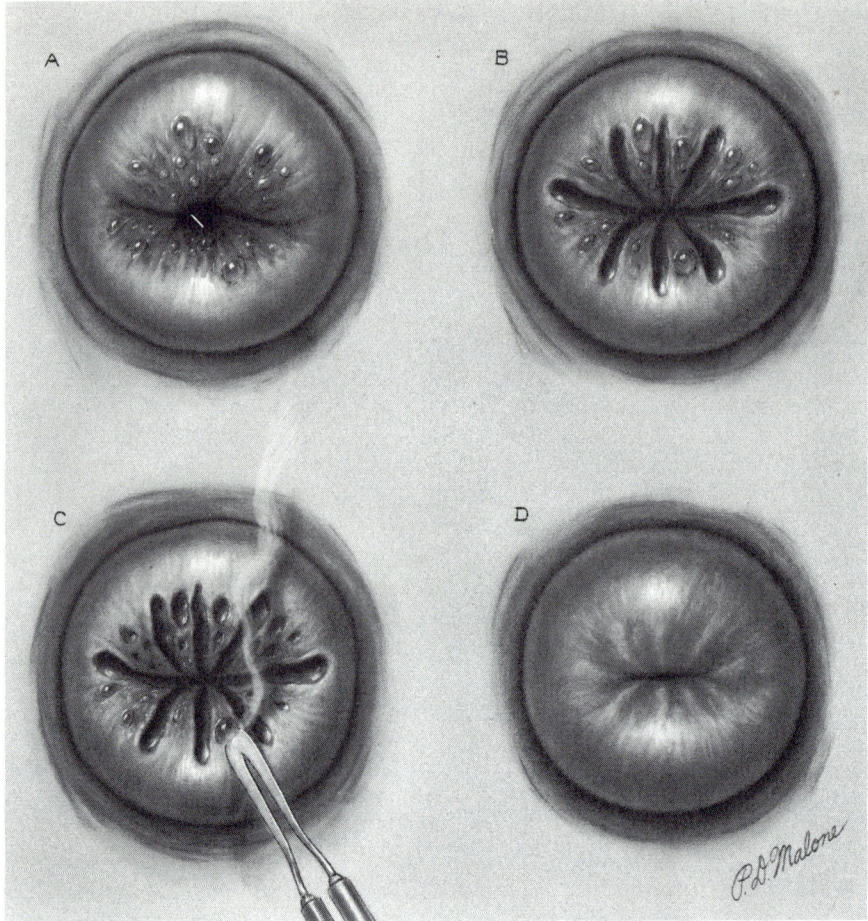

FIG. 20-13. Cauterization of cervix. (A) Indicates infected cervix with many nabothian cysts. (B) Indicates radial cautery marks. (C) Cysts are destroyed individually with cautery blade. (D) Appearance of cervix 6 months after cauterization.

normal-looking cervix (Fig. 20-13 D). If an ectropion of the cervix was present, the scars formed by the longitudinal strokes of the cautery tend to draw the lips inward. On the whole, the properly cauterized cervix will usually present an ultimate picture more nearly normal than the cervix upon which trachelorrhaphy or tracheloplasty has been done.

CONIZATION OF THE CERVIX

With the invention of the electrosurgical apparatus, conization of the cervix came into vogue, being used extensively in some clinics and very conservatively in others. We have definitely been on the conservative side, but we believe that the procedure is of value, provided that it is used with proper indications. Since our series of "hot" conized cervices is too small to be of any statistical value, we prefer to evaluate the results from a clinic in which the procedure has been used more extensively. Miller and Todd have reported on a series of 899 conizations done from 6 months to 3 years before the follow-up study. Of these, 747 were done before and 152 after the menopause. No immediate serious complications occurred in the 899 cases. Strictures of the cervix, sufficiently severe to necessitate return for dilation, occurred in

6.46 per cent; probable strictures, as judged by answers to questionnaires, occurred in 2.47 per cent. Usually the strictures that were treated were mild, but there were some in which the entire canal was obliterated by dense scar tissue. Miller and Todd also concluded from a small series of cases in which pregnancy followed conization that the effect on pregnancy was in general harmful. The harmful effect was chiefly in the direction of premature labor and abortion rather than cervical dystocia, as might have been anticipated. Eighteen per cent of the women who became pregnant had premature labor, and in 13.6 per cent the pregnancy ended in abortion.

Very occasionally we have found conization of the cervix a useful procedure in connection with subtotal hysterectomy. Since today total hysterectomy is an almost routine procedure, it is seldom used. However, there is the occasional case in which hysterectomy is done for salpingitis and for myomata, in which total hysterectomy is extremely difficult. Discretion may be the greater part of valor, and the operator may wisely settle for a subtotal hysterectomy. Hot conization of the cervix will eliminate the infected cervix and a troublesome discharge.

As discussed in Chapter 33 on carcinoma in situ, we frequently do cold conizations to establish a diagnosis of that disease. Cervical cauterization, especially in the nulliparous woman, can result in stenosis, and therefore it should not be done unless there is a sound reason on a pathologic basis.

Technic

The technic of "hot" conization is very simple. Hospitalization is desirable but not absolutely necessary. We usually administer Pentothal Sodium intravenously and place the patient in the lithotomy position. The cervix is exposed with a proper speculum, grasped with a tenaculum and drawn toward the outlet. The tip of the instrument is placed against the external os, and the combined cutting and coagulating current is turned on. The wire cuts into the cervix to the desired depth, and the instrument is twisted, thus enucleating a cone of endocervix and leaving a base of coagulated tissue that is usually quite dry (Fig. 20-14). As after cauterization, about 6 weeks is usually required for sloughing and complete epithelialization. A small gauze wick is placed in the cervical canal for 24 hours unless hysterectomy is to follow conization immediately. The patient is advised to use a daily cleansing douche, beginning about the 4th day after the conization, for at this time a blood-tinged discharge usually begins. She is advised to return for observation every 2 weeks. At the time of observation the cervical ulcer is swabbed with Merthiolate solution (1-1,000), and a small sound is passed through the cervical canal. If a tendency to stenosis is noted, larger Hegar dilators are passed. We believe that this follow-up is most essential in the prevention of subsequent stricture. At the end of about 6 weeks the coned-out area is usually covered with healthy-looking mucosa, and most of the cervical discharge has disappeared.

AMPUTATION OF THE CERVIX

The operation of amputation of the cervix is rarely done by the authors except in combination with certain operations for prolapse, such as the Manchester, the Interposition, and the Richardson Composite operations. It has long since been abandoned as the usual method of treating cases of chronic cervicitis with or without cervical laceration.

To justify our present attitude toward amputation it is necessary to view the operation historically. It was first widely practiced by the French surgeons as a routine means of treating prolapse. Marion Sims, in 1866, advocated the operation for prolapse and also for inflammatory disease of the cervix. He did the operation in young as well as older women and did not believe that it interfered with subsequent pregnancies. T. A. Emmet stated categorically that the operation had no effect on fertility, pregnancy, or labor. Important as these men

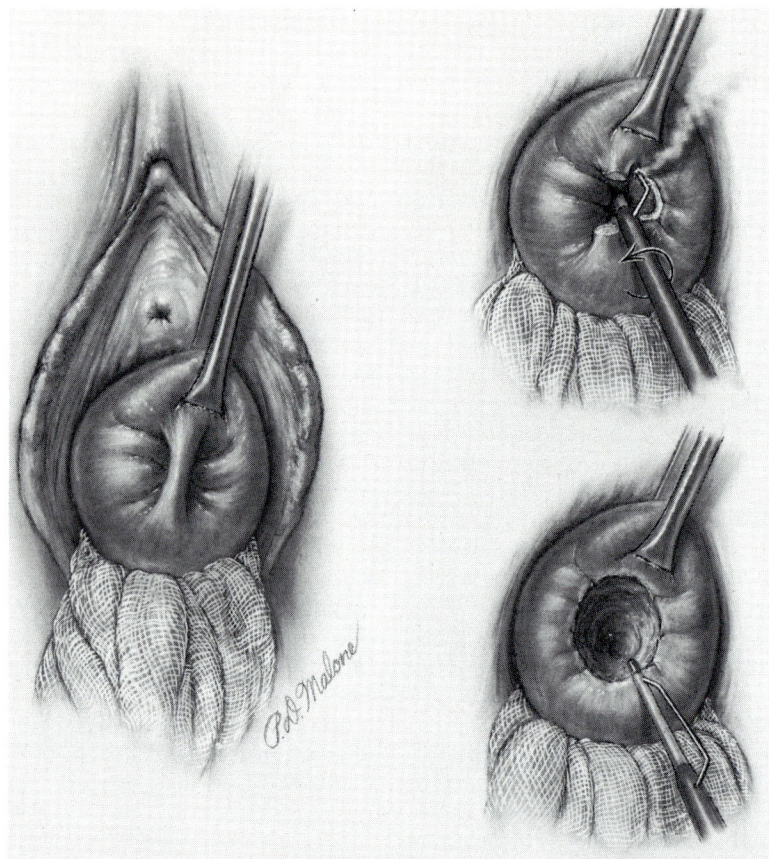

Fig. 20-14. Conization of cervix. (*Left*) Shows condition of lacerated cervix. (*Top*) Electrosurgical coning instrument is inserted into cervical canal and rotated. (*Bottom*) Showing cervix from which cone of tissue has been removed.

were in their chosen field during their epoch, it is apparent that their fondness for this operation was not based upon knowledge of the subsequent obstetric histories of their patients.

Audebert, in 1898, was one of the first to direct attention to the ill effects of cervical amputation. In a comparison between prenancies in the same women before and after cervical amputation he found a great increase in abortions, premature labors, and dystocia. Veador Leonard, in 1914, in an extensive analysis of the after-effects of cervical amputation on 128 women at the Johns Hopkins Hospital, found that four fifths of them who might have been expected to become pregnant remained sterile. Of those who became pregnant, 50 per cent had premature interruption of pregnancy, and of those proceeding to term, an even larger percentage had difficult labors. Carrying the idea of sterility to the extreme, Zoefgen even recommended high cervical amputation for sterilization.

A study of the subject which was made by J. J. Fisher in 1951 reviewed the pregnancies of women after cervical amputation. Before the operation 91 per cent of the pregnancies of these women had gone to successful conclusion, whereas after amputation only 21.5 per cent of the pregnancies ended successfully. The cesarean section rate went up from 0 to 57 per cent; the only surviving babies in the series were delivered by section. Vaginal delivery when attempted was characterized by either a prolonged first stage or an increased latent period between rupture of the membranes and the inauguration of labor.

From the above studies it is clear that amputation of the cervix in women who may subsequently become pregnant is to be condemned strongly. However, there is a selected group of cases in which the operation can be done to advantage; these are essentially women at or near the menopause, in whom there is marked cervical laceration, accompanied by severe infection and, in some instances, a tendency to polyp formation. In those women the question of childbearing need not be considered, and amputation or conization is the procedure of choice.

Every surgeon who has had experience in cervical operations, dating back a quarter of a century, is acquainted with the relative frequency of postoperative cervical hemorrhage and with the difficulty of controlling this at times. When hemorrhage occurs, it is usually from 7 to 14 days after the operation, at the time when the catgut begins to give way. As a rule, control of the bleeding is not easily accomplished by suturing the friable, vascular postoperative cervix. Because healing after such a secondary operation is tardy and accompanied by infection, the end result leaves much to be desired.

In 1916 Sturmdorf published his method of tracheloplasty. His operation is not a cervical amputation; indeed, one of the virtues claimed for it is this fact. Hence, he advocates it as the operation of choice in the childbearing period. The operation consists of coring out the infected glandbearing tissue that lines the cervical canal and of relining the canal with a flap of mucous membrane dissected free from the vaginal portion of the cervix. The typical Sturmdorf operation is done with much less frequency than formerly, since cervices that require a destruction of the glands of the endocervix are now treated in most clinics by the cautery or by electrosurgical conization; both of these procedures are discussed elsewhere in this chapter. In rare cases, however, in which cauterization has failed and in which there is a great excess of discharge from large numbers of intracervical glands, Sturmdorf conization may prove to be a curative procedure. It is also an excellent method of obtaining complete biopsy material from the region of the external os. We have adopted and applied the Sturmdorf principle of covering the raw surface with a flap of mucosa to the operation of amputation of the cervix and believe that it is superior to other types of amputation. The procedure described is usually less bloody than the average amputation, and postoperative hemorrhage is rarely encountered. The absence of postoperative hemorrhage is due to the fact that the flap of mucosa has healed to the raw surface of the shortened cervix by the time the catgut has become weakened.

Technic: Low Amputation of the Cervix

The operation is carried out more readily if the cervical canal is dilated before proceeding with the operation.

Step 1. A circular incision is made around the cervix (Fig. 20-15 A). The mucous membrane covering the vaginal portion of the cervix is dissected back. The point at which this incision is made depends upon the length of the cervix and the height at which the amputation is desired. The amount of mucosa freed must be estimated by the operator as sufficient to cover the shortened cervix.

Step 2. A suture of No. 1 chromic catgut is placed in both sides of the cervix to ligate the cervical branch of the uterine vessels (Fig. 20-15 B). If these sutures are well placed, there is usually very little bleeding when the amputation is done.

Step 3. Amputation of the cervix (Fig. 20-15 B). Usually no vessels need be ligated individually, but if there is a very active bleeder, it is best to transfix it, using No. 0 chromic catgut. A simple ooze from the cut surface is controlled by the apposition of the mucosal flap.

Step 4. Covering of the shortened cervix with the mucosa flaps (Fig. 20-15 C). Either the anterior or the posterior flap

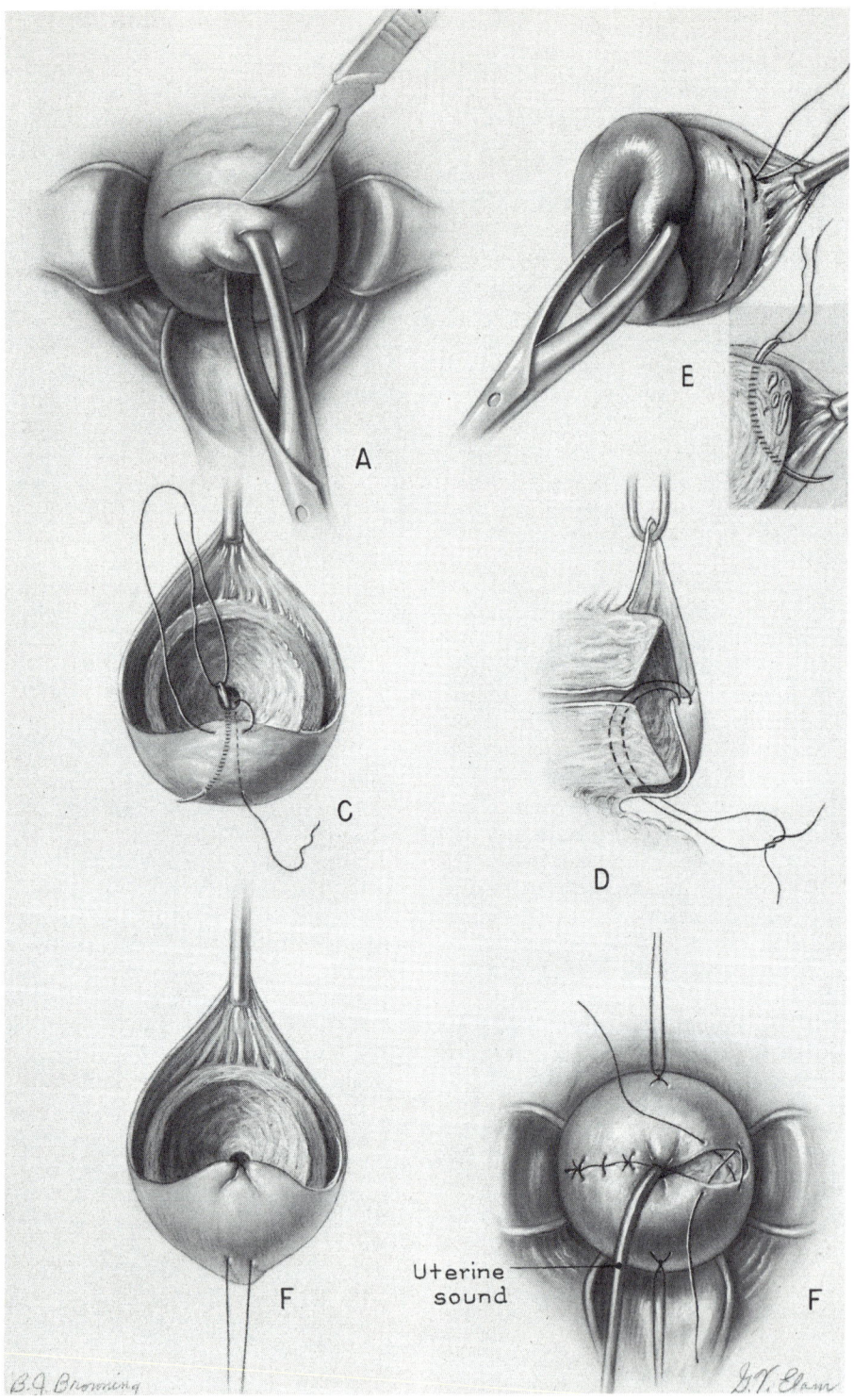

FIG. 20-15. Low amputation of cervix. (A) Circular incision through the mucosa. (B) Flaps of mucosa have been dissected back. Cervical branches of uterine vessels are ligated. The dotted line indicates level of amputation. (C) Mattress suture is being placed as in Sturmdorf tracheloplasty. (D) Demonstrating method of action of suture in drawing the flap into the canal. (E) The lower flap has been pulled into position. (F) Anterior and posterior flaps have been drawn into the canal. Lateral mucosa wounds are being sutured.

may be apposed first, depending on convenience. This is done by means of a mattress suture of No. 1 chromic catgut on a large cervical needle. The method of placing this suture is best demonstrated by observing Figure 20-15 D and E. The suture first picks up the anterior flap of mucous membrane in the midline. The suture is then carried into the shortened cervical canal, piercing the shortened cervix anteriorly and emerging into the vagina as the flap is pulled downward. Then the other end of the suture is threaded, and, in a similar manner, the needle is carried into the cervical canal and out, parallel with the first half of the suture. This mattress stitch is repeated on the posterior lip of the cervix. The edges of the mucosa flaps laterally are approximated and sutured with figure-of-eight or interrupted sutures, as is necessary. In making these lateral sutures it is well to take a bite in the subjacent portion of the cervix in order to obliterate dead space and thus ensure hemostasis. At the conclusion of the operation the cervical canal should be identified and proved patent by the insertion of a Kelly clamp or a uterine sound (Fig. 20-15 F).

Technic: High Amputation of the Cervix

When the cervix is markedly elongated, the above-described technic of low amputation will not remove sufficient cervix to accomplish the desired end. High amputation of the cervix is often part of the Manchester operation, or simple high amputation with cystocele repair may be the combination of procedures necessary to give the patient complete relief of her symptoms.

The amount of cervix desired to be removed is decided upon, and a circular incision is made through the mucosa, estimating the amount of mucosal flap needed to cover over the shortened cervix. The flap is dissected free around the circumference of the cervix (Fig. 20-16). In the elongated cervices, upon which this operation is most often done, the bases of the broad ligaments are often much elongated. Therefore the broad ligament base is clamped with an

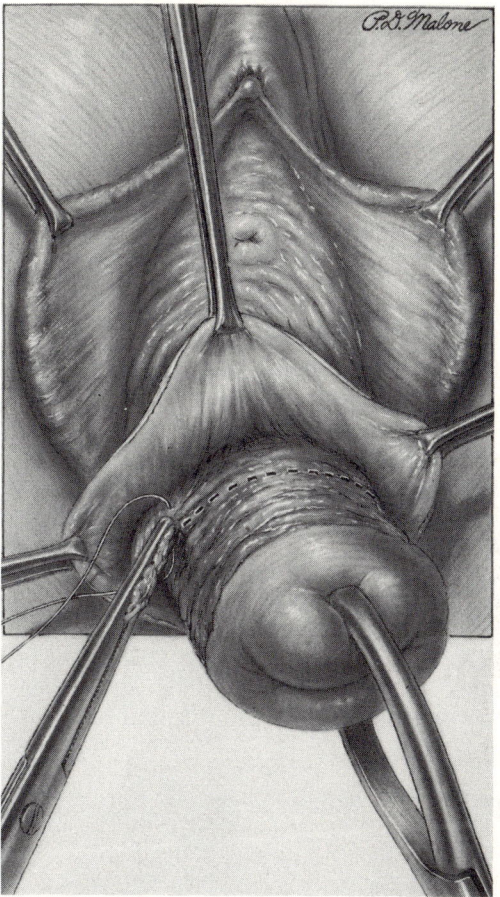

Fig. 20-16. High amputation of cervix. The lowermost portion of the broad ligament has been clamped and cut. It is about to be sutured with No. 1 chromic catgut.

Ochsner clamp, parallel with the side of the cervix, and cut. The ligament containing the cervical branch of the uterine vessels is transfixed with a suture of No. 1 chromic catgut. If the cervix is greatly elongated, a second bite of broad ligament may be taken. In placing the suture it is well to bite well into the side of the cervix. If this is done, the amputation is relatively dry, and no further hemostasis is necessary in most cases than that effected by the suturing of the flaps over the cut surfaces of the shortened lips. This step is repeated on the opposite side. If a Manchester operation is to be done, the bases of the broad ligament are brought together in front of the shortened cervix. Covering of the shortened cervix is carried out as described and illustrated in low cervical amputation.

Technic: Sturmdorf Tracheloplasty

A circular incision is made about the rim of the cervix, and by blunt and sharp dissection a flap of mucosa is freed about the entire cervix. Mayo scissors and the handle of a scalpel are excellent instruments for this maneuver. Figure 20-17 A shows the flap completely free.

The region of the external os is grasped with an appropriate instrument. In the illustration a Jacobs clamp is used for this, but this is too large an instrument in some instances, and an Ochsner clamp or even an Allis clip may fit the individual case better.

A cone or core is dissected out of the cervix as shown in Figure 20-17 B. The apex of the cone should be at approximately the level of the internal os. Thus most of the endocervical glands are removed. A small-bladed scalpel is well suited to this task.

The next step is the relining of the cervical canal with the previously prepared mucosa flaps. It is our custom to utilize first the posterior flap. No. 1 chromic catgut, threaded on a large cutting needle, is best suited for the so-called Sturmdorf stitch, which is in reality simply a mattress suture. The posterior flap of mucosa is first picked up in the midline near the edge. One end of the suture is carried up into the cervical canal with the cutting needle and out through the posterior lip of the cervix, as the mucosa flap is pulled forward. Then the other end of the suture is threaded into the cutting needle, and the process is repeated. The two ends of the suture should emerge on the posterior surface of the cervix about 5 or 6 mm. apart (Fig. 20-17 C).

When this suture is pulled taut, the posterior mucosa flap is pulled well into

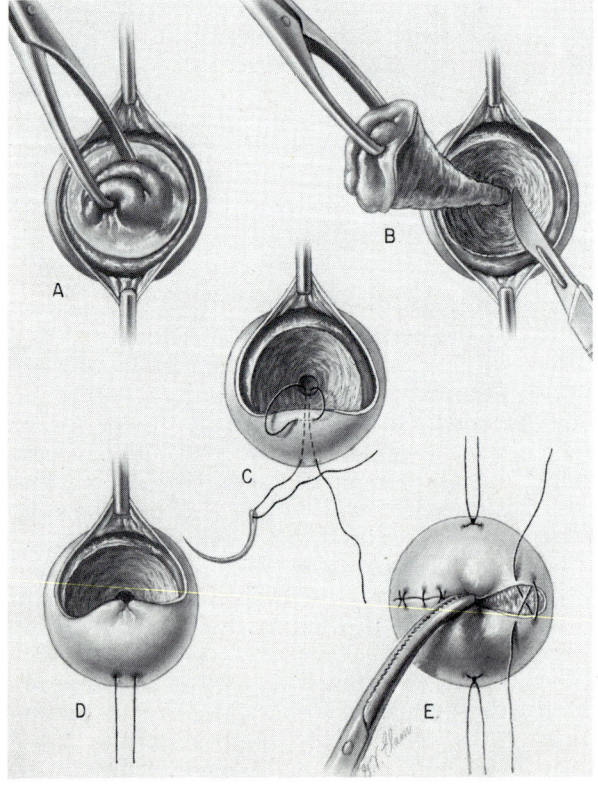

Fig. 20-17. Sturmdorf tracheloplasty. (A) The circular incision has been made, and mucosal flaps are freed. (B) A cone containing the endocervix is excised. (C) Mattress suture has been placed to cover the posterior lip with mucosal flap. (D) Mattress suture has been pulled tight, drawing the mucosal flap into the cervical canal. (E) Mattress sutures are tied. Lateral mucosa edges are approximated.

the newly made cervical canal (Fig. 20-17 D).

This process is repeated on the anterior lip.

Sufficient mucosa is excised from the flaps laterally so that a neat closure may be effected. In some instances none need be excised; in other instances there is considerable redundancy. Approximation of the mucosa edges laterally is usually done with interrupted or figure-of-eight sutures of No. 0 chromic catgut. For the sake of hemostasis a bite is taken in the subjacent cervical tissue (Fig. 20-17 E).

SCHRÖDER AMPUTATION

Amputation of the cervix in a manner described by Schröder is still a favorite method in some clinics. It consists essentially of amputation of the anterior and the posterior lips after making a transverse incision, dividing the cervix up to the level at which amputation is desired. Each lip is then amputated in a transverse V-manner, after which the tissues are approximated with interrupted catgut sutures. The authors prefer the method of amputation previously described in this chapter, covering the raw area with a mucosa flap by using the Sturmdorf mattress suture. However, there is one condition in which the Schröder amputation of a single lip is an excellent procedure. When the anterior lip is greatly hypertrophied, bringing it low in the vagina, without actual descent of the uterus, its removal may be desirable. The Schröder amputation of the anterior lip serves very well for this. This condition may accompany a cystocele, and the Schröder hemiamputation combined with a radical repair of the cystocele leaves a very neat operative accomplishment. Hemiamputation by the Schröder method is shown in Figure 20-18.

TRACHELORRHAPHY

The operation of trachelorrhaphy as described and practiced by Emmet was among the commonest of gynecologic operations of several decades ago. Now

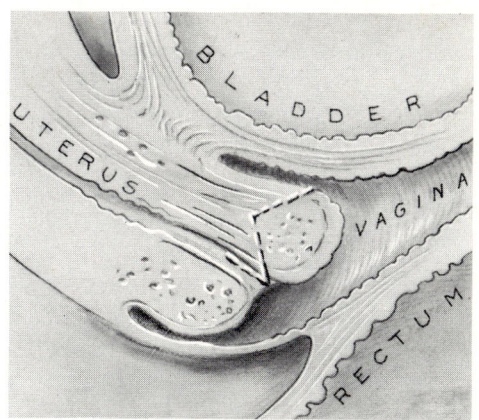

FIG. 20-18. Hemiamputation of cervix, Schröder method. Dotted lines show incisions.

it has been almost completely replaced by the other procedures discussed in this chapter. It consists essentially of denudation of the old laceration and suturing the denuded surfaces together (Fig. 20-19). It has the disadvantages of not removing all of the infected tissue that is responsible for the leukorrhea, and, from the standpoint of cancer prophylaxis, it does not remove all of the tissue about the external os which is most vulnerable to cancer. Surgically, there is the disadvantage that postoperative hemorrhage is not uncommon. At the conclusion of the operation the sutured cervix appears very neat, and the surgeon might compliment himself on his attainment. If hemorrhage occurs, it does so usually from the 10th to the 14th postoperative day. To attempt to control this by resuturing is difficult, because of the friable condition of the tissue at that time. If the hemorrhage is controlled by packing, the pack spreads the lips of the cervix further apart, and then slow secondary healing takes place. Viewing such a cervix after healing, one sees a much worse-looking cervix than was present before the operation, and nothing will have been accomplished. The cauterized cervix will usually appear infinitely more normal after it has completely healed.

In the past 25 years the senior author has performed a single trachelorrhaphy.

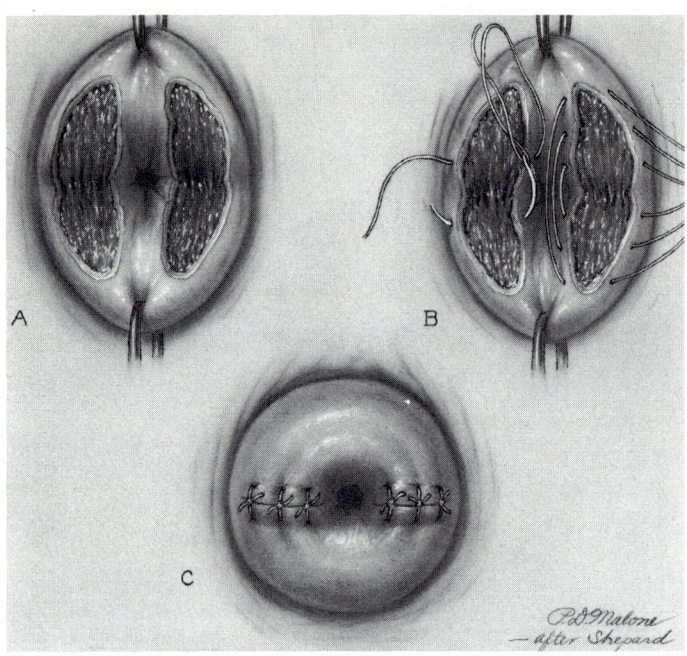

FIG. 20-19. Trachelorrhaphy. (A) Mucosa has been denuded from lateral tears. (B) Denuded surfaces are approximated with interrupted catgut sutures. (C) Sutures have been tied, restoring cervix to a normal appearance.

The indication was a very deep cervical tear in a woman who had had several premature labors at about 7 months. The deep laceration of the circular cervical musculature was thought to be a possible cause of the patient's inability to carry the child to term. Following the repair, the patient went to term with the next pregnancy. Because of the possibility of a rare indication for the operation, the technic is described here, but the operation today is chiefly of historical interest.

TECHNIC: TRACHELORRHAPHY

Since most cervical lacerations are of a transverse bilateral nature, the usual trachelorrhaphy is done by excising a V-shaped piece of tissue on each side, denuding the bilateral defects (Fig. 20-19 A). Interrupted sutures of No. 1 chromic catgut are taken so as to approximate the denuded areas (Fig. 20-19 B). When the sutures are tied, the cervix is restored to practically a nulliparous appearance (Fig. 20-19 C).

BIBLIOGRAPHY

Audebert, J. L.: Étude sur la grossesse et l'accouchement après l'amputation de col. Amer. Gynec. Obstet., 49:20, 1898.

Curtis, A. H.: Pathology and treatment of chronic leukorrhea. Surg. Gynec. Obstet., 37:657, 1923.

———: Chronic pelvic infections. Surg. Gynec. Obstet., 42:6, 1926.

———: Obstructive lesions of the uterus and their complication. Surg. Gynec. Obstet., 60:930, 1935.

Emmet, T. A.: Laceration of the cervix uteri as a frequent and unrecognized cause of disease. Amer. J. Obstet. Gynec., 7:442, 1874.

———: Surgery of the cervix in connection with the treatment of certain uterine diseases. Amer. J. Obstet. Gynec., 1:339, 1869.

Fisher, J. J.: The effect of amputation of the cervix uteri upon subsequent parturition. Amer. J. Obstet. Gynec., 62:644, 1951.

Hunner, G. L.: The treatment of leukorrhea with the actual cautery. J.A.M.A., 46:191, 1906.

———: The cautery treatment of cervicitis: a historical summary. Journal-Lancet, 55:59, 1935.

Hunter, J. W. A.: Conservation of the cervix uteri in operations for prolapse, new operative technic. Brit. Med. J., 2:9991, 1939.

Leonard, V. N.: The postoperative results of trachelorrhaphy in comparison with those of amputation of the cervix. Surg. Gynec. Obstet., *18*:35, 1914.

Meyer, R.: Die Epithelentwicklung der Cervix und Portio Vaginalis Uteri und die Pseudoerosio congenita. Arch. Gynäk., *91*:579, 1910.

———: Die Erosion und Pseudoerosion der Erwachsenen. Arch. Gynäk., *91*:658, 1910.

———: Development of stratified epithelium from mucous cells at portio vaginalis uteri after erosion. Zbl. Gynäk., *47*:946, 1923.

Miller, N. F., and Malcolm, R. L.: An evaluation of common cervical lesions. Amer. J. Obstet. Gynec., *35*:990, 1938.

Miller, N. F., and Todd, O. E.: Conization of cervix. Surg. Gynec. Obstet., *67*:265, 1938.

Novak, E.: Pathologic diagnosis of early cervical and corporeal cancer with special reference to the differentiation from pseudomalignant inflammatory conditions. Amer. J. Obstet. Gynec., *18*:449, 1929.

Scheffey, L. C.: Definitive methods for the prompt diagnosis and management of pelvic malignancy — a prophylactic approach. First Asiatic Congress of Obstetrics and Gynecology, Tokyo, Japan, 1957.

Schröder, R.: Die Anatomie der chronischen Cervixgonorrhöe. Zbl. Gynäk., *55*:3429, 1931.

Sims, M.: Amputation of cervix. Trans. Med. Soc. New York, 1861.

Sturmdorf, A.: Tracheloplastic methods and results: A clinical study based upon the physiology of the mesometrium. Surg. Gynec. Obstet., *22*:93, 1916.

Te Linde, R. W.: Amputation of the cervix with application of the Sturmdorf flap principle. Surg. Gynec. Obstet., *43*:513, 1926.

———: Cancerlike lesions of the uterine cervix. J.A.M.A., *101*:1211, 1933.

Zoefgen, W.: Sterilisierung durch hohe Cervix Amputation. Zbl. Gynäk., *60*:737, 1936.

21

Dilatation of the Cervix and Curettage of the Uterus

DILATATION OF THE CERVIX

INDICATIONS

Dilatation of the cervix is carried out as a preliminary step to curettage of the uterine cavity. As a therapeutic measure it is done for acquired or congenital cervical stenosis, for dysmenorrhea, for sterility in connection with the Rubin's test, to permit the introduction of intracervical and intra-uterine radium, and as a part of other operations on the cervix, such as trachelorrhaphy and amputation.

The reason for cervical dilatation in most of the procedures mentioned above is quite obvious. In connection with dysmenorrhea and sterility there is room for controversy, and a discussion of the subject is in order.

It is a recognized fact that many cases of dysmenorrhea are not cured by cervical dilatation. Because of frequent failures some gynecologists have almost abandoned it as a part of their therapeutic amamentarium. We do not subscribe to this totally pessimistic point of view. In most instances it is impossible to detect those cases of dysmenorrhea that will be relieved by cervical dilatation. Often the operation must be done as a therapeutic test, but fortunately it is such a minor procedure that one is justified in performing it on that basis. Those cases of dysmenorrhea that occur in parous women may be eliminated immediately. If the dilatation resulting from the birth of the child has not relieved the menstrual pain, surely surgical dilatation will not do so. In the nulliparous woman who suffers most during the latter days of her period, there is little chance of relief by dilatation. In the nulliparous woman who suffers most just before the onset of the flow or during the early part of the flow, there is a possibility of relief from cervical dilatation. However, this is by no means certain, for this history is the commonest of all in dysmenorrheic women, not all of whom are relieved by cervical dilatation.

When acute anteflexion of the uterus is present, often there is an associated narrowing at the internal os, and dilatation gives relief in a fair percentage of such cases. There is no way of telling with certainty which women will experience relief and which will not. It is our clinical impression that about one third of the cases are relieved permanently of the greater part of their menstrual pain; one third are helped to some degree or temporarily, with a gradual recurrence of pain after some months; and about one third receive no help whatever. We make it a rule to acquaint the patient with these facts before proceeding with the operation and permit her to come to her own decision on whether or not her menstrual pain is sufficiently severe to justify an operation with this chance of success.

In sterility cases a slight dilatation of the cervix is usually necessary in nulliparous women in order to introduce the Rubin's cannula. Following the completion of the tubal insufflation, it is our custom to dilate the cervical canal thoroughly. We believe that benefit can be derived from this and base our belief on two observations. Before the era of Rubin's test, dilatation and curettage were done frequently for sterility. Although the results of this procedure were not as good as they are today by combining cervical dilatation with tubal insufflation, a certain percentage of the women with a long history of sterility became pregnant. Furthermore, one frequently sees pregnancy take place promptly after Rubin's test when the tubes were found open at a very low pressure. It is our opinion that such results are probably due, in most instances, to the cervical dilatation rather than to the passage of gas through normally patent tubes.

TECHNIC: CERVICAL DILATATION

The patient is placed on the table in the lithotomy position, and the vagina and the perineum are cleaned up with the usual technic. The cervix is grasped with a 4-pronged tenaculum (Fig. 21-1, *left*) and gently drawn to the outlet. A sound (Fig. 21-1, *right*), is passed through the cervical canal into the uterine cavity. This gives one exact confirmatory information on the position of the uterus and

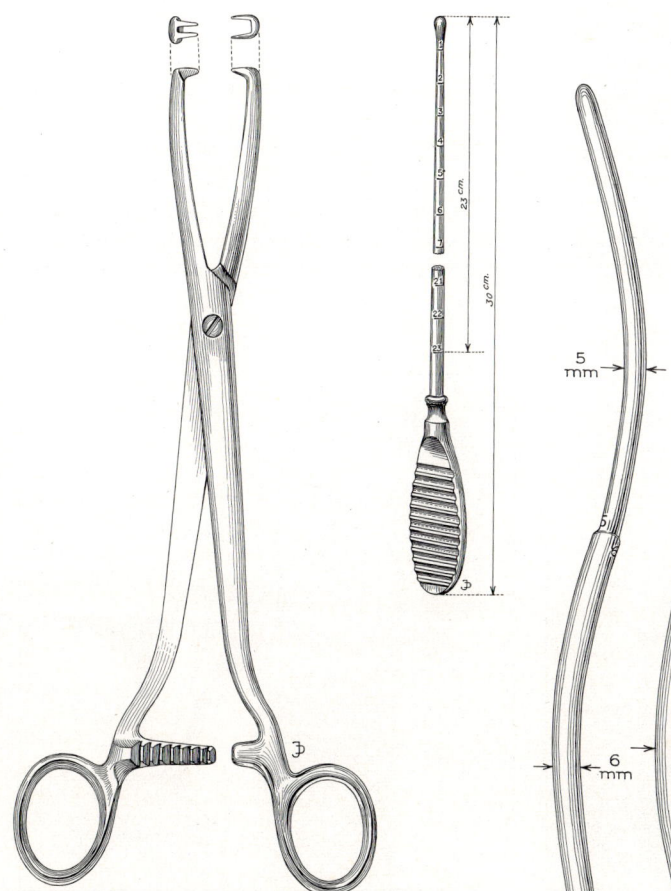

FIG. 21-1. (*Left*) Straight Jacobs clamp, used for pulling down cervix when performing curettage and for grasping cervix in doing subtotal hysterectomy. (*Right*) Uterine sound.

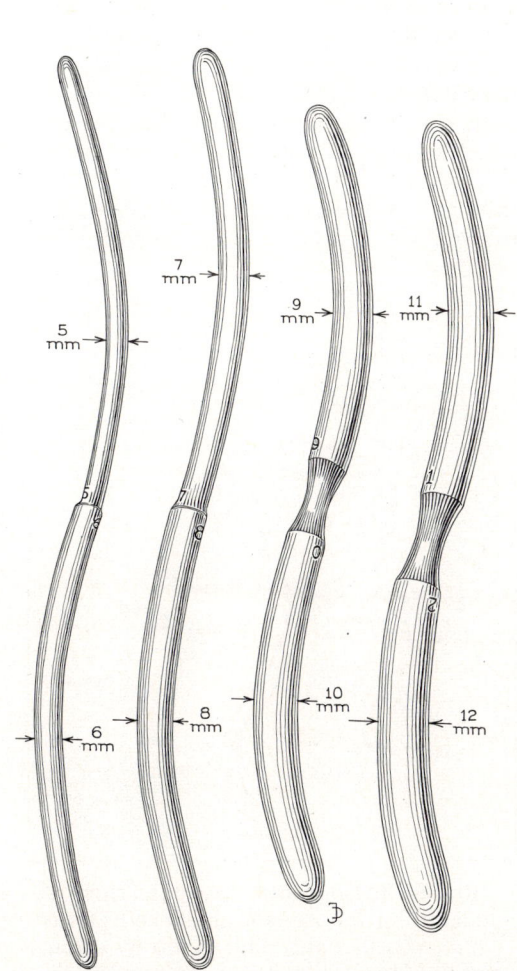

FIG. 21-2. Graduated Hegar dilators.

of the angulation between the cervical canal and the uterine cavity. An idea of the degree of stenosis of the cervical canal can also be detected in this manner.

Dilating the cervical canal is begun with a small Hegar dilator (Fig. 21-2). The uterine wall may be perforated by the improper use of a Hegar dilator; usually this is due to lack of knowledge or disregard of the position of the uterus. When acute anteflexion is present, the dilator may perforate posteriorly (Fig. 21-3). When retrodisplacement exists, the perforation usually takes place anteriorly (Fig. 21-4). (This complication may be avoided by sounding the uterine cavity prior to dilatation of the cervix.) It is rare that the dilator perforates the fundus except when there is a much atrophied postmenopausal uterus. After the small Hegar dilator is passed, successively larger ones are used. For ordinary curettage, dilatation to No. 8 or No. 9 Hegar suffices. When dilatation is done for dysmenorrhea or sterility, we prefer to carry the dilatation up to No. 10, but this is not always possible. When the internal os is dilated with difficulty, we generally use the Goodell dilator also (Fig. 21-5), stretching the os until the Hegar dilator of the next larger size can be passed. The Goodell dilator is a powerful instrument, and it must be used carefully. The danger is less of perforation, as with Hegar dilators, but of splitting the side of the cervix. If this occurs and results in appreciable bleeding, the laceration should be sutured.

When dilatation of the cervix is done for removal of placental tissue, dilatation up to No. 11 and No. 12 Hegar is often necessary to permit the introduction of a large blunt curette and placental forceps. We do not use the Goodell dilator on the soft pregnant or recently pregnant cervix because of the danger of tearing it, with resultant cervical incompetence.

CURETTAGE OF THE UTERUS

INDICATIONS, CONTRAINDICATIONS, AND ANESTHESIA

Curettage of the uterus is the most frequent of gynecologic operations and is generally regarded as a simple and

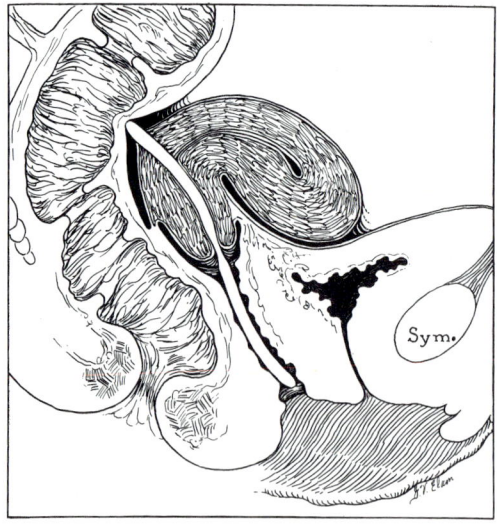

FIG. 21-3. Illustrating the possibility of puncture of the acutely anteflexed uterus which was thought to be in retroposition, and the Hegar dilator was erroneously directed posteriorly.

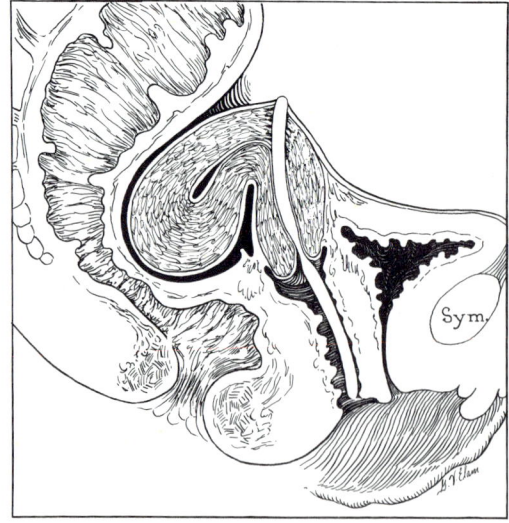

FIG. 21-4. Illustrating the possibility of puncture of the retroflexed uterus which was thought to be in anteposition, and the Hegar dilator was erroneously directed anteriorly.

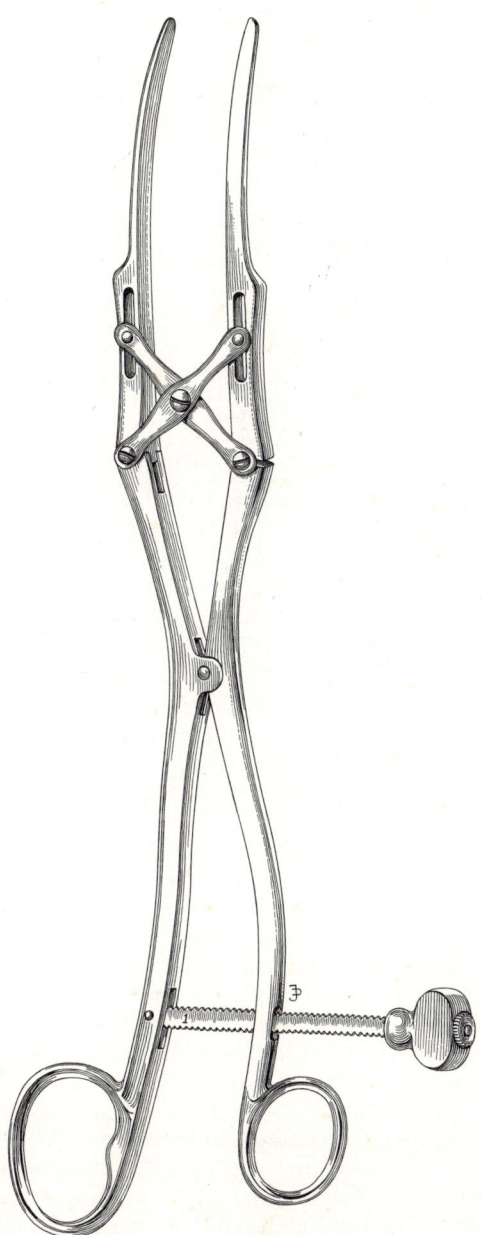

Fig. 21-5. Goodell dilator.

harmless procedure. Like most simple procedures, it may be done correctly or incorrectly. Nor is it entirely devoid of danger. A curettage done under proper aseptic technic carries with it very little risk, but if proper precautions are disregarded, complications, and even death, may result.

The chief purpose of curettage of the uterus is the removal of endometrial or endocervical tissue for histologic study in those cases in which there has been abnormal uterine bleeding. Thus a diagnosis of endometrial carcinoma may be made or excluded. When the bleeding is of a functional nature, a knowledge of the type of endometrium is of value in future therapy; in sterility cases a curettage done premenstrually will give definite information on ovulation during the current month. Curettage of the cervical canal is indicated when carcinoma of the endocervix is suspected in the intact uterus, in evaluating the possible spread of endometrial adenocarcinoma to the endocervix, or when bleeding takes place from a cervical stump.

In some instances curettage may be of great value therapeutically. The benefit to be derived from curettage in dysfunctional bleeding is discussed below. Certainly it is of great value for the temporary relief of profuse uterine bleeding. The endometrial polyp (Fig. 21-6) may be removed successfully by the curette or by polyp forceps, and it is our opinion that many cases of so-called dysfunctional uterine bleeding which are cured permanently by a single curettage are actually instances in which a polyp was removed by the curette. One of the chief therapeutic uses of the curette is the removal of retained placental tissue following abortion or full-term delivery.

The chief contraindication to curettage is infection. Acute cervicitis, acute salpingitis, and acute vaginitis all constitute conditions under which curettage should be avoided. Curettage of the infected endometrium should be avoided, also, but at times it must be done for the removal of retained placental tissue. Indeed, the endometritis associated with retained products of conception will fail to get well until the foreign material is cast off spontaneously or is removed by the curette. Frequently, curettage must be done through a chronically infected cervix; this is a safe procedure if proper precautions are taken to sterilize the vagina and the cervical canal.

Pentothal Sodium is the anesthetic that we have used for curettage almost ex-

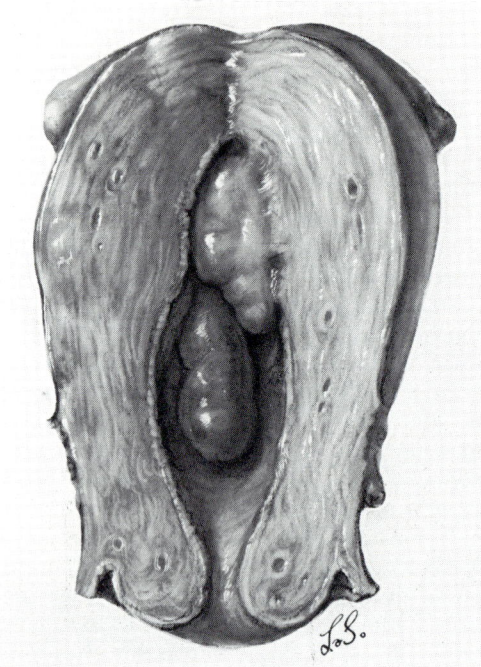

Fig. 21-6. Opened uterus, showing 2 separate endometrial polyps.

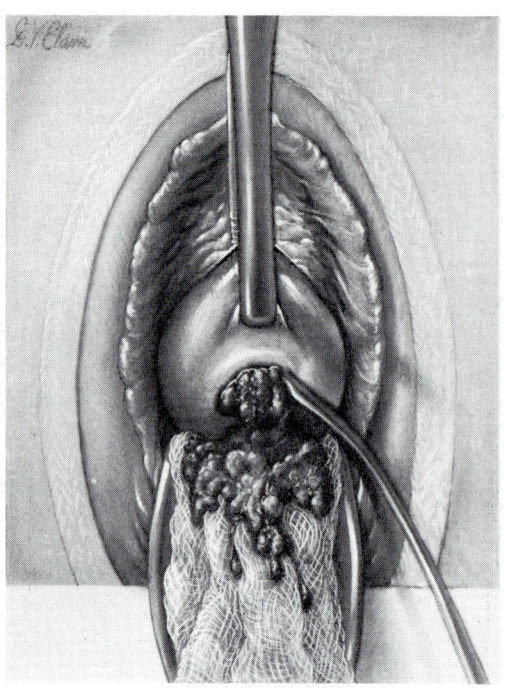

Fig. 21-7. Method of collecting curettings and blood on gauze.

clusively during the past several years. It is rapid in action, approaches almost complete safety if used properly, and recovery from it is almost entirely devoid of unpleasant effects. Of course, cyclopropane or nitrous oxide may be added at the discretion of the anesthetist. Also, relaxing agents may be used when further relaxation is necessary for a proper examination under anesthesia. On rare occasions, in feeble old women who have required curettage for postmenopausal bleeding, we have performed the operation with no other anesthetic than hypodermic administration of a sedative combined with a paracervical block.

Technic: Curettage of Uterus

After anesthetization, the patient is put in the lithotomy position, and the vagina is cleaned up with the usual technic. The cervical canal is then swabbed out with a small cotton pledget soaked in alcohol. This little refinement in technic we believe to be important, for the cervical canal is open to the flora of the vagina, and no matter how thoroughly the vagina may be cleaned up, the cervical canal remains contaminated unless special attention is given to it. The uterine cavity is always initially sounded in order to get an idea of its size and to confirm the impression of its position as received from examination under anesthesia. The cervical canal is dilated with Goodell and/or Hegar dilators as described in the previous section. A dilatation up to No. 9 or 10 Hegar is sufficient for the usual diagnostic curettage. A gauze sponge is placed within the vagina along the posterior retractor so that the blood and the endometrium removed from the uterus may fall upon it (Fig. 21-7). A small, bluntly serrated curette (Fig. 21-8) is then introduced into the uterus, and in a systematic manner the entire uterine cavity is curetted. The anterior, the posterior, and the lateral walls are scraped gently but firmly, and finally the top of the cavity is scraped with a side-to-side movement (Fig. 21-9).

The cervical canal should be curetted prior to curettage of the endometrial cavity if there is any suspicion of its being the site of malignancy or polyps. The Gusberg curette is a small, specially shaped instrument which is particularly useful in curetting the endocervix. The differential curettage of the endocervix, separate from the endometrium, is important in the diagnosis of endometrial carcinoma which may have extended to the endocervix (see endometrial carcinoma in Chapter 36, Carcinoma of the Corpus Uteri). Patients with postmenopausal bleeding are particular candidates for a differential curettage.

The unclotted blood is absorbed quickly by the gauze sponge, leaving the relatively clean endometrium to be placed in the small, wide-mouthed sterile bottle that is always on the instrument table. The curettings are placed immediately in the fixative, and the specimen is sent to the laboratory.

In addition to scraping the uterus, the curette is useful in exploring the uterine cavity for irregularities in its contour, such as may be caused by a submucous fibroid. In this way one may discover small fibroids that are entirely undetectable through bimanual palpation. Also in our clinic it has become a routine procedure to biopsy the cervix thoroughly whenever a curettage is done.

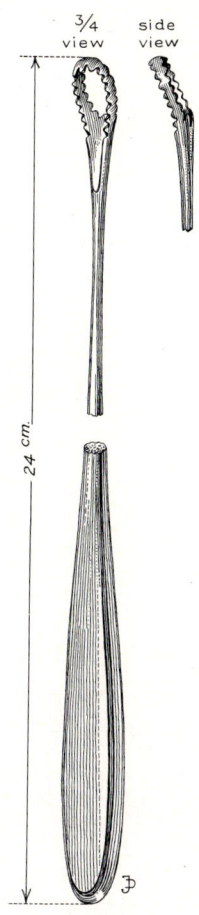

FIG. 21-8. Small serrated curette for routine curettage.

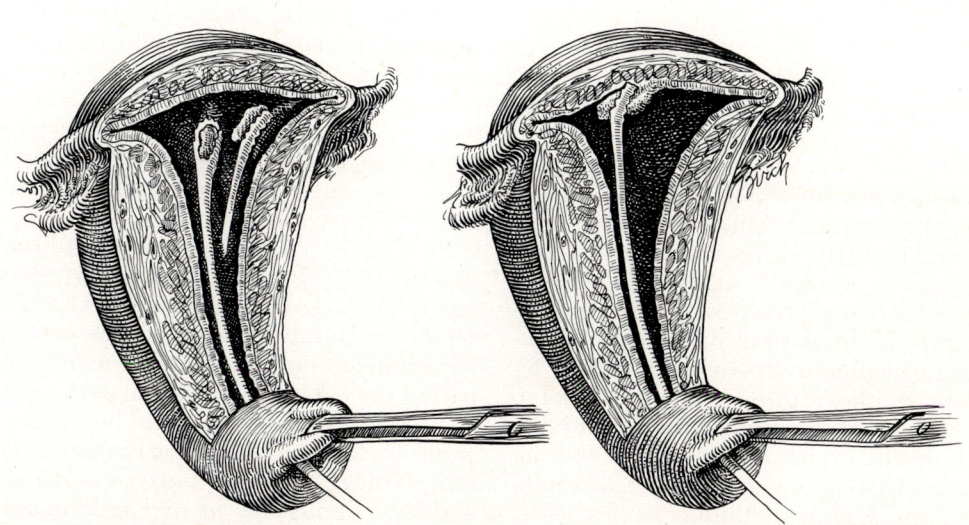

FIG. 21-9. Method of curetting uterine cavity systematically. (*Left*) Anterior, posterior, and lateral walls of cavity are curetted systematically. (*Right*) Then the top of cavity is curetted thoroughly.

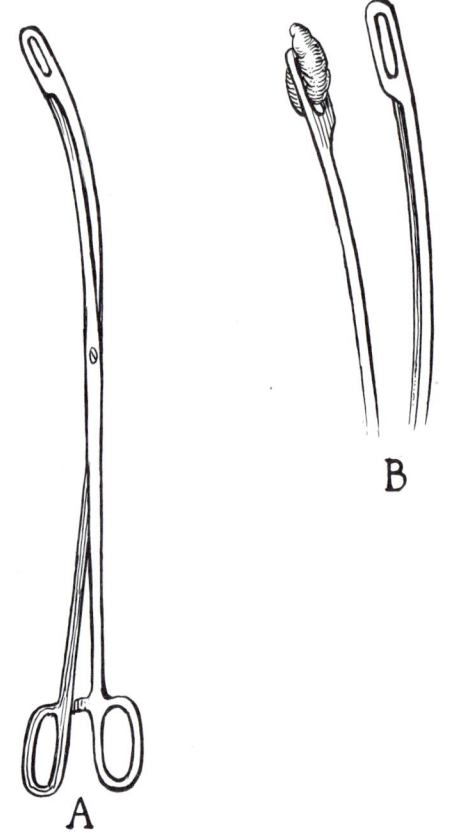

FIG. 21-10. (A) Ureteral stone forceps, an excellent instrument for removal of endometrial polyps. (B) Shows polyp which was missed at curettage, grasped in forceps.

This is discussed further in the chapter on carcinoma in situ.

It is important to explore the uterine cavity with a forceps at each curettage. One of the easiest things to do is to miss an endometrial polyp with an ordinary curette. As a result, many unnecessary hysterectomies have been done because of supposed persistent or recurrent functional bleeding following a curettage. By means of the routine use of the polyp forceps such operations may be avoided. It is easier to identify and remove an endometrial polyp if the uterine cavity is explored with the stone forceps (Fig. 21-10 A) *before* curetting the cavity. In a 28-month period on our service during which the forceps were used routinely, Josey found that the diagnosis of endometrial polyp was made 130 times. In 83 of these cases the polyp was removed by forceps (Fig. 21-10 B). Although the sessile form of submucous myoma is diagnosed easily by noting an irregularity of the uterine wall with the curette, the pedunculated variety, like the endometrial polyp, may escape detection because of its narrow stalk. Often such fibroids may be grasped with the polyp forceps. Likewise, often a congenital septum may be detected with the forceps.

When curettage is done as a curative measure for removal of placental tissue, a large, blunt, smooth curette is used to lessen the chances of perforation. The larger and softer the uterus, the larger should be the curette used, and the more careful should one be to avoid perforation. When large masses of placental tissue are present, the ovum forceps are most useful when used in conjunction with the curette.

PERFORATION OF THE UTERUS

If the position and the consistency of the uterus are carefully noted through bimanual examination under anesthesia before curettage is undertaken, perforation will rarely occur. When the position of the uterus is not known to the operator, perforation may occur with remarkable ease. Also in the senile atrophic uterus, perforation may be done with extremely slight force of the sound or the curette. Perforation is discovered by failure of the sound or the curette to encounter resistance at the point that it normally should do so, as judged by the palpated size of the uterus.

Perforation of the uterus by a small curette in performing an ordinary diagnostic curettage is usually not a serious accident. Curettage may not necessarily be stopped, but one should avoid that part of the cavity at which the perforation occurred. The patient should be watched carefully for signs of hemorrhage or infection. If signs of hemorrhage develop, the abdomen should be opened and the uterine wound sutured. If signs of infection develop after operation, penicillin therapy should be intensified and fortified

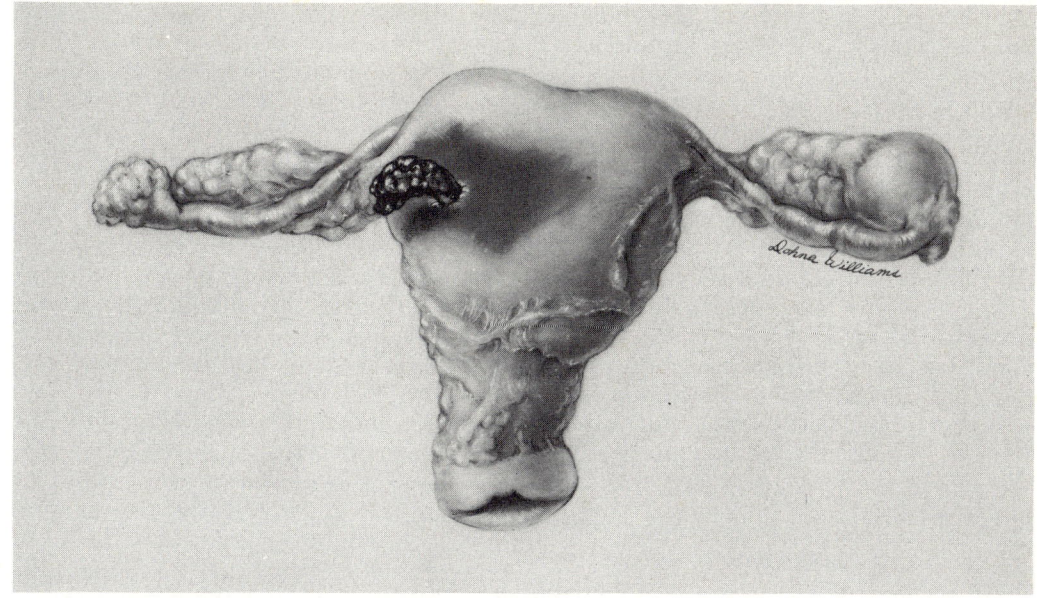

Fig. 21-11. Demonstrating result of punctured uterus. Specimen removed directly after puncture.

with streptomycin. The patient should be watched for localization of the infection. If this occurs, the abscess should be drained. It is a rarity for either serious hemorrhage or infection to occur.

Figure 21-11 shows a uterus removed immediately after a perforation. This uterus was removed because the gross character of the curettings indicated malignancy. There was only a small blood clot found at the site of the perforation. Recently, Word *et al.* analyzed 70 accidental uterine perforations. Among these, 7 unplanned hysterectomies were done on unprepared patients. In none did the findings in the peritoneal cavity warrant hysterectomy. In fact, it only compounded the error. Fifty-five patients were treated conservatively, and only 1 developed a complication in the form of a pelvic abscess, which was drained by colpotomy.

When perforation of the large, boggy, postabortal or puerperal uterus is done by a large curette or placental forceps in removing placental tissue, there is danger of injury to gut, prolapse of gut into the wound, hemorrhage and/or infection. The treatment that should be given and the procedures that should be followed are discussed in Chapter 22, Abortions.

DYSFUNCTIONAL UTERINE BLEEDING

Since one of the most common indications for dilatation and curettage is for control of dysfunctional uterine bleeding, it is important that this entity be discussed in greater detail. As defined in our clinic, dysfunctional uterine bleeding includes any abnormal uterine bleeding in the absence of infection, gestation, or tumor within the uterus. According to this definition, such bleeding is primarily the result of alterations in the normal blood levels of estrogen and progesterone, with resultant abnormal stimulation and shedding of the endometrium. Similarly, an organic lesion may be present in the generative organs outside the uterus when the bleeding from the uterus is entirely dysfunctional in nature. Indeed, this is the case in some instances when bleeding is associated with granulosa and theca cell tumors of the ovary. It is also the case when abnormal bleeding is associated with a corpus luteum retention cyst of the ovary. However, in the vast majority of cases of dysfunctional uterine bleeding, no gross pathologic lesion is present in the ovary. Hamblen excludes by definition those cases in which the bleeding is associated with some obvious endocrine disorder. By his definition, bleeding associated with hypothyroidism would be excluded; by our definition it would be included.

There is also some confusion in the literature as to the proper name for this condition. Most authors currently prefer the term *dysfunctional bleeding,* since in a strict sense normal menstruation is a form of functional bleeding. In the past the term *functional bleeding* was generally used.

Symptoms

Dysfunctional uterine bleeding, occurring most frequently during menarche and menopause, may appear as almost any type of abnormal bleeding. Menorrhagia is common. It may be an increase in the profuseness of the menstrual flow, an increase in duration, or both. A frequent history is that of a gradual increase in profuseness and duration, the periods becoming longer and longer until they finally merge with one another, and the bleeding is continuous. Periods of several weeks of amenorrhea between bleeding spells are common. Intermenstrual spotting or profuse bleeding may also be of a functional nature, and even menopausal bleeding falls in this category. However, the vast majority of cases of postmenopausal bleeding have an organic basis, and they should be considered as of organic origin until proved to be otherwise. Nevertheless, at times postmenopausal dysfunctional bleeding is associated with ovarian neoplasms, especially those of the feminizing type.

Dysfunctional bleeding in general should be looked upon as a disease of the two extremes of the reproductive life. Its years of greatest incidence are those between 40 and the menopause, although we have seen it frequently at all ages of menstrual life. Of special note are those cases occurring in girls of the "teen"age. We have noted it as early as 12 years and much earlier when associated with granulosa cell tumors of the ovary. When bleeding is noted before the age of normal puberty, the possibility of a feminizing tumor always should be considered, although this is one of the more infrequent causes of precocious puberty.

Pathophysiology

The pathologic endometrial picture associated with dysfunctional uterine bleeding has been studied extensively. One obtains from the literature the impression that many gynecologists formerly assumed that dysfunctional bleeding was invariably associated with enodmetrial hyperplasia. This point of view is no longer tenable, for there is now overwhelming evidence that any type of endometrium may be found with this clinical syndrome. Keene and Payne found hyperplasia present in 60 per cent of their cases of functional bleeding. Jones, in a study made in our laboratory, found hyperplasia present in 63 per cent of the cases (Fig. 21-12). There was secretory endometrium in 17 per cent of Jones's cases and nonsecretory endometrium of the interval, postmenstrual, or atrophic type in the remaining 20 per cent. Thus, in at least 17 per cent of this series, normal cyclic changes were taking place in the endometria, and it is probable that many which showed the postmenstrual type of endometrium would have shown secretory glands had they been curetted later in the cycle. In addition, the time interval between the onset of abnormal bleeding and curettage may be sufficient to permit ovulation from a subsequent unimpaired cycle. This may confuse the histologic pattern regarding the ovulatory or anovulatory character of the bleeding. That dysfunctional bleeding can be associated with an exaggerated progestational picture or even decidual-like picture was shown by the study of Henricksen and Te Linde. In examining curettings and uteri removed for bleeding, they found several endometrial specimens in which there were full or partial decidual-like changes. In some of these there was conclusive evidence that neither intra- nor extra-uterine preg-

FIG. 21-12. Endometrial hyperplasia from a dysfunctional bleeder.

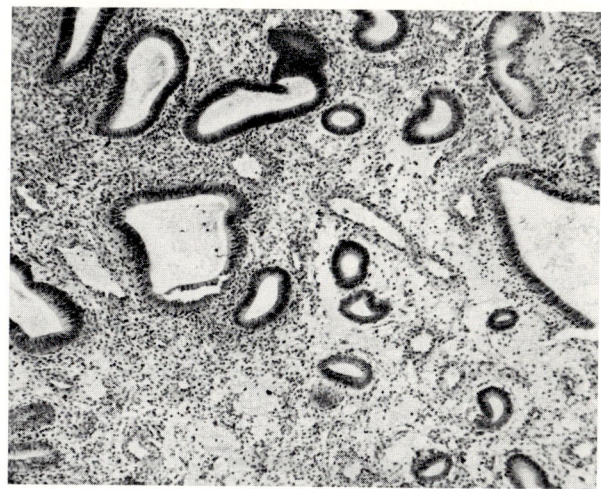

nancy was present; in others there was strong presumptive evidence.

Since dysfunctional bleeding may be present in association with such a variety of microscopic pictures, it is obvious that the bleeding is not inherently bound up etiologically with the microscopic picture. The physiologic mechanism of the excessive and/or irregular flow is related to the variation in the circulating levels of blood steroids which influence the frequency and duration of endometrial shedding.

PATHOLOGY OF ENDOMETRIAL HYPERPLASIA

Since hyperplasia is one of the most frequent conditions of the endometrium associated with dysfunctional bleeding, and since a thorough acquaintance with its pathology is so essential, its gross and microscopic pictures are discussed here in some detail. The condition was first described by Cullen in 1900, and the name *hyperplasia* was suggested by Welch, who concluded that the condition represented a true hyperplasia of the glandular and the stromal elements. In the original case described by Cullen a great quantity of endometrial tissue was obtained by curettage. We have seen repeatedly as much tissue at curettage as when endometrial carcinoma is present. In fact, many a surgeon, inexperienced in pathology, has proceeded with hysterectomy on the assumption that he was dealing with malignancy. Yet there is usually a difference, grossly, between hyperplastic and neoplastic endometrium; the former is spongy and the particles smoothly rounded, whereas when such a quantity of tissue is obtained from a carcinomatous endometrium, the fragments are friable and often necrotic-appearing. In some instances in which we have had the opportunity of examining the entire uterus, we have found a polypoid overgrowth of the endometrium thoughout the cavity of the corpus, which ends abruptly at the internal os. In contrast with this, endometrial carcinoma does not respect physiologic barriers, and if it is present in the lower portion of the endometrial cavity, it probably will invade the cervical canal. In some specimens the excessive endometrium is built up into a localized polyp-like structure, and the remainder of the endometrial surface is relatively smooth. However, in other cases the endometrium may be of normal thickness and appearance. In these cases no excess of endometrium is obtained on curettage, and the particles of endometrium do not differ when seen without the microscope from those of normal endometrium. This endometrium, which is not increased grossly, may have as hyperplastic a microscopic picture as the endometrium that is characterized by a great excess of tissue.

Etiology

From our knowledge of the histology of the various endometrial pictures associated with dysfunctional bleeding, it is obvious that the endocrinologic disturbance responsible for all cases of such bleeding is not identical. From the standpoint of etiology, the *anovulatory* type, showing the endometrial picture of hyperplasia or nonsecretory endometrium, is the most frequent, accounting for 80 to 85 per cent of all cases. The more infrequent *ovulatory* type, which includes the remaining 15 to 20 per cent, is the most difficult to define etiologically, as well as to treat.

Both types are related to a hypothalamic-pituitary-ovarian dysfunction which is caused by an imbalance in the gonadotrophin-release mechanism of the hypothalamic nuclei. Such an imbalance may interfere with cyclic ovulation, which produces unopposed estrogen stimulation of the endometrium. Formerly it was generally accepted that the abnormality was a state of hyperestrogenism. That such a simple state of affairs does not always exist is evident from the fact that one cannot demonstrate in every case an excess of estrogenic hormones in the urine or the blood. Furthermore, Burch *et al.* has offered abundant evidence from animal experimentation to indicate that endometrial hyperplasia may result from various degrees of ovarian insufficiency. Such evidence suggests that the duration of estrogen stimulation, rather than the quantity of this hormone, is the most important feature of anovulatory bleeding.

Studies by Schröder provide some of the earliest evidence of anovulation as one of the major factors in dysfunctional bleeding. His study of the ovaries and the endometrium confirmed the absence of corpus luteum formation in association with endometrial hyperplasia, suggesting continuous, unopposed estrogen stimulation of the endometrium.

Many factors are associated with anovulatory bleeding which require a thorough investigation for proper treatment of this entity. These include (1) psychogenic factors, hypothalamic dysfunction and pituitary abnormalities; (2) endocrine disturbances with abnormal steroid metabolism of adrenal or ovarian origin (including the Stein-Leventhal syndrome and functioning ovarian tumors); (3) nutritional deficiencies, metabolic disease (including thyroid dysfunction and diabetes), acute and chronic disease; and (4) physiologic changes of the ovary at menarche and menopause.

The *ovulatory* type of dysfunctional uterine bleeding is more difficult to explain and is more commonly associated with anatomic defects of the uterus than any other factor. However, in the absence of such factors as endometrial polyps, submucous or intramural myomata, this pattern of bleeding must be considered dysfunctional. A persistent corpus luteum cyst (Halban's disease) and the phenomena of irregular shedding as described by McClennan are explanations for this type of uterine bleeding.

Treatment of Dysfunctional Uterine Bleeding

In considering the treatment of dysfunctional bleeding, one always should bear in mind that the condition is one in which spontaneous remissions are frequent. It is well to keep this foremost in one's mind for two reasons: (1) as encouragement to the physician and the patient in those cases that resist conservative therapeutic measures, and (2) as a basis for evaluating therapeutic measures. Often much credit has been given to different forms of therapy when the remissions were obviously spontaneous.

All cases of dysfunctional bleeding require a diagnostic curettage for study of the endometrium. For the group in the years when cancer is more prevalent, this is particularly important and never should be neglected; in the 'teens, curettage may be deferred at times until therapy has been given a trial. In performing this curettage, it is our belief that it should be done under general anesthesia rather than with the suction curette on the unanesthetized patient. When the patient is anesthetized, the curettage is apt to be done more thoroughly, and thoroughness is essential from the standpoint of ruling out malignancy and of obtaining the greatest therapeutic value from the procedure. The therapeutic value of uterine curettage when used as the only method of treatment for dysfunctional bleeding is reportedly effective in 40 to 60 per cent of the cases. Our own results with curettage have been reported by Jones and Te Linde, and demonstrate that 42 per cent of such patients require no further treatment.

If bleeding recurs in the younger patient, our experience with repeat curettements has been rewarding. In general, two or three such procedures are performed prior to resorting to more definitive surgery. In the older group after the age of 40, we have resorted to hysterectomy somewhat earlier than in the younger age group.

In a disease that is obviously the result of an endocrine dysfunction, it is natural that attempts should be made to correct the disorder by means of endocrine substitutional therapy. The hormonal treatment as carried out in the clinic at Johns Hopkins Hospital is outlined by Dr. Georgeanna Jones as follows:

Anovulatory functional (dysfunctional) uterine bleeding, associated with an estrogenic or hyperplastic endometrial pattern, can often be successfully controlled by progesterone substitution therapy while efforts are being made to establish an etiologic diagnosis (Fig. 21-13). The synthesis of many new, effective progestational compounds has made a number of satisfactory therapeutic regimens available, but certain facts must be understood in order to obtain successful clinical results.

Progesterone is not a hemostatic agent and exerts its action only on withdrawal, thus producing a chemical type of curettage. Therefore, if the patient is bleeding at the time therapy is instituted, bleeding will not be controlled until 6 to 8 days after cessation of therapy. Consequently, appropriate steps must be taken to cover this lag period: bed rest if symptoms are severe enough to warrant it, iron therapy and reassurance. If the patient is not bleeding at the initiation of treatment, a menstrual period can be expected within 2 to 4 days after cessation of progesterone therapy.

The basic method of treatment is a single injection of 25 mg. of progesterone in oil (water suspensions are irritating and cause severe local reactions) given once every 28 days for 3 cycles as suggested by Holmstrom. 17-Hydroxy-progesterone-caproate (125 mg., Delalutin, Squibb) can be substituted for progesterone, but in our experience it offers no advantages. If the patient is bleeding at the initiation of treatment, it is wise to cover the initial injection with additional oral therapy over a 3-day period; 25 or 30 mg. daily of ethisterone is adequate for this purpose. Ethisterone can also be used without intramuscular progesterone, and this method has the advantage of reducing the number of office visits necessary. A 5-day course of 25 or 30 mg. of ethisterone daily, repeated every 28 days for 3 cycles, is given. Approximately 2 per cent of patients with anovulatory bleeding show an atrophic endometrial pattern. In this group of patients, it will be necessary to give adjunctive estrogen: 1 mg. of stilbestrol or its equivalent, during the 3 weeks prior to progestational therapy.

The 19-nortestosterone derivatives are potent progestational agents and are reported to be hemostatic in action. These substances—two of the most popular are norethynodrel (Enovid) and norethindrone (Norlutin)—are also most effective as pituitary gonadotrophin suppressors. They are synthetic compounds and have diversified hormonal activities, showing both progestational and androgenic action. Norethynodrel is also estrogenic, and the commercial preparation (Enovid) has additional estrogen supplied. Southam reports that the 19-nortestosterone compounds will arrest bleeding within 24 hours, if given in amounts of between 10 and 30 mg. daily. This dosage can be continued for 3 weeks and then discontinued, allowing the patient to menstruate. Although expedient, the inherent danger in the use of these drugs is that real pathology may be obscured, as it is reported that bleeding due to thrombocytopenia, endometrial polyps, fibroids and conceivably carcinoma of the endometrium can be controlled equally as well as functional bleeding. However, 19-nortestosterone can also be used as progestational substitution therapy, in which case only 2.5 mg. daily during a 5-day period is adequate to relieve symptoms.

It should be emphasized again that progestational therapy is substitutional and rarely if ever initiates ovulation. Functional bleeding is subject to spontaneous remissions; thus 40 per cent of the patients will not require further treatment after an initial 3-month therapy

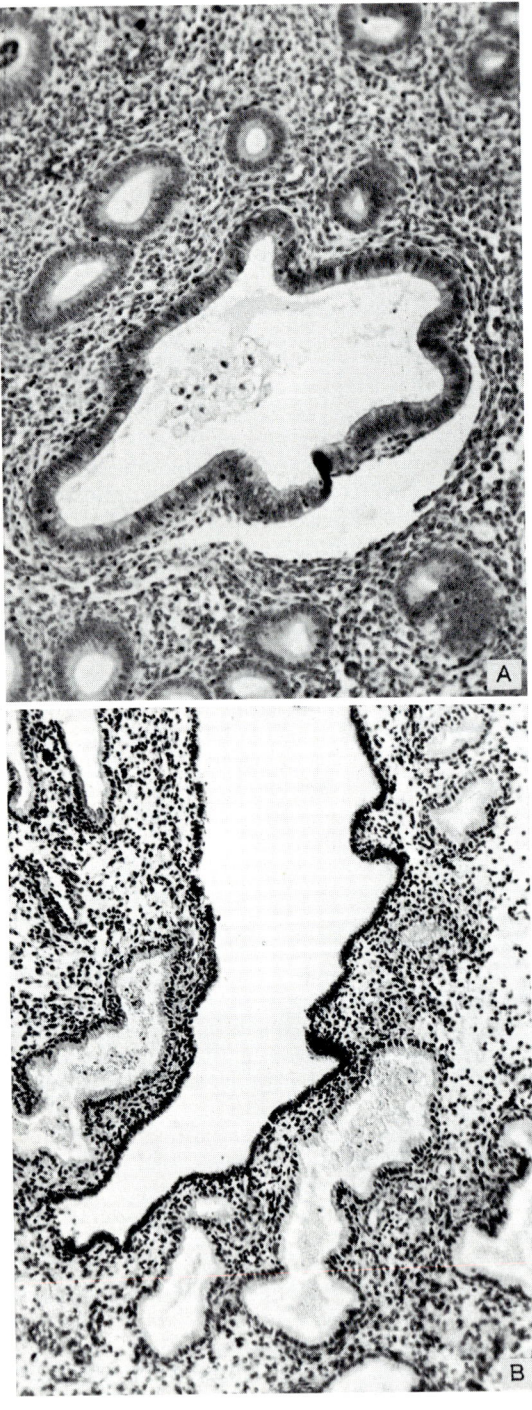

Fig. 21-13. (A) Endometrial hyperplasia before treatment. (B) Same endometrium changed to secretory type following progesterone therapy.

period. While the symptoms are being controlled hormonally, diagnostic procedures should be undertaken to clarify the underlying etiologic factor and institute specific therapy as indicated. Such therapy would include, in addition to specific treatment of organic disease, nutritional replacement; thyroid in adequate dosage when there is definite laboratory evidence of hypothyroidism; and propylthiouracil or surgery if hyperthyroidism is present; good diabetic regulation for the diabetic patient; reassurance and mild sedation for the emotionally disturbed patient with psychiatric care when indicated. If polycystic ovaries are found, a Wedge resection operation must be performed.

Should the patient fail to respond to curettage or endocrine therapy, more radical therapy, primarily hysterectomy, should be considered in proportion to the age of the patient and her desire for future childbearing. Although a hysterectomy may be considered as an admission of therapeutic defeat, it is frequently an expeditious method of resolving a refractory and recurrent type of dysfunctional uterine bleeding. In general, the ovulatory type of bleeding responds the poorest to replacement hormonal therapy and has the highest incidence of recurrence. With persistent bleeding following repeat curettement and cyclic hormonal therapy, hysterectomy may be required. If other conditions are present that should be corrected surgically, such as relaxed vaginal outlet, rectocele, cystocele, or uterine descensus, we recommend vaginal hysterectomy as the treatment of choice. For patients under the age of 40, who have failed to respond to repeated curettements and hormonal therapy, we perform hysterectomy with conservation of ovarian tissue. In patients below the age of 30, resort to radical treatment is to be strongly avoided. If endocrine therapy fails, one almost always can control the hemorrhage temporarily by repeated curettage, or by the continuous, uninterrupted use of increasing amounts of progestational agents for 3 months or longer. In most instances, persistence in these conservative measures is rewarded eventually with remission of the bleeding and often a return to a normal menstrual cycle.

Although rarely used, intracavitary radium or x-ray castration is an effective method of producing ovarian castration in those cases in which surgery is contraindicated, and conservative therapy has failed. The usual dosage of radium is 2,000 to 2,400 mg. hrs. in a single application. While many authors have found no definite proof of an increased incidence of pelvic malignancy in such irradiated patients, the experience of Palmer and Spratt of 9.5 per cent malignancy rate in 746 patients so treated is of major concern to the clinician. This method of treatment is reserved for the seriously ill patient in whom uterine hemorrhage can be controlled by no other method.

The recent use of clomiphene in inducing ovulation appears promising but is effective only for the specific treatment of hypothalamic dysfunction. While the precise mechanism of action of the drug remains uncertain, the increase in FSH and LH excretion from the anterior pituitary suggests a direct effect on the gonadotrophin-releasing factors in the hypothalamus. The usual recommended dose is 50 mg. daily for 5 days, although a dose of 100 mg. daily may be given if there is failure of response. Kistner has produced ovulatory cycles in 70 per cent of patients treated, but discontinuing the drug after treatment for 3 to 6 months is frequently associated with the recurrence of anovulatory cycles. In addition, ovarian enlargement, hot flushes, pelvic discomfort, and multiple ovulation are frequent side-effects of this treatment.

BIBLIOGRAPHY

Bergman, P.: The clinical treatment of anovulation. Int. J. Fertil., 3:27, 1958.

Burch, J. C., Williams, W. L., and Cunningham, R. S.: Etiology of hyperplasia. Surg. Gynec. Obstet., 53:338, 1931.

Charles, D., Barr, W., and McEwan, H. P.: Use of clomiphene in dysfunctional uterine bleeding due to endometrial hyperplasia. J. Obstet. Gynaec. Brit. Comm., 71:66, 1964.

Copeland, W. E., Nelson, P. K., and Payne,

F. L.: Intrauterine radium for dysfunctional uterine bleeding: Long-term follow-up study. Amer. J. Obstet. Gynec., 72:416, 1956.

Cullen, T. S.: Cancer of the Uterus. p. 497. New York, Appleton, 1900.

Halstrom, E. G.: Progesterone treatment of anovulatory bleeding. Amer. J. Obstet. Gynec., 68:1321, 1954.

Hamblen, E. C.: Endocrinology of Woman. pp. 424-443. Springfield, Ill., Charles C Thomas, 1949.

Hunter, R. N., Ludwick, H. V., Motley, J. F., and Oaks, W. W.: The use of radium in treatment of benign lesions of uterus: A critical 20-year survey. Amer. J. Obstet. Gynec., 67:121, 1954.

Jones, G. E. S., and Te Linde, R. W.: An evaluation of progesterone therapy in the treatment of endometrial hyperplasia. Bull. Johns Hopkins Hosp., 71:282, 1942.

——: Survey of functional uterine bleeding with special reference to progesterone therapy. Amer. J. Obstet. Gynec., 57:854, 1949.

Josey, W. E.: Routine intrauterine forceps exploration at curettage. Amer. J. Obstet. Gynec., 11:108, 1958.

Keene, F. E., and Payne, F. L.: Treatment of functional uterine hemorrhage. Amer. J. Obstet. Gynec., 34:688, 1937.

Kempers, R. D., Decker, D. G., and Lee, R. A.: Induction of ovulation with clomiphene citrate. Obstet. Gynec., 30:699, 1967.

Kistner, R. W.: Induction of ovulation with clomiphene (Clomid). S. African J. Obstet. Gynec., 5:25, 1967.

McClennan, C. E., and Rydell, A. H.: Extent of endometrial shedding during normal menstruation. Obstet. Gynec., 26:605, 1965.

Narula, R. K.: Endometrial histopathology in dysfunctional uterine bleeding. J. Obstet. Gynec. of India, 17:614, 1967.

Norris, H. J., and Taylor, H. B.: Postirradiation sarcomas of the uterus. Obstet. Gynec., 26:689, 1965.

Novak, E.: Relation of hyperplasic of endometrium to so-called functional uterine hemorrhage. J.A.M.A., 75:292, 1920.

Palmer, J., and Spratt, D.: Pelvic carcinoma following irradiation for benign gynecologic disease. Amer. J. Gynec., 72:497, 1956.

Paloucek, F. P., Randall, C. L., Graham, J. D., and Graham, S.: Cancer and its relation to abnormal vaginal bleeding and radiation. Obstet. Gynec., 21:530, 1963.

Radman, H. M., and Korman, W.: Uterine perforation during dilatation and curettage. Obstet. Gynec., 21:210, 1963.

Schröder, R.: Anatomische Studien zur normalen und pathologischen Physiologie des Menstruationzyklus. Arch. Gynäk., 104:27, 1915.

Sippe, G.: Endometrial hyperplasia and uterine bleeding. J. Obstet. Gynaec. Brit. Comm., 69:1015, 1962.

Southam, A. L., and Richart, R. M.: The prognosis for adolescents with menstrual abnormalities. Amer. J. Obstet. Gynec., 94:637, 1966.

Swartz, D. T., and Jones, G. E. S.: Progesterone in anovulatory uterine bleeding: Clinical observations. Fertil. Steril., 8:103, 1957.

Stander, R. W.: Irradiation castration. Obstet. Gynec., 10:223, 1967.

Te Linde, R. W., and Henriksen, E.: Decidualike changes in the endometrium without pregnancy. Amer. J. Obstet. Gynec., 39:733, 1940.

Word, B.: Current concepts of uterine curettage. Postgrad. Med., 28:450, 1960.

Word, B., Gravler, L. C., and Wideman, G. L.: The fallacy of simple uterine curettage. Obstet. Gynec., 12:642, 1958.

22

Abortions

ELEANOR DELFS, M.D.*

Abortions occur frequently enough to be a major health problem, involving a large number of women in illness and many hospital admissions. Exact incidence is uncertain due to failure to report many early and uncomplicated abortions and concealment of some induced abortions. It is not possible to divide the abortions accurately between spontaneous and induced, but some approximations may be derived. Traditionally, it has been taught that 10 per cent of pregnancies terminate in spontaneous abortion but recent studies indicate a higher figure. Erhardt's data, derived from records of practicing obstetricians, and Warburton's and Fraser's data, derived from special genetic records, both showed 15 per cent. Because of their population composition, these studies probably minimize induced abortions.

A different approach to incidence is the ratio of abortions to live births in hospital admissions. Lash, Webster, and Barton, in a Cook County Hospital survey of 22,287 abortions under 20 weeks' gestation, found a ratio of 1:4.1 (20% abortions). State of Illinois hospitals had a ratio of 1:10.3, which mirrors the difference between urban and nonurban populations, as has been noted in earlier reports. The difference between the incidence as derived from hospital admissions and the spontaneous abortion history data noted above should approximate the induced abortions, that is, about 5 per cent of conceptions. If this seems low, it may be emphasized that the figure is derived from a large urban public hospital, which would be expected to have a maximum number of induced abortions. If it is assumed that 20 per cent of all pregnancies abort and annual births are 3.6 million, it can be anticipated that there will be 900,000 abortions each year in the United States. Allowing for underreporting, the number is probably somewhat over 1 million.

The recorded mortality due to abortions may not be entirely accurate, as a few deaths may be attributed to other causes for concealment, but the number of deaths has unquestionably decreased greatly in the past 2 to 3 decades. In 1965 there were 1,189 maternal deaths in the United States, of which 235 (19.8%) were due to abortions. In 1940 there were 1,815 deaths attributed to abortions, almost 8 times the recent number. Reduction in mortality has not been uniform in all areas. Gold, in a review of the mortality in New York City from 1951 through 1962, found the percentage of abortion deaths rising from 26.1 to 42.1 per cent of total maternal deaths; however, the ratio of abortion deaths per 10,000 live births remained steady, varying up and down between 6.0 and 7.3, an indication of decreases in other causes of maternal death not exhibited to the same extent by abortion deaths. Induced abortion and its mortality have always been

---

* Professor, Department of Gynecology and Obstetrics, Marquette School of Medicine.

higher in large urban centers than elsewhere. With the rapid extension of improved contraceptive facilities into these areas, there should be further improvement in abortion statistics. Such a change is already occurring in some cities.

Although mortality from abortion has been greatly reduced, there is still a considerable morbidity with residual chronic pelvic pain, sterility, ectopic pregnancy, surgical removal of pelvic organs, and neuroses as late results of abortion in many women.

TERMINOLOGY

Abortion is the expulsion of the product of conception in the first 20 weeks of gestation or with a fetus under 500 gm. (actually a 500-gm. fetus is usually closer to 22 weeks gestational age). Such a definition is reflected in the collection of data by U.S. Vital Statistics and World Health Organization classification of perinatal mortality. Termination of pregnancy between the 20th and 28th week (500-1,000 gm.) is classified as immature delivery and is essentially an obstetric problem.

Spontaneous abortion is, as the name signifies, one which occurs without outside initiation, either medical or instrumental.

Induced abortion is brought about by outside means. It may be *legitimately* induced therapeutically or *illegally* induced, in which case it is often spoken of as a criminal abortion.

A *complete abortion* is one in which the entire ovisac is expelled spontaneously in 1 or 2 stages. An *incomplete abortion* is one in which a part of the fetus, the placenta, or the decidua remains in the uterus. When uterine contractions and bleeding have begun, signifying beginning detachment of the ovisac, the term *threatened* abortion is used. When, in the judgment of the physician, the detachment of the ovisac has reached a stage in which nothing can prevent its expulsion, the abortion is considered *inevitable*.

Habitual abortion refers to repeated abortion in the same individual, the term usually being limited to those cases with 3 or more consecutive abortions.

Missed abortion is a term applied to those cases in which the entire ovisac is retained for some time after the death of the fetus. Litzenberg arbitrarily placed a limit of 2 months after the death of the fetus as the borderline between abortion and missed abortion.

Any of the above types of abortion may become *infected*. The infection may remain within the confines of the uterus or spread into extra-uterine tissues.

THERAPEUTIC ABORTION

LEGAL AND MEDICAL CONSIDERATIONS

There has been concern recently about variability in abortion laws and diversity of medical opinion regarding proper standards of medical practice. Important changes have occurred in mortality, management, and indications in abortion which make reassessment desirable. The termination of pregnancy before viability is a serious procedure with legal, ethical, moral, and religious aspects as well as the strictly medical considerations of indications and risks which cannot be ignored.

Berthelson and Ostergaard reviewed 23,666 therapeutic abortions in Denmark and found a mortality rate of 0.7 per 1,000 operations and nonfatal complications in 3.2 per cent. Many of these procedures were done for eugenic and humanitarian reasons in healthy women; hence these figures are probably minimal. When therapeutic abortion is contemplated in women with serious organic disease, the risk of mortality is much greater and must be weighed carefully.

Roemer has classified the abortion laws of different countries in five categories, with selected countries illustrating each:

1. Laws authorizing abortion on demand: U.S.S.R., Bulgaria, and Hungary.
2. Laws authorizing abortion on social grounds: Japan, Poland, Czechoslovakia, and Yugoslavia.
3. Laws authorizing abortion on socio-

medical grounds: Iceland, Sweden, Denmark, and Norway.

4. Laws authorizing abortion on medical grounds: Syria, Honduras, Switzerland, England, several American states.

5. Laws authorizing abortion only to save the life of the woman: majority of American states, Western Australia, Venezuela, Chile, and France.

The United States is one of the most conservative countries with regard to therapeutic abortion. The impetus to change U.S. abortion laws has centered in several general areas:

1. Liberalization in restrictive states to permit therapeutic abortion when medical conditions threatening the life or health of the mother exist. The majority of states permit abortion only if maternal life is threatened, and very few allow termination on the probability of fetal abnormality. Uniformity of state laws for strongly medically indicated cases would eliminate many problems. Probably most physicians and the majority of laymen would subscribe to such change in laws.

2. Aim to decrease criminal abortion with the availability of legalized abortion. Such expectation may not be realistic. Tietze has pointed out that illegal abortion has not disappeared in countries where legal abortion is available on request; in Hungary legal abortions exceed live births (rates are 17.8 and 13.1), but an illegal abortion rate of 3.3 to 4.4 has persisted for years. Czechoslovakia and Sweden likewise continue to have many illegal abortions in spite of the availability of legal abortion in both countries.

3. Increased utilization of therapeutic abortion as a population control measure. This is not the medically optimal method since it carries risks of mortality and morbidity and is wasteful of personnel and hospital facilities to accomplish what could be better achieved by contraception. The availability of easy abortion makes for proliferating demand as contraceptive efforts are frequently discontinued. After Japan legalized abortion on social grounds, the rate rose from 137 abortions per 1,000 live births in 1950 to 682 per 1,000 in 1958, with a decrease in efforts to avoid pregnancy (Roemer).

Abortion on demand, which is implied in the last two areas, is controversial in the United States and is probably favored by only a minority of physicians and laity. Several legal and medical organizations have proposed standards for implementation throughout the country. A policy statement passed by the American Medical Association in 1967 follows:*

The American Medical Association is opposed to induced abortion except when:
1. There is documented medical evidence that continuance of the pregnancy may threaten the health or life of the mother, or
2. There is documented medical evidence that the infant may be born with incapacitating physical deformity or mental deficiency, or
3. There is documented medical evidence that continuance of a pregnancy, resulting from legally established statutory or forcible rape or incest, may constitute a threat to the mental or physical health of the patient;
4. Two other physicians chosen because of their recognized professional competence have examined the patient and have concurred in writing; and
5. The procedure is performed in a hospital accredited by the Joint Commission on Accreditation of Hospitals.

The American College of Obstetrics and Gynecology has adopted a similar policy. It is stressed that these are recommendations, not laws, and the gynecologist must be familiar with the current laws in his state. His judgment and that of his consultants will dictate his management of cases within the applicable legal boundaries.

Concurrently with demands for liberalizing abortion laws, the actual therapeutic abortion rate has fallen steadily over the past 2 decades due largely to improved management of medical complications. Gold and his co-workers, reviewing therapeutic abortions in New York City for 20 years ending in 1962, reported a rate of 1.8 per 1,000 live births, down from 5.1 in the early 1940's. In a survey of 522,600 deliveries, Hall found a rate of 2.0 per 1,000 deliveries. Tietze, with data of the Professional

---

* American Medical Association Policy on Therapeutic Abortion. J.A.M.A., *201*:544, 1967.

Activities Survey for 1963–65 summarizing over 1 million deliveries, found a rate of 1.9 per 1,000. The indications for the procedure have shifted in many regions from predominantly organic medical complications to psychiatric conditions. In 1945 Kuder and Finn reported a series with indications which were representative of conservative practice at the time: medical diseases, 83.9 per cent; obstetric and gynecologic complications, 7.2 per cent; neuropsychiatric, 5.7 per cent; and miscellaneous, 3.2 per cent. Tietze in the recent study of 2,007 therapeutic abortions quoted above showed indications:

	Per Cent
Psychiatric	34
Medical (somatic) disease	27
Rubella	22
Not stated	17

Russell and Moore found similar indications of maternal medical disease, 41 per cent; psychiatric disease, 32 per cent; and fetal involvement (mostly rubella), 27 per cent. Within the maternal medical disease category the distribution was:

	Per Cent
Cardiovascular	24
Renal	12
Malignancies	12
Diabetes	5
Neurologic	3.5
Gastroenterology	3.5
Tuberculosis	3
Other	37

Detailed evaluation of all individual indications cannot be given here, but some general principles are outlined which present the philosophy of the author regarding the commoner indications. In most medical complications treatment can be directed advantageously toward the disease without disturbing the pregnancy. A few diseases may be aggravated by pregnancy; somewhat more frequently a disease may have reduced the function of an organ so that there is no reserve to meet demands of pregnancy, and decompensation threatens. There should be consultation on all therapeutic abortions, preferably by a specialist in the disease involved, to assist in evaluating the extent of disease and the risk.

Chronic Hypertensive Vascular Disease. Mild and moderate disease is compatible with pregnancy. Very high blood pressures (e.g., 180-200/120 or above), particularly with high diastolic levels and fixed status, are hazardous to mother and fetus. If there are advanced eyeground changes, signs of renal impairment, or enlargement of the heart, the risk is great, and therapeutic abortion is justified; indeed, this is one of the most valid indications for the operation. If in addition there is history in a previous pregnancy of cardiac failure or severe superimposed pre-eclampsia, the indication is strong. Chesley found 71 per cent recurrence of superimposed pre-eclampsia.

Cardiac Disease. Need for therapeutic abortion has decreased with improved management of rheumatic fever, which has reduced heart damage, and improvement in function by cardiac surgery in some rheumatic and congenital lesions has decreased the problem further. The most important aspect in prognosis is the functional capacity of the heart, which can be designated advantageously by the New York Heart Association Classification I to IV. Ninety per cent of cardiacs seen in pregnancy are Class I and Class II (Mendelson) and generally do well if carefully supervised. Class III patients need marked restriction of activities, and many require extended hospitalization. Bunim and Appel found that one third of Class III cardiacs will fail during pregnancy unless preventive steps are adequate; 65 per cent with a history of previous failure will fail during pregnancy. Those at especially high risk may warrant therapeutic abortion if seen early in pregnancy. Unfavorable factors are age over 35 years, history of previous failure, increased pulmonary pressure, and serious rhythm disturbances, particularly auricular fibrillation. A different point of view has been expressed by Gorenberg and Chesley and by O'Driscoll, Coyle, and Drury, who have concluded from a large series that abortion is not necessary.

Both groups had remarkably low mortality, but results were dependent upon patient cooperation and protracted hospitalization, conditions impossible to achieve at times. Class IV patients cannot tolerate operative procedures and are best treated medically until compensation can be improved.

In some high-risk cardiacs who have lesions suitable for surgical correction, particularly mitral stenosis, heart operation may be an alternative to therapeutic abortion, prolonged hospitalization, or poor response. Many obstetricians and cardiologists have been opposed to cardiac surgery during pregnancy except in unusual circumstances, but this attitude may be altered somewhat with improved technics. Recently Ueland collected 514 cases of valvulotomy during pregnancy with maternal mortality of 1.7 per cent.

Open heart surgery and repair of congenital lesions during pregnancy have had very limited use and are not favored except in special situations. Many women with congenital heart lesions do well in pregnancies. Those with functional capacity too limited to meet the pregnancy load should have therapeutic abortion. Following later cardiac surgery in the nonpregnant state, pregnancies can often be carried successfully.

Renal Disease. The need for therapeutic abortion in renal disease is determined largely by the functional capacity of the kidneys rather than the nature of the disease process. If function is inadequate to prevent nitrogenous retention or has little reserve above that level, the maternal risk is too high to be acceptable. Associated hypertension increases the hazard. Therapeutic abortion based on such a functional limitation is applicable to a variety of pathologic lesions, including chronic glomerulonephritis, chronic pyelonephritis, polycystic kidneys, lupus nephritis, and diabetic glomerulosclerosis.

Pulmonary Disease. Early termination of pregnancy is rarely demanded by pulmonary disease except where the respiratory reserve is so minimal that pregnancy changes will exceed it. Advanced emphysema, bronchiectasis, or severe chronic asthma may occasionally reach such a limit. Postpneumonectomy patients do not need abortion if the remaining lung has good function. Pulmonary tuberculosis is rarely an indication now except possibly in far advanced disease with limited functioning lung tissue or drug resistance. The course of the disease is not significantly altered by therapeutic abortion, as shown by Schaefer, Douglas, and Dreishpoon.

Malignancies. It may be stated that generally pregnancy and malignancies of all types develop independently with little reciprocal effects. Treatment may be similarly independent in most cases. In advanced malignancies when only palliation is possible, abortion is pointless and removes a possible source of emotional support and purpose which the pregnancy may give. When the malignancy is amenable to treatment, this should be carried out without disturbance of the pregnancy unless its presence interferes with access to the tumor. Malignancies of cervix, uterus, or ovaries in early pregnancy must be treated definitively without regard to the pregnancy. Carcinoma of the breast was formerly considered an indication for therapeutic abortion, but current data does not support this view. Westberg in a country-wide study in Sweden concluded that the prognosis depended on the stage of the disease and the adequacy of therapy rather than the presence of pregnancy, though the latter delayed diagnosis at times. Holleb and Farrow, following women with radical mastectomy in the first trimester, found as good survival in those delivering at term as those subjected to therapeutic abortion. Prognosis was dependent upon presence or absence of node metastases at operation. Byrd and his co-workers had 5-year survival of 76 per cent of patients with radical mastectomy during pregnancy without therapeutic abortion.

Psychiatric Disease. It has been pointed out by Rosen that therapeutic abortion for this indication involves a preponderance of well-to-do, educated, middle and upper class women. More cultural, ethnic, and religious aspects complicate the problem, and psychiatry is able to offer less objective diagnostic and prognostic criteria than are available in most somatic diseases. There are some questions that require forthright answers: (1) Is there established, serious psychiatric illness, is it chronic or progressive, was it clearly established before the onset of pregnancy? (2) Will life or health be threatened if pregnancy continues, i.e., will the patient commit suicide or will the illness be worsened? (3) Will the psychiatric condition be worsened by therapeutic abortion?

Many conservative clinicians in the past have required evidence of psychiatric disease present before the pregnancy for consideration of therapeutic abortion. Such a requirement minimizes ambivalence, simulation, and social pressures influencing decisions.

Threat of suicide is not supported by the data. Höök followed up 248 women refused legal abortion and found no suicides or attempted suicides and only 11 per cent who had had illegal abortions. Several Swedish studies show no suicides in women denied abortion. The effect of pregnancy on ultimate mental health of psychiatric patients is problematic. Simon points out that predicting development or exacerbation of a psychotic episode is very difficult, and that there is no data proving that therapeutic abortion alters the long-term prognosis. Arén and Amark studied 142 women with mental illness to whom abortion was granted but not carried out. On follow-up several years later, 89 per cent had done well; the remaining 11 per cent had continued with some difficulties. They concluded that in general the seriousness of illness had been overestimated and abortion recommended too freely.

The possibility that psychiatric illness may be initiated or aggravated by therapeutic abortion has been reported in some cases, but this risk may have been exaggerated. Ekblad found 11 per cent of patients transitorily disturbed after therapeutic abortion but only 1 per cent incapacitated for work. Simon and Senturia made a critical review of reported series and found the data inconclusive. In their own carefully designed prospective study, they came to the conclusion that women with good mental health meet the problem of medically necessary therapeutic abortion with only transient mild depression. Serious psychiatric illness following abortion was related to pre-existing psychiatric disease and only rarely precipitated by abortion.

In summary, it is hard to avoid the conclusion that the treatment for psychiatric disease is psychotherapy rather than therapeutic abortion. If pregnancy represents a threat to such a patient, contraception or sterilization will usually solve that problem. There should be a declining indication for abortion in this area as for the other (somatic) medical complications.

Fetal Indication. There is no specific recognition of potential fetal malformation as an indication for therapeutic abortion in most states. Rubella is the major factor in this category. Warkany and Kalter reviewed 15 prospective studies of rubella infection in the first 12 weeks of pregnancy and found congenital malformations in 16.9 per cent. Incidence declined after 10 weeks and was not above that of the control group after 12 weeks. Many physicians consider abortion proper for rubella in the high-risk period if parents are unwilling to accept the risk. However, a number of normal fetuses are bound to be sacrificed, and the legal status remains ambiguous. Fortunately this unsatisfactory situation will be resolved when rubella immunization becomes available in the near future.

Methods of Therapeutic Abortion

Having concluded that the interruption of pregnancy is necessary, one must decide which is the best method in the particular case. There is often much justifiable controversy over this. The decision depends on several factors such as the duration of the pregnancy, parity, the condition for which the interruption is done, the condition of the patient at the time of interruption, the desirability of combining sterilization with abortion, and the wisdom of doing other gynecologic surgery at the same time. In the following discussion it is assumed that the gynecologist concerned is capable of carrying out the best operative procedures.

The surgical methods of termination of pregnancy therapeutically before the period of viability may be listed as follows:

1. Ordinary dilatation and curettage, utilized only before the patient has missed her 2nd period.
2. Cervical dilatation with the Hanks or Hegar dilator and removal of products of conception with blunt curette and ovum forceps or sponge holder. This method is utilized up to the 12th week.
3. Evacuation by uterine aspiration with a blunt hollow curette and negative pressure. This method can be used up to 12 weeks.
4. Preliminary gauze packing of the lower uterine segment and subsequent removal of products of conception by fingers and/or instruments. This method is utilized occasionally with patients from 12 to 14 weeks pregnant.
5. Injection of the uterus with hypertonic saline or glucose supplemented, if necessary, with intravenous oxytocin infusion. This method is applicable after 14 to 16 weeks.
6. Hysterotomy or hysterectomy. These procedures are commonly used after 14 weeks, and in some instances before, when abortion is to be combined with sterilization.

Before performing a therapeutic abortion it is wise to give penicillin, beginning approximately 24 hours before the operation: 600,000 units given twice on the day preceding the operation and the same dosage on the morning of the operation is adequate; 600,000 units twice daily for 3 days after the surgery is a wise precaution. If the patient should be febrile, the antibiotic therapy is increased.

Blood should be typed and crossmatched in case of need for transfusion, and intravenous glucose solution should be started before operation. Oxytocin, 10 units, may be added to the infusion to firm the uterine wall, if needed.

The method of choice is dilatation and curettage done with the usual Hegar or Hanks dilators and the ordinary small serrated curette if the pregnancy is interrupted before 6 weeks (before missing the 2nd period). If done with careful aseptic technic, it is almost as safe a procedure as the ordinary diagnostic curettage on the nonpregnant uterus. When the pregnancy has progressed beyond this time, the dangers attending cervical dilation and instrumental emptying of the uterus are increased. For the first 12 weeks of pregnancy, dilatation of the cervix with metal dilators is to be preferred to preliminary gauze packing.

In dilating the cervical canal preliminary to emptying the uterine cavity, sterile technic must be carried out meticulously. The vagina must be cleansed and sterilized with special care, and the cervical canal should be cleansed with alcohol swabs. Another precaution, which is important when the cervical canal of the pregnant uterus is to be dilated, is to examine the patient carefully under anesthesia to learn the exact position of the uterus. Perforation of the soft uterus with the dilators is easily done if the operator persists in forcing the dilator in a direction other than that of the cervical canal. Dilatation should be carried to a sufficient degree to permit the free use of the necessary instruments in the uterine cavity and the removal of the products of conception. During the first 6 weeks of pregnancy dilatation to 1 cm. or slightly more is all that is necessary, but at the end of the 3rd month dilatation to 2 cm. is sometimes required. When the dilator is introduced, one must guard against permitting it to slip suddenly with great force past the resistant internal os. The Hanks dilators have ridges to prevent introduction beyond a certain point, but the Hegar dilator can be used with equal safety if the operator has this precaution in mind, as he should at all times when working on the pregnant uterus (Fig. 22-1).

When the pregnancy has advanced beyond the 12th week, we are apt to empty the uterus by hysterotomy but occasionally, especially in parous women, emptying it through the cervix seems to be advisable. In such cases cervical dilatation by preliminary gauze packing may be safer and more satisfactory than dilatation with metal dilators. To one who is surgically minded, the idea of packing the lower uterine segment with gauze and then entering the uterine cavity a day later is repellent. However, this method is used by a great many professional abortionists who have a remarkably low incidence of clinical infection, and it is safer than forcing rapid dilatation with metal dilators when pregnancy has advanced beyond the 12th week.

The method of emptying the uterus after the cervix has been dilated depends chiefly on the duration of the pregnancy. As stated above, during the very early weeks of pregnancy the ordinary small serrated curette is effective and safe. In these early cases a little more than the usual care must be exerted in using the small curette if the uterus shows appreciable softening. Also, care should be taken to curette the entire cavity completely, for it is possible to miss an early ovum in spite of a reasonably thorough curettage. Later, up to the 12th week, the ovum forceps, the sponge holder, and the large blunt curette are the best instruments for removing the products of conception. An injection of oxytocin just before curettage is a worthwhile precaution. The large blunt curette is introduced, and the uterine cavity is curetted gently (Fig. 22-2). One can usually get an idea of the force with which one may safely curette by the consistency of the uterus noted on bimanual examination and by the sensation imparted through the curette as the uterine wall is stroked. Often little tissue comes away with the curette, but the products of conception are loosened, and the ovum forceps is then used to remove them. It is best not to attempt to tear the ovum from the sides of the cavity with the ovum forceps, for it is possible in attempting this to tear away pieces of the myometrium and even perforate the uterus (Fig. 22-3). In some instances when the pregnancy is not far advanced, the regular ovum forceps may be too large to pass easily through the

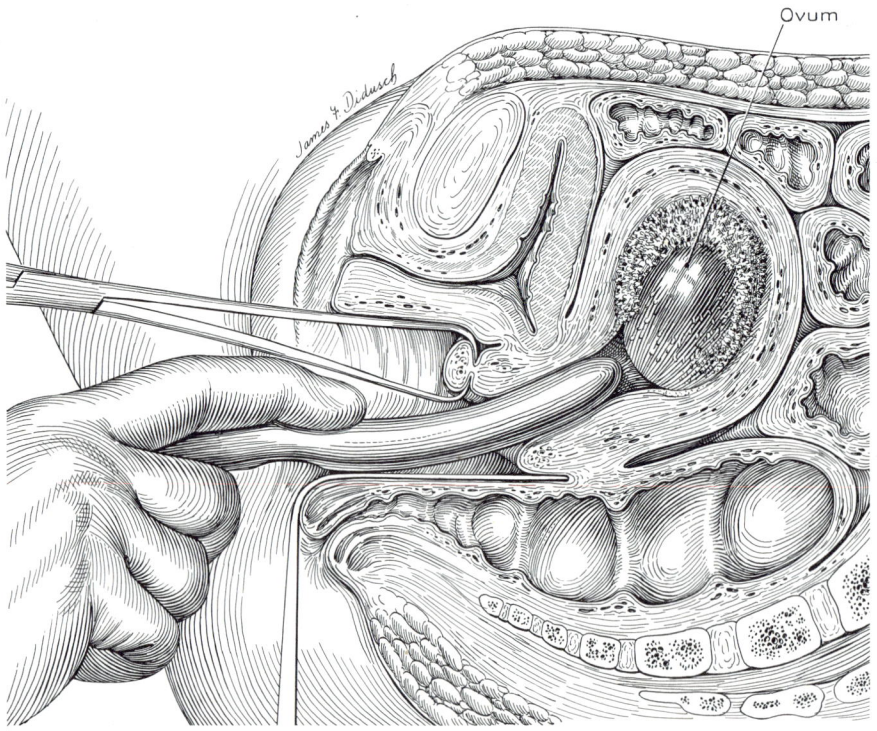

FIG. 22-1. The cervix is dilated with a Hegar dilator.

Therapeutic Abortion   433

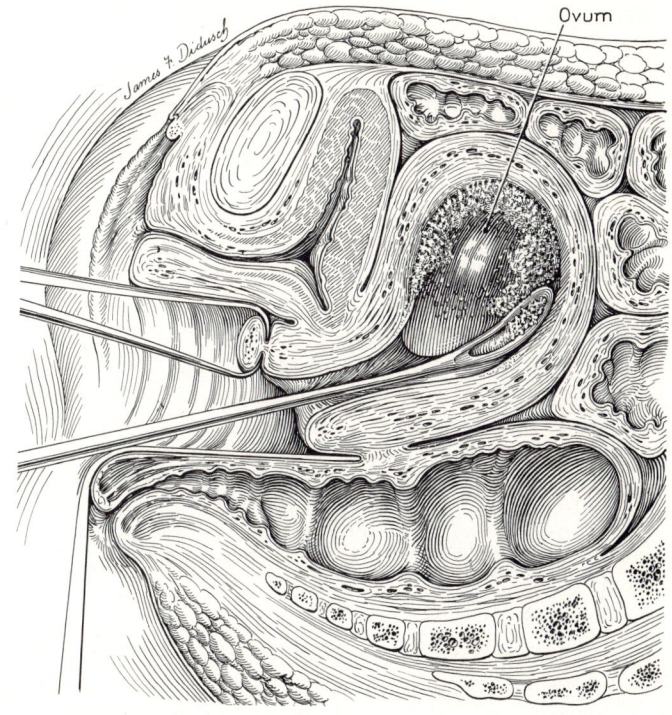

Fig. 22-2. The ovisac is detached from the uterine wall with a blunt curette.

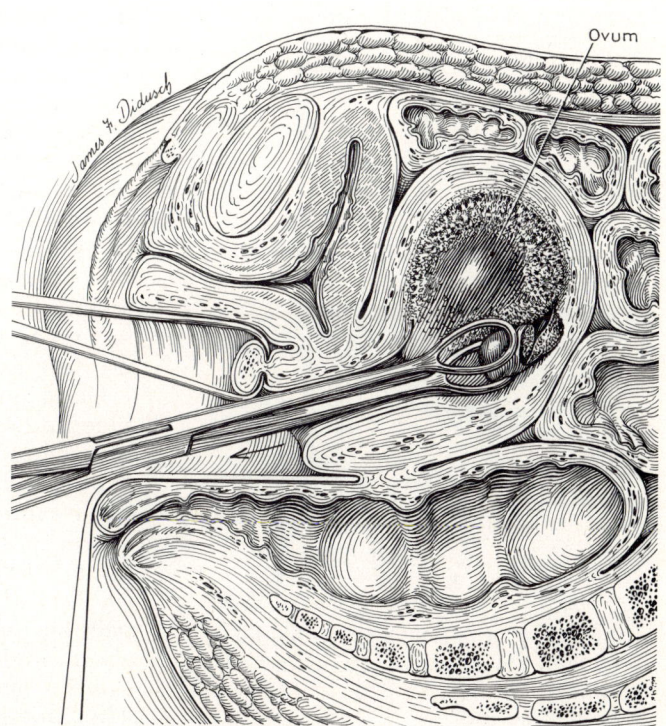

Fig. 22-3. A piece of myometrium is torn away with the instrument.

internal os and be manipulated readily. Then the ordinary sponge holder may be found to be a most useful instrument for removing the embryo and the membranes.

One of the greatest difficulties in performing a therapeutic abortion is to determine when the operation has been completed. When the operator feels that he has removed all the products of conception completely by the above maneuvers, a sponge holder is wrapped with a dry gauze sponge as shown in Figure 22-4, and the walls of the uterine cavity are rubbed with it. Often particles of placental tissue will be found adherent to it.

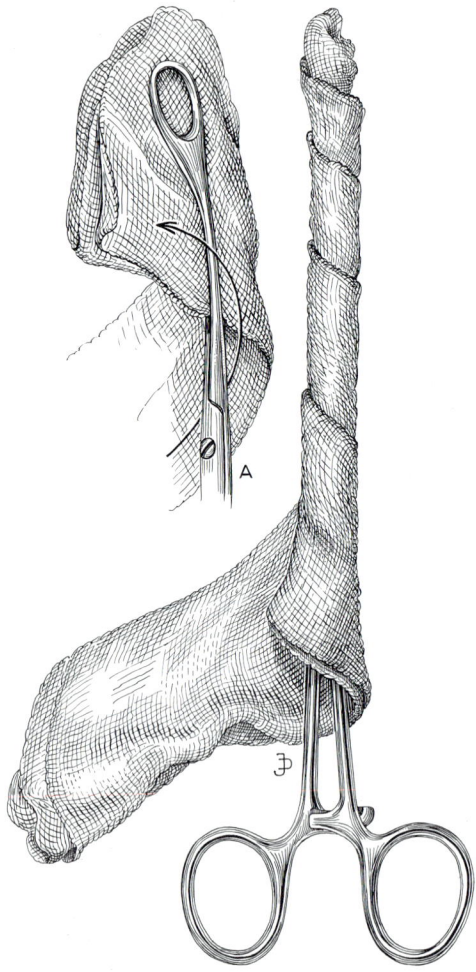

FIG. 22-4. A curved sponge holder covered with gauze is an excellent and soft instrument for freeing placental remnants from uterine wall.

Often after the 10th week, loosening of the membranes can be done best with 1 or 2 fingers introduced through the widely dilated cervix. Removal of the products of conception is usually not very successful with 1 or even 2 fingers, but after loosening these products digitally, they can be removed readily with the ovum forceps or the sponge holder.

The question of packing the uterine cavity arises after its instrumental emptying. There are only two reasons for considering it: the control of hemorrhage and the removal of particles of membrane or fetus that have not come away with the instruments. In our experience, packing is seldom necessary for the control of hemorrhage. As soon as the operator believes that he has completed the operation, an ampule of oxytocin is given, or the infusion rate is increased. If the bleeding does not seem to be under control after giving the oxytocin ample time to act, the uterine cavity may be packed tightly with a gauze strip from 1 to 3 inches in diameter, depending on the size of the uterine cavity. It is removed at the end of 12 hours. Occasionally, in spite of every effort, it is apparent that the entire product has not been removed instrumentally. A pack then may be inserted, to be removed at 12 hours when the remaining particles may come away with the pack.

After a therapeutic abortion the patient is kept in the hospital 4 to 5 days. Even when the pregnancy is only of a few weeks' duration, the operation should not be considered as lightly as an ordinary diagnostic curettage. Some danger of infection is ever present, even when the greatest aseptic care is exercised.

Occasionally, persistent or profuse bleeding indicates that evacuation of the uterus has not been complete, and one is confronted with the possible necessity of further intra-uterine instrumentation. *The second entrance of the uterine cavity is attended with much greater danger than the first.* It is in performing abortions on patients who have been attempting to abort themselves that criminal abortionists most often get into difficulties. The slight infection introduced at the first attempt is usually well walled off, but the breaking down of the leukocytic wall by the second instrumentation permits millions of organisms to enter the lymphatics and the bloodstream. Even when the temperature is normal, one must assume that some infection exists in the uterine cavity for several days following an abortion done under the best aseptic conditions. Therefore one should postpone as long as possible a second attempt to empty the uterus completely. Hemorrhage is the symptom that eventually may force a second operation, but by repeated transfusions one is often able to keep up the hemoglobin and avoid, or at least defer, entering the uterine cavity again. When the second operation becomes unavoidable, the patient is thoroughly treated prophylactically with a chemotherapeutic agent for 24 hours before the operation is done, unless extreme hemorrhage does not allow this much time. In that case chemotherapy is instituted immediately after operation.

Evacuation by uterine aspiration is a relatively new procedure but has had wide use, especially in eastern Europe, where it is apparently displacing the use of dilatation and curettage for therapeutic abortions before the 12th week. It can also be used for evacuation of incomplete and missed abortions and hydatidiform mole.

The method is outlined by the diagram in Figure 22-5. The aspiration curette is a metal or rigid plastic tube with smooth beveled tip and bent to adapt to cervix and corpus, with a small hole near the base for finger control of negative pressure. Sizes varying from 6 to 12 mm. bore allow adaptation to the duration of pregnancy. Pressure tubing connects to a trap specimen bottle with gauze screen to separate tissue from fluid. This in turn connects to a dry trap joined to a source of vacuum. A suitable electric pump is necessary as suction of 18 to 25 inches of mercury (or 0.4 to 0.8 kg. per cm.²) is necessary. (An assembly of aspirator, traps, and pump is now available commercially.)

The aspiration curette and tubing are sterilized, and the perineum and vagina are prepared and draped as for curettage. General anesthesia is used when much dilatation is needed; paracervical block may be used for some cases. Vladov reported that 40 per cent of his early abortions were done with practically no dilatation and no anesthesia. The exact position of the uterus is determined and its cavity sounded. The cervix is grasped with a tenaculum and dilated to the desired size of suction curette (about 1 mm. for each week of pregnancy). The curette is introduced with suction off; ergotrate, 1 mg., or oxytocin is given intravenously; and the uterus is palpated for firmness. The suction is then turned on and controlled by the finger on the opening at the base. The curette aperture is moved systematically over the uterine wall to remove all of the product. The procedure is completed in 3 minutes by an experienced operator. Curettage to check completeness of evacuation has been reported to yield very little additional tissue in most cases.

Kerslake and Casey have reviewed reports covering 1,728 cases and added their own experience. Several series reported no uterine perforations, others an incidence varying from 0.09 to 0.7 per cent. Blood loss was reported significantly less, postoperative infection and complications less, and hospital stay

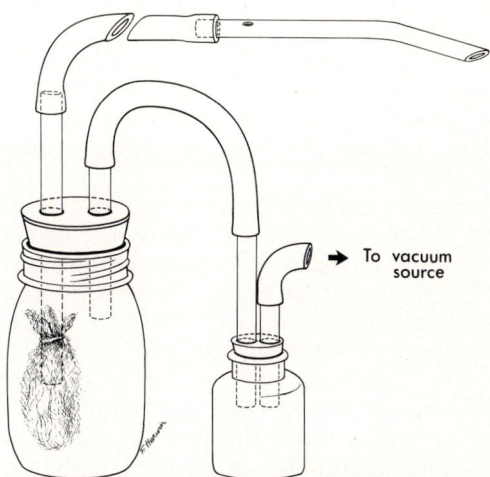

FIG. 22-5. Uterine aspiration system. (Courtesy of Dr. C. J. Eaton, University of Michigan Medical Center)

shorter than with termination by dilatation and curettage.

Termination of pregnancy after 12 weeks has been done occasionally by packing the cervix with sterile gauze and completing by dilatation, ovum forceps, and manual evacuation 24 hours later. This carries hazard of infection and perforation and had best be replaced by hypertonic injection, hysterotomy, or hysterectomy in most cases.

The hypertonic injection method is especially applicable to the patient with pregnancy beyond the 14th week who is a bad risk for laparotomy. It does not permit sterilization, but this can be handled by some other means or at a later time if the condition improves. The patient is prepared by emptying the bladder, is placed on the table in slight Trendelenburg position, and the abdomen is cleaned as for laparotomy. Amniocentesis is done, using local anesthesia and a 6- or 7-inch 18-gauge needle with stylet. The needle is placed in the lower midline above the bladder but well below the top of the fundus to avoid the bowel. After the stylet is removed and the syringe is attached, aspiration of 100 to 200 cc. of fluid is done, depending on the duration of pregnancy. The fluid is replaced with the same volume of 20 per cent sodium chloride solution or 50 per cent glucose in water solution. There is a latent period of 18 to 48 hours with a mean time of about 32 hours before evacuation occurs. The actual labor is usually short, once it begins, but can be augmented with oxytoxin if necessary. The hypertonic saline can cause serious cardiorenal reactions if it gets into the maternal circulation; this can be especially serious in a patient with cardiac or chronic hypertensive vascular disease. The glucose injection has been followed by fatal infections in a few cases (Peel, Briggs, and MacDonald *et al.*).

The termination of pregnancy after the 12th week is best done by hysterotomy or hysterectomy if the patient is able to tolerate laparotomy and particularly when sterilization is indicated as well. Even for pregnancies of less than 12 weeks, if sterilization is indicated and the patient is a satisfactory operative risk, the single definitive hysterotomy and sterilization is the procedure of choice.

Whenever laparotomy is to be done for termination of pregnancy and sterilization, the matter should be discussed with the patient. Although saving the uterus in a sterile woman would not appear to be important, the preservation of the menstrual function may be excessively important in the minds of some women. The medical condition of the patient may dictate the shortest possible procedure, which for many operators would be hysterotomy and tubal sterilization. Fibroids in the pregnant uterus may make hysterectomy the desirable method of accomplishing the desired ends. When hysterectomy is done, the total operation is preferable and usually can be carried out quite as simply as on the nonpregnant woman. However, it should be borne in mind that these patients are not robust, and total hysterectomy should not be persisted in if the risk of added operating time outweighs the advantages of removing the cervix.

Most conditions that are serious enough to require therapeutic abortion are also mandatory for sterilization. Indications and methods of tubal ligation are discussed in Chapter 19. The Pomeroy operation is quickly done without blood loss. The Irving procedure is only slightly more complicated and has a higher success rate.

Technic: Abdominal Hysterotomy for Termination of Pregnancy. A low midline incision is made as for the usual pelvic laparotomy. If the pregnancy is early, the uterus is delivered out of the abdomen. If it is advanced, the operation may be done without delivering the uterus. It is not justifiable to enlarge the incision sufficiently to deliver a greatly enlarged uterus. Moist gauze packs are used to keep the blood from running into the abdominal cavity.

An incision is made through the anterior uterine musculature, and the uterine cavity is entered. In order to elevate the anterior wall and steady the uterus, a traction suture of catgut is placed at either end of the incision (Fig. 22-6). An

FIG. 22-6. Abdominal hysterotomy for therapeutic abortion. (A) The uterus has been opened, and the fetus has been delivered. (B) The myometrium has been sutured with interrupted sutures. (C) The serosa is approximated with continuous suture of fine catgut.

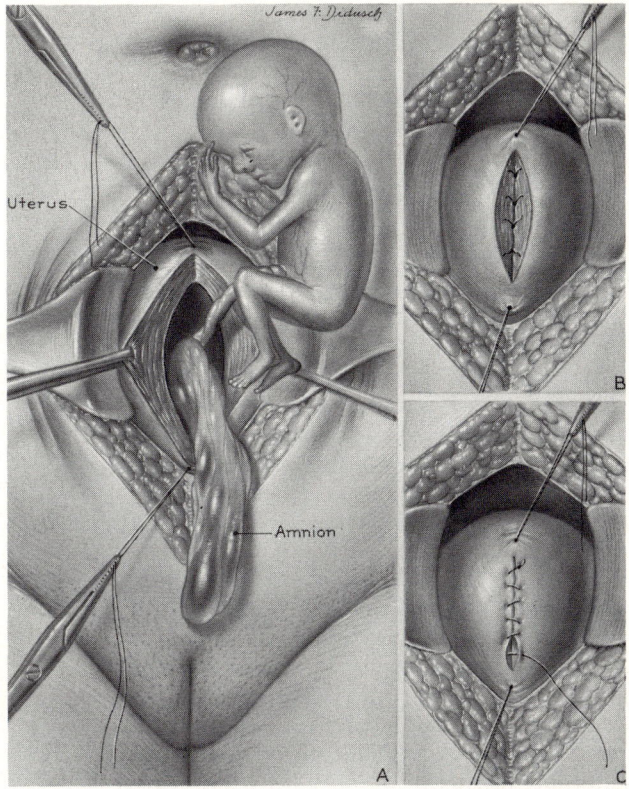

attempt is made to shell out the complete sac intact from the uterine cavity. In the more advanced pregnancies often this is not accomplished. The fetus and the ruptured amnion are delivered, and then the placental tissue (Fig. 22-6 A). An ampule of ergotrate is then given intravenously. Ten units of oxytocin may be added to the intravenous drip.

Closure of the uterine incision is done in 2 or 3 layers. The musculature is first approximated with interrupted or figure-of-eight sutures of No. 0 chromic catgut which do not enter the uterine cavity (Fig. 22-6 B). The second layer closes the serosa and the superficial musculature with a continuous Cushing stitch of No. 0 chromic catgut (Fig. 22-6 C).

HABITUAL ABORTION

The term *habitual abortion*, referring to 3 consecutive abortions, is supported by long usage, but its reliability as a statistical indicator of future outcome has been challenged. Nevertheless, if deficiencies can be found and rectified, the expectation for successful pregnancy increases. Some women have an occasional surviving infant interspersed in a series of abortions, so that they do not fit the definition, but they have disturbed reproduction and warrant search for etiologic factors. *Recurrent abortion* may be a more inclusive term.

In searching for factors responsible for recurrent abortion, consideration of the patterns of abortion and the pathology of the abortus is useful. Unfortunately, the product is often not evaluated, and the patient knows little about her previous losses. Recurrent abortions may be due to:

1. Defective gametes (sperm or ovum).
2. Deficiencies in uterine environment, which may involve:
   a. General support—nutritional and metabolic;

b. Specific support—hormone influences on endometrium and myometrium;
c. Anatomical factors—myomata, congenital uterine anomalies, cervical incompetence;
d. ? Psychological factors.

Abortions due to gamete deficiency are usually poor with villi only, possibly an empty sac or a small stunted ovum. Inadequate endometrium at implantation or soon afterward may likewise cause this type of early defective product. Late deficiency of myometrial support is usually associated with a well-formed fetus. Lack of metabolic support from low thyroid function is most often associated with an early defective product but occasionally results in a late abortion of a well-formed fetus. Years ago Delfs and Jones related the pathology of the abortus to patterns of physiologic deficiency, and subsequent experience has fortified this concept. Anatomic factors are generally associated with well-formed fetuses. The same should be true of psychologic factors if, indeed, they have any etiologic role.

Investigation of recurrent abortion should begin with a detailed history of previous pregnancies, including their duration, symptoms, onset and sequence of bleeding, pain, and membrane rupture during the actual abortion, and information about the abortus. Whether a fetus was present or absent, normally formed and sized for dates, and alive or dead at delivery gives clues to areas of deficiency. This should be followed by a general medical history, physical examination, and laboratory studies as outlined. It is important to cover all areas as many patients have multiple factors, and all should be corrected, if possible. Ideally, these patients should be evaluated in the nonpregnant state with study continued through pregnancy, particularly in the early months. If the patient is pregnant when first seen, it is desirable to make all studies that can be done during pregnancy, as information gained may be helpful in future pregnancies even if the current pregnancy cannot be salvaged.

INVESTIGATION OF RECURRENT ABORTION

Examinations

Preconceptional Study:
History—general and detailed reproductive; dietary evaluation.
Physical examination.
Diagnostic tests:
   Urine—sugar, albumen, microscopic (culture, if indicated).
   Blood—Hemoglobin, WBC and differential.
      Sedimentation rate.
      Serologic test for syphilis.
      Blood typing—patient and husband.
   Glucose tolerance test.
   Thyroid function tests—PBI, T_3 uptake, etc.
   Luteal phase evaluation:
      Basal body temperature, 3 to 4 months.
      Pregnanediol excretion, 7 to 9 days postovulation.
      Endometrial biopsy, 7 to 9 days postovulation.
   X-ray—chest.
      Hysterogram (special attention to internal os).
   Semen examination of husband.

Postconceptional Study:
   Serum chorionic gonadotrophin.
   Pregnanediol excretion.
   PBI (if indicated).

Definite or Probable Factors

When examinations are complete, definite or probable factors should emerge for correction.

Defective Gametes. Such deficiencies are suspected when abortions have occurred in the first 10 to 12 weeks with absent or poor embryos. The etiology of poor gametes is unknown. Carr demonstrated abnormal chromosomes in 22 per cent of 400 abortions. Such studies may be of importance in the future but are not yet generally available clinically.

Semen examination gives some indication of the adequacy of the male gamete. The author has seen several recurrent aborters in whom no abnormality was demonstrated except defective sperm in the husband. Joël judged sperm defect to be the etiologic factor in 17 per cent of 114 habitual aborters whom he studied.

There is no test for normality of the ovum, but after implantation the normality of the young trophoblast can be checked by assay for chorionic gonadotrophin. If this is very low for the duration of pregnancy, it indicates a poor product, and further therapy is not given.

Early blighting of the implantation may occur if the endometrium is not well supported, and this factor needs to be corrected before assuming that failure is in the sperm or ovum.

Deficiencies in Environment. The environment of the embryo or fetus in utero is dependent upon general physiologic and specific hormonal factors.

GENERAL NUTRITIONAL SUPPORT. Many animal experiments attest the importance of good nutrition in fetal development. Warkany reviewed the human data and found convincing relationship between diet and successful pregnancy. The patient with abortion history should have a high quality diet with ample protein and balanced vitamins and iron. Many women will benefit from vitamin B supplementation to meet the increased need of early pregnancy. Calories should be allocated to adjust the weight up or down toward the ideal before pregnancy is undertaken. Overweight women frequently have poor quality diets needing correction. If the glucose tolerance test is abnormal, diet should be adjusted accordingly.

THYROID. Association of decreased thyroid function and recurrent abortion has been known for years. Delfs and Jones found thyroid deficiency in 55 per cent and the sole deficiency in 32 per cent of recurrent aborters. They noted correlation of thyroid deficiency with poorly developed products usually lacking a fetus. In a few women there may be later abortions of formed fetuses, suggesting that more than one pathway may be involved. In individuals with repeated abortion history, PBI of 4.0 or below is indication for therapy even without clinical signs as the reproductive process is one of the most sensitive indicators of hypothyroidism. Very early in pregnancy the PBI normally rises so that a PBI of 6.0 mcg. per cent is the lower limit for pregnant women. Dessicated thyroid (or equivalent amounts of other preparations) is satisfactory, with dosage usually between 32 and 128 mg. Very large amounts are not required or desirable. Supplementary therapy should be given at least 3 to 4 months before pregnancy is attempted.

PROGESTERONE. This hormone is a major support of pregnancy originating from two sources, the corpus luteum and later the placenta, and having two functions, the preparation and maintenance of the endometrium and augmentation of the myometrial growth with diminution of contractility.

Luteal Phase and Early Pregnancy. Adequacy of the corpus luteum function can be evaluated by basal body temperature chart supplemented by determination of 24-hour pregnanediol excretion and endometrial biopsy, both determined between days 7 and 9 after ovulation. If progesterone is ample, usually all of these tests will be normal; if it is inadequate, some or all tests may show deficiency. If the endometrium is poorly prepared, implantation may not take place, or very early abortion may occur; if deficiency is less severe, blighting may occur, followed later by abortion. Such luteal phase deficiency must be corrected during cycles when pregnancy is being planned by giving progesterone from the 3rd day after ovulation (temperature chart). Progesterone in oil, 15 mg. I.M. daily, or its equivalent supports a good progestational endometrium. Medroxyprogesterone acetate (Provera), 5.0 to 7.5 mg. daily by mouth, may be used.

When the menstrual period is missed, assay of chorionic gonadotrophin and pregnanediol determination are done. If the gonadotrophin is normal, suggesting a normal product, progesterone support is continued. Some guide to dosage is indicated by pregnanediol values, the aim being to follow the rising curve of normal pregnancy. Supplement for the first trimester of 25 to 50 mg. of progesterone daily or its equivalent will usually be sufficient. (Hydroxyprogesterone caproate [Delalutin], 125 mg. I.M. twice weekly, or medroxyprogesterone acetate [Provera], 15 to 30 mg. daily by mouth, may be used.) Aborters with a history of early abortions only, who have normal pregnanediol values after pregnancy is well established, may be gradually withdrawn from supplemental progesterone after the 4th month.

Late (Placental) Progesterone Deficiency. Beyond the 2nd to 3rd month most of the progesterone is produced by the placenta and functions chiefly on the myometrium, augmenting growth and decreasing contractility. Inadequacy of placental progesterone may result in midtrimester abortion or premature labor. Characteristically in this type of loss the fetus is normally formed and may even be born alive. Women with this deficiency will require supplenentation until 35 to 36 weeks, when the fetus has good expectation of survival. Daily progesterone of 50 to 100 mg. I.M. or its equivalent— e.g., hydroxyprogesterone caproate (Delalutin), 250 mg. 2 or 3 times weekly— would be average support, but occasional patients may require 200 mg. progesterone or more daily. For episodes of threatening labor in late months of pregnancy, larger amounts, up to 400 to 600 mg. daily, may be needed to control the acute situation. Pregnanediol excretion may be helpful in determining needed dosage if hydroxyprogesterone caproate is being used, as it is not excreted as pregnanediol. It must be remembered that this medication is metabolized slowly and is without effect until about 24 hours after injection; hence it cannot be relied upon in acute threats. Progesterone is better in such situations. Intravenous infusion of 10 per cent ethyl alcohol in dextrose solution may be used as a sedative in the acute threats of labor, but it does not give support for physiologic deficiency as does progesterone.

Anatomic Factors. Uterine myomas, uterine anomalies, and cervical incompetence have been implicated as anatomic causes of recurrent abortions.

MYOMATA usually are not a cause of abortion unless they are submucous in location, and the placenta is implanted over the myoma. Even then, unless there is serious deficiency of blood supply, the pregnancy may accommodate very well. Only after complete investigation and elimination of other possible causes of abortion should myomectomy be undertaken and then only between pregnancies.

DOUBLE UTERUS may be associated with abortion and premature labor but not regularly so. In an unselected series of patients with uterine anomalies admitted to an obstetric service, two thirds had no difficulties or histories of previous losses (Jones, Delfs, and Jones). In a study series of women with double uterus who presented because of recurrent abortions, more than a third had demonstrable endocrine deficiencies which responded to therapy, and pregnancies were successful. One third eventually had unification operations, with 50 per cent having successful pregnancies subsequently. Operation should be reserved for patients with a history of well-formed fetuses who have been well investigated and no other factors found. The author has treated a few patients with double uterus and a history of repeated midtrimester losses with supplementary progesterone on the rationale of promoting uterine growth and reducing irritability in the distorted corpus. The pregnancies continued close to term with successful outcome, but further study of this therapy would be desirable.

INCOMPETENT CERVIX is a term which includes two different concepts: the first is a cervix with a demonstrable anatomic defect due to previous laceration through the internal os; the second is a somewhat less concrete concept of a congenital deficiency in the cervix which permits excessively early, silent effacement and dilatation occurring in the midtrimester or early 3rd trimester of pregnancy, that is, changes which resemble the normal condition at the onset of labor at term.

The first type is very rare and requires

careful hysterogram to corroborate the diagnosis. It is properly treated by excision of the scar and plastic repair in the nonpregnant state. Lash and Lash have described a procedure of this type.

The second type is certainly not common, as Barter *et al.* found only 19 such cases among 35,000 obstetric cases. The diagnosis cannot be made with any confidence unless thorough investigation of reproductive failure as outlined above is carried out.

The Shirodkar-Barter cerclage operation has been rather widely used for the congenital type of case in recent years. The procedure is illustrated in Figures 22-7 to 22-14. It is usually done in preselected patients between 14 and 18 weeks of pregnancy when the possibility of first trimester abortion of poor products is past. Some do the procedure at later stages of pregnancy when by examination the cervix is found to be dilating, but results are often disappointing when there is much effacement, or dilatation is 3 cm. or more. It should never be undertaken if there is any evidence suggesting ruptured membranes, amnionitis, bleeding, or uterine irritability. Subsequent to the cerclage the occurrence of rupture of membranes, infection, or labor pains requires *immediate* removal of the suture as a few cases of fatal infection and of ruptured uterus have occurred as complications.

The place of this operative procedure in reproductive failure is difficult to assess with certainty. The considerable literature on the subject is hard to evaluate because many series have reported little if any physiologic study before or after the operation, and many patients have been given supplementary progesterone therapy following surgery. The author has depended much more on the physiologic study and treatment outlined

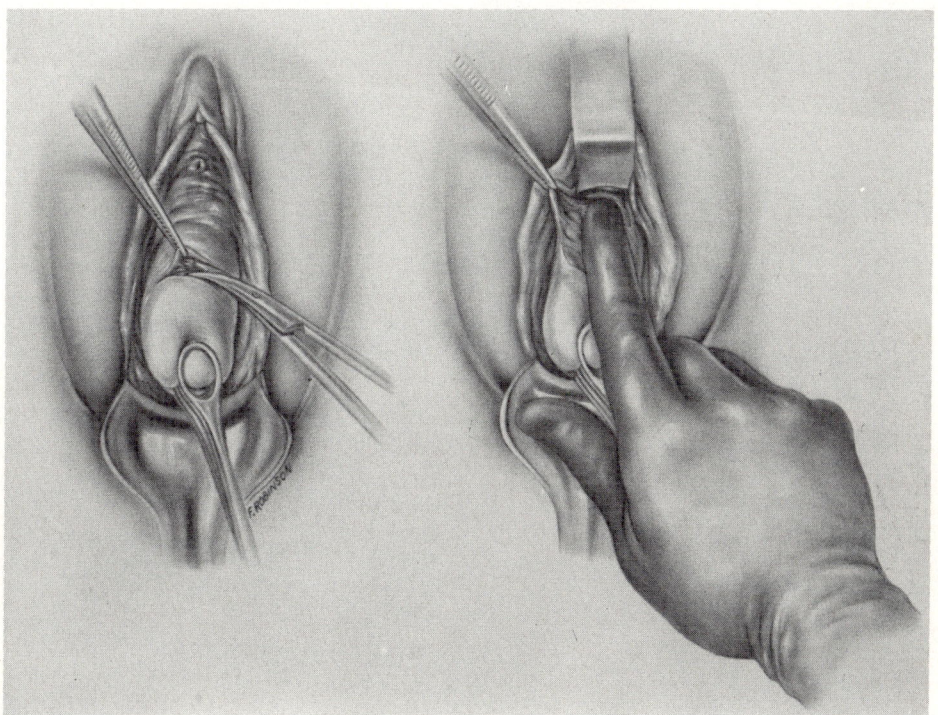

Fig. 22-7 (*Left*). A transverse incision is made through the vaginal mucosa at its junction with the cervix.
Fig. 22-8 (*Right*). The bladder is advanced. This is necessary so that the ribbon suture may be placed high enough to be of value.
(Figs. 22-7 to 22-14 from Dr. R. H. Barter and the Ethicon Co.)

442 Abortions

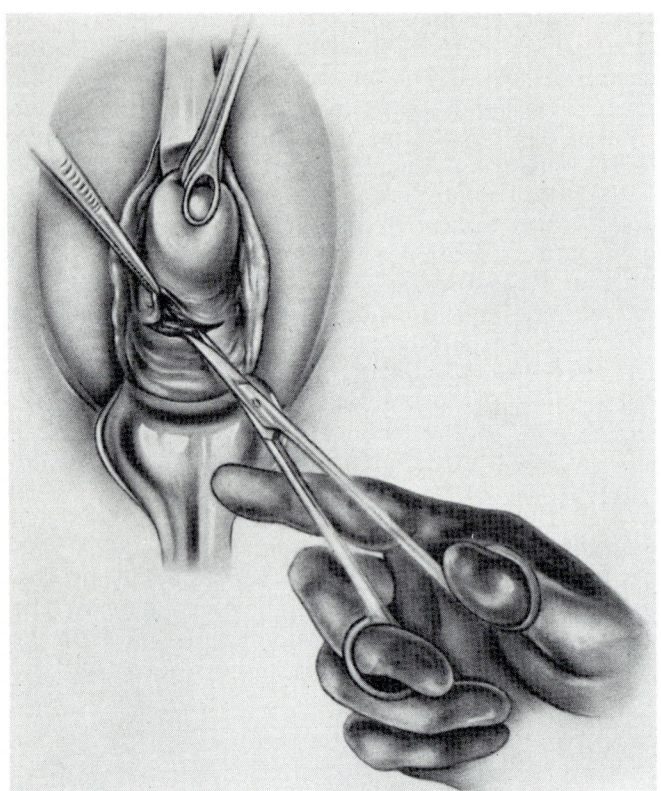

Fig. 22-9. A transverse incision is then made through the vaginal mucosa, posteriorly as it is reflexed onto the cervix.

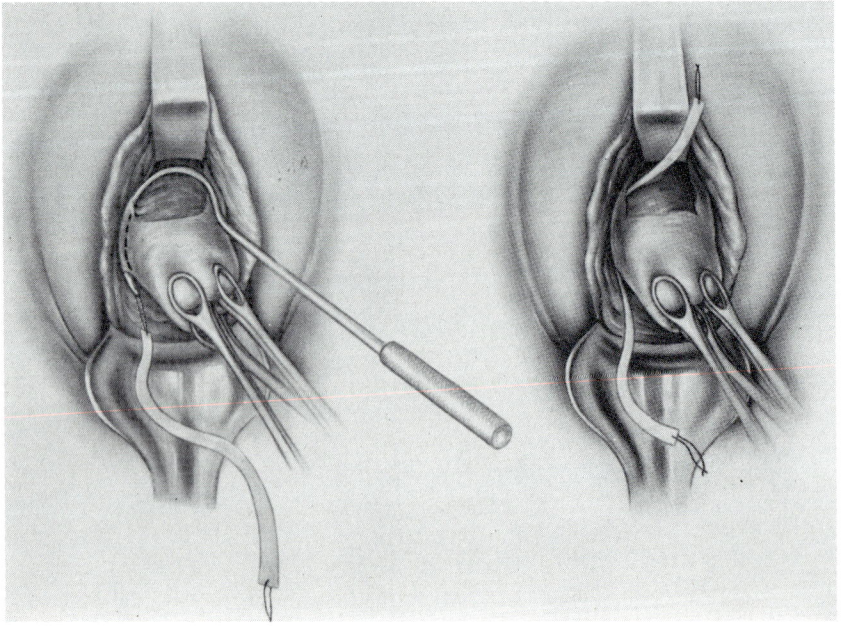

Fig. 22-10. (*Left*) An aneurysm needle is introduced beneath the mucosa and is made to emerge posteriorly. The encircling ligature strip is then pulled upward under the mucosa on the right. (*Right*) Shows the ligature in place on the right side.

FIG. 22-11. A mirror image aneurysm needle is then inserted on the left, and the other end of the ligature is brought anteriorly beneath the mucosa.

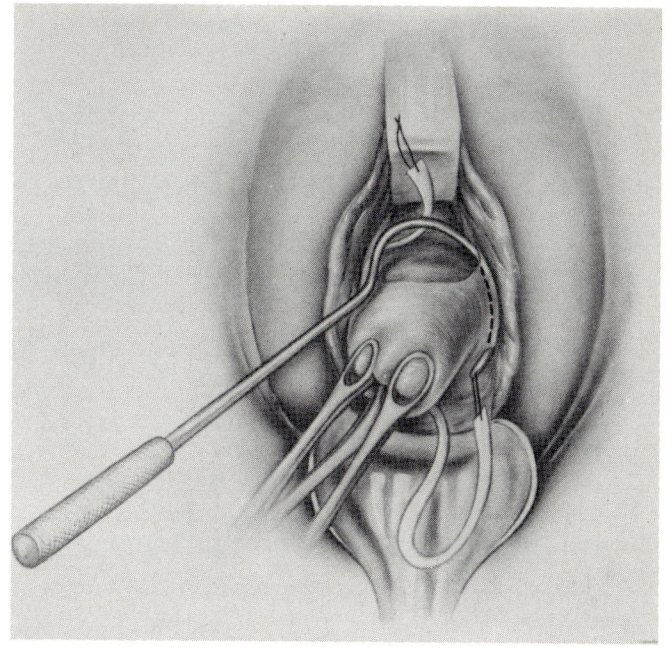

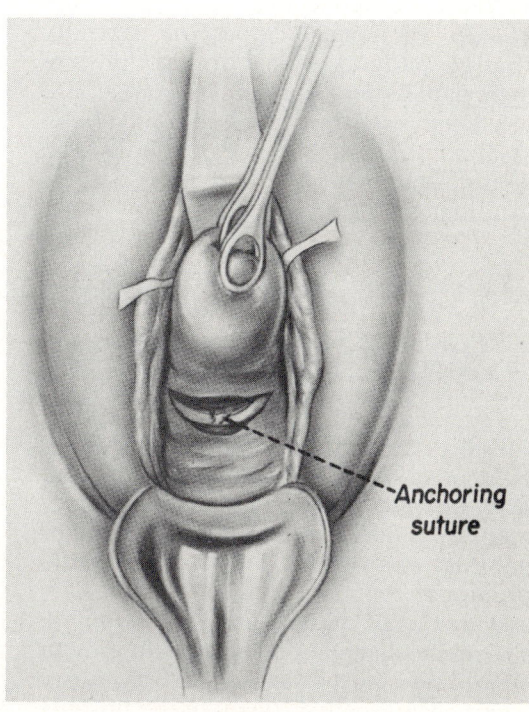

FIG. 22-12. Shows the ligature anchored posteriorly by 2 fine silk sutures.

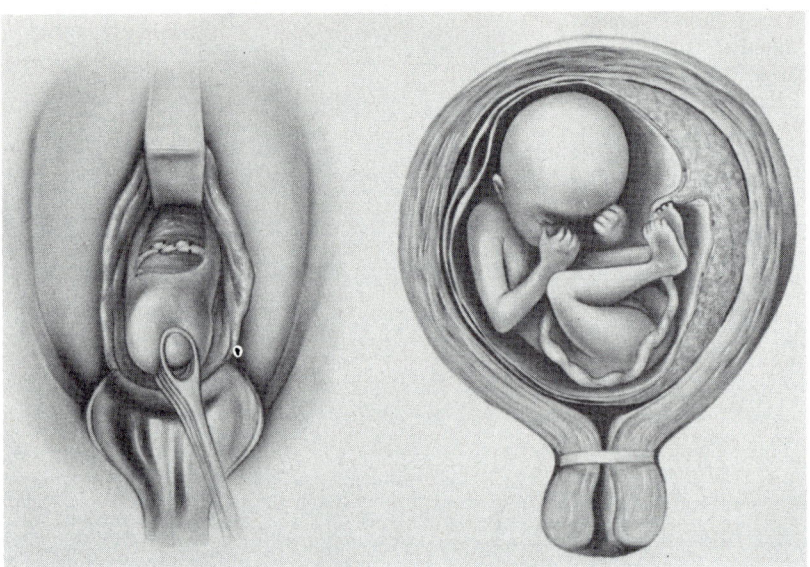

Fig. 22-13 (*Left*). Shows the encircling ligature in place, after having been looped once, pulled tightly to close the cervix. The cervix should not admit the tip of the finger after the ligature has been tightened. The ligature is anchored anteriorly with fine silk.

Fig. 22-14 (*Right*). Shows the level at which the encircling ligature should be at the completion of the operation.

above for the late aborter, with results at least as good (over 75 per cent success) as those reported for the surgical approach. In a small group of carefully studied patients presenting no physiologic deficiencies, the cerclage procedure has been used but has frequently been disappointing in the very patients who would seem to be the most logical candidates.

TREATMENT OF UNINFECTED, AFEBRILE ABORTIONS— THREATENED, INEVITABLE, COMPLETE, AND INCOMPLETE

Threatened abortion presents with a variable amount of bleeding without pain or with mild cramps. The patient may be put at rest and given supplementary progesterone, as outlined under habitual abortion. If symptoms subside promptly, the pregnancy may continue, and moderate activity may be resumed. Frequent observation for uterine growth should be made, as missed abortion may occur occasionally if death of the product has already taken place when symptoms are manifested and treatment initiated.

When, in the opinion of the physician, the abortion is inevitable, the ideal treatment is to complete it as soon as possible and in the most conservative manner. This should be done to prevent continued bleeding and to reduce the possibility of infection ascending into the uterine cavity through the patulous cervix. There is often room for difference of opinion on whether or not an abortion has passed from the threatened to the inevitable stage. There is no single criterion upon which the decision may be made, and often the greatest clinical judgment is required. Prolonged and profuse bleeding is the most significant sign that the pregnancy cannot be saved. However, it is difficult to state how profuse and how prolonged bleeding must be in order to indicate that the abortion is inevitable. Everyone with wide experience can recall cases in which, after great blood loss, a pregnancy has continued. However, when hemorrhage is alarming, one is justified in assuming that the abortion is inevitable. As a general rule it may be stated that if treatment causes no cessation of the bleeding within a week, the abortion is certain. Again, there are many exceptions to this rule.

Cramp-like pains, occurring at regular intervals and continuing after treatment, suggest that the time has come to help in the expulsion of the fetus. When the cervix has been dilated sufficiently to admit a finger, especially in the nulliparous woman, the chances of saving the fetus are poor. A slight dilatation of the parous cervix is less significant.

If the hemorrhage does not necessitate immediate emptying of the uterus, often a pregnancy test may be of value. If negative, it is conclusive; but if positive, one should bear in mind that sufficient chorion to give a positive test may remain alive for a week or more after fetal death.

The differentiation between an infected and an uninfected case is important but may be equally difficult. Any case in which there is an elevation of temperature to 100° F. after hydration must be considered infected. However, the absence of fever does not exclude infection, and an ovisac plugging the cervical canal may give rise to fever without manifest bacterial infection. Nevertheless, an elevation of temperature is probably the most reliable single sign of infection. Leukocytosis is also significant. Most important is the history, and every effort must be made to learn the true facts. If there is a history or evidence of previous instrumentation, the chances for intra-uterine infection are so great that the case must be considered and treated as though there were intra-uterine infection.

When it is concluded that abortion is inevitable and uninfected, the uterus should be emptied promptly. Evacuation by medical means is the simplest treatment for those in whom it can be achieved (about one third of cases). A course of oxytocin injections I.M., 5 units (0.5 cc.) every half hour for 4 to 6 doses, is sometimes promptly effective. An alternate method is an intravenous infusion of 10 units of oxytocin in 500 cc. of glucose in water. Expulsion usually occurs in 1 to 6 hours, and tissue should be examined for completeness. If it appears to be complete, cramps cease, and bleeding subsides, the uterus can be assumed to be empty. After 1 or 2 days of rest in the hospital limited activity may be permitted. An occasional patient may have recurrence of active bleeding due to unrecognized retained fragments of tissue and require curettage later, but this is an innocuous procedure with a smaller and firmer uterus after some involution has taken place.

If the medicinal method does not succeed promptly, or if evacuation is incomplete or fragmented, or if there is excessive bleeding during oxytocin administration, it should be abandoned immediately in favor of surgical completion. Blood for transfusion should be available before attempting either medicinal or surgical procedures.

If a part or all of the products of conception are retained in the uninfected uterine cavity, it must be completely emptied with appropriate instruments. There is general agreement among gynecologists and obstetricians concerning this. However, there is disagreement on the method by which this is best accomplished. There is much prejudice, in general, against the use of the sharp curette. Some of this is justifiable, but the aversion which some obstetricians have to it is unfounded. For example, in very early pregnancy and when placental tissue of later pregnancy has been retained for weeks or even months, the uterus is often little, if any, larger or softer than the nonpregnant organ. The safe and most effective instrument for removing such products of conception is the ordinary serrated curette, such as is used for diagnostic curettage. On the other hand, many a soft pregnant uterus has been perforated with such a curette.

Sometimes, one need only place a speculum in the vagina and remove a large piece of placental tissue protruding from the cervix (Fig. 22-15). Generally speaking, in early pregnancy when the cervix is firm, much cervical dilatation is

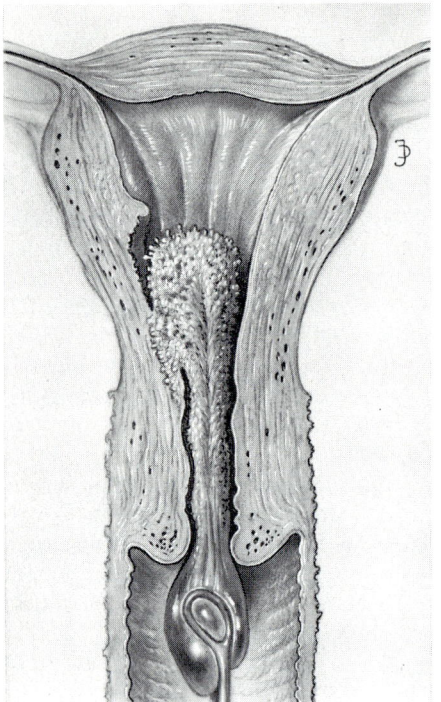

Fig. 22-15. Fetal membranes protruding from the cervix are removed with a sponge holder, which does not enter cervical canal.

impossible. Evacuation by instruments is the method of choice in such cases. To attempt to dilate such a cervix to the point at which a finger can be introduced might result in serious laceration. Furthermore, the single finger introduced through a tight cervix is incapable of sufficient maneuvering to remove the ovisac or the placental remnants. In pregnancy advanced beyond 12 weeks, when sufficient cervical dilatation is attained, the placental tissue can often be loosened with the finger (Fig. 22-16) and removed with a sponge stick (Fig. 22-17). As a rule one should remember that the larger and softer the uterus, the blunter should be the instrument selected, and the greater the care with which it should be used. What has been said regarding the dangers of operative procedures in emptying the uterus per vaginam in therapeutic abortions is equally applicable in the treatment of incomplete abortion.

A new and promising surgical approach to incomplete abortion is the uterine aspiration method described under therapeutic abortion. This has the advantage of requiring less dilatation and instrumentation; hence it presents a smaller risk of perforation of the uterus. Blood loss is usually minimal, and the leukocytic barrier in the endometrium is less disturbed. Peretz and his co-workers carried out successful evacuations in 375 women with incomplete abortions, 68 per cent of whom required no dilatation of the cervix and no anesthesia. Eaton used the method in 178 cases and checked results by curettage; 81 patients with early incomplete abortions were found to have no residual tissue; 97 patients with late abortions beyond 12 weeks showed 40 per cent to have some residual tissue after uterine aspiration; 41 patients with septic abortions were evacuated without any serious complications.

TREATMENT OF INFECTED ABORTIONS

The patient with infected abortion presents a special problem which should not be underestimated even though it does not appear serious at first sight. Elevation of temperature over 100° F. is indicative of some infection, and over 101° F., a serious involvement. History or suspicion of intra-uterine interference adds to potential hazard. White blood count and differential may add corroboration and give some evidence of patient response.

Careful sterile pelvic examination will aid in diagnosing the extent of infection. If tenderness is absent or limited to the uterus, infection is probably contained within the uterine cavity and myometrium. Parametrial thickening and tenderness indicate beginning extension; cul-de-sac and forniceal tenderness suggests involvement of pelvic peritoneum. Lower abdominal tenderness and guarding means spread into the abdominal peritoneum. If there is significant fever, blood culture should be made. Speculum examination should be done and culture,

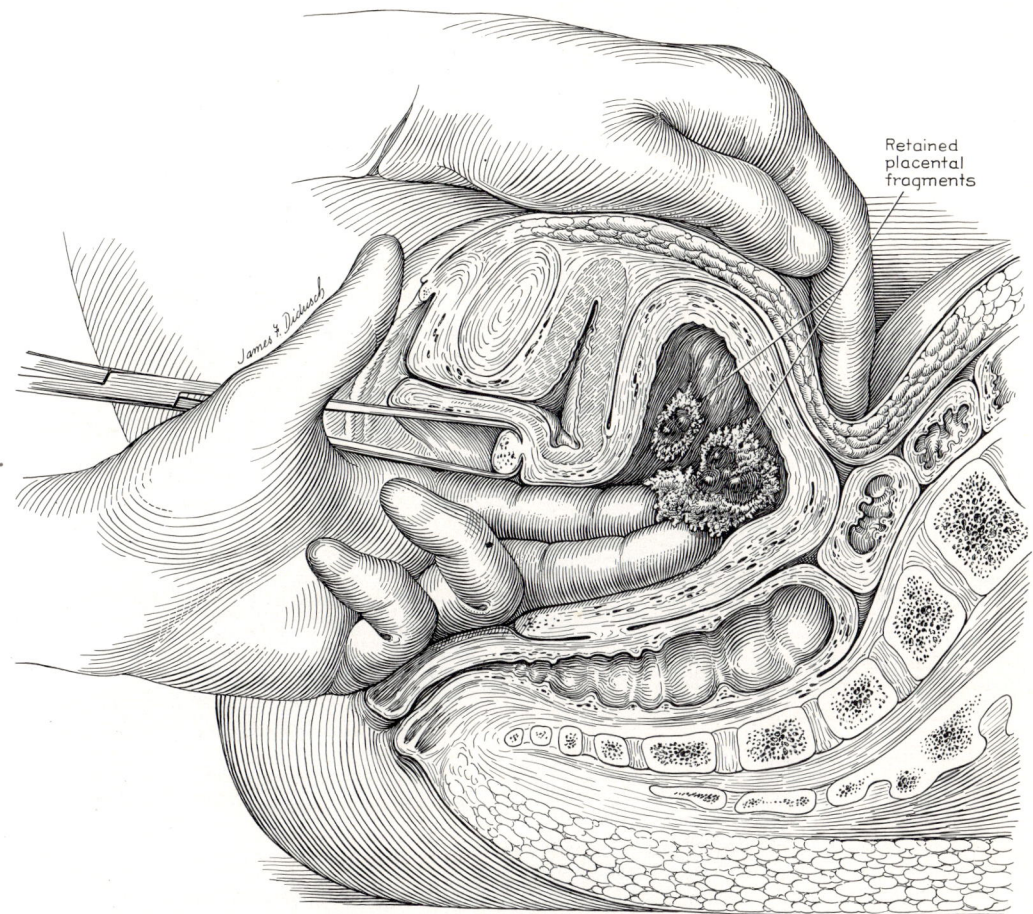

Fig. 22-16. Digital removal of retained placental fragments.

sensitivity tests, and smear taken from the cervical canal. Gram stain of the smear should be examined at once, as it may make an early presumptive diagnosis of *Clostridium welchii* or *E. coli* infection, which may dictate therapeutic use of antitoxin and choice of antibiotics. If tissue presents in the cervix, it is extracted with sterile sponge stick, but the uterine cavity is not instrumented. When there is suspicion of intra-uterine manipulation, x-ray of the abdomen and lower chest should be taken to rule out foreign bodies and air under the diaphragm, as either is evidence of perforation and requires immediate laparotomy.

All infected abortion cases must be monitored for temperature, pulse, blood pressure, and urinary output at frequent intervals. Broad antibiotic coverage should be started at once. If the temperature is under 101° F., with no spread of infection beyond the uterus, moderate antibiotic dosage such as penicillin, 600,000 units every 6 hours, and streptomycin, 0.5 gm. I.M. every 12 hours, will usually eliminate the infection. If the patient is ill with temperature over 101° F., rapid pulse, or signs of infection beyond the uterus, or if there is history of interference, massive therapy should be started, using 5 million units of penicillin in 1,000 cc. of glucose in water intravenously and 1 gm. of streptomycin intramuscularly. Glucose solution should be continued to give at least 3,000 cc. with 15 million units of penicillin in the first 24 hours, and 1 gm. of streptomycin every 12 hours. Dosage may be reduced after 2 to 3 days if response is prompt. If improvement is not satisfactory, suitable changes may be made in accord with

448 Abortions

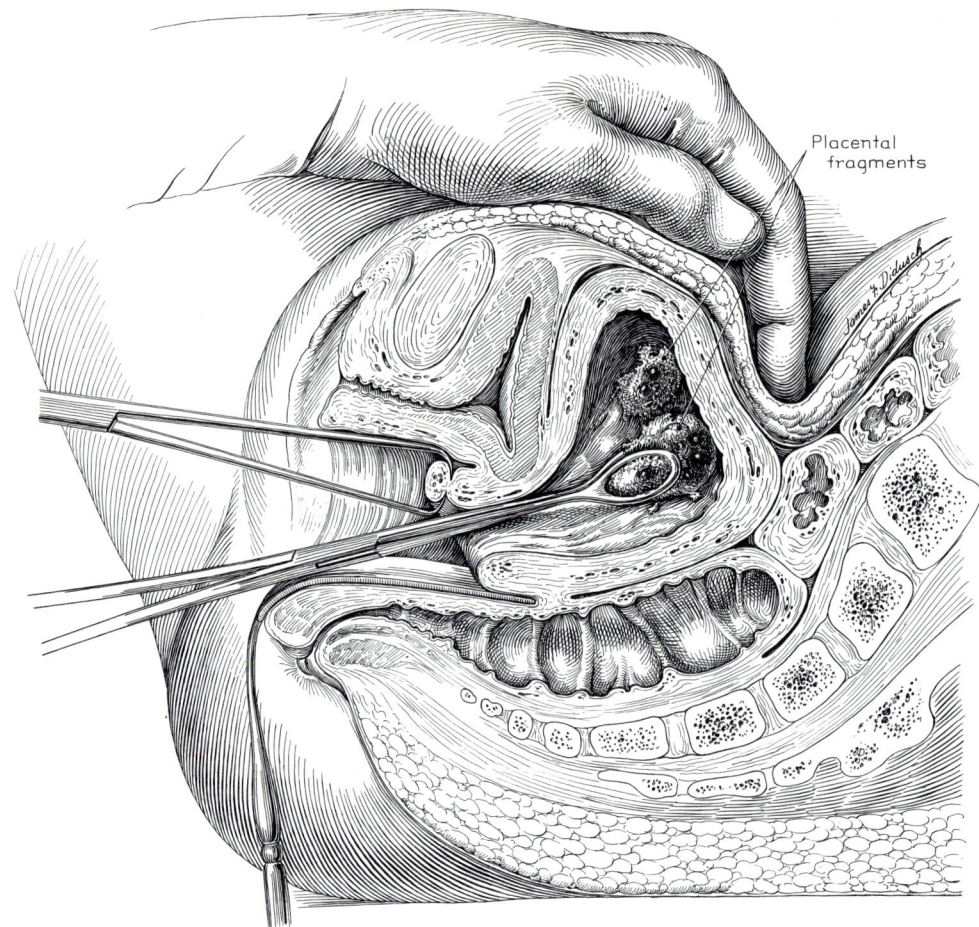

FIG. 22-17. Removal of placental fragments from uterus with sponge holder.

cultures and sensitivities. Blood replacement in anemic patients helps to combat infection. Curettage for completion of the abortion is deferred until the patient has been afebrile for at least 48 hours unless massive bleeding forces an earlier procedure. In the latter case uterine aspiration or manual evacuation is the preferred procedure.

Over a number of decades both before and after the advent of antibiotics, there have been several reversals of opinion on early versus later evacuation of the uterus in infected abortion. There is a very extensive literature on both sides of the subject, but the current trend is toward greater dependence on antibiotic and supportive treatment, with deferred operative measures.

Most patients with infected abortion will respond well to the regime outlined above. A small number, perhaps 2 per cent, will develop septic shock with falling blood pressure and decreasing urinary output. They become extremely ill and have a poor prognosis. The subject of septic shock is discussed in Chapter 11. Some other patients may have extra-uterine spread of infection before therapy is instituted and may have protracted chronic courses.

EXTRA-UTERINE SEPTIC INFECTION

Septic abortion, in which the infection has passed beyond the confines of the uterus, presents a problem in therapy quite different from that of infected abortion in which the infection is limited to the uterus. Whereas there is considerable justifiable difference of opinion on the advisability of intra-uterine manipulation in the latter type of case, almost everyone is in agreement that intra-uterine instrumentation is contraindicated when there is extension beyond the uterus. In order to consider treatment intelligently, a short review of the pathology is desirable.

Pathology

The organisms that penetrate beyond the uterine wall are in the vast majority of cases streptococci, but staphylococci and the Welch bacilli may also be the primary invading agents. Most of the streptococci are anaerobic; the incidence of hemolytic streptococci was found by Brown and Hunt to be only 1.8 per cent. However, the importance of hemolytic streptococci as a factor in mortality must be stressed, since in 57.1 per cent of their fatal cases the hemolytic streptococcus was isolated. All of the above-mentioned organisms have the ability to invade tissues and have been labeled by Curtis as the "cellulitis" group. As a result of invasion by these organisms, cellulitis, salpingitis, peritonitis, thrombophlebitis, septicemia, and distant embolic abscesses may form (Fig. 22-18).

At the beginning of the inflammatory process within the uterine cavity, an attempt is made to limit its extension by the outpouring of leukocytes which, with the aid of fibrin, form a wall in the endometrium and the myometrium. In the majority of cases, this barrier and the antibodies in the blood are successful in preventing the spread of the infection, but in certain cases the organisms penetrate the leukocytic wall and enter the myometrium. In addition to intra-uterine infection, organisms enter the cervical tissues through fresh lacerations. If the penetration is not halted, the organisms pass through the musculofibrous wall of the corpus and the cervix, and the parametrial and the paracervical tissues are invaded. Exudate pours into these tissues, and they become greatly thickened.

This process is subperitoneal and may be unilateral or bilateral. As it advances, all the connective tissue surrounding the uterus, the rectum, the bladder, and the ureters thickens, and these organs become solidly fixed. The infection may advance upward along the course of the ureter to the perinephric region or downward into the paravaginal tissues. The cellulitis, which is thus formed, may persist as such or break down into abscesses. The cellulitis is of ligneous consistency and even when abscesses do result, the walls may be formed by thick "cellulitis" tissue that gives no clue to the liquefied interior. Abscess may form low in the broad ligament and be palpable per vaginam, or it may form in the upper part of the ligament and be present above Poupart's ligament.

In addition to the ability of these organisms to penetrate tissue, they also may travel along the surface of the endometrium and out through the tubal lumina. Pyosalpinges form from streptococcal and staphylococcal infections, which may be indistinguishable grossly from neisserian pus tubes. The statement is frequently made in the literature that tubal infections resulting from abortions are of the peritubal type. This is frequently true as the result of the tube's becoming involved from broad ligament

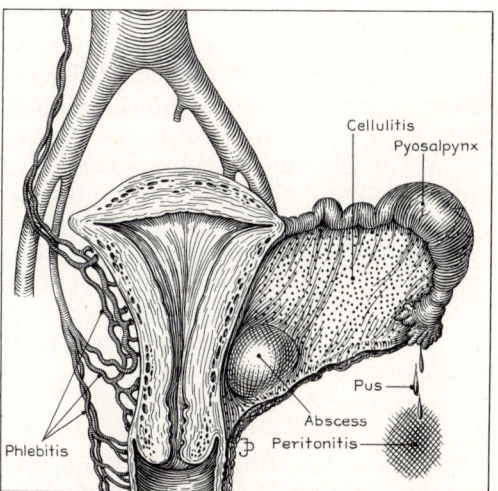

Fig. 22-18. Diagram illustrating methods of extension of abortive infection.

cellulitis or from peritonitis. However, a true endosalpingitis from extension of infection from the uterine cavity has often been demonstrated.

Organisms passing through the tubes enter the peritoneal cavity, and peritonitis results. Such peritonitis may be limited by adhesions to the pelvis, where localized abscesses can form in the cul-de-sac or elsewhere. More often, however, the peritonitis becomes generalized. The tendency to general peritonitis is much greater than with neisserian infection. The peritoneum may also become infected with lightning speed as a result of perforation of the infected uterus by a surgical instrument. In addition, the peritoneum may be infected via the lymphatics from infection in the subperitoneal spaces. In a similar manner the ovary may become abscessed through the lymphatics.

Extension of the infection by the venous route is one of the most serious complications. Fortunately, this occurs in a relatively small percentage of the cases. Brown and Hunt, for example, obtained positive blood cultures in only 8 of 500 cases of abortion. Nevertheless, it is noteworthy that of the 7 women who died in their series, 5 had positive blood cultures. It should be considered, however, that showers of cocci may enter the bloodstream from time to time and be missed on culture. In some of the cases a septic thrombophlebitis occurs in the pelvic veins, which may be considered as a defense mechanism against the invading organisms. When the thrombosis extends to the femoral veins, the typical picture of phlegmasia alba dolens results. In other cases there are no thromboses, and the organisms enter the blood freely from the infected uterus and extrauterine tissues. Abscesses may occur in almost any distant part of the body as a result of hematogenous dissemination of the infection.

TREATMENT

When dealing with septic abortion, one of the first things to ascertain is whether or not the infection has extended beyond the confines of the uterus. The signs of peritonitis should be looked for. Palpation of the lower abdomen for adnexal enlargement or for broad-ligament abscess, presenting above Poupart's ligament, should be done. However, the most revealing procedure is the pelvic examination, made with a sterile glove. First, a 2-finger examination is made; then the index finger is left in the vagina, and the middle finger is inserted into the rectum. Broad-ligament induration can best be palpated by the combined vaginal and rectal examination. Broad-ligament and adnexal thickening and tenderness are definite indications of extension of the infection beyond the uterus. These examinations should be gentle and not repeated oftener than is necessary to keep one informed on the progress of the disease.

The patient is put at rest in semi-Fowler's position. Nourishment and fluids are maintained by intravenous administration of glucose solution. If there is abdominal distention from peritonitis, a duodenal or Wangensteen suction system is instituted. While intravenous glucose is being given, penicillin, 5 to 15 million units each 24 hours, may be administered in the glucose. Later it may be given intramuscularly or by mouth as the patient's condition improves. Streptomycin, 1.0 gm. I.M. every 12 hours, may be given for broader coverage. Antibiotics are continued as long as the temperature remains elevated. The patient is often anemic in the early stage of the disease, due to recent hemorrhage. Later, progressive anemia develops as a result of blood destruction by the infection. Repeated transfusions help the patient to combat the infection; often they are lifesaving.

If the patient shows steady improvement, she should not be disturbed by frequent pelvic examinations. If she does not improve, gentle abdomino-vagino-rectal examinations should be made as often as the physician thinks necessary to keep informed of the course of the disease. Dissemination of the pelvic infection can result from rough examinations, which should be scrupulously avoided. Evidence of localization of the infection as abscesses in the peritoneal cavity, the cul-de-sac, or the broad ligament should be carefully noted, and the abscesses should be drained without delay.

Fortunate is the patient with peritonitis in whom there is localization of an abscess in the cul-de-sac, where drainage by colpotomy is easy and effective. When there is evidence of localization of an abscess higher in the abdomen, it should be drained through a small incision directly over it.

When the infection is limited to the subperitoneal spaces and the cellulitis breaks down to form an abscess, recovery is hastened by drainage. Figure 22-19 illustrates the usual sites of abscess formation. If the abscess points in the base of the broad ligament, it can be drained ideally by posterior colpotomy (Fig. 11-3). If the broad-ligament abscess is present above one of the inguinal ligaments, it can be felt by abdominal palpation. A small muscle-splitting incision

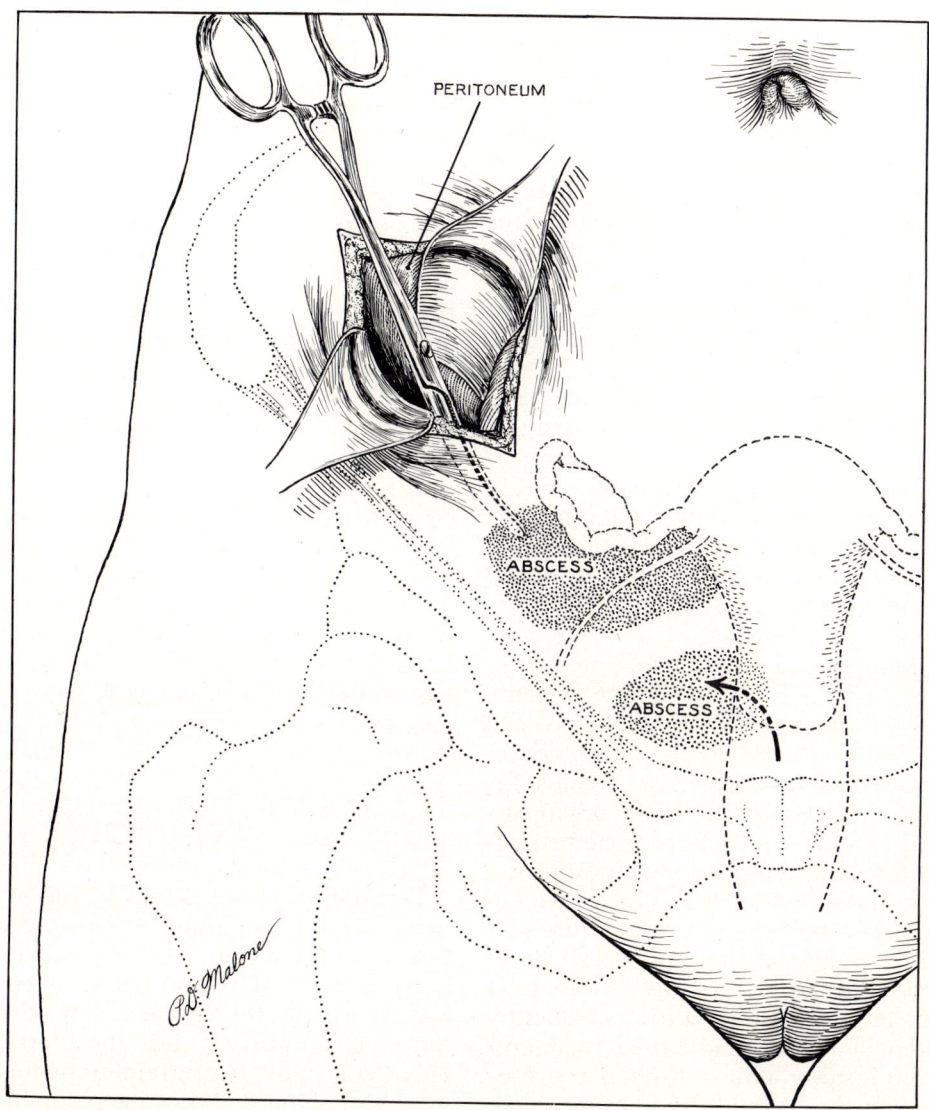

FIG. 22-19. Illustrating two possible methods of drainage of broad ligament abscesses. (A) Extraperitoneal abdominal route. (B) Vaginal route.

is made over it, down to the preperitoneal space. Then a long Kelly clamp is inserted downward and inward toward the abscess cavity (Fig. 22-19). The drainage tract is enlarged with the finger, and cigarette drains are inserted into the abscess cavity.

When acute cellulitis persists and the temperature remains septic, diathermy treatments are instituted, which may hasten the breaking down of the inflamed tissue into an abscess. The question of whether or not an abscess has actually formed is, at times, difficult to solve. Even a fairly large abscess may be encased in a thick rigid capsule of cellulitis tissue, and no fluctuation will be palpable. If spiking fever persists, we believe that it is justifiable to penetrate into such indurated tissue either via the cul-de-sac or the abdominal route. Not infrequently one will be rewarded by finding pus, but if unsuccessful, the breaking into the cellulitis tissue, well walled off between the leaves of the broad ligament, will do no harm. Even if no pus is found, drains are inserted, and eventually the tissues may break down along the drainage tract. Drainage from such cellulitis tissue is often of long duration, but ultimate resolution probably is hastened.

The treatment of thrombophlebitis is discussed in Chapter 4, Postoperative Care and Complications, and the same principles of treatment apply to postabortive phlebitis.

Chronic postabortive infection in the adnexa and the broad ligaments presents a special therapeutic problem. It has been shown by Curtis that streptococci often persist in the pelvic tissues for months and even years. If the organisms persist in such virulence as to be responsible for daily temperature elevations, a course of antibiotics should be instituted. Even when there is no temperature elevation, the aim of therapy should be to restore the pelvic organs to as near normalcy as possible. Often persistently thickened adnexa and broad ligaments may be restored almost to their previous condition by regular diathermy treatments, provided that they are carried out religiously for weeks or even months. Surgical measures should be deferred much longer than in neisserian disease. Streptococci live much longer in the tissues than gonococci, and there is greater danger of dissemination of virulent organisms by surgical trauma. Since the tubal inflammation often takes the form of perisalpingitis, the tubes have a much greater chance of remaining patent. If future pregnancies are desired, one should be ultraconservative with regard to surgery, in the hope that the lumina of the tubes will be preserved. It is truly remarkable what may be accomplished if diathermy and douching are persisted in. Pelves which are almost solid with cellulitis may, with great patience, often be restored ultimately to an almost normal condition.

However, in spite of prolonged conservative treatment, surgery is required in a small percentage of these women to restore health. Chronic infection of the cervix frequently follows abortions and requires surgical attention. The resulting adherent uterus, adnexal and intestinal adhesions may be responsible for persistent pain. Chronic abscess in the ovary or in the tube and the ovary may interfere with normal health. Functional bleeding, due to disturbed ovarian function, may be sufficiently troublesome to require surgery. Rarely, the freeing of adhesions about the tubes may be justified because of sterility. The best surgical procedure must be decided upon at the operation. Hysterectomy, salpingectomy, and cervical cauterization are all procedures that may be required to restore the patient to health.

PERFORATION OF THE PREGNANT UTERUS

Perforation of the uterus is one of the more frequent complications of emptying the pregnant womb. The real incidence is, of course, difficult to learn. Since the fault is usually the operator's, most cases fail to find their way into the literature. However, most well-trained gynecologists will admit that they have punctured one or more pregnant uteri in the course of their careers. Among the less experienced the incidence must be much greater.

Prevention requires careful consideration, for the condition has a high mortality. First, an exact preoperative knowledge of the size, the consistency, and the position of the uterus will reduce the chances of perforation. Also, one should make certain that the bladder is completely emptied by catheter so that the uterus is not displaced by a full bladder. Sufficient dilatation of the cervix to permit the easy handling of instruments or to permit the use of the finger in loosening the membranes is an important factor in lessening the possibility of perforation. One should measure carefully the depth of the uterus with a uterine sound at the beginning of the operation and avoid passing dilators or other instruments beyond that depth. The use of the ovum forceps only for removal of loosened pieces of tissue, rather than forcibly tearing the sac from the wall, is wise because a piece of myometrium can easily be torn away (Fig. 22-3) and an instrument passed through the weakened spot.

The prompt recognition of the perforation is of the utmost importance. The passage of an instrument beyond the depth of the uterine cavity is diagnostic. When the operator suspects that he has perforated the uterus, he is justified in carefully and slowly passing a blunt uterine sound through the suspected perforation to determine with certainty whether or not the wall has been perforated. The appearance of intestines within the grasp of the ovum forceps is sad but certain evidence that the uterus has been perforated and the intestines brought through the opening, with probable injury to the intestinal wall. Evidence of internal hemorrhage following the instrumentation is also diagnostic. This does not usually become evident until after the patient has left the operating room.

From the standpoint of treatment, accidental perforation of the uterus can be grouped into three categories:

1. Perforation while doing a clean therapeutic abortion.

2. Perforation while completing an incomplete abortion.

3. Perforations previously done, often by an abortionist or the patient, whose sterile technic is open to question.

The treatment of perforation of a clean pregnant uterus during a therapeutic abortion differs with the instrument with which it is done, the site of perforation, and other circumstances. When the cervix is perforated with a dilator, the opening should be closed at once. Anteriorly, the bladder can be dissected up from its cervical attachment, and the rent in the uterus can be exposed and sutured. If the bladder has been entered, it should be closed with 2 layers of fine chromic catgut. If the perforation is in the posterior wall of the cervix, the cul-de-sac should be opened through the posterior fornix. By means of retractors the wound can be exposed and sutured.

When the perforation is through the corpus uteri, a decision must be made whether to open the abdomen immediately or treat the patient expectantly. Opinion is divided. Our own view is that if the perforation is done with a curette or a uterine sound and if it is a reasonable supposition that the intestines have not been injured, the patient may be treated expectantly. By a "reasonable supposition that the intestines have not been injured" we mean that if there is simply the passage of a sound or a curette further than the limits of the uterus and the instrument is withdrawn promptly, it is unlikely that there is any injury to the bowel wall. If, on the other hand, the operator has reason to believe that he has curetted the contents of the abdominal cavity, he must recognize the possibility of intestinal injury and perform an immediate laparotomy. If the perforation is done with a sponge holder or ovum forceps, there is less likelihood of intestinal injury, and the treatment may be expectant. If bowel is brought out of the cervix with an instrument, it should be pushed back into the uterine cavity, and the abdomen should be opened immediately.

Expectant treatment is begun in the operating room. The pulse and the blood pressure should be taken repeatedly. While the patient is thus observed, preparation for laparotomy is begun so that, if it becomes necessary, there will be no delay. If the pulse and the blood pressure remain unaltered, and if the operator feels that it is unlikely that he has injured the bowel, the patient is sent to the recovery room. Ten units (1 cc.) of oxytocin is given, and a course of ergotrate started, and the patient is placed in Fowler's position. Penicillin is given immediately, 600,000 units every 6 hours. Streptomycin also is given intramuscularly in a dosage of 1 gm. every 12 hours. If the patient develops signs of internal hemorrhage or peritonitis, a laparotomy is done without delay.

On opening the abdomen the question of closing the opening in the uterus versus hysterectomy must be considered. The age of the patient and the desirability of more children are important factors in making the decision. Often sterilization is desirable for the very reason that the abortion was done. Because of the condition of the patient, a rapid hysterectomy is advisable, and the surgeon must decide whether or not to do a total or subtotal operation. He must take into consideration his own operating ability as well as the patient's condition in making the decision. When local infection has developed as a result of the perforation, hysterectomy is usually preferable, but when there is general peritonitis and the patient's condition is poor, simple suturing of the perforation is wiser. If there has been injury to the bowel, it, of course, must be repaired. Drainage down to the perforated area is advisable. Dependence is then chiefly on antibiotics to overcome the infection.

When there is no infection, and preservation of the childbearing function is desirable, suturing the uterine rent, thus controlling hemorrhage, is permissible.

When perforation is done in completing an incomplete abortion, one should proceed on the assumption that an infected uterus has been punctured, because an incomplete abortion is usually infected even though there are no clinical signs to indicate it. Whereas formerly we advocated immediate laparotomy in such cases, we feel justified today in watchful waiting while treating the patient intensively with antibiotics. If observation indicates that there is either continuing hemorrhage or spreading infection, laparotomy should be done. Hysterectomy will usually be indicated, but occasionally the youth of the patient and the desire for future children may tempt one to close the perforation rather than perform hysterectomy. It should be recalled that in dealing with incomplete abortions the situation with regard to future pregnancies is generally quite different than in dealing with therapeutic abortions.

When one sees, in consultation, a case of suspected perforation that has been previously instrumented by a colleague, an abortionist, or the patient herself, the question that first arises is whether one is dealing with a uterus that actually has been perforated or with a simple infected abortion. If possible, the previous operator should be questioned for evidence, but often he is not accessible. The history of sudden collapse during the instrumentation, or the sudden development of signs of severe infection or hemorrhage after the instrumentation is suggestive of perforation. Abdominal x-ray may show air under the diaphragm or occasionally a foreign body in the abdomen. Such history and findings, especially if augmented by abdominal distention, muscle spasm, and tenderness, are indications for immediate institution of intensive antibiotic therapy and laparotomy. If perforation of the uterus or ruptured abscess is found, definitive surgery is done. If, as occasionally may happen, there is no perforation, hematoma, or ruptured abscess but rather spreading or generalized peritonitis, dependence should be on antibiotic therapy, as such an advanced extra-uterine infection is not benefited by further surgery.

BIBLIOGRAPHY

American Medical Association Policy on Therapeutic Abortion. J.A.M.A., 201:544, 1967.

Arén, P., and Amark, C.: The prognosis in cases in which legal abortion has been granted but not carried out. Acta Psychiat. Scand., 36:203, 1961.

Barter, R. H., Dusbabek, J. A., Riva, H. L., and Parks, J.: Surgical closure of incompetent cervix during pregnancy. Amer. J. Obstet. Gynec., 75:511, 1958.

Bengtsson, L. M.: Missed abortion. The etiology, endocrinology and treatment. Lancet, 1:339, 1962.

Berthelsen, H. G., and Ostergaard, E.: Techniques and complications in therapeutic abortion. Danish Med. Bull., 6:105, 1959.

Briggs, D. W.: Induction of labor with hypertonic glucose. Brit. Med. J., 1:701, 1964.

Brown, T. K., and Hunt, G. A.: Bacteriologic study of 500 consecutive abortions with treatment and results. Amer. J. Obstet. Gynec., 32:804, 1936.

Bunim, J. J., and Appel, S. B.: A principle for determining prognosis of pregnancy in rheumatic heart disease. J.A.M.A., 142:90, 1950.

Byrd, B. F., Jr., Bayer, D. S., Robertson, J. C., and Stevenson, S. E.: Therapy of breast cancer in pregnancy. Ann. Surg., 155:940, 1962.

Calderone, J. S. (ed.): Abortion in the United States. New York, Paul B. Hoeber, 1958.

Carr, D. H.: Chromosome studies in spontaneous abortions. Obstet. Gynec., 26:308, 1965.

Chesley, L. C.: Toxemia of pregnancy in relation to chronic hypertension. Western J. Surg., 64:284, 1956.

Curtis, A. H. (ed.): Obstetrics and Gynecology. Philadelphia, W. B. Saunders, 1933.

Delfs, E., and Jones, G. E. S.: Endocrine patterns in abortions. Obstet. Gynec. Surv., 3:680, 1948.

Driscoll, M. K., Coyle, C. F. V., and Drury, M. J.: Rheumatic heart disease complicating pregnancy. The remote prospects. Brit. Med. J., 2:767, 1962.

Eaton, C. J.: Uterine aspiration for evacuation of the pregnant uterus. J.A.M.A., 207:1887, 1969.

Ekblad, M.: Induced abortion on psychiatric grounds. Acta Psychiat. Scand., Suppl. 99, pp. 1-238, 1955.

Erhardt, C. L.: Pregnancy losses in New York City, 1960. Amer. J. Pub. Health, 53:1337, 1963.

Gold, E. M., Erhardt, C. L., Jacobziner, H., and Nelson, F. G.: Therapeutic abortions in New York City: A 20-year review. Amer. J. Public Health, 55:964, 1965.

Gorenberg, H., and Chesley, L. C.: Rheumatic heart disease in pregnancy; the remote prognosis in patients with "functionally severe" disease. Ann. Intern. Med., 49:278, 1958.

Hall, R. E.: Therapeutic abortion, sterilization and contraception. Amer. J. Obstet. Gynec., 91:518, 1965.

Holleb, A. I., and Farrow, J. H.: The relation of carcinoma of the breast and pregnancy in 283 patients. Surg. Gynec. Obstet., 115:65, 1962.

Höök, K.: Refused abortion. Acta Psychiat. Scand., 39:168, 1963.

Jaffin, K., Kerenyi, T., and Wood, E. C.: Termination of missed abortion by the induction of labor in midpregnancy. Amer. J. Obstet. Gynec., 84:602, 1962.

Joël, C. A.: The etiology of habitual abortion with consideration of the male factors. Gynaecologia, 154:257, 1962, and Obstet. Gynec. Surv., 18:623, 1963.

Jones, G. E. S., and Delfs, E.: Endocrine patterns in term pregnancies following abortion. J.A.M.A., 146:1212, 1951.

Jones, H. W., Delfs, E., and Jones, G. E. S.: Reproductive difficulties in double uterus. Amer. J. Obstet. Gynec., 72:865, 1956.

Kerslake, D., and Casey, D.: Abortion induced by means of the uterine aspirator. Obstet. Gynec., 30:35, 1967.

Kuder, K., and Finn, W. F.: Therapeutic interruption of pregnancy. Amer. J. Obstet. Gynec., 49:762, 1945.

Lash, A. F., and Lash, S. R.: Habitual abortion: The incompetent internal os of the cervix. Amer. J. Obstet. Gynec., 59:68, 1950.

Lash, A. F., Webster, A., and Barton, J. J.: A survery of over 20,000 abortions at the Cook County Hospital, 1961-1965. Trans. Amer. Assoc. Obstet. Gynec., 79:110, 1968.

MacDonald, D., O'Driscoll, M. K., and Geoghegan, F. J.: Intra-amniotic dextrose—a maternal death. J. Obstet. Gynaec. Brit. Comm., 72:452, 1965.

Mendelson, C. L.: Cardiac Disease in Pregnancy. Philadelphia, F. A. Davis, 1960.

Peel, J.: Letter to editor. Brit. Med. J., 2:1397, 1962.

Peretz, A., Grunstein, S., Brandes, J. M., and Paldi, E.: Evacuation of the gravid uterus by negative pressure (suction evacuation). Amer. J. Obstet. Gynec., 98:18, 1967.

Roemer, R.: Abortion law: The approaches of different nations. Amer. J. Public Health, 57:1906, 1967.

Rosen, H.: Therapeutic Abortion. New York, Julian Press, 1954.

———: Abortion. In The Encyclopedia of Mental Health. Vol. I. New York, F. Watts, 1963.

Russell, K. P., and Moore, J. G.: Maternal medical indications for therapeutic abortion. Clin. Obstet. Gynec., 7:43, 1964.

Schaefer, G., Douglas, R. G., and Dreishpoon, I. H.: Tuberculosis and abortion. Amer. Rev. Tuberculosis, 70:49, 1954.

Shirodkar, V. N.: Contributions to Obstetrics and Gynecology. Edinburgh, E. & S. Livingstone, 1960.

Simon, A.: Psychiatric indications for therapeutic abortion and sterilization. Clin. Obstet. Gynec., 7:67, 1964.

Simon, N. M., and Senturia, A. G.: Psychiatric sequellae of abortion: Review of the literature. Arch. Gen. Psychiat., 15:378, 1966.

Simon, N. M., Senturia, A. G., and Rothman, D.: Psychiatric illness following therapeutic abortion. Amer. J. Psychiat., 124:59, 1967.

Tietze, C.: Abortion in Europe. Amer. J. Public Health, 57:1923, 1967.

———: Therapeutic abortions in the United States. Amer. J. Obstet. Gynec., 101:784, 1968.

Ueland, K.: Cardiac surgery and pregnancy. Amer. J. Obstet. Gynec., 92:148, 1965.

Vital Statistics of the United States, 1965. Vol. II, Mortality. Washington, D.C., U.S. Govt. Printing Office, 1967.

Vladov, E.: The vacuum aspiration method of interruption of early pregnancy. Amer. J. Obstet. Gynec., 99:202, 1967.

Warburton, D., and Fraser, F. C.: Spontaneous abortion risks in man: Data from reproductive histories collected in a medical genetics unit. Amer. J. Human Genet., 16:1, 1964.

Warkany, J.: Maternal nutrition during pregnancy and its relationship to reproductive failure. In La Prophylaxie en Gynécologie et Obstétrique. Geneva, Georg et Cie., 1954.

Warkany, J., and Kalter, H.: Congenital malformations. New Eng. J. Med., 265:993, 1046, 1961.

Westberg, S. V.: Prognosis of breast carcinoma for pregnant and nursing women: A clinical-statistical study. Acta Obstet. Gynec. Scand., 1 (Suppl. 4):239, 1946.

23

Congenital Absence of the Vagina

Congenital absence of the vagina is fortunately a rare malformation. Counseller found the condition occurring once in 4,000 female admissions at the Mayo Clinic. In the vast majority of women born without vaginas there is also the congenital absence of the uterus. Nevertheless, among 26 patients of Counseller's who were laparotomized, 4 had anatomically normal tubes, ovaries, and uterus. Three had developed hematosalpinx, and 3 endometriosis. Underdeveloped uteri and bicornuate uteri are encountered occasionally, but in the majority of cases nothing can be felt in the usual position of the uterus, or there is simply a slight midline thickening in the broad ligament. Almost all of these patients have normal ovaries and fully developed secondary sexual characteristics. In our personal experience we never have seen a woman with a congenital absence of the vagina who was not typically feminine physically.

We have seen a few women with congenital absence of the vagina who were quite unconcerned about their condition, who had no interest in matrimony and no desire to have the condition corrected. However, this attitude is very unusual, and the majority of these individuals have a normal reaction to the opposite sex and intend to marry if possible. The knowledge of the physical defect may give them a feeling of inferiority. The individual with absent vagina is usually brought to the gynecologist at the age of 14 or 15 when the failure of the menses to appear gives the mother concern. Frank recommended the formation of an artificial vagina by his nonsurgical method early in life, for there is little, if any, tendency of a vagina thus formed to contract. He believed that the establishment of a vagina early in life helped to combat the feeling of inferiority sometimes present in these girls. We cannot concur in this, believing that the optimum time for the correction of the condition is about 6 months before contemplated marriage.

Wharton has called attention to the frequency with which absence of the vagina is associated with congenital malformations of the urinary tract. Congenital absence of one kidney, ectopia of the unilateral kidney, horseshoe kidney, and duplication of the ureter have all been described. In fact, among 41 patients of Counseller's group who were investigated urologically, only 20 had normal urinary tracts. Hence, it would seem advisable to make intravenous urograms on all women with congenital absence of the vagina, if for no other reason than to give the patient an exact knowledge of her condition.

Many ingenious operations have been devised for the formation of an artificial vagina.

During the past decade our experience has crystallized our ideas so that we believe there is only one method of dealing with the complete congenital absence of the vagina, namely, the McIndoe operation. The others are described briefly because of their historical interest.

Among the older operations is that of Baldwin, in which a double loop of ileum was resected and brought down to function as a vagina. The operation carried with it a mortality which was too high to justify it. Today with antibiotic sterilization of the intestinal tract, it could be done with a much lower mortality, but still it is not justifiable because such excellent results can be obtained with the safer McIndoe procedure. In addition, the intestinal mucosa often secreted a very irritating and disagreeable discharge.

Schubert utilized the lower segment of the rectum, transplanting it anteriorly for use as a vagina. This operation also carried a high mortality; there was often damage to the rectal sphincter and frequently a resulting fecal fistula.

At the present time Shirodkar utilizes a segment of the sigmoid and claims excellent results. He believes that the mucous secretion of the sigmoid is an advantage in serving as lubrication to the vagina. In our opinion utilization of a segment of the large bowel is unjustified in view of the simplicity of the McIndoe operation. We have never had a complaint of dryness of the artificial McIndoe vagina.

The formation of an artificial canal lined by the labia minora, as described by Graves, was practiced with some success but is much more complicated than the modern skin-grafting method.

The multistage Frank-Geist "satchel-handle" operation, in which pedicle flaps obtained from the inner aspect of the thigh were utilized, has also been abandoned because of its multistage complicated technic.

FRANK NONSURGICAL METHOD OF MAKING AN ARTIFICIAL VAGINA

In 1938 Robert Frank described a method of formation of an artificial vagina without operation. In 1940 he reported remarkably satisfactory results in 8 cases treated by this method. His follow-up study showed that a vagina formed in this manner remains permanent in depth and caliber, even in patients who have neglected dilatation for more than a year.

Our results in a few cases in which we attempted this method have not been very satisfactory. Great persistence and cooperation are necessary on the part of the patient, which are not usually obtainable; and even in some cases in which complete cooperation is had, the cavity fails to materialize. If an occasional patient desires to attempt this rather tedious exercise, we have no objection to her trying it. Hence, the technic is described. In case of failure, a surgical procedure can be done later.

Technic

The first step is important. A narrow pyrex tube, 0.8 cm. (5/16 inch) in outside diameter, is introduced by the physician in the center of the hymenal region, in a direction backward and inward, with the patient in the lithotomy position (Fig. 23-1). The patient is carefully taught to perform this maneuver 3 times daily for at least a half hour for 1 week. This is important in order to stretch the mucosa so that further measures do not distort and dilate the urinary meatus. After the first week, the patient is taught to insert the tube downward and inward as before, but when this position has been attained, to change the direction of insertion in a line paralleling the normal axis of the vagina. The tube is held in place for one half hour in the morning and one half hour in the evening. Usually in from 2 to 4 weeks a sufficient depression permitting the retention of a 3-inch-long tube has been attained. The shorter tube, as soon as it can be introduced for its full length, is kept in place throughout the night by a small pad of cotton and an appropriate T-binder. Within 6 to 8 weeks, the full length of the vagina, 2½ to 2¾ inches, has been reached. The patients are warned not to apply excessive force, which is manifest by spotting, indicating injury of the delicate mucosa lining.

It is now time to use a tube 1.5 cm. (5/8 inch) in diameter, inserted for the length of 7 cm. and kept in place every night for 8 to 10 hours. When this tube is admitted readily, the final size 2 cm. (3/4 inch) is used until marriage. In the earlier cases, still larger tubes were used but appear to be unnecessary. Exof execution and does not require the skill in plastic surgery necessary for the successful accomplishments of the older procedures then in vogue. Wharton described the operation as follows:

This is simplicity itself. A common feature in all operations for the construction of the vagina is the dissection of the space between the bladder and the rectum. This step in the operation can usually be finished easily in 10 or 15 minutes. Into this newly created space, one introduces the vaginal mold covered by a condom, and that completes the operation.

The operative procedure is usually very easy. As Baldwin said, the creation of the space between the bladder and rectum can usually be done by blunt dissection, after the incision is made in the external mucous membrane or across the dome of the rudimentary vagina. One needs only to follow the plane of cleavage furnished by the fibroareolar tissue between the layers of subvesical and perirectal fascia (Figs. 23-2 and 23-3). There is very little danger of perforating either the rectum or bladder, if one follows this layer. In case of doubt one can orient himself by a sound in the urethra or a finger in the rectum.

One can easily perforate the bladder, however, if this plane of cleavage has been replaced by scar tissue, due to a former operation. The author experienced this accident once.

There are two rather important details to observe in preparing the vaginal space. In the first place, the space must be larger than one expects it to be eventually. It may contract during convalescence; it is hardly likely to enlarge. The contracture may be due to slipping of the mold, to pressure of surrounding organs or to compression of the mold. The vaginal space should be large in all dimensions. The second item concerns hemostasis. One encounters significant blood vessels usually only at two points, at the level of the broad ligament on each side. These ligaments are rather resistant and may require incision in each lateral wall. At this point, the vaginal vessels leave the uterine arteries and veins and may require ligation. These vessels, however, are small and do not compare with the vessels found in the normal vaginal plexus.†

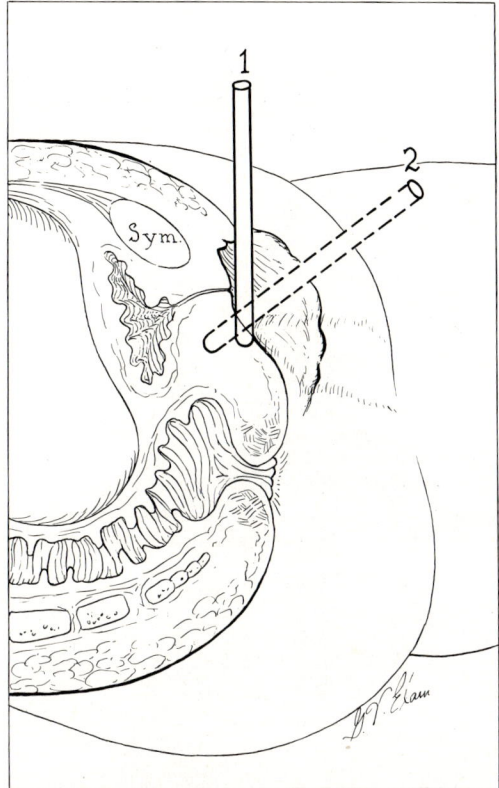

FIG. 23-1. Frank nonoperative method of making vagina. Diagram showing method of making pressure with test tubes. Tube 1 is directed backward and inward for the first week. Tube 2 is directed in normal vaginal axis after the first week.

amination of all these patients shows a normal vulva and introitus. The vagina readily admits two fingers to the depth of 6½ to 7 cm. (2½ to 2¾ inches) from the fourchette. The canal is lined with soft, resilient mucous membrane, and a standard vaginal speculum can be introduced and opened without discomfort to the patient.*

WHARTON OPERATION FOR CONSTRUCTION OF A VAGINA

In 1932 Wharton devised an operation based on the remarkable proliferative power of the vaginal mucosa. It is simple

---

* Frank, R. T.: The formation of an artificial vagina without operation. Amer. J. Obstet. Gynec., 35:1054, 1055.

† Wharton, L. R.: A simple method of constructing a vagina. Ann. Surg., *107*:843, 1938.

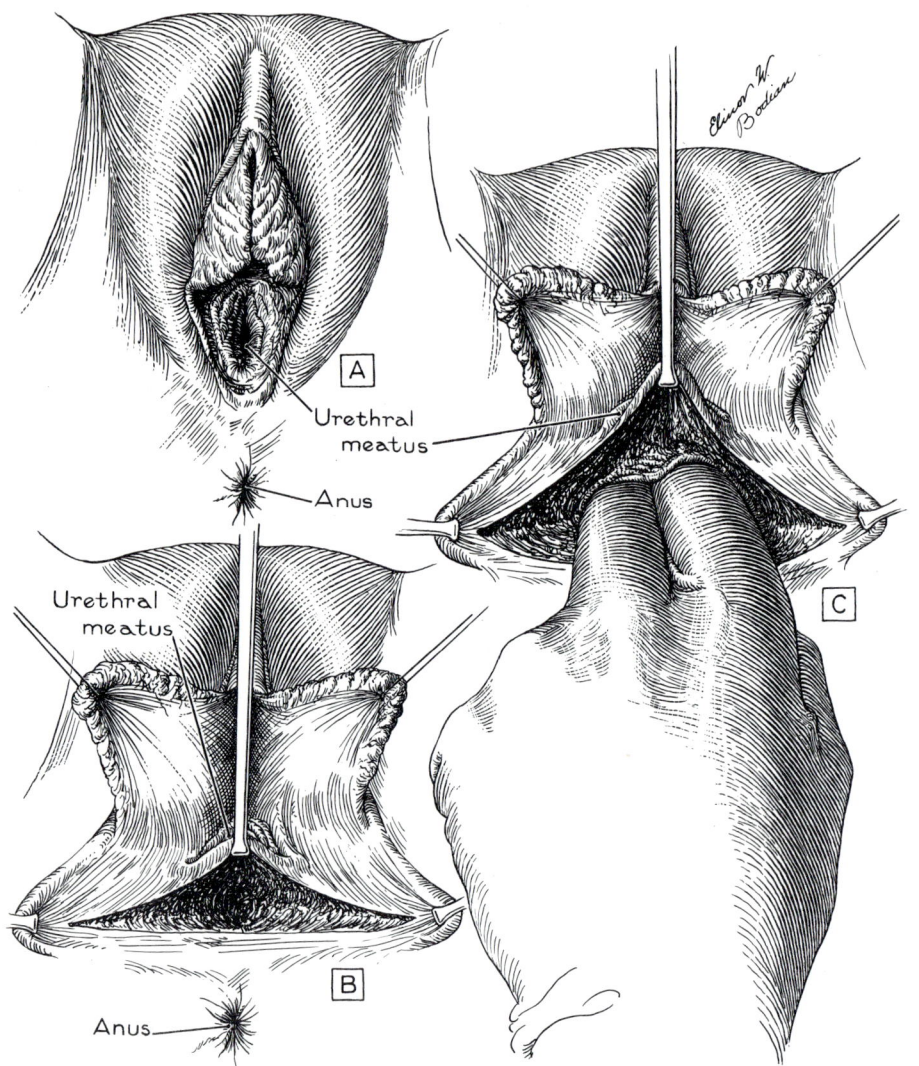

Fig. 23-2. Wharton operation for congenital absence of the vagina. (A) Indicates preoperative condition, showing dilated urethral meatus. (B) Shows transverse line of incision between the urethra and the anus. (C) Indicates method of dissecting space between the urethra and the rectum, using two fingers and alternately opening and closing them.

Like the other methods mentioned above, the Wharton operation is chiefly of historical interest. The method of dissecting the space for the mold, however, is exactly like that used in the McIndoe operation, which in the opinion of the authors supersedes all others.

McINDOE OPERATION

In 1938 McIndoe described an operation very much like that of Wharton with the additional step of skin grafting the newly formed vaginal cavity with a split-thickness skin graft, held in place with a vaginal mold. The operation has been done extensively in this country by Counseller with a high percentage of success. In the last 20 years we have used it exclusively with practically perfect results.

Before the operation is begun, it is important to distinguish between a congenitally absent vagina and uterus and

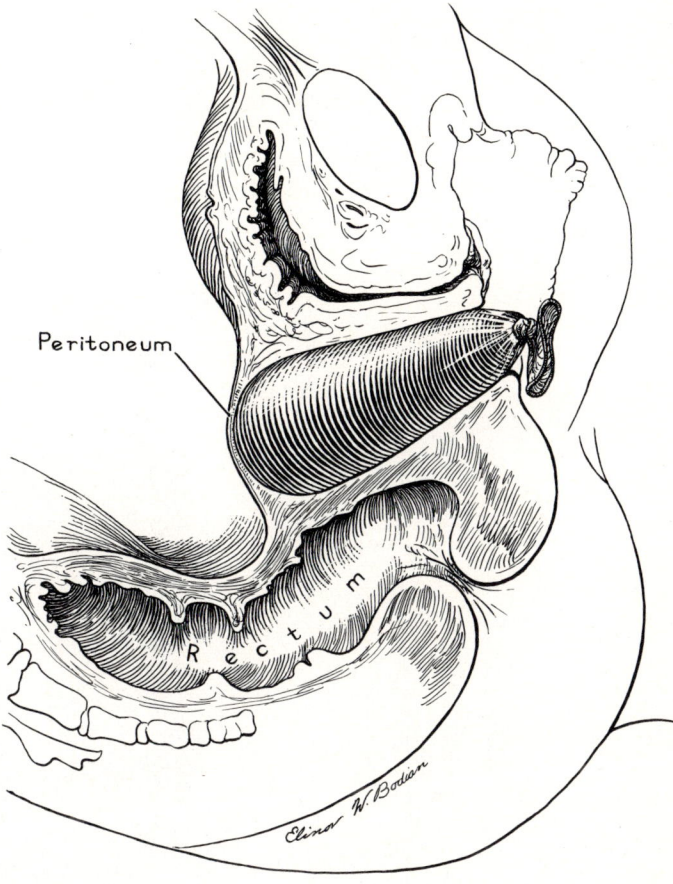

FIG. 23-3. Wharton operation for congenital absence of the vagina. Space has been completely dissected to the peritoneum. Rubber-covered balsa-wood mold is in place. In this instance skin-grafting was not used.

an imperforate hymen. This can usually be done by pelvic examination. When the vagina and the uterus are congenitally absent, on rectal examination the urethra can easily be felt through the anterior rectal wall. This will be even more striking if a sound is placed in the urethra while the rectal examination is made. On the other hand, if one is dealing with an imperforate hymen, the cervix and the corpus will be felt through the rectum, and often a hematocolpos will be felt if the patient is past puberty. In the rare cases in which the vagina is absent but the uterus present, the uterus will also be palpable. In some instances a small space before the cervix can be felt, distended with blood. In those cases there will be a history of recurring monthly pain as the patient attempts to force out the menstrual blood, most of which will be forced out of the tubes in a retrograde manner, causing peritoneal irritation.

Technic

First, a split-thickness skin graft is cut from the superiormedial aspect of the patient's thigh of proper size to cover the vaginal form (Fig. 23-4 A). Because of the resulting scar, a few patients have requested that the graft be taken from the buttock. The Reese dermatome is a convenient instrument for taking the graft, but an experienced graft-cutter can cut a satisfactory graft freehand. The outer surface of the graft is placed between two layers of moist gauze. The thigh wound is then dressed with petrolatum gauze and covered with sterile gauze. This wound is not dressed until the vaginal form is removed 2 weeks later.

The patient is placed in the lithotomy position, and an incision is made through the mucosa of the vaginal vestibule as shown in Figure 23-4 B. The space between the urethra and the bladder anteriorly and the rectum posteriorly is then dissected until the undersurface of the peritoneum is reached (Fig. 23-4 B). This step may be made safer by inserting a sound or a catheter in the urethra. Bleeders are clamped in the cavity and tied with very fine catgut. It is essential to have the cavity dry to prevent hemorrhage beneath the graft. Separation of the graft from its bed means the inevitable death of the graft in that area.

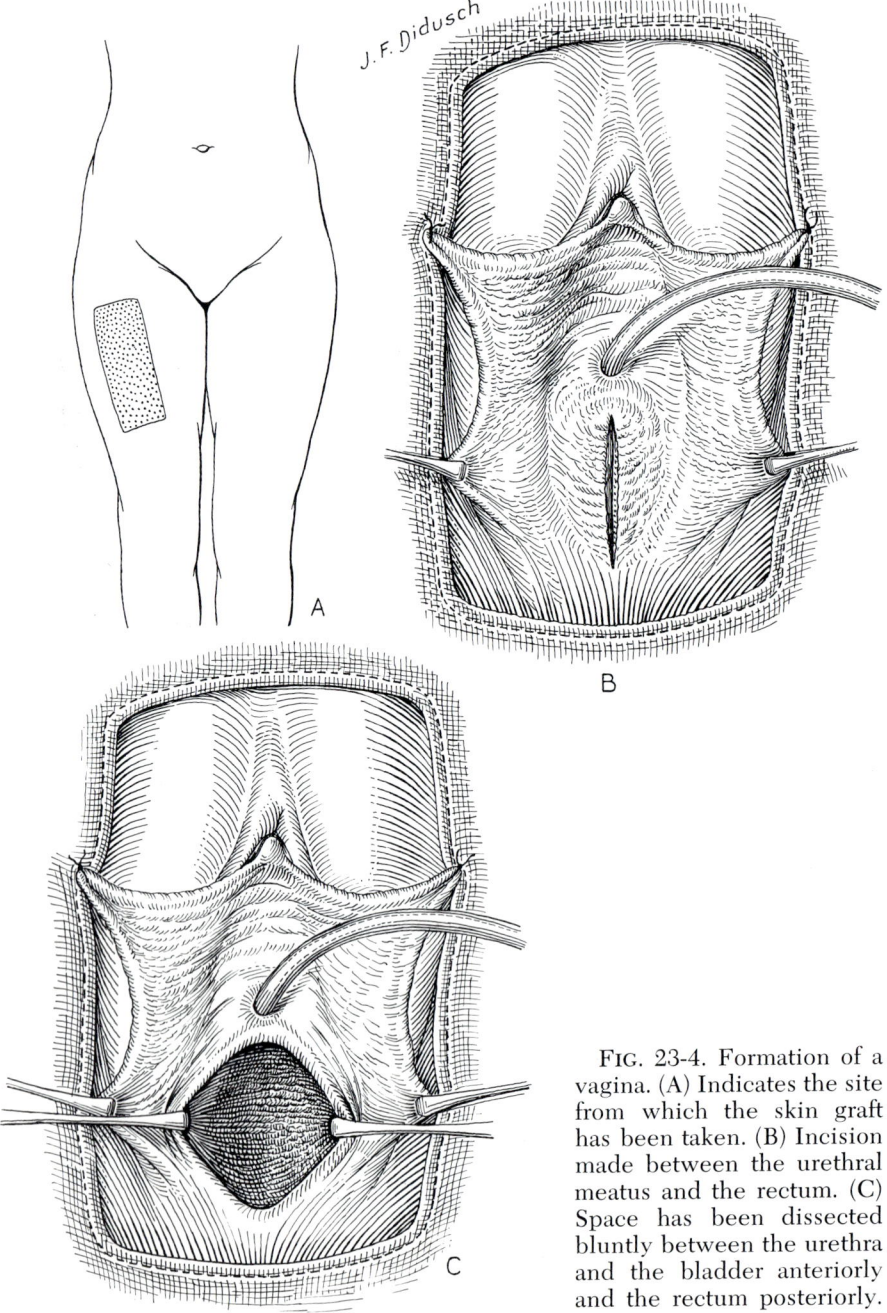

FIG. 23-4. Formation of a vagina. (A) Indicates the site from which the skin graft has been taken. (B) Incision made between the urethral meatus and the rectum. (C) Space has been dissected bluntly between the urethra and the bladder anteriorly and the rectum posteriorly.

Partial Absence of the Vagina   467

sinus tract with the dimple on the opposite side (Fig. 23-12 A). A probe could be introduced into the sinus tract for about 2 cm., but there was no induration along the tract, and only pliable areolar tissue was encountered in dissecting the space between the vagina and the rectum. After continuing this dissection for about 3 cm. the cervix could be palpated, but it was apparently covered with a membrane, the under surface of which was visible (Fig. 23-12 B). It was obvious that this membrane had to be opened in order to expose the cervix. The danger of opening the bladder and the rectum was recognized. With a mushroom catheter in the bladder which could be moved about, the limits of the bladder could be recognized. An assistant inserted his gloved finger beneath the drapes into the

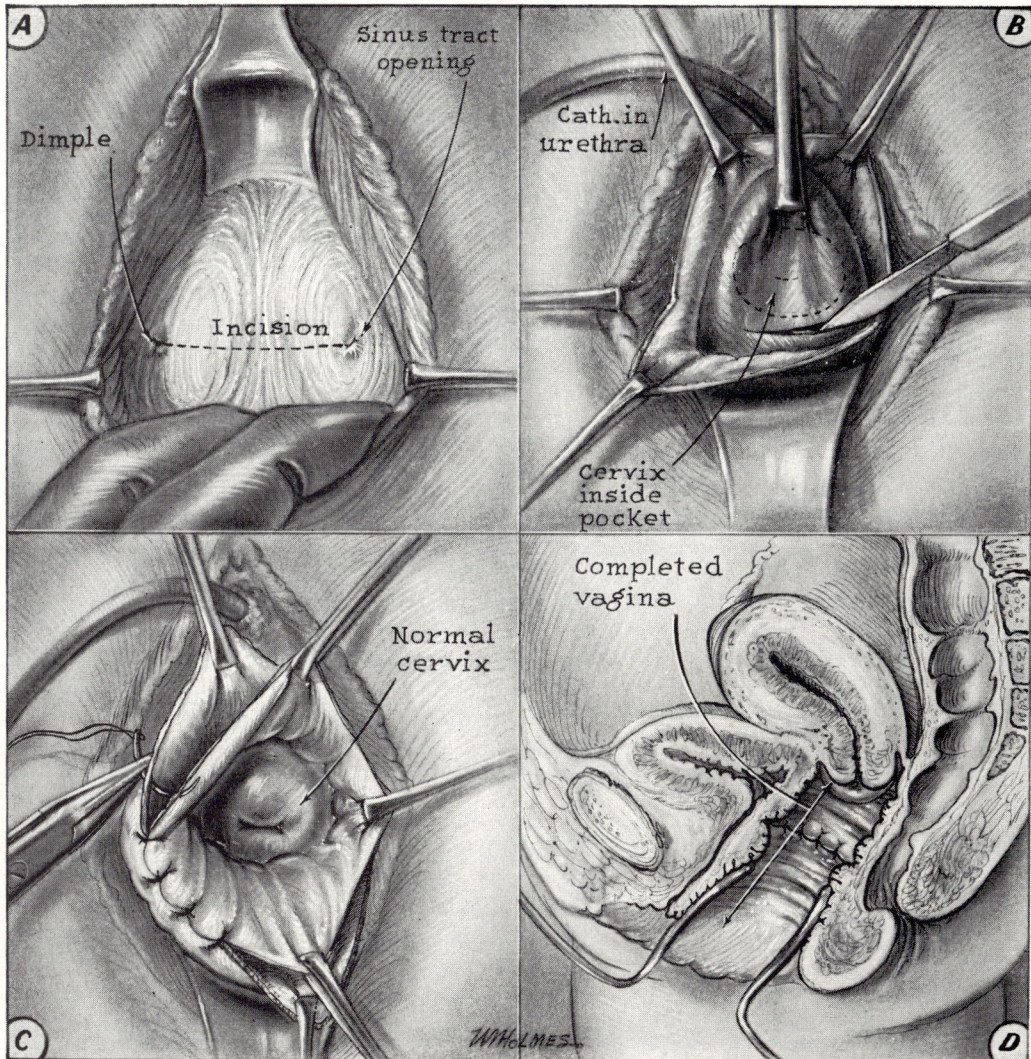

FIG. 23-12. (A) Showing upper end of a short vagina, with sinus tract opening through which the patient menstruated; also showing incision through mucous membrane. (B) Areolar tissue has been dissected through to the pocket of mucosa which covered the cervix. The mucosa is being incised. (C) An anastomosis is being made between the lower vagina and the upper vagina. (D) Showing completed vagina. It is slightly shorter than normal but of normal caliber.

rectum so that the anterior rectal wall could be recognized at all times. An incison was then made through the mucosa, just posterior to the cervix as shown in Figure 23-12 B. The small upper vaginal cavity was thus entered, and the cervix was exposed. The opening in the upper vagina was enlarged until it equalled the opening in the vault of the lower vagina. The edges of the upper and the lower cavities were then anastomosed, using interrupted sutures of No. 00 chromic catgut (Fig. 23-12 C). Figure 23-12 D shows the completed anastomosis with a vagina which is of normal caliber but slightly shorter than the normal average.

BIBLIOGRAPHY

Baldwin, J. F.: The formation of an artificial vagina by intestinal transplantation. Ann. Surg., *40*:398, 1904.

———: Formation of an artificial vagina by intestinal transplantation. Amer. J. Obstet. Gynec., *56*:639, 1907.

Bryan, A. L., Nigro, J. A., Counseller, V. S.: One hundred cases of congenital absence of vagina. Surg. Gynec. Obstet., *88*:79, 1949.

Frank, R. T.: The formation of an artificial vagina without operation. Amer. J. Obstet. Gynec., *35*:1053, 1938.

———: The formation of an artificial vagina without operation (intubation method). New York J. Med., *40*:1669, 1940.

Frank, R. T., and Geist, S. H.: The formation of an artificial vagina by a new plastic technic. Amer. J. Obstet. Gynec., *14*:712, 1927.

Graves, W. P.: Method of constructing an artificial vagina. Surg. Clin. N. Amer., *1*:611, 1921.

McIndoe, Archibald: Treatment of congenital absence and obliterative conditions of vagina. Brit. J. Plast. Surg., *2*:254, 1950.

Schubert, G.: Über Scheidenbildung bei angeborenem Vaginaldefekt. Zbl. Gynäk., *45*:1017, 1911.

Shirodkar, V. N.: Personal communication.

Thompson, J. D., Wharton, L., Sr., and Te Linde, R. W.: Amer. J. Obstet. Gynec., *74*:397. 1957.

Wharton, L. R.: A simple method of constructing a vagina; report of four cases. Ann. Surg. *107*:842, 1938.

24

Malpositions of the Uterus, Cervical Stump and Vagina

RETRODISPLACEMENT OF UTERUS

HISTORY

The recognition and the surgical correction of retrodisplacement of the uterus form an interesting chapter in the development of gynecology. In 1955 Frederic Fluhmann wrote a review of the subject, and in this brief historical sketch we have drawn heavily from his work. He who fails to heed the mistakes of the past is apt to repeat them. With this in mind we have considered it worthwhile to sketch briefly this history.

During the early part of the 18th century retrodisplacement of the uterus became identified as an obstetric complication. In 1774 William Hunter described at autopsy a uterus impacted in the hollow of the sacrum during the 5th month of pregnancy which was dislodged with difficulty. During the 18th century retrodisplacement was considered an acute complication of pregnancy, occurring during the 4th and the 5th months of pregnancy and often resulting in death. Death resulted, too, from fatal injuries dependent upon forceful attempts at displacement. Denman in 1782 considered overdistention of the bladder the chief cause of the condition and recommended repeated catheterization as the essential treatment.

In Howard Kelly's review of the subject he calls the early part of the 19th century the "pessary period." It was then that retrodisplacement became recognized in the nonpregant state, and many ingenious instruments and technics were devised for bringing the uterus forward and holding it there. Churchill in 1857 described the symptoms as greater menstrual flow, pelvic engorgement, greater tendency to abortion, a sensation of depression and falling of the womb, pain, difficult and frequent urination, dull backache, a sense of pressure in the rectum, pain down the thighs, leukorrhea, and interference with general health. Even then Nauche stated that the condition could exist without symptoms, but unfortunately no one heeded him. Although J. Marion Sims was a strong advocate of the use of pessaries, he cited several instances of vaginal ulceration, vesicovaginal and rectovaginal fistula resulting from their use. He believed that no one who did not possess mechanical ingenuity should attempt to insert a pessary. He himself shaped each pessary individually to the vagina using "block tin or gutta percha softened with a little lead."

In the latter part of the 19th century there began what Fluhmann calls the "dark ages of operative furor." Alexander and Adams are credited with doing the first abdominal uterine suspensions. Alexander performed his first one in 1881, and Adams in 1882, but the latter recorded the operation first in the literature. The operation soon attained great popularity, and numerous modifications were described. Kelly in 1914 collected over 50 types of suspension, and in 1925 Crossen collected 110. Three years later Hadden collected 120. There was a veritable orgy of operating. Alexander became so enthusiastic about uterine suspension that on one occasion he was asked to demonstrate the operation for some visiting surgeons. He sent 4 assistants north, south, east and west throughout Liverpool to find a suitable case. They returned empty-handed, saying that in all Liverpool they could find no woman who had not had the Alexander operation performed on her. Howard Kelly stated that he personally had done over 1,000 suspensions, and Barton Cook Hirst reported "hundreds." In the Woman's Hospital in New York, George Ward reported 3,357 abdominal suspensions among 22,625 gynecologic operations. By that time, and even before, skeptics were raising some questions. Scanzoni wrote in 1850, "My decided conviction is that the mechanical treatment of this affection of retrodisplacement . . . is either useless or positively mischievous." Although J. Montgomery Baldy devised a method of uterine suspension, he wrote, "Like the poor, the subject seems to be always with us. There come periods of quiescence in its discussion, but nothing, however, conclusively leads us near the goal. . . . We should not discuss the treatment of retrodisplacement but treatment of conditions with which retrodisplacements of the uterus occur as an incident."

In 1914 there was a symposium on the subject in Philadelphia. At that time Baldy said, "In my opinion nine-tenths of the operations performed on women for retrodisplacement are uncalled for. . . . Dr. Cragin is such an old and warm friend that I would hate to tell him what I thought of him for doing 200 retrodisplacement operations in a single year. . . . If you recall the fact that Kelly has performed about 1,000 operations for retrodisplacements before he discovered that the several procedures he was following were incompetent, you will wonder with me what in the world became of those 1,000 women. . . . I am sorry to say it but it looks to me as though the possible number of retrodisplacement operations performed in this country is limited only by the number of females in existence."

In spite of these freely expressed critical attitudes, Aldridge in 1940 stated, "Retroversion of the uterus will probably always be one of the more common gynecological conditions requiring treatment and surgical intervention for the cure of symptoms in some cases."

Within the past 3 or 4 decades there has been a gradual reduction in the number of operations done. In our clinics it is a rarity to open an abdomen primarily for a uterine suspension.

What factors have brought this about? In the first place, on the face of it, it would seem unlikely that a condition which occurs in 20 to 30 per cent of the population would require correction. Another factor which contributed to the rejection of the suspension operations was the failure of many operative procedures to hold the uterus in position. But more important still was the failure of relief of symptoms even when the uterus was held in perfect position. Then, too, there were a few serious postoperative complications. Finally, a better understanding of physiology and endocrinology in relation to infertility and abortions has made gynecologists less anxious to perform uterine suspension. A better understanding of the orthopedic causes of low back pain has also kept many women from unnecessary surgery.

Fluhmann concludes his historical review with an expression of his own views on the subject of uterine suspension: "It is not necessary for adequate gynecologic practice. At most it occasionally may play a secondary role to other procedures such as peritonization of the pelvis, conservative treatment of endometriosis, correction of certain vascular disorders and plastic reconstruction of the fallopian tubes."

With this historical background, we shall attempt to express our personal view in the present chapter.

ANATOMIC CONSIDERATIONS

Before discussing the correction of the retrodisplaced uterus, the anatomic structures and the mechanism by which the uterus is held in its normal position of anteflexion and anteversion should be reviewed. The portio vaginalis points postero-inferiorly, and the corpus is bent with a wide obtuse angle on the cervix, so that when the woman is erect, the corpus lies practically horizontally, resting loosely upon the bladder. There are minor variations in the direction of the axis of the cervix and the corpus which must be considered to be within normal limits. There are also physiologic displacements due to distention of the bladder or to pregnancy; during the latter part of pregnancy the uterus becomes a practically vertical organ.

The fibromuscular tissue lying beneath the peritoneum and attached to the cervix forms certain ligaments which play an important part in maintaining the uterus in anteposition. The tissue within the lower portion of the broad ligament, extending from either side of the cervix to the side of the pelvis, forms the ligamentum transversalis colli (Mackenrodt), the so-called cardinal ligament. The 2 cardinal ligaments have as their chief function the maintaining of the cervix at its normal level. They are discussed more fully when uterine prolapse is considered, but uterine retrodisplacement cannot be considered independent of prolapse. As retrodisplacement plays an important part in the descent of the uterus, so descensus causes the corpus to fall back from its normal position. Beneath peritoneal folds, on either side of the cul-de-sac of Douglas, are 2 fibromuscular structures, usually well developed, the uterosacral ligaments. They are attached to the posterolateral surface of the cervix and proceed backward on either side of the rectum, to be inserted into the periosteum of the sacrum, thus holding back the cervix. The uterus is normally an organ of some rigidity. If the cervix is held backward and the corpus lies forward, the intra-abdominal pressure falls upon the posterior surface of the horizontal corpus and maintains it in anteposition. If the uterosacral ligaments are congenitally inadequate or have become so through childbirth, the cervix moves forward. Under such conditions the uterus, swinging on a more or less fixed transverse axis at about the level of the internal os, moves backward, and the intra-abdominal pressure falls on the anterior surface of the corpus, aggravating the retrodisplacement.

The round ligaments also serve an important purpose in holding the uterus in anteposition; advantage is usually taken of this in correcting surgically its malposition. Upon opening the abdomen and inspecting the normal pelvis, it is obvious that the round ligaments do not tautly hold the fundus forward. How then can the round ligaments play such an important role in maintaining the anteposition? It is because of their function in bringing the fundus back to anteposition after its physiologic displacement. If the uterosacral ligaments hold the cervix back and the round ligaments replace the corpus to its forward position after displacement from a distended bladder or pregnancy, intra-abdominal pressure will maintain it there.

Another factor in keeping the uterus in normal position is the tonus of the musculature of the uterus itself. When the tonus is firm, the corpus is easily maintained forward by the mechanism described above. However, when the musculature is flabby, coils of intestine which have worked into the vesicouterine pouch may force the body backward on the cervix in a hinge-like manner. Once the retroflexion is begun, it can be completed easily by intra-abdominal pressure upon the anterior uterine surface. As a matter of fact, in most cases of retrodisplacement there is a combination of retroversion and retroflexion, although either may exist independently.

The term *retrocession* has been applied to a posterior displacement of the entire uterus while the normal anteflexion of corpus onto body persists. In fact, the anteflexion may be exaggerated beyond the normal, even when the uterus as a whole lies back. Retrocession is usually congenital and often associated with a uterus of subnormal size. Frequently, the cervix is much longer than normal, while a small corpus is acutely anteflexed on it.

SYMPTOMATOLOGY IN RELATION TO TREATMENT

In considering the treatment of retrodisplacement of the uterus, it is essential to consider the symptomatology. At the onset it must be emphasized that in the majority of cases retroversion gives rise to no symptoms at all. In another large group of cases the symptoms are slight and do not justify an abdominal suspension. It is generally estimated that 1 out of 5 women has a congenitally retrodisplaced uterus. One of the commonest findings in making routine pelvic examinations is retrodisplacement of the uterus in women who are completely free of symptoms, and it is our opinion that such uteri should not be suspended. Occasionally, one hears the opinion expressed by surgeons that retrodisplacement, even though asymptomatic, may lead to "degeneration of the ovaries." We do not share this view and have seen no pathologic evidence to support it. This opinion, together with a desire to operate, has resulted in subjecting great numbers of women to needless suspensions, so that even today many suspensions are performed which could be avoided. How common it is to encounter women who have had uterine suspensions for backache of orthopedic origin, frequency of urination, or symptoms of a general neurasthenic nature that have no relation to the position of the uterus and are only exaggerated by useless surgery! One should consider seriously, in all cases in which uterine suspension is contemplated, whether or not the symptoms of which the patient complains are due to the misplaced uterus; this may be difficult, and the best clinical judgment is necessary in order to arrive at a proper decision. It should be remembered that the operation is never an emergency, and one can afford to observe the patient for a time before making a final decision. In most cases the therapeutic test of holding the uterus in position for a few months with a Smith-Hodge pessary can be used to advantage. Unfortunately, it is not always possible to hold a uterus in position by means of a pessary; when it is possible, frequently one can determine by the relief obtained whether or not a suspension is indicated.

In general, it may be said that an uncomplicated, retroposed uterus is less apt to be responsible for symptoms than one complicated by other intrapelvic disease. Among the conditions commonly associated with and frequently a factor in the cause of retrodisplacement are: salpingitis, endometriosis, ovarian tumors, myomata, and childbirth injuries. Often these conditions are responsible for symptoms which, in themselves, necessitate surgery, but frequently complete relief will not be obtained without a proper suspension of the uterus, together with the correction of the other pelvic lesions. It should not be lost sight of, however, that even the complicated retrodisplaced uterus may be asymptomatic. How frequently an adherent retroverted uterus is encountered with the residue of an old salpingitis, without causing the patient any discomfort!

In order to evaluate the symptoms with reference to treatment, a consideration of individual symptoms is in order.

Backache and Bearing-Down Abdominal Discomfort. For many years the question of the relation of retrodisplacement of the uterus to backache has been a controversial one. It is true that innumerable retroverted uteri have been suspended because of backaches for which they were not responsible. This has induced some gynecologists to take the view that an uncomplicated, retrodisplaced uterus cannot cause backache. Our experience has not forced us to such an extreme position. Gratifying results obtained by suspending uteri in certain selected cases strongly contradict such a view. Lynch found backache to be present in half of the patients with retroversion. However, this does not indicate that half of the women with retrodisplacement suffer from backache as a result of the position of the uterus. The percentage is obviously much smaller. Lynch relieved backache in 81 per cent of the patients upon whom he operated.

Sacral or lumbosacral backache and bearing-down abdominal pain are considered together, because when these are due to retrodisplacement, they usually occur together and appear to the patient to be inseparable. Often she describes her discomfort by bringing her hands around from her back into the lower quadrants in order to indicate bearing-down discomfort. The backache and the abdominal discomfort are usually dull in nature and increase as the day goes on. If the patient complains of backache before she arises in the morning, and particularly if she gets relief on becoming active, one can be quite sure that the position of the uterus is not responsible for the pain. Such a clinical picture is often seen as a result of a mild lumbar arthritis in which the patient has less discomfort as she "loosens up." When one is doubtful about the etiologic relationship between the position of the uterus and the backache, the patient should be examined orthopedically. If the orthopedist fails to find a definite cause for the back discomfort, the therapeutic test of the pessary is invaluable. If the uterus is held up with the pessary and the backache is relieved, only to return when the uterus falls back after the pessary is removed, one can be quite sure that a suspension will give relief.

Disturbances of Menstruation. Any type of disturbance of menstruation may be present with retrodisplacement of the uterus, but in most instances the position of the uterus has no etiologic relationship to the disturbance. For example, amenorrhea, polymenorrhea, hypomenorrhea, and oligomenorrhea of endocrine origin occur with the retroverted as well as with the anteverted uterus, and a correction of the uterine malposition will have no curative effect on the menstrual disorder. Likewise, one is never justified in explaining intermenstrual bleeding on the basis of retrodisplacement. Also, menorrhagia or hypermenorrhea usually can be explained as attributable to another cause, although in some instances the retrodisplacement is responsible for the increased menstrual flow. The passive venous congestion of the uterus lying in the cul-de-sac may cause increased bleeding from the denuded menstrual endometrium. We have repeatedly seen a reduction of excessive menstrual flow following a uterine suspension.

Often it is difficult to judge the relation of dysmenorrhea to retrodisplacement. So-called idiopathic or essential dysmenorrhea is no respecter of uterine position and is found to occur in the anteverted as well as in the retroverted uterus. On the other hand, there is no doubt, judging from the relief obtained by suspension in some cases, that retrodisplacement of the uterus may cause dysmenorrhea. It is probable that marked retroflexion of the uterus, affording poor drainage of the menstrual flow, is more apt to be a factor in dysmenorrhea than when retroversion exists alone. The menstrual discomfort may take the form of cramps or sacral backache. Since it frequently is difficult to evaluate the relation of uterine position to menstrual pain, the therapeutic test of the pessary is again useful here.

Sterility. The finding of a uterus in retroposition in a woman complaining of sterility is no indication that the position of the uterus has any relation to the sterility problem. In such cases, a thorough investigation of the sterility must be made in both the male and the female, without regard for the retroposition. It is our opinion that sterility is slightly greater in women with retrodisplacement than in those without. It is possible that the edematous endometrium, seen at times in a large boggy, retroposed uterus, may not afford suitable soil for implantation of the fertilized ovum. However, this opinion is very difficult to prove. One is seldom, if ever, justified in undertaking uterine suspension for the relief of sterility alone.

Abortion. It is doubtful that retroposition is ever responsible for abortion before the 12th week of pregnancy. One sees many unexplained early abortions about which it is impossible to make statements regarding their etiology. It is our opinion that these early abortions are no more common in women with retroposed uteri than in others. When abortions occur repeatedly from about the 3rd or the 5th month and are associated with retroposition of the uterus, one may question the position of the uterus as a cause. This is particularly true when the uterus is acutely retroflexed, so that its spontaneous rise above the sacral promontory is difficult. In such cases where the uterus becomes wedged in the pelvis, uterine suspension may be justifiable, but if the patient is pregnant at the time of consultation, the uterus should be put in position and held there by pessary until the first trimester of pregnancy is past.

Nervous Symptoms. The general nervous constitution of the patient should be taken into consideration when suspension is contemplated. The question frequently resolves itself into this: Is the patient by nature a neurotic individual who is capitalizing on the fact that she has a malplaced uterus, or are her nervous symptoms the result of chronic, pelvic discomfort which has made her irritable and nervously exhausted? Often the answer is difficult, and frequently a period of careful observation is desirable before coming to a final conclusion.

Indications for Suspension

We do not quite agree with Fluhmann that suspension of the uterus is not necessary for adequate gynecologic practice. There are some young women in whom the symptoms of the retroversion are clear-cut and severe. Most of these are parous women, and often there is slight descensus accompanying the retrodisplacement. We prefer to have such women complete their families, and then we would advise a vaginal hysterectomy and whatever vaginal plastic operation may be indicated. Such advice may not always be agreeable to the patient, but she demands relief from her very troublesome discomfort. Under such conditions, we believe that there is still a place for intra-abdominal suspension of the uterus.

In our clinic we believe it to be indicated frequently in connection with conservative operations such as those done for endometriosis tubal pregnancy, or plastic operations on the tubes for relief of infertility. To leave a uterus in the cul-de-sac while doing the above conservative procedures would be to do incomplete surgery and often not give complete relief.

Choice of Operations

An abdominal suspension of the uterus after the menopause is seldom indicated unless the primary indication for opening the abdomen is the removal of some lesion—for example, a benign ovarian cyst. In most of such instances the opposite ovary and the uterus should be removed. In choosing the best operation in premenopausal women one must consider the likelihood and the desirability of future pregnancies. In the young women in whom future pregnancies are expected, we have found the modified Gilliam suspension to be most satisfactory. We have seen no evidence that it is detrimental to subsequent pregnancies, and we believe that pregnancy does little harm to a properly performed suspension of this kind. Many surgeons have reported satisfactory results with other types of suspensions, and we have no doubt that their results justify their claims. Among the most used in this country are the Olshausen and the Baldy-Webster. We prefer the modified Gilliam to the Olshausen because it is more nearly correct anatomically. This is not a mere academic preference, for by shortening the round ligaments through the internal inguinal ring, there is left no opening lateral to the point of attachment to the abdominal wall, as there is in the Olshausen, through which loops of intestine may become strangulated. We prefer the modified Gilliam to the Baldy-Webster because in the Gilliam operation the distal and weaker part of the round ligaments are reefed in, allowing the proximal stronger portions to serve in bringing the uterus forward. On the other hand, in the Baldy-Webster the stronger proximal portions of the ligaments are sutured to the posterior surface of the uterus, leaving the weaker distal portions to serve as the functioning portions of the ligaments.

The Alexander-Adams extraperitoneal shortening of the round ligaments in the inguinal canals has been almost completely abandoned in this country, although it is still in use in some European clinics; it is a blind operation, and its only advantage lies in the fact that it is extraperitoneal. Before the days of dependable aseptic surgery this was a great advantage, but today the danger of operative infection of the peritoneal cavity is negligible. The operation precludes the possibility of visual examination of the pelvic organs and correction of any accompanying lesions in the pelvis.

Regardless of the type of round-ligament suspension employed, there are cases in which simple round-ligament shortening will not adequately hold the uterus in anteposition. In those cases additional procedures are necessary. One of the more essential of these is shortening of the uterosacral ligaments. This is especially valuable in cases in which some descensus is present or when the cervix is markedly anterior. Another valuable procedure is the suturing of the bladder peritoneum at a point on the anterior uterine wall higher than its normal reflexion. At times, after shortening the round ligaments, the fundus still has a tendency to sag backward. The pull of the advanced bladder peritoneum is frequently sufficient to bring the center of gravity of the uterus forward and thus permit the intra-abdominal pressure to be exerted on the posterior surface.

Recently Durfee has suggested the use of mersilene tape for use in connection with abdominal suspension of the uterus and reports 28 cases without recurrence. In a rare case with atrophic round ligaments this might be useful. However, reporting 28 cases would indicate to us that he is performing intra-abdominal suspensions too often, when some other procedure would be the operation of choice.

When the patient has had all the children that she desires and particularly when an extensive vaginal plastic operation is indicated, the best "suspension" may be a vaginal hysterectomy. There is little reason for saving the uterus when it is necessary to operate upon a woman over 40 for symptomatic retroversion. The removal of the uterus will relieve the symptoms of retroversion and at the same time ensure against future trouble due to functional bleeding or uterine neoplasm. An additional reason for hysterectomy is afforded when dysmenorrhea is a prominent sympton.

Technic: Modified Gilliam Suspension of Uterus

A short midline incision is usually made, although a modified Pfannenstiel incision is also quite satisfactory. The uterus is brought forward, and a catgut traction suture is placed about one round ligament. The point at which this suture is taken should be such that when both ligaments are withdrawn for suture to the inside of the rectus sheath, the uterus will be in good position. The exact point can be determined only by trial and error, but the average distance is about 3 or 4 cm. from the uterine cornu (Fig. 24-1 A).

An Ochsner clamp is placed on the edge of the fascia at the level of the anterior superior spine of the ilium. A small Kelly clamp is placed on the peritoneal edge at the same level. The belly of the rectus is then separated from its sheath by blunt and sharp dissection (Fig. 24-1 B).

A long Kelly clamp is used to circumvent the belly of the rectus at the point where it has been freed, and the peritoneum is pushed up by the nose of the clamp at the internal inguinal ring. An assistant snips the peritoneum over the point of the clamp as the jaws are separated slightly (Fig. 24-1 C). The point of the Kelly clamp thus enters the peritoneal cavity. The catgut which was previously placed about the round ligament is now placed in the jaws of the long Kelly clamp, and the clamp is withdrawn. This maneuver brings the round ligament out of the peritoneal cavity through the internal inguinal ring, and a loop is brought between the rectus muscle and its sheath (Fig. 24-1 D). The loop is sutured to the under surface of the fascia

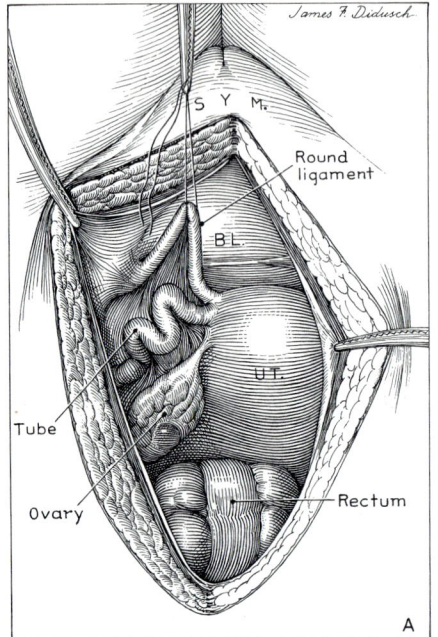
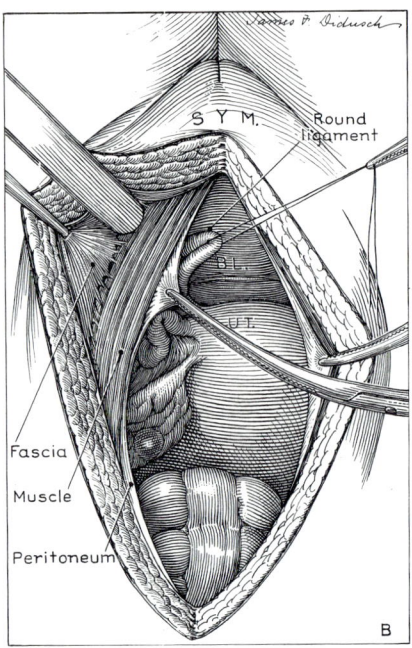
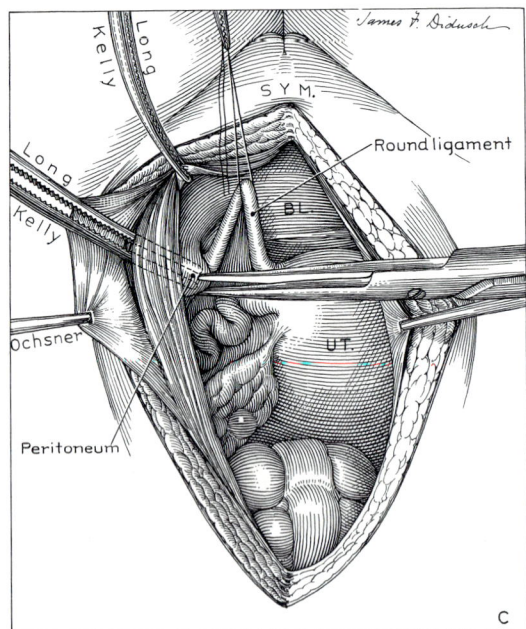

Fig. 24-1. Modified Gilliam suspension of uterus. (A) A traction suture of catgut has been placed about the round ligament at an appropriate point. (B) The rectus sheath is dissected from the belly of the muscle. (C) A long Kelly clamp has been passed around the belly of the rectus, through the internal inguinal ring. The peritoneum is being cut over the nose of the clamp so that it may enter the peritoneal cavity.

with linen or silk sutures. In placing these interrupted sutures care should be taken not to encircle the entire ligament and thus strangulate it, but rather to take substantial bites into the substance of the ligament on both sides and at the end of the loop (Fig. 24-1 E).

This procedure is repeated on the opposite side.

After the suspension has been done as

Retrodisplacement of Uterus

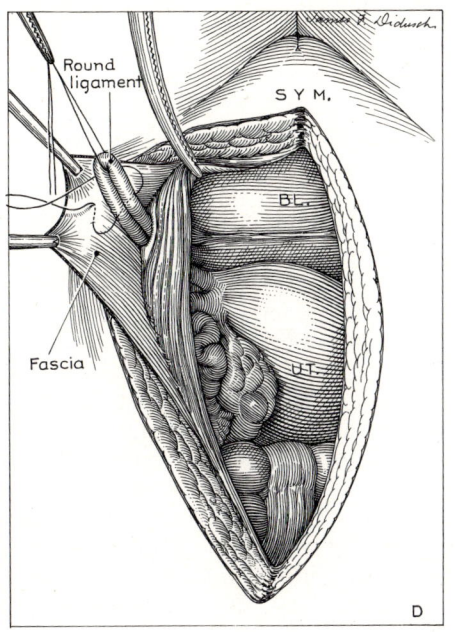
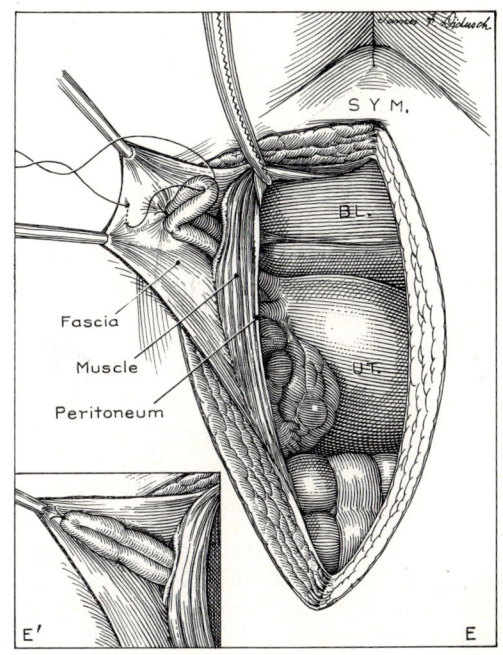
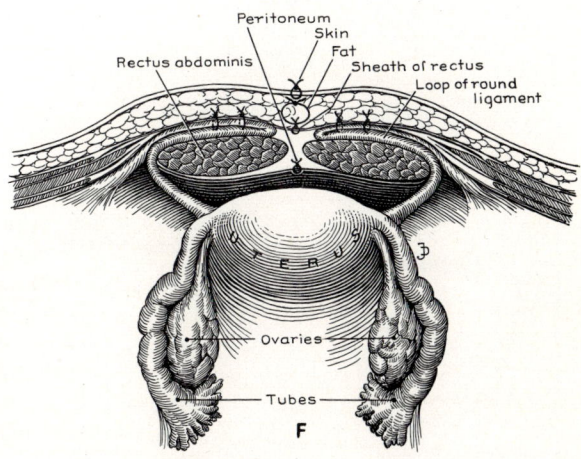

FIG. 24-1 (*Continued*). Modified Gilliam suspension of uterus. (D) The traction suture has been grasped by the Kelly clamp and withdrawn through the internal ring. The round ligament is being sutured to the inside of the rectus sheath with medium silk or Pagenstecher linen. (E) Another suture is anchoring the round ligament to the fascia. The inset shows how the round ligament has been sutured to the fascia. None of the sutures encircles the round ligament. (F) Transverse section showing final result.

described, the hand should be introduced into the abdomen to ascertain that there is no loop of round ligament lateral to the point where the ligament has been withdrawn from the peritoneal cavity. Such a loop can exist when the round ligament has been withdrawn at a point medial to the internal ring, or when all of the lateral segment of the ligament has not been withdrawn from the abdomen. If such a condition is found, it should be corrected to prevent strangulation of a loop of bowel between the ligament and the abdominal wall.

After completing the modified Gilliam suspension one should make certain that the standard suspension satisfactorily suspends the uterus. If it does not, additional methods of supporting the uterus should be utilized. We have found advancement of the bladder peritoneum on the anterior uterine wall and shortening of the uterosacral ligaments of great value. One should also make sure that a knuckle of tube has not been drawn into the internal inguinal ring, as may happen when the traction suture is placed too close to the uterus. This may cause sterility or predispose to ectopic pregnancy. The final result of the suspension is shown in Figure 24-1 F.

Technic: Advancement of Bladder Peritoneum

It is not uncommon to find, after performing any type of round-ligament suspension, that the fundus is not quite sufficiently far forward to permit intra-abdominal pressure to act upon its posterior surface and thus hold the uterus in good anteposition. Often the additional forward placement necessary can be accomplished by advancing the bladder peritoneum to a higher level on the anterior surface of the uterus. This may be done by cutting the peritoneum at its normal reflexion from the uterus onto the bladder, and suturing it to the uterus at a higher level.

There is another method of bladder advancement, which we prefer when it is done in connection with a Gilliam suspension. After shortening the round ligaments by the method just described, the bladder peritoneum is frequently thrown into a transverse fold slightly in front of its normal reflexion onto the uterus; this fold may be sutured to the anterior surface of the uterus well above the normal reflexion without cutting the peritoneum. The suturing may be done with continuous or interrupted sutures of medium silk or linen (Fig. 24-2). The peritoneal surfaces, thus approximated, heal together, and often the added tilt forward which the uterus receives is sufficient to maintain it in good position. We never have noted any bladder discomfort or disturbance from carrying out this procedure.

Technic: Shortening of Uterosacral Ligaments

Shortening of the uterosacral ligaments is accomplished very easily if exposure is adequate. The uterus may be held forward by the hand of an assistant or by means of an abdominal retractor. It is well to have the pelvis free of intestines. If they do not fall back into the abdomen as a result of good anesthesia, they should be packed back with moist gauze. Using medium silk or linen suture material on a round needle, the uterosacral ligaments are brought together and sutured to the posterior surface of the cervix in the midline just below the level of their insertion into the uterus. If further shortening is desired, a second similar suture is taken above the first (Fig. 24-3). Since the ureters lie in close proximity to the lateral aspect of the uterosacral ligament, care must be taken to avoid kinking or ligating the ureter

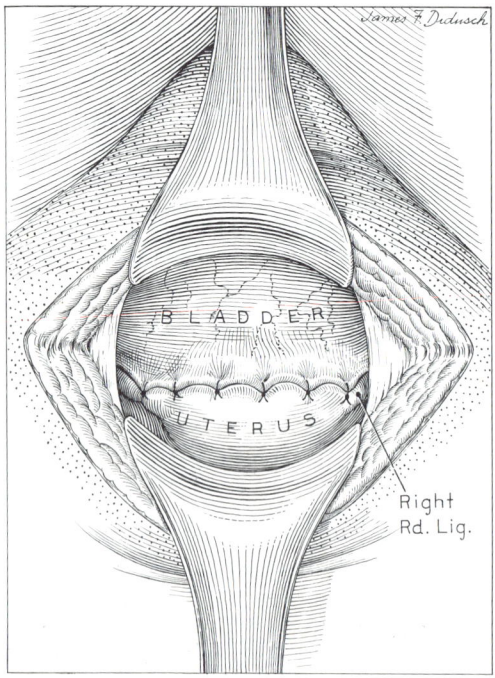

FIG. 24-2. Advancement of bladder peritoneum onto fundus of uterus. Interrupted sutures of medium silk have sutured a fold of bladder peritoneum high on the fundus of the uterus.

during this plication procedure. The more vigorous the plication of the ligaments, the greater is the chance of injury to the ureter. The holding of the cervix posteriorly is important in keeping the fundus forward; it also aids in preventing descensus.

VENTROFIXATION IN RELATION TO RETRODISPLACEMENT

Ventrofixation, hysterorrhaphy, and hysteropexy were terms applied to the earliest operation in which an attempt was made to suspend the retroplaced uterus. The interest of this operation is now historical. Howard Kelly, who was one of the first to attempt the operation, said in his *Operative Gynecology*:

I just called attention to this mode of relieving retroflexion in Germany in the spring and summer of 1886, when I also secured notes of unpublished cases similarly treated by Dr. Brennecke of Madgeburg, Professor Werth of Kiel, and Professor Sänger of Leipzig, which were published with an original case of my own. Professor Olshausen of Berlin, who had the subject under consideration at that same time, was the first to publish a paper on it, October 23, 1886. My own paper, entitled "Hysterorrhaphy" and describing a case operated upon April 25, 1885, was read before the Philadelphia Obstetrical Society, November 4, 1886, and published in the *American Journal of Obstetrics*, January, 1887.

Figure 24-4 shows the technic. It is shown as a matter of historical interest in the evolution of uterine suspension.

PROLAPSE OF UTERUS

GENERAL CONSIDERATIONS

The subject of the best treatment of uterine prolapse and its allied conditions is still one to evoke discussion and disagreements in gynecologic circles. In many clinics in this country vaginal hysterectomy is done routinely and is considered to be the answer to all degrees of prolapse. In others the Manchester operation, with modifications, is thought to be the universal answer. The interposition operation has lost greatly in popularity. It is rare today to encounter a gynecologic surgeon who would advocate a combined procedure of vaginal plastic and intra-abdominal suspension. Doing the entire operative procedure via the vagina represents real progress as illustrated by the results, which are far better than those obtained in former years when combined procedures were common.

In our opinion one should not approach the subject with a fixed plan. Each case should be treated as an individual problem. Indeed, the surgeon should be privileged to modify his plans as he proceeds with the operation and evaluates the structures as they are encountered during the dissection. The most important factors to be kept in mind in evaluating an individual for type of operation are:

The age and the general physical condition of the patient.

The desirability of preserving menstruation.

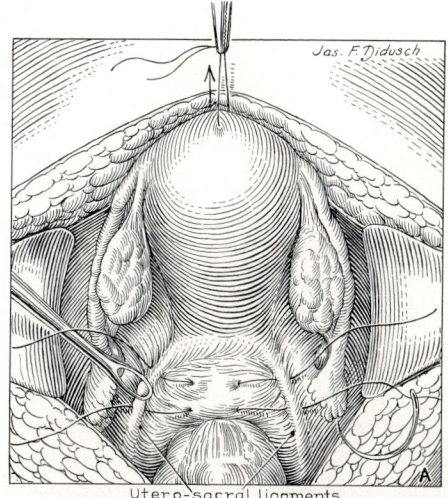
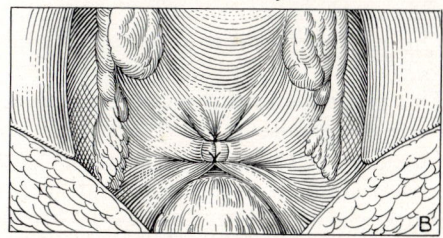

FIG. 24-3. Shortening of uterosacral ligaments. (A) Interrupted sutures of medium silk or Pagenstecher linen are passed through the uterosacral ligaments and the posterior surface of the cervix. (B) Sutures have been tied, thus shortening the ligaments.

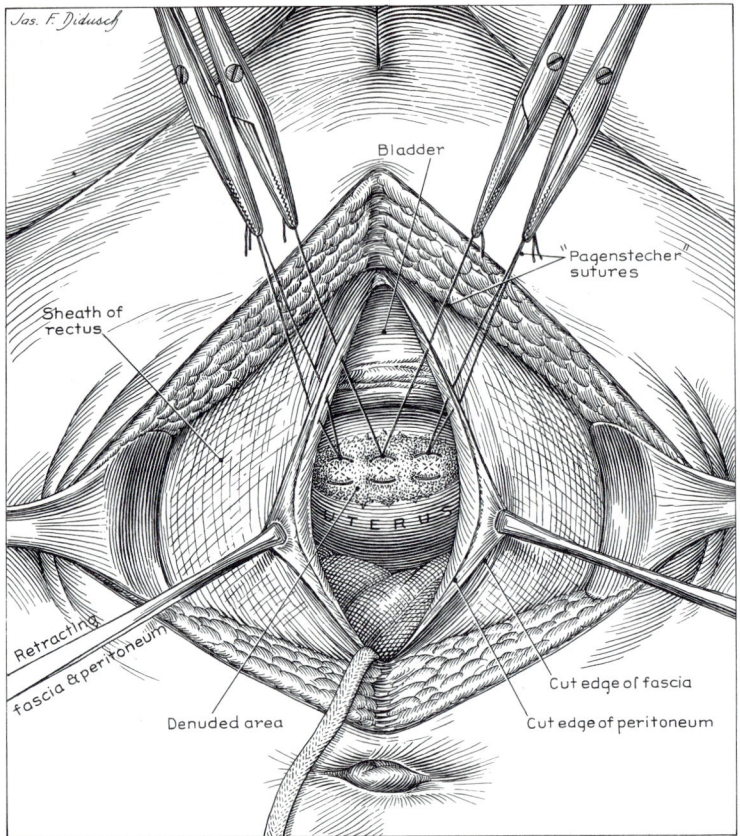

FIG. 24-4. Ventral fixation of uterus. Fundus is scarified. Three figure-of-eight Pagenstecher sutures are placed in the fundus. Two are brought out laterally through the peritoneum, the muscle, and the fascia. These are tied with the peritoneum open. The middle suture is brought out through the peritoneum and the fascia, one thread on either side. This suture is pulled up and tied as the peritoneum is closed.

The desirability of preserving the childbearing function.

The degree of descensus.

The condition of the cervix and the corpus uteri.

The presence and the degree of cystocele.

The presence and the degree of rectocele or enterocele.

All of these factors will be considered in discussing the various operative procedures described in this book for the cure of prolapse and allied conditions.

As we express our opinion on the various operations, we realize fully that there is room for honest difference of opinion on this subject. Without doubt, in many cases equally satisfactory results may be obtained by more than one method. If this were not true, there would not be such strong adherents of the different types of procedure. It is assumed that each surgeon who strongly defends a particular operation does so believing that that procedure is giving satisfactory results in his hands. There is no doubt that the skill of the individual operator, in a particular operation, is a great factor in his results. *But no matter how skillful a surgeon may become in a favorite procedure, he never should permit his enthusiasm for it to overcome his judgment as to its indication.*

ANATOMIC CONSIDERATIONS

In discussing the cure of prolapse of the uterus it is advisable to consider first the supporting structures that have failed to hold the uterus in correct position and how best to utilize them in restoring the uterus and the vagina to their normal positions, or in supporting that portion of the uterus which is permitted to be retained and the vagina.

The structures concerned in maintaining the uterus in normal position are:

1. The round ligaments.
2. The uterosacral ligaments.
3. The bases of the broad ligaments (cardinal ligaments, ligamentum transversalis colli, Mackenrodt).
4. The fascia lying between the anterior vaginal wall and the bladder (subvesical fascia or pubovesicocervical fascia).
5. The fascia lying between the posterior vaginal wall and the rectum.
6. The floor of the pelvis (the levator ani muscles).

Round Ligaments. The function of the round ligaments is to draw the uterus forward to its normal anatomic position after it has been displaced backward physiologically by bladder distention or pregnancy. Once returned to its normal position forward, the intra-abdominal pressure on the posterior surface of the uterus holds it forward. Increased intra-abdominal pressure, such as that caused by straining at hard work or defecation, causes slight temporary descent of the anteposed uterus. If the supports of the uterus are adequate, the uterus promptly returns to its former level. When the uterus is retroposed, or when the round ligaments fail to bring it forward after physiologic displacement backward, intra-abdominal pressure tends to force the uterus downward into the vagina like a piston in a cylinder. If the other supporting structures are sufficiently firm, the uterus may be maintained at its normal level despite the mechanical disadvantage of retrodisplacement, but a greater strain is put on the other supporting structures than when the uterus is anteverted.

Uterosacral Ligaments. The uterosacral ligaments, which are part of the endopelvic fascia lying subperitoneally, extend from the cervix back to the sacrum; they hold the cervix back and also aid in holding it up. Congenitally long ligaments, or ligaments which have lost their tonus as the result of pregnancy, permit the cervix to be displaced forward and downward; this allows the corpus to be displaced backward until the axis of the uterus and that of the vagina coincide. Intra-abdominal pressure then tends to force the uterus down in the vagina.

Broad Ligaments. The bases of the broad ligaments are also part of the endopelvic fascia and play an extremely important role in maintaining the uterus at its normal level. These cardinal ligaments, attached to the sides of the intra-abdominal portion of the uterine cervix, fan out laterally as they approach the sides of the pelvis to which they are attached. One must assume a congenital factor of weakness of these ligaments in some cases of prolapse, for occasionally one sees them greatly attenuated in women who have neither done much physical work nor borne any children. However, in most cases in which the cardinal ligaments fail, childbearing and physical work play a major role. The softening effect of the pregnancy hormones, the weight of the pregnant uterus and the increased intra-abdominal pressure of hard work all tend to stretch the cardinal ligaments and permit the uterus to drop to a permanently lower level.

Fascial Sheath. The normal nulliparous vagina is maintained in position as a semirigid structure by a strong fascial sheath which encases the mucosa. Anteriorly, this pubovesicocervical fascia lies between the bladder and the vagina and stretches from its origin at the symphysis pubis beneath the bladder to be inserted into the anterior wall of the cervix. The upper part of this fascia is easily seen when the bladder is dissected down in performing an abdominal total hysterectomy. Posteriorly, similar rectovaginal fascia separates the vagina from the muscular wall of the rectum, giving support to the vaginal tube and preventing the anterior rectal wall from bulging into the vagina. When these fascial structures are torn and stretched by childbirth, the vaginal wall becomes redundant and flabby; rectocele and cystocele develop. The weight of the uterus, especially if it is retroverted, aggravates the sagging of the vagina, and when prolapsus becomes complete, the vagina may become entirely everted.

Muscular Floor of the Pelvis. Finally, there is the muscular floor of the pelvis to be considered. This forms the foundation upon which the vaginal tube rests and hence the foundation upon which the uterus rests ultimately. Tearing and separation of the pubococcygeal fibers of the levator muscles weaken this floor and widen the aperture through which the vagina and eventually the uterus may descend. For a better understanding of the factors concerned in prolapse of the uterus the reader is referred to the diagrams shown in Figures 24-5 and 24-6.

All of these structures play a part in holding the uterus in its normal position; some or all of them are utilized in the various operations described below, designed to restore support to the pelvic structures.

THE MANCHESTER (DONALD OR FOTHERGILL) OPERATION

In 1888 Donald, of Manchester, began treating prolapsus uteri by the combination of anterior and posterior colporrhaphy and amputation of the cervix. For over half a century this operation has been performed continuously in Manchester by a number of gynecologists upon "all patients with prolapsus uteri, irrespective of age, social position or parity." Before Fothergill modified the operation, the procedure was to amputate the cervix by the Schröder method and to follow this by an anterior colporrhaphy. Fothergill made the incision for the anterior repair triangular in shape with the base at the cervix and then carried the incision around the cervix to perform the amputation. This exposed the bases of the broad ligaments to better advantage than by the method previously employed and facilitated the approximation of these supporting structures in front of the cervix. This operation, with

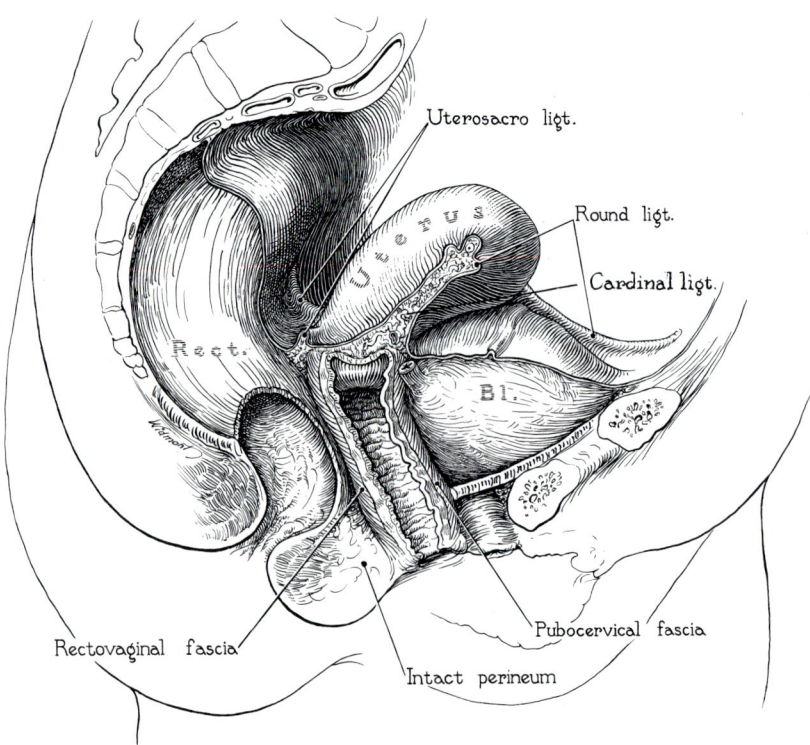

FIG. 24-5. Indicating normal supports of uterus.

slight variation, has been done by different members of the Manchester staff since 1888. Descriptions of its technic, which have appeared in the literature, vary as to detail. The operation as done in this clinic is described in this volume. The fundamental principles underlying the procedure are exactly as in the operation described by Shaw from the Manchester Clinic in 1933, but certain details differ slightly.

In 1933 Shaw reported on 549 patients who had been treated for prolapse by this method. His reports were obtained by questionnaire; no attempt was made to describe anatomic results. Ninety-six per cent were reported as completely cured, a figure which compares favorably with the best reports on any method of treating prolapse. In spite of this report we are not convinced that the operation is the one of choice in "all patients with prolapse uteri, irrespective of age, social position or parity." It is our opinion that the Manchester operation is a satisfactory procedure when (1) there is a cystocele associated with a prolapse of first or second degree; (2) childbearing need no longer be considered; and (3) when the uterus is not in marked retroposition or when the retrodisplaced uterus is a small atrophic structure and not contributory to the patient's symptoms. The operation is particularly satisfactory under the above conditions when much of the apparent prolapse is due to cervical elongation.

We believe that there is a definite objection to the operation when future pregnancy is likely, because of the amputation of the cervix. Leonard found that, following cervical amputation, the incidence of sterility was abnormally high; premature delivery between the 6th and the 8th months increased, and cervical dystocia was common. Shaw's own results would seem to condemn the operation during the childbearing period. Only 27 of the 549 women of his reported group subsequently had children. Since admittedly the operation was done on women "regardless of age," there must have been a goodly proportion of young women in the group. The small number who subsequently bore children appears to indicate a high incidence of either sterility or abortion. Shaw relates further that of the 27 who had children "only 5

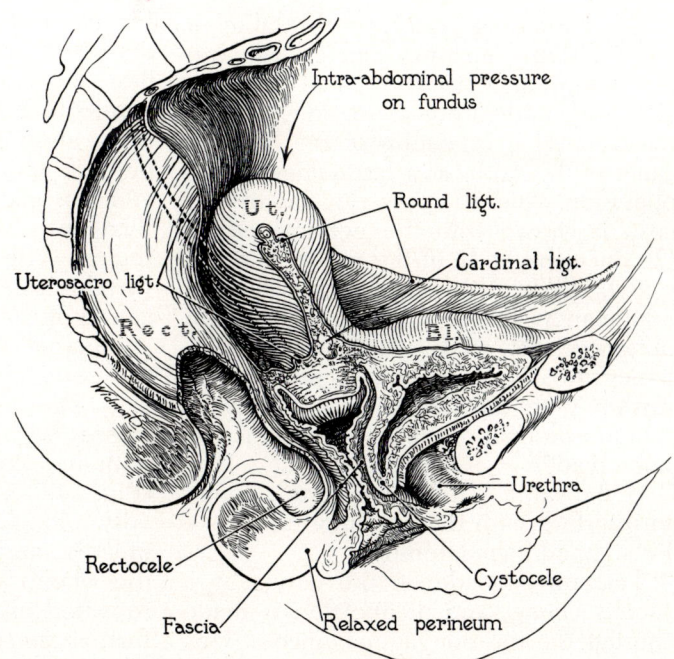

Fig. 24-6. Indicating how failure of normal supports permits descent of uterus, as well as cystocele and rectocele formation.

showed any signs of recurrence." The recurrence of the prolapse in 18.5 per cent of the women who bore children would seem to us to contraindicate the operation in women in whom future pregnancy is probable. The late Dr. Hunter, while a member of the University of Manchester staff, regarded the operation as contraindicated when further childbearing was a consideration.

We must confess that we never have used this operation for complete procidentia, because it scarcely seems logical that a simple anterior colporrhaphy, with suturing of the cardinal ligaments in front of the cervix coupled with cervical amputation and posterior colporrhaphy, can support the completely prolapsed uterus. In our opinion, other methods described in this chapter will give stronger support.

Except for the Le Fort operation, the Manchester operation has one advantage over most of the other vaginal procedures for cure of uterine prolapse. It is simpler and usually can be done in less time and with less shock. Hence in elderly or in otherwise frail women, in some instances it may be used with great advantage.

Technic

The patient is placed on the table in the lithotomy position and cleaned up for operation with the usual technic. Dilatation and curettage are done for two reasons: (1) a dilatation of the cervical canal is desirable at a later stage of the operation when the posterior flap of mucosa is drawn into the cervical canal; (2) since the body of the uterus is to be saved, it is well to make certain that no malignancy exists. If the endometrium obtained looks at all suspicious of malignancy grossly, it is best to proceed no further with the operation until microscopic examination of the curettings has been made.

If the labia minora are long enough to interfere with the operation they may be stitched back laterally.

Traction is made on the cervix by a Jacobs clamp, and an incision is made through the anterior vaginal mucosa. This incision may be made in the midline from cervix to urethral meatus, dissecting beneath the mucosa with the curved scissors as illustrated in the operation for cystocele, or a more-or-less triangular piece of vaginal mucosa may be excised as practiced by Shaw of the Manchester Clinic. Our usual practice is to make a midline incision connecting with a transverse incision at the cervix, excising the excess of mucosa later. In the illustrations the operation is done through this inverted-T incision, but the initial incision is not shown, since it is identical with that illustrated in the cystocele operation.

The flaps of vaginal mucosa are dissected laterally, and the bladder is dissected up from its attachment to the cervix. In the beginning the separation of the bladder from the cervix must be done by sharp dissection, but usually after a few "snips" with the scissors the bladder may be freed from the uterus by blunt dissection with the finger up to the vesico-uterine reflexion of the peritoneum. The bladder is held up anteriorly with a thin-bladed retractor as illustrated in Figure 24-7 A.

The transverse cervical incision through the mucosa is then carried posteriorly, completely circumcising the cervix. The posterior flap of mucosa is dissected free from the cervix until a flap has been mobilized sufficiently ample to cover easily the posterior lip of the shortened cervix. Having freed the mucosa about the cervix both anteriorly and posteriorly, the base of the broad ligament is exposed in the paracervical region. The tissue in this region is of variable thickness. If there is great elongation of the cervix, the structure may be attenuated markedly. Contained in it is the cervical branch of the uterine vessels. The fibrous tissue is clamped, en masse, with an Ochsner clamp parallel with and close to the cervix, cut and tied (Fig. 24-7 A). When the cervix is markedly elongated so that a great length must be amputated, two tandem bites of the clamp may be necessary. This is repeated on the opposite side. To sever further the cervical blood supply, a suture ligature of No. 1 chromic catgut is placed through the side of the cervix bilaterally, just above the point of intended amputation.

The cervix is amputated as indicated by the dotted line in Figure 24-7 A, and the shortened posterior lip is covered with the posterior flap of mucosa, using a mattress suture of No. 1 chromic catgut. The exact method of placing this suture is indicated on page 404 under "cervical amputation."

The ligated broad ligament bases are then drawn together and sutured in front of the shortened cervix. It is well to bite into the anterior cervical wall with this suture in order to fix the ligaments in this position (Fig. 24-7 B).

Beginning beneath the urethra, the pubocervical fascia, which has been freed from the lateral mucosa flaps, is approximated in the midline with interrupted mattress sutures of No. 0 chromic catgut as indicated in Figure 24-7 C. This fascia covers over, successively, the urethra, the base of the bladder, the lower portion of the uterus, and finally at least part of the broad ligaments that have been approximated previously in the midline. The lower sutures are made to bite into the anterior surface of the lower portion of the body of the uterus.

Figure 24-7 D shows the fascia approximated and the excess of vaginal mucosa being excised. The mucosa is then sutured in the midline with interrupted sutures of No. 0 chromic catgut. It is usually advantageous to suture the cervical end of the mucosal incision first. In doing this, a bite is taken into the anterior lip of the shortened cervix, as illustrated in Figure 24-7 D. One or two lateral sutures are necessary to cover the cervix completely. Figure 24-7 E shows the completed operation.

Posterior colporrhaphy is then done with appropriate technic to cure the relaxed outlet, the rectocele, and/or the enterocele as indicated in the individual case.

THE WATKINS TRANSPOSITION OPERATION

This operation for cystocele and uterine prolapse was first done by Thomas J. Watkins in 1898 and was reported by him the following year. Freund was the first (1895) to deliver the uterus into the vaginal canal for the cure of uterine prolapse and cystocele. He delivered the uterus through an incision in the posterior vaginal fornix and sutured the anterior vaginal wall to the posterior surface of the uterus, and the posterior vaginal wall to the anterior surface of the uterus. He then made an opening through the fundus of the uterus for drainage. The fundus was left uncovered in the vagina. Fritsch modified Freund's operation by denuding an area on the anterior vaginal wall and suturing the posterior wall of the uterus to it, after the uterus had been delivered anteriorly. A T-shaped incision was made on the posterior vaginal wall, and two flaps of mucosa were dissected free. These flaps of mucosa were reflected over the fundus of the uterus and sutured there. Wertheim modified Fritsch's procedure by delivering the uterus through an incision in front of the cervix and scarifying the anterior wall of the vagina and the posterior wall of the uterus. Then the two scarified areas were sutured together with catgut. Schauta and Wertheim later reported an operation very similar to that described by Watkins, and frequently the Watkins operation has been called the Wertheim operation. As a matter of historical record, Watkins published his operation in 1899, before Wertheim's report of his modification of Freund's operation and 3 years before Wertheim's assistant, Bucura, reported on the results of the Wertheim-Freund operation. Hence we shall refer to the operation under consideration as the Watkins transposition operation. It is generally known throughout this country as the *interposition operation*, but Watkins preferred the term *transposition*, since the uterus and the bladder are transposed.

This operation was formerly used extensively for uterine prolapse and cystocele, and in most instances the results were very satisfactory. Our results were reviewed independently by Shaw, Brady, and Everett for 3 different eras.

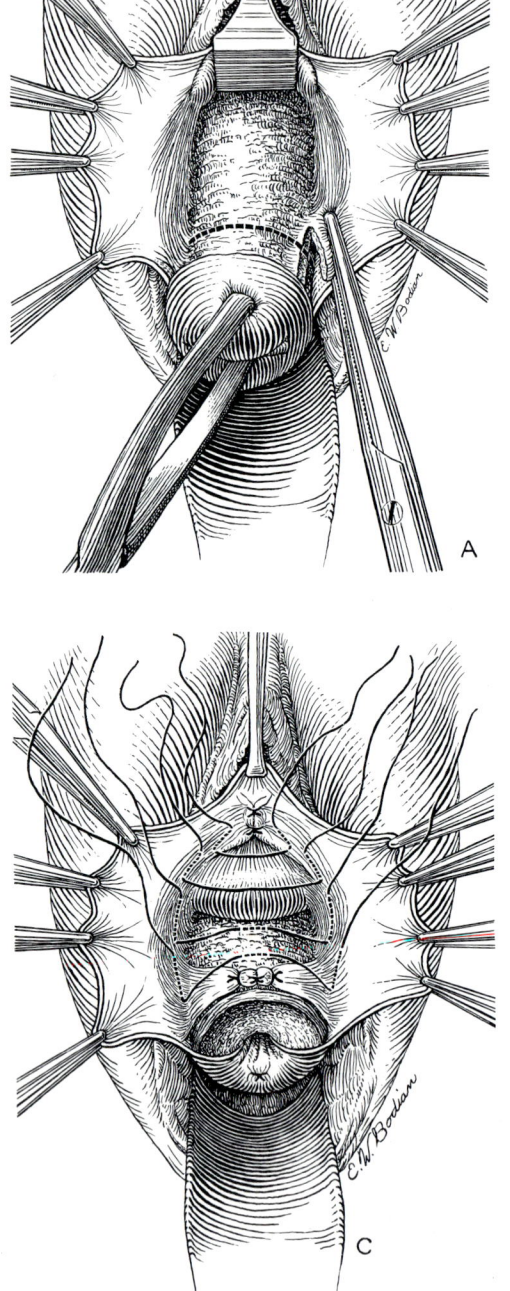

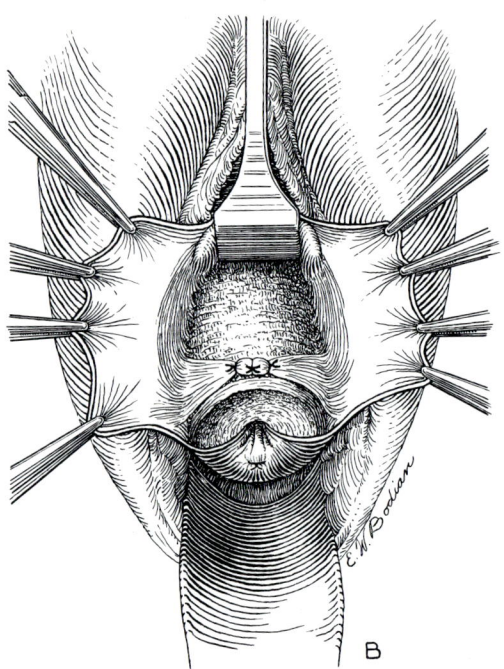

Fig. 24-7. Manchester operation for uterine prolapse and cystocele. (A) The bladder has been dissected up from the cervix. The incision has been carried through the mucosa around the cervix, and the mucosa dissected free from the cervix. The bases of the broad ligaments are thus exposed. The left has been clamped and cut. The dotted line indicates where the cervix is to be amputated. (B) The cervix has been amputated, and the posterior lip has been covered with a flap of mucosa. The bases of the broad ligaments have been sutured to the anterior surface of the cervix. (C) Pubovesicocervical fascia is being approximated in the midline beneath the urethra, the base of the bladder, and the cervix. Note that the lower sutures bite into the anterior wall of the cervix.

Their combined figures gave evidence of recurrence in 3.5 per cent of the cases. Everett could find no evidence for the belief that an advanced degree of prolapse is a contraindication to the transposition operation, for in his series all cases with complete procidentia were cured. Through extensive personal ex-

Prolapse of Uterus 487

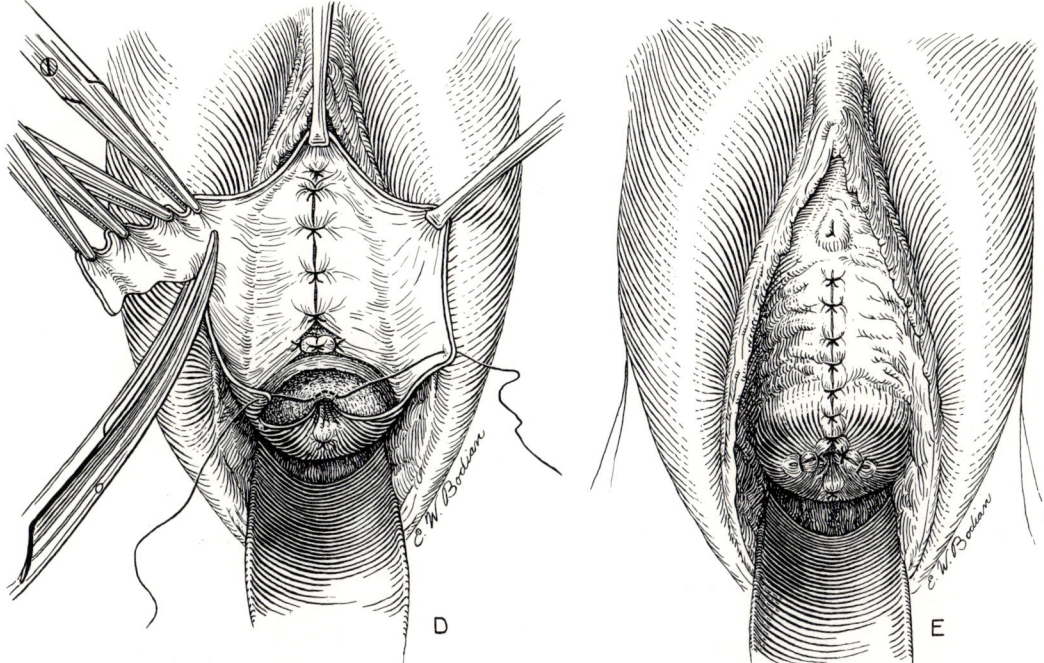

Fig. 24-7 (*Continued*). Manchester operation for uterine prolapse and cystocele. (D) The fascia approximation has been completed. Excess vaginal mucosa is being excised. The first suture has been placed through flaps of the mucosa, biting into the cut surface of the shortened cervical lip to cover it with mucosa. (E) The operation on the anterior wall has been completed. It is to be followed by a posterior colporrhaphy.

perience with this operation we have had only 2 cases in which the results were not satisfactory. Failure to amputate the cervix, which seemed to be unnecessary at the time of the operation, was the cause of the unsatisfactory results in these 2 instances. Subsequently, the cervices became elongated and protruded. Since this experience we have routinely amputated the cervix, even though it has not appeared elongated, and the results have been remarkably and uniformly successful. We have found the operation especially useful when a very large cystocele is present, and when the uterus is of the proper size to serve as an adequate plug in supporting the bladder. When the uterus is an extremely small postmenopausal structure and the cystocele is large, one may bring the pubovesical-cervical fascia completely together in the midline in front of the small uterus or perform a vaginal hysterectomy or a Spalding-Richardson operation. As performed by most surgeons, the transposition operation is a lesser procedure than the vaginal extirpation of the uterus and, hence, less shocking to the aged or to the patient who is otherwise a poor surgical risk.

Obviously, pregnancy should not follow this operation. If it is done on a woman in whom pregnancy is possible, the tubes should be cut and ligated. Aside from the question of pregnancy, we dislike the operation on young women because if fixes the anterior vaginal wall to the uterus, and the vagina is less pliable than after a Spalding-Richardson composite operation or a vaginal hysterectomy. The anterior vaginal wall is also shortened appreciably in some instances, and the resultant vagina is less satisfactory as a functioning organ. Disease of the corpus uteri is a definite contraindication to the operation, although often small myomata can be excised and the uterus transposed quite satisfactorily. Even the possibility of *subsequent* disease is a disadvantage in young women who have many years ahead of them during which myomata or functional bleeding may develop. The operation always should be preceded by a diagnostic curettage in order to exclude the possibility of interposing a corpus containing endometrial carcinoma. There always remains the possibility of subsequent development of a corpus carcinoma, and this must be considered a point against the operation. Fortunately, such a possibility is rare. A uterus subject to functional bleeding should not be transposed. For technical reasons there are times when a large fibrotic organ cannot be interposed successfully. In short, we consider the interposition operation a satisfactory procedure for the cure of prolapse of the uterus up to third degree in women approaching or past the menopause, when the uterus is healthy, bearing in mind the contraindications mentioned above. It is of special value when there is an accompanying large cystocele and a uterus that has not become too atrophic or too large to serve as an effective support for the base of the bladder. We also prefer it to the vaginal hysterectomy or the Spalding-Richardson composite operation when the general condition of the patient dictates a shorter operation. However, often an equally good result can be obtained by the use of a still simpler and shorter operation under such circumstances, namely, the Manchester operation. Because we believe there is the occasional woman with a large cystocele and moderate descensus, with a uterus of exactly the proper size and poor pubocervical fascia in which the transposition operation serves very well, we have included it in this chapter.

Technic

The patient is put in the lithotomy position, and a posterior retractor is placed in the vagina. The anterior lip of the cervix is grasped with a Jacobs clamp, and the cervix is drawn toward the outlet.

An inverted T-shaped incision is made. Customarily, we first make the cross bar of the T through the vaginal mucosa at its reflexion onto the anterior lip of the cervix. Then, using a curved scissors, a tunnel is made beneath the vaginal mucosa in the midline by alternately opening and closing the scissors and keeping the curved end of the scissors directed toward the mucosa. After tunneling for a few centimeters, the mucosa is cut in the midline, the tunneling is continued, and the mucosa is cut again. This is continued until the urethral meatus is reached, as indicated in the portrayal of the cystocele operation on page 536.

The mucosa flaps are dissected laterally, thus exposing the base of the bladder. The attachment of the bladder to the cervix is then cut, and the bladder is pushed upward. Soon a plane of free cleavage is encountered, and the finger can be easily pushed up to the vesico-uterine fold of the peritoneum (Fig. 24-8 A).

Next, a narrow retractor is placed in this dissected space, and the bladder is held upward. This usually exposes the undersurface of the peritoneum of the vesico-uterine fold. If the peritoneum is not seen readily, the uterus may be pulled down by placing figure-of-eight sutures in the anterior surface of the lower portion of the uterus and making traction. When the peritoneum is visualized, it is incised. It is a good plan to place a catgut suture on the peritoneal edge for later identification. Following this, the narrow retractor is introduced into the peritoneal cavity, and the anterior surface of the uterus is exposed.

Amputation of the cervix is usually best done at this stage of the operation, because getting rid of the cervix often facilitates delivering the fundus. The technic of cervical amputation used here is similar to that described on page 404 in Figure 20-15; or, if a high amputation is desirable, the technic described on page 405 in Figure 20-16 is used. Only the posterior lip of the shortened cervix is covered over with a flap of mucosa at this stage (Fig. 24-8 B). The anterior lip is covered at the final stage of the operation.

Next, the fundus is delivered through the peritoneal opening. We have found the Lahey thyroid clamps to be especially well adapted for this. They bite into the uterus with the several teeth; hence they are not as apt to tear out as is the ordinary tenaculum. When these clamps are not available, it is our habit to deliver the uterus by successive figure-of-eight sutures in a hand-over-hand manner as shown in Figure 24-8 B.

If the operation is done on a premenopausal woman, cornual resection of the tubes should be done for sterilization as indicated in the inset in Figure 24-8 C. The tube is ligated with No. 0 chromic catgut and is cut about a centimeter from the uterine cornu. It is excised at the cornu, and the cornual wound is closed with figure-of-eight sutures of No. 0 chromic catgut.

The opening in the peritoneal cavity is closed by using a few interrupted sutures of No. 0 chromic catgut to attach the peritoneum to the posterior surface of the delivered uterus (Fig. 24-8 C).

The fundus of the uterus is then sutured beneath the pubic rami as indicated in the inset in Figure 24-8 D, using No. 1 chromic catgut. A single ample bite of tissue into each uterine cornu and into the tissues beneath the pubic rami completes this fixation of the uterus. It is not necessary to carry the subpubic sutures into the periosteum of the pubis, as suggested by some surgeons. The uterus can only heal to the tissues with which it is in contact; hence nothing is to be gained by including the periosteum in the suture. In order to prevent the trigone from slipping out from behind the fundus, it is our custom to place a mattress suture through the fundus and to carry it out through the vaginal mucosa just behind the urethral meatus as in Figure 24-8 D.

The excess of vaginal mucosa is excised as is shown by the dotted line in Figure 24-8 D. Closure of the anterior vaginal incision is done with interrupted sutures of No. 0 chromic catgut. Each of these sutures picks up a bit of the subjacent uterus to obliterate dead space (Fig. 24-8 E). The final one of these sutures covers the anterior lip of the shortened cervix. The redundant mucosal edges laterally in the region of the cervix are approximated with figure-of-eight sutures of No. 0 chromic catgut.

The sagittal section of the completed operation (Fig. 24-8 F) shows the position of the uterus at the conclusion of the operation. From this diagram one sees how impossible it is for the cystocele to recur when the uterus is adherent to the anterior vaginal wall. It is also apparent that the direction of the axis of the uterus has been altered so that it can no longer descend into the vagina as a plunger in a cylinder.

THE VAGINAL HYSTERECTOMY

Although vaginal hysterectomy is an extremely useful operation in selected cases, we do not believe that it is the final answer to all cases of prolapse. We realize that this statement is not in agreement with the views of many excellent gynecologists, such as Heaney, Allen, Edwards, Aldridge, and the Mayo group. However, the experience of this clinic has not been identical with theirs, and our opinion is based chiefly on our own observations. When the operation is done for extreme prolapse with eversion of the vagina, our results were not very satisfactory even though anterior and posterior colporrhaphy were done. Although the reports from some clinics where vaginal hysterectomy is done routinely do not agree with our experience, the senior author has seen many cases of vaginal prolapse following vaginal hysterectomy done elsewhere.

It must be remembered that in those clinics from which much better results are reported, the operation is done in a great percentage of the instances for conditions other than prolapse. Therefore it is to be expected that the ultimate anatomic results would be better so far as vaginal support is concerned. Nevertheless, Danforth, who was an ardent advocate of vaginal hysterectomy, reported unsatisfactory results in 12.5 per cent of those cases *in which the operation was done for prolapse*. When prolapse of the vagina does occur following vaginal hysterectomy, it should be remembered that the condition is one of the most difficult to cure with the preservation of a func-

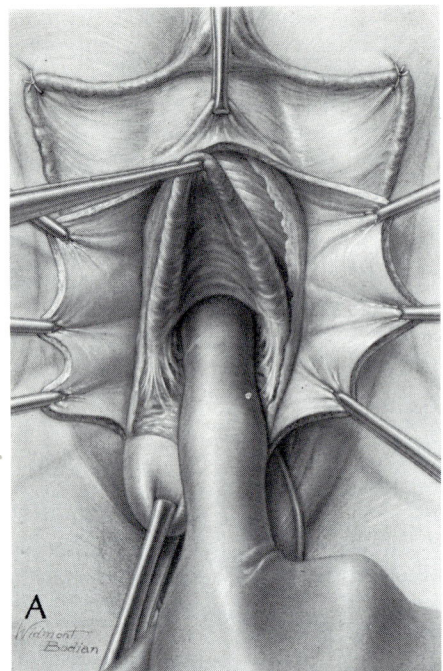
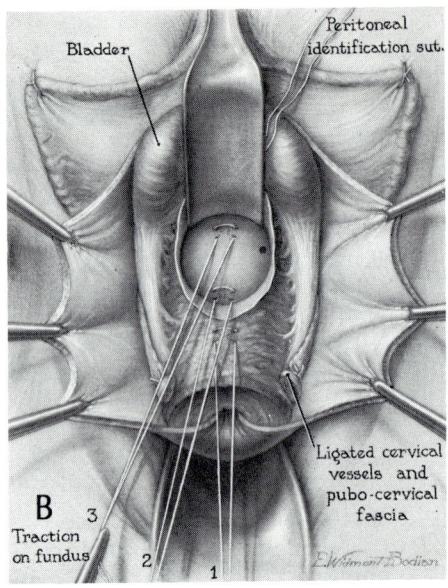
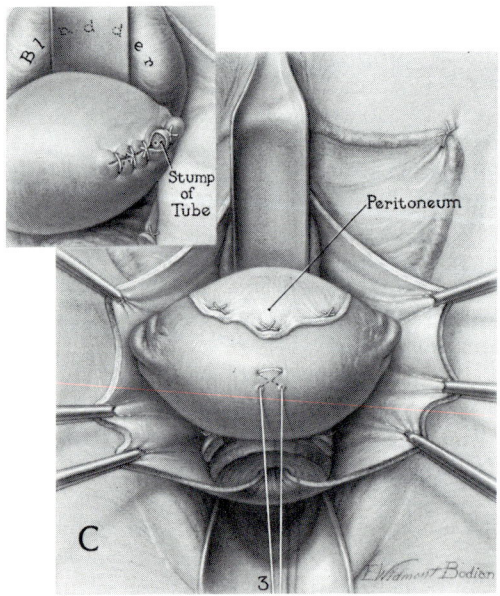

FIG. 24-8. Watkins transposition operation. (A) An inverted T-shaped incision has been made, and the flaps of the bladder mucosa have been dissected laterally, as illustrated in the operation for cystocele. The bladder is now being separated from its uterine attachment. (B) The cervix has been amputated, and the posterior lip has been covered with a flap of vaginal mucosa. The vesico-uterine fold of peritoneum has been incised, and the uterus is being delivered by traction sutures. (C) The peritoneal flap has been sutured to the posterior aspect of the uterus, thus closing the peritoneal opening. The inset shows the cornual resection of the tube for sterilization.

tioning vagina. We reserve the vaginal hysterectomy in the cure of marked prolapse for those cases in which disease of the uterus makes its removal desirable, such as small myomata, functional bleeding, and unexplained postmenopausal bleeding. In spite of our skepticism for the operation as a cure-all for uterine prolapse, we are most enthusiastic about the operation in properly selected cases for some other conditions, which are discussed in Chapter 8, Myomata Uteri.

Heaney Technic

The performance of a vaginal hysterectomy is facilitated by the use of a proper operating table. When the patient is in the lithotomy position, the hips should come just to the edge of the table so that the hanging speculum may

Prolapse of Uterus 491

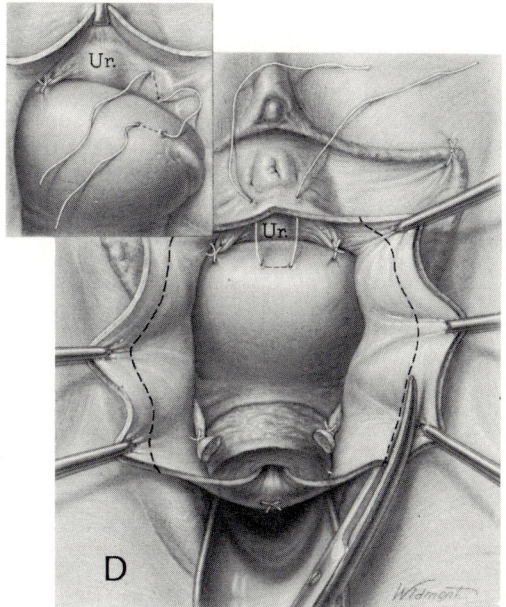
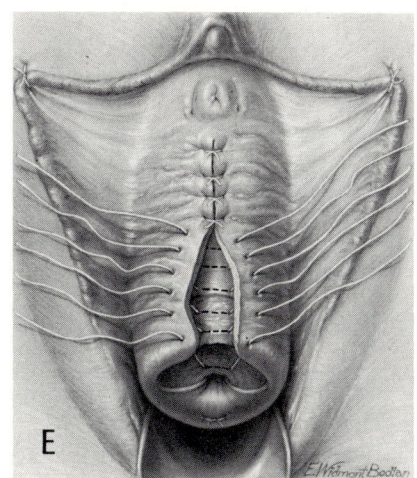

Fig. 24-8 (*Continued*). Watkins transposition operation. (D) The inset shows the fundus being sutured beneath the pubic rami. The larger picture shows the fundus sutured in place. An additional mattress suture has been placed in the midline to prevent prolapse of the urethra or the trigone. Excess vaginal mucosa is being trimmed off. (E) Closure of the vaginal incision with interrupted sutures. With each suture a bit of subjacent tissue is picked up to obliterate dead space.

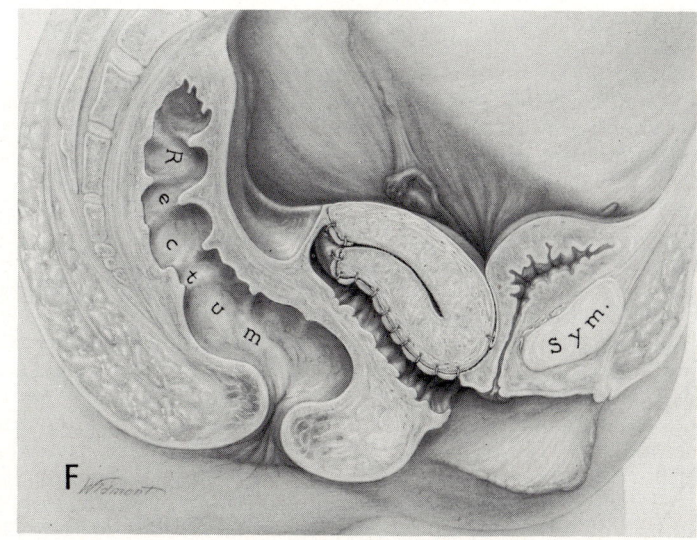

Fig. 24-8 (*Continued*). Watkins transposition operation. (F) Shows transposed uterus fixed in its new position. Increased intra-abdominal pressure serves only to press the fundus more snugly against the urethra, which is supported by the fundus.

swing free. If the patient is down too far, the axis of the vagina points upward, and vision is obscured. Narrow delicate instruments also contribute to ease in operating vaginally. Heavy cumbersome tools may make access to the uterus through a virginal vagina impossible. In addition, a well-focused spotlight is essential.

After the patient has been anesthetized and placed in proper position, the vulva and the perineum are thoroughly washed, as is also the vagina, with soap and water; the bladder is completely emptied with a catheter and the operative field is swabbed with dilute tincture of iodine or Lugol's solution, the excess of which is removed by alcohol.

The labia, when long, should be stitched back out of the way (Fig. 24-9 A). If the introitus is too tight, a small midline episiotomy will overcome the difficulty. A narrow vaginal fornix is a more serious obstacle to easy operating.

The cervix is seized with a bullet forceps and is pulled strongly into view. If it is badly eroded or cystic, it should be well sterilized with a cautery. Two cubic centimeters of obstetrical pituitary extract are injected into the paracervical tissues or vaginal walls (Fig. 24-9 A). This will reduce the bleeding to a minimum. A transverse incision is made through the mucosa of the vaginal wall just above the portio but below the attachment of the bladder (Fig. 24-9 A). A sound passed into the bladder will demonstrate how low the bladder lies.

If a cystocele is to be corrected, the vaginal wall is carefully freed from the bladder in the center of this incision. Then curved scissors are introduced between the vaginal wall and bladder with the curve forward. The vaginal wall is easily separated from the bladder by shoving the closed scissors carefully forward toward the urethra, then spreading the blades, shoving forward again with closed blades and opening again until under the urethra. The flaps are now freed laterally from the bladder, partly by blunt dissection with gauze and by the scissors until as much is loosened as is to be removed. The redundant mucosa is now cut away, and all bleeding points accurately controlled. If the urethra is to be tightened, it is done at this time and the mucosa over the urethra sutured with interrupted No. 2 ten-day chromic catgut, which is used throughout the entire operation. The rest of the anterior colporrhaphy is completed after the removal of the uterus.

The bladder is now freed from the anterior surface of the uterus up to the plica vesico-uterina (Fig. 24-9 B, C). Usually this can be accomplished by blunt dissection with gauze. If a previous plastic operation has been performed in this region, adhesions may make blunt dissection impossible, and sharp dissection may become necessary. One must be careful then that the dissection is carried out rather toward the uterus than toward the bladder. If the bladder is entered, great care must be used in loosening the rest of the bladder from its attachment so as not to widen the opening. As soon as the bladder is loosened, the hole in the bladder is repaired by interrupted No. 0 chromic sutures through the bladder mucosa, followed by a line of similar sutures through the muscularis of the bladder.

At the completion of the operation, an indwelling rubber catheter is to be inserted; this catheter is of the umbrella type if a hole in the bladder was repaired, or a hollow two-wing Malecot type if a urethroplastic operation was done. The umbrella type remains in the bladder with less discomfort and rarely slips out, but its removal may undo the urethroplastic repair; while the Malecot may be removed by stretching out the head by the use of a sound. While separating the bladder from the anterior wall of the uterus it should also be separated at its urethral attachments for about an inch on each side.

The free peritoneal fold in front is now looked for, incised (Fig. 24-9 D), and a narrow-bladed retractor inserted into the peritoneal cavity to hold the bladder and the ureters forward (Fig. 24-9 E). Occasionally, the uterus remains too high to make the plica vesico-uterina readily accessible, or a tumor low down on the cervix interferes at this point. If the bladder cannot be pushed up easily enough and delay is encountered in getting in to the anterior cul-de-sac, puttering may cause damage; in such an event one should cease work here and attempt to enter the posterior pouch. Pull the cervix strongly forward and make a transverse incision through the vaginal mucosa, at the height of the posterior fornix (Fig. 24-9 G), joining the anterior to the posterior incisions by cutting on each side of the cervix through the mucosa (Fig. 24-9 G). Do not plunge boldly into the cul-de-sac; the rectum may be injured. After cutting through the mucosa, push it back with the finger or by sharp dissection until the peritoneum is seen (Fig. 24-9 H). Then incise it and introduce a narrow right-angled retractor similar to the one used in front (Fig. 24-9 J). Occasionally, difficulty is met in entering the posterior space. Persistence at this stage adds to the chance of injury to the rectum.

Pushing back the mucosa in the attempt to see the peritoneum exposes each sacro-uterine ligament. These should now be seized separately and extraperitoneally by a narrow, curved, grooved clamp with distal teeth similar to a gallbladder clamp. The ligament is then cut on the uterine side, and the clamp is replaced by a fixation ligature (Fig. 24-9 J, K, L, M). Loosening of the sacro-uterines usually allows the uterus to descend sufficiently so that both cul-de-sacs, previously not accessible, may now be entered.

Having now placed a retractor in both the anterior and the posterior cul-de-sacs, they are held as widely apart as possible and to the left side of the patient so as to expose the left broad ligament. The left sacro-uterine ligament having been cut and ligated with catgut, both strands are held by a hemostat and cut long so that they may be identified later as holding the sacro-uterine ligament. The left uterine vessels can now be seen; they are similarly clamped, cut, and replaced by a fixation suture of catgut (Fig. 24-9 N). In successive similar steps the broad ligament on the left is disposed of as high as possible. When further progress on the left cannot be made, the retractors are slipped to the right of the patient, and the right sacro-uterine is cut (Fig. 24-9 O) and ligated, and the double strand of catgut held in a hemostat. In similar steps the uterine vessels are disposed of, and the right broad ligament is severed from the uterus as high as exposure allows.

It may happen that, after both uterine vessels are tied off, further progress in the vaginal removal of the uterus, for one cause or another, is impossible; in such an event the cervix is to be amputated, all bleeding points closed with interrupted catgut, the abdomen opened, and the operation completed from above. This impasse need cause no apprehension. This combined operation has been performed many times to avoid contaminating the abdominal cavity from the infected cervix of a uterus which could not possibly be removed vaginally, or for other causes.

When the broad ligaments have been loosened high on each side, the uterine body, if not adherent and not too large, presents itself at the posterior opening, where it may be hooked by a bullet forceps and partially pulled outside the pelvis (Fig. 24-9 P). The upper portion of the broad ligament, the uterine end of the tube, the suspensory ligament of the ovary, and the round ligament on the left side can now all be identified. These are clamped (Fig. 24-9 Q) and cut, and the clamp is replaced by a ligature in the same way as the lower parts of the broad ligaments were treated, except that where the sacro-uterine ligament was left with two strands of catgut to identify it, the uppermost ligature on each broad ligament is left with a single strand (Fig. 24-9 R). After the left side of the uterus is freed, the right is loosened by a similar technic. The uterus is now inspected to see whether any pathologic processes exist that would make advisable the removal of otherwise normal appendages.

If the body of the uterus is too large to remove intact, cutting the cervix off may allow its easy delivery. If still too large, a morcellation must be done. This is made easier by keeping up continuous traction. No piece should be cut loose unless the uterus is held against possible retraction into the abdominal cavity. While doing a morcellation the upper portions of the broad ligaments should be found as quickly as possible for, after the communicating branches of the ovarian vessels are securely ligated, then the fear of excessive bleeding may be dismissed.

When the uterus has been removed, a small pack is introduced, the tape of which is held by a hemostat, to hold back the intestines. The appendages are now inspected by drawing them into the operative field and are left or removed as seems advisable. It is rare that they cannot be inspected and examined or operated upon as easily through the vaginal incision as by the abdominal route, opinions of inexperienced operators to the contrary notwithstanding. If a morcellation was done, the pelvis should be palpated for possible fibroid nodules that may have been shoved off and left behind.

The abdomen is now ready for closure. If an anterior repair was started, this is now completed, using interrupted catgut sutures so as not to shorten the anterior vaginal wall. When this is completed, closure proceeds as in a simple vaginal hysterectomy. A suture is passed through the right edge of the anterior mucosal incision, which takes several superficial bites of the denuded posterior wall of the bladder up to the peritoneal incision which the suture includes (Fig. 24-9 S). The narrow right-angle retractor is again inserted anteriorly so that the peritoneum is picked up in successive bites out to the round ligament and the tubo-ovarian stump, around which the suture is passed so as to ligate doubly the ovarian vessels. Then the suture is passed in bites from the upper to the lower part of the broad ligament, passing from the posterior surface of the broad ligament anteriorly so as to catch the peritoneal edges and thereby

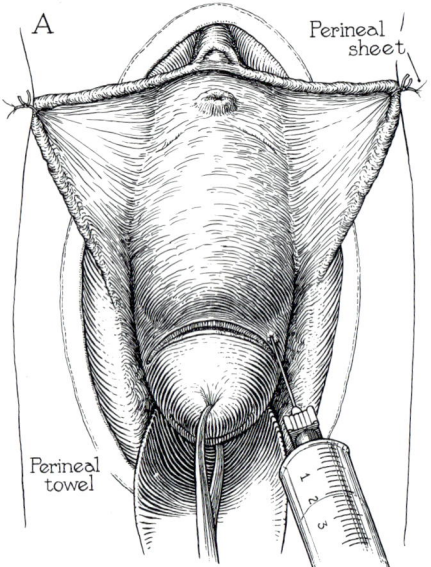
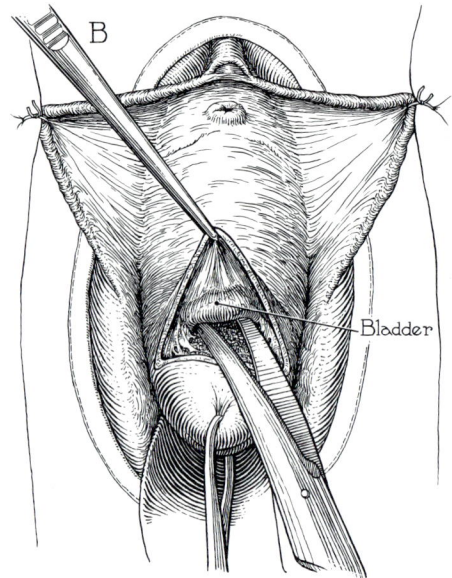
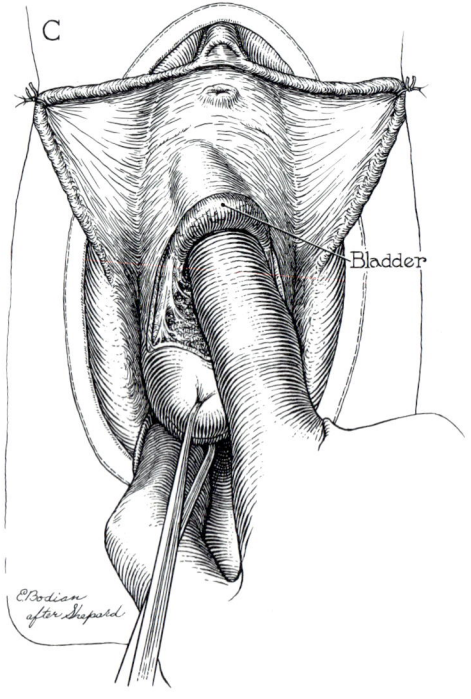

Fig. 24-9. Heaney technic for vaginal hysterectomy. (A) The labia minora are sutured back. Dilute Neo-synephrine is injected. The incision is made. (B) The bladder is dissected from the uterus with sharp dissection. (C) The bladder is separated up to the plica vesico-uterine by blunt finger dissection.

Prolapse of Uterus 495

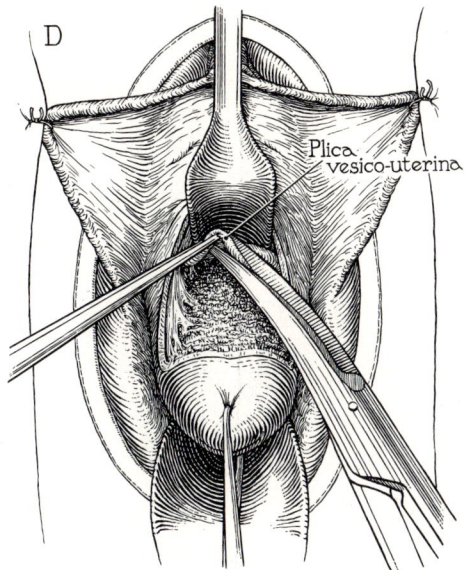

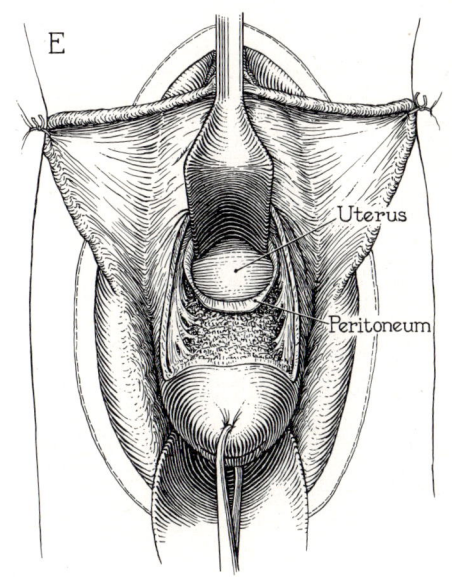

FIG. 24-9 (*Continued*). Heaney technic for vaginal hysterectomy. (D) The plica vesico-uterine is incised. (E) A retractor is introduced into the peritoneal cavity. (F) The pelvis is explored with the index finger.

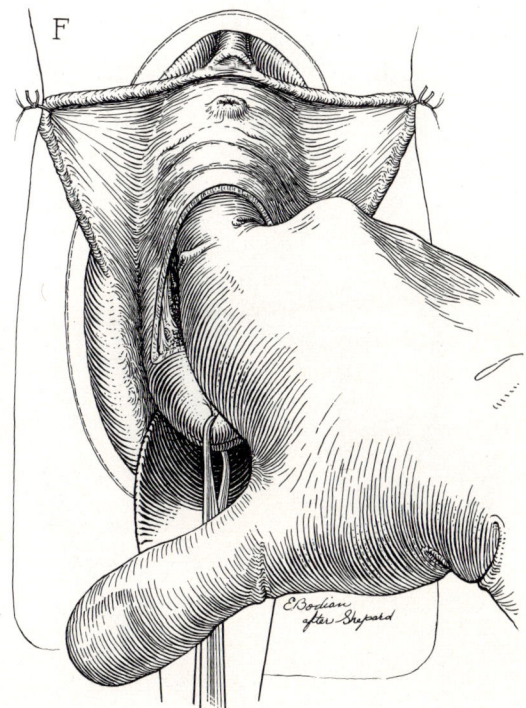

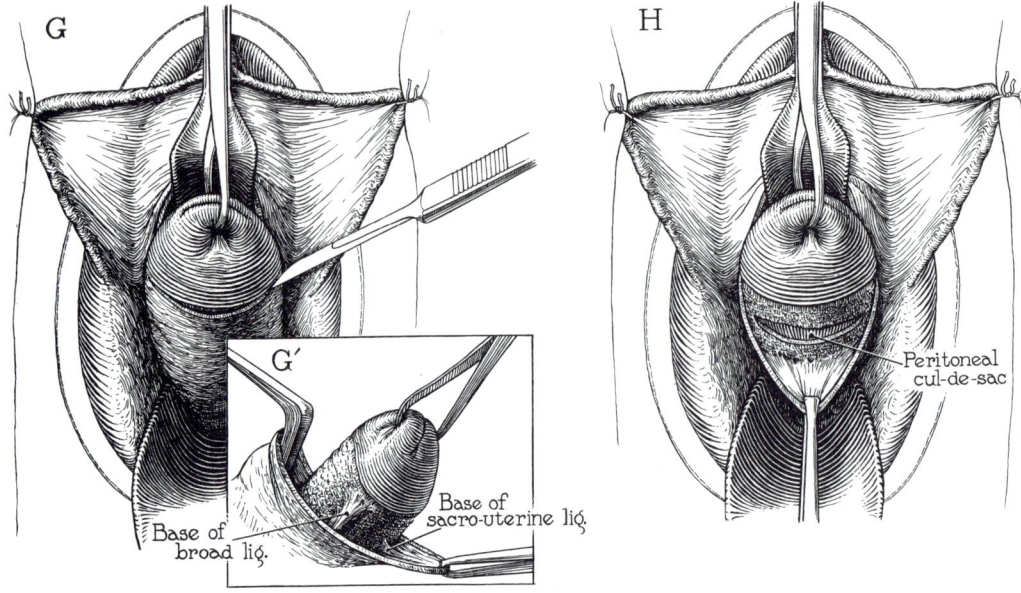

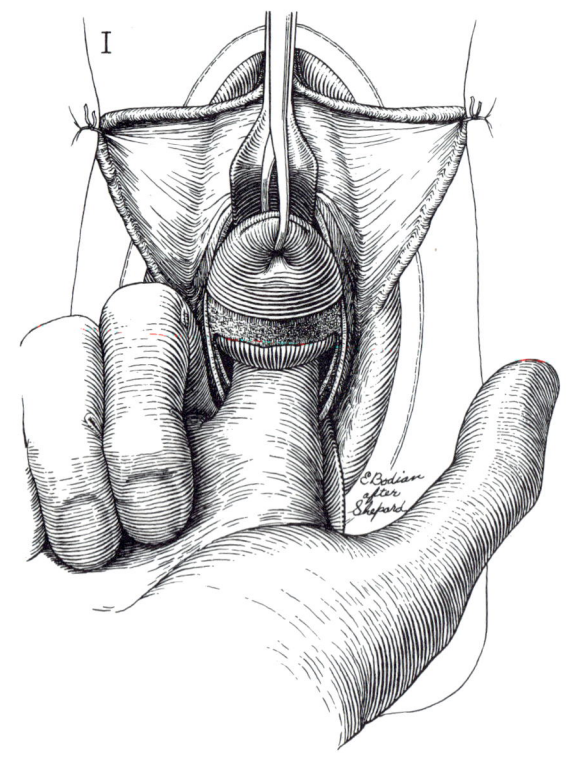

Fig. 24-9 (*Continued*). Heaney technic for vaginal hysterectomy. (G) Posterior transverse mucosal incision. (G′) The sacro-uterine ligament and the base of the broad ligament are exposed. (H) The peritoneum of the cul-de-sac is exposed. (I) The cul-de-sac is explored.

Prolapse of Uterus

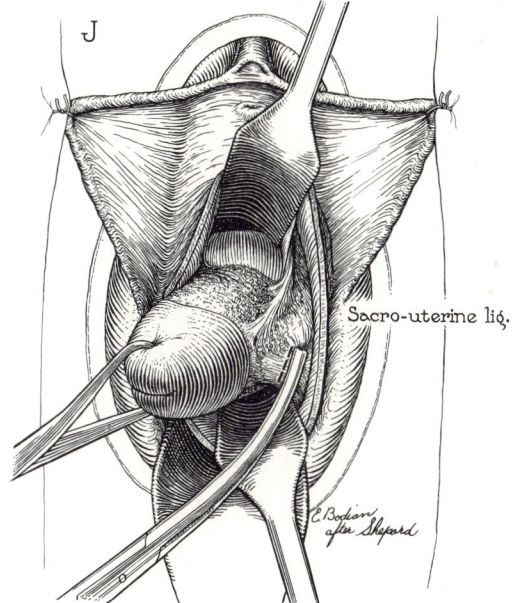

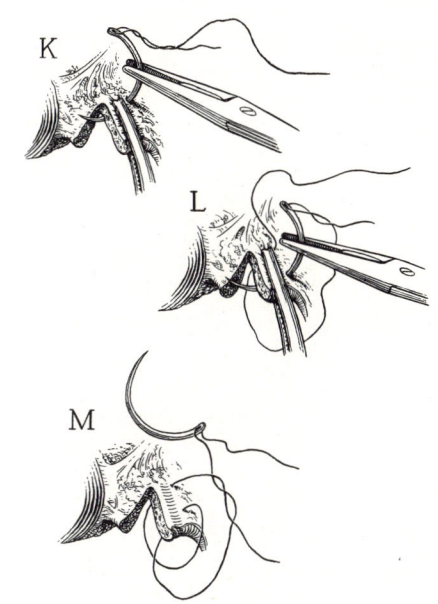

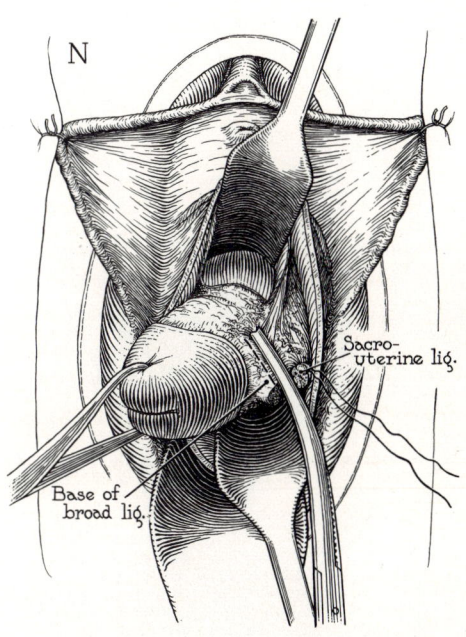

FIG. 24-9 (*Continued*). Heaney technic for vaginal hysterectomy. (J) The left sacro-uterine ligament is clamped. To be cut at dotted line. (K, L, M) Transfixion of the sacro-uterine ligament. (N) The base of the broad ligament with the uterine vessels is clamped. To be cut at dotted line.

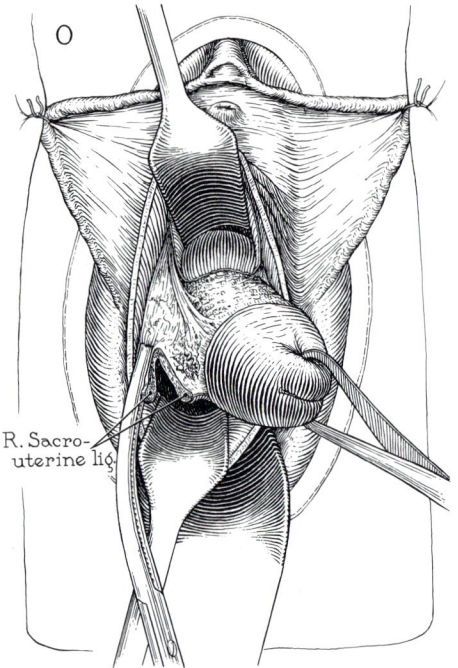
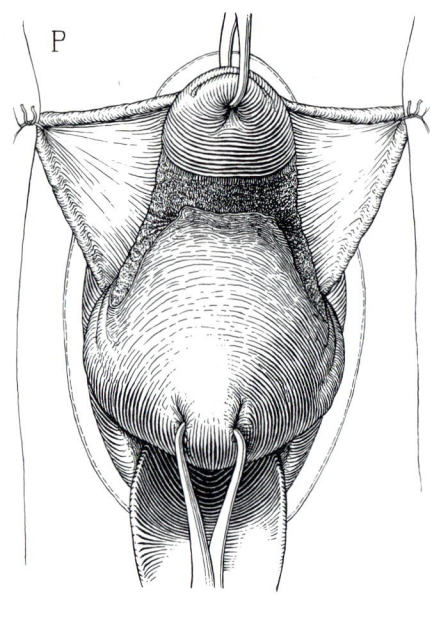
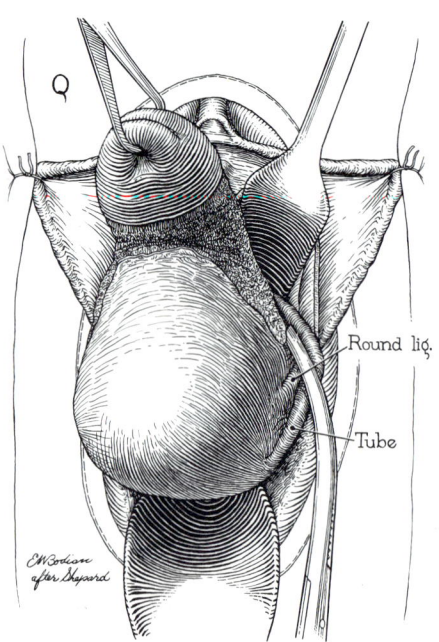

Fig. 24-9 (*Continued*). Heaney technic for vaginal hysterectomy. (O) The right sacro-uterine is clamped and cut. (P) The fundus of the uterus is delivered. (Q) The upper portion of the broad ligament, including the tube, the ovarian ligament, and the round ligament, is clamped.

Prolapse of Uterus 499

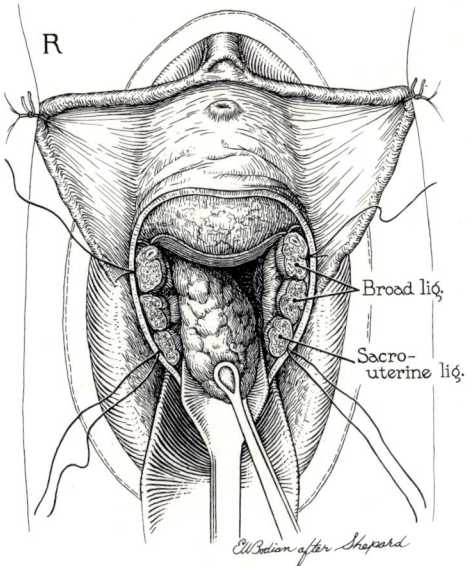

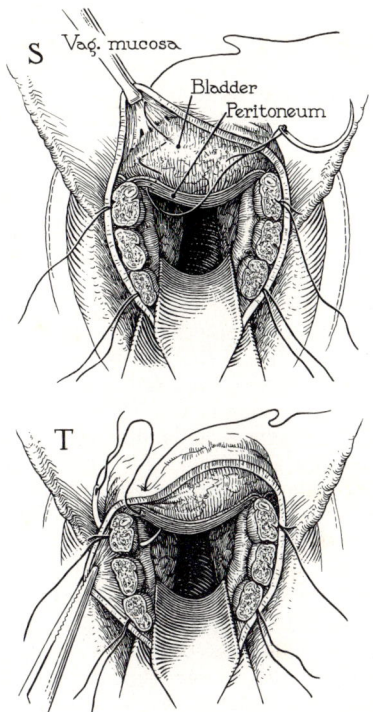

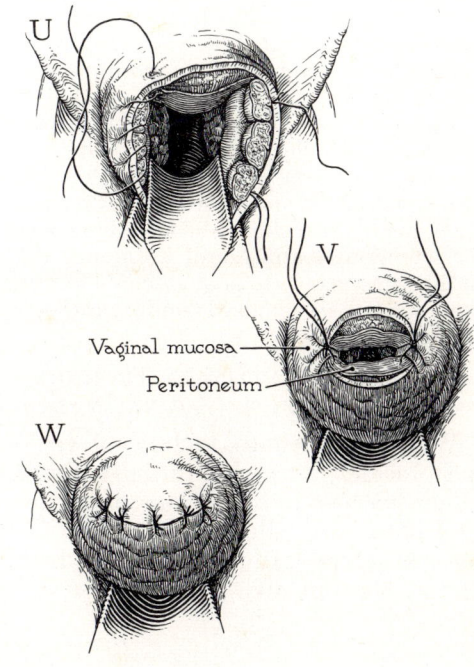

Fig. 24-9 (*Continued*). Heaney technic for vaginal hysterectomy. (R) Showing cut surface of the broad and the sacro-uterine ligaments. The ovary is examined. (S) Beginning closure. (T) Closing suture picks up the broad ligament. (U) A ligature is placed and is about to be tied. (V) Similar ligatures are placed and tied on both sides. (W) The vaginal vault is completely closed.

perform a peritoneal toilet (Fig. 24-9 T, U). When the suture reaches the level of the stump of the uterine vessels, it passes around it in such a way as to relegate these vessels. The suture then picks up the peritoneum of the posterior incision and is passed around the sacro-uterine ligament and then out into the posterior fornix. Then this suture is tied. It has doubly ligated all vessel stumps, and attached the round and broad and sacro-uterine ligaments to the vaginal vault so as to hold up the vault of the vagina. In addition, it has performed the peritoneal toilet on the right side of the pelvis and has closed the right side of the vaginal incision.

A similar suture is started on the left side which duplicates exactly the steps described for the right side (Fig. 24-9 V). Before tying this second suture, the peritoneal pack is removed. Two or three interrupted sutures, which in turn pick up the anterior mucosal edge, the anterior peritoneum, the posterior peritoneal edge, and the posterior mucosa, complete the operation (Fig. 24-9 W). Considerable bleeding occurs from the posterior flap, and this incision is longer than the anterior so that these anteroposterior sutures usually take two or three bites of the posterior flap for each one in the anterior incision. This makes a smoother closure and controls the troublesome oozing from the posterior incision. If a tendency to prolapse exists, the sacro-uterine ligaments are sewn together before closing the vaginal vault. The operation is completed by performing repair of the posterior pelvic floor, if advisable.

The patient is allowed out of bed on the 7th day, at which time perineal sutures and the retention catheter, if one was used, are also removed. If an indwelling catheter was used, the bladder should be tested once daily for retention of urine until it empties itself, in the same way as is done immediately after the operation when no indwelling catheter is used.*

TE LINDE-MATTINGLY TECHNIC OF SUSPENSION OF VAGINAL VAULT

While the Heaney technic of vaginal hysterectomy was used initially in many clincs, various modifications of the original procedure (illustrated in Fig. 24-9) have developed. In the previous editions of this text our own technic, as used at Johns Hopkins, was not included and is presented briefly at this time to illustrate our method of vaginal vault suspension and peritonization.

Figure 24-10 A shows the initial steps of the vault suspension following removal of the uterus. The three ligamentous supports are visible on either side of the vault, including the tip of the broad ligament, the cardinal ligament in the center, and the uterosacral ligament. The suspension is performed prior to placing the peritoneal suture. After entering the pelvis through the lateral vaginal mucosa, the continuous suture of No. 1 chromic catgut is placed through the tip of the broad ligament, distal to the tied ligature, to avoid pulling off the suture on the pedicle (Fig. 24-10 B). A deep suture in the cardinal ligament, as shown in Figure 24-10 C, provides one of the main supports to the vaginal vault. The uterosacral ligament is held firmly on stretch so that a deep bite may be taken in this structure (Fig. 24-10 E), following which the suture is brought through the lateral vaginal mucosa to complete the suspension on one side of the vault. Figure 24-10 F demonstrates the completed suspension on both sides, and the sutures are held untied until the peritoneal suture is placed.

In recent years it has been our preference to plicate routinely the uterosacral ligaments and cul-de-sac together to prevent the subsequent development of an enterocele. Figure 24-10 G illustrates one technic of a posterior culdoplasty which we have found effective. The initial suture a has been placed, includes the uterosacral ligaments, and has incorporated the cul-de-sac peritoneum. Suture b includes the same structures but at a slightly higher level. One or more similar sutures may be placed higher in the cul-de-sac in cases in which there is marked redundancy or early enterocele formation. Figure 24-10 H illustrates similar plication sutures, which originate through the vaginal mucosa of the posterior fornix. As shown by suture c, the suture passes through the pelvic peritoneum and picks up the individual uterosacral ligaments, without including the

---

* Heaney, N. Sproat: Technic of vaginal hysterectomy. Surg. Clin. N. Amer., 22:73, 1942.

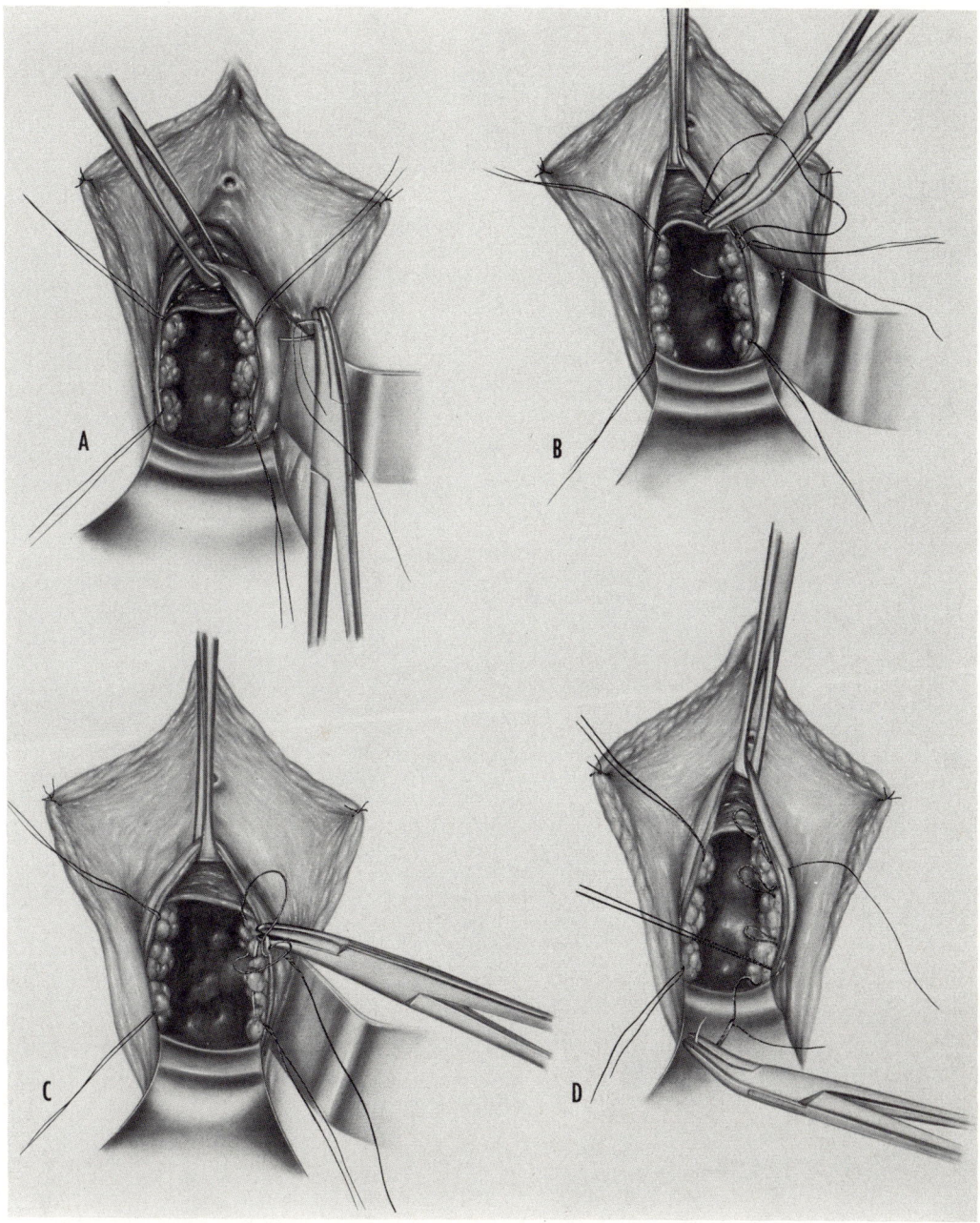

Fig. 24-10. Te Linde-Mattingly technic of suspension of vaginal vault. (A) Suspension of vault, showing the three ligamentous supports on each side of the vagina, the top of the broad ligament, the cardinal ligament, and the uterosacral ligament. A continuous suture (No. 1 chromic) is placed through the lateral vaginal wall. (B) Continuous suture includes the tip of the broad ligament or infundibulopelvic ligament, following which the retention suture on this ligament is cut. (C) The cardinal ligament is firmly incorporated in the suspension suture. (D) Suture of the uterosacral ligament completes the ligamentous support of the vaginal vault.

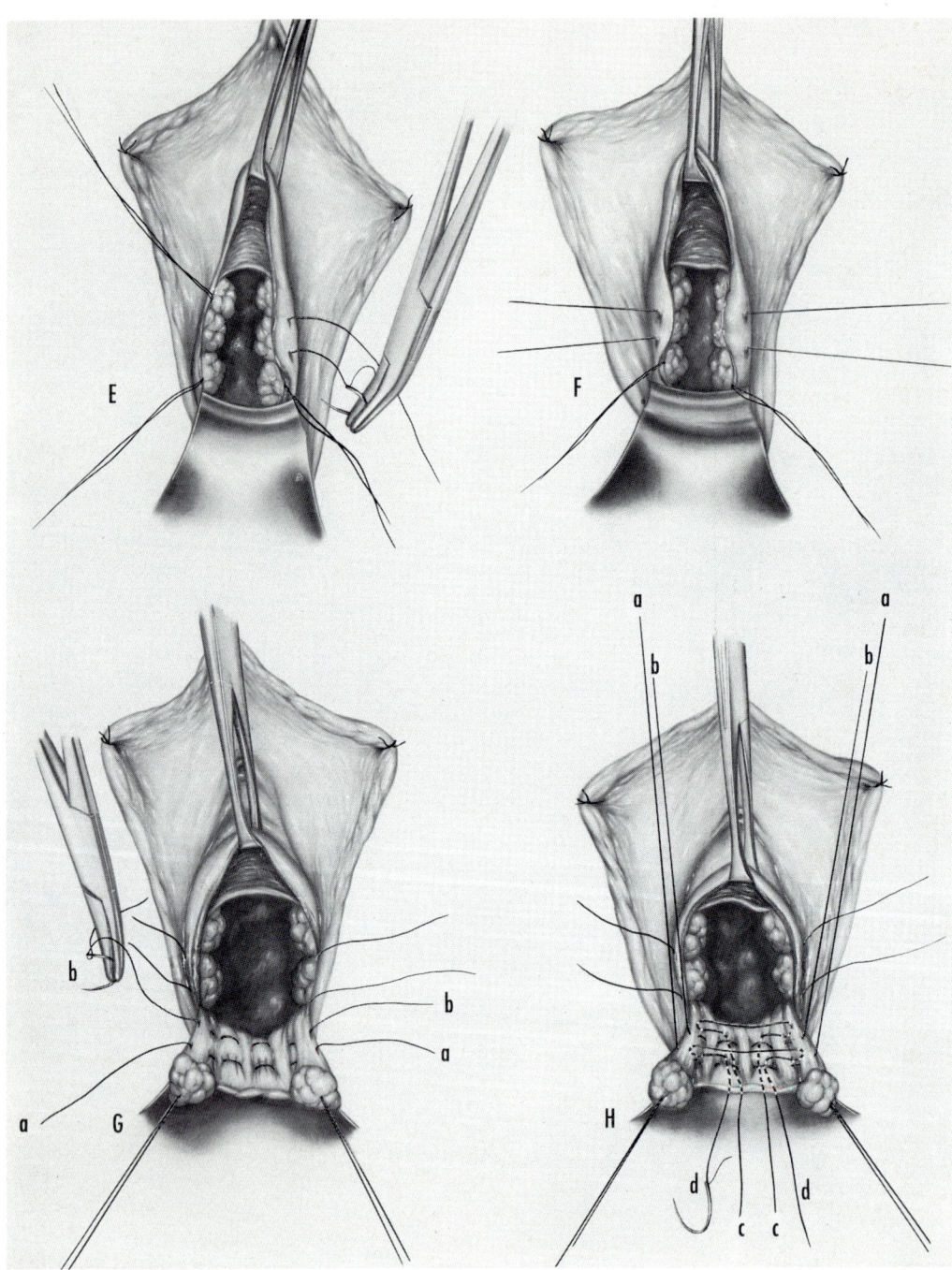

FIG. 24-10 (*Continued*). Te Linde-Mattingly technic of suspension of vaginal vault. (E) The suspension suture is continued through the vaginal mucosa, and the suture is not tied until the purse-string suture of the peritoneum has been placed. (F) Both suspension sutures have been completed and are held untied. (G) Posterior culdoplasty, showing internal sutures which incorporate the uterosacral ligaments with the peritoneum of the cul-de-sac. (H) Posterior culdoplasty, showing both interior and exterior sutures. Sutures which begin in the posterior fornix, exterior to the peritoneal cavity, are passed through the vagina and peritoneum and pick up each uterosacral ligament before passing back into the vagina. Sutures are not tied until purse-string peritoneal suture is placed.

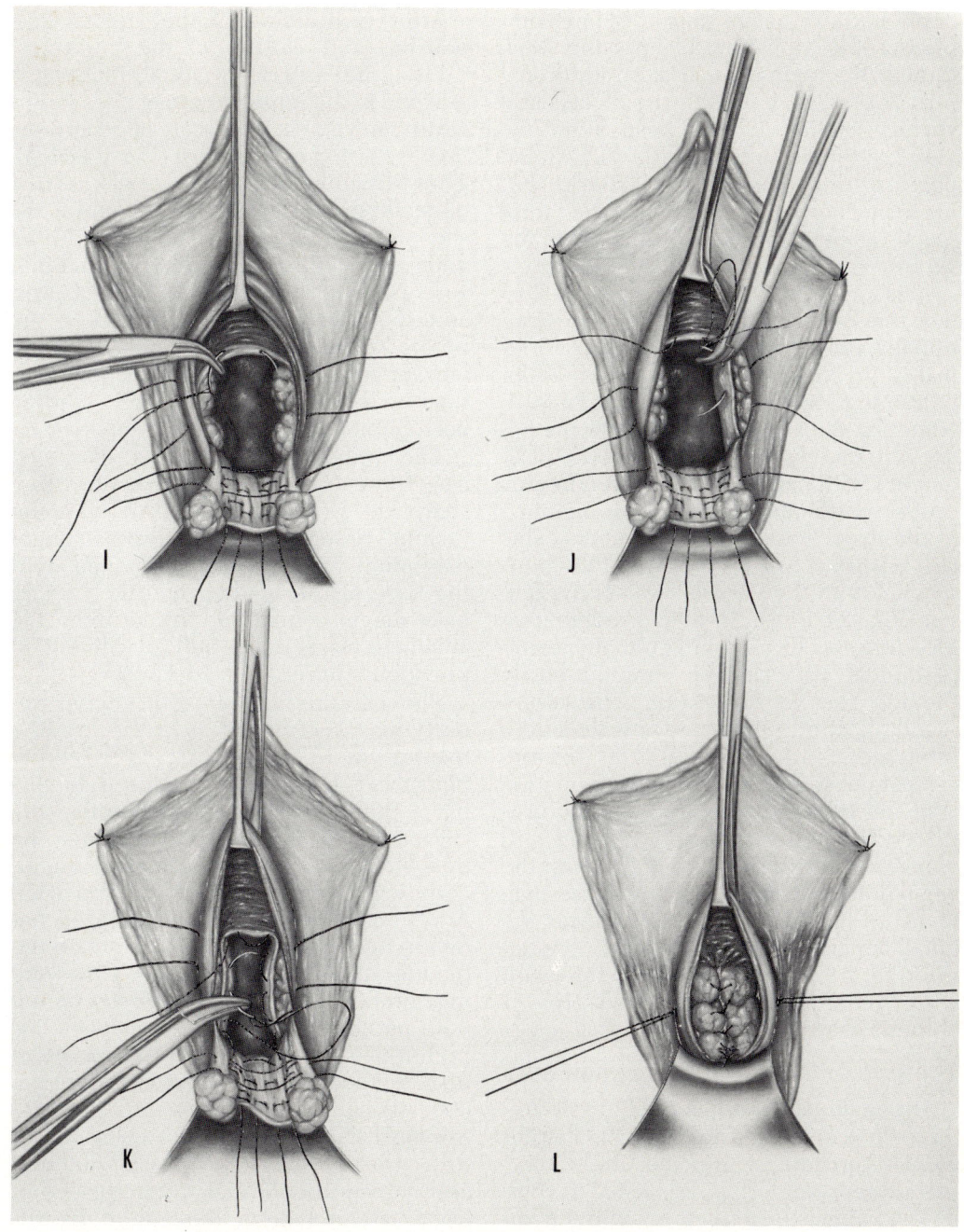

Fig. 24-10 (*Continued*). Te Linde-Mattingly technic of suspension of vaginal vault. (I) Beginning of purse-string suture to close peritoneal cavity; vault suspension sutures and culdoplasty sutures remain untied until peritoneal cavity is completely closed. (J) Continuation of purse-string suture, showing free margin of peritoneum which will extraperitonize the adjacent ligaments and prevent postoperative hemorrhage into peritoneal cavity. (K) Peritoneal stitch nearing completion, showing purse-string suture placed *above* culdoplasty sutures. (L) Purse-string suture completed and tied; culdoplasty sutures have been tied; supporting ligaments remain extraperitoneal and are included in vaginal vault suspension sutures, which are tied *before* tying purse-string suture (to permit replacement of a suspension suture if broken).

peritoneum of the cul-de-sac, before completing the plication by passing back through the vaginal mucosa. An additional plication stitch d is shown, placed at a slightly higher level. These latter vaginal sutures will provide additional depth to the vagina in the posterior fornix by anchoring the mucosa to the uterosacral ligaments in the midline when the sutures are tied.

This procedure is completed by closing the peritoneal cavity with a continuous purse-string suture which originates in the center of the bladder peritoneum as shown in Figure 24-10 I. Note that the suture incorporates the entire circumference of the pelvic peritoneum with particular care taken to pick up the peritoneum *behind* the ligatures of the major vessels and ligaments. This will ensure complete closure of the peritoneum with the vessels *outside* the pelvis (Fig. 24-10 J). Should postoperative bleeding occur, it will remain extraperitoneal and can be drained easily through the vaginal vault. The uterosacral plication sutures are now tied, both internally and externally to ensure against subsequent enterocele formation (Fig. 24-10 K). The uterosacral sutures placed through the posterior fornix will elongate the vagina by anchoring the vaginal mucosa to the uterosacral ligaments (Fig. 24-10 L). The anterior vaginal repair is initiated at this point, prior to transverse closure of the vault with figure-of-eight sutures of No. 1 chromic catgut.

Technic of Anterior Colporrhaphy

Although the subject of cystourethrocele is discussed in detail in Chapter 25, Urethrocele, Cystocele, and Stress Incontinence of Urine, it is usual to combine a vaginal husterectomy with an anterior vaginal repair. These procedures are usually combined because of the major use of the vaginal hysterectomy today for the treatment of relaxed vaginal outlet. It is advisable, therefore, that the technic of an anterior colporrhaphy be included with this discussion of vaginal hysterectomy.

After completion of the vaginal suspension and closure of the peritoneal cavity, the anterior vaginal mucosa is grasped in the midline with Allyse clamps while the vaginal wall is elevated approximately 4 to 5 cm. forward (Fig. 24-11 A). The Mitzenbaum scissors are inserted beneath the mucosal surface, and a tissue plane is developed in the midline with scissor dissection. The vaginal mucosa is retracted laterally with clamps, and the dissection is continued to the region of the urethral meatus. It is important not to traumatize the meatus as this will delay spontaneous voiding postoperatively.

The pubovesical fascia is dissected free from its vaginal attachment with a sharp knife (Fig. 24-11 B). An avascular "white" tissue plane provides easy finger dissection with an opened sponge until the base of the bladder and the urethra have been completely freed from the attached fascia to permit placement of plication sutures (Fig. 24-11 C).

The paraurethral plication of the underlying fascia begins near the urethral meatus where Kelly sutures are securely placed. A Kelly clamp is used to displace the underlying urethra so that the suture of No. 0 chromic catgut may be tied without causing necrosis of an incorporated portion of the urethral wall. Additional Kelly sutures are placed beneath the urethra to the region of the bladder neck (Fig. 24-11 E). Here one may prefer to plicate the sphincter region with permanent sutures, as has been our preference for many years in cases of urinary incontinence. Two or three No. 000 silk sutures are placed at the urethrovesical junction, with one such suture directly over the vescial junction and one additional such suture placed in front of and behind the initial silk suture. If the urethrocele is quite large a second row of plicating chromic sutures may be used, but one must use caution to avoid snugging the urethra too tight and delaying voiding.

The plication continues beneath the base of the bladder, imbricating the vesical fascia for support of the cystocele. Usually, the separated fascial margins of the urogenital diaphragm can be visualized and are easily approximated in the midline. Although the most posterior portion of the bladder fascia, frequently called the "bladder pillars," should be plicated, it is most important to avoid overcorrection of the cystocele. If one inadvertently elevates the bladder base too high in attempting to achieve better fascial support, it is quite possible to produce a direct runoff type of urinary incontinence which may be more symptomatic than was present prior to surgery. After completing 1 or 2 plication layers, (Fig. 24-11 F), the excess vaginal mucosa is excised to the region of the urethral meatus. While care must be taken to avoid removing too much vaginal mucosa, particular effort must be made to avoid removing part of the labia minora in this part of the procedure (Fig. 24-11 G). The vaginal mucosa is approximated in the midline with interrupted chromic No. 0 sutures, which anchor the mucosa to the underyling fascia (Fig. 24-11 H). This anchoring suture will obliterate the dead space beneath the mucosa and will eliminate the need to pack the vagina at the end of the procedure.

The Spalding-Richardson Composite Operation for Uterine Prolapse and Allied Conditions

In 1937 Edward H. Richardson described an operation for uterine prolapse and associated conditions which has been used in this clinic frequently since. Because of his dissatisfaction in some respects with the various current methods of curing uterine prolapse, Richardson devised this composite operation which utilizes principles and technics of various procedures already in use. It consists essentially of cervical amputation, corpus removal at any level desired, the utilization of the isthmic portion of the uterus with its broad and uterosacral ligament attachments for interposition and finally the approximation in the midline of the pubocervical fascia beneath the urethra, the base of the bladder, and the retained portion of the uterus.

The Richardson plan has as its objective:

(1) Riddance of the hypertrophied and diseased vaginal portion of the cervix. (2) Extirpation of the corpus uteri, together with the tubes and the ovaries if indicated. (3) Optional destruction or excision of any remaining cervical canal epithelium. (4) Minimal trauma and devitalization of structures, later to be utilized for reconstruction purposes. (5) Preservation of an assured and adequate blood supply to these several units. (6) Total ablation of associated enterocele through high obliteration of the cul-de-sac of Douglas. (7) Rational utilization of all supporting structures that experience has demonstrated to be helpful and dependable, namely: the pubocervical fascia; the basal portions of the broad ligaments with their extraordinarily strong cervical attachments; the uterosacral and the round ligaments; the fascia of the rectovaginal septum, as well as the muscles and the fascial layers of the pelvic floor and the perineum. (8) Re-establishment of a vagina of normal depth and caliber. (9) Restoration of normal anatomic relationship.

Richardson made no claim of originality for any of the multiple procedures used in his operation but stated that it was a *composite* operation that utilizes many operative steps already in use independently for various conditions in gynecologic surgery. Richardson's operation was presented before the American Gynecological Society in 1937 and was published in the *American Journal of Obstetrics and Gynecology* in November of that year. In 1942 Richard W. Te Linde and Edward H. Richardson, Jr., reported on the first 5 years' experience with this operation in the Johns Hopkins Clinic. On reading this article Ludwig Emge communicated with Richardson and called to his attention the fact that a similar operation had been described by Spalding in 1919. On reading Spalding's and Richardson's descriptions it is apparent that both authors described independently practically identical operations; both were activated by the shortcomings of the other operations in vogue for uterine prolapse; and both

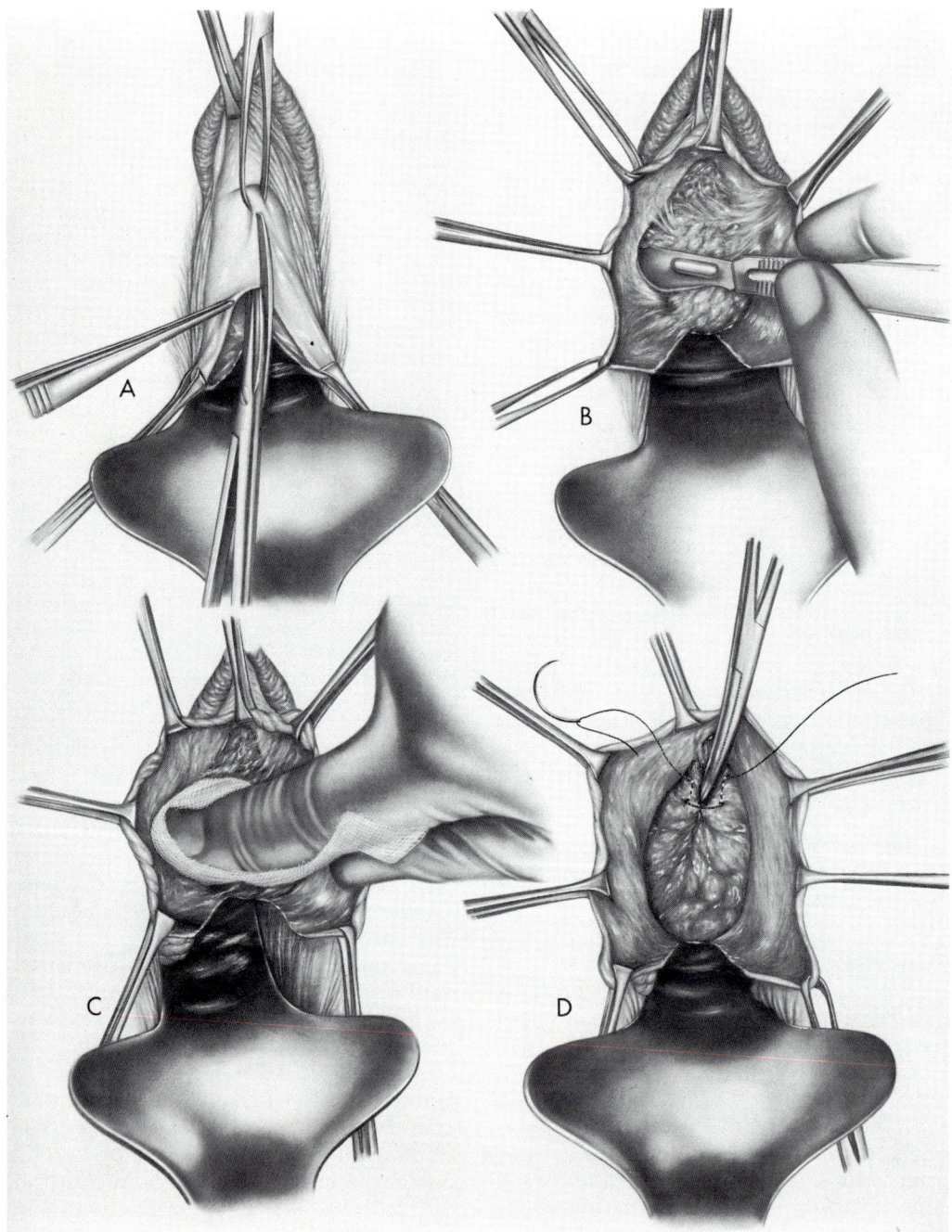

Fig. 24-11. Technic of anterior colporrhaphy. (A) Shows the initial midline dissection of the vaginal mucosa from the underlying fascia. (B) The pubovesico-cervical fascia is incised from the vaginal mucosa by sharp knife dissection. (C) A sponge over the index finger is used to free bluntly the fascia beneath the bladder and rectum from the mucosa. (D) Kelly plication sutures are begun.

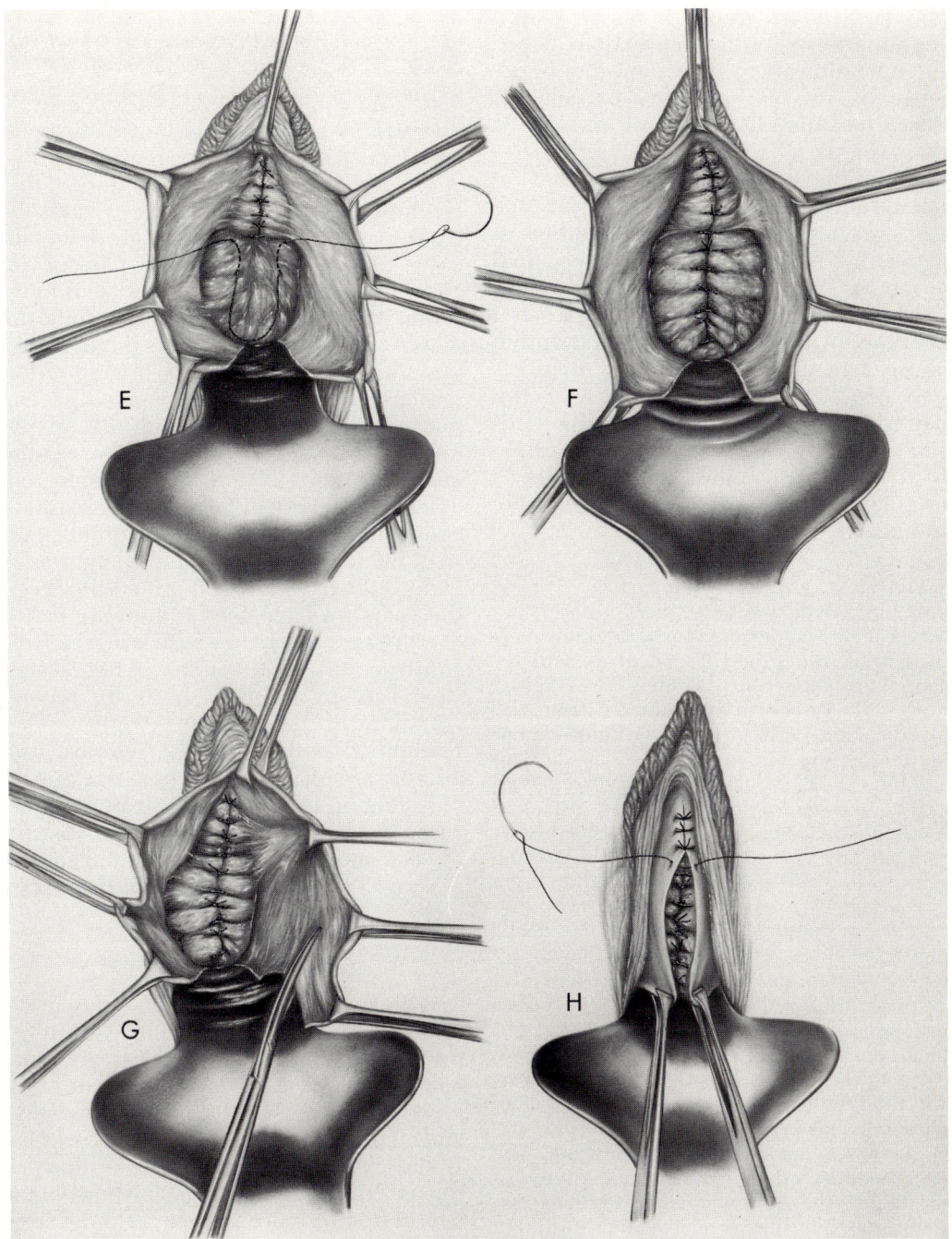

FIG. 24-11 (*Continued*). Technic of anterior colporrhaphy. (E) Kelly plication sutures continued to the vesical neck. Note that a Kelly clamp is used with each plication stitch to depress the underlying urethra or bladder. (F) After completing the plication sutures beneath the base of bladder, the excess mucosa is excised (G). Care must be taken to avoid excising the medial part of the labia minora. (H) The mucosa margins are then approximated in the midline with interrupted sutures which include the underlying fascia.

emphasized the same points in claiming superiority for their operations. Since the operation was worked out independently by the two authors, we suggest that it be called by their joint names. To those of us who use the operation frequently the remarkable fact is that an operation which has the merit of this one has escaped the general attention of gynecologists since Spalding's original article in 1919. Spalding's article is published under the title, "A Study of Frozen Sections of the Pelvis with Description of an Operation for Pelvic Prolapse." Perhaps the anatomic aspects of the paper eclipsed the surgical. Richardson's plan as carried out in this clinic is given later in some detail. Spalding's original technic is presented concisely in his own words as follows:

The fascia, overlying the cystocele, is exposed by a deep transverse incision across the cervix at the bladder junction. If this incision is superficial, the strong fascial plane will remain attached to the bladder. The vaginal wall with the fascia is separated from the bladder rather widely laterally. Before opening the peritoneum, the bladder is pushed up and the vaginal portion of the cervix removed as a cone according to the method of Hegar. A stitch is placed on either side of the cervix to ligate the vaginal branches of the uterine vessels, and the posterior half of the cervix is covered by a vaginal flap. The next step consists in opening the peritoneum and lifting the bladder away with a broad Doyen retractor. The fundus of the uterus is delivered as in an interposition operation; the round ligaments are cut and tied with long catgut ligatures; the broad ligaments are clamped, close to the uterus, as far as the internal os and the fundus of the uterus removed by amputation. This exposes the sacro-uterine ligaments which are shortened if necessary. The stumps of the broad ligaments are sutured to the cervix and the cut round ligaments carried through the cervical canal and sutured to the inferior surface of the cut cervix. The mucous lining of the cervix is removed previous to this procedure. This pulls the cervix high and gives some support to the lateral walls of the bladder when removing the retractor. The fascia in the anterior vaginal wall is now dissected and overlapped as described by Neel and Rawls, and sutured to the stump of the cervix. This completely closes the bladder hernia. The mucosa is sutured by means of a few interrupted catgut sutures over the fascia and the anterior half of the cervix.*

It is now more than 30 years since this operation was first described. It has not had wide acceptance. One reason for this is the fact that the vaginal hysterectomy is simpler and easier. This does not necessarily mean that it is the best for all cases of prolapse. With the passage of years the senior author has had an opportunity to follow his private patients on whom this operation was done many years ago. To evaluate any operation for prolapse, a long-term follow-up is necessary. The long-term results of this operation have been excellent, and we retain our initial enthusiasm for it in selected cases. It is a more difficult and more time-consuming operation than the others, but with modern anesthesia and blood transfusions we have found it quite safe. Over the years we have used it more for cases of extreme prolapse in which marked reconstruction of the vagina is necessary. It affords an excellent basis for reconstruction of the anterior vagina. The remaining portion of the uterus also affords an excellent anchor for purse-stringing an enterocele. Also in extreme cases of prolapse the remaining isthmus of the uterus may be advantageously anchored to the periosteum of the pubic arch.

Technic

With the patient in the lithotomy position and after the usual vaginal cleansing, the anterior lip of the cervix is grasped, and the cervix is drawn to the outlet. A mucosa clip grasps the urethral meatus, and slight traction is made on it anteriorly. If the cystocele is large, the midline of the anterior vaginal wall is grasped with a succession of mucosa clips from the urethral meatus to the cervix so that the mucosa may be put on a stretch. A transverse incision is made through the re-

---

* Spalding, Alfred B.: A study of frozen sections of the pelvis with description of an operation for pelvic prolapse. Surg. Gynec. Obstet., 28:534-536, 1919.

flexion of the anterior vaginal mucosa onto the cervix about 1 or 2 cm. from the external os. The point of a Mayo scissors is inserted beneath the mucosa in the midline, and the anterior vaginal wall is separated from the bladder in the midline by alternately opening and closing the scissors. The mucosa clips are removed successively as each is reached. As each segment of 3 or 4 cm. is separated, the vaginal mucosa is cut in the midline, ultimately forming the usual inverted T-shaped incision, as in the first step of the cystocele operation. For demonstration of this, the reader is referred to the illustrations of cystocele operation.

Next, the bladder is dissected up from its attachment to the cervix. In order to do this, sharp dissection is first necessary (Fig. 24-12 A); but after the intimate attachment of the bladder to the cervix has been cut, often the rest of the dissection up to the vesico-uterine fold of peritoneum can be done with blunt dissection by the finger.

The edges of the vaginal flaps that have been grasped with mucosa clips are spread out by assistants, and the pubo-vesico cervical fascia is dissected from each flap (Fig. 24-12 B). In the midline this fascia is quite thin, but laterally it is usually quite sturdy.

Next, the cervix is amputated. Different technics are permissible for this, but we prefer the technic as described elsewhere in this volume, performing either a high or a low amputation, depending upon the length of the cervix. The posterior lip of the shortened cervix is covered with a flap of mucosa which has been dissected free and then drawn into the canal with a mattress suture as in the Sturmdorf tracheloplasty (Fig. 24-12 C). The cervical amputation is much less bloody if the cervical branches of the uterine vessels are first ligated bilaterally.

The vesico-uterine pouch of peritoneum is incised as indicated by the dotted line in Figure 24-12 B, and the fundus is delivered. We have found that the Lahey thyroid clamps used in a hand-over-hand manner are admirably suited for this. If the fundus is so large that it is brought forth with difficulty, a wedge-shaped piece may be excised as in Figure 24-12 C, or if a myoma is conveniently situated in the anterior wall, a myomectomy may be done.

The uterine end of the round ligament, the tube, and the ovarian ligament are triply clamped en masse, cut and doubly ligated with No. 1 chromic catgut (Fig. 24-12 D). This is repeated on the opposite side. A supravaginal amputation is done at the desired level. Before making the amputation, the ascending uterine vessels are clamped and ligated below the point of amputation as shown in Figure 24-12 E. It is well to make this a V-shaped cut, as is done in abdominal supravaginal hysterectomy, to facilitate closure. Closure of the stump is done with interrupted or figure-of-eight stitches of No. 1 chromic catgut as shown in Figure 24-12 E. The cut ends of the tubes, the round and the ovarian ligaments are sutured to the stump as indicated in Figure 24-12 F.

The isthmic portion of the uterus which remains is shown in the diagram in Figure 24-12 G. It will be noted that it has an ample blood supply. The uterosacral and the portion of the broad ligaments containing the uterine vessels are attached to this remaining segment, and these structures are utilized in building up support for the vagina.

The edge of peritoneum formed by incising the vesico-uterine peritoneal pouch is then sutured to this remaining portion of the uterus (Fig. 24-12 H). It is well to suture this posterior to the incision line in the uterine musculature so that in case there is any postoperative hemorrhage, the bleeding will be external and not intraperitoneal. Since the description of this operation as given in the first edition of this book and as illustrated in this volume, we have made one alteration in technic. The lowest portion of the broad ligaments, which are clamped, cut, and sutured, as illustrated in our description of the Manchester operation, are brought together and sutured to the anterior surface of the remaining isthmic portion of the uterus, exactly as in performing the Manchester

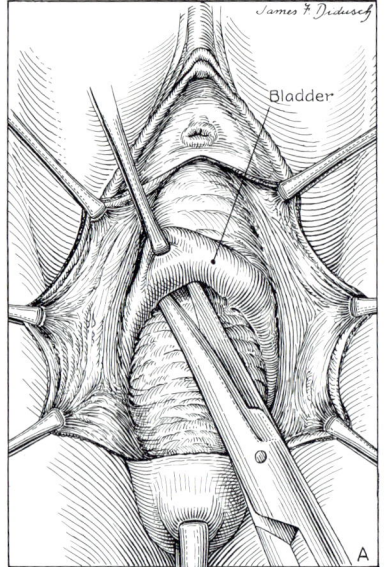
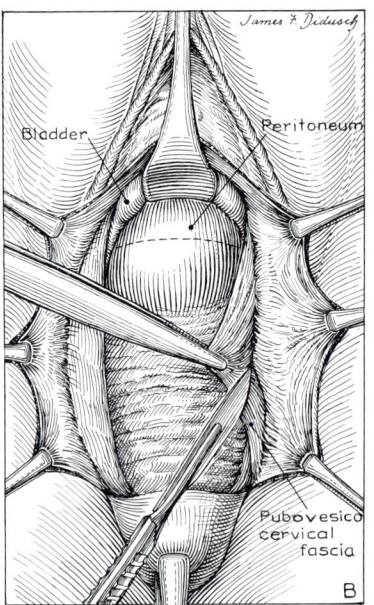
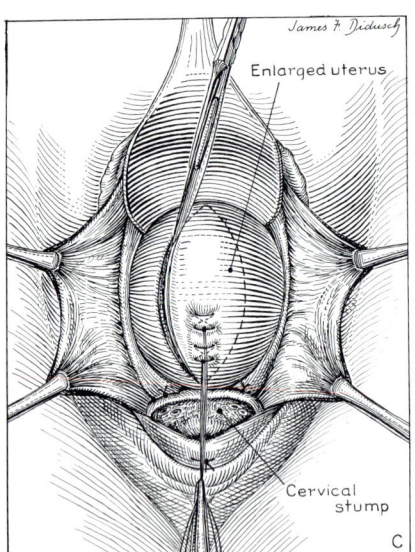
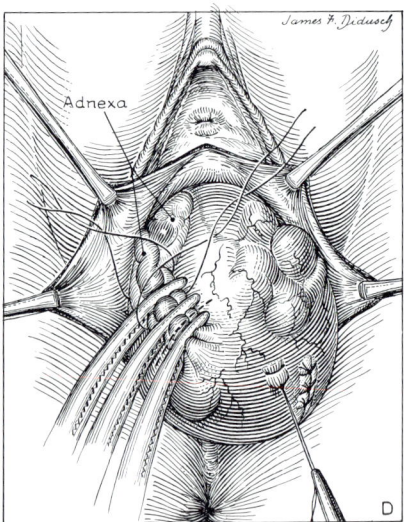

FIG. 24-12. Spalding-Richardson operation for uterine prolapse. (A) An inverted T-shaped incision has been made, and flaps have been dissected lateralward. The bladder is being dissected free from its attachment to the cervix. (B) The vesico-perineal fold of peritoneum has been exposed. The transverse dotted line shows the line of incision. The fascia is being dissected from the flaps of the vaginal mucosa. (C) The fundus is being delivered by traction sutures. Because of its large size in this case, a wedge-shaped piece of myometrium is being excised. The cervix has been amputated. (D) The corpus is completely delivered. The round ligament, the tube, and the ovarian ligament are clamped en masse, cut as indicated by dotted line, and doubly ligated.

Prolapse of Uterus 511

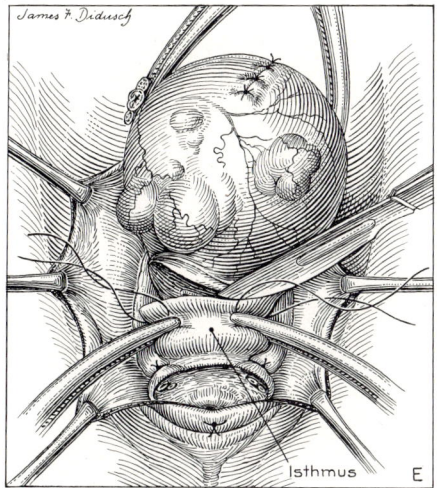
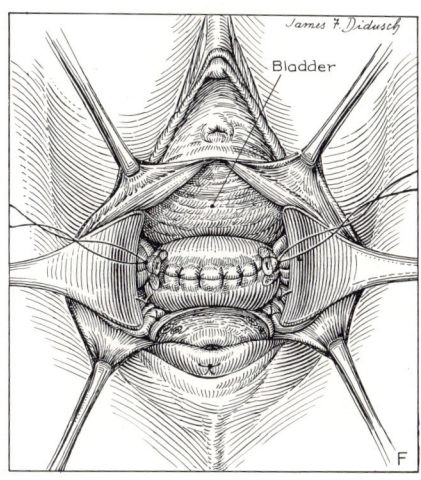
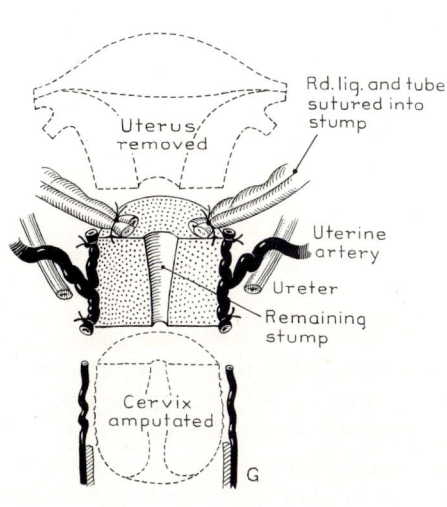
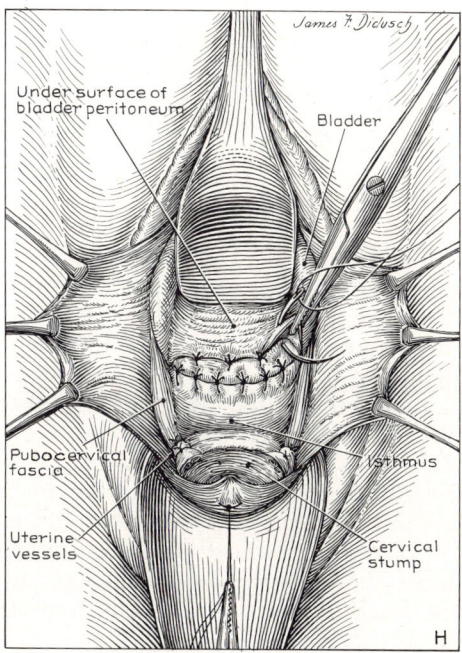

FIG. 24-12 (*Continued*). Spalding-Richardson operation for uterine prolapse. (E) The corpus is being amputated from the cervix. Uterine vessels are ligated as indicated by sutures. (F) The incision in the upper portion of the cervix is closed with interrupted sutures. The tubes, the ovarian ligaments, and the round ligaments are sutured to the cervix. (G) Diagram indicating the portion of uterus that remains. Note that the blood supply is intact. (H) The peritoneum is sutured to the isthmus of the uterus posterior to the suture line in the uterus.

512 Malpositions of the Uterus, Cervical Stump and Vagina

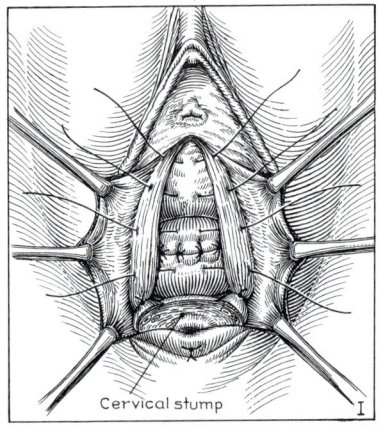

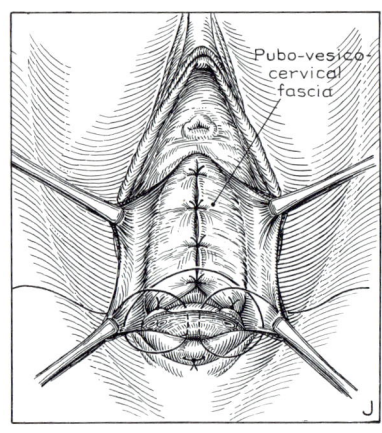

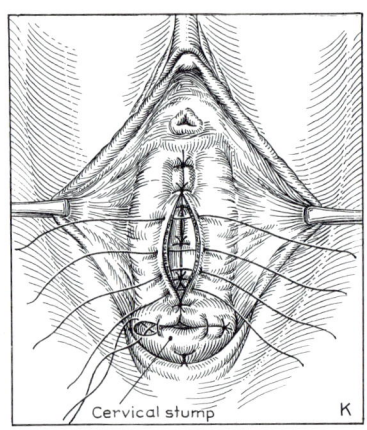

Fig. 24-12 (*Continued*). Spalding-Richardson operation for uterine prolapse. (I) Pubovesicocervical fascia is to be approximated beneath the urethra, the base of the bladder, and the cervical stump. (J) Fascia has been completely approximated, and the anterior lip of the shortened cervix is about to be covered with the split flap of vaginal mucosa. (K) Showing final sutures approximating the vaginal mucosa which has been trimmed to appropriate proportions.

operation. We now regard this step as one of the most important, for it draws the isthmus upward and backward. Thus the advantage of a Manchester operation is attained without the disadvantage of the retained corpus.

The pubovesico cervical fascia is then brought together in the midline by interrupted sutures of No. 0 chromic catgut, beginning beneath the urethra, continuing beneath the base of the bladder and finally covering the stump of the uterus (Fig. 24-12 I, J).

The anterior lip of the shortened cervix is then covered over with vaginal mucosa flaps which have been trimmed down to the proper size for closure (Fig. 24-12 J). The suturing of the vaginal mucosa laterally over the cervix and of the midline incision completes the operation (Fig. 24-12 K).

The pelvic floor and the rectocele are then repaired as indicated by the degree of relaxation and the size of the rectocele. If an enterocele is present, it likewise is repaired.

Vaginal Plastic Operations Combined With Modified Gilliam Suspension of Uterus

As previously stated in this chapter, the author does not favor a vaginal plastic operation combined with a round-ligament suspension for uterine prolapse. Only when the desired end cannot be accomplished entirely by the vaginal route do we resort to the combination of operations. In doing this, we realize fully that an operation that hangs up the prolapsed uterus is less satisfactory than those that build up support from below. However, on occasion one must consider future pregnancies. The vaginal hysterectomy, the transposition operation of Watkins, and, to a lesser degree, the Manchester operation are not compatible with future pregnancies. Occasionally, one encounters a young woman with marked descensus of the uterus, vaginal relaxation, rectocele and/or cystocele. If the symptoms of these conditions are not too severe, such a patient should be advised to complete her family and then have the most suitable operation done. Sometimes a pessary can be utilized to advantage for symptomatic relief for a year or two, until after the desired children are born. However, the symptoms of the relaxed condition and prolapse may be so distressing that operation is advisable without long delay. The only procedures possible under such circumstances are a combination of the necessary plastic operation and some type of round-ligament suspension. In doing the vaginal plastic operation in such cases it is possible to plicate the bases of the broad ligaments much as is done in the Manchester operation, omitting the cervical amputation. A modified Gilliam suspension by the round ligaments, close to the uterine cornua, does as well as any type of suspension. Shortening of the uterosacral ligaments also helps to maintain the uterus at the proper level. For the technic of vaginal plastic operations and the Gilliam suspension, see the sections devoted to those subjects.

Ventral Fixation of Uterus or Cervical Stump for Prolapse

Ventral fixation of the whole uterus or a part thereof is rarely the proper method of treating uterine descensus. However, in unusual circumstances the procedure may be used to advantage. In brief, ventral suspension is indicated when prolapse of the uterus occurs in elderly women in whose abdomen there is a lesion which requires laparotomy and upon whom a minimum of surgery for relief of both conditions is indicated. A large ovarian tumor may be responsible for the prolapse by pushing the uterus down in the vagina. Smaller ovarian tumors, although having no etiologic relationship to the prolapsed uterus, require laparotomy because of the possibility of malignancy. If, on inspection at laparotomy, the ovarian tumor is benign, simple salpingo-oophorectomy may be all that is required for its eradication. Then a quickly performed ventral fixation of the uterus of the elderly woman will often relieve the symptoms of prolapse with a minimum of surgery. When there are marked prolapse and great elongation of the cervix, fixation of the fundus may not elevate the cervix sufficiently to relieve the patient. Amputation of as much of the corpus as necessary may be done, and the rest may be fixed to the abdominal wall. In some instances all of the corpus must be removed and the cervix fixed to get the required elevation.

The technic of ventral fixation of the uterus is described on page 480. The technic of ventral fixation of the cervical stump or vagina in connection with vaginal prolapse is described on pages 524 to 525.

The Le Fort Operation

The original Le Fort operation, as described by its author, consisted of a denudation of a long narrow triangle on the posterior wall of the vagina and a similar one on the anterior wall. The bases of these triangles were just below the cervix, and the apices were at the outlet. The closure was brought about by the complete approximation of these denuded areas.

The operation is performed rather frequently in some clinics, but in our opinion it should be done only when there is some good reason why one of the usual operations for prolapse which will give a functioning vagina cannot be carried out. Its use is restricted to elderly widows or to women who, with their husbands, have no further interest in marital relations. We are inclined to regard it as an admission on the part of the surgeon that he is unable to cure the prolapse by some procedure which would leave a functioning vagina; yet there are rare cases in which it is very useful. Its virtue lies in the fact that it is perhaps the least shocking of any of the procedures used for the cure of prolapse, and that it can be done safely, under local anesthesia if necessary, in elderly women who might otherwise be condemned to a pessary. Regardless of the age of the patient, the closure of the vagina should never be done without a complete understanding on the part of the patient as to the termination of her sex life. A disadvantage to the typical Le Fort operation lies in the fact that occasionally partial urinary incontinence results, due to the pull of the posterior vaginal wall on the anterior wall that is intimately attached to the urethra and the trigone. This disadvantage can be avoided by closing only the upper portion of the vagina, stopping short of the area which underlies the vesical trigone and the urethra. In fact, in recent years we have practically abandoned the typical operation in favor of closing only the upper two thirds of the vagina. If there is a urethrocele, an oval area of mucosa is denuded beneath th urethra and closed longitudinally. Then the levators are approximated very tightly, leaving only enough opening for urination.

Technic

With the patient in the lithotomy position, the cervix is drawn outward as far as possible. In the cases in which the Le Fort operation is done, this more or less completely everts the vagina.

The area to be denuded anteriorly is marked out with the scalpel as indicated by the dotted line in Figure 24-13 A. Sufficient mucosa should be left laterally to form a canal for drainage of cervical secretions. The area to be denuded extends to within 2 cm. of the tip of the cervix and to within 2 cm. of the urethral meatus.

The mucosa is denuded from the anterior vaginal wall by a combination of sharp and blunt dissection (Fig. 24-13 B).

An area of mucosa of equal size and shape is denuded from the posterior vaginal wall (Fig. 24-13 C).

The mucosal edges are approximated transversely below the cervix with interrupted sutures of No. 0 chromic catgut (Fig. 24-13 D).

Beginning at the top, the denuded areas are approximated with as many rows as necessary of interrupted sutures of No. 0 chromic catgut (Fig. 24-13 E, F, G).

Finally, the mucosal edges are approximated with interrupted sutures of No. 0 chromic catgut (Fig. 24-13 H). Mucosa-lined tunnels left on both sides are demonstrated by the Kelly clamps in Figure 24-13 H.

GOODALL-POWER MODIFICATION OF LE FORT OPERATION

Goodall and Power have modified the Le Fort operation to permit fairly satisfactory coitus and thus increase the scope of the operation. It is our opinion that there exist few indications for this modification. In almost all cases of prolapse in younger women, where coitus is of considerable importance, some other type of operation can be done that results in a better vagina. However, in rare conditions when there have been previous unsuccessful attempts at cure and the structures appear to be so poor that cure with a normal vagina seems to be hopeless, this operation may be desirable. It consists essentially of closure of the upper portion of the vagina by approximating triangular denuded areas. If the anterior wall below the level of vaginal closure is redundant, the mucosa may be excised as shown in Figure 24-14. Then an appropriate posterior perineal repair is done.

Technic

With the patient in the lithotomy position, traction is made on the cervix which, in the type of case in which this operation is done, practically everts the vagina. A triangular area of the vagina is denuded of mucosa with the base of the triangle about a centimeter from the cervix. If the vagina is short, this triangular area should not be over one third the length of the vagina. If the vagina is long, it may be one half the length of the vagina (Fig. 24-14 A).

Mucosal edges of triangle bases are approximated with interrupted sutures of No. 0 chromic catgut (Fig. 24-14 B).

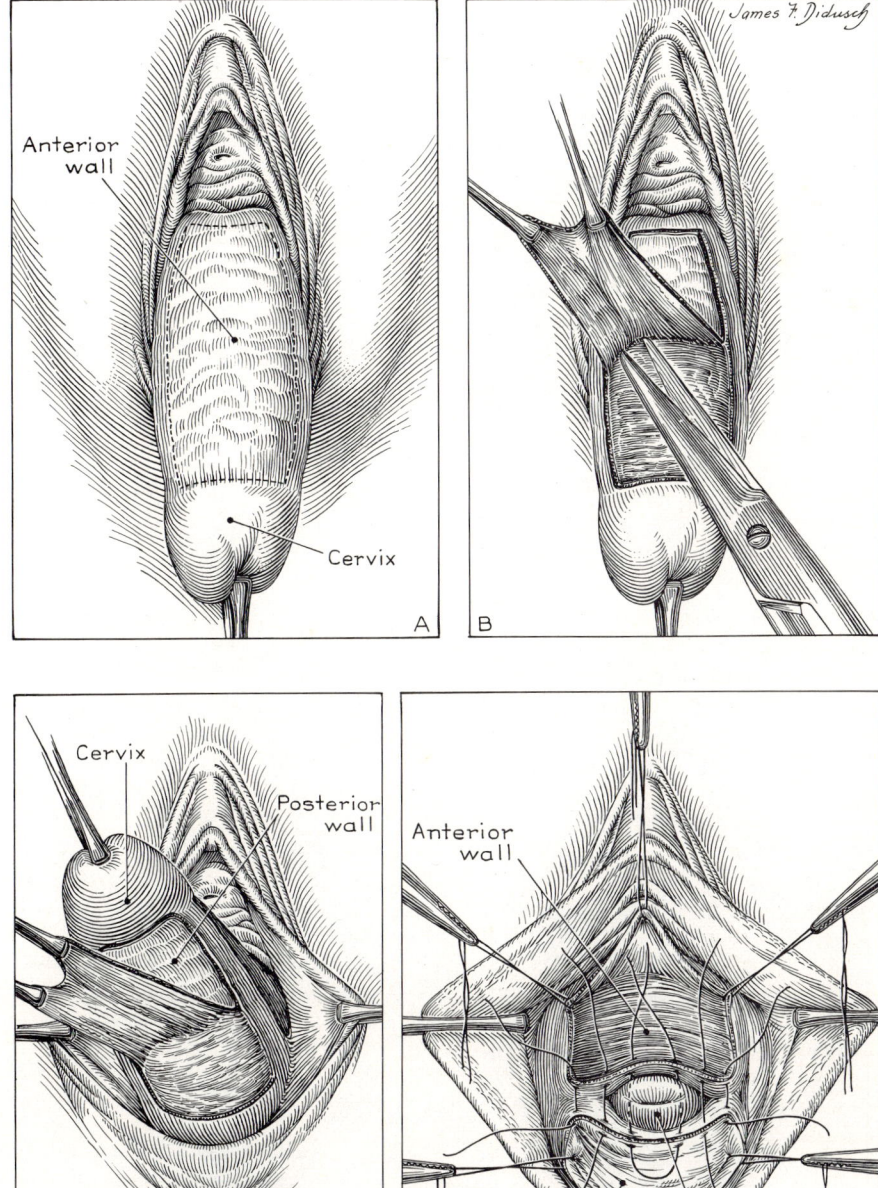

FIG. 24-13. Le Fort operation for uterine prolapse. (A) Dotted line indicates incision in anterior vaginal wall. (B) Flap outlined is being excised. (C) A similar flap is being excised from posterior vaginal wall. (D) The vaginal mucosal edge is being approximated beneath the cervix.

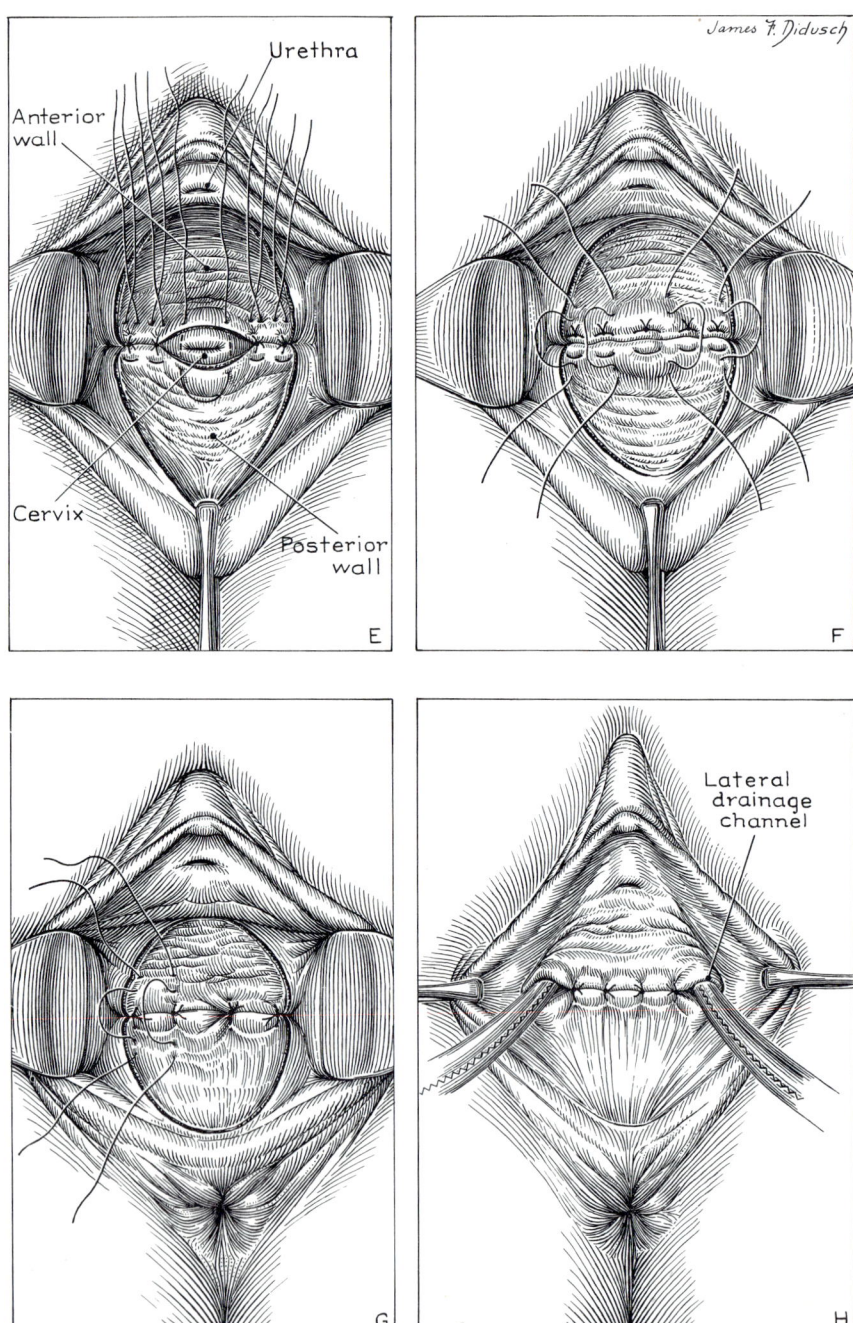

FIG. 24-13 (*Continued*). Le Fort operation for uterine prolapse. (E, F, G) The denuded areas on the anterior and the posterior walls are approximated by several layers of interrupted sutures of No. 0 chromic catgut. (H) Finally, the mucosal edges are closed. Note the tunnels left on either side, demonstrated by Kelly clamps.

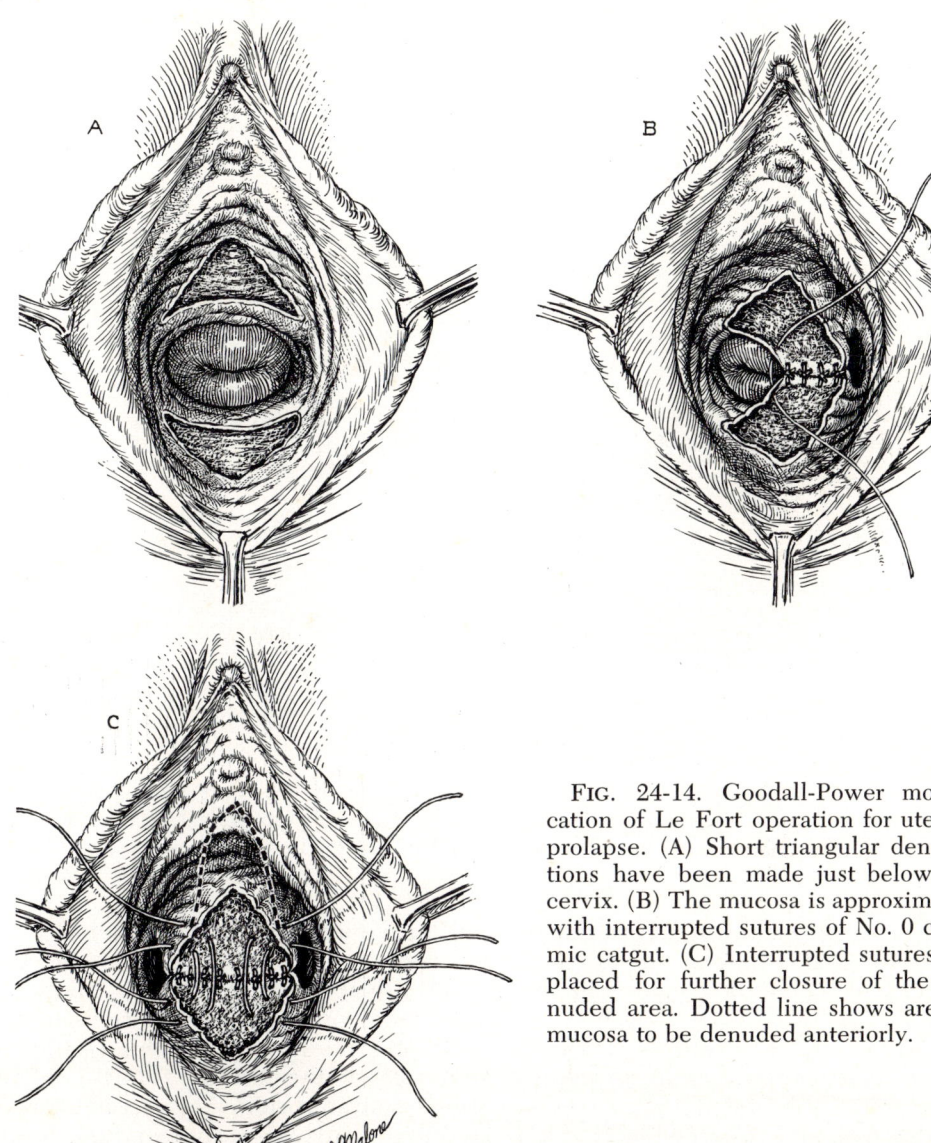

FIG. 24-14. Goodall-Power modification of Le Fort operation for uterine prolapse. (A) Short triangular denudations have been made just below the cervix. (B) The mucosa is approximated with interrupted sutures of No. 0 chromic catgut. (C) Interrupted sutures are placed for further closure of the denuded area. Dotted line shows area of mucosa to be denuded anteriorly.

Interrupted sutures of No. 0 chromic catgut are placed laterally, as indicated in Figure 24-14 C. These sutures pick up the mucosa and also some of the adjacent raw surface so that when they are tied, there will be no dead space. Before these sutures are tied, the anterior vaginal wall is opened up for repair of the cystourethrocele. An area of mucosa is removed as indicated in Figure 24-14 C. The pubocervical fascia is dissected free from the mucosa and brought together in the midline as in the usual cystocele operation. The lateral sutures are tied at this stage, and the anterior mucosal wound is closed with interrupted sutures of No. 0 chromic catgut.

An area of mucosa is denuded posteriorly, as indicated in Figure 24-14 D. The levator muscles are approximated with interrupted sutures of No. 0 chromic catgut.

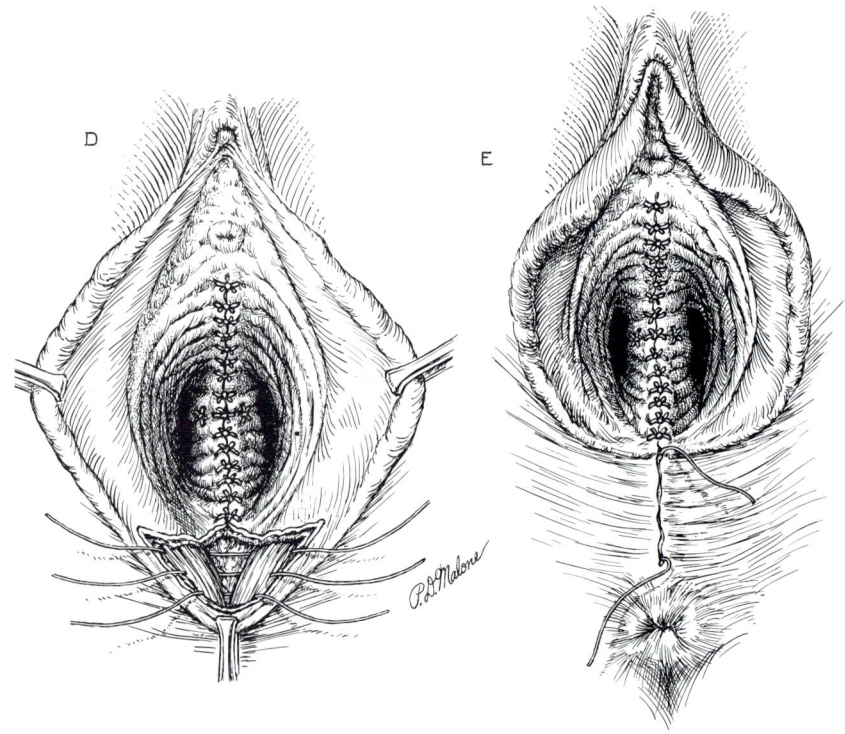

Fig. 24-14 (*Continued*). Goodall-Power modification of Le Fort operation for uterine prolapse. (D) The upper vagina has been closed by approximating denuded triangular areas. A cystocele has also been repaired. The perineum is being repaired. (E) Completed operation.

Finally, the perineal wound is approximated with a continuous subcuticular suture of No. 0 chromic catgut (Fig. 24-14 E).

The vagina which results is single in the lower portion and double in the upper part. The obliterated upper vagina gives the patient a fixation point upon which the cervix rests. In the lower portion of the vagina, the anterior and the posterior walls have been restored, and the resulting vagina, although it has been shortened, is fairly satisfactory as to function.

PROLAPSE OF THE VAGINA, WITH OR WITHOUT CERVIX, FOLLOWING HYSTERECTOMY

General Considerations

Slight vaginal prolapse, too slight to make the patient conscious of it, not infrequently occurs following hysterectomy. More or less complete vaginal prolapse rarely occurs following abdominal or vaginal panhysterectomy, and more rarely still following subtotal removal of the uterus. Today, when subtotal hysterectomy is becoming less frequent, prolapse of the cervical stump is indeed a rarity. The reason for the occurrence of prolapse more frequently after total hysterectomy is probably the fact that when any type of total extirpation of the uterus is done, there must be some crushing of the cardinal and the uterosacral ligaments, whereas when subtotal removal is performed, the amputation usually is done above the level of these ligaments. Failure to utilize properly the ligamentous supports in rebuilding the upper pelvic floor is a major factor in the occurrence of prolapse of both the cervix and the vagina after hysterectomy. The occurrence of this condition following removal of the uterus may also be due to failure to recognize and deal with some degree of descensus, relaxed outlet, rectocele, cystocele, or enterocele at the time of the hysterectomy. These conditions, which represent a failure of the undersupports of the uterus, may be symptomless at the time of hysterectomy and later give rise to symptoms. This is not to say that all symptomless vaginal relaxations should be repaired when hysterectomy is done. Many of the relaxations of both the anterior and the posterior walls never will require correction, but their presence should be noted, and when it is felt that more support to the cervix or the vagina is necessary than can be given by the intra-abdominal suspension, the support should be augmented by the indicated vaginal plastic operation.

Senile changes in the tissues of the vagina and the ligamentous supports undoubtedly are factors in some cases of vaginal prolapse. Hence, no matter how meticulous a job is done for vaginal support at the time of the primary operation, probably there will always be a very small irreducible number of women who develop vaginal prolapse.

Even today a few cases of vaginal prolapse are encountered following abdominal hysterectomy for uterine prolapse. This procedure alone has no place in the treatment of genital prolapse, and properly trained surgeons recognize this.

Protrusion of a mass from the vaginal outlet is the symptom that usually brings these women with prolapse of the vagina or the cervix to seek relief. Walking and sitting may become difficult for them. Cystocele, rectocele and/or enterocele associated with the vaginal or cervical prolapse may produce the usual symptoms due to these herniations.

TREATMENT

The treatment of vaginal prolapse depends first of all upon an evaluation of the anatomic condition. Then one must consider the age and the general physical condition of the patient and her views on further sexual activity. In the woman who is a very poor operative risk, a pessary is occasionally satisfactory, but sometimes marked vaginal relaxation associated with complete inversion of the vagina prevents the use of a pessary. Often this condition occurs in elderly women who have no interest in further sexual life. In those women, complete or partial colpocleisis can be done with a minimum of operative shock and quite a satisfactory result to the patient. When the cervix is still present, a Le Fort operation or a modification of it, such as that described by Goodall and Power, may be done. When the cervix has been removed, a colpocleisis is quite satisfactory in this group of elderly women (Fig. 24-15).

To preserve a functioning vagina, surgical ingenuity may be put to a severe test. There is no single operation that will be adequate in all cases. Careful preoperative planning to suit the individual case is desirable, but, in spite of the most meticulous preoperative plans, improvising at the operating table is often necessary. One can only use the supporting structures at hand, and their quality is often not apparent until they are inspected at operation. In some instances the supports of the vagina can be so utilized that the entire surgical job can be done from below. However, in many instances a combination of vaginal plastic procedures and some kind of abdominal suspension are necessary for a satisfactory result. Usually, when vaginal prolapse occurs after either total or subtotal operation, a cystocele, a rectocele and/or an enterocele will be found to be present. These conditions occur in various combinations. We have seen well-preserved anterior and posterior vaginal walls with a hernia defect at the vaginal vault through which an enterocele sac protrudes. We have also seen only a cystocele present with an intact posterior wall. Likewise, a rectocele may be present with a well-supported bladder. In any case, one can be certain that the restoration of the vagina to a semirigid tube greatly increases the chances of a lasting cure.

Pratt and Symmonds have divided their cases into 3 groups and such a division is very useful when planning the surgical attack.

The first type consists of a relatively pure enterocele, with or without rectocele, that develops behind a well-supported anterior vaginal wall. This type usually occurs after a vaginal hysterectomy and probably represents a neglected enterocele or potential enterocele. Such cases can usually be cured by dissecting out the enterocele sac, obliteration of the cul-de-sac, and proper repair of the rectocele.

The second type includes a moderate prolapse of the vaginal vault combined with enterocele, cystocele, and rectocele. In these cases there is a general laxity of the urogenital support, and usually they can be cured by a vaginal approach. This consists of dissection of the enterocele with high ligation of the sac, approximation of the uterosacral ligaments, and fixation of the uterosacral and the cardinal ligaments to the vaginal vaults as should be done in vaginal hysterectomy. Then appropriate anterior and posterior colporrhaphy should be done. If on completion of these procedures the operator is not satisfied with the vaginal support, some type of abdominal fascia support can be added. These vaginal procedures often result in some shortening of the vagina.

The third and most difficult type to repair is complete vaginal inversion. Perhaps *eversion* would be a better descriptive term, for the entire vagina is everted from the introitus. Many of the women with this condition are in the age group when a functioning vagina is of little importance. Colpocleisis can be done and in our hands has given very satisfactory results. However, when a functioning vagina is desired, cases often require a dissection and an obliteration of the enterocele, a rebuilding of the anterior and the posterior vaginal walls, and perineorrhaphy, combined with some type of abdominal suspension. Abdominal suspension alone in these cases is usually quite unsatisfactory. Also, the tissues which one has to work with below are usually inadequate. Hence, the combined procedures usually offer the best chance of success.

We are presenting herewith some operations which we have found useful, but the operator must select the proper procedures and suit them to the individual case. Often he must improvise and approach the operation with an open mind, being willing to change his planned approach as the operation proceeds.

Williams and Richardson described a similar operation, using bilateral strips of fascia from the aponeurosis of the external obliques.

Several of these operative procedures will be described and portrayed in detail, since it is the opinion of the author that no single operation fits all cases of vaginal prolapse. Therefore it is essential that the surgeon be familiar with several technics in order to choose wisely the best procedure for the individual case.

The operator should be warned not to become too enthusiastic about his result until a few years have elapsed. The immediate result appears good in almost all cases, but a few years of wear and tear are required before the ultimate result can be evaluated.

Technic: Complete Colpocleisis for Prolapse of Vagina Following Total Hysterectomy

An incision is made about the circumference of the vaginal outlet in the region of the carunculae myrtiformes, as indicated in Figure 24-15 A. The mucosa of the anterior vaginal wall is dissected free up to the top of the vagina (Fig. 24-15 B). The posterior vaginal mucosa is then dissected free, and thus all of the vaginal mucosa is removed (Fig. 24-15 C).

The method of closure of the vagina depends on its caliber. If the vagina is small, it is closed with a succession of purse-string sutures of No. 0 chromic catgut as indicated in Figure 24-15 D, E. If the caliber of the vagina is too large to be closed conveniently with purse strings, it is closed with a series of continuous sutures placed transversely. The vaginal mucosa is closed vertically with interrupted sutures of No. 0 chromic catgut (Fig. 24-15 F). In performing this colpocleisis it is well to bear in mind that if the closure of the vagina is carried out completely to the vaginal outlet, the sphincter of the bladder may be handicapped in its closure. Therefore it is advisable to close the vagina only to about 4 cm. from the urethral meatus and not quite as completely as illustrated in Figure 24-15.

Technic: Operation for Prolapse of Vagina Following Total Hysterectomy, Using Preserved Fascia Lata of Ox (Grant-Ward)

An incision is made from umbilicus to symphysis, and the peritoneal cavity is entered. The intestines are packed back,

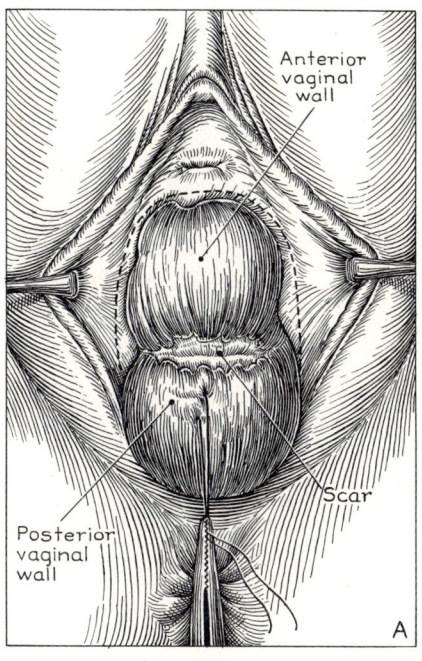
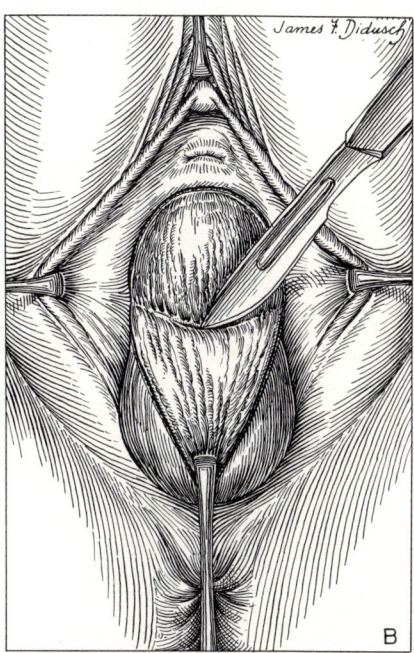
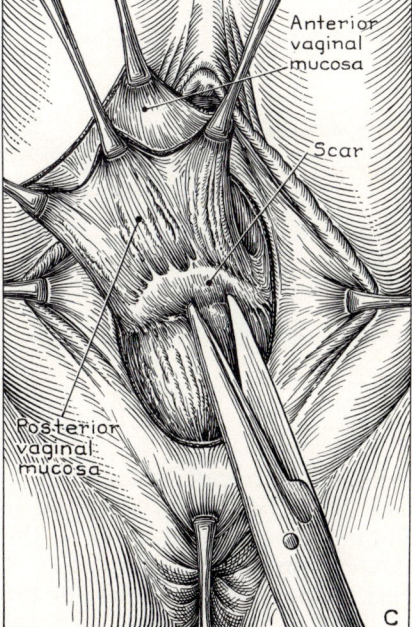

FIG. 24-15. Colpocleisis for vaginal prolapse following total hysterectomy. (A) Dotted line indicates incision, encircling vaginal vestibule. (B) The anterior vaginal wall is dissected free. (C) The posterior vaginal wall is dissected free.

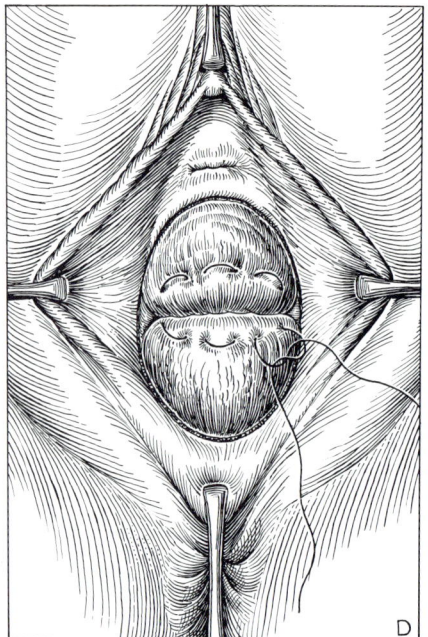
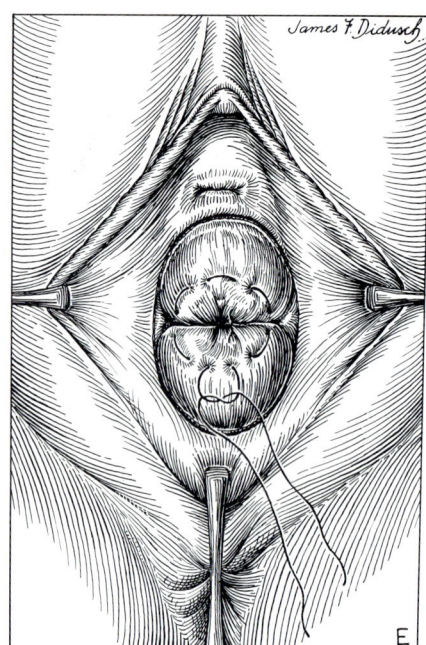
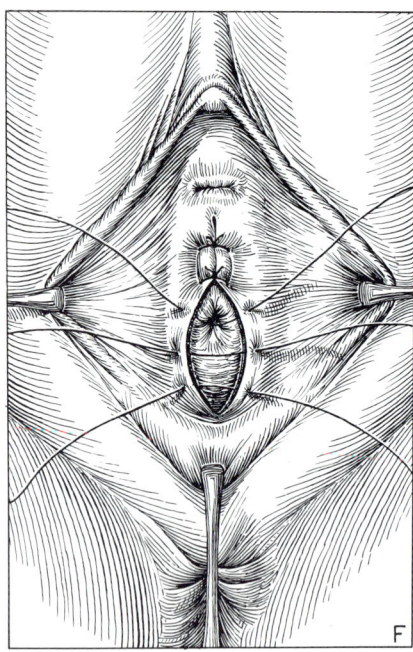

Fig. 24-15 (*Continued*). Colpocleisis for vaginal prolapse following total hysterectomy. (D) The vagina is closed with successive purse-string sutures, placed from above, downward. (E) The second purse-string suture is placed. (F) The last purse string has been tied, and the mucosa is approximated with interrupted sutures.

if necessary, and the pelvic region is exposed.

One strong suture of preserved ox fascia lata in a Koontz fascia needle is placed through the vaginal vault on the right side as illustrated in Figure 24-16 A. The fascia is then worked beneath the peritoneum laterally and anteriorly to the region of the internal abdominal ring. It is made to pierce the rectus muscle and the sheath, which is exposed by dissecting the fat from it laterally from the midline incision.

The fascia is carried under the peri-

Prolapse of the Vagina, With or Without Cervix, Following Hysterectomy

toneum by running the large needle under the peritoneum for its full length, then bringing it out and reinserting it in the large needle hole, continuing subperitoneally. This is carried out step by step until the fascial strip has been brought to the desired point. The small openings in the peritoneum made by the needle leave practically no raw surface. They can be seen in Figure 24-16 B.

The other end of the first suture, attached to the vaginal vault, is then threaded onto a Koontz fascia needle, and in a similar subperitoneal manner it is carried anteriorly under the peritoneum of the bladder to the symphysis region. It is made to pierce the rectus muscle and its sheath and is then anchored to the anterior surface of the fascia. The ends of the fascia strips are sutured to the fascia with fine black-silk sutures.

This procedure is repeated on the opposite side, so that finally the vagina is supported by 4 fascial strips.

In using Koontz preserved fascia lata of the ox, it must be remembered that this preserved tissue does not become an integral part of the host, unless it is embedded in a vascular area to permit its organization by fibroblasts growing from the adjacent tissue. The preserved fascia acts as a scaffolding on which this tissue grows.

The burying of the fascial strips beneath the peritoneum also prevents them from extending like guy ropes across the peritoneal cavity to entrap a loop of bowel.

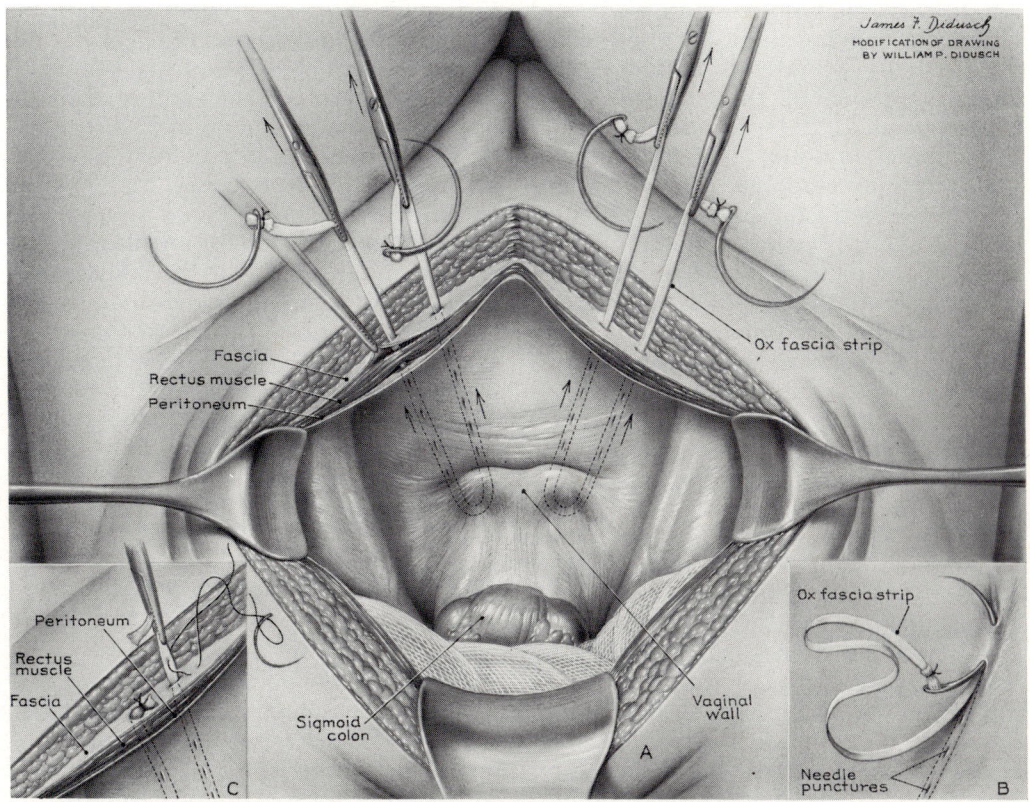

FIG. 24-16. Grant Ward operation for suspension of prolapsed vagina with preserved fascia strips. (A) Position of fascial strips beneath peritoneum and through abdominal wall structures. (B) Method of placing fascia beneath peritoneum. (C) Method of suturing fascial strips to outer surface of rectus sheaths.

Technic: Williams and Richardson Method for Suspension of Prolapsed Vagina With or Without Cervical Stump

The vaginal vault is elevated by packing the vagina tightly with gauze, leaving the end long so that it can be removed during operation without disturbing the drapes. A Pfannenstiel incision is made through the skin and subcutaneous tissues from a point about 3 cm. medial to the anterior superior iliac spine to a similar point on the opposite side. The external oblique aponeurosis is cleaned carefully for a space at least 3 cm. wide throughout the length of the incision. A strip of the external oblique aponeurosis 1.5 cm. wide is dissected free, the inferior margin of which must be carefully determined so that it splits the fibers of the aponeurosis about 1 cm. above the border of the external inguinal ring. The strips are then detached from the linea alba and laid aside, leaving them attached to the muscle belly laterally (Fig. 24-17). The medial portions of the strips will, of course, contain re-enforcing fiber from the internal oblique. The Pfannenstiel incision is next completed, and the rectus muscles are retracted laterally. The apex of the previously packed vagina is identified and pulled up with a figure-of-eight traction suture, after which the vaginal pack is removed. Using a large Kelly clamp, the internal oblique and transversus abdominis muscles are perforated at the attached ends of the fascial strips, which should be slightly above the abdominal inguinal ring. The tip of the clamp is insinuated between the leaves of the broad ligament along the course of the round ligament. The peritoneum is perforated at the lateral fornix of the vagina, and the tip of another Kelly clamp is grasped and drawn back through the tunneled path to the perforation in the rectus muscle. With this second clamp the free end of the fascial strip is grasped and drawn extraperitoneally to the lateral fornix of the vagina and attached thereto with interrupted sutures of medium fine silk. When repeated on the opposite side, a musculofascial sling is formed which pulls the fornices of the vagina upward and laterally. Enterocele of any degree should receive adequate attention at this time. Closure of the abdominal wound completes the operation. No difficulty has been encountered in closing the defect left by the excised strip of fascia.

Technic: Fixation of Vaginal Vault to Anterior Abdominal Wall

After doing whatever repair work is found necessary per vaginum, the operator may be dissatisfied with the suspension of the vagina. Fixation of the vaginal vault by the following technic may be of value. The vagina must be long enough and mobile enough to reach the abdominal wall; if not, the Grant-Ward or Williams-Richardson technic would be preferable.

A low midline incision is made, and 2 strips of fascia about 1 cm. in width are cut from the rectus sheath as shown in Figure 24-18 A.

After entering the peritoneal cavity the vagina which has been packed with gauze is identified. The vault is denuded of peritoneum as shown in Figure 24-18 B. If the bladder is adherent over the vault, it is dissected free and pushed anteriorly.

Large cutting fascia needles which have been threaded with the fascial strips are then used to suture the dome of the vagina to the undersurface of the rectus sheath (Fig. 24-18 C). The ends of the fascial strips are tied down to the anterior rectus sheath with nonabsorbable sutures such as silk or mersilene (Fig. 24-18 D). The fascial incision is then closed with figure-of-eight sutures of No. 1 chromic catgut.

Technic: Use of Inert Suture Materials in Marked Vaginal Prolapse With Enterocele

With the advent of inert suture materials such as mersilene in strap form, another weapon is available which may prove valuable in curing this difficult condition. It must be emphasized that no single operation is applicable to all these cases. The operation described below has proven satisfactory in the hands of Mattingly. It is applicable to cases of

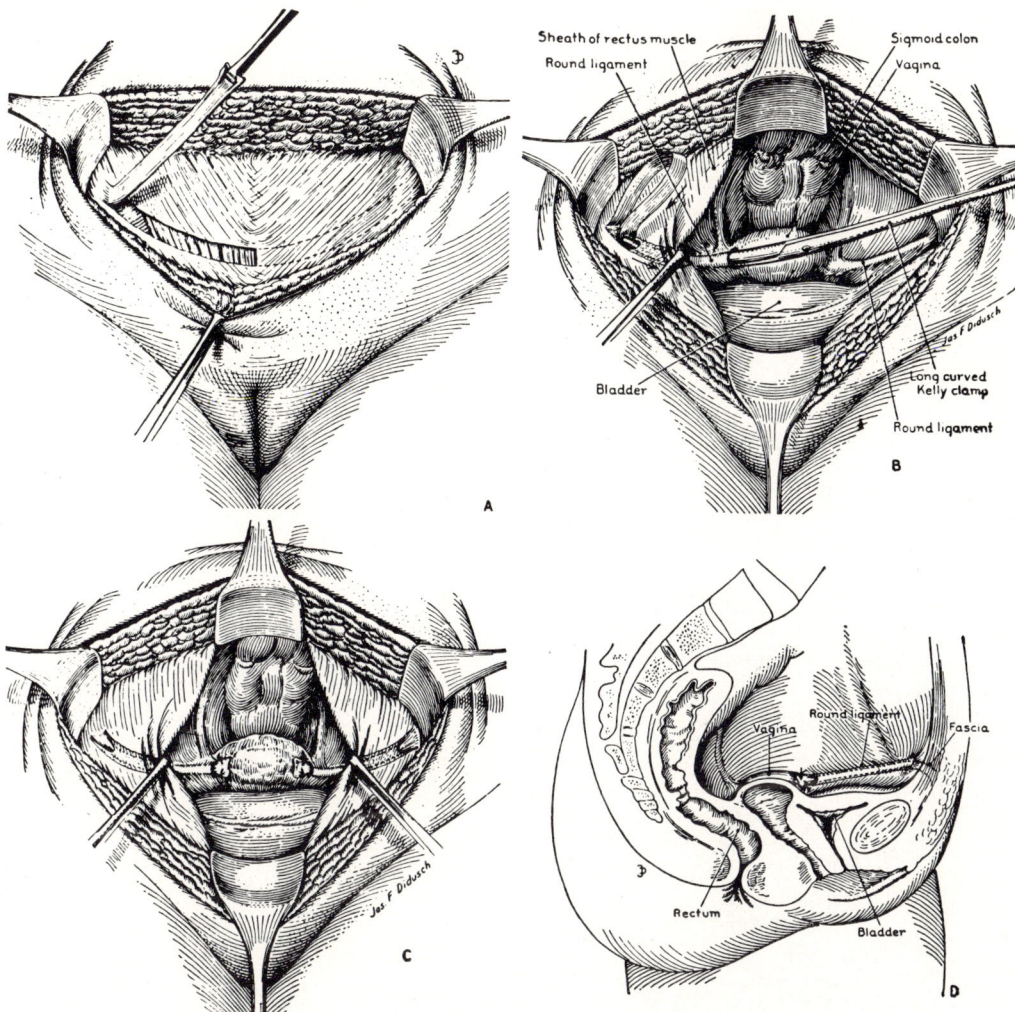

Fig. 24-17. (A) A transverse incision has been made through the fat, and a suitable area of fascia has been cleaned of fat. One fascial strap has been dissected free. (B) A tunnel is made through the leaves of the broad ligament beneath the round ligament. The muscles are perforated with the tip of the clamp, and the end of the strap is grasped. (C) The fascial straps have been drawn between the leaves of the broad ligaments and sutured to the corners of the vagina. (D) Sagittal view, showing mechanism by which vagina is held in place.

marked vaginal prolapse with enterocele.

Figure 24-19 outlines a combined procedure of ventral suspension of the vaginal vault with a mersilene strap and an abdominal culdoplasty. Identification of the vault is facilitated by packing the vagina with gauze prior to the laparotomy. After reflecting the peritoneum and base of the bladder from the apex of the vault, a long Kelly clamp, including the mersilene strap, is advanced beneath the peritoneum along the lateral pelvic wall to the region of the base of the broad ligament, lateral to the lower ureter. The peritoneum is opened at this point and the tape introduced into the paravaginal space. The tape is sutured to the midportion of the vault, utilizing mersilene suture material, and again anchored at

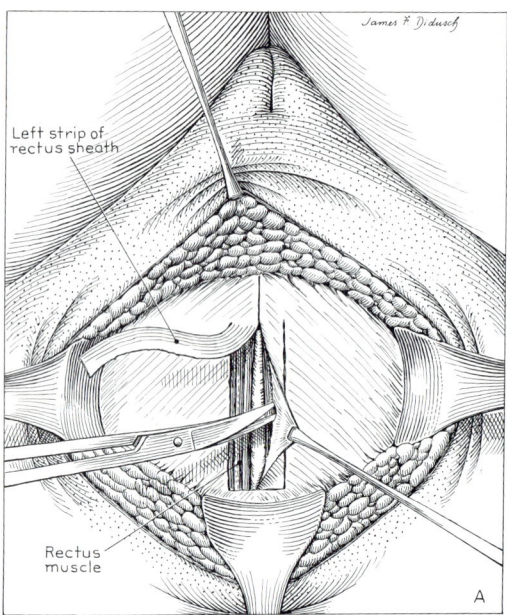

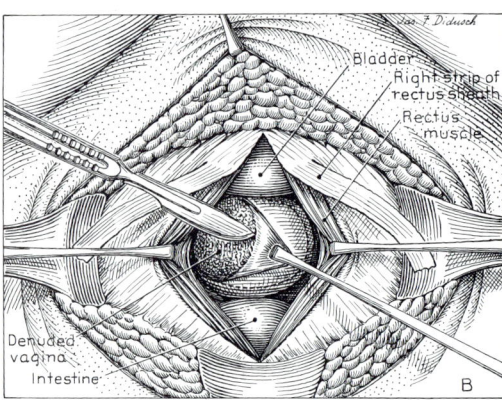

Fig. 24-18. (A) Two narrow strips of fascia are cut from either side of the midline incision. (B) The top of the vagina is denuded of serosa.

the lateral angle of the vault. The opposite half of the vault is supported in an identical manner, and the peritoneum is closed over the mersilene sling, completely extraperitonizing the permanent material. Traction is then exerted on the straps until maximum support of the vault is obtained, and the straps are then sutured to the fascia of the anterior rectus sheath.

Prior to suturing the mersilene straps to the anterior fascia, the cul-de-sac is completely obliterated by concentric rows of purse-string sutures, utilizing silk or other permanent material. The parietal peritoneum of the sacrum is approximated by successive sutures to the parietal peritoneum of the right lateral pelvic wall, and the visceral peritoneum of the rectosigmoid and rectovaginal septum. It is necessary to place the purse-string sutures as high as possible toward the promontory in an effort to prevent the cul-de-sac from re-forming and to avoid the effect of intra-abdominal pressure from the small bowel against the vault and rectovaginal septum. Such a "peritoneal hammock" has proven to be most effective in holding the bowel out of the lower pelvis as well as giving additional fibroblastic support to the suspended vault. Care must be taken to avoid disturbing the ureter as the overlying peritoneum is plicated.

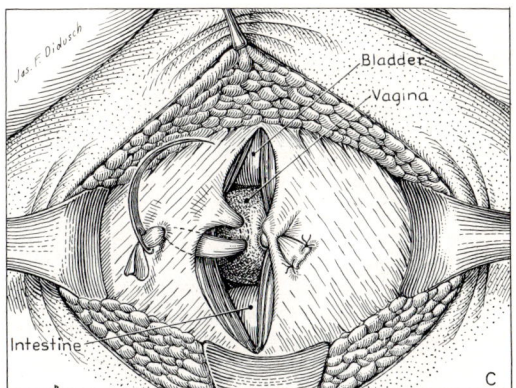
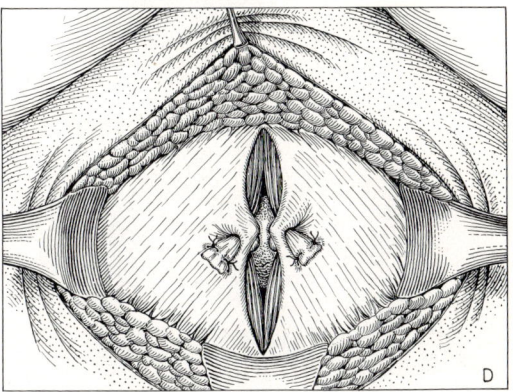

FIG. 24-18 (*Continued*). (C) Using a large fascia needle, the denuded top of the vagina is sutured to the undersurface of the rectus sheath. (D) Fascia strips are sutured to the outer surface of the rectus sheath with silk sutures.

THE USE OF PESSARIES

One of the oldest appliances used in medicine is the vaginal pessary. With the advent of modern surgery, the use of pessaries became less prevalent and less important; yet today the proper use of pessaries in selected gynecologic cases is an accomplishment that every gynecologist should master.

Only 3 types of pessaries remain in general use today of the great assortment that was manufactured in the past. These are the Smith-Hodge, the ring, and the Menge types.

THE SMITH-HODGE PESSARY

The Smith-Hodge pessary is used to hold the retroposed uterus in anteposition. It should be remembered that this pessary does not bring the retrodisplaced uterus forward. It simply holds it in position after it has been brought forward manually.

Indications. It has been stressed earlier in this chapter that most uteri in retroposition are asymptomatic and require no treatment. This is equally true whether one is considering surgery or the use of pessaries. The use of the pessary to hold the uterus forward is indicated under the following conditions:

1. *As a therapeutic test* when there is doubt as to whether the position of the uterus is responsible for the symptoms of which the patient complains. After the uterus is held in good position for a few months, the patient should be relieved of her symptoms, if they are dependent upon the retrodisplacement. If the response to this treatment is equivocal, the pessary may be removed and left out for a time to see whether or not the symptoms become aggravated. By observation on the part of the patient and the physician the possibility of relief by suspension usually can be ascertained in this way.

2. *To hold the uterus in anteposition*

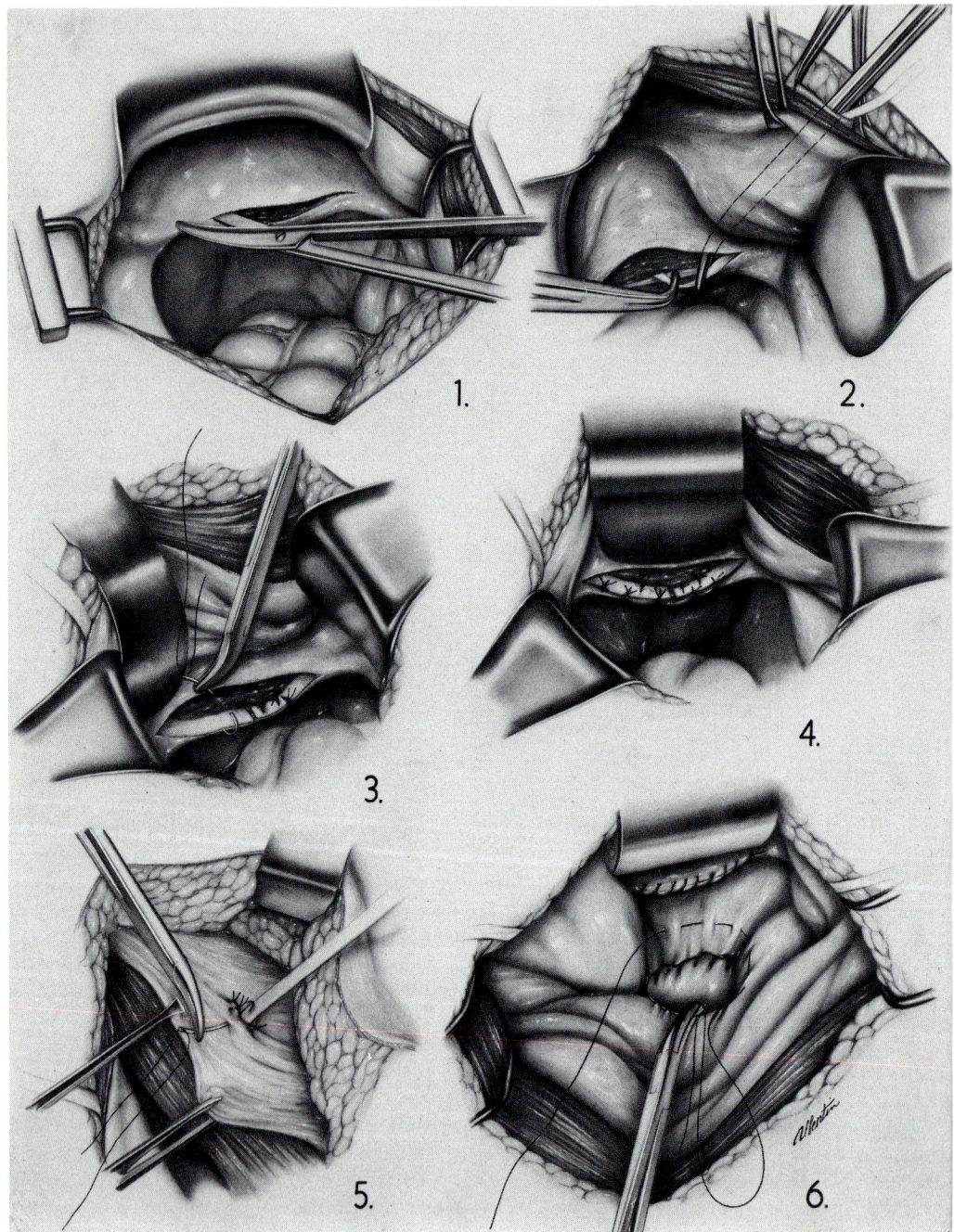

FIG. 24-19. Procedure for combining ventral suspension of the vaginal vault with abdominal culdoplasty.

1. Excision and reflection of bladder peritoneum from vaginal vault.
2. Retroperitoneal insertion of mersilene strap from anterior abdominal wall to vaginal vault.
3. Suture of mersilene straps to vaginal vault.
4. Completed fixation of mersilene straps to vaginal vault.
5. Suture of mersilene strap to anterior rectus fascia along lateral margin of rectus muscle.
6. Serial plication of redundant cul-de-sac.

during early pregnancy. When during early pregnancy the uterus is in deep retroposition, and particularly when there is a high degree of retroflexion, the inability of the fundus to rise above the sacral promontory can be responsible for abortion, usually between the 3rd and the 4th months. The holding of such a pregnant uterus in anteposition to the end of the 4th month by means of a Smith-Hodge pessary is particularly indicated when there is a history of repeated abortions.

3. *To give temprary relief* from symptoms of retrodisplacement when surgical correction is to be deferred. A common reason for deferring surgical treatment may be the desire for more children before a corrective operative procedure is done, which may be performed more advantageously after completion of the family when a vaginal hysterectomy may often be combined with vaginal plastic operation. Suspension operations may also be deferred for economic reasons or because of compelling duties.

4. *Occasionally because of sterility.* If after thorough investigation of the infertile couple all is found in order except a marked retrodisplacement, suspension of the uterus on the rather remote chance that it will relieve the sterility scarcely seems to be justified. The doubtful benefit of maintaining the uterus in good position may be attained by the use of the Smith-Hodge pessary.

5. *During the puerperium or after abortion.* Shortly after delivery or abortion, the retrodisplaced uterus may give rise to rather severe low backache and bearing-down pelvic discomfort. Often this can be relieved by holding the uterus forward with a pessary. The improvement in the circulation of the uterus in good position for several weeks may remain after removal of the pessary. Even if the uterus does become retrodisplaced after removal of the pessary, the smaller organ in the cul-de-sac often gives rise to no symptoms.

Contraindications. Using the Smith-Hodge pessary is contraindicated in the presence of vaginitis. This contraindication applies equally to other types of pessaries, for the presence of a foreign object within the vagina prevents the healing of the inflammatory process. Also, the pessary should be excluded when acute cervicitis is present, but there is no contraindication with the usual case of chronic cervicitis. Acute salpingitis also obviously contraindicates the pessary. When chronic salpingitis or endometriosis is present and the uterus is bound in the cul-de-sac, it is quite useless to attempt to hold it forward by means of a pessary.

Replacing the Retrodisplaced Uterus. The first essential step before inserting the pessary is the replacement of the uterus into normal anteposition. This usually may be attained with the greatest of ease, but on occasion it may be extremely difficult. Simply pushing the cervix posteriorly with one or two fingers in the vagina may cause the fundus to come forward. This maneuver may be augmented by pressure on the abdomen in an attempt to work the abdominal hand into the pelvis behind the uterus. The fundus is pushed forward at the same time that the cervix is pushed posteriorly (Fig. 24-20). When the cervix is short, it may be difficult to sustain pressure against the anterior lip. In such cases pressure on the posterior fornix may draw the cervix back. Another maneuver which is useful when the finger slips off the cervix is to grasp the anterior lip with a

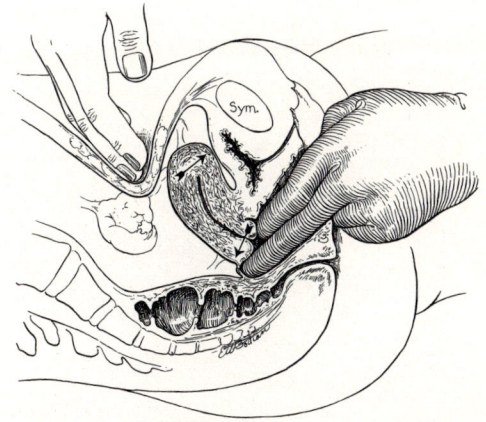

Fig. 24-20. Showing method of replacing uterus into anteposition. The vaginal fingers push the cervix postero-inferiorly. Pressure is exerted on the posterior surface of the fundus with the abdominal hand.

tenaculum and exert pressure posteriorly by this means.

One of the most useful procedures is to insert the index finger into the vagina and the middle finger in the rectum. While the index finger presses the cervix back, the middle finger is made to boost the fundus forward. Pressure is made with the abdominal hand in an attempt to bring the fundus forward (Fig. 24-21).

Insertion of the Pessary. After replacement of the uterus into its correct position it is often well to have an assistant maintain gentle pressure on the anterior abdominal wall to prevent its slipping back. With the operator's left hand the labia are spread and the broad end of the lubricated pessary is brought in apposition with the outlet. The pessary should be pressed into the vagina obliquely as this represents the greatest diameter of the vaginal outlet. As soon as the broad end of the pessary passes the levator muscles, it is rotated so that it lies transversely, and the cross bar is pushed behind the cervix (Fig. 24-22). The pessary thus makes pressure on the posterior vaginal fornix, which in turn holds the cervix back (Fig. 24-23). If the cervix is held posteriorly, the uterus, being a semirigid structure, remains in antepo-

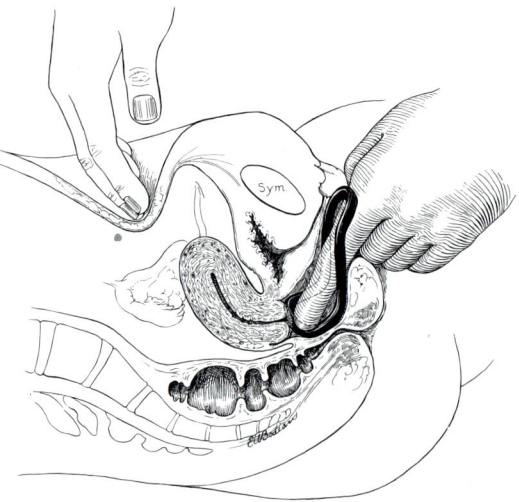

FIG. 24-22. The Smith-Hodge pessary has been introduced into the vagina. The cross bar is being depressed to place it behind the cervix.

sition by virtue of the intra-abdominal pressure on the posterior surface.

The pessary should be large enough to remain in place without dropping from the introitus and without shifting within the vagina. It should be large enough to press gently against the suburethral vaginal mucosa and thus have a point of counterpressure in order to exert moderate pressure on the posterior fornix. On the other hand, if it presses too tightly against the urethra, the patient may be unable to void. It should not be so tight as to be uncomfortable or produce pressure necrosis and ulceration of the mucosa.

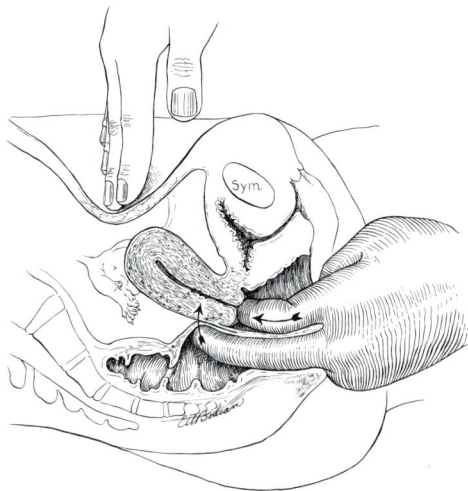

FIG. 24-21. Showing method of replacing uterus anteriorly. With the index finger in the vagina the cervix is pushed posteriorly. With the rectal finger the uterus is boosted anteriorly.

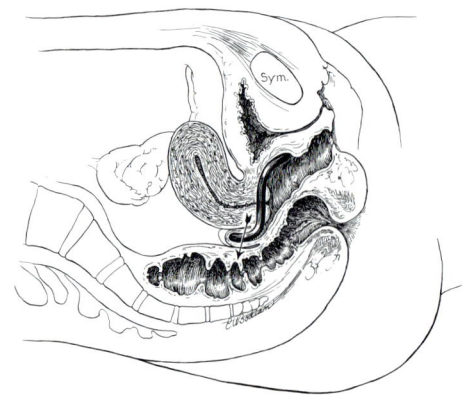

FIG. 24-23. Showing mechanism of holding uterus in anteposition by Smith-Hodge pessary.

Often the pessary can be shaped to fit the vagina of a particular individual by modifying its shape after dropping it momentarily into boiling water. By this method it may be narrowed, lengthened, widened, shortened, or its curves modified so as to be moulded more nearly to the shape of the vaginal cavity.

After the pessary has been fitted, the patient is asked to walk about the examining room for a few minutes to determine whether or not she is comfortable. Then she is asked to get on the table again, and the position of the pessary and the uterus is checked. It is our custom to have the patient return in a week to determine if she is comfortable. The position of the pessary and the uterus is checked again, with the patient on the examining table. If all is well, the woman is asked to return every 4 months in order that the vaginal mucosa may be inspected and the position of the uterus checked. Removal of the pessary may not be necessary if all is well. While wearing the pessary the patient is asked to take a daily cleansing douche.

The Ring and the Menge Pessaries

Admittedly, the best cure for prolapse and cystocele is surgery. However, palliation is indicated not infrequently. In young women who desire more children it is desirous to relieve symptoms temporarily by means of the pessary until another pregnancy is completed; then radical and often sterilizing surgery may be done with satisfactory results. There is also a rather large group of elderly women who are very poor surgical risks, due to cardiac and/or renal disease, diabetes, etc., who suffer from prolapse and cystocele of varying degree.

The ring pessary may be used quite satisfactorily for cystocele and slight descensus. It is inserted obliquely into the vagina and twisted as soon as it passes the levators so that it lies obliquely as shown in Figure 24-24. If the outlet is sufficiently narrow to permit the pessary to remain in place, the cervix is supported, and the anterior vaginal wall is placed on stretch sufficiently to prevent the cystocele from protruding.

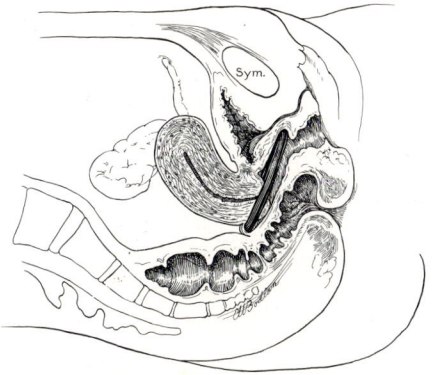

Fig. 24-24. Ring pessary is in place, keeping the redundant anterior vaginal wall from prolapsing.

When there is a marked prolapse, the ring pessary seldom supports the uterus sufficiently to take care of the condition. Then a pessary of the Menge type is the one of choice. The knob which fits into the cross bar is detachable, and the ring is inserted without it. After the ring is adjusted transversely in the vagina, the knob is inserted and turned to lock into position. The cervix thus rests in the ring, and the knob maintains the ring in a transverse position (Fig. 24-25). The knob is held in its downward position by the levators, the urethra, and the rectum; these structures prevent it from being deflected laterally, anteriorly, or posteriorly.

As with other types of pessaries, daily douches and return visits to the gynecologist's office at 3-month intervals are required.

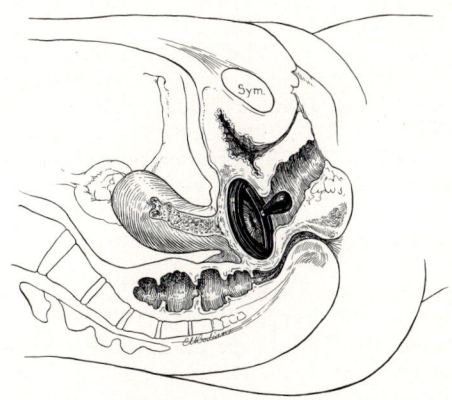

Fig. 24-25. Menge pessary is in place, preventing the cervix from descending.

BIBLIOGRAPHY

Adams: Cited by W. P. Graves. *In* Graves, W. P.: Gynecology. Philadelphia, W. B. Saunders, 1916.

Aldridge, A. A.: Retrodisplacements of the uterus in relation to pregnancy. Amer. J. Obstet. Gynec., *40*:361, 1940.

Alexander, W.: Quoted by A. H. Curtis. *In* Curtis, A. H. (ed.): Obstetrics and Gynecology. Philadelphia, W. B. Saunders, 1937.

Baldy, J. M.: Prolapse of the uterus. Trans. Amer. Gynec. Soc., 27:25, 1912.

———: The treatment of uterine displacements. Surg. Gynec. Obstet., *8*:421, 1908.

Bissell, Dougal: Vaginal hysterectomy for prolapse. Surg. Gynec. Obstet., *78*:138, 1919.

Brady, Leo: Results with the Watkins interposition operation in the treatment of prolapsus uteri. Surg. Gynec. Obstet., *43*:476, 1926.

Bucura, Constantin: Über die plastische Verwendung des in die Scheide gestürzten Uterus-körpers bei Prolapsen. Z. Geburtsh. Gynäk., *45*:422, 1901.

Churchill, F.: The Diseases of Women. Philadelphia, Blanchard & Lea, 1857.

Cullen, T. S.: Use of sutures as tractors in vaginal operation for prolapsus. Amer. J. Obstet. Gynec., *4*:544, 1922.

Danforth, W. C.: The place of vaginal hysterectomy in present-day gynecology. Amer. J. Obstet. Gynec., *36*:787, 1938.

Donald, A.: A short history of the operation of colporrhaphy, with remarks on the technic. J. Obstet. Gynaec. Brit. Emp., *28*:256, 1921.

Durfee, R. B.: Management of genital organ prolapse. Clin. Obstet. Gynec., *9*:1047, 1966.

Everett, Houston S.: End-result with the Watkins interposition operation. Surg. Gynec. Obstet., *61*:403, 1935.

Fluhmann, C. F.: The rise and fall of suspension operations for uterine displacement. Bull. Johns Hopkins Hosp., *96*:59, 1955.

Fothergill, W. E.: Anterior colporrhaphy and amputation of the cervix combined as a single operation for use in the treatment of genital prolapse. Amer. J. Surg., *29*:161, 1915.

Freund, H. W.: Über Moderne Prolapsoperationen. Zbl. Gynäk., *25*:441, 1901.

Fritsch, H.: Prolapsoperation. Zbl. Gynäk., *24*:49, 1900.

Gilliam, D. T.: Round-ligament ventrosuspension of the uterus: A new method. Amer. J. Obstet., *41*:299, 1900.

Goff, J. Riddle: An improved and perfected operation for the relief of extreme cases of procidentia, cystocele and rectocele. Amer. J. Obstet. Gynec., *42*:611, 1910.

Goodall, J. R., and Power, R. M. H.: A modification of the Le Fort operation for increasing its scope. Amer. J. Obstet. Gynec., *34*:968, 1937.

Graves, W. P.: Olshauser operation for suspension of the uterus. Surg. Gynec. Obstet., *52*:1028, 1931.

Heaney, N. Sproat: Vaginal hysterectomy – its indications and technic. Amer. J. Surg., *48*:284, 1940.

———: Technic of vaginal hysterectomy. Surg. Clin. N. Amer., *22*:73, 1942.

Hirst, B. C.: A modification of the Alexander operation. Surg. Gynec. Obstet., *20*:599, 1915.

Kelly, H. A.: Hysterorrhaphy. Amer. J. Obstet., *20*:33, 1887.

———: History of retrodisplacement of the uterus. Surg. Gynec. Obstet., *20*:598, 1915.

Leonard, V. N.: The postoperative results of trachelorrhaphy in comparison with those of amputation of the cervix. Surg. Gynec. Obstet., *18*:35, 1914.

Lynch, F. W.: The frequency and meaning of backache in gynecology. Amer. J. Obstet. Gynec., *12*:719, 1926.

Mayo, Charles H.: Uterine prolapse with associated pelvic relaxation. Surg. Gynec. Obstet., *20*:235, 1915.

Neel, J. C.: The etiology and treatment of cystocele. Surg. Gynec. Obstet., *29*:320, 1919.

Olshausen, R.: Über ventrale Operation bei Prolapsus und Retroversio Uteri. Zbl. Gynäk., *10*:698, 1886.

Rawls, Reginald M.: Cystocele: Review of the literature. Trans. Amer. Gynec. Soc., *43*:133, 1918.

Richardson, Edward H.: An efficient composite operation for uterine prolapse and associated pathology. Amer. J. Obstet. Gynec., *34*:814, 1937.

Schauta, F.: Über Prolapsoperationen. Gynäk. Rundschau., *3*:729, 1909.

Schauta, F., and Wertheim, E.: Quoted by Watkins. *In* Treatment of cases of extensive cystocele and uterine prolapse. Surg. Gynec. Obstet., *2*:659, 1906.

Shaw, Henry N.: Results in interposition

operation for procedentia and prolapse of the uterus. Surg. Gynec. Obstet., 34:394, 1922.

Shaw, William F.: The treatment of prolapsus uteri, with special reference to the Manchester operation of coloporrhaphy. Amer. J. Obstet. Gynec., 26:667, 1933.

Spalding, Alfred B.: A study of frozen sections of the pelvis with description of an operation for pelvic prolapse. Surg. Gynec. Obstet., 29:529, 1919.

Symmonds, R. E., and Pratt, J. E.: Vaginal prolapse following hysterectomy. Amer. J. Obstet. Gynec., 79:899, 1960.

Te Linde, Richard W., and Richardson, Edward H., Jr.: End results of the Richardson composite operation for uterine prolapse. Amer. J. Obstet. Gynec., 45:29, 1943.

Ward, George G.: Problem of the cystocele. Amer. J. Obstet. Gynec., 79:593, 1919.

——: Ox fascia lata for reconstruction of round ligaments in correcting prolapse of vagina. A.M.A. Arch. Surg., 36:163, 1938.

Watkins, T. J.: The treatment of cystocele and uterine prolapse after the menopause. Amer. J. Obstet. Gynec., 15:420, 1899.

——: St. Luke's Hospital Reports. Chicago, 1906.

——: Treatment of cases of extensive cystocele and uterine prolapse. Surg. Gynec. Obstet., 8:471, 1909.

——: Transposition of the uterus and bladder in the treatment of extensive cystocele and uterine prolapse. Amer. J. Obstet. Gynec., 65:225, 1912.

Webster, J. C.: A satisfactory operation for certain cases of retroversion of the uterus. J.A.M.A., 37:913, 1901.

Williams, G. A., and Richardson, A. C.: Transplantation of external oblique aponeurosis: An operation for prolapse of the vagina following hysterectomy. Amer. J. Obstet. Gynec., 64:552, 1952.

Wertheim, E.: Zur plastischen Verwendung des Uterus bei Prolapsen. Zbl. Gynäk., 23:369, 1899.

25

Urethrocele, Cystocele, and Stress Incontinence of Urine

Urethrocele and cystocele should be discussed together, for although either may occur independently, some degree of one is usually present with the other. Also, some descent of the uterus is often associated with these two conditions, but not invariably so. Therefore most cystocele repairs are done in connection with operations for descensus. However, there are cases in which it is advisable simply to repair a urethrocele or cystocele. This is particularly true in elderly women who have symptoms wholly dependent upon the cystocele and/or urethrocele who are not the best operative risks, and on whom it is advisable to do the least surgery compatible with relieving her symptoms.

URETHROCELE AND CYSTOCELE

Urethrocele is a protrusion downward of the urethra from its attachment just beneath the symphysis pubis. It results from inability of the musculofibrous tissue to give it normal support. Childbirth injuries to the urogenital trigone and the pubovesicocervical fascia are chiefly responsible for the condition, although it is seen occasionally in a nulliparous woman. Injury to the above structures may be so great as to result in the formation of a urethrocele immediately after childbirth, but in many instances the supporting structures are left in sufficiently good condition to support the urethra for a time. Years later, with the natural loss of tone of supporting tissue and the stress and strain of work, the urethra may prolapse and the symptoms of urethrocele develop.

Sometimes a urethrocele alone may cause such bulging that the patient will consult the doctor relative to this protrusion. Aside from the bulging there may be no inconvenience, but the most uniform symptom of urethrocele is stress incontinence of urine. In the lesser degree of this, the patient spurts a few drops of urine on coughing, sneezing, or straining. There is usually a tendency for this slight degree of incontinence to become aggravated with the passage of time, and occasionally there results a complete incontinence when the patient is standing. Usually, even in these extreme cases, there is little or no difficulty when the patient is lying down. The defect in the mechanism causing this type of incontinence is due to the inability of the circular, constricting urethral muscle fibers to contract normally when the urethra is pulled downward with the prolapsed vaginal wall (Fig. 25-1). If one observes the closing of the normal urethra through a cystoscope, the circular, camera-shutter-like action of the normal sphincter is obvious. When the vaginal mucosa bulges downward on straining, it pulls with it the undersurface of the urethra and the internal sphincter. Thus the normally round urethral lumen is converted into an oval, and the circular muscles cannot function effectively. For further consideration of stress incon-

Urethrocele and Cystocele 535

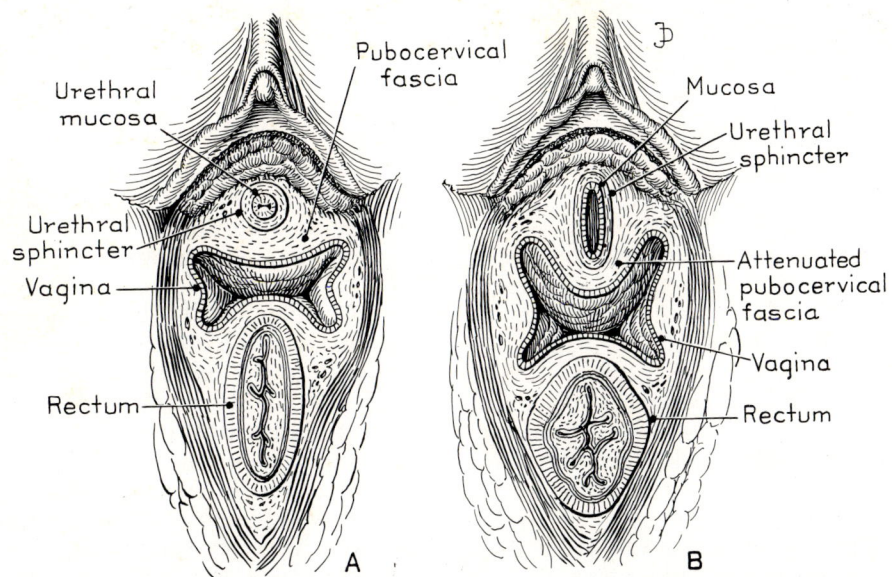

Fig. 25-1. (A) Schematic representation of camera-shutter-like action of normal urethral sphincter. (B) Schematic representation of failure of urethral sphincter to close on straining after development of urethrocele.

tinence of urine, see discussion on the subject later in this chapter.

Cystocele is a herniation of the bladder, causing the anterior vaginal wall to bulge downward. Like urethrocele, it is usually the result of childbirth injury. The child's head may stretch and separate the pubococcygeal fibers of the levator ani muscles, and this permits a general sagging of the vaginal walls. However, the most important factor in the formation of cystocele is incompetency of the pubovesicocervical fascia. This broad structure extends as a sheet downward from the cervix between the vaginal wall on one side and the bladder and the urethra on the other. As with urethrocele, cystocele may develop shortly after delivery, but often it does not appear for a decade or more after childbirth. The deterioration of tissue with age, as well as with the strain of daily life, is undoubtedly a factor in the formation of a cystocele years after childbirth. One rarely sees a cystocele in a nulliparous woman.

When there is a cystocele of considerable size, the woman may complain of a bearing-down sensation in the vaginal region, and often there is the annoying feeling of a bulging, protruding mass. She frequently believes this to be her "womb," when the protrusion is actually the cystocele. Coupled with this there is often, although not always, an urgent and frequent desire to urinate when standing or walking. These urinary symptoms may be present when the urine is quite free from infection, but the absence of infection must be proved by the microscopic examination of a catheterized specimen of urine and not taken for granted. Frequently, the urine is infected as a result of incomplete emptying of the bladder when a large cystocele permits the lowermost portion of the bladder to drop to a level below that of the internal sphincter. Cystitis, developing from this, aggravates the vesical irritability, which often is already present without infection. When such an infection is present, bacterial cultures should be complemented with antibiotic sensitivity studies and the appropriate antibiotic agent used to clear up the infection before surgical treatment of the cystocele is undertaken. A pessary may be used to support the bladder while this chemotherapy is in progress, thus reducing the amount of residual urine and increasing the probability of successful eradication of the infection. When the infection has been long-standing, it may fail to clear up preoperatively, and much time may elapse after operation before the bladder becomes free of infection and the patient free of bladder irritability.

TREATMENT

The treatment of urethrocele and cystocele is surgical. Occasionally, when surgery is contraindicated or must be deferred, the patient can be made comfortable with a ring pessary. Since cystocele and urethrocele so frequently occur together, the operations for both conditions are often combined. The most essential step in the cure of these two conditions is restoring support to the urethra and/or the bladder by proper use of the pubovesicocervical fascia. The technic of the operation for cystocele follows. The technic of the operation for urethrocele is given in connection with stress urinary incontinence, since this is the symptom for which operation is done most often.

TECHNIC: REPAIR OF CYSTOCELE

The patient is placed on the table in the lithotomy position, and traction is made on the anterior lip of the cervix by means of a Jacobs clamp. An inverted T-shaped incision is made through the anterior vaginal wall. The transverse cut is first made at the reflexion of the vaginal mucosa onto the anterior lip of the cervix. A curved Mayo scissors is then inserted through this transverse incision and made to tunnel upward (Fig. 25-2 A). If there is no urethrocele, it is best to stop the incision short of the urethra, for the scar which forms about the sphincter region occasionally keeps the sphincter from closing normally, and partial incontinence may result. The plane of cleavage which the scissors enters is

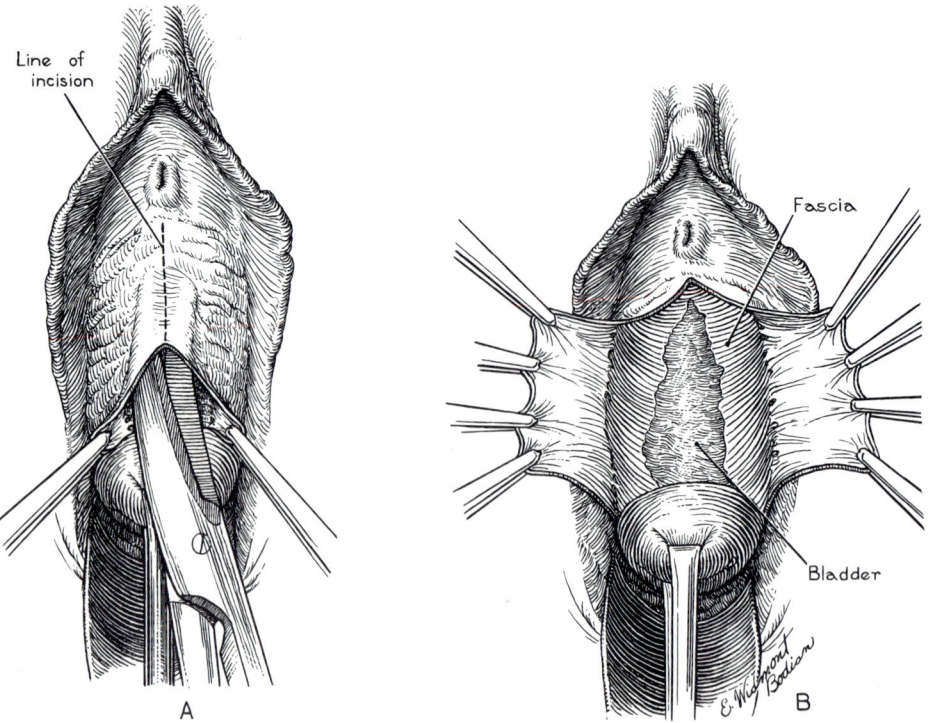

FIG. 25-2. Radical repair of cystocele. (A) An inverted T-shaped incision is made through the anterior vaginal wall. Vaginal mucosa is separated from the bladder by alternately opening and closing curved scissors. (B) Flaps of mucosa have been dissected laterally. The fascia has been dissected from the mucosa and left attached to the bladder.

between the pubovesicocervical fascia and the bladder. After the tip of the scissors has passed a few centimeters, the mucosa is cut in the midline. The alternate tunneling and cutting are continued until the urethral meatus is reached if there is also a urethrocele.

The edges of the vaginal mucosa are grasped with Kocher clamps and retracted. Using the scalpel, a separation of the pubovesicocervical fascia from the mucosa flaps is started. Then the dissection is continued with gauze. In this way the fascia is left attached to the bladder, except for an area in the midline (Fig. 25-2 B). This ensures a good blood supply to both the fascia and the subjacent bladder.

The bladder is picked up with a smooth forceps and separated from its attachment to the cervix. After a few snips with the scissors the bladder can usually be pushed up with the gloved finger (Fig. 25-2 C).

Holding the bladder up with a slender retractor causes the lateral portions of the fascia to stand out as pillars. The fascia pillars are brought together in the midline and sutured to the cervix by 2 or 3 interrupted sutures of No. 0 chromic catgut (Fig. 25-2 D).

After completion of this step, the bladder will be well advanced from its former low attachment to the cervix. The closure of the remainder of the hernial gap is completed by bringing together the fascia in the midline, beneath the base of the bladder (Fig. 25-2 E). If there

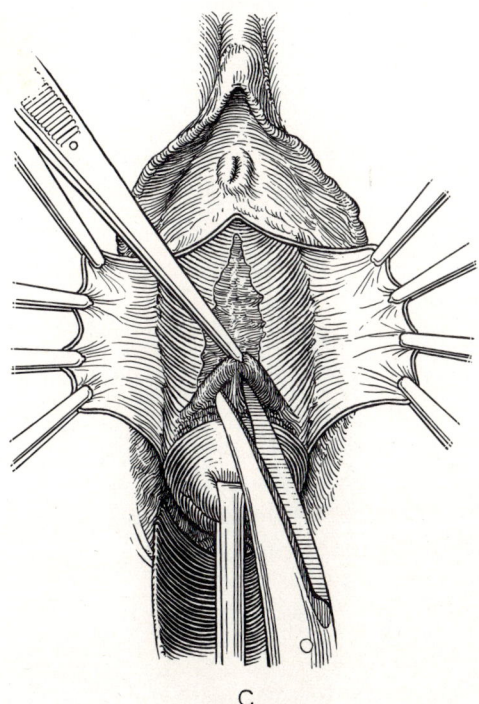
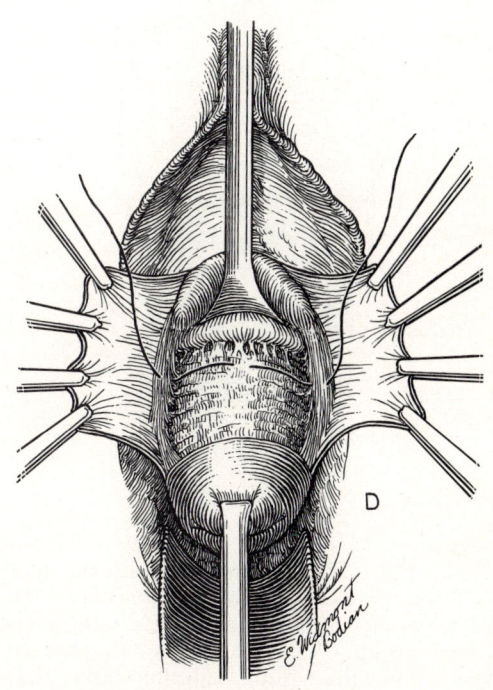

FIG. 25-2 (*Continued*). Radical repair of cystocele. (C) Attachment of bladder to cervix is being cut. After a few snips with the scissors the bladder usually can be dissected up by blunt dissection. (D) The bladder has been well advanced, exposing pillars of pubovesicocervical fascia. The first suture has been placed which will approximate pillars in front of cervix.

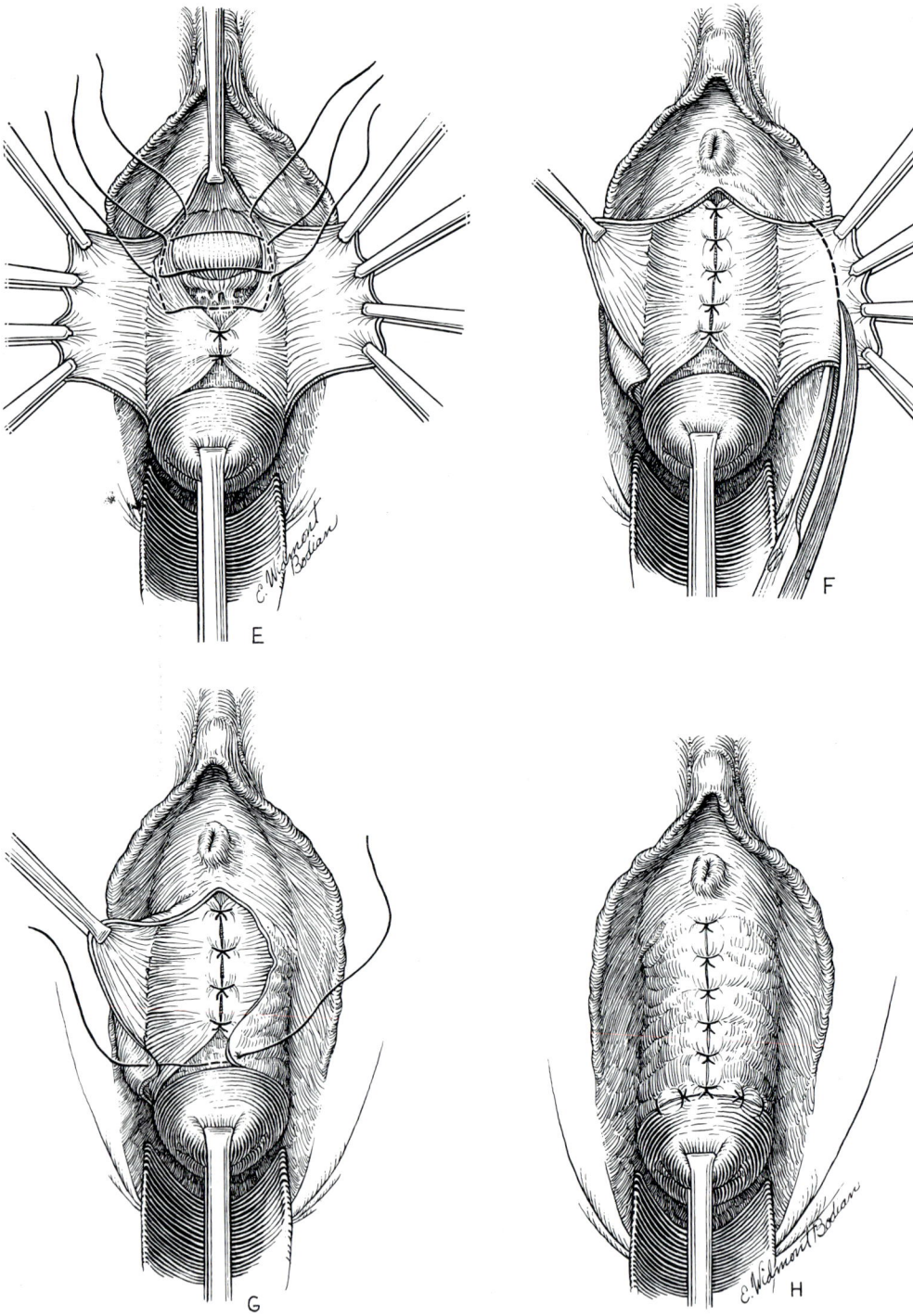

Fig. 25-2 (*Continued*). Radical repair of cystocele. (E) Sutures have been placed for approximation of pubovesicocervical fascia over cervix, bladder, and urethra. (F) Fascia has been completely approximated, and excess of vaginal mucosa is being excised. (G) First suture is being placed for approximation of vaginal flaps. Note that it bites through the anterior wall of the cervix. (H) Operation completed.

Urethrocele and Cystocele 539

is the co-existence of a urethrocele, the fascia is approximated in the midline beneath the urethra.

Figure 25-2 F shows the entire hernial opening strongly closed with broad sheets of fascia. The excess of mucosa of each vaginal flap is excised.

In making the final closure of mucosa, often it is wise first to approximate the mucosa at the cervical end. In doing this a bite is taken in the cervix in the midline (Fig. 25-2 G). The fixing of the mucosa at this point, leaving the suture long and making traction, serves to line up the edges of the incision for closure. The operation is completed by approximating the mucosal edges with interrupted sutures of No. 0 chromic catgut in the midline and laterally at the cervix (Fig. 25-2 H).

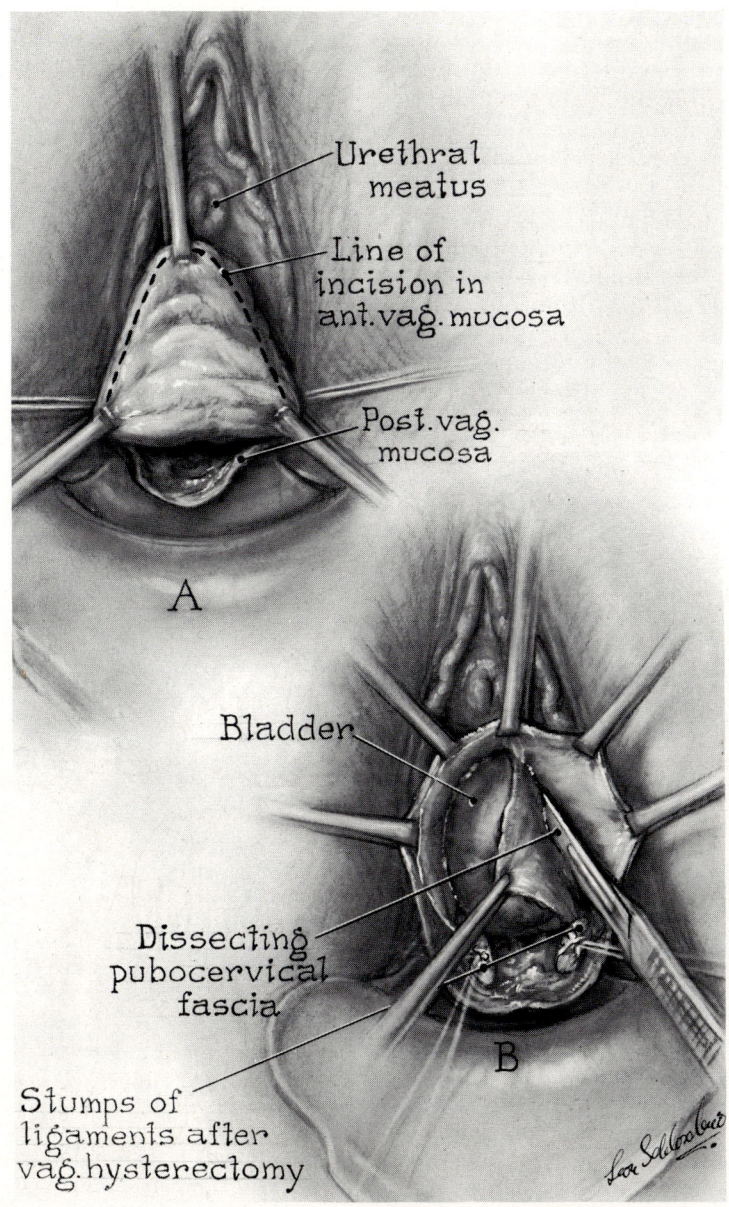

FIG. 25-3. (A) Incision is made as shown in dotted line, and this mucosa is denuded. (B) The pubocervical fascia is dissected free from the mucosa laterally.

REPAIR OF CYSTOCELE WITH VAGINAL HYSTERECTOMY

In repairing a cystourethrocele at the time of vaginal hysterectomy, it is done in the routine manner as described elsewhere in this chapter, except that there is no cervix to "bite" into, in approximating the pubocervical fascia. There are instances in which there is no urethrocele, and it may be advantageous to do the high cystocele repair "in reverse," from the apex of the vagina downward.

Technic. After completing the hysterectomy and suturing the ligament to the vagina, the peritoneum is closed. An inverted V-shaped incision is made with the broad base of the triangle formed by the transverse incision at the top of the vagina (Fig. 25-3 A). After denuding the mucosa from this area, the pubocervical fascia is dissected free from the mucosa on either side as shown in Figure 25-3 B.

The stumps of the ligaments are brought together as shown in Figure 25-4 A, biting into the posterior vaginal wall, thus obliterating the space through which an enterocele might form. The pubocervical fascia is then approximated in the midline with sutures as shown in Figure 25-4 B. Figure 25-5 A shows all these sutures tied except the last one, and the assistant is inverting the bladder wall as the final suture is tied. Thus the fascial support of the bladder is restored. Further trimming of the vaginal mucosa is done as necessary, and the vagina is closed longitudinally with interrupted sutures, as shown in Figure 25-5 B.

STRESS INCONTINENCE OF URINE

The most frequent form of incontinence of urine in women is that known as stress incontinence. Usually it first manifests itself by the escape of a few drops of urine following unusual exertion. There

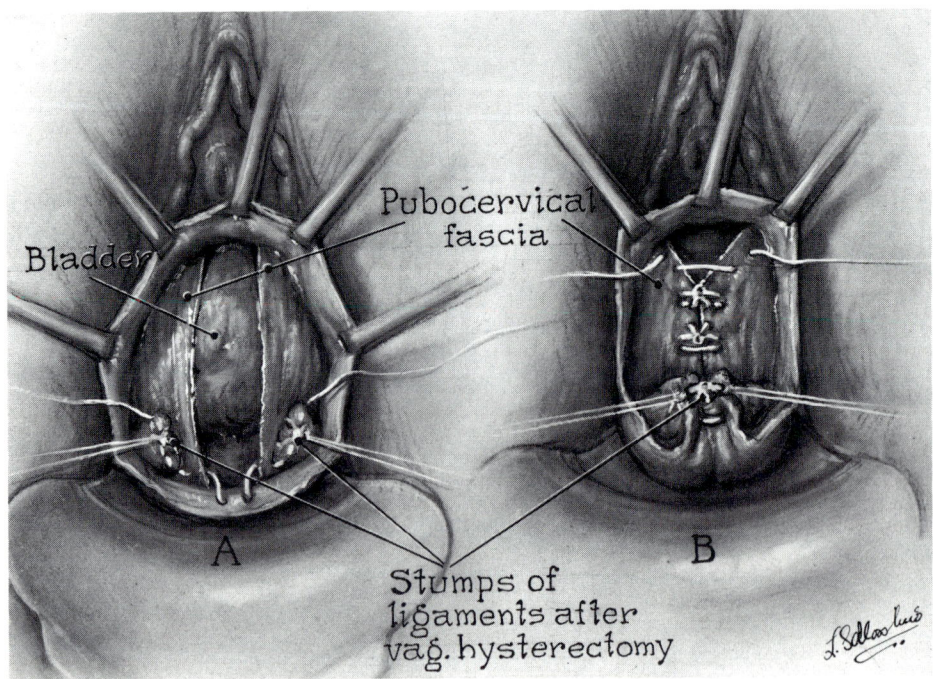

FIG. 25-4. (A) The stumps of the uterine ligaments which were previously sutured to the vagina are brought together, biting into the posterior flap of mucosa to obliterate the space and prevent an enterocele. (B) Pubocervical fascia is being brought together in the midline, with mattress sutures of No. 0 catgut.

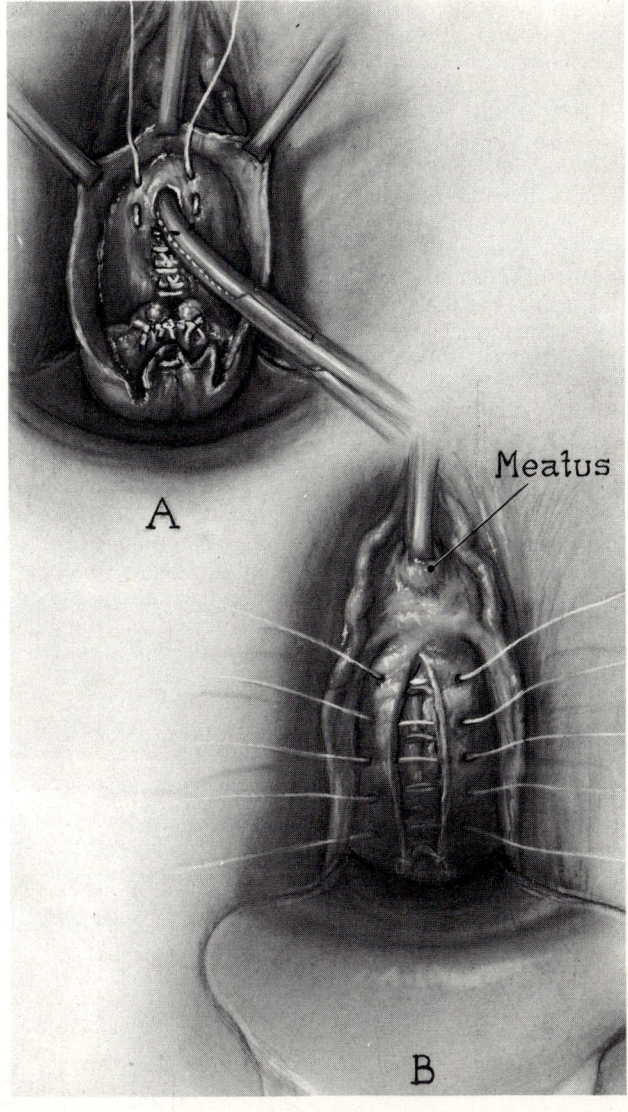

FIG. 25-5. (A) The last opening in the fascia is closed, inverting the bladder with a Kelly clamp. (B) After excising any redundant mucosa, the vaginal incision is closed with interrupted catgut sutures in the midline.

is a tendency for the incontinence to become exaggerated, and soon there is a gushing of urine on coughing, sneezing, laughing, stooping, or even walking. If it is not treated, the incontinence may become almost complete. Howard A. Kelly first wrote about the condition in 1913 and described a method of treating it which has proved to be quite satisfactory; we continue to use it today with some modifications. We shall quote directly from Kelly's original article:

There is a peculiar form of incontinence of urine in women which either follows child-birth or comes on about middle age and is not associated with any visible lesion of the urinary tract. Sometimes the most suggestive picture that can be seen by a cystoscope is a gaping internal sphincter orifice which closes sluggishly. In the incontinence which comes on at about 40 years or over the patient usually first notices the occasional escape of a few drops of urine as she makes some unusual exertion. This grows worse until, at last, a little urine runs out whenever she coughs, laughs, sneezes, lifts anything or steps up high. The condition may finally become so bad that the underclothes are constantly wet and soiled with the malodorous secretions.

For a long time surgeons have tried to relieve this condition by a variety of operations, some of them more or less bizarre, designed to act upon the external urethral orifice by contracting it, or to resect the vagina at the internal orifice, or to kink the urethra, or in one way or another to compress it. The operations rarely succeed. I have seen many patients subjected to them, but none relieved.

The key to successful treatment lies at the internal orifice of the urethra and in the sphincter muscle which controls the canal at this point. For the past 10 or 12 years I have been operating constantly upon patients suffering from this minor distressing incontinence and I have succeeded in relieving every case where there had not been a destruction of the tissues at the urethral orifice, that is, where there had been no vesicovaginal fistula with sloughing.

The operation which I do is as follows (Fig. 25-6): A Pezzer catheter is introduced into the urethra; the tube ought to be small, not over 5 mm. in diameter. With the patient in the lithotomy position, the posterior wall of the vagina is retracted, and the area at the neck of the bladder is brought down with either forceps or four guy sutures.

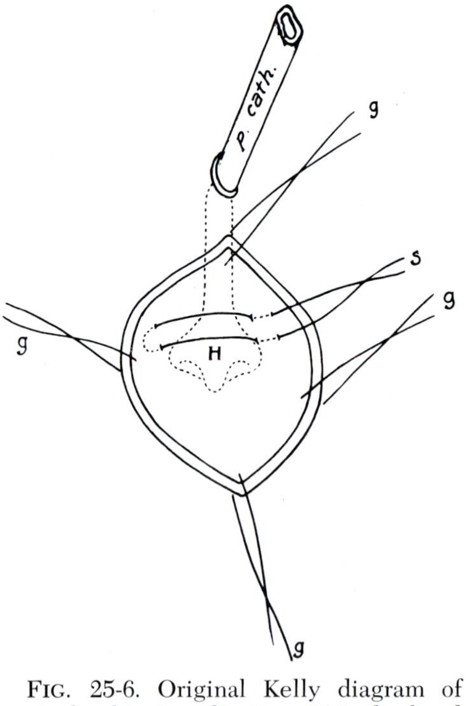

The next step is to slit the vaginal wall down to the urethra and the bladder in the median line for about 1½ to 2 inches. The neck of the bladder should fall at about the center of the incision. The position of the neck is easily determined at all times by moving the catheter to and fro and feeling its head, which presses close up against the urethra. The utmost care should be taken not to cut the urethra or the bladder at any step of the operation. After making this median incision the vagina is further dissected off on both sides with tissue forceps and dissected away from a distance of 2 to 2½ cm. around the neck of the bladder. This dissection may be made with blunt-pointed scissors which push their way into the tissues, separate the bladder from the vaginal walls, and then cut the connecting fibrils. The dissection should be deepest at the neck of the bladder.

When the detachment of the vagina from the bladder is completed, the finger should be able to grasp at least one half or two thirds of the neck of the bladder, including continuous urethra. Sometimes the bladder wall is so thin that its mucosa shines through.

The next step is to suture together the torn or relaxed tissues at the neck of the bladder, using 2 or 3 mattress sutures of fine silk or linen passed from side to side. The first suture taking in about 1½ cm. of tissue is tied at once, when the succeeding suture may be passed outside this, further contracting and bringing together the tissues at the neck (Fig. 25-6). This is the principal part of the operation, and when done the mushroom catheter ought to be pulled out, the head of the catheter escaping with a little jump as it clears the tightened reconstructed sphincter at the neck of the bladder. The more or less redundant vaginal walls, which have been detached in order to expose the sphincter area, are now resected so that the remaining tissues can be snugly brought together from side to side, so as to support the vesical area operated upon and avoid any dead space between bladder and vagina. I prefer to do this suturing with a continuous fine catgut suture in one or two layers.*

Fig. 25-6. Original Kelly diagram of vesical sphincter plication. H is the head of the catheter marking the neck of the bladder; gggg are the guy sutures holding the wound open; S is the suture at the neck of the bladder reuniting the sphincter muscle.

In 1914 Kelly and Dumm reported on 20 cases upon whom the senior author had operated. In 16 the operation was successful.

---

* Kelly, Howard A.: Incontinence of urine in women. Urol. Cutan. Rev., *17*:291, 1913.

The above quotation is from a paper which we regard as a milestone in the history of the treatment of stress incontinence. However, since the publication of this paper, we have made some observations which we regard as important to an understanding of the different types of stress incontinence which should be recognized in order that they may be treated effectively.

The most important point to be clearly established before resorting to any type of surgery is to determine definitely that one is dealing with stress incontinence and not incontinence of the urge type. This is not always easy. A careful history is essential to make certain of the type. Urgency amounting to incontinence is commonly the result of an irritating lesion somewhere in the urinary tract. Hence with a history of this type a complete urologic study whould be made. Cystitis trigonitis, urethritis, or an inflammatory lesion from the upper tract feeding pus into the lower tract can be responsible. Also, it must be admitted that urgency and even incontinence may be present on a nervous basis without any demonstrable lesion in the urinary tract; whether a lesion is identified or not, one thing is certain, the condition will not be cured surgically. If both types of incontinence are present, it should be made clear to the patient that surgery will not cure the urge incontinence. There are tests that have been described to demonstrate stress incontinence, but there is a very simple method which generally supplies the answer. With the patient on the examining table with her bladder full, she is asked to cough. This produces a spurt of urine of variable volume, depending on the degree of incontinence. The examiner's index finger is then placed beneath the urethra touching it but making no pressure. If a strong cough does not produce leakage, one can be quite certain that he is dealing with stress incontinence, and there is an excellent chance of cure by plication.

The cases of true stress incontinence may be divided into four groups:

1. Those cases associated with a urethrocele or cystourethrocele.

2. Those cases following childbirth or previous surgery of the anterior vaginal wall but unassociated with demonstrable urethrocele or cystourethrocele.

3. Those cases occuring in nulliparous women, in which no defective innervation to the urethra or the bladder can be demonstrated.

4. Cases resulting from improper use of the resectoscope upon the vesical neck.

The cases associated with urethrocele or cystourethrocele form the largest group and, fortunately, in this group the operative results are almost uniformly successful. The mechanism whereby the vesical sphincter fails to remain closed when the woman increases her abdominal pressure is dependent upon the sphincter fibers of the vesical neck and the urethra being pulled down with the vaginal wall. Thus the concentric closure of the circular fibers is prevented (Fig. 25-1). In this group it is important to bring together the pubovesicocervical fascia in the midline to support the urethra and the bladder base after the sphincter fibers of the vesical neck and the urethra have been tightened. In fact, many of such cases could be cured by a properly performed operation for cystourethrocele without a sphincter plication, but if there is an appreciable degree of incontinence, plication more certainly assures success. It is our custom, in all of the cases in which we plicate for incontinence, to plicate from the internal sphincter region forward for the entire length of the urethra. Circular muscle fibers are found for the full length of the urethra and may be used to advantage in restoring bladder control.

In the second group of cases, where there is no demonstrable urethrocele or cystourethrocele, the incontinence depends upon scarring which has resulted from the obstetric injury or previous surgery of the anterior vaginal wall. If one does a sufficient number of operations for cystocele on women without preoperative stress incontinence, sooner or later one will encounter a case in which stress incontinence follows the surgery. As a result of scar tissue forming in the sphincter region, the muscle is prevented from closing normally. When the sphincter action is observed from within through a cystoscope, incomplete and irregular closure may be observed, because the sphincter is prevented from a normal concentric closure by the scars. One also may see this same picture through the cystoscope in cases of the first group after an unsuccessful attempt at repair. In repairing this condition we have had some success by dissecting more completely around the circumference of the urethra, perhaps two thirds of the way, leaving only the superior attachment of the urethra intact before plicating the urethra. In this manner an attempt is made to release scars which prevent complete sphincter closure. However, one is not always successful in restoring continence by this operation, and in recent years we have treated this group of cases with some type of Goebell-Stoeckel operation, especially if the incontinence is marked.

There is a third group of women who have stress incontinence, who have had no children and in whom no faulty nervous mechanism can be demonstrated. These women are usually elderly, but on rare occasions we have seen the condition in young, nulliparous women. In elderly women there is apparently a loss of muscle tone, although the cause of this is not clear. In this nulliparous group a plication of the sphincter and the urethra for its full length is done with success in some instances, but the results are not as satisfactory as in the group in which the incontinence results from childbirth. Therefore in this group we have recently performed a Goebell-Stoeckel type of operation as the primary procedure when the incontinence is marked.

There is yet a fourth group of women who have stress incontinence resulting from the use of the resectoscope on the female vesical neck. Caulk reported on the treatment of contracture of the vesical neck in women by means of the cautery punch. Later, Folsom became very enthusiastic about the procedure for a condition which he referred to as female prostatism. From his writings one gets the impression that he considered female prostatism almost as frequent as the disease in the male. He even regarded some of the tissue removed by the resectoscope as being histologically consistent with prostatic tissue. The senior author had the opportunity of examining some of this tissue and could not concur in this diagnosis. As a result of his writing, urologists have more and more been using the resectoscope in the region of the vesical sphincter, chiefly in cases of chronic urinary infection associated with some residual urine. In our experiences in female urology at Hopkins we have failed to find the need of using the resectoscope at the vesical neck in women except in a few cases of neoplastic involvement from pelvic malignancy. However, we have encountered valves in the female urethra in children with persistent urinary tract infections as reported by Brack which are removed successfully by the resectoscope. Urologists have been using the resectoscope with increasing frequency, and we as gynecologists are seeing an increasing number of incontinent women from this procedure. In some instances the incontinence is of the stress type, and in others it is constant and almost complete. In a few cases there have actually been fistulas at the sphincter region. In 1948 Everett reported 5 cases of incontinence resulting from this procedure, and we have seen several more since then.

Technic: Operation for Urethrocele and Plication of Vesical Sphincter for Stress Incontinence of Urine

Figure 25-7 A shows the urethrocele for which this operation is done. The bulging is confined to that part of the vagina beneath the urethra and the trigone of the bladder. There is no herniation whatever of the bladder beyond the region of the trigone.

After making a midline incison through the vaginal mucosa extending from the urethral meatus as far back as the urethrocele extends, the flaps of mucosa are dissected laterally. Beginning less than a

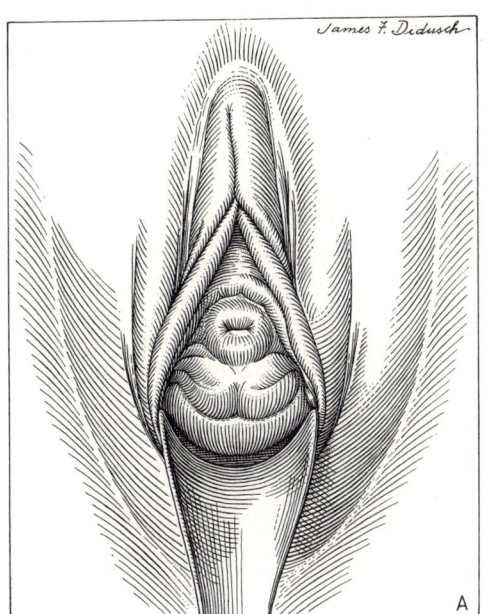
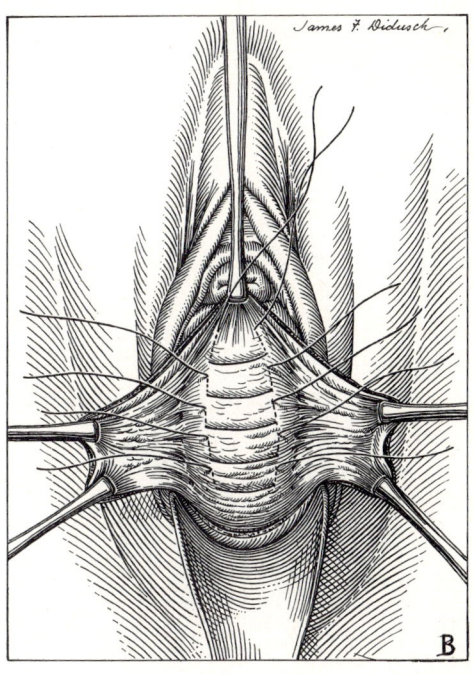
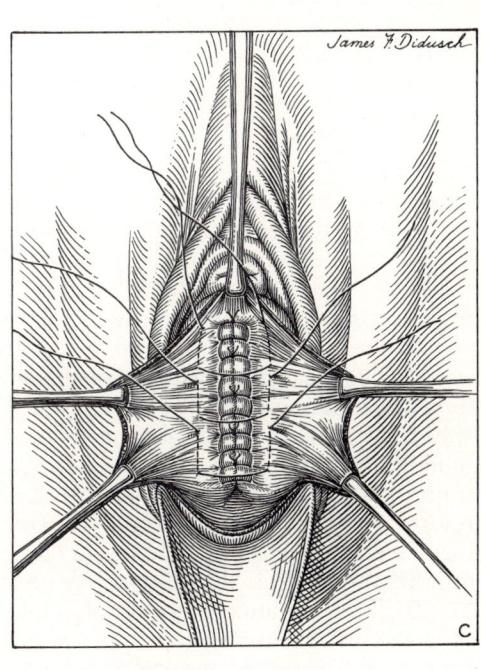

Fig. 25-7. Operation for urethrocele and stress incontinence of urine. (A) Shows urethrocele which was responsible for the stress incontinence. (B) A midline vaginal incision has been made about 4 cm. in length extending back from urethral meatus. Mattress plication stitches have been placed. (C) The entire urethra and sphincter region has been plicated with mattress sutures of medium silk. These sutures narrow the urethra and tighten the sphincter. A second row of slightly coarser stitches is placed through the fascia.

centimeter from the urethral meatus, a succession of mattress sutures is taken as indicated in Figure 25-7 B. These bites of tissue are taken on each side of the urethra and parallel with it. For these delicate sutures, medium silk and a thin curved needle should be used. The sutures are carried back to the trigonal region, past the point of junction of the urethra and the bladder. This internal sphincter region is usually about 3 or 4 cm. from the urethral meatus. It may be

546 Urethrocele, Cystocele, and Stress Incontinence of Urine

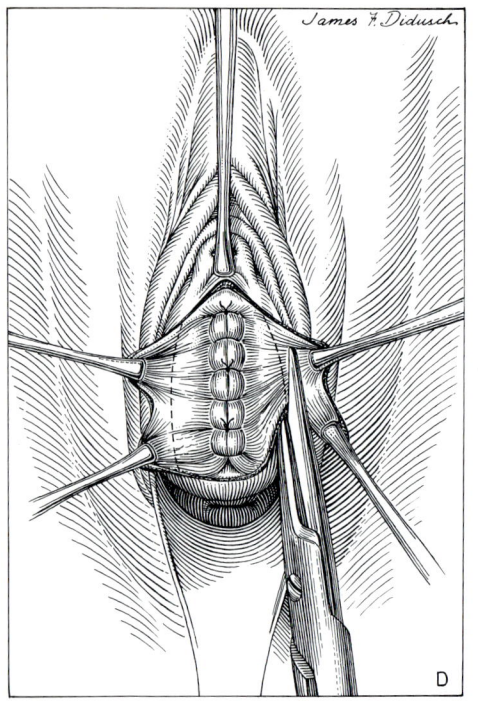 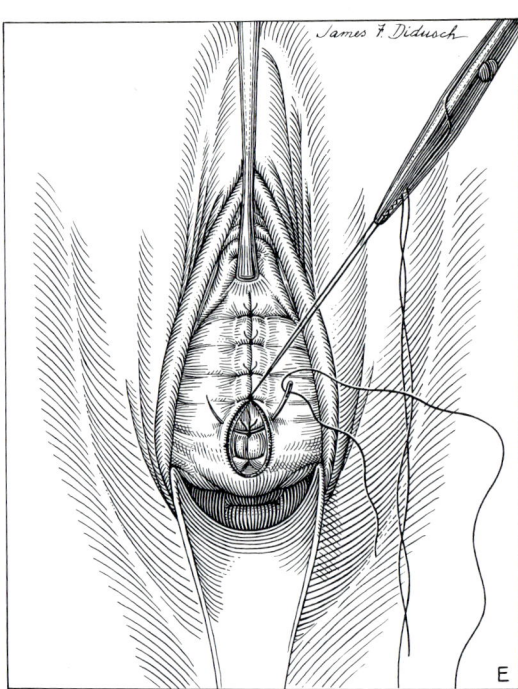

Fig. 25-7 (*Continued*). Operation for urethrocele and stress incontinence of urine. (D) The fascia sutures have been tied, giving support to the urethra. Excess of mucosa is excised. (E) Vaginal incision is closed in the midline.

located exactly by inserting a Foley catheter in the bladder and withdrawing it, noting the point where it meet obstruction. After the internal sphincter region has been identified, the catheter should be withdrawn before tying the sutures, because its presence in the urethra interferes with the tightening of the sphincter and the urethral tube. It is our practice to tighten the entire urethral tube in addition to the internal sphincter region as originally described by Kelly, for there are circular muscular fibers around the urethra throughout its entire length, and advantage should be taken of these in improving the sphincter action. As these sutures are tied, the tissue between them is inverted by an assistant who makes slight pressure over the urethra in the midline with a Halsted clamp inserted from above as each suture is tied.

After this first layer of mattress sutures has been tied, a second row of mattress sutures is placed as indicated in Figure 25-7 C. This second layer approximates fibers of the pubovesicocervical fascia and forms a support upon which the urethral tube rests. No. 00 chromic catgut is used for this, and larger bites of tissue are taken than when placing the first row of plicating sutures (Fig. 25-7 C). If, as in the case illustrated, 5 bites are taken to plicate the span of the urethra and the sphincter, perhaps the fascia covering that same span can be brought together in 3 bites.

After this second layer has been tied, the excess of vaginal mucosa is excised (Fig. 25-7 D). Then the mucosa is approximated in the midline with interrupted stitches of No. 00 chromic catgut (Fig. 25-7 E). It is a good plan to pick up a bite of the subjacent fascia with a few of these sutures to close any possible dead space beneath the mucosa.

This operation may be done alone or in combination with the operation for cystocele.

RESULTS

The plication operation as above described has been used extensively by us with generally good results. Ninety per cent of the patients reported complete continence; 5 per cent were improved; and 5 per cent unimproved.

When this follow-up was done, many of the patients had been operated upon several years before, but others only recently. Counseller found that the percentage of successes declined to 70 with the passage of time. We have no figures on this phase of the subject, but it is true that it is not uncommon to encounter patients who have developed some degree of leakage after years of continence from plication. In this connection we should mention Kegel's reported success with perineal exercises. He has devised and used a perineometer, an instrument for registering muscle contractions and restoring tone to the vagina. Our experience with this has not been great or very successful. We have not found many women very enthusiastic about practicing perineal contraction for 20 minutes 3 times a day as recommended by Kegel. Our patients have preferred to have the relative minor surgical procedure done with an excellent prospect of success.

BIBLIOGRAPHY

Bissell, D.: Cystocele: Overlapping of the fascia of the posterior vaginal wall for cure of rectocele. Amer. J. Obstet., 78:1, 1919.

Brack, C. B., and Guild, H. G.: Urethral obstruction in the female child. Amer. J. Obstet. Gynec., 76:1105, 1958.

Caulk, J. R.: Contractures of vesical neck in the female. J. Urol., 6:341, 1921.

Counseller, V.: Urinary incontinence in women. Amer. J. Obstet. Gynec., 45:479, 1943.

Curtis, Arthur H. (ed.): Obstetrics and Gynecology. vol. 3, p. 53. Philadelphia, Saunders, 1933.

Everett, Houston S.: Gynecological and Obstetrical Urology. Baltimore, Williams & Wilkins, 1944.

———: A condemnation of resectoscopic procedures upon the female vesical neck. Urol. Cutan. Rev., 52:80, 1948.

Folsom, A. I., and Obrien, H. A.: The female urethra. J.A.M.A., 128:408, 1945.

Kegel, A. H.: Progressive resistance exercise in the functional restoration of the perineal muscles. Amer. J. Obstet. Gynec., 56:238, 1948.

Kelly, Howard A.: Operative Gynecology. vol. 1, p. 375. New York, Appleton, 1909.

———: Incontinence of urine in women. Urol. Cutan. Rev., 17:291, 1913.

Kelly, H. A., and Dumm, W. M.: Urinary incontinence in women, without manifest injury to the bladder: A report of cases. Surg. Gynec. Obstet., 18:444, 1914.

Pawlick, Karl: Beiträge zur Chirurgie der weiblichen Harnröhre; I. Herstellung der Kontinenz der weiblichen Blase. Wien. med. Wchnschr., 33:769, 1883.

26

Urinary Incontinence Not Curable by Sphincter Plication

JOHN H. RIDLEY, M.D.*

Although a great majority of cases of stress incontinence of urine can be cured by plication of the sphincter and the urethra, as described previously, there are some failures, and one must look to another method for curing them. Especially is failure apt to result in those cases unrelated to childbirth injury in which the poor sphincter musculature has insufficient tone to control the urine when the intravesical pressure is raised. Often failure with the plication operation in good hands is the result of previous bungling attempts, with resulting scar tissue, making it impossible for the sphincter to contract adequately, regardless of how tightly it is plicated.

Congenital absence of sphincter mechanism associated with a completely formed urethral tube is rare but does occur. In such cases it is possible that circular musculature is present but uninnervated; however, there is no demonstrable evidence of other neurologic defects. Such cases cannot be cured by sphincter plication; consequently, some other type of mechanism for urinary control must be devised.

In another group of cases the urethra is congenitally defective or absent due to variable degrees of epispadias. The formation of a urethral tube is of no value unless some sphincter mechanism can be devised.

Destruction of all or part of the urethra by obstetric injury necessitates the construction of, or the repair of, a urethra, but often in such cases one is unable to repair the sphincter musculature sufficiently to restore continence.

Finally, there is a group in which the incontinence depends upon faulty innervation. The commonest congenital defect in the nervous mechanism is found in connection with spina bifida. Among the acquired lesions are cord tumor, tabes dorsalis, transverse myelitis, multiple sclerosis, and traumatic lesions of the cord. It is important to obtain as much data as possible upon the exact nature of the nerve defect in order to attempt intelligent correction. Kennedy devised an instrument for taking urethrograms which demonstrates the degree of sphincter failure. Barnes obtained satisfactory information by using a device simpler than Kennedy's. It was formed from 2 finger cots connected with a reservoir of strong sodium iodide. The bladder is filled with 180 cc. of 8 per cent sodium iodide solution, after which the balloon is placed in the urethra. The pressure in the balloon is maintained at 35 cm. of water. Weakness of the urethral sphincters is demonstrated by their inability to compress the balloon. This can be demonstrated by roentgenograms. By varying the pressure in the balloon and noting the ability of the sphincter to compress it, the exact degree of sphincter action is demonstrated.

One should be very careful in selecting

---

* Associate Clinical Professor, Department of Obstetrics and Gynecology, Emory University.

cases for surgery with neurologic disease. Cystometric studies should be made to determine the intravesical pressure, since increased intravesical pressure may give rise to incontinence when the sphincter mechanism is normal. If sphincter tone is demonstrated to be normal, and if the intravesical tone is increased, obviously no surgical procedure directed at the sphincter will be of any value. Also, if a cystogram shows reflux up the ureters, indicating faulty valve action at the ureterovesical junction, probably it is poor judgment to attempt to give that individual a vesical sphincter. We have learned from experience with a few such cases that obstructing the outlow of urine from the bladder may result in too much back pressure on the kidneys and predispose the patient to recurring attacks of pyelitis. On two occasions we were forced to break down the newly formed sphincter to stop the recurring attacks of pyelitis. Of course, in all neurologic cases an attempt should be made to correct the underlying condition, but unfortunately this is often impossible.

In all of the above groups of cases the surgeon must seek elsewhere than the vesical neck and the urethra to create a mechanism effective in the control of the urine. Many operations have been devised, none of which has been universally successful, although some can be used to advantage in certain cases. A short summary of these attempts may be useful to the student of incontinence of urine in women.

HISTORICAL DEVELOPMENT OF OPERATIVE PROCEDURES

In 1907 Giordano utilized a portion of the gracilis muscle to encircle the urethra. Deming in 1926 reported that he restored continence by this means in a woman in whom a urethral tube had been constructed previously because of epispadias.

In 1910 Goebell described an operation in which he dissected free the pyramidalis muscles, brought them down posterior to the symphysis, and encircled the urethra near its junction with the bladder. He suggested crossing the muscles if their length permits. He reported one case in which this operation was done after constructing a urethra in a child suffering from epispadias. A second operation of this type was done on a 2-year-old child who was incontinent following an operation for meningocele. In both cases the results were reported as satisfactory. An obvious difficulty with this operation lies in the fact that the pyramidalis muscles vary greatly in their development and may be too short to encircle the urethra.

In 1911 Squier utilized the transversus perinei and the levator ani muscles to restore continence to a man whose sphincter had been cut at a previous surgical operation. He reported success. Taussig also utilized the right levator ani muscle in a case in which the urethra had been destroyed at delivery. A flap of vaginal mucosa was turned forward for the formation of a new urethra. A portion of the right levator ani muscle, which had been dissected free, was transposed beneath the base of the bladder and sutured to the left pubic fascia. A purse-string suture was placed about the urethra, picking up the levator fibers so that when the purse-string was drawn tight, muscle fibers were drawn in a crescentic form beneath and partially around the urethra.

In 1914 Frangenheim utilized the pyramidalis muscle with an attached strip of fascia from the sheath of the rectus to encircle the male urethra. The strap was brought down retropubicly around the urethra and was sutured to itself. The operation was done for incontinence following a perineal injury with stricture formation. The result was reported as perfect.

In 1917 Stoeckel combined the use of the pyramidalis muscle and the fascia strip with a plication at the sphincter region. He first dissected from the midline a strip of fascia with the pyramidalis muscles attached. The distal portion of the strip was split and brought down retropubicly to the urethral region. The split ends were made to encircle the urethra and were sutured together below the urethra. He reported 2 cases treated successfully. In the first case a fistula had resulted from a vaginal cesarean section. After closure of the fistula the patient was still incontinent. By combining sphincter plication with the use of the pyramidalis muscle and the fascia strip, the patient was cured. The second case was one of a urethrocystocele associated with incontinence. The combination operation resulted in cure.

In 1932 Norman Miller modified the technic of the Goebell-Frangenheim-Stoeckel operation by bringing the pyramidalis muscle with an attached fascia strap down to and beneath the urethra anterior to the symphysis. Apparently the object of this modification was to avoid the possibility of retropubic hemorrhage, particularly from the paraurethral venous sinus frequently encountered at the bladder neck. However, it should be noted that the bleeding encountered by Miller's procedure may be most troublesome about the clitoris. In addition, the fascia strap was placed too far forward of the urethrovesical junction to be most effective. Thus the procedure never gained wide acceptance. As will be described subsequently, we have encountered only very little difficulty from bleeding in the process of placing the fascia strap retropubically.

In 1933 Price reported the cure of urinary incontinence in a girl with congenital absence of the sacrum and the coccyx and without innervation of the sphincter. He used a sling of autogenous fascia lata which he brought around the urethra retropubically and then attached both ends to the rectus muscle. The principles of this technic with subsequent modification have been used as a most dependable procedure and will be described in detail later in this chapter.

In 1942 Aldridge devised a modification in which he combined some of the points of the Goebell-Frangenheim-Stoeckel procedure with those of Price's. Making a transverse lower abdominal incision, he developed strips of aponeurosis from the rectus sheath on both sides. He directed his incisions for the procurement of these fascia strips outward and upward, paralleling the fibers of the aponeurosis (Fig. 26-1). The fascia straps were detached laterally and the free ends brought down through the rectus muscles, then retropubicly, finally passing

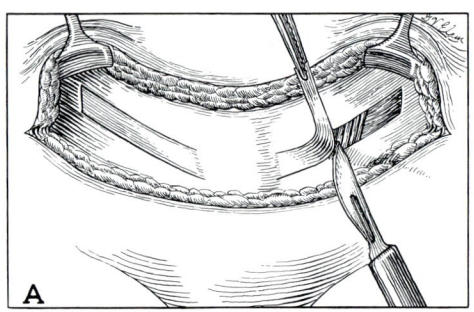

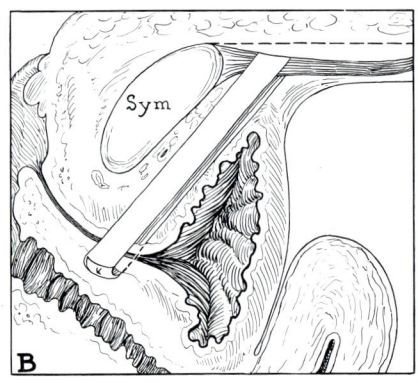

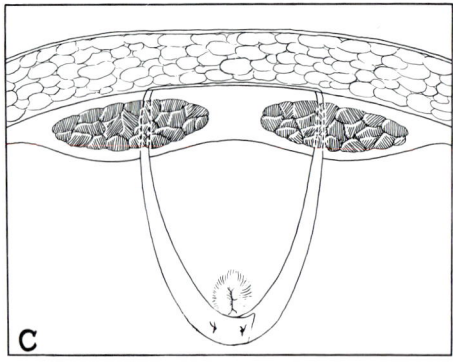

Fig. 26-1. Aldridge modification of Goebell-Frangenheim-Stoeckel operation for urinary incontinence. (A) The fascial strips are being separated through a Pfannenstiel incision. (B) The fascial strips are shown in position around the posterior portion of the urethra. Dotted line indicates position of rectus muscles when contracted. (C) Diagram indicating sling-like action of the fascial strips.

beneath the urethra. He depended upon the elasticity of the rectus muscle to afford the proper pull on the urethra.

In 1949 Wilfred Shaw, of London, described an operation in which a broad strip of fascia lata is transplanted beneath the entire length of the urethra and bladder base. Holes are drilled through the pubic bones bilaterally, and the ends of the fascial slings are pulled through these holes. The ends of the sling are sutured with catgut to the tendinous tissue in the vicinity of the holes, with the desired amount of tension on the sling. He reports 51 persons operated upon by this method, with 1 death. Thirty-five of these patients with simple stress incontinence were cured.

In the same year Marshall, Marchetti, and Krantz reported an entirely new operation which they had carried out on 50 patients, 38 with the usual type of stress incontinence, 25 of whom had had a total of 40 standard gynecologic operations without relief. The procedure consisted of simple operative elevation and fixation of the vesical neck and the urethra by suturing them to pubic periosteum and rectus muscles by the suprapubic route with chromic catgut. Figure 26-10 demonstrates the operation quite clearly. They report 82 per cent of the cases as having excellent results. Later refinement of technic and preoperative evaluation of the patient have improved these results.

In search for the perfect material to be used in the sling procedure, operators have used practically every conceivable type, and, as yet, no completely satisfactory agent has been found. Generally speaking, the autogenous materials, such as fascia, have functioned most dependably and with least tissue reaction. The use of foreign tissues such as ox fascia or collagen has not proven satisfactory. The use of the synthetic polyester fibers such as dacron (mersilene) at first seemed to be the final answer because of the availability of the material and the facility with which it could be used. However, contrary to the success reported for its use in other areas of the body, it has proved to be unsatisfactory and is condemned in its use in the sling procedures. Williams and Te Linde in 1962 reported with guarded enthusiasm the use of mersilene in the sling procedure, but later condemned its use as longer periods of observation were made. Ridley in 1966 reported its use in 17 cases with 4 subsequent rather serious complications. Thus it has been concluded that this material is unsatisfactory and is condemned for further use.

The more recent literature is replete with many modifications of the three basic technics for correction of stress urinary incontinence: (1) the Kelly repair-plication procedure (described fully in preceding chapter), (2) the sling procedure, and (3) the urethral repositioning (urethropexy) procedure. Only time and experience will serve to evaluate them; however, the general principles of correction of stress urinary incontinence remain the same despite the passing parade of various procedures. As the understanding of stress urinary incontinence increases, the likelihood of a much more successful procedure increases, but thus far there remains the apparently irreducible number of failures resulting from any procedure. Individual surgeons will select the type of procedure in which they are most proficient and successful, and will use this specific procedure in the great majority of their cases. However, surgeons should not limit the choice of procedure inflexibly and try to fit all cases into one particular type of operation to the exclusion of the others.

More recent contributions have been by Green, Ball, Ingelmann-Sundberg, Pereyra, and Gunther. However, the percentage of failures and the incidence of complications remains about constant. In this chapter our recommendations will be based upon our experience.

CHOICE OF OPERATION

When the surgeon considers whether surgery is indicated and what is to be his choice of operation, there are many facets to be considered. In particular and within the scope of this chapter, which is concerned primarily with cases in which stress urinary incontinence has not been cured by sphincter plication, he must consider why the first efforts have failed. Although the expected percentage of success, whether it be cured or tolerably improved by the Kelly plication, is appreciably high, the failures must nevertheless be cared for by more sophisticated study and procedures. It is believed that the Kelly plication technic, with its simplicity, safety, and degree of success, should in the great majority of cases be the first effort. There is an exception to this rule, however, in those cases of incontinence in women, often elderly, without anterior vaginal wall relaxation. In these cases the incontinence is apparently due to poor sphincter muscle tone and tissue weakness as a result of advancing years. Little or nothing can be expected from tightening these poor muscles. Hence, in such cases which are sufficiently severe to require correction, we have proceeded directly with the sling procedure.

The Johns Hopkins Hospital through the years, and with periodic updating of the records, shows roughly 90 per cent cured, 5 per cent improved, and 5 per cent failure. Other clinics of large patient loads have reported from 70 per cent to 85 per cent success. It seems that overall we may expect from 80 per cent to 85 per cent success with the properly done Kelly plication. Counseller, Brewer, and others have noted that the rate of success will gradually decline as years pass from the time of the performance of the plication, suggesting recurring tissue failure. Hence it becomes obvious that we must find muscular support elsewhere than from the damaged sphincter to give these women continence. Green and others have stressed the importance of the urethrovesical angle in relation to incontinence. More recent studies by Greenwald, Thornburg, and Dunn have cast doubt on the importance of this angle. They found the same demonstrable deformities in approximately 65 per cent of 17 patients who had no stress incontinence. Our own experience coincides more nearly with that of Greenwald, Thornburg, and Dunn.

We have seen various types of angles in women with incontinence and with perfect control. The percentage of "normal" and "abnormal" angles in patients with and without control are such as to cause us to conclude that the angle is not the essential factor. It is true that by plication and by the sling the angle is changed, but we are induced to believe that this is incidental, and that the factor which restores continence is the suburethral support in the region of the urethrovesical junction.

Our conclusions, however, do not mitigate the importance and necessity of a thorough evaluation of the condition preoperatively. Of greatest importance is the history, making certain that we are dealing with true stress incontinence rather than incontinence due to excessive urge. The knowledge of the type of previous surgery is important. Previous surgery often results in excessive scar tissue in the operative region, which is apt to make the contemplated surgery more difficult, but it does not rule out a further attempt, as we have cured many women with badly scarred urethras by means of a sling. Hence it is of interest to note that a large percentage of women with stress incontinence were cured empirically years before we had the more complete understanding of the phenomenon that we have today.

In not a few instances it is well to combine one of the strap procedures with cystocele repair and plication of the suburethral fascia. When this is done, it is well to complete first the placing of the fascial strips beneath the urethra and then to bury them beneath the suburethral fascia. In this manner the transplanted fascial strips are less liable to infection from the vagina than if they lie more superficially.

When there is a scar of a previous midline incision, one should not choose an operation requiring the use of a midline fascial strap. Similarly, when the lateral fascia is scarred by a broad rectus or McBurney scar, the Aldridge lateral straps should be avoided. When a urethra has been made previously by a plastic operation and sphincter action is to be attempted, it is unwise to cut into the suburethral vaginal mucosa for fear of entering the urethral lumen. In such instances a single long strap of fascia from the midline or fascia lata may best be used in a U-shaped manner as indicated in Figure 26-8, so that a tunnel is made between the vaginal and the urethral mucosa with a small thin-bladed knife.

Our experience and results with the Marshall-Marchetti-Krantz procedure have been favorable, and in many instances in which concomitant intra-abdominal pathology exists, it has been first choice, thus sparing a combined abdominovaginal procedure. It should be noted here that in the event of failure of the Marshall-Marchetti-Krantz procedure, our choice for the "ultimate effort," regardless of what other procedures have failed previously, is the sling procedure. This conclusion has also been put forth by Marchetti and Green. We have had a great number of successes with the sling after Marshall-Marchetti-Krantz operation failures, but we should not like to give the impression that we consider only the sling procedure after the Marshall-Marchetti-Krantz failures. In most instances we proceed to the sling procedure following plication failures unless intra-abdominal pathology necessitates an abdominal incision. With increasing experience and success with the fascia lata sling and with the Aldrige modification using the abdominal aponeurosis, we have favored the Goebell-Frangenheim-Stoeckel procedure more and more. Our results have been quite successful except in some neurologic cases in which the operation was done early in our experience against indication which we now more readily recognize through more careful preoperative screening.

PREOPERATIVE EVALUATION OF THE BLADDER

Regardless of what choice is made to try to correct the case of intractable stress urinary incontinence, there seems to be the irreducible minimum which defy correction. Some of these can be identified by careful screening, and operation upon these types is obviously contraindicated. The most serious condition which can indeed be aggravated by the improper choice of procedure is the atonic or otherwise neurologicly impaired bladder. On all cases of stress urinary incontinence in which any procedure other than the simple Kelly plication is contemplated, it has been our routine to perform a cystometrogram to evaluate the bladder dynamics and capacity. This procedure is done without anesthesia and can be performed satisfactorily in the office. Whereas a Lewis Recording Cystometer is desirable, it is not absolutely necessary to have one to evaluate the bladder properly. Ridley has shown a simple technic for evaluation of the bladder as an office procedure. Again we emphasize that a careful history should be taken, particularly noting any previous surgery of the genitourinary tract and the exact subjective complaints of the patient.

The patient is allowed to void, and this specimen is saved for chemical analysis. With the patient on the examining table in dorsolithotomy position, the vulva and urethral meatus are properly prepared, using an aqueous solution of Zephiran 1:750 (benzalkonium chloride), and a medium-sized straight metal catheter is carefully inserted into the urethra. By experience it can be noted what the degree of inclination of the urethra is to the axis of the symphysis; if the catheter passes into the bladder horizontally or with the inserted tip inclined upward, the relationship of the urethra to the symphysis axis is roughly normal, and the urethra is probably continent. Conversely, if the inserted tip points downward and away from the horizontal, it can be assumed that the urethra has rotated downward from the axis of the symphysis, suggesting ineffectual urethral support. In this type of deformity we would expect improvement with proper supporting reconstruction such as we have obtained with the sling procedure. This is only an approximation, but we find that it makes it unnecessary to perform routine chain cystourethrograms. The amount of residual urine is measured as the catheterization is completed. This amount of urine—and there is usually sufficient amount under any circumstances—is saved for microscopic examination, culture, and sensitivity tests. Next, a Foley No. 20 F with a 5-cc. balloon is inserted for tests of bladder capacity and dynamics. This catheter is connected to a graduate flask hanging about 36 inches above the symphysis, and increments of 50 cc. of normal saline lightly tinted with methylene blue are allowed to gravitate into the bladder. The patient is not apprehensive or uncomfortable if a detailed explanation has been given to her of the planned procedure. Allowing 10 seconds between influx of the increments of normal saline, a careful record is kept of how much saline is allowed to flow in. The end point of the test comes when the patient has a true urgency and is just beginning to have spasm for micturition. A note is made of the amount of saline used, and the bladder is now promptly allowed to begin to drain. It has been determined that if the patient will tolerate only 150 cc. or less of the saline solution, we are dealing usually with urge incontinence, a bladder of chronic spasm (Hunner's ulcer), or of decreased capacity due to fibrosis. Any amount over 300 to 600 cc. is classified as normal, and amounts over 600 cc. suggest bladder atony or some neurologic impairment.

To test further for the amount of stress urinary incontinence, approximately 250 cc. of the saline is allowed to remain in the bladder, and the Foley catheter is removed. The patient is now asked to give a firm cough while the urethra and evidence of leakage are being observed with the patient in the lithotomy and standing positions. The Marchetti or "stress" test of evaluation of the anterior vaginal wall without compression of the urethra is done. The vaginal mucosa in the region of the urethrovesical junction is infiltrated with a wheal of local anesthetic agent just lateral to the midline on either side. This area is grasped with an Allis clamp on either side of the urethra to avoid compression, and the structures are gently thrust upward and backward to a more retropubic position. It is possible also similarly to reposition the urethrovesical junction retropubicly with the index and middle fingers without compression of the urethra to make the Marchetti test. The patient is now asked to cough firmly again. If there is no longer any leakage with this effort, one may assume that repositioning the urethra by supporting it with a sling or by retropubic urethropexy should improve or cure the stress incontinence. All of this evaluation can be done easily and quickly at one appointment. If the patient has a history of chronic or recurring urinary tract infection or lithiasis, or if the bladder studies just completed are not within normal limits, then the whole urinary tract must be further evaluated by excretory and retrograde urography and endoscopy.

The choice of operation for the correction of stress urinary incontinence must be even more refined if there exists extraordinary scarring from previous surgery, neoplasm, or treatment thereof, or congenital deformities. Search for irregularities of closure and anatomy

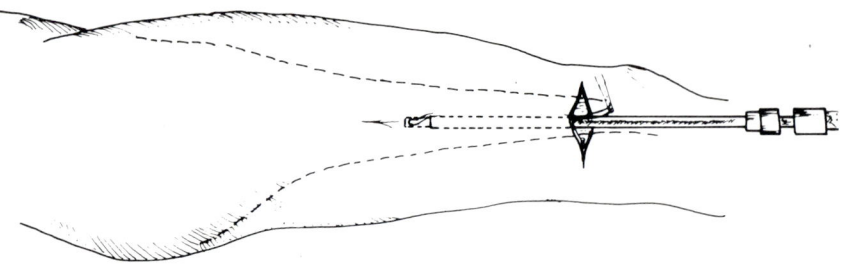

Fig. 26-2. Method of getting fascial strip.

through the air cystoscope, water cystoscope, or by indirect air cystoscopy may be helpful in determining this.

Another example is the aged patient who has undergone previous colpocleisis for procedentia in whom a suprapubic approach could not effectively elevate the urethra and bladder neck, but the sling procedure could.

Still another example is one in which the patient has had previous surgery for construction of a congenitally or surgically absent urethra, or in which there has been a successful repair of a vesicovaginal or vesicourethrovaginal fistula. The sling procedure using a split fascia lata strap (transected and bilateral) would be chosen. The technic of these procedures among others which were considered most useful are given in detail below.

OPERATIVE PROCEDURES

Technic: The Goebell-Frangenheim-Stoeckel Procedure Using the Fascia Lata Strap

This technic has become the more dependable, the easiest, and thus the most frequently used by us as the years have gone by. Procurement of the fascia lata is quick and simple:

The patient is placed on the table in the supine position, with either thigh surgically prepared by shaving and cleaning. The site of incision is optional depending on the patient's desire for a less likely visible scar or the gynecologist's desire for the easiest approach to and procurement of the fascia. The incision just above the lateral condyle of the femur has been used most frequently (Fig. 26-2). A 2- to 3-inch incision is made at right angles to the direction of the fibers of the fascia lata. The fascia is stripped of fat as well as possible with the gauzed finger, and the fascia is split by 2 incisions 1 cm. apart in the direction parallel to the course of the fibers (Fig. 26-3). This strap is now transected 1 cm. superior to its inferior attachment, and this free end is threaded through the eye of the Masson fascia stripper (other equally simple fascia strippers are available) (Fig. 26-3). The fascia stripper is then thrust firmly and evenly cephalad beneath the skin until it can go no further. The strap thus excised is cut by sliding the sheath over the inner tube of the

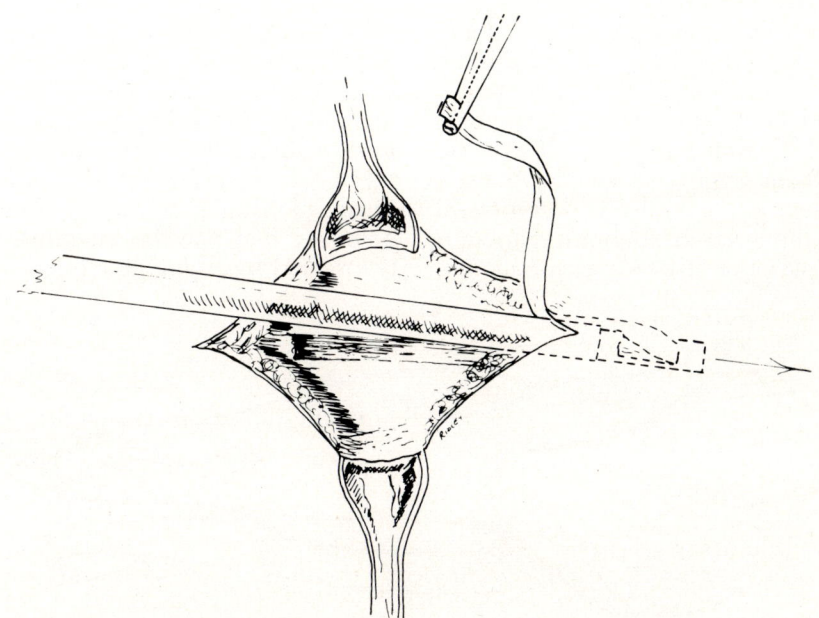

Fig. 26-3. Method of action of Masson fascial stripper.

stripper and the strap removed. An additional strap of fascia lata can be taken at the same time if there is any doubt about the sufficiency of the first excision. The fascial defect within sight beneath the incision is closed with 2 or 3 interrupted sutures of 000 chromic catgut and the skin closed per routine. An elastic compression bandage may be applied over the thigh if there is any evidence of bleeding, which is exceedingly rare in this procedure.

It is here emphasized that the procurement of the fascia strap is easy and quick. It can be done through either the incision described above or one just inferior to the greater trochanter of the femur. Because the fascia lata fibers fan out from below upward (Fig. 26-4), it is thought that the strap cut from below upward is one of more uniform width and strength, thus facilitating its removal. Only rarely will the patient complain of any pain in the thigh postoperatively, and no complications have been encountered. On the contrary, however, there is a chance, although relatively infrequent in the Aldridge technic, that the patient may develop an incisional hernia at the sites where the fascia straps have been developed from the anterior abdominal aponeurosis (Fig. 26-1).

The patient is now changed to a dorsolithotomy position and appropriately cleaned and draped, in order that a combined field of the lower abdomen and perineum is simultaneously accessible. A 7- to 10-cm. transverse incision is made 3 cm. above the symphysis down to the fibers of the anterior abdominal aponeurosis. If previous lower abdominal incisions have been made, the underlying fascia may be somewhat distorted or obscured by scarring, but with care it can be identified. Two small slit-like incisions about 1 cm. in length are made 2 cm. above the symphysis and 2 cm. to either side of the midline and parallel to the direction of the aponeurotic fibers. With finger dissection or blunt instrument dissection, the muscle bellies of the rectus abdominis are split, and the finger is thrust into the space of Retzius to either side of the midline. The wound is lightly packed with a wet saline sponge and the operative site shifted to the vagina.

The anterior vaginal wall is incised in the midline about 1 cm. posterior to the external urethral meatus over the entire length of the urethra. The incision is carried to the level of the cervix if anterior colporrhaphy is also needed. The sphincter area may be more easily determined by an indwelling balloon catheter. The subjacent vaginal fascia is dissected and developed as described in the section on colporrhaphy. One of the great advantages of the sling procedure is that any necessary vaginal surgery can be done in conjunction with the vaginal portion of the operation. In some cases Kelly plication sutures are well taken concomitantly. Again by the use of finger dissection, a shallow tunnel is developed on either side of the urethra marked by the indwelling No. 16 F balloon catheter, beneath and posterior to the inferior surface of the pubic rami. Most of the potentially troublesome bleeding that may be encountered here is avoided by blunt dissection reflecting

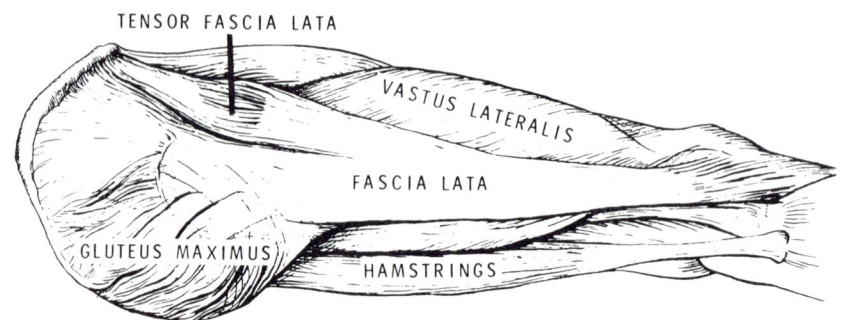

Fig. 26-4. Fanning of fascia lata.

the tissues from lateralward to medialward toward the bladder neck.

A uterine dressing forceps with a medium blunt end is of proper curvature for gently thrusting retropubicly from above downward. The tip of the clamp (Fig. 26-5 D) is passed through the slit-like openings of the anterior aponeurosis retropubicly downward until the instrument tip can be palpated in the shallow retropubic tunnel on that side of the urethra. The tip still closed is gently thrust through this resisting tissue, the urogenital diaphragm, to present into the vaginal incision. A small slit over the point of the clamp with a scalpel may be necessary to facilitate this passage. The tip of the clamp with the concave curve toward the symphysis is pressed gently against the posterior surface of the bone as it is passed downward, thus minimizing the chance for injury to the bladder or opening the venous sinuses which lie in the space of Retzius near the bladder neck. By using this technic and gentle pressure, bleeding is unlikely to occur. If it does, it is usually of venous origin and can be controlled by gentle pressure. The tip of the strap of fascia lata is grasped through the vaginal incision and drawn retropubicly. It is attached firmly with 2 or 3 sutures of 3-0 silk to the anterior sheath of the rectus, thus also closing securely the slit-like incision previously made.

The process of the passage of the uterine dressing forceps (or long Kelly clamp) retropubicly into the vaginal field is repeated on the other side, and the other free end of the strap of fascia lata is drawn upward, without twisting, to be attached to the anterior abdominal aponeurosis at the contralateral incision previously made. Thus a continuous sling is formed beneath the urethra, and appropriate tension is applied before this strap of fascia lata is firmly attached to the abdominal fascia. The operator must check to be sure that the strap has been passed *beneath* the urethra near its juncture with the bladder, and that no injury has occurred before final fixation of the strap is done.

"Appropriate" tension of the sling beneath the urethra must be more fully described. The most frequent mistake of the beginner or less experienced operator to get the sling *too tight*, thus truly obstructing the urethra. It is only necessary to support the bladder neck. There can be no hard and fast rule about what tension to apply on the strap, but it can be safely said that gentle support is desired rather than obstructing or distorting force.

With the patient in this dorsolithotomy operating position, it may be valuable to note what relative inclination the urethra has to the horizontal. As has been mentioned in preoperative evaluation of the bladder, a rough estimate of correct anatomic position may be gotten by inserting a straight metal catheter into the bladder. It has been noted that proper supportive tension of the sling will bring the catheter tip at least to horizontal or above the horizontal with a retropubic inclination. A further test is made by filling the bladder with 300 or 400 cc. of sterile water and applying gentle suprapubic pressure. There should be no leakage. Usually there is little or no obstruction to the passage of the metal catheter through the urethra after fastening the sling, but on withdrawal one might feel a slight jump as the catheter tip passes the point of support by the sling. Again we say "gentle support" rather than obstructing force. This support is actually augmented and the so-called angle further corrected by gravity as the patient later assumes a sitting or an erect position.

The abdominal incision is closed, and after the necessary vaginal repair work is completed, the vaginal incision is closed. The balloon retention catheter is left in the bladder and the vagina packed with Iodoform gauze for 24 hours.

TECHNIC: ALDRIDGE MODIFICATION OF THE SLING OPERATION

This operation is similar in principle to that just described using the fascia lata strap. However, the fascia sling is developing bilaterally from a portion of the anterior abdominal aponeurosis, parallel to Poupart's ligament and of sufficient length laterally to accommodate any depth of the symphysis and be joined beneath the urethra.

The patient is placed on the table as described in the previous operation, except that the abdomen is draped for a transverse incision.

A semicircular transverse lower abdominal incision is made through the panniculus; the aponeurosis is cleared of fat over an area about 1 inch wide; and bleeding is controlled.

The strips of fascia are cut on either side of sufficient length to be carried down retropubicly and encircle the urethra. The length of these strips, naturally, must be estimated and will vary, depending on the width of the symphysis pubis; but if they are carried up to the level of the anterior superior spines of the ilia, they will be of sufficient length, even though the symphysis is quite wide. The strips will be composed of the aponeurosis of both external and the internal oblique in the medial half, but the aponeurosis of the internal oblique laterally is replaced by muscle. Therefore the distal portion of the strap will be composed of external oblique fascia only. The straps are separated from the subjacent muscle and thus mobilized down to their bases. The medial end of each strip is left attached at about 1.5 cm. from the midline (Fig. 26-1). The incisions in the aponeuroses are then closed with continuous sutures of No. 0 chromic catgut; the fat is approximated with interrupted sutures of No. 000 chromic catgut; and the skin is closed with continuous fine silk, leaving a small unclosed space at the midportion of the incision. The fascia strips are placed in this space and covered with moist sponges. The closed portion of the abdominal wound is covered with sterile towels.

The operator is then seated for the vaginal portion of the operation. The labia minora are sutured laterally for good exposure, and a posterior retractor is placed in the vagina. An Allis clip is placed in the urethral meatus, and a second one in the midline on the vaginal wall about 6 cm. back from the first. A midline incision is then made through the vaginal mucosa, extending from about 1 cm. from the urethral meatus back for about 5 cm. The vaginal mucosa is dissected laterally.

Any dissection made lateral to the urethra must be done cautiously and with the fingertip, as described in the previous operation. The index finger of the left hand is placed to the patient's left side of the urethra with the indwelling balloon catheter. Then with a long uterine dressing forceps in the right hand, the space of Retzius is traversed from above downward until the tip is felt below. The handle of the clamp is kept pressed to the abdomen as the point is passed downward, thus enabling the operator more surely to keep its point gently against the periosteum of the posterior surface of the pubic bone and symphysis and so protect the bladder. If difficulty is encountered in the fascial plane of the urogenital diaphragm lateral to the urethra, a small cut with the scalpel directly over the tip of the clamp allows it to perforate. As the tip of the dressing forceps presents into the vaginal field, it is grasped by the tip of a similar clamp and pulled upward until the lower clamp can be made to grasp the free end of the fascial straps developed from the anterior abdominal aponeurosis. Now the free end of the fascia is drawn downward retropubicly into the vagina. The process is repeated on the patient's right side, the aponeurotic strips being carried downward to present into the vagina. The ends of the straps are overlapped slightly, and any excess is trimmed away after these ends have been securely joined with 3 or 4 interrupted sutures of medium silk. Care is taken to get the proper amount of tension on the straps to give the patient continence. This is tested by distending the bladder through a smooth metal catheter and making moderate supra-pubic pressure. If a cystourethrocele repair is to be done, it is completed at this point, and the fascia strips are buried beneath the suburethral fascia. The excess of mucosa is excised, and the vaginal wound is closed with interrupted sutures of No. 0 chromic catgut. The small midportion of the abdominal wound is then closed.

In only two instances has the author perforated the bladder, but no postoperative complications were encountered with the use of adequate drainage by indwelling catheter and suprapubic rubber drain. The two cases had been previously operated upon by the Marshall-Marchetti-Krantz procedure, and there was obliterative scarring in the space of Retzius. Both cases are now counted among the successful sling procedures.

TECHNIC: GOEBELL-FRANGENHEIM-STOECKEL PROCEDURE (ORIGINAL TECHNIC)

The technic of the original sling operation has been modified as years have passed, but the original technic may be chosen under certain circumstances in which the Aldridge modification is contraindicated or the operator does not choose to use the strap of fascia lata. Procurement of the fascia is here also done before the vaginal portion, and the abdominal incision is closed to minimize

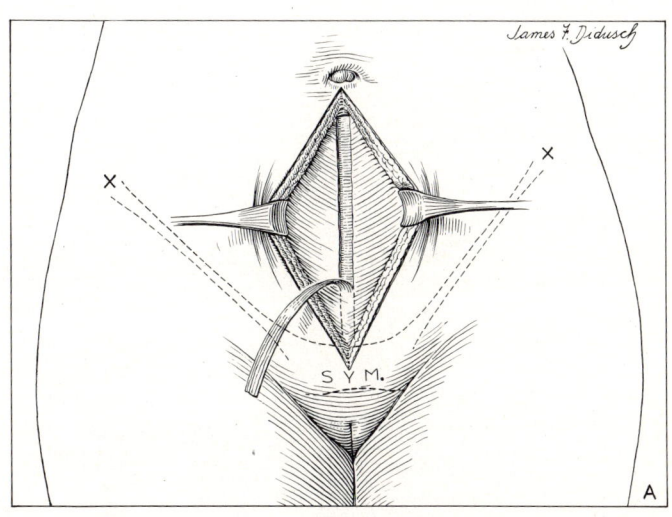

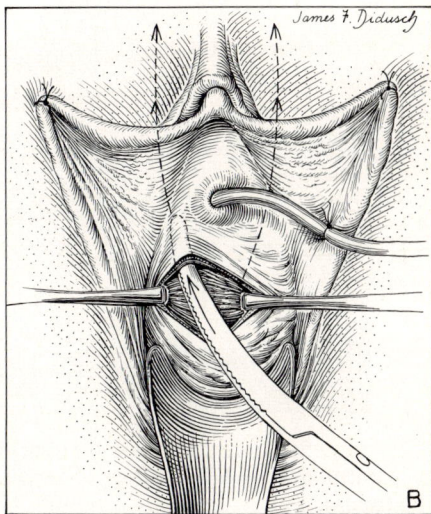

FIG. 26-5. Goebell-Frangenheim-Stoeckel operation for urinary incontinence. (A) A midline incision has been made, and a strip of fascia is excised. (B) A midline incision has been made through the vaginal mucosa, and the flaps dissected laterally. Arrows indicate direction of retropubic tunnels.

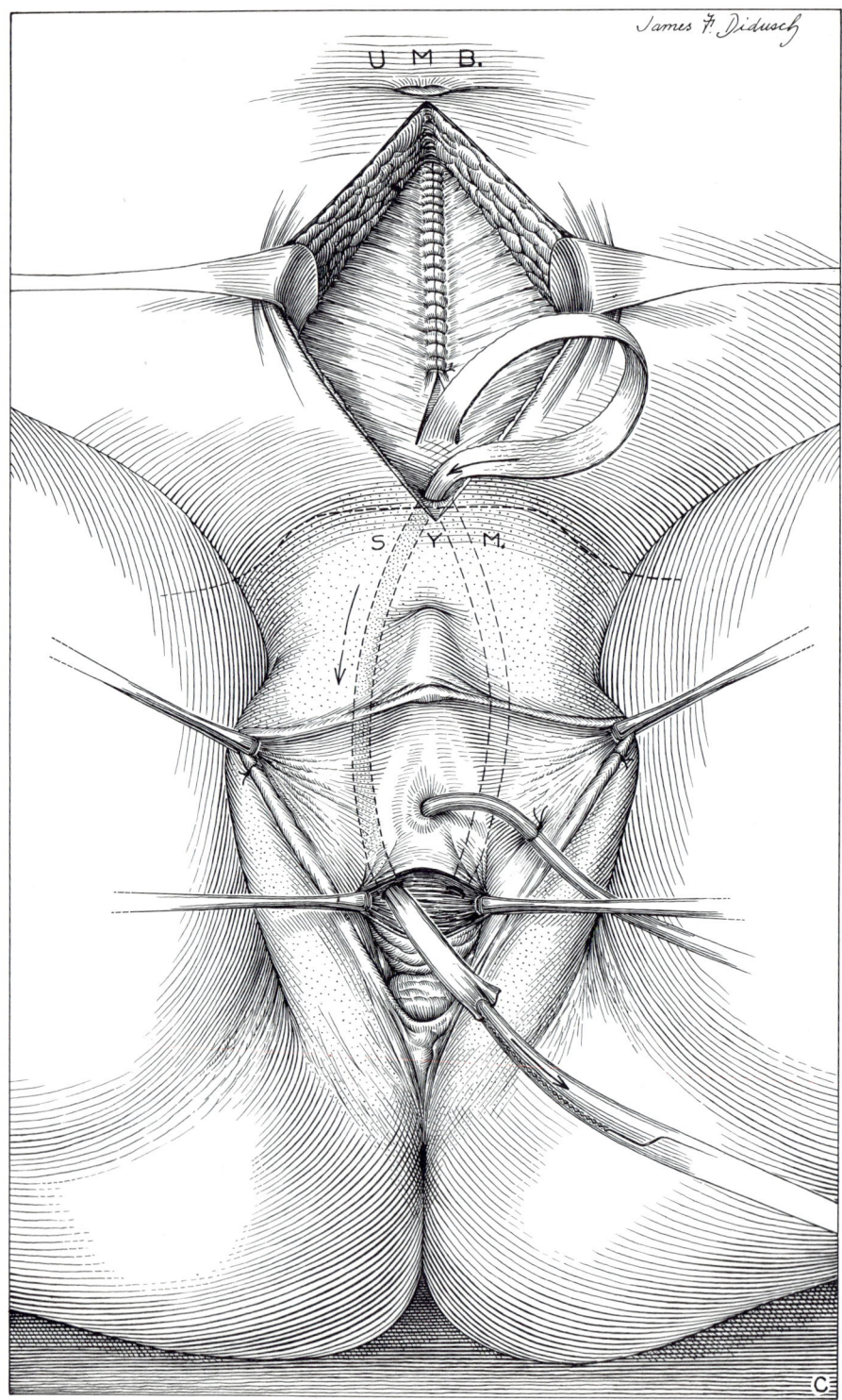

FIG. 26-5 (*Continued*). Goebell-Frangenheim-Stoeckel operation for urinary incontinence. (C) The strap of fascia has been brought down through one retropubic tunnel.

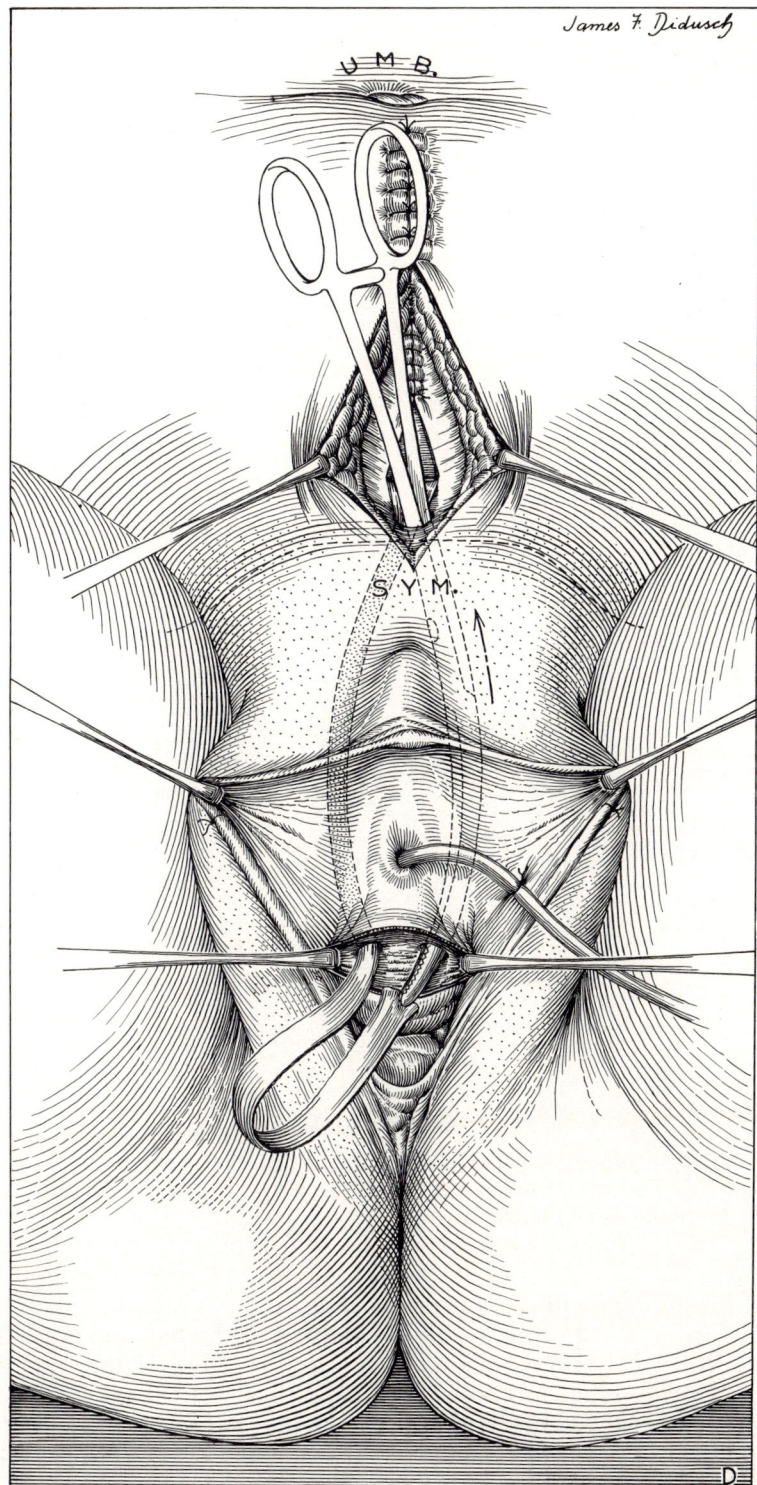

Fig. 26-5 (*Continued*). Goebell-Frangenheim-Stoeckel operation for urinary incontinence. (D) The strap of fascia is being drawn up through the other tunnel, thus encircling the urethra.

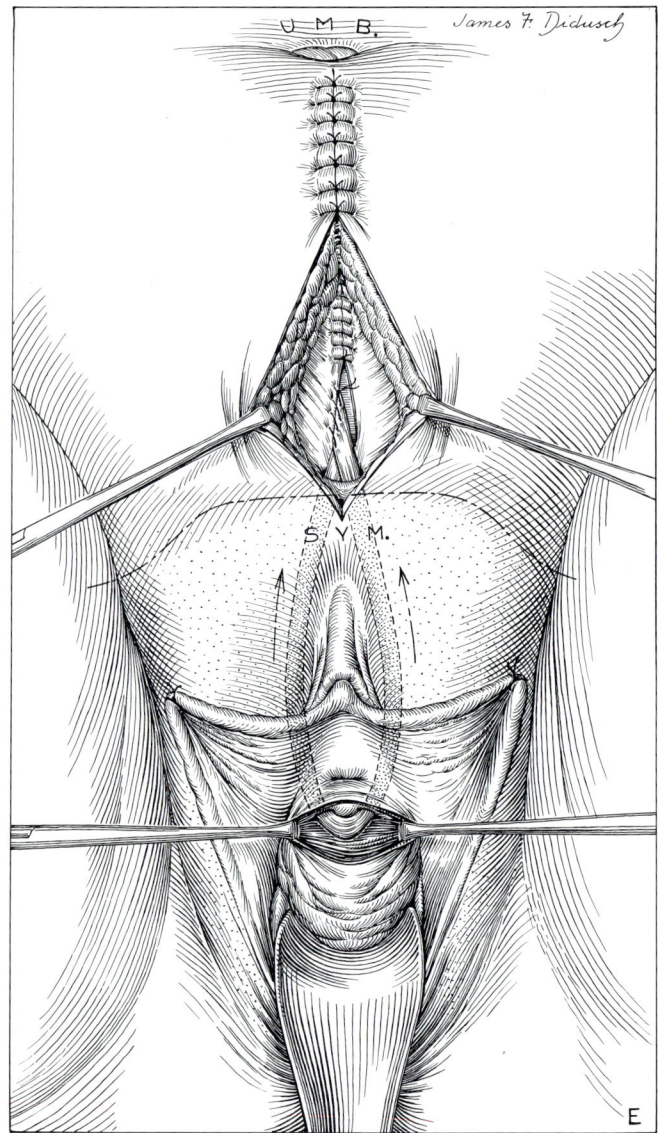

Fig. 26-5 (*Continued*). Goebell-Frangenheim-Stoeckel operation for urinary incontinence. (E) The strap has been drawn to the proper tension and sutured with medium silk to the fascia of the rectus.

the chance for contamination from the vagina.

A midline incision through the skin and the fat is made from umbilicus to symphysis. The sheath of the rectus is cleaned of fat for 1 or 2 cm. on either side of the midline. A strip of fascia, fully 1 cm. in width, is freed in the midline, leaving it attached to the lower end (Fig. 26-5). The pyramidalis muscles will be seen on the posterior surface of the lower portion of the flap and are left in situ.

At this stage of the operation it is a good plan to close the fascia incision and also the subcutaneous fat and skin, except at the lower end, in order to minimize the chances of infection of the midline incision. The skin incision is not shown closed in Figure 26-5 C for the purpose of orientation, but it is our custom to have closed the fascia and the skin, except at the lower end, at this stage of the operation.

The technic of delivery of the fascia sling is similar here to that described in the two previous operations. The long strap developed from the midline is passed through the rectus muscle on one side 2 cm. from the midline and delivered into the vaginal incision on the same side of the urethra, passed *beneath* the urethra and brought up through the space of Retzius to the anterior abdominal aponeurosis, where it is attached with the proper tension. The midline excision of the fascia may be from the symphysis to the xiphoid, giving a continuous strap, or may be a broader one from the symphysis to the umbilicus, split, and brought down on either side of the urethra as described in the Aldridge modification.

Technic: The Transected Sling Modification

Ridley has described this variation of the basic technic of using the fascia lata sling permitting the creation of adequate support for the bladder neck where a midvaginal incision or dissection is not feasible. For example, we are confronted at times with an ordinarily unworkable situation such as previous successful closure of a urethrovaginal or urethrovesicovaginal fistula; or the presence of a previously constructed urethra which was either congenitally absent or deformed by hypospadias (Fig. 26-6) or surgically absent from previous accident or slough; or the very thin avascular vaginal membrane which is encountered in the end results of postirradiation scarring.

The strap of fascia lata is procured as described previously in this chapter, and the suprapubic exposure of the anterior aponeurosis is accomplished and the structure slit. Careful blunt dissection is made through the space of Retzius down to the lateral aspects of the bladder neck. One-cm. incisions are made approximately 1 cm. lateral to the midline of the urethra and through the subjacent fascia and scar tissue. The point of the uterine

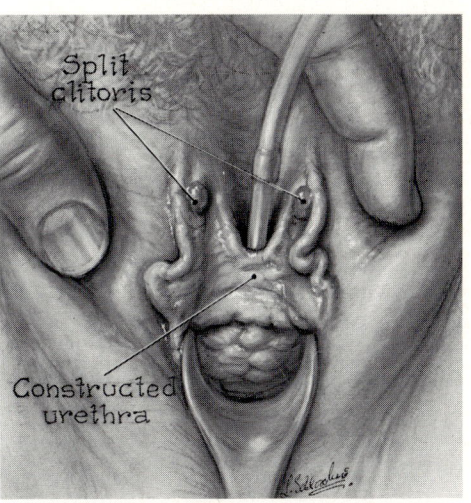

Fig. 26-6. Shows a reconstructed urethra in a woman with epispadias. After construction of the urethra there was no continence, but a secondary sling operation gave her continence that has persisted in spite of 3 childbirths through the vagina.

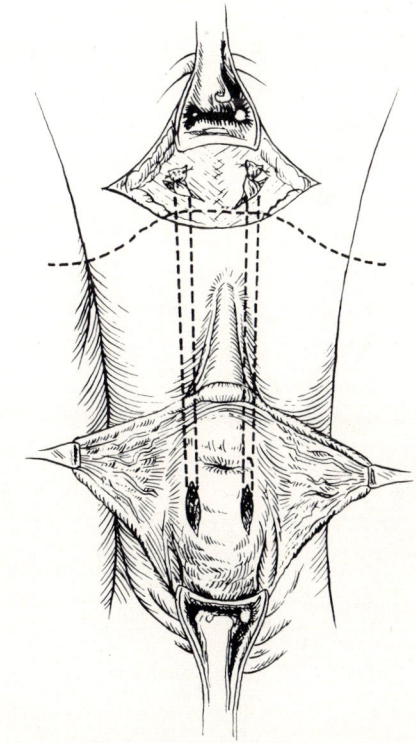

Fig. 26-7. Method of utilizing fascia strips by suturing them on either side of the urethra, a desirable method when the septum is so thin as to endanger perforation into the urethra if an attempt is made to bring the strap beneath it.

dressing forceps is directed as described previously, lateral to the urethra, with its indwelling balloon catheter, through the small vaginal slit-like incision. The strap of fascia lata is brought through the incision, fastened to the anterior abdominal aponeurosis, and carried beneath the urethra into the other vaginal incision and up to the other side of the anterior abdominal aponeurosis. Thus the sling is formed, and proper tension is applied and the ends fastened abdominally. However, the vaginal portion of the sling is still exposed, but the urethra has not been exposed or injured. The intact vaginal mucous membrane overlying the urethra has not been opened. The fascia strap is now firmly fixed with medium silk to the subjacent vaginal fascia and scar tissue beneath each of the small lateral vaginal incision (Fig. 26-7). The subtending portion of the strap which is exposed is trimmed away, and the vaginal incisions are closed. Three such cases have been done with excellent results, the time postoperative varying from 2 to 4 years.

In some cases such as those described above in which the urethrovaginal septum is very thin due to previous surgery, Te Linde has advocated tunneling through the septum carefully, using a small-bladed knife and carrying the sling through the tunnel with an aneurysm needle (Fig. 26-8). This may result in perforation of the mucosa of the urethra or vagina, and it is probably better in cases in which the septum is very thin to cut the sling and fasten the ends at the points of the two lateral incisions, as described above. In some cases with a thin scarred suburethral area, an area of thickened and more normal mucosa can be found slightly posterior to the ure-

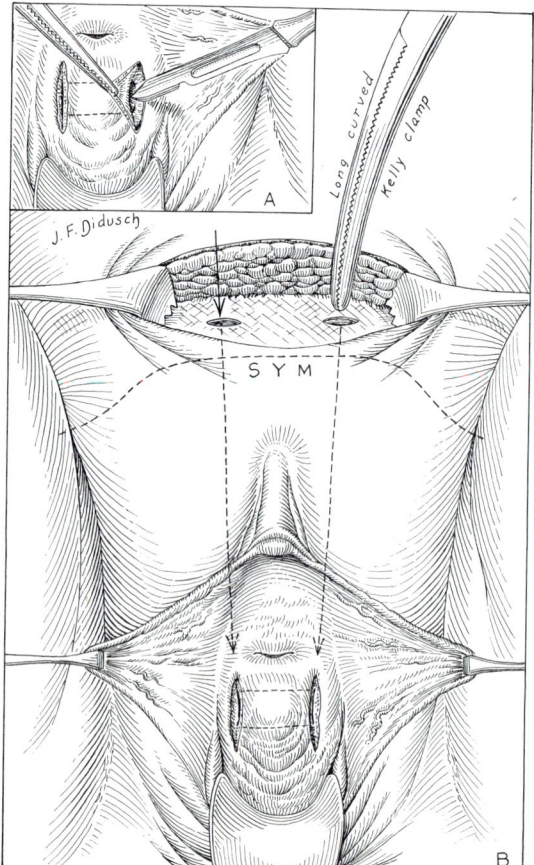

FIG. 26-8. Modified Goebell-Frangenheim-Stoeckel operation, using strip of fascia lata. (A) Two short slits are made on either side of the urethra, and a transverse tunnel is made between the urethral and the vaginal mucosa. (B) A short transverse suprapubic incision has been made, and the fascia has been punctured to permit the passage of a long Kelly clamp.

thra, just beneath the trigone. By using this area for placing the sling either through a tunnel or after denuding the vaginal mucosa through a midline incision, continence may be obtained (Fig. 26-9).

TECHNIC: THE MARSHALL-MARCHETTI-KRANTZ OPERATION

The technic of this procedure has been fundamentally unchanged since originally described by its authors in 1949. However, as time has passed, there have been a few changes such as those in suture placement and types of material, and a few variations in the method of accomplishing the retropubic fixation of the urethra and bladder neck. In our experience this procedure, as compared with the sling procedure, has been used approximately in the ratio of 1:4.

Currently we have found the following technics of the Marshall-Marchetti-Krantz procedure quite satisfactory. The anesthetized patient in supine position is given a pelvic examination, and a final check is made on previous pelvic findings, particularly of any intra-abdominal pathology. A No. 24 F Foley catheter with a 30-cc. bulb is inserted into the bladder. Although a Pfannenstiel incision is the preferred approach to the space of Retzius, this is not always feasible if the intra-abdominal portion of the operation demands the lower midline approach. When there must be an intra-abdominal procedure performed, this is usually completed and the peritoneum securely closed before dissection into the space of Retzius is begun. This is usually done by blunt dissection, which is more desirable to avoid bleeding; however, if there is distortion or obliteration by scarring of disease or previous surgery, sharp dissection must be used. Whatever oozing or bleeding is encoun-

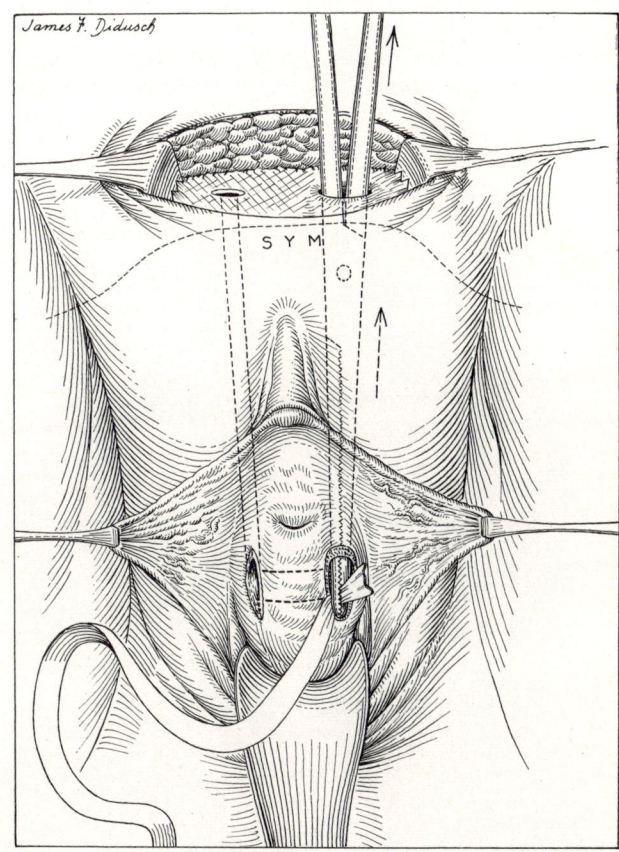

FIG. 26-9. Modified Goebell-Frangenheim-Stoeckel operation. Retropubic tunnel has been made with a Kelly clamp, and the fascia lata strip has been grasped. It is to be withdrawn and sutured to fascia.

tered can usually be controlled by pressure, individual ligature, or careful fulguration. Adequate exposure in this rather limited space may be difficult to obtain, particularly in the more obese individuals. The dissection is carried down toward the inferior aspect of the symphysis to within 1 cm. of the external urethral meatus. A vaginal pack that has been placed preoperatively may aid in demarcating the vaginal walls lateral to the urethra. Even more satisfactory, when feasible, is to have the surgeon insert 2 fingers into the introitus and elevate the anterior vagina and bladder neck so that the sutures may be more easily and accurately placed. The catheter demonstrates the urethra and the balloon indicates the bladder neck and trigonal area. The sutures of No. 1 chromic catgut—three in number, on either side—are taken; each suture is taken (1) into the submucosa of the vaginal wall lateral to the urethra, (2) into the wall of the urethra, and (3) into the periosteum of the symphysis. The No. 4 Mayo (round) needle is thrust rather deeply into the vaginal wall, delicately into the urethral wall, and firmly into the periosteum (Fig. 26-10 A). It has been found that even the medium round (taper point) needle will occasionally tend to "cut-out" of the periosteum. If this portion of the suture is placed firmly with a thrust which accurately follows the curvature of the needle, it will gain a satisfactory purchase. These lateral sutures are placed, tied, and cut in pairs from below upward. A final suture is placed proximal to the bladder neck over the balloon by taking a bite lateral to midline on the left, a bite in the midline at the bladder neck, and a bite lateral to the midline on the right. This final suture is then fixed to the top of the symphysis or the fascial tendons of the rectus muscles. It is usually not necessary to use any more sutures than those mentioned to obliterate the space of Retzius for the retropubic vesicourethral suspension. Additional sutures for security may be placed, however, in the anterior dome of the bladder to anchor this further to the posterior aspect of the anterior abdominal wall (Fig. 26-10 B). A small Penrose drain is placed on either side of the midline in the operative area and the wound closed per routine. The No. 24 F Foley catheter

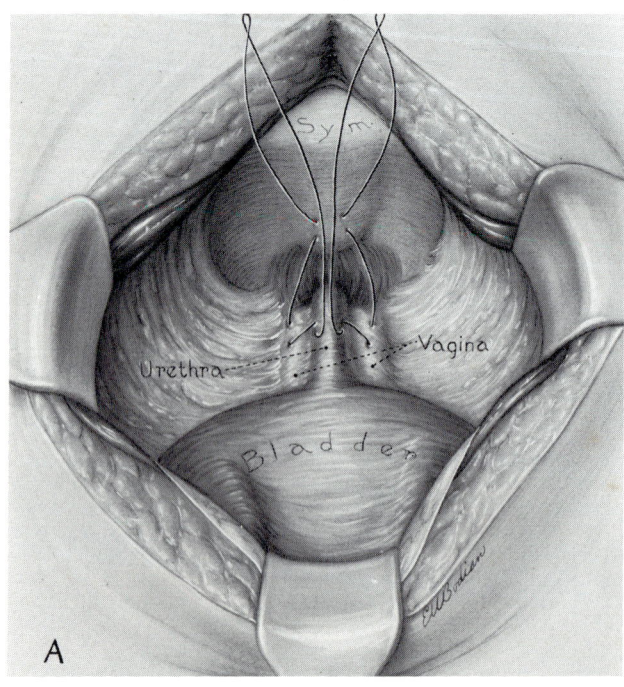

Fig. 26-10. Marshall-Marchetti operation. (A) Exposure of retropubic space, showing introduction of first stitches.

with the 30-cc. balloon is replaced with a No. 20 F Foley catheter with a 5-cc. balloon.

Inspection of the vagina following this procedure reveals that the cystourethrocele no longer exists, the entire vaginal wall together with the urethra being markedly elevated. The Foley catheter is left attached to the thigh by adhesive tape. The catheter is left in the bladder for 7 days.

POSTOPERATIVE CARE

The postoperative care of the bladder after any of these procedures may be difficult and disturbing both for the patient and the operator. When one considers that there is practically always some derangement of bladder function and urinary tract infection from inadequate drainage or previous manipulations, one can see that there is an increased likelihood of trouble. In the older patients, who comprise the majority of the group presenting themselves for these types of operations, urinary tract infection and altered bladder dynamics are very common. Previous or recurrent cystocele and prolapse have allowed residual urine to become chronically contaminated and never completely responsive to chemotherapy. Preoperative evaluation procedures, although meticulously and carefully done, frequently introduce infection or light up a quiescent infection in the urinary tract. Although an effort will have been made to try to correct the infection preoperatively, one realizes that trouble postoperatively is more probable.

If obvious infection is known to be present at the time of surgery, the drug of choice, having been previously determined by sensitivity and culture studies, is given without interruption until the bladder is emptying itself well postoperatively, and the urine is free from infection. The use of prophylactic chemo-

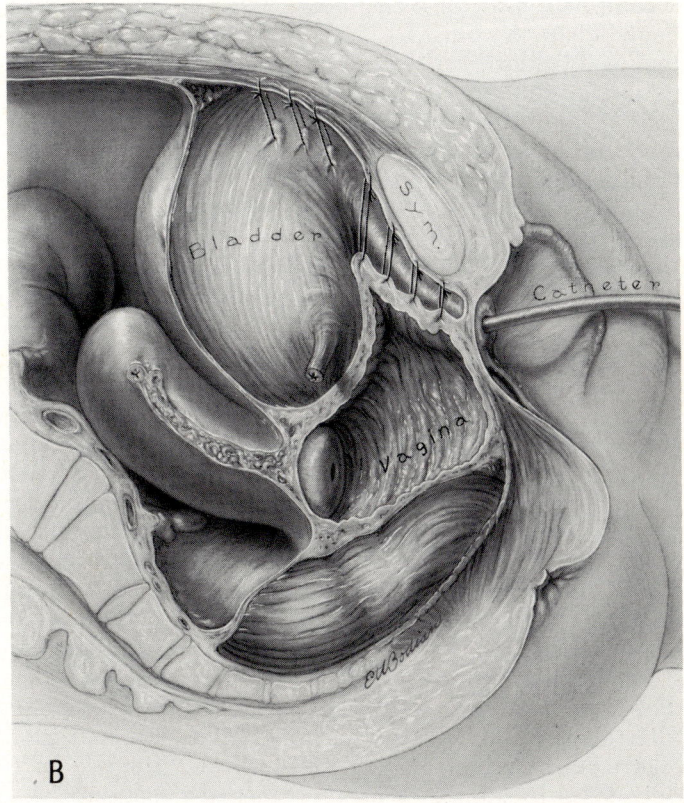

Fig. 26-10 (Continued). Marshall-Marchetti operation. (B) Off-center sagittal view, showing how sutures have been placed.

therapy is optional, but some feel that if chemotherapy is not already underway, it is wise to start a course of sulfisoxazole (Gantrisin) or another drug of similar spectrum, to be continued after the catheter is removed and until the urine is free from pus. The vaginal pack (Iodoform) is removed the morning following the operation, and the suprapubic drains, in the cases of the Marshall-Marchetti-Krantz procedures, on the 3rd or 4th postoperative day. The removal of the catheter both for the sling procedure or the retropubic suspension procedure is usually done on the 3rd postoperative day, allowing the patient to get to the bathroom to try to void. Early ambulation is of definite value. It is important to impress upon the patient that at first she may be completely unable to void or void only in small amounts. If she is not reassured by this explanation, she may become apprehensive and then her state of anxious tension will hamper prompt recovery. Prior to operation an explanation is given to her of just what the procedure sets out to accomplish, and by what means this is done. Then she must be made to realize that a bladder "weakened for such a period of time preoperatively" will require some time to recover strength and function. Mild tranquilizing drugs are of definite benefit. If the bladder residual is decreasing and is no more than 100 cc., the catheter is left out permanently. Urecholine, 10 to 20 mg. by mouth may be given 3 or 4 times per day for a week to help reduce bladder residual and to increase muscular tone. Even so, follow-up studies have shown that the incidence of residual urine with pyuria of 60 cc. or more was found in 22 per cent of 36 cases after 6 months following the sling procedure. Further follow-up shows that this gradually improves with proper chemotherapy and bladder stimulation. Similar observations have been reported following the retropubic urethrovesical suspension.

In the past 3 years suprapubic bladder drainage by a small polyethylene or Silastic tube has made the postoperative care of the bladder much easier and reduced the incidence of urinary tract infection. It is now used routinely in practically all of these described procedures.

RESULTS

In our hands the sling procedure has been more successful although it is difficult to make direct comparisons of these various types of procedures. This is chiefly due to the fact that the indications for the operation vary from one gynecologist to another. When such a corrective procedure is performed as the primary effort, the degree of success is, as expected, higher than if this same procedure is done following one or more previous but unsuccessful surgical attempts. As an example, Burch in 1968 reported 93 per cent success rate in 143 cases using the Cooper's ligament modification of the Marshall-Marchetti-Krantz procedure, but it is noted that 92 per cent of the patients had had no previous surgery for correction of stress urinary incontinence, not even a Kelly plication procedure. On the other hand, in a recently reported series by the author of 53 cases in which the sling procedure was used, all but 4 of the patients had undergone one or more previous surgical attempts, including vaginal repairs with Kelly plication sutures, 6 Marshall-Marchetti-Krantz procedures, and 1 sling operation. The final results after observation of at least 6 months were 88 per cent cured, 8 per cent tolerably improved, and 4 per cent failures.

As time passes, the percentage of cures tends to be rather constant after the use of the fascial sling, whereas "late" failures or less than satisfactory results will gradually rise for several years after the use of the Kelly plication procedure. The retropubic retrovesical suspension procedure has a tendency to permanent stability, as reported with the sling procedures.

Seven of the procedures in 53 reported cases of the sling operation had had previous transurethral resection of the bladder neck in an attempt to cure incontinence in the female. Two of these 7 patients had resulting vesicourethro-

27

Surgical Conditions of the Urethra

URETHRAL CARUNCLE

Urethral caruncles are benign polypoid growths presenting at the urinary meatus and usually originating from the posterior wall (Fig. 27-1 A). In some instances they are attached by a small pedicle; in others they are sessile. Usually they are single, but multiple caruncles arising from the same general area do occur. Because of their vascularity, they are deep red in color and often raspberry-like in appearance.

Histologically, there are 3 types: papillomatous, angiomatous, and granulomatous. The papillomatous is by far the most common type. They are covered with stratified squamous or transitional epithelium and have a scanty connective tissue and vascular framework. The angiomata are composed of dilated vessels with a small amount of connective tissue between the vessels. It is only fair to say that there is some doubt whether these represent true angiomata, or whether their predominant vascularity represents dilatation due to partial strangulation of the veins. Since there are often abrasions of the epithelium, there is frequently polymorphonuclear or round-cell infiltration. The least common caruncles are composed of granulation tissue and are inflammatory in origin.

Whether urethral caruncles that are benign may undergo malignant change is a question which has often been considered. There are several instances reported in the literature of carcinoma of the urethral meatus which are said to have been preceded by a urethral caruncle. The difficulty in judging these statements is that biopsies of the preceding "caruncles" are lacking. It is quite possible that the lesion was malignant from the beginning, simulating a caruncle.

Urethral caruncles are often incidental findings on routine pelvic examination and are entirely asymptomatic. However, there may be pain on urination, and the pain may be excruciating. We never have been able to distinguish histologically between the sensitive and the nonsensitive caruncles. A blood-tinged discharge or frank bleeding may be the complaint. There is very little difficulty at diagnosis in most instances. The tumors are soft on palpation, whereas carcinoma at the meatus is indurated and infiltrating.

Small caruncles may be entirely destroyed by monopolar fulguration (Fig. 27-1 B). If the caruncle is larger, the pedicle may be severed with the surgical diathermy knife, and the base is thoroughly destroyed with the desiccating current. There is often a tendency for urethral caruncles to recur, but much less tendency when they are removed as suggested above than when they are clipped off with the knife or the scissors. Sometimes, with recurrent caruncles, the distal portion of the urethral floor requires resection. This is done as in the resection

Gunther, R. E.: Letter to Editor. Obstet. Gynec., *31*:295, 1968.
Ingelman-Sundberg, A.: Partial denervation of the bladder. Acta Obstet. Gynec. Scand., 38:487, 1959.
——: Urinary incontinence in women excluding fistulas. Acta Obstet. Gynec., Scand., *31*:266, 1951-52.
Jeffcoate, T. N. A., and Francis, W. J. A.: Urgency incontinence in the female. Amer. J. Obstet. Gynec., *94*:604, 1966.
Kennedy, W. T.: Incontinence of urine in the female: Some functional observations of the urethra illustrated by roentgenograms. Amer. J. Obstet. Gynec., *33*:19, 1937.
Marchetti, A. A., Marshall, V. F., and O'Leary, J. F.: Suprapubic vesicourethral suspension and urinary stress incontinence. Clin. Obstet. Gynec., 6:195, March 1963.
Marchetti, A. A., Marshall, V. F., and Shultis, L. D.: Simple vesicourethral suspension: A survey. Amer. J. Obstet. Gynec., *74*:57, 1957.
Marshall, V. F., Marchetti, A. A., and Krantz, K. E.: The correction of stress incontinence by simple vesicourethral suspension. Surg. Gynec. Obstet., 88:509, 1949.
Miller, N. F.: Surgical treatment of urinary incontinence in the female. J.A.M.A., 98:628, 1932.
O'Leary, J. A.: Osteitis pubis in vesicourethral suspension. Obstet. Gynec., *24*:74, 1964.
Pereyra, A. J., and Lebherz, T. B.: Combined urethrovesical suspension and vaginourethroplasty for correction of urinary stress incontinence. Obstet. Gynec., *30*:537, 1967.
Price, P. B.: Plastic operations for incontinence of urine and of feces. Arch. Surg., 26:1043, 1933.
Ridley, J. H.: Indirect air cystoscopy. Southern Med. J., *44*:114-121, February 1951.
——: Surgical treatment of stress urinary incontinence in women. J. Med. Assoc. Georgia, *44*:135, 1955.
——: Appraisal of the Goebell-Frangenheim-Stoeckel sling procedure. Amer. J. Obstet. Gynec., 95:714, 1966.
Stoeckel, W.: Uber di Verwendung der Muculi Pyramidales bei der operativen Behadlung der Incontinentia Urinae. Zbl. Gynäk., *41*: 11, 1917.
Squier, J. B.: Postoperative urinary incontinence: Urethroplastic operation. M. Rec., *79*:868, 1911.
Taussig, F. J.: A new operation for urinary incontinence in women by transposing the levator ani muscles. Amer. J. Obstet. Dis. Women & Child., 77:881, 1918.
Wharton, L. P., Jr., and Te Linde, R. W.: An evaluation of fascial sling operation for urinary incontinence in female patients. J. Urol., 82:76, 1959.
Williams, T. J., and Te Linde, R. W.: The sling operation for urinary incontinence using Mersilene ribbon. Obstet. Gynec., *19*:2, 241, February 1962.

Failure of the operator to recognize urge incontinence or decreased bladder capacity for various causes will result in a failure or less than satisfactory result with his procedure. Again, proper preoperative study is emphasized.

Two patients with failure of all efforts to correct an intractable stress urinary incontinence had developed such scarring from previous injury, surgery, or disease that the tissues were unyielding and unworkable. Thus scarring can be another most important factor, giving either complete or partial failure. In each of these patients, previous efforts had included both the Marshall-Marchetti-Krantz procedure and the sling procedure. However, considerable scarring should not deter another trial of a sling procedure, for we have had considerable success in several. Neither of these patients chose to have the ultimate effort, the diversion of the urinary stream into the intestinal tract.

Chronic pulmonary disease such as bronchiectasis, emphysema, asthma, giving an intractable cough, is a frequent cause of failure of repair. It would be ideal to say that with control of the cough, one can expect improvement of the stress urinary incontinence, but this is too frequently not possible.

We have outlined in this and the preceding chapter the methods by which we attempt surgically to correct stress urinary incontinence. With a basic understanding of the three fundamental procedures, one should choose the method or improvise as the particular case demands. It is difficult to say with certainty which procedure is the best, and the experience of the operator should influence the decision to some degree. We have favored the Goebell-Frangenheim-Stoeckel procedure in most cases of previous failure because of its simplicity, dependability, and paucity of complications. However, it is not done to the exclusion of the other procedures, many of which should be in the armamentarium of the well-trained gynecologist, who should be comprehensively equipped to deal with all the problems and vagaries of stress urinary incontinence.

BIBLIOGRAPHY

Aldridge, A. H.: Transplantation of fascia for relief of urinary stress incontinence. Amer. J. Obstet. Gynec., 44:398, 1942.

Ball, T. L., Knapp, R. C., Nathanson, B., and Lagasse, L. D.: Stress incontinence. Amer. J. Obstet. Gynec., 94:997, 1966.

Ball, T. L., and Wright, K. L.: Stress incontinence, complication and sequellae of the Marshall-Marchetti operation. Pacif. Med. Surg., 73:290, 1965.

Barnes, A. C.: Roentgenologic study of urethral sphincter strength in female. J. Urol., 47:694, 1942.

Brewer, J. I.: Personal communication.

Burch, J. C.: Cooper's ligament urethrovesical suspension for stress incontinence. Amer. J. Obstet. Gynec., 100:764, 1968.

Christensen, B. C., and Ostergaard, E.: Result of operations for stress incontinence: A study based on patients operated on during the years 1952-1960. Acta Obstet. Gynec. Scand., 42:367, 1964.

Counseller, V. S.: Surgical correction of stress incontinence—methods and techniques. J. Int. Coll. Surg., 24:330, 1960.

Cramer, H.: Fundamental and technical facts concerning Goebell's operation for urinary incontinence. Zbl. Gynaek., 53:342, 1929.

Deming, C. L.: Transplantation of the gracilis muscle for incontinence of urine. J.A.M.A., 86:822, 1926.

Everett, H. S.: A condemnation of resectoscopic procedures upon the female vesical neck. Urol. Cutan. Rev., 52:80, 1948.

Frangenheim (Cöln): Zur Operativen Behandlung der Inkontinenz der männlichen Harnröhre. Verhandlungen der deutschen Gesellschaft für Chirurgie, 43rd Congress, p. 149, 1914.

Goebell, R.: Zur Operativen Beseitigung der angeborenen Incontinentia vesicae. Z. Gynäk. Urol., 2:187, 1910.

Green, T. H., Jr.: Development of a plan for the diagnosis and treatment of urinary stress incontinence. Amer. J. Obstet. Gynec., 83:632, 1962.

Greenwald, S. W., Thornberry, J. R., and Dunn, L. J.: Cystourethrography as a diagnostic aid in evaluation of stress incontinence. Obstet. Gynec., 29:324, 1967.

vaginal fistulas which were successfully repaired before the sling procedure was performed. The practice of transurethral resection of the bladder neck to cure stress urinary incontinence in the female is strongly and justifiably condemned by the gynecologist, but the practice is still sometimes used. Everett pointed out the dangers of the practice, and subsequent observations have corroborated his findings and substantiated his conclusions.

Osteitis pubis has not been a complication postoperatively in the use of the sling procedure; however, there have been cases reported although few in number—3.5 per cent by Ball—following the Marshall-Marchetti-Krantz procedure. In these few cases the discomfort may be distressing and last for as long as 3 months, but clears up completely without sequellae.

Recent evaluation and publications of the Marshall-Marchetti-Krantz procedures on the Ob-Gyn Service at Georgetown University Hospital reveals classification and results as in Table 26-1.

Most of the severe cases were those in which patients had had one or more previous procedures for incontinence (85% of them through the vaginal route). Marchetti states that the Marshall-Marchetti-Krantz procedure is being performed more and more as a primary procedure for correction of stress urinary incontinence. The overall success rate, including the mild, moderate, and severe cases operated on primarily or secondarily, is 89.2 per cent. We are not completely in accord with this view. Our primary attack is usually the Kelly plication, especially if a cystocele is present.

In a recent publication of appraisal of the sling procedure, the author reported 85 per cent cure, 11 per cent improved, and 4 per cent failures in 53 cases. In this series of cases, 36 done by one operator, the strap was of autogenous fascia lata. Thirty-two of the 36 cases had had one or more previous procedures with failures, including the Marshall-Marchetti-Krantz and the sling procedure itself. It was found that the space of Retzius, now scarred by previous surgery, was more amenable to the lesser amount of dissection of the Goebell-Frangenheim-Stoeckel procedure than the larger amount of dissection needed for proper performance of the Marshall-Marchetti-Krantz procedure.

ANALYSIS OF FAILURES

Even the best conceived and best executed procedures for correction of stress urinary incontinence will have a certain percentage of failures, and analysis of these failures can teach the operator what to be aware of on a future effort.

A most common cause of failure is improper choice of the type of procedure to be done. It has been pointed out in the discussion of the preoperative studies of the bladder and patient that much unnecessary trouble can be avoided if the neurologicly impaired bladder is detected. This is most important because such weakness of detrusor power is only aggravated by any operative procedure that causes any obstruction at the bladder neck, whether this obstruction be simply a constriction by plication, or a repositioning of the bladder neck and urethra by the sling procedure, or the retropubic vesicourethral suspension. Careful preoperative study of bladder capacity and dynamics will rule out this pitfall.

TABLE 26-1

Classification	Per Cent	Patients	Failed	Success Within Category
Mild	11%	20	0	100%
Moderate	54%	101	11	89%
Severe	35%	66	14	79%

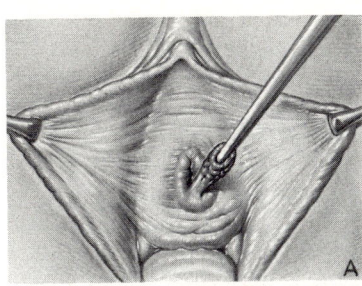 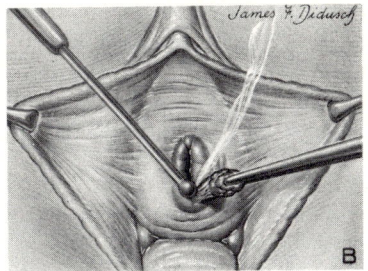

FIG. 27-1. Destruction of urethral caruncle with high-frequency fulguration.

described in this chapter for urethral prolapse, but only the inferior half of the circumference of the urethra is excised.

URETHRAL PROLAPSE

Slight eversion of the mucosa at the urethral meatus is common and seldom gives rise to symptoms. Real prolapse of the mucosa of the urethra is rare. It is characterized by a sliding outward of the urethral mucosa through the meatus. Then it becomes cyanotic, edematous, and even infarcted (Fig. 27-2). The symptoms vary greatly. Prolapse may cause no discomfort and only be detected when a bloody discharge occurs as the result of the breaking down of the congested tissues. Other patients complain of sudden, severe, and continuous pain with frequency of urination and tenesmus.

The cause of urethral prolapse is not known. Emmet thought that during parturition the child's head pressed forward the loose tissue about the neck of the bladder and lacerated the periurethral fascia. This scarcely seems to be a likely explanation, for the cases are most prone to occur at the extremes of life. Emmet's explanation would seem to be more suitable for the formation of urethrocele. Keefe reports the age incidence as 60 per cent below 15 years; 12 per cent between 15 and 40 years; and 28 per cent over 40 years. We have observed it only in infants and elderly women. In infants it usually is preceded by a severe coughing or crying spell. Paroxysms of coughing also seem to be related to its occurrence in some of the elderly women. From the frail nature of the elderly women in whom we have seen the condition, it would seem reasonable to believe that the loss of tone and elasticity of tissues, due to age, is a factor in its formation.

The treatment may be palliative or surgical. Occasionally, the edematous mass of tissue may be reduced, but even if this maneuver is successful, recurrence is common. Hot, moist compresses give temporary comfort.

Several surgical procedures have been suggested. The procedure advocated by Kelly and Burnam is illustrated in Figure 27-3. The prolapsed mucosa is amputated by a circular incision, as shown in Figure 27-3 A. The cut edges are then sutured with No. 000 chromic catgut, as shown in Figure 27-3 B. Amputation with the electrosurgical knife is more advantageous than excision with the scalpel.

Livermore was the first to advocate treatment of urethral prolapse with fulguration. He fulgurated the 4 points of the compass for a few seconds each and

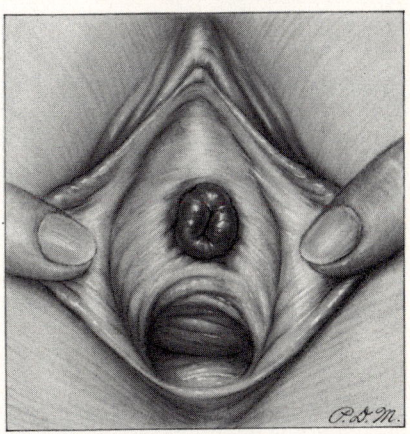

FIG. 27-2. Prolapsed urethra.

574 Surgical Conditions of the Urethra

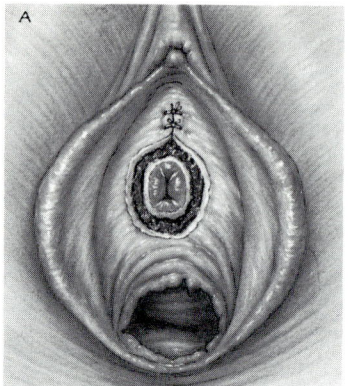 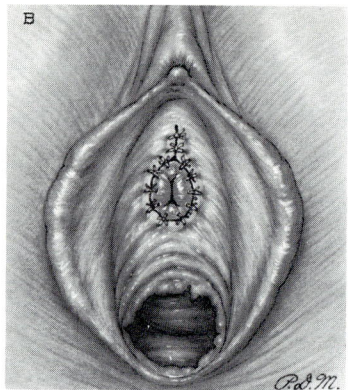

FIG. 27-3. Whitehead type of operation for urethral prolapse. (A) The prolapsed mucosa has been excised. (B) Completed operation.

reported success. When the prolapse is not too marked, the scarring produced in this manner would seem to be effective, but if there is extensive prolapse with infarction, all of the prolapsed tissue must be removed or it will slough. In such cases circumcision is preferable to fulguration.

CYSTS OF SKENE'S DUCTS

On rare occasions the lumen of one of Skene's ducts may become occluded, and a retention cyst may result. The etiology of this occlusion must be inflammatory, but we have observed it in women in whom there was no suggestion of neisserian infection in the history or the physical findings. Figure 27-4 A shows the typical picture with the resultant deformity of the urethral meatus.

The cysts should be excised even though, when small, they may be asymptomatic. The reason for this is the fact that the larger they become, the greater will be the difficulty in dissecting the cyst from the displaced urethra, and the more danger there will be of injuring it. A glass catheter is first inserted into the

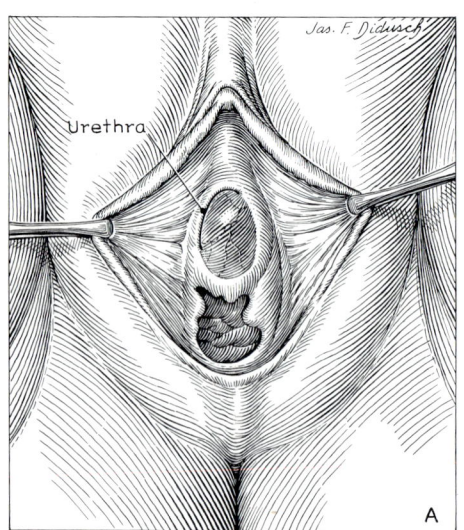 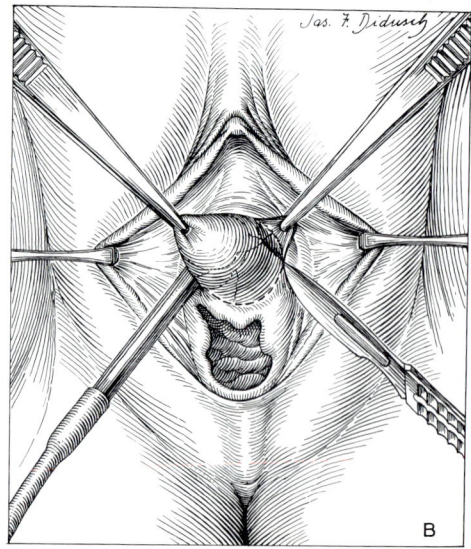

FIG. 27-4. Excision of Skene's cyst. (A) Shows preoperative condition. (B) Glass catheter has been inserted in the urethra to identify it. Dotted line indicates incision encircling cyst.

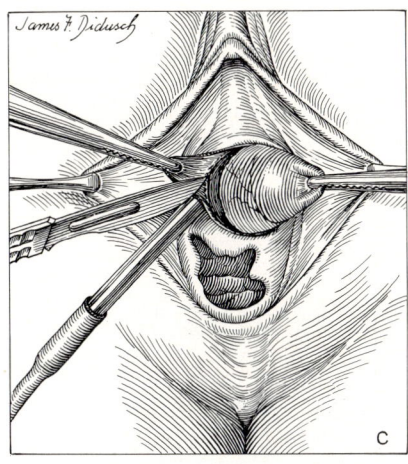
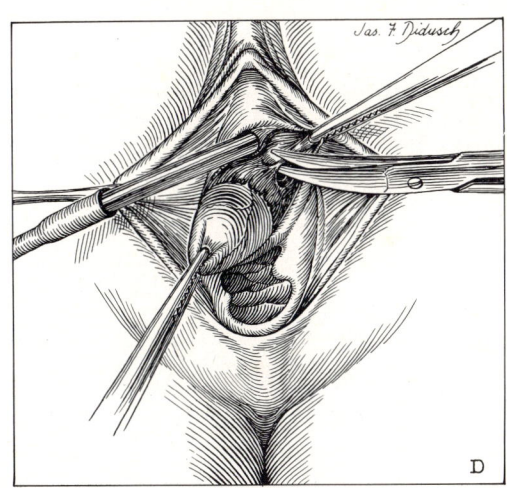
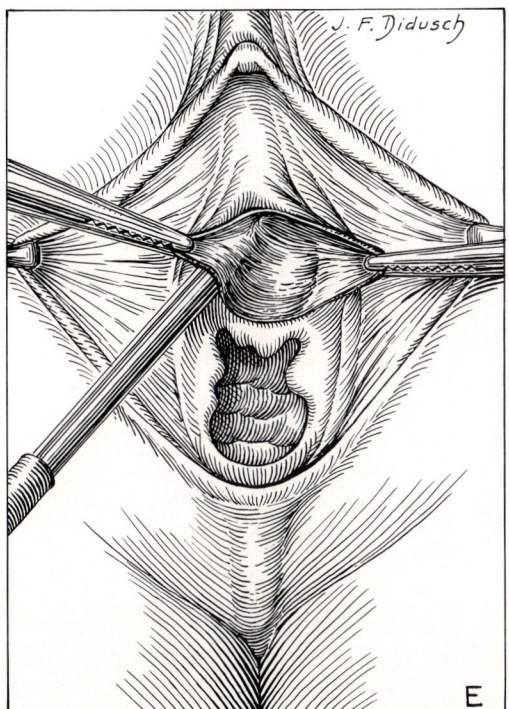
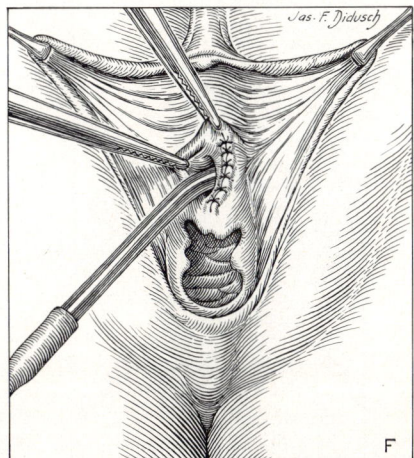

FIG. 27-4 (*Continued*). Excision of Skene's cyst. (C) The cyst is freed with sharp dissection. (D) The incision has been completed about the cyst. (E) The cyst has been completely removed, leaving the urethra intact. (F) The mucosa has been approximated with No. 000 chromic catgut in interrupted sutures.

urethra, and a circular incision is made about the base of the protruding cyst (Fig. 27-4 B and C). With careful dissection the cyst is freed from its bed as shown in Figure 27-4 D, bearing in mind constantly the danger of injury to the delicate urethra. In Figure 27-4 E the cyst has been completely removed. The raw surfaces are approximated with No. 000 chromic catgut, any redundant mucosa is excised, and the mucosal edges are sutured together with interrupted sutures of the same fine chromic catgut (Fig. 27-4 F).

SUBURETHRAL CYST

Suburethral cysts, such as the one shown in Figure 27-5 A, are of unknown etiology. It is unlikely that the cyst shown here arose from Skene's gland for it was exactly in the midline, a short distance within the vagina, and did not displace the meatus. It interfered with coitus but otherwise gave rise to no symptoms. Its

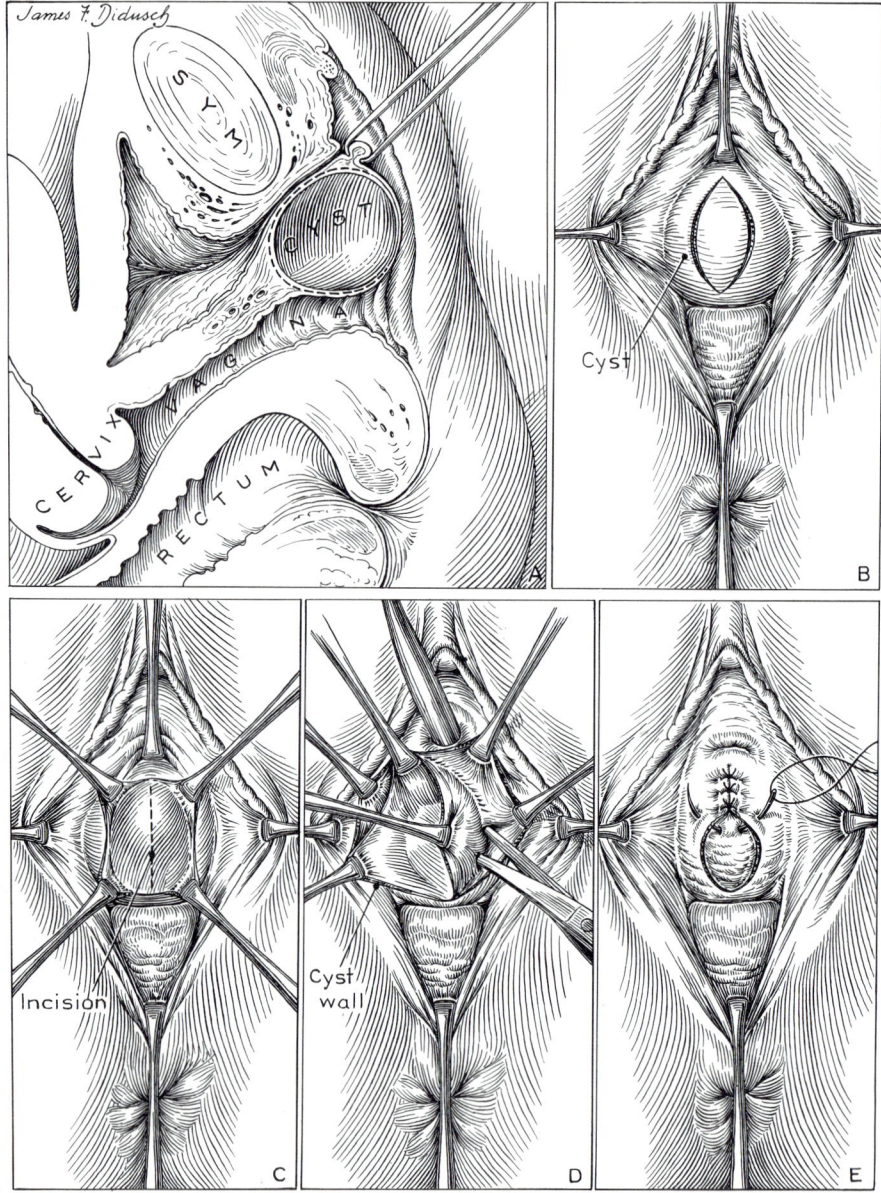

FIG. 27-5. Excision of a suburethral cyst. (A) Sagittal section showing relation of the cyst to the vagina and the urethra. (B) Incision is made through vaginal mucosa beneath the cyst. (C) The vaginal mucosa has been dissected from the cyst wall. The dotted line indicates the incision in the cyst wall. (D) With the cyst open, the wall is dissected free from the subjacent urethra. Note Hegar dilator in the urethra. (E) The cyst has been removed without injury to the urethra. The mucosa is being closed with interrupted sutures of fine chromic catgut. Each suture takes a bite of the subjacent periurethral tissue.

excision is shown in Figure 27-5. Figure 27-5 B illustrates the vaginal mucosal elliptical incision which is designed to remove the excess vaginal mucosa. Then the wall of the cyst is deliberately incised, as shown in the dotted line in Figure 27-5 C. A Hegar metal dilator is placed in the urethra, in order to identify if easily at all times during the operation. Then the cyst wall is excised with sharp dissection (Fig. 27-5 D). The vaginal mucosal incision is closed with interrupted sutures of No. 00 chromic catgut, each stitch picking up a bit of the subjacent tissue but avoiding the urethral lumen (Fig. 27-5 E).

DIVERTICULUM OF THE URETHRA

The subject of diverticulum of the urethra in the female is scarcely a new one, the first case having been reported in 1805 by Hey, who stated that he had treated his first case in 1786. The second case to find its way into the literature was that of Foucher in 1857. Priestley reported the third case in 1867. Lawsen Tait described a case of "saccular dilatation of the urethra" in 1875. The first reports were of single cases, whereas later reports of multiple cases appeared, such as that of Hunner in 1938. He stated that he had seen probably 12 to 15 cases of urethral diverticulum, including 3 with calculi in the sac.

In spite of these reports the condition has not been generally recognized by the profession, and there is no doubt that many women are unnecessarily suffering from it today, even though they have repeatedly consulted gynecologists and urologists. It seems apparent that whenever the condition is called to the attention of the profession by an article in the literature, more cases are diagnosed. Then after a lapse of time the cases seem to be overlooked again. This point is well illustrated by our experience at the Johns Hopkins Hospital. During the 19-year period, 1931–49, 22 cases were diagnosed and treated at the Hopkins Hospital. The cases were reviewed and published by Wharton and Kearns in 1950. In the succeeding 5-year period through 1954, 41 cases were diagnosed. Since then, being more alert to the possibility and with better diagnostic methods, we are encountering urethral diverticula with increasing frequency.

They are usually small but vary in size from 3 mm. to 8 cm. in diameter. Some of the larger ones burrow along the entire length of the urethra. It is possible that the majority of these cysts begin as neisserian urethral infections which break through into the suburethral tissue and form an abscess cavity that ultimately becomes lined with epithelium. The gonococcus is seldom cultured, but this does not exclude it as the primary agent. The usual organisms cultured are *Escherichia coli*, gram-positive cocci, and diphtheroids. However, the diverticulum shown in Figure 27-6 never had shown evidence of inflammation clinically, and the excised wall was not inflamed, as revealed by microscopic examination. The lining was epithelium, identical with that of the normal urethra. It became apparent during the patient's first pregnancy and hence could not have been the result of obstetric injury. It would seem that a congenital cause must be ascribed to such a diverticulum. Many causes have been considered to be responsible for urethral diverticula, but there is no proof of any of them. In 1941 Parmenter described 8 cases and suggested various acquired etiologies such as trauma from childbirth, infection of urethral gland with sealing off of communication with the urethra and subsequent re-establishment of communication, instrumentation of the urethra, urethral stone, and urethral stricture. In addition, he considered several congenital causes such as origin from Gartner's duct, faulty union of prima, folds, cell nests, wolffian duct, and vaginal cysts that have ruptured into the urethra.

The symptomatology is variable. Among 66 cases studied by Lawrence Wharton, Jr., and Te Linde, in 44 the chief complaint was dysuria; frequency was complained of 29 times, and urgency 14 times. A lump in the vagina, intermittent

578   Surgical Conditions of the Urethra

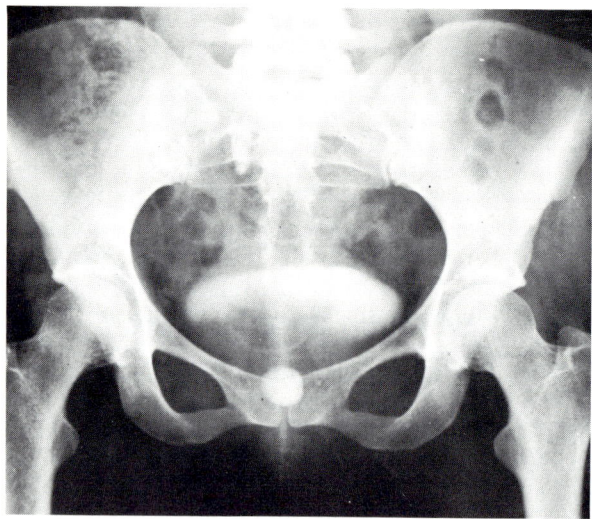

FIG. 27-6. Showing urethral diverticulum filled with contrast medium. The bladder is partially filled.

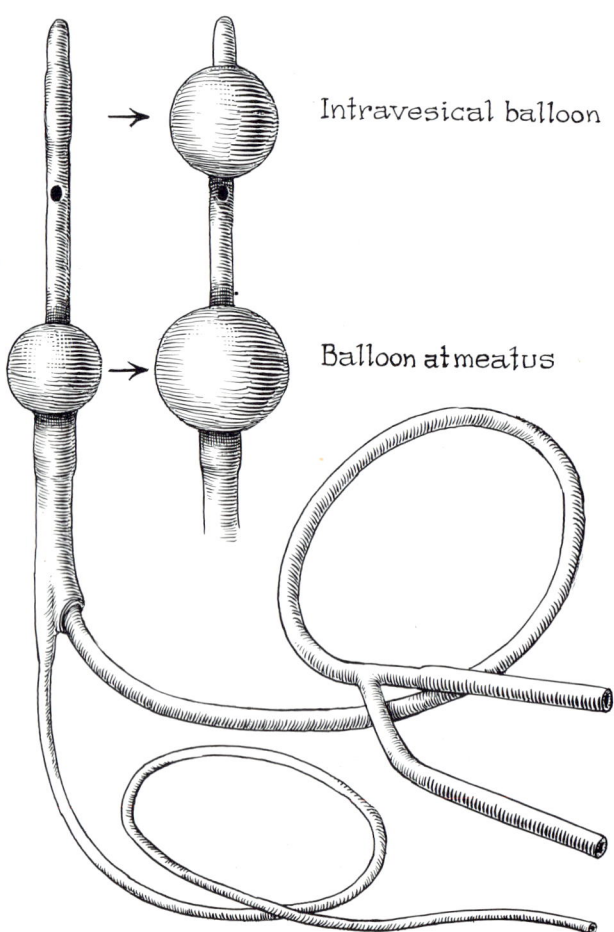

FIG. 27-7. Special catheter for injecting medium for urethrogram. The distal balloon is deflated, and the catheter is introduced. The proximal balloon is movable and is pressed against the meatus to trap the contrast medium in the urethra.

discharge from the urethra, hematuria, dyspareunia, and pain on walking were also complained of. Pus was found in the catheterized urine specimen in 35 cases. This would seem to be dependent upon the position of the orifice. If it is sufficiently close to the outer end of the urethra, there may be no leakage of pus back into the bladder. It is probable that this may explain the absence of symptoms of "cystitis" in a fairly large percentage of the cases. On examination of the urethra through the cystoscope, often an opening can be demonstrated, but some of the openings are extremely small, and usually there is edema due to inflammatory swelling, so visualization may be difficult or impossible. The diagnosis is usually firmly established by the demonstration of the diverticulum by roentgenograms. This is accomplished by the use of a special catheter devised by Davis and Cian and pictured in Figure 27-7. Figure 27-8 shows such a catheter in the urethra and the diverticulum being filled with Salpix under pressure. By its use the urethra may be blocked off at either end and distended with Salpix (see Fig. 27-8). Figure 27-6 shows a roentgenogram of a diverticulum demonstrated in this manner. The important thing to remember is the possibility of a urethral diverticulum in cases of intractable cystitis. The palpation of a suburethral mass in such cases is extremely suggestive of diverticulum. Pressure on the mass may cause the escape of urine or pus from the meatus.

The treatment consists of complete excision of the wall and closure of the defect in the urethra. Figure 27-9 A shows the diverticulum protruding into the vagina. Its smooth vaginal covering is seen in contrast with the rough mucosa of the rest of the vaginal wall. In order to avoid injury to the urethra, it is advisable to open into the cavity of the diverticulum. A midline incision is made through the vaginal mucosa and the wall of the diverticulum (Fig. 27-9 A). The edges of the incision are retracted, and the interior of the cavity is inspected.

The opening into the urethra usually is easily seen, especially if a glass or metal

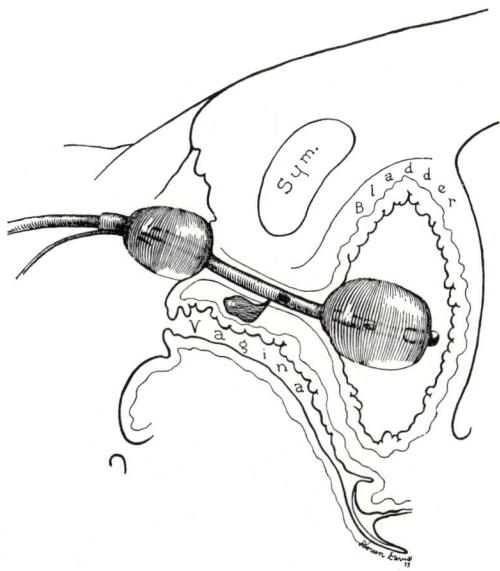

FIG. 27-8. Apparatus used for positive pressure urethrography. (Davis, H. J., and Cian, L. G.: Positive pressure urethrography: a new diagnostic method. J. Urol., 75:753, 1956)

urethral catheter has been passed (Fig. 27-9 B). Under sight, the rather thick mucosa of the diverticulum is separated from the vaginal mucosa and is trimmed off. The urethral defect is closed with interrupted mattress sutures of No. 00 chromic catgut, which invert the edge into the urethral lumen (Fig. 27-9 D). After trying these sutures, they are buried with another row of mattress sutures by approximating the suburethral fascia (Fig. 27-9 E). Finally, the vaginal mucosal incision is closed with interrupted sutures of fine chromic catgut.

An indwelling catheter is usually inserted and left in until the morning of the 5th day. The patient is allowed to go to the toilet to void and usually can. The trauma of repeated catheterizations should be avoided if possible. If the patient is unable to void for a day after removal of the catheter, it is probably better to replace the indwelling catheter for a few more days. If the diverticulum has been removed from the distal portion of the urethra so that there has been little trauma to the vesical sphincter region, we frequently omit the indwelling catheter

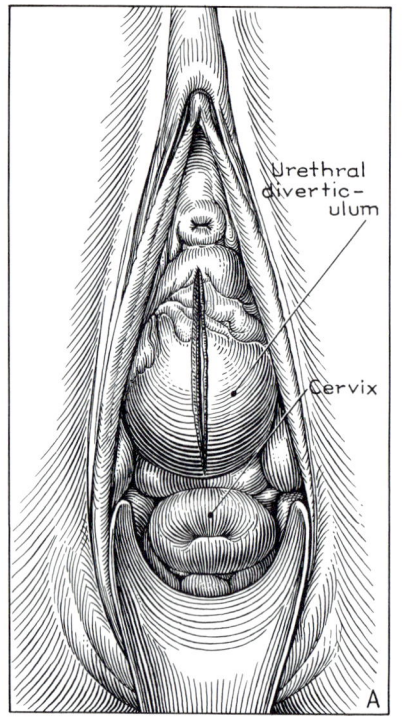 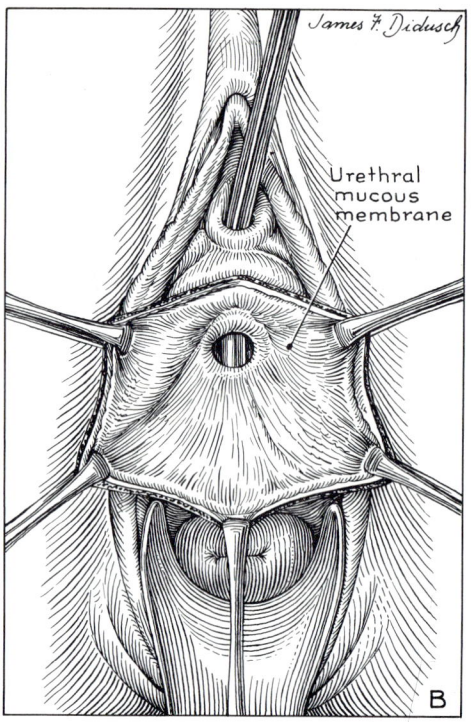
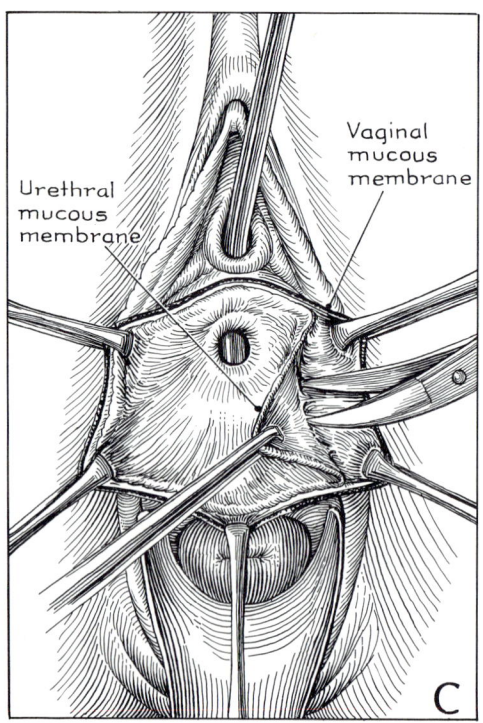 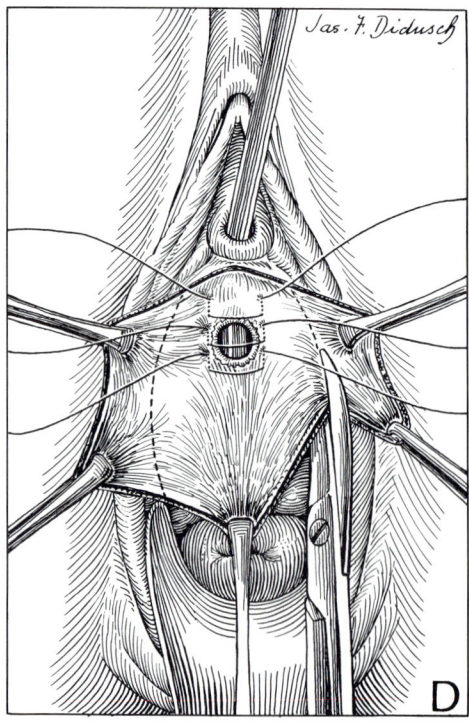

Fig. 27-9. Diverticulum of the urethra. (A) Incision is made through the vaginal mucous membrane and the wall of the diverticulum. (B) The diverticulum is laid wide open, demonstrating communication with the urethra. (C) The mucosa lining the diverticulum is being completely removed. (D) The communicating opening is closed with mattress sutures, and excess of vaginal mucosa is being excised.

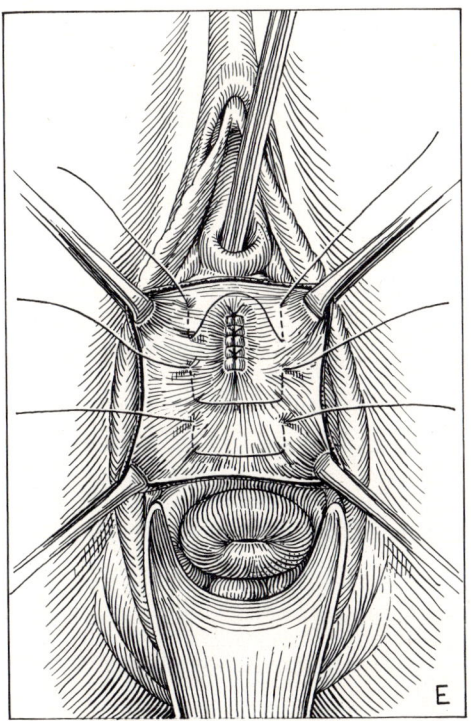 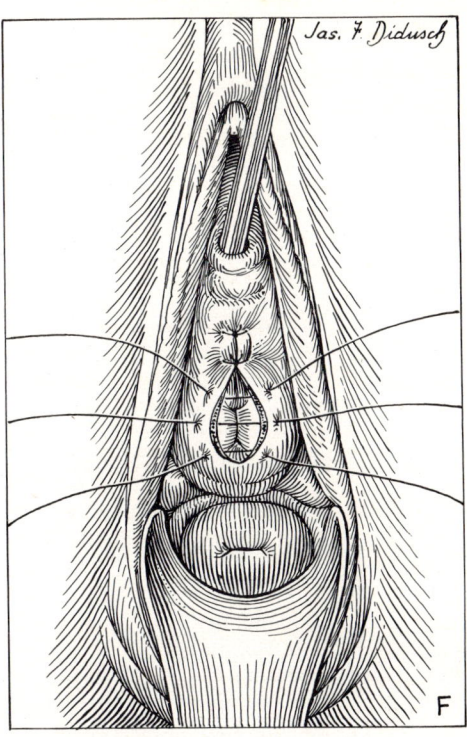

FIG. 27-9 (*Continued*). Diverticulum of the urethra. (E) First line of closure is reinforced with a second one, using interrupted mattress sutures of No. 0 chromic catgut. (F) Mucosa is closed with interrupted sutures of No. 0 chromic catgut.

and permit the patient to be up to void, which she usually does from the onset.

The results of excision of urethral diverticula are usually satisfactory. Three of our 66 cases developed urethral strictures. These were delicate and easily broken down by urethral dilatation, giving permanent relief. An occasional small urethral fistula occurs which is easily repaired if it causes incontinence. In the distal part of the urethra, such a fistula gives no incontinence and need not be repaired.

Edwards has advocated splitting the urethra for its full length in order better to visualize excision of the sac. In most cases, in our opinion, this is not necessary. Recently our experience with suprapubic drainage by a Silastic tube has proven ideal for these cases.

CARCINOMA OF THE URETHRA

Although malignant lesions of the female genital tract are discussed in detail in Part Four of this text, the rare malignancy of the female urethra frequently mimics the clinical symptoms of urinary tract infection and incontinence. Because of this fact, this lesion is presented in this section of the text to re-emphasize the importance of a complete urinary tract work-up prior to surgical correction of urinary incontinence. When urinary tract symptoms other than incontinence are present, such an investigation should include an intravenous pyelogram; catheterized urine specimen for microscopic analysis, culture, and antibiotic sensitivities; water cystoscopy with direct vision of urethra and bladder; and cystometry.

Carcinoma of the female urethra is fortunately a rare condition. In an extensive review of the literature McCrea found only 546 cases of urethral malignancy reported. Of these, 504 were carcinoma, 23 sarcoma, and 19 melanomas. The carcinomas were chiefly of the epidermoid type; but occasionally an adenocarcinoma, apparently arising from the paraurethral glands, is encountered. In 1966 Hassin and MacNiel reported the

TABLE 27-1. CARCINOMA OF FEMALE URETHRA

Case No.	Intra-urethral Radium	Contra-urethral Radium	X-ray Abdominal	X-ray Perineal
1	None	2,708 mg. hrs. (2 treatments)	900 r each of 4 ports 200 kv.	1,800 r 200 kv.
2	1,200 mg. hrs. (4 treatments)	2,400 mg. hrs. (1 treatment)	None	None
3	1,200 mg. hrs. (4 treatments)	2,000 mg. hrs. (2 treatments)	None	2,000 r at 200 kv.
4	775 mg. hrs.	1,175 mg. hrs. (2 treatments)	2,100 r each of 2 ant. ports 400 kv.	None
5	None	1,100 mg. hrs. (2 treatments)	2,000 r 200 kv. each of 2 large ports	None
6	600 mg. hrs. (2 treatments)	None	1,000 r at 200 kv. single abdom. port	None
7	None	1,600 mg. hrs. (2 treatments)	1,600 r 400 kv. single port	None
8	None	1,200 mg. hrs. (1 treatment)	None	None
9	1,200 mg. hrs. (4 treatments)	None	2,500 r each 4 fields 400 kv.	None
10	2,383 mg. hrs. (2 treatments)	1,907 mg. hrs. (2 treatments)	1,100 r each 4 fields 400 kv.	500 r 250 kv. single field
11	900 mg. hrs. (3 treatments)	1,188 mg. hrs. (1 treatment)	None	None

TABLE 27-2. CARCINOMA OF FEMALE URETHRA

Case No.	Age	Path. Diagnosis	Clinical Type	Treatment
1	62	Epidermoid car., transitional	Vulvo-urethral	Radium, x-ray, and surgery
2	55	Epidermoid car., transitional	Urethral	Radium
3	62	Intraepithelial car. of urethra	Vulvo-urethral	Rad. and x-ray
4	53	Epidermoid car., spinal cell	Vulvo-urethral	Rad. and x-ray
5	61	Urethral caruncle with malig. degen.	Vulvo-urethral	Rad. and x-ray
6	52	Epidermoid car., transitional	Urethral	Rad. and x-ray
7	76	Carcinoma urethra	Urethral	Rad. and x-ray
8	59	Epidermoid car., transitional	Vulvo-urethral	Rad. Excis. caruncle
9	62	Epidermoid car., transitional	Urethral	Rad., x-ray, and surgery
10	48	Epidermoid carcinoma	Urethral	Rad. and x-ray
11	67	? Carcinoma in polyp	Urethral	Radium

49th case, having found only 48 in the world literature. The symptoms of progressively severe dysuria, urinary frequency, urgency, and stranguria are usually followed by frank hematuria and retropubic pain.

Since urethral malignancy is so rare and since results are often unsatisfactory, there is no standard therapy. The treatment depends upon the size, position, and type of lesion. Very small lesions have been reported as cured by partial excision of the urethra. On the other hand, extensive excision with inguinal lymph gland dissection and diversion of the urine has been done for more advanced lesions. Even with operations falling into the exenteration category, the results are frequently disappointing.

In many instances irradiation would appear to be superior to surgery, although the reported series of irradiation, surgery, and a confirmation are so small that it is impossible to draw generalized conclusions. Wineland reports a 16 per cent 5-year survival in 25 cases treated by irradiation alone. From the Hopkins clinic Brack has reported on 11 cases treated in various ways with irradiation. Table 27-1 gives his method of treatment in some detail, and Table 27-2 gives the treatment according to clinical and histologic types.

From the available literature one can only conclude that despite the individual consideration which must be given to each case, and the best of judgment, one cannot expect a very high salvage.

BIBLIOGRAPHY

Brack, C. B., and Bickerson, R. J.: Carcinoma of the female urethra. Amer. J. Roentgen., 79:472, 1958.

Davis, H. J., and Cian, L. G.: Positive pressure urethrography: a new diagnostic method. J. Urol., 75:753, 1956.

Edwards, Eugene A., and Beebe, Robert A.: Diverticula of the female urethra. Obstet. Gynec., 5:729, 1955.

Hassin, A. B., and MacNiel, A. T.: Primary carcinoma of the paraurethral glands. Brit. J. Surg., 53:689, 1966.

Keefe, J.: Prolapse of the female urethra. J.A.M.A., 69:17, 1935.

Livermore, G. R.: Treatment of prolapse of the urethra. Surg. Gynec. Obstet., 32:557, 1921.

McCrea, L. E.: Malignancy of the female urethra. Urol. Survey, 2:85, 1952.

Parmenter, F. J.: Diverticulum of the urethra. J. Urol., 45:479, 1941.

Wharton, L. R., and Kearns, W.: Diverticula of the female urethra. J. Urol., 63:1063, 1950.

Wharton, L. R., Jr., and Te Linde, R. W.: Urethral diverticulum. Obstet. Gynec., 7:503, 1956.

28

Vesicovaginal and Urethrovaginal Fistulas

HISTORY

The subject of vesicovaginal fistula dates from antiquity. Mahfouz of Cairo described a vesicovaginal fistula found in a mummy estimated to be about 4,000 years old. Since the literature contains many historical sketches of the subject, no attempt at such a review will be made here, but reference will be made to a few of the milestones in the development of our present operative knowledge. No one man is responsible for this knowledge; it has been acquired step by step through the tireless efforts of surgeons dating back to the 17th century. Before that time the condition was considered hopeless, and one sees references even as late as the middle of the 18th century to the treatment of these fistulas by the wearing of a pulverized toad in a little bag over the pit of the stomach. The more practical-minded of those times devoted their efforts to making receptacles to catch the urine, thus making the life of the victim more endurable.

The first real surgical contribution was made by a Hollander, H. Van Roonhuyse, whose contributions were far in advance of his time and apparently were overlooked by many later writers who fumbled about with much-less-rational methods. In 1672 Van Roonhuyse recommended:

The placing of the patient in a position appropriate for lithotomy.

The satisfactory exposure of the fistula by a retracting speculum.

The thorough denudation of the margins of the fistula.

The approximation of the denuded edges by means of quills thrust through the edges of the wound and held in place by silk threads.

The dressing of the wound with balsam and absorbent vaginal dressings.

The patient kept quiet in bed until the parts had healed.

There is no report of Van Roonhuyse's successes and failures, but Johannas Fatio, of Basel, reported on 2 cases successfully operated upon by him in 1675 and 1684. He states that he employed the "method of the skilled physician, Van Roonhuyse."

In the early 19th century some workers used caustics to freshen up the edges, and hooks and other devices to draw the edges together, but little real surgical progress was made until 1839, when George Hayward, at the Massachusetts General Hospital, reported some cases in which he described the important technical point of detaching the vagina from the bladder. Then came ether anesthesia, and it probably was used for the first time for this operation by Hayward in 1847. In 1846 Metzer, of Prague, described using an instrument very much like the Sims's speculum. In 1847 John Mettauer, of Virginia, first used twisted metal (lead) sutures. In 1852 Wutzer, of Bonn, reported curing 11 out of 35 patients. He was the first to use suprapubic drainage.

In 1845 Jobert de Lamballe described his incision for relieving tension on the suture line. It consisted of a transverse vaginal incision anterior to the cervix, whereby the bladder could be freed from the cervix. Gustav Simon, who was a pupil of Jobert and appreciated the value of easing the tension on the suture line, attempted to do this by the use of tension sutures instead of incisions.

Marion Sims's first paper on vesicovaginal fistula appeared in 1852, and it is generally conceded that he is the father of surgery for vesicovaginal fistula in America. There is no doubt that he attained greater success than anyone up to his time. It is interesting to note, however, that his operation was not new. Each step had been used and described before by the surgeons mentioned above and by others. The only innovation which Sims contributed was the use of silver wire. This was, in truth, one of the greatest contributions, and Sims guarded his priority with such jealousy that he devoted most of his anniversary oration before the New York Academy of Medicine, in 1857, to defending it. He declared it to be "the most important contribution as yet made to the surgery of the present century."

In 1893 L. Von Dittel first described the transperitoneal approach, dissecting the bladder from the uterus and the vagina and closing the opening in the bladder from above. The following year Mackenrodt made a contribution to the technic which was of greatest importance. He incised the vagina in the midline across the fistula and then, with knife and forceps, split the margins of the fistula so as to separate completely the bladder from the vaginal wall. He then closed the bladder and vaginal incisions separately. This procedure described by Mackenrodt approximates broad raw surfaces for healing and more nearly approaches our modern methods than any technic previously described.

In 1896 Kelly described a method of closing a large bladder defect by freeing the bladder from the cervix "all the way up to the peritoneum, and widely on both sides by blunt dissection.... The part of the bladder freed from its attachments behind was now easily drawn forward and accurately applied to the immovable anterior third." In the communication describing this procedure Kelly mentioned preoperative ureteral catheterization in order to avoid injury of the ureters, a procedure which we have found to be invaluable. In 1914 Latzko described a technic suited to cases of vesicovaginal fistula resulting from total hysterectomy. It consists of obliteration of the vaginal vault with approximation of broad areas of denuded tissue. In 1942 he reported upon 31 cases of vesicovaginal fistula treated by this method with cure of 29, improvement in one case, and failure in another. Latzko's contribution has been a truly great one, and in recent years its value has been magnified by the fact that there have appeared so many fistulas resulting from total hysterectomy. Since using his technic for the closure of these postoperative fistulas we have not had a failure.

ETIOLOGY

Vesicovaginal fistulas (Fig. 28-1), as seen today, fall chiefly into 3 groups: (1) those resulting from obstetric injury; (2) those resulting from operative accidents, chiefly during abdominal panhysterectomy; (3) those resulting from extension of carcinoma of the cervix or the radium treatment of this disease; and (4) a small miscellaneous group. Formerly, those following obstetric injury formed the largest group, but the improvement in obstetric methods has greatly reduced their number. The increased popularity of total hysterectomy has resulted in a great increase in operative fistulas. Contributions by Norman Miller and by Holden have noted this fact, and our experience coincides with theirs. In 1956 Everett and Mattingly reviewed the 149 cases of fistula operated upon at the Johns Hopkins Hospital between the years 1933 and 1953. Classified from the standpoint of etiology they are as follows:

	CASES
Obstetric injury	28
Gynecologic surgery	65
Carcinoma of cervix and its radiation therapy	48
Miscellaneous	8

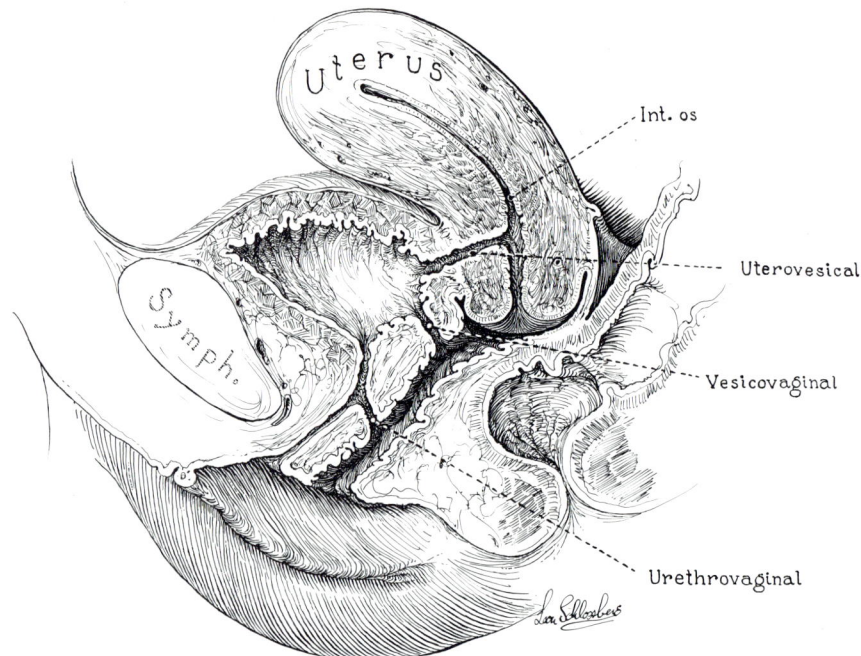

Fig. 28-1. Diagrammatic sagittal section showing locations of vesicocervical, vesicovaginal, and urethrovaginal fistula.

The 3 principal types mentioned above are so grouped from an etiologic standpoint, but also they fall naturally into the same groups when considered from the point of view of cure. The obstetric fistulas should be repaired by the vaginal route in most instances. Those resulting from total hysterectomy are usually very high in the vagina. They, too, may often be approached best by the vaginal route, but rarely are best repaired transperitoneally. Those formed by the breaking down of carcinomatous tissue in the vesicovaginal region are often not repairable. When the fistula is the result of a radium burn or of the destruction of carcinomatous tissue in the vesicovaginal septum by radium or x-rays, the closure is usually very difficult, due to reduced blood supply and excessive scar tissue. Before attempting the cure of such a fistula, multiple biopsies should be taken from the edges of the fistula and the cervix to establish the fact that all carcinomatous tissue has been destroyed.

SYMPTOMS AND DIAGNOSIS

The successful treatment of vesicovaginal fistula depends upon an exact diagnosis; it is impossible to discuss treatment without reference to diagnostic signs and procedures. With a small fistula the urinary leakage may be slight and, in some instances, dependent upon the position of the patient. Women with such a fistula may void a good quantity of urine, whereas, with larger fistulas, sufficient urine does not collect in the bladder to permit voiding. With marked incontinence the vulva usually becomes reddened and excoriated, and urinary salts may collect on the parts. Pustules frequently form on the vulva and the thighs. The odor of decomposing urine may be so offensive as to be disgusting to the patient and repulsive to others.

Most vesicovaginal fistulas are painless. If the patient complains of pain and has had a previous operative attempt, one should consider the possibility of a buried nonabsorbable suture with calculus formation (Fig. 28-2). But fistulas resulting from irradiation can cause severe pain. Graham has reported 10 such cases with progressive pain, aggravated by movement or sitting. The areas of these fistulas are very tender, and often anesthesia is required for a satisfactory examination. The vagina and labia have

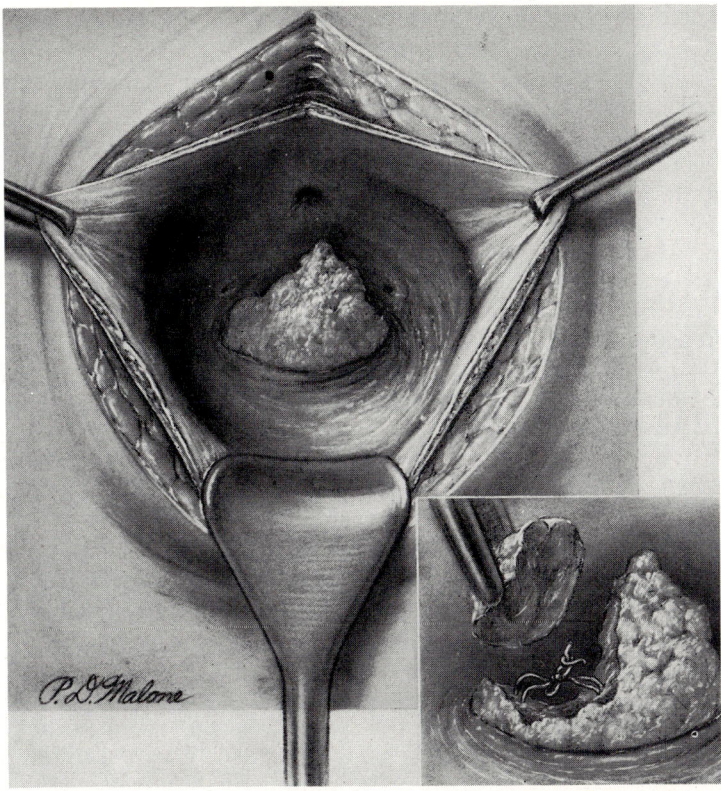

FIG. 28-2. Demonstrating calculus formation about silver-wire suture, erroneously used in interior of bladder.

greenish-gray deposits, and in many cases there is necrotic tissue along the margins of the fistula. Bacteria in the vagina split urea and produce an alkaline medium in which crystals form. However, all irradiation fistulas fortunately do not fall into this painful pattern.

The diagnosis usually lies between vesicovaginal fistula and incontinence due to weakness of the sphincter. When the loss of urine is due to weakness of the sphincter, urine usually can be seen to spurt from the meatus when the patient, with her bladder full, is asked to cough. When the fistula is large, it is easily palpated through the vagina or seen with the patient in the knee-chest, the Sims lateral, or the lithotomy position. If no fistulous opening can be readily demonstrated, often it may be found by filling the bladder with a weak solution of methylene blue and then inspecting the anterior vaginal wall. If no point of leakage is discovered by this method, two clean sponges are placed in the vagina, and the patient is allowed to walk about, the sponges being removed later and inspected for stains. Using two sponges not only will reveal the presence or absence of a fistula but will give information on the site of the fistula.

The air method of Kelly is admirably adapted for cystoscopic examination of these patients. This always should be done in order to ascertain the size and the position of the fistula and particularly its relation to the ureteral orifices and the vesical sphincter. When the cystoscopic examination is made with a water cystoscope, difficulty is experienced in filling the bladder when the opening is large. With the air method, the bladder expands satisfactorily, even in the presence of a large fistula. However, with either water or air cystoscopy, small fistulas are often seen with great difficulty from within the bladder.

When a urinary fistula develops postoperatively, the diagnosis lies between vesicovaginal and ureterovaginal fistula. Needless to say, an exact differentiation is necessary before considering treatment. If the bladder is distended with methylene blue solution, and the urine in the vagina is unstained, the communication is with the ureter. This should be confirmed by cystoscopy, which will show the ureteral orifice on the affected side failing to spurt urine. Usually a catheter will meet with an obstruction when the tip reaches the point of ureteral injury.

Also intravenous urography should be a routine part of the preoperative investigation. A hydroureter and/or hydronephrosis suggests a ureteral fistula, but it can also be the result of scarring on the edge of a bladder fistula in the region of the ureteral orifice. In any case, the urogram should be a matter of record for the protection of the surgeon. The discovery of a hydroureter or hydronephrosis postoperatively may be blamed upon the operator. Proof of its presence before operation may vindicate the surgeon.

TREATMENT
General Principles

Specific examples of the different types of operations as done in our clinic will be described later in detail. Some of the principles which we believe to be important are enumerated here:

1. It is an advantage to have the tissues in as good condition as possible before attempting the operation. In the case of postoperative or postdelivery fistulas, generally 6 months should elapse from the time of injury before attempting the repair. This important point, which Hunner emphasized frequently, is disregarded all too often, and attempts at repair are made too early when the condition of the tissues makes success impossible. One always should remember that every unsuccessful attempt at closure produces scar tissue and makes future attempts that much more difficult. Hot sitz baths, warm irrigations with potassium permanganate solution, 1:8,000, and weak vinegar douches are useful procedures for the removal of incrustations from the tissues and getting the tissues in good condition for surgery.

2. The choice of the approach to the operative field is all-important. We have come more and more to the conclusion that almost all vesicovaginal fistulas should be closed per vaginam. This is surely true for the fistulas resulting from obstetric injuries. It is equally true for the postirradiation fistulas. Formerly, we attacked transperitoneally many of the postoperative fistulas situated at the apex of the vagina. The adaptation of the Latzko technic to such fistulas has almost done away with the transperitoneal approach. In recent years we have attacked such fistulas transperitoneally only in those rare instances in which many previous vaginal operations have resulted in so much vaginal scarring as to make the fistula inaccessible through the vagina. We do not consider the virginal outlet a disadvantage to the vaginal approach because an outlet can be enlarged readily by a unilateral or bilateral Schuchardt incision (Fig. 28-3). We recognize the fact that some excellent surgeons, such as Pfaneuf, recommend the transvesical approach to fistulas and treat them successfully by that method. However, we believe that it is certainly not a method of approach of the usual fistula. We have operated upon an unusual fistula transvesically, resulting from a spicule of bone perforating the bladder at the time of an automobile accident. The more experience we have with various types of fistulas, the more we have concluded that one should not close one's mind to any avenue of approach, and that each case should be considered individually.

When the vaginal approach is used, exposure may best be accomplished at times by putting the patient in the lithotomy position; in others, in the Sims lateral; and in others, in the knee-chest posture. The great majority of our fistulas are repaired in the lithotomy position. Dropping the head of the table and elevating the buttocks often facilitates exposure.

3. Preoperative cystoscopic examina-

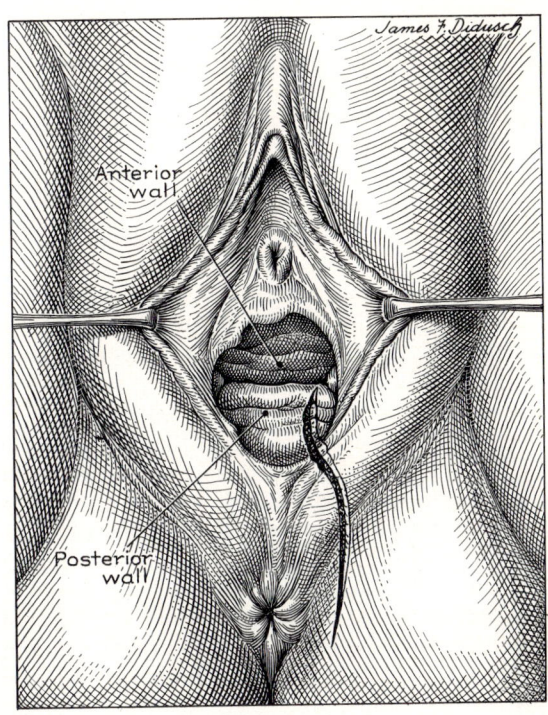

FIG. 28-3. Schuchardt's incision.

tion is of great advantage. If the surgeon is skilled in cystoscopy, the examination is best done by him so that he can ascertain the relation of the ureteral orifices to the fistula. As stated above, the direct air cystoscope is admirably adapted to this examination, because no matter how large the fistula, the bladder will expand when the patient is in the knee-chest posture. The indirect water method is disadvantageous, due to rapid escape of the water in case the fistula is large. When the fistula is near one or both ureteral orifices, either or both of them should be catheterized preoperatively to prevent the inclusion of the orifice or the intravesical portion of the ureter in a suture.

4. A wide area of denudation should be made about the fistulous opening, and the bladder should be sufficiently mobilized to prevent closure without tension. Wide denudation is particularly important in the closure of postirradiation fistulas, because the scar tissue surrounding the fistula is poor in blood supply, and healing is at a great disadvantage. Therefore it is desirable to approximate as broad surfaces as possible to enhance the chance for healing. Also, the farther one dissects away from the fistulous opening, the better the blood supply becomes.

The first row of fine catgut sutures should not enter the bladder but should be taken parallel with the edge of the fistulous tract so as to invert the edge into the bladder. If possible, the first row of sutures should be reinforced by a second one. Usually, interrupted sutures are preferable to a continuous suture. Silver-wire sutures which approximate the mucosal edges should pick up the subjacent tissue to obliterate the dead space. Wire sutures never should be buried in the closure, and under no circumstances should they enter the bladder. If they do, a calculus will form around them (Fig. 28-2).

5. Separate closure of the vaginal incision with interrupted sutures of silver wire or fine catgut greatly increases the chance of success. The silver wires may be left in from 14 to 16 days without showing evidence of infection. If the vaginal flaps are sufficiently mobile to

permit, it is desirable not to have the bladder and the vaginal suture lines superimposed one on the other.

6. There should be no absolute rule regarding postoperative drainage of the bladder. In simple cases when the closure has been done with good tissues, and particularly when the operative region has been some distance from the vesical sphincter, a retention catheter may be left in the bladder only over night until the patient is completely alert following the anesthetic. The next morning it may be removed and the patient permitted to get up to void. She should be catheterized immediately for residual urine following voiding. If she empties her bladder down to a residual of 100 cc., further catheterization may be omitted. In slightly more difficult cases an indwelling Foley catheter is left in the urethra. However, in the very difficult cases, especially those in which several previous operations have resulted in failure, double drainage is an excellent plan. Many a good surgical repair of a fistula has been ruined by a nurse who permitted the bladder to become distended—a consequence of the urethral catheter's becoming obstructed. Establishment of drainage either per vaginam (Fig. 28-4) or suprapubically (Fig. 28-5) adds very little to the operation and greatly increases the chances of success. We prefer a therapeutic vesicovaginal fistula to suprapubic drainage. Such a fistula should not be made through scar tissue but if made through normal tissue, the artificial opening will close spontaneously soon after the catheter has been removed. If the anterior vaginal wall does not permit a therapeutic fistula because of the extent of the operative closure or because of scar tissues, suprapubic drainage through a mushroom catheter is quite satisfactory.

7. When the fistula is large and difficult of closure, the patient should remain in bed for 14 days. Patients with small fistulas without much scar tissue about them may be up in a few days without endangering the success of closure. We never have insisted on the patient's remaining in a prone position. If adequate drainage

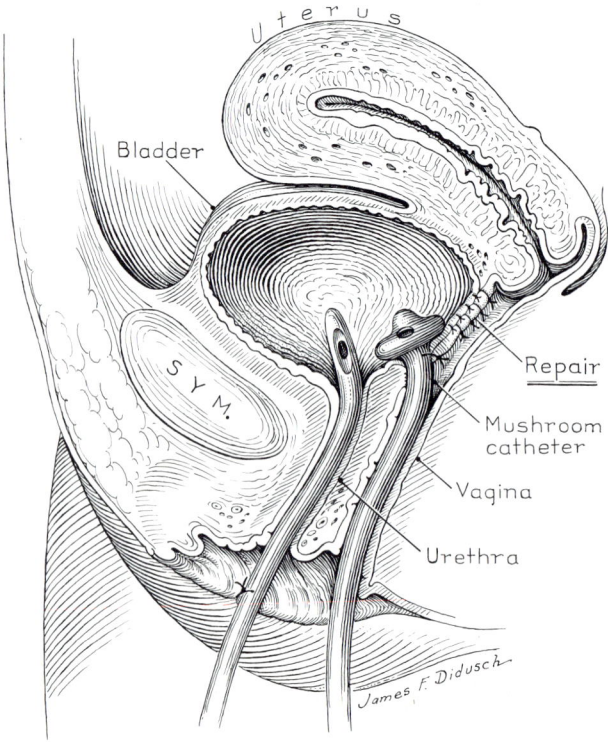

FIG. 28-4. Demonstrating double bladder drainage through the urethra and the surgical vesicovaginal fistula. The surgical fistula in this case was made just above the trigone.

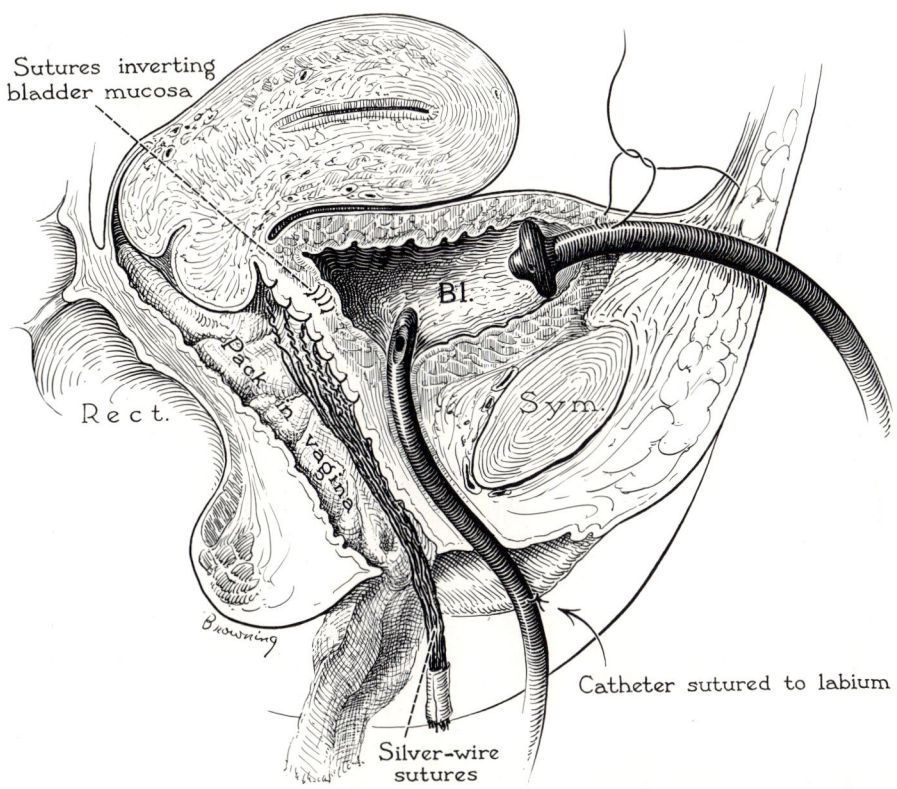

FIG. 28-5. Double bladder drainage through urethra and suprapubic cystotomy.

is established so that the bladder does not become distended, it makes little difference in what position the patient lies.

8. Only when the closure of a vesicovaginal fistula is considered to be absolutely impossible, should one consider diversion of the urinary stream. The painful postirradiation fistulas, such as those previously mentioned, described by Graham, fall into this group. In former years we transplanted the ureters into the sigmoid, but experience has taught us that transplantation into functioning bowel usually shortens the patients life. This is usually due to the development of hydronephrosis and pyelonephritis, with the attending disturbances of the chemical constituents of the blood. There are exceptions to this rule but they are rare. We now reserve sigmoidal implantations for cases in which we believe the patient's lifetime is limited by the presence of malignancy. A good example of this would be a fistula resulting from irradiation of advanced cervical cancer when cure is very unlikely. When a fistula is the result of benign disease or injury but impossible of closure, we believe that the implantation of the ureters into an isolated ileal loop is the procedure of choice. We would also prefer this method for an irradiation fistula resulting from the treatment of cervical cancer when the chances of permanent cure of the malignancy seem good.

9. Special delicate, long, narrow instruments greatly facilitate operative work on fistulas in the vagina. A few examples of these are shown in Figures 28-6 to 28-8.

10. Very rarely a minute vesicovaginal fistula may be closed by fulgeration. Falk and Orkin have reported success in 5 of 10 attempts and Hyman in 4 of 8 cases. They emphasize that the tract should be free from infection and the vesicovaginal septum should not be too thin. If this rule is not observed, fulgeration may increase rather than decrease the caliber of the opening.

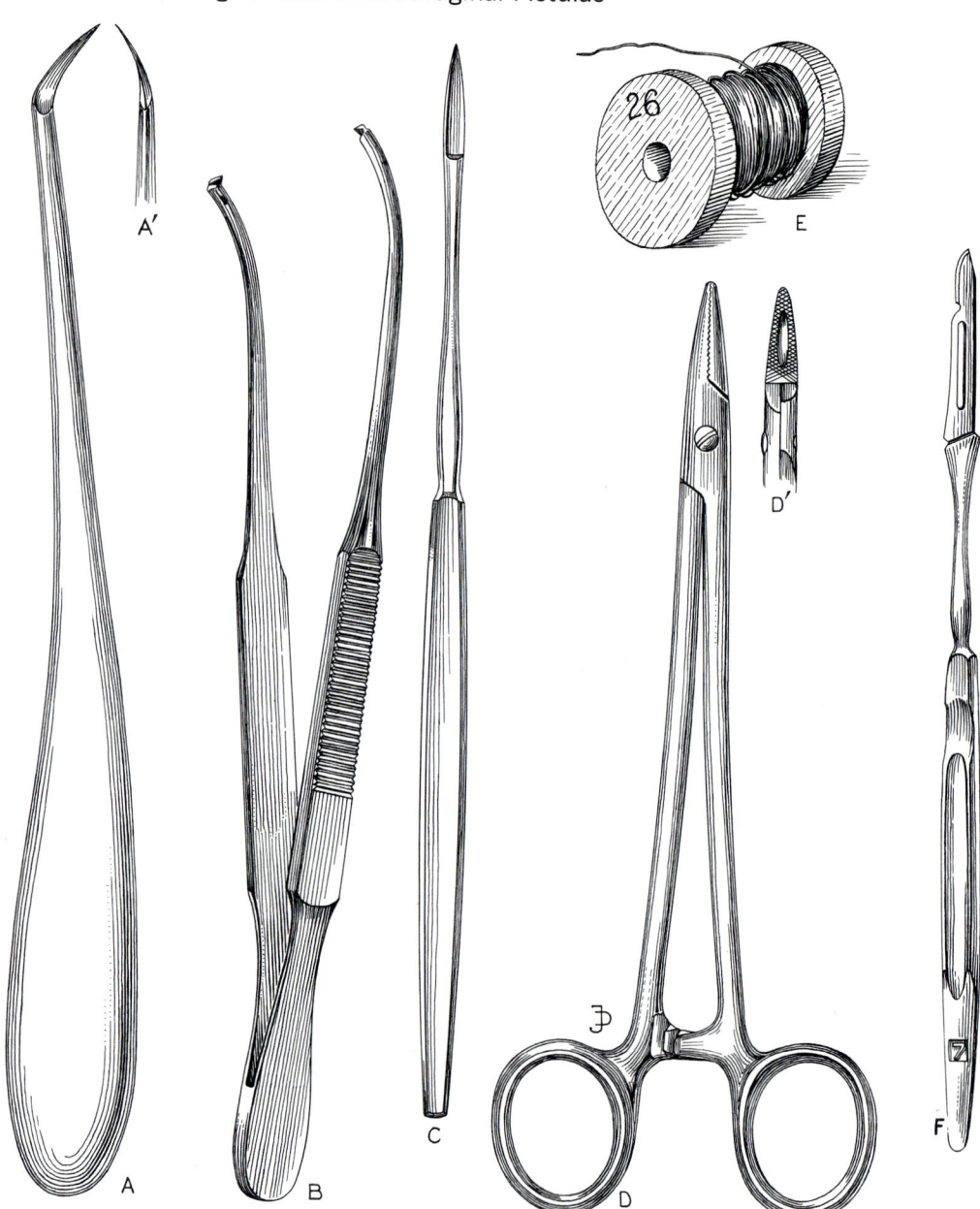

Fig. 28-6. Useful instruments for repair of vesicovaginal fistulas. (A) Curved, long-handled knife, very serviceable for denuding vaginal mucosa from around fistula, high in the vagina. (B) Long, curved, mousetooth forceps, useful for working high in the vagina. (C) Slender, small-bladed, long-handled knife, useful for working deep in vagina. (D) Mayo type needle holder. (E) Number 26 silver wire. (F) Small-bladed, slender Bard-Parker knife, extremely useful in repairing vesicovaginal fistulas.

Technic: Closure of Small Vesicovaginal Fistula

A small vesicovaginal fistula may be closed by the simple technic shown in Figure 28-9. The particular fistula pictured here resulted from too deep fulguration, by a urologist, of an elusive ulcer of the bladder. The patient also had stress incontinence of urine from a re-

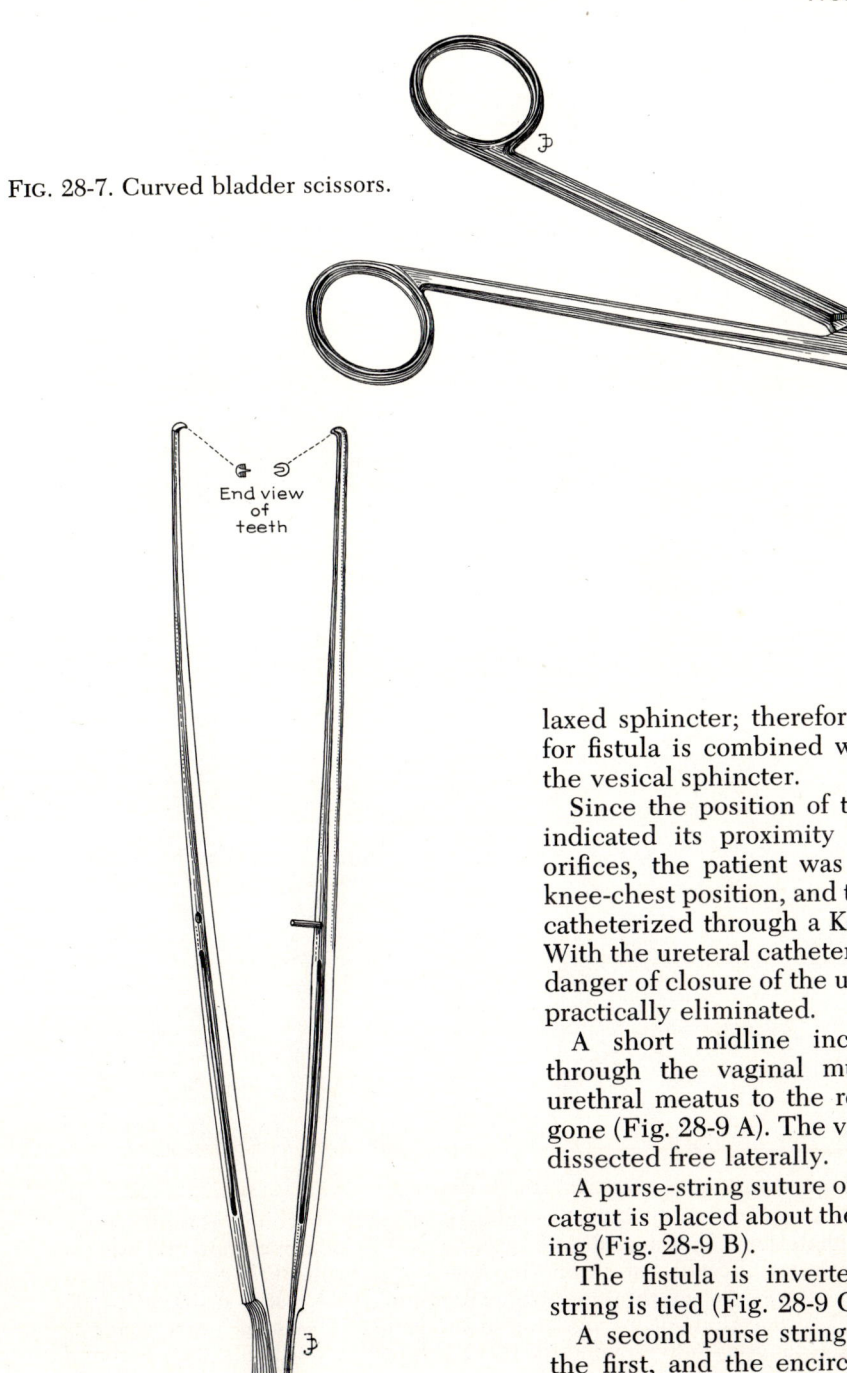

FIG. 28-7. Curved bladder scissors.

FIG. 28-8. Long, thin, mousetooth forceps admirably suited for vesicovaginal fistula work.

laxed sphincter; therefore the operation for fistula is combined with plication of the vesical sphincter.

Since the position of the small fistula indicated its proximity to the ureteral orifices, the patient was first put in the knee-chest position, and the ureters were catheterized through a Kelly cystoscope. With the ureteral catheters in the ureters, danger of closure of the ureteral orifice is practically eliminated.

A short midline incision is made through the vaginal mucosa from the urethral meatus to the region of the trigone (Fig. 28-9 A). The vaginal mucosa is dissected free laterally.

A purse-string suture of No. 00 chromic catgut is placed about the fistulous opening (Fig. 28-9 B).

The fistula is inverted as the purse string is tied (Fig. 28-9 C).

A second purse string is placed about the first, and the encircled tissue is inverted (Fig. 28-9 D).

The urethral and vesical sphincter region is then plicated as indicated in Figure 28-9 E to H.

The mushroom catheter that had been previously placed in the bladder to help localize the sphincter is left in to keep the bladder collapsed for 10 days.

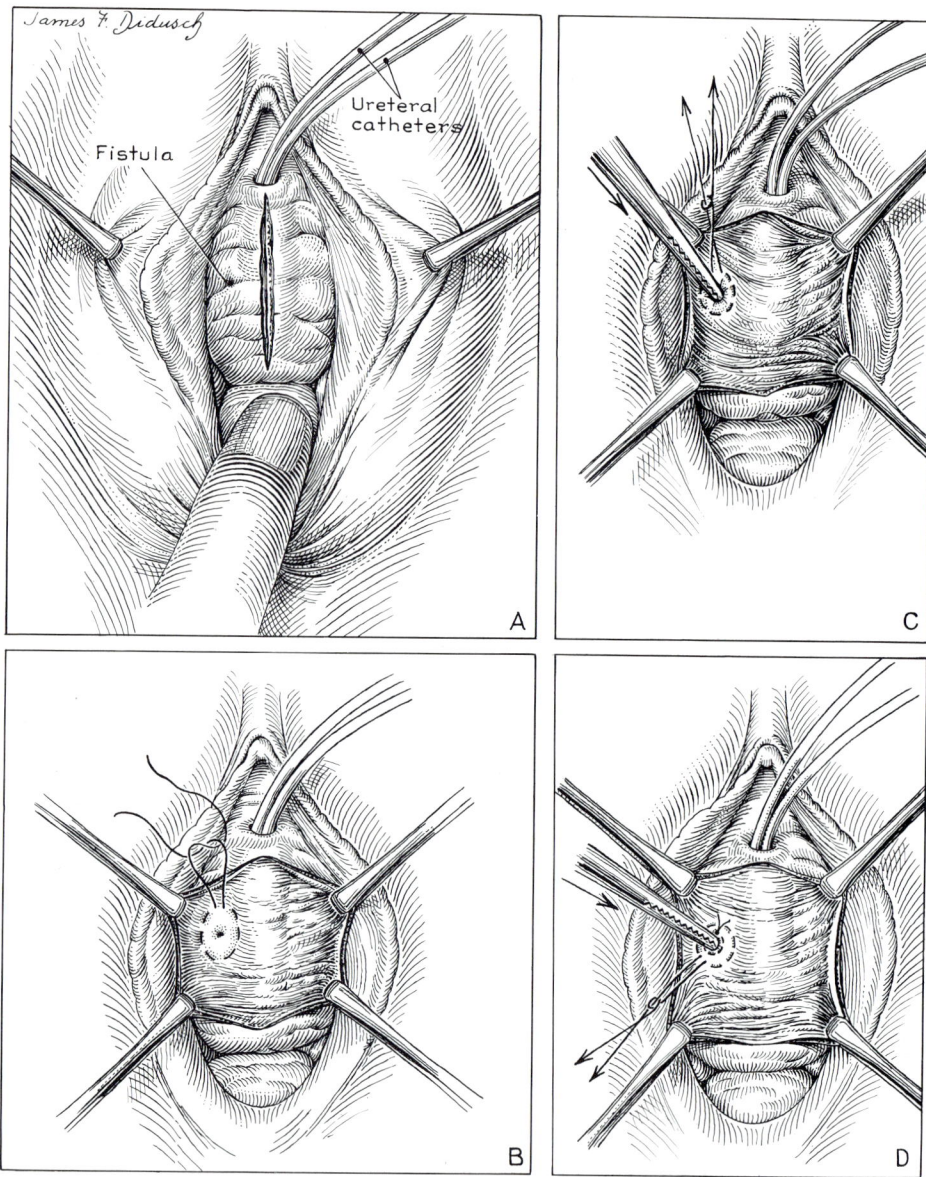

FIG. 28-9. Closure of a very small vesicovaginal fistula at the trigone. (A) Both ureters have been catheterized for their identification. Since in this operation the vesical sphincter was to be plicated also, a midline incision is made through the anterior vaginal wall to expose the urethral and trigonal region. (B) A purse string of No. 00 chromic catgut is placed about the opening of the fistula. (C) As the purse string is tied, the tissue is inverted into the bladder. (D) A second purse string is placed around the first.

TECHNIC: STANDARD OPERATION FOR CLOSURE OF SIMPLE VESICOVAGINAL FISTULA

This simple technic is used in closing an easily exposed fistula in which there is no excess of scar tissue. It represents a more or less typical closure, if there is such a thing as a typical closure in a condition in which there is such great variation. The simple fistula for which this

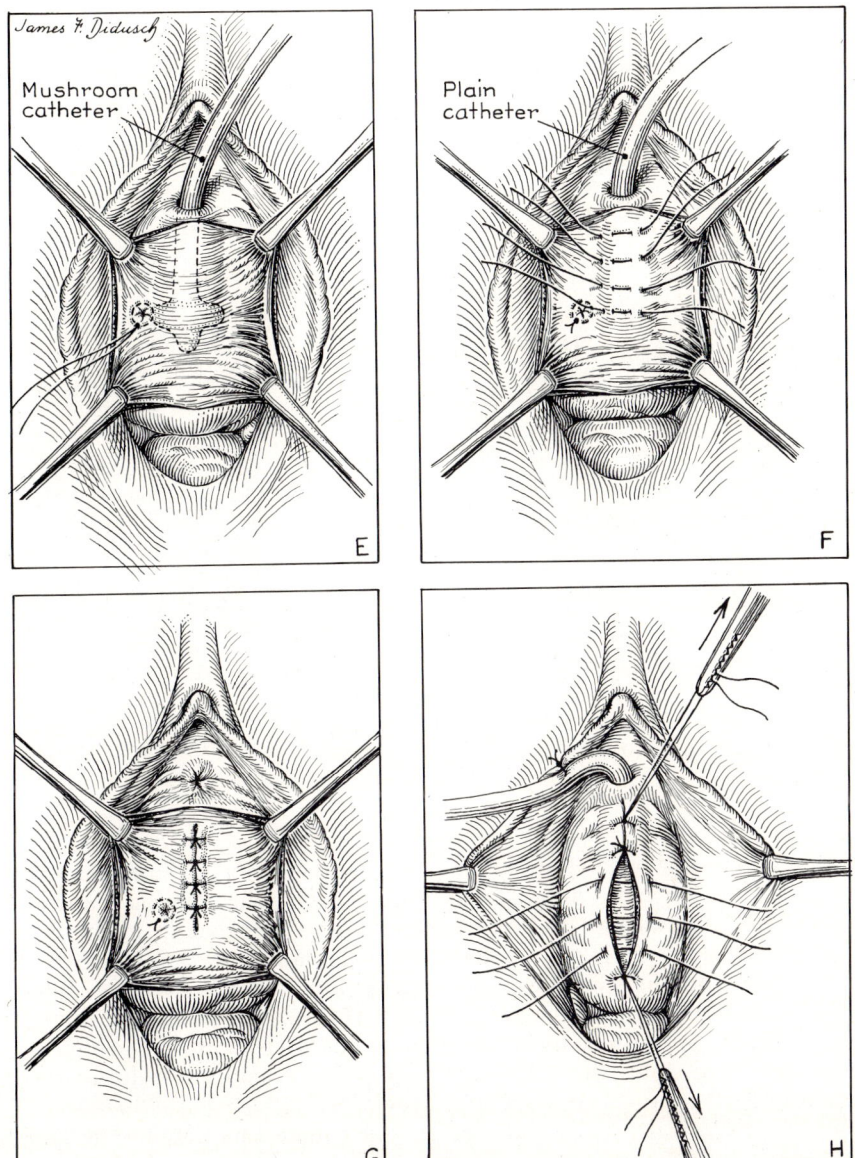

Fig. 28-9 (*Continued*). Closure of a very small vesicovaginal fistula at the trigone. (E) Demonstrates mushroom catheter head at the vesical sphincter. (F) Plication stitches have been taken at the vesical sphincter region and along the urethra. (G) The sphincter has been sutured, and the fistula closed. (H) Excess of vaginal mucosa has been excised, and vaginal flaps have been united in the midline. The vaginal and vesical closures are not superimposed on each other.

operation is done is shown in Figure 28-10 A.

Since the fistula is close to the trigone, the ureters are first catheterized. An incision is made about the fistulous opening, and the vaginal mucosa is dissected free from the bladder for sufficient distance to mobilize enough bladder wall for a double line of closure. Usually a zone of about 1 cm. is sufficient (Fig. 28-10 B).

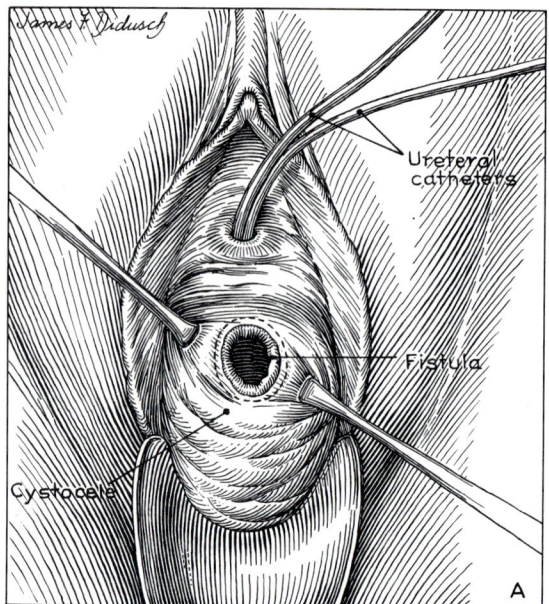 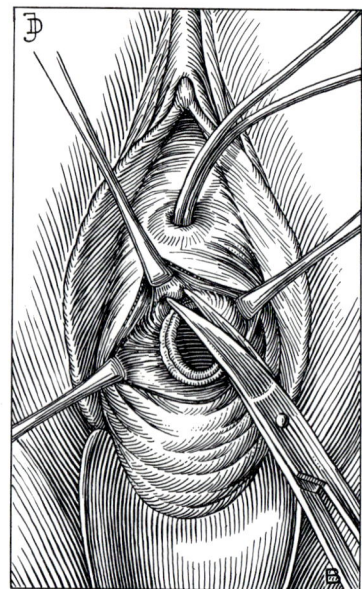

Fig. 28-10. Standard operation for closure of a simple vesicovaginal fistula. (A) Ureters have been catheterized to prevent encirclement of a ureter with a suture. An incision about the fistulous opening is marked by the dotted line. (B) The vaginal mucosa is dissected back from the fistulous opening for a sufficient distance to mobilize the bladder wall about the fistula.

Beginning at one end of the opening, a continuous suture of No. 00 chromic catgut is placed as indicated in Figure 28-10 C. These stitches are taken parallel to the edges of the opening, well into the bladder wall, but not through the mucosa. When the suture is pulled tight, the edges are inverted into the bladder. When complete, it is tied, and a second similar one is placed, inverting the first (Fig. 28-10 D).

At this stage of the operation the closure is tested by introducing into the bladder about 200 cc. of sterilized milk through a glass catheter. The advantage of milk over methylene blue is that it does not stain the tissues in case leakage occurs. If the suture line is not watertight, the weak point is further reinforced with interrupted sutures, mobilizing more bladder if necessary.

The vaginal mucosa is trimmed, if redundant, and closed with interrupted sutures of No. 00 chromic catgut. This closure is made in the direction that gives the least amount of tension. In the case illustrated, the vaginal suture line is made at a right angle to the suture line of the bladder wall (Fig. 28-10 E). It is desirable not to have the suture lines superimposed, the one on the other, but it is not wise to close the mucosa under excessive tension in order to accomplish this.

An indwelling catheter is usually left in the bladder for about 12 days. In simple cases such as this, no secondary bladder drainage is necessary.

Figure 28-11 demonstrates the closure of a large but simple vesicovaginal fistula, extending from the cervix to the bladder trigone. This fistula was the result of the administration of Pituitrin during the second stage of labor. The uterus was ruptured, and the tear extended through the cervix and into the vagina and the bladder. Closure was easily effected after a waiting period of 6 months, when the tissues were in excellent condition.

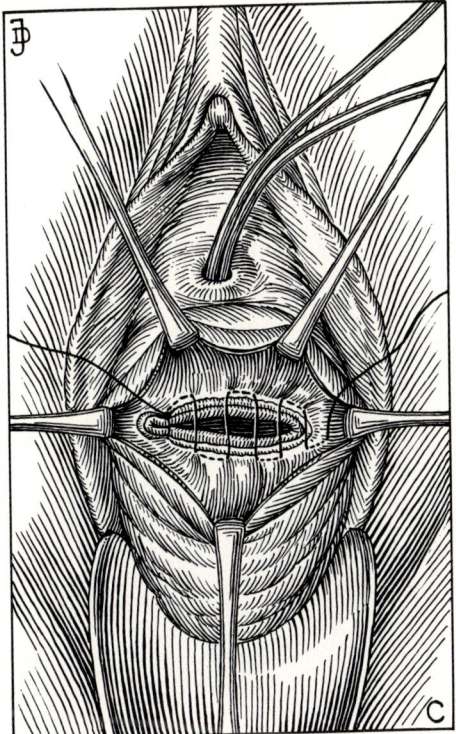
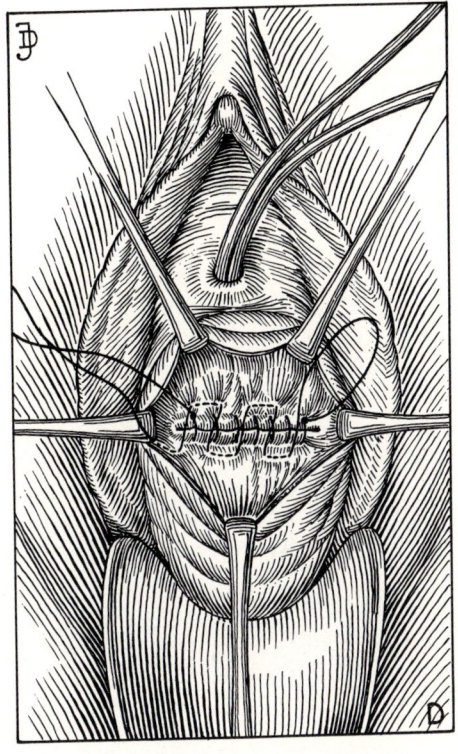
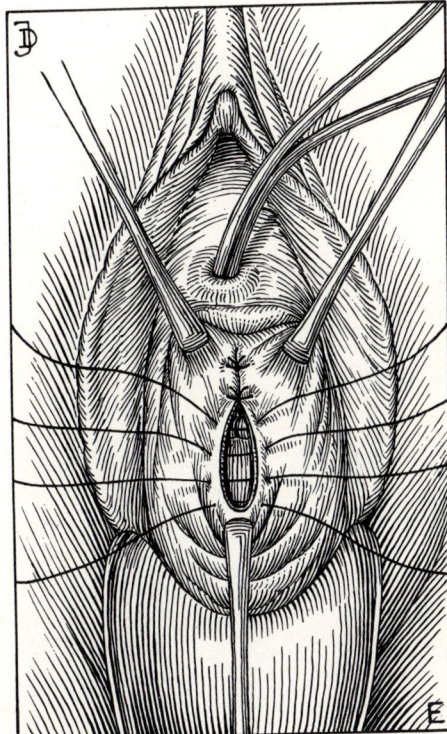

FIG. 28-10 (*Continued*). Standard operation for closure of a simple vesicovaginal fistula. (C) The first suture line is placed as a continuous suture of No. 00 chromic catgut, inverting tissue into the bladder. (D) A second suture line is placed, inverting the first. (E) The mucosa has been trimmed and is closed at right angles to the other sutures with interrupted sutures of No. 0 chromic catgut. A mushroom catheter has been placed in the bladder.

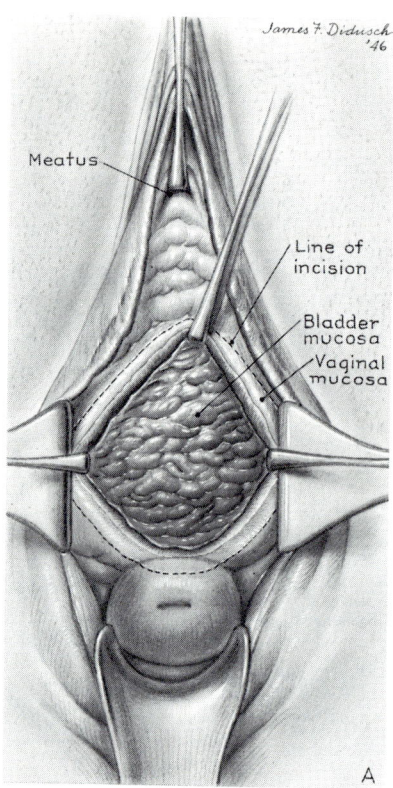
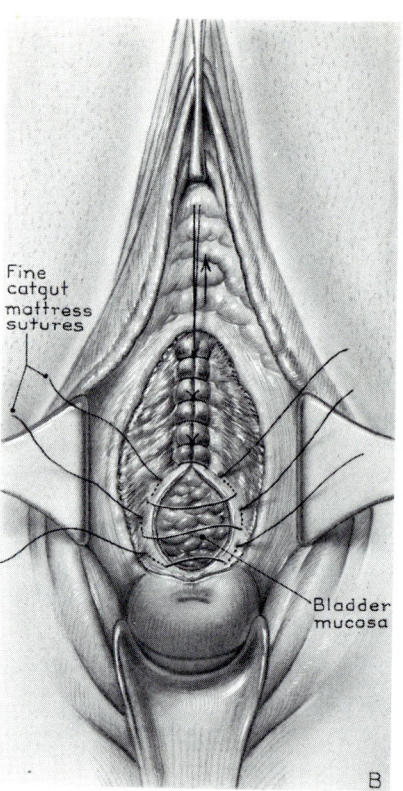
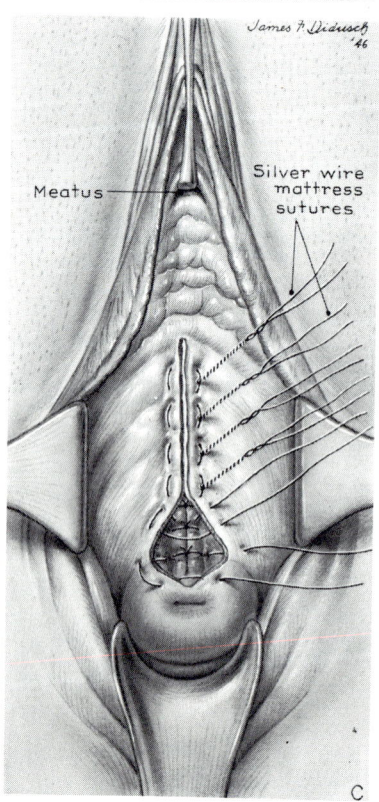

FIG. 28-11. (A) Large vesicovaginal fistula extending from cervix almost to meatus. (B) First row of mattress sutures has been placed, inverting edge into bladder. (C) Vaginal mucosa being closed with silver-wire mattress sutures, everting edge into vagina.

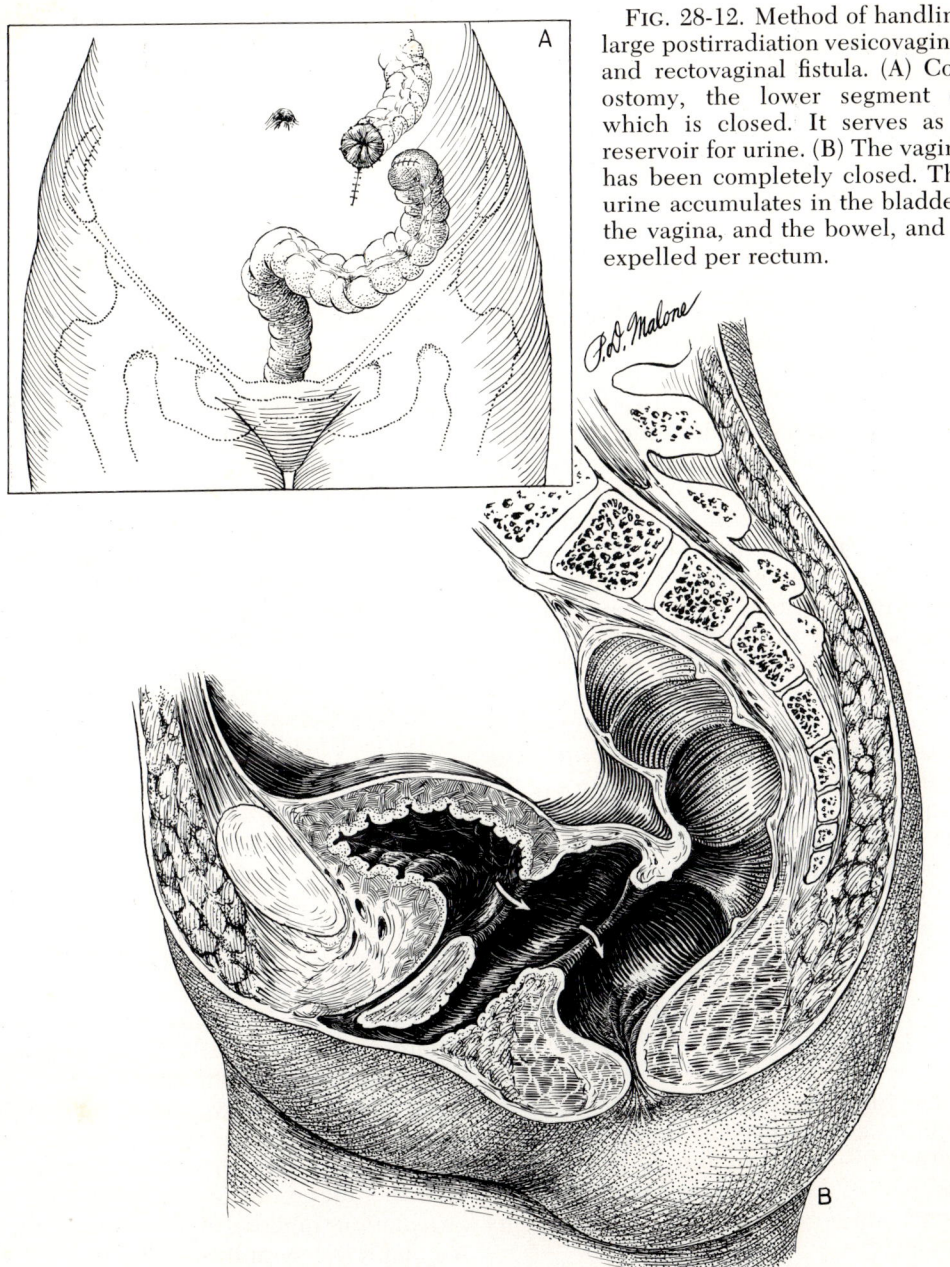

FIG. 28-12. Method of handling large postirradiation vesicovaginal and rectovaginal fistula. (A) Colostomy, the lower segment of which is closed. It serves as a reservoir for urine. (B) The vagina has been completely closed. The urine accumulates in the bladder, the vagina, and the bowel, and is expelled per rectum.

Technic: Operation for Large Vesicovaginal and Rectovaginal Fistulas, Following Irradiation for Advanced Carcinoma of the Cervix

The fistulas for which this operation was done occurred 12 years after irradiation following total abdominal hysterectomy for carcinoma of the cervix. There was practically a complete loss of the vesicovaginal and rectovaginal septa. Several biopsies, taken from the edges of the fistulas, showed no cancer. The patient was miserable from the leakage of both urine and feces, and the vulva and the thighs were markedly excoriated. Her ultimate condition with a permanent colostomy and voiding urine per rectum was eminently satisfactory to her, in comparison with her original pitiful state.

A permanent colostomy was established by bringing a loop of the sigmoid out through a lower-right rectus incision (Fig. 28-12 A).

Having diverted the feces from the vulval region, the patient was put on sitz baths, and the condition of the skin of the vulva and the thighs was greatly improved. Then the vagina was completely closed. The insides of the labia majora were denuded, and the labia minora and the clitoris were excised. The raw surfaces acquired in this way were brought together with many interrupted, buried sutures of No. 0 chromic catgut, and the skin was closed with a continuous subcuticular stitch. For 10 days a rectal tube was left in the rectum to drain off the urine while the labia were healing together. After several weeks the upper end of the lower segment of bowel was closed to prevent reflux of urine when the patient reclined. Thus the bladder, the vagina, and the rectum were made a reservoir for urine (Fig. 28-12 B). The patient had complete urinary control and voided per rectum at intervals of 2 to 3 hours.

Technic: Operation for Restoration of Urethra and Urinary Continence

The following operation is designed for certain cases of urinary incontinence resulting from destruction of the urethra and part of the sphincter from childbirth injury, surgery, or from a granulomatous lesion.

A U-shaped flap of vaginal mucosa is dissected free and held forward, thus exposing the undersurface of the trigone and sphincter region of the bladder (Fig. 28-13 A, B). Rather deep interrupted stitches of medium silk are taken in the sphincter region, which, when tied, tighten the internal orifice (Fig. 28-13 C).

The flap of mucosa is drawn downward and an area about 6 or 7 mm. in width is denuded forward on either side for a distance equal to the length of the flap (Fig. 28-13 D).

The edge of the flap is held forward with a smooth dissecting forceps and curled under, so that the raw surface of the flap may be sutured to the anterior denuded area (Fig. 28-13 E). Interrupted sutures of No. 00 chromic catgut are used. This is repeated on the other side, thus forming an epithelial-lined tube to serve as a urethra.

The wound is closed by approximating the mucosal edges with interrupted sutures of No. 0 chromic catgut (Fig. 28-13 F). This buries the newly constructed urethra and completely closes the wound (Fig. 28-13 G).

In order to direct the urine and permit healing of the newly constructed urethra, a surgical vesicovaginal fistula is made at a higher point, and a mushroom catheter is inserted (Fig. 28-13 G).

Another Operation for Formation of Urethra and Restoration of Urinary Continence

The operation above described has served well in a few cases of absent urethra, but since the last edition of this book we have performed a few successful operations by a different method described below. The choice between the 2 operations depends upon where the most well-vascularized vaginal mucosa is available. In the preceding operation there was no redundant mucosa in the urethral region due to scarring, but there was ample well-vascularized vaginal mucosa beneath the base of the bladder. Therefore a flap was turned forward. In the technic about to be described there was ample mucosa in the urethral region beneath the symphysis. Therefore it was used to roll up a cylinder to serve as a urethra. After performing this operation successfully on 2 women who had lost their urethras as a result of sloughing after plastic surgery, the senior author found a description of the identical operation by Falk and Tancer, who reported 3 successful cases.

Technic. A U-shaped incision is made surrounding the vesical opening and extending forward to the area of the meatus

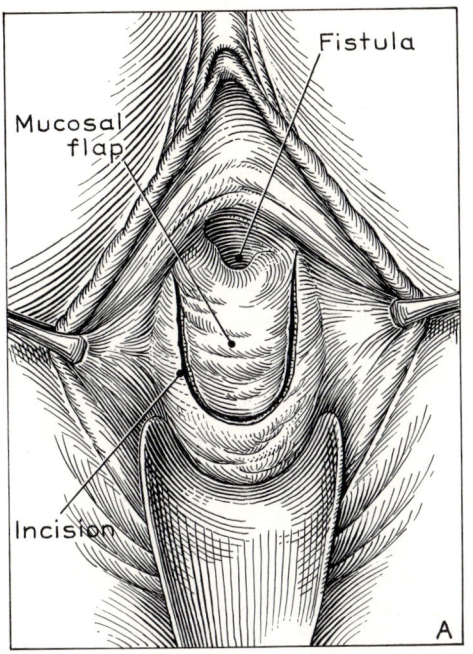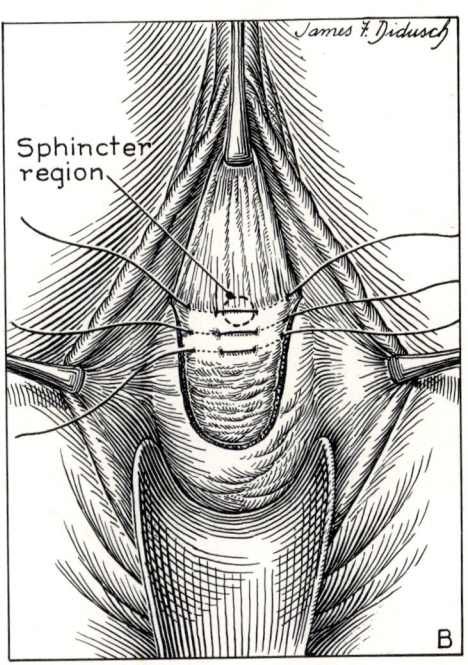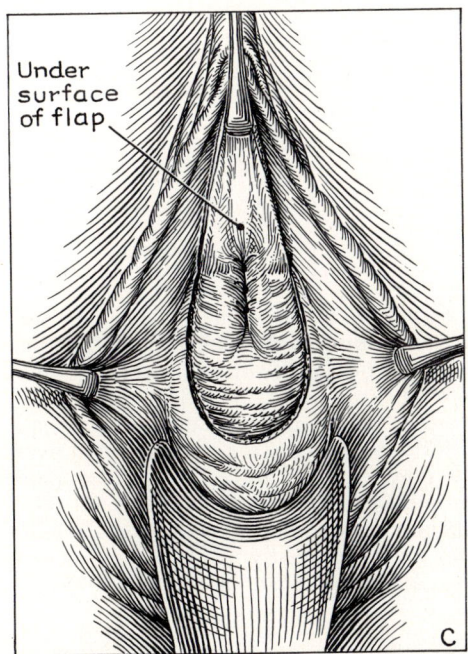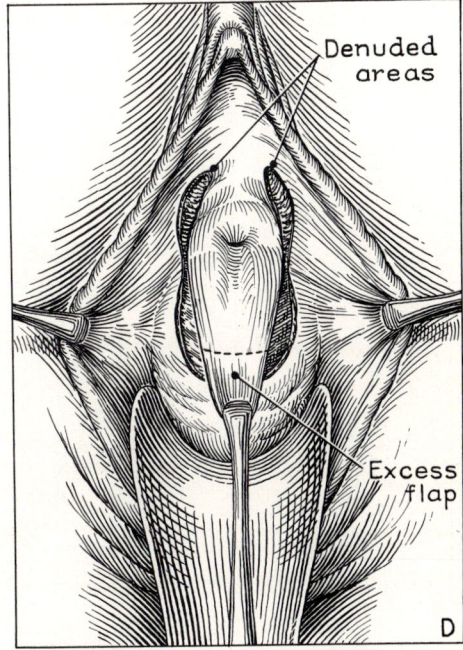

Fig. 28-13. Plastic operation for formation of urethra and repair of sphincter. (A) A U-shaped incision is made through the vaginal mucosa. (B) The mucosal flap has been freed and pulled forward. Three interrupted sutures of medium silk are placed to tighten the sphincter region. (C) The sphincter sutures have been tied, inverting the tissue. (D) The mucosal flap has been pulled downward, and areas have been denuded anteriorly on both sides.

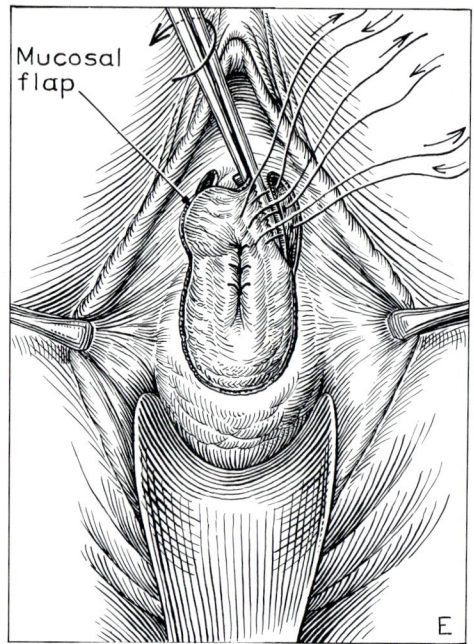
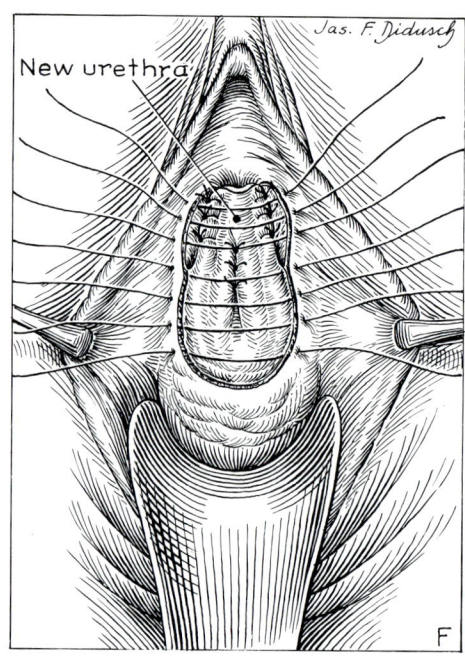
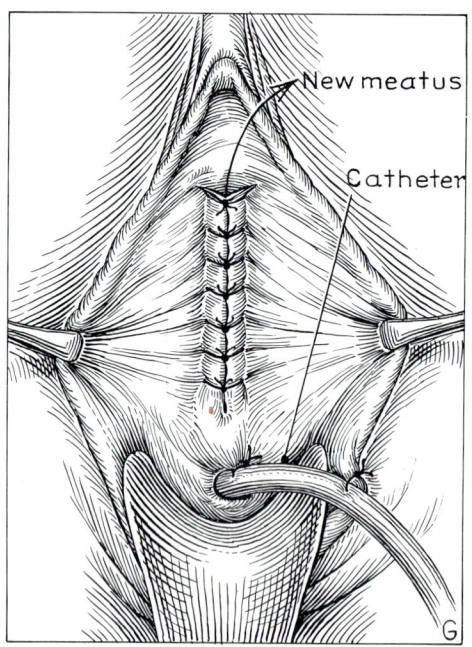

FIG. 28-13 (*Continued*). Plastic operation for formation of urethra and repair of sphincter. (E) The flap is sutured anteriorly with No. 00 chromic catgut, rolling the flap inward so as to approximate raw surfaces. (F) Mucosal edges are approximated over the newly formed urethra with interrupted sutures of No. 00 chromic catgut. (G) The bladder is kept empty by means of a catheter in a surgically made vesicovaginal fistula, placed posterior to plastic work.

(Fig. 28-14 A). The bladder urine is diverted through a catheter in the cystotomy wound. Flaps of mucosa are dissected free as shown in Figure 28-14 B. The flaps are rolled up to form a tube, being sutured with interrupted No. 00 chromic catgut (Fig. 28-14C). This tube is formed around a Foley catheter which has been placed in the bladder. Then the tube is buried by suturing together the pubovesicocervical fascia with interrupted sutures in the midline (Fig. 28-14 D). In the

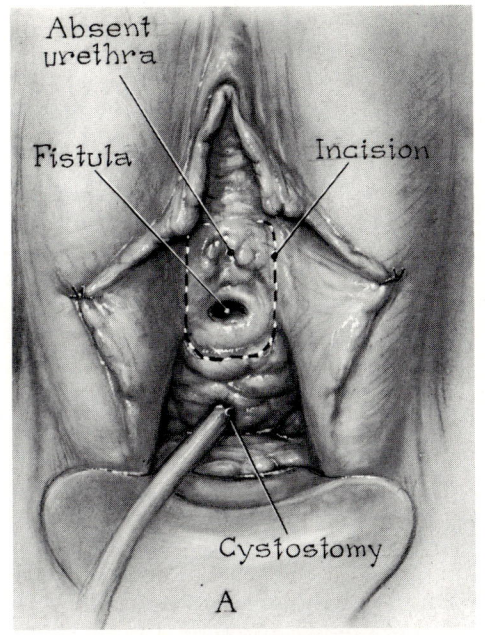
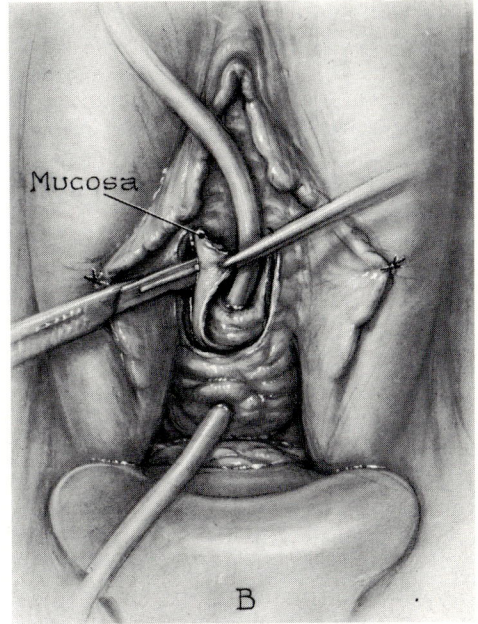
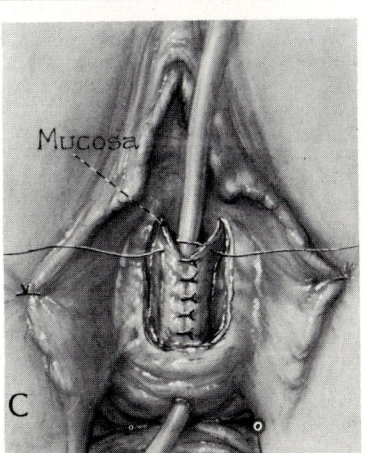
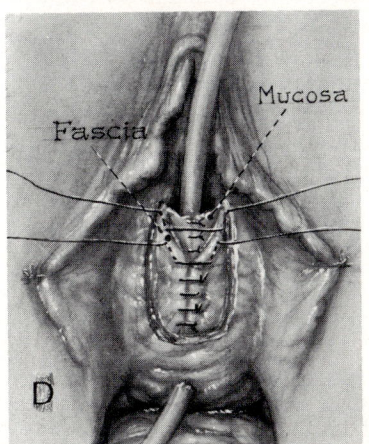
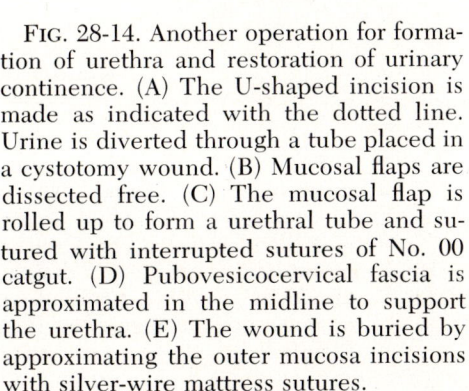
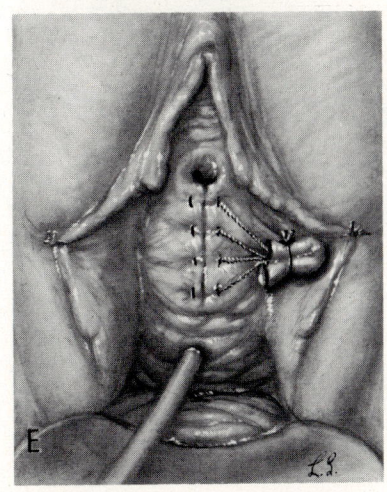

FIG. 28-14. Another operation for formation of urethra and restoration of urinary continence. (A) The U-shaped incision is made as indicated with the dotted line. Urine is diverted through a tube placed in a cystotomy wound. (B) Mucosal flaps are dissected free. (C) The mucosal flap is rolled up to form a urethral tube and sutured with interrupted sutures of No. 00 catgut. (D) Pubovesicocervical fascia is approximated in the midline to support the urethra. (E) The wound is buried by approximating the outer mucosa incisions with silver-wire mattress sutures.

sphincter region the structures are tightened with as many sutures as are thought necessary in an attempt to give sphincter action. The outer incision edges are then approximated with mattress sutures of No. 26 silver wire, which sutures are tightened to the proper tension by twisting (Fig. 28-14 E).

Technic: Operation for Urethrovesicovaginal Fistula

The fistula for which this operation was done resulted from obstetric injury which caused a rather large defect in the anterior vaginal wall, the base of the bladder, and the first portion of the urethra (Fig. 28-15 A).

The first step in the operation is the insertion of a mushroom catheter through a vaginal cystotomy made above the fistula, to divert the urine from the operative area (Fig. 28-15 B).

The vaginal mucosa is dissected free from around the fistula. This dissection is carried sufficiently far laterally to denude enough tissue to permit double closure of the opening (Fig. 28-15 C).

Using interrupted sutures of No. 00 chromic catgut, the urethral and the bladder musculature is closed over a small Hegar dilator which has been placed through the urethral meatus and into the bladder (Fig. 28-15 D).

The first row of sutures is reinforced by a second row of interrupted sutures of No. 00 chromic catgut (Fig. 28-15 E). These sutures invert the first row and bring together the subvesical and suburethral fascia. They also augment the sphincter action at the internal sphincter region and along the entire urethra.

Finally, the edges of the mucosal wound are trimmed, and the mucosal wound is closed with interrupted sutures of No. 00 chromic catgut (Fig. 28-15 F).

One of the most important steps in this operation is the diversion of the urine from the urethra by means of the mushroom catheter through the cystotomy wound. By means of this, it is unnecessary to use a catheter in the urethra, which would have the undesirable effect of keeping the newly constructed sphincter dilated and also would act as a foreign body in proximity to the sutures.

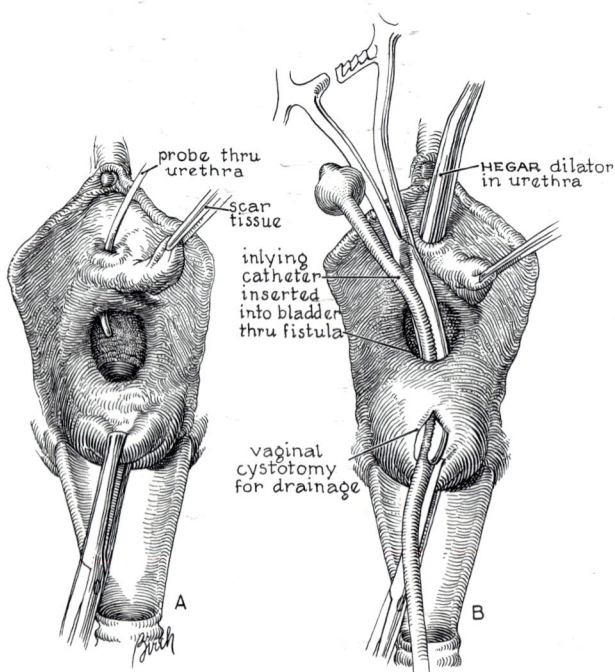

Fig. 28-15. Repair of vesico-urethrovaginal fistula. (A) Indicates defect in vaginal urethral and bladder walls. (B) A vaginal cystotomy is done for drainage above the fistulous opening, and a mushroom catheter is being inserted.

FIG. 28-15 (*Continued*). Repair of vesicourethrovaginal fistula. (C) Vaginal mucosa flaps are dissected free laterally. (D) Bladder and urethral walls are approximated with interrupted sutures of No. 00 chromic catgut. These sutures do not pierce the mucosa of the bladder or the urethra but invert the bladder and the urethral edges.

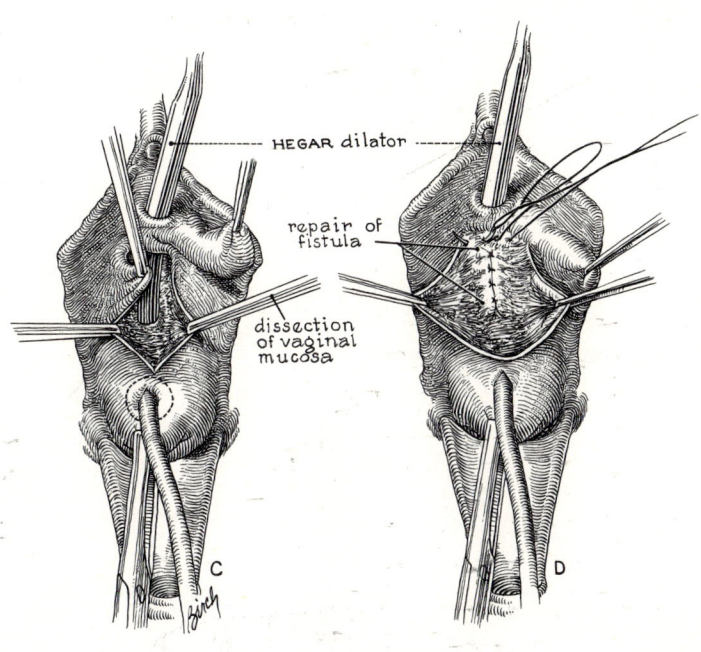

FIG. 28-15 (*Continued*). Repair of vesicourethrovaginal fistula. (E) Submucosal stitches approximate the fascia, thus reinforcing the first row of sutures and approximating broad surfaces for healing. (F) After the excess of mucosa is excised, the edges of the mucosa are sutured with interrupted sutures of No. 0 chromic catgut. (G) Completed operation.

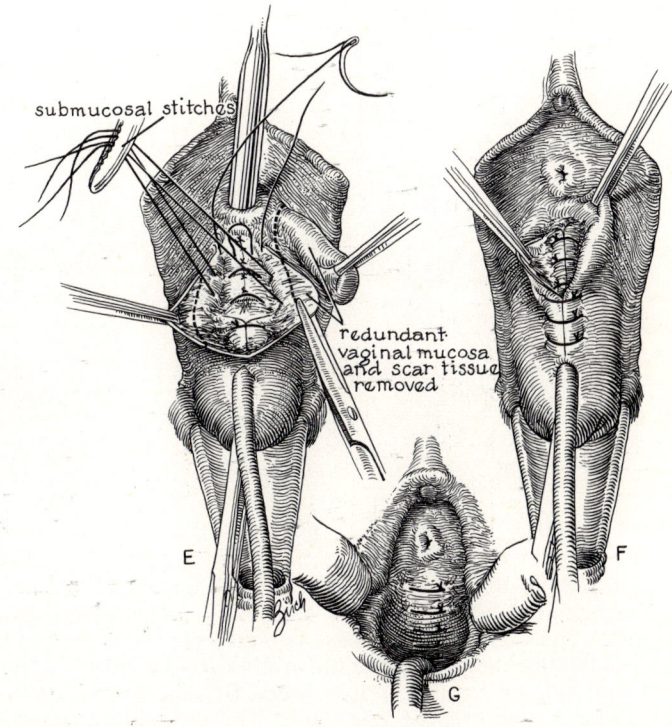

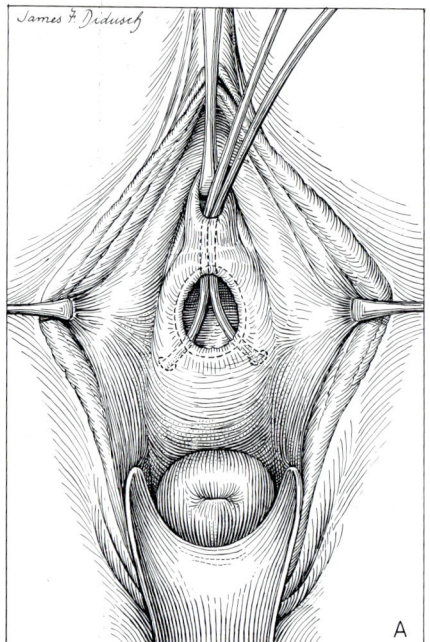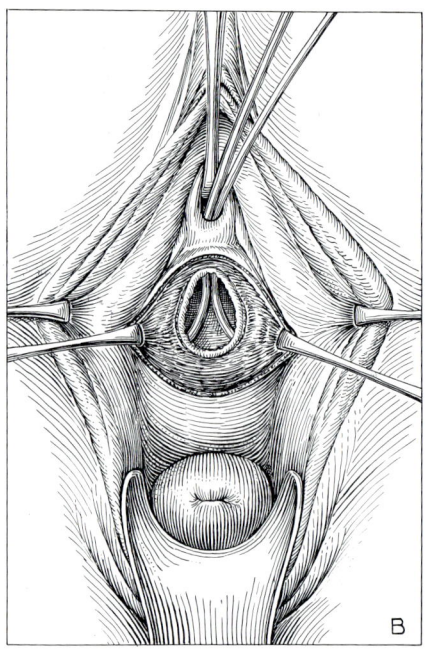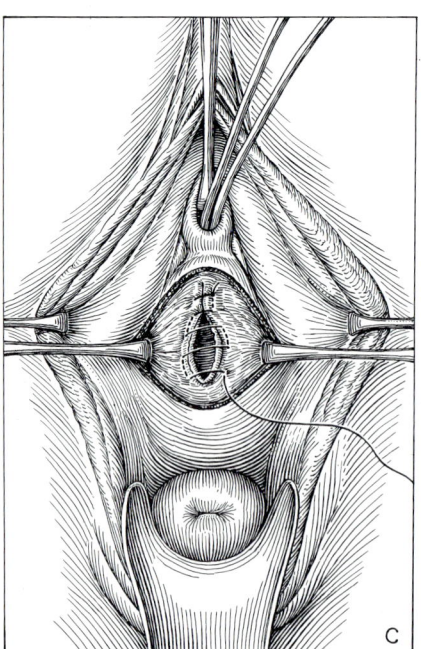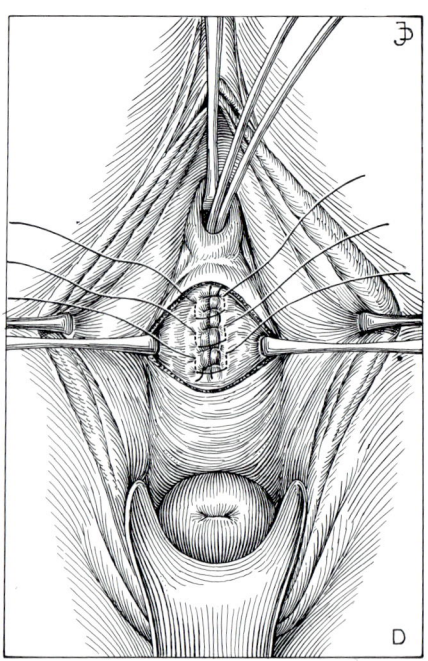

FIG. 28-16. Repair of vesicourethrovaginal fistula, involving sphincter. (A) Demonstrates fistula. Both ureters have been catheterized. Dotted line indicates incision. (B) The vaginal mucosa has been dissected from around the fistula, exposing the base of the bladder and part of the urethra. (C) The fistula is closed with a continuous Cushing stitch of No. 00 chromic catgut. (D) The first suture line is reinforced with mattress sutures of No. 00 chromic catgut. These stitches further tighten the sphincter by drawing the subvesical fascia together.

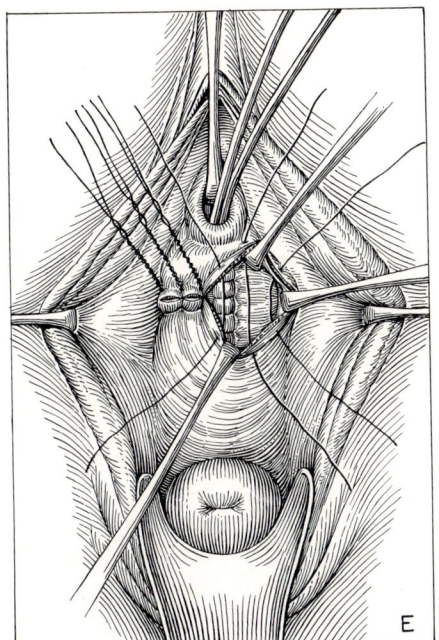 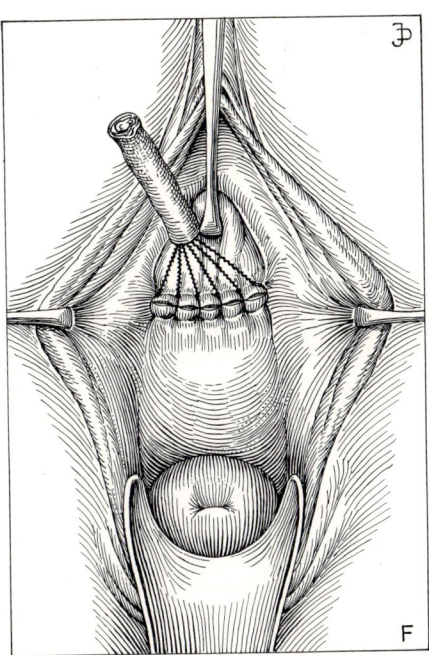

Fig. 28-16 (*Continued*). Repair of vesicourethrovaginal fistula, involving the sphincter. (E) The vaginal mucosa is closed transversely, at right angles to subjacent suture line. (F) Fistula closed. The final closure is with No. 26 silver wire. The mucosa is everted as wires are closed by twisting.

Technic: Another Type of Operation for Repair of Urethrovesicovaginal Fistula, Involving Sphincter

This operation was performed successfully to cure a vesicourethrovaginal fistula, resulting from childbirth. A third of the urethra was destroyed and also a portion of the trigone. The sphincter muscles at the vesical orifice were destroyed, and the ends were retracted.

Because the bladder defect was in close proximity to the ureteral orifices, both ureters were first catheterized with No. 7 catheters, using the Kelly air cystoscope. These catheters were left in place until the operation was completed.

The patient was placed on the table in the lithotomy position, and the fistula was exposed as shown in Figure 28-16 A. A circular incision was made through the bladder mucosa about the edge of the opening, as indicated by the dotted line in Figure 28-16 A. The vaginal mucosa was dissected free from the base of the bladder and the vesical end of the urethra (Fig. 28-16 B).

The defect in the bladder and the urethra was closed from side to side with a continuous Cushing suture of No. 00 chromic catgut (Fig. 28-16 C). The longitudinal closure was chosen for this fistula in order to approximate the retracted sphincter ends. This suture passed into the bladder musculature but not through the mucosa. When pulled taut, the margins of the fistula were inverted into the bladder. This suture line was reinforced with a second one of interrupted mattress sutures of No. 00 chromic catgut as shown in Figure 28-16 D. These sutures passed through the subvesical fascia and musculature and thus further approximated the retracted sphincter muscle fibers.

The vaginal mucosa could be closed with least tension transversely (Fig. 28-16 D). This was most fortunate, for it permitted closure in 2 layers, without necessitating the superimposition of one suture line upon the other. The vaginal mucosa was everted as it was closed with interrupted sutures, using No. 26 silver wire. The wires were twisted until the mucosa was approximated rather loosely. If twisted too tightly, they will cut through the mucosa. The ends of the wires were cut to even length, twisted together and covered with adhesive tape to prevent pricking the patient (Fig. 28-16 E).

Because the sphincter had been sutured as tightly as possible, it was advisable not to keep the urethra and the sphincter fixed in an open position with a large catheter. Therefore, a No. 12 male rubber catheter was placed in the urethra, and the bladder also was drained suprapubically with a No. 30 mushroom catheter. The importance of double drainage cannot be stressed too strongly in a case such as this. The chances of having a workable sphincter are infinitely better if a cure is effected at the first attempt at repair. If this first attempt should fail and the fistula be cured at a subsequent operation, the scar tissue in the sphincter region would be a great liability in the functioning of the repaired sphincter.

The silver-wire sutures were removed on the 14th postoperative day. Healing was firm, and the patient was obviously cured of the fistula. Hence the urethral and the suprapubic catheters were removed at that time. Then the patient was permitted up and voided normally; suprapubic drainage ceased in a few days.

Technic: Latzko Operation for Vesicovaginal Fistula Following Total Hysterectomy

This operation is applicable after a total hysterectomy has been done. Since the fistulas resulting from this operation are almost always small and high in the vagina, the shortening of the vagina caused by the approximation of the anterior and the posterior vaginal walls is slight.

Usually the fistula may be brought into operating range by traction sutures. If there is difficulty in accomplishing this, the vagina may be made shallower by a lateral episiotomy or a true Schuchardt incision (Fig. 28-3). At times the incision may also be conveniently drawn downward with a Young prostatic retractor. An oval incision is made for a radius of about 1 cm. about the fistulous opening (Fig. 28-17 A).

The vaginal and everted vesical mucosa, if present, is cut off as shown in Figure 28-17 B and C. The denuded areas are brought together with interrupted mattress sutures of No. 00 chromic catgut as shown in Figure 28-17 D. After placing this first line of sutures the bladder is filled with sterile milk and tested for leakage. Even if the first suture line apparently closes the fistula, at least one more similar suture line is placed. If there is any doubt about the blood supply of the approximated tissues, a third suture line may be placed. This may require further denudation of the vaginal mucosa. In fact, it is often advisable not to denude at the beginning of the operation as wide an area as may ultimately be necessary. Avoiding early complete denudation often prevents blood loss which may be extremely annoying to the operator and depleting to the patient. After the last catgut suture has been placed, the mucosa is closed with silver wire (Fig. 28-17 F and G). In the average postpanhysterectomy fistula the vagina will not be closed more than 1 or 2 cm. If several previous unsuccessful attempts at closure have been made and much scar tissue surrounds the fistula, considerable vaginal length may have to be sacrificed, but this is a relatively small sacrifice when compared with the incontinence.

Technic: Utilization of Latzko Method for Closure of Large Postirradiation Vesicovaginal Fistula

Although the sine qua non for the use of the Latzko technic always has been that the patient's uterus be removed previously, we have found an extension of its use in the cure of some large postirradiation fistulas which otherwise would be incurable. In some instances the cervical cancer has been completely cured and the cervix totally eradicated by irra-

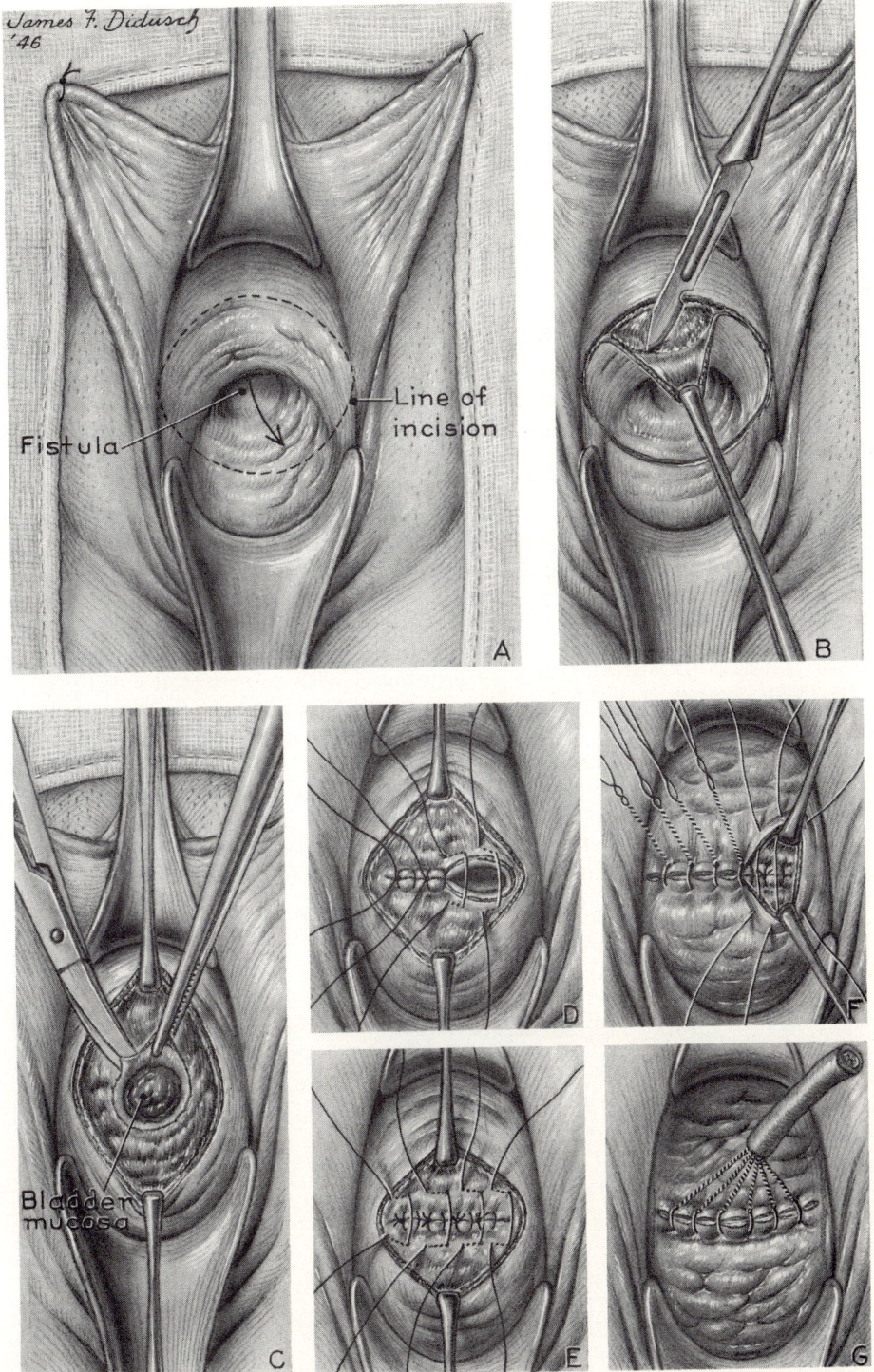

FIG. 28-17. (A) Line of incision. Mucosa within dotted line is to be removed. (B) Mucosa is being removed by sharp dissection. (C) Vaginal mucosa has been removed. (D) First layer of mattress sutures being placed. (E) Second layer of mattress sutures placed. (F) Vaginal mucosa being closed with silver wire. (G) Completed operation. Ends of wires have been twisted together and covered with rubber tubing.

diation, but the patient is left with a large vesicovaginal fistula. The extreme scarring so fixes the tissues that closure of the fistulous opening is out of the question. One should first make certain by biopsy that no carcinoma remains in the region of the cervix or on the margins of the fistula. If the biopsies are negative for cancer, and if at least 3 years have elapsed since the irradiation therapy, it is justifiable to consider relieving the patient of the great distress of incontinence. The fistula is closed by denuding a broad area of both anterior and posterior vaginal walls below the fistula and suturing them together with several layers of interrupted catgut sutures. Including the obliterated cervix in the bladder has proved to be quite innocuous. Although this procedure is applicable in only a small percentage of irradiation fistulas, it has given complete relief to a selected few women.

Technic: Transabdominal Closure of Vesicovaginal Fistula

The fistula for which this operation was done resulted from an abdominal total hysterectomy. In most instances, such a fistula can be closed to advantage by the Latzko method. In this instance, however, 6 previous unsuccessful attempts at closure had been made, and excessive scarring so fixed the vagina that exposure from below seemed to be extremely difficult. A urinary calculus had lodged in the fistula, and a severe cystitis resulted (Fig. 28-18 A). The stone was first removed.

Through a low midline incision the pelvis is inspected with the patient in an exaggerated Trendelenburg position. The intestines are packed back into the abdomen. The bladder is found adherent to the apex of the vagina at the site of the fistula. The peritoneum is cut at its attachment to the vagina and dissected free. It is left attached to the bladder. In making this dissection, it should be borne in mind that the flap of peritoneum is to be used later to bring down between the bladder and the vagina. After freeing the peritoneal flap, the dissection is carried down until the vagina and the bladder in the fistula area are completely separated. Then the vagina is closed with interrupted sutures of No. 0 chromic catgut. The bladder, which has been sufficiently mobilized, is closed with 2 layers of sutures as shown in Figure 28-18 B. It should be noted that these sutures do not pass through the bladder mucosa, and that they invert the edges into the bladder cavity. After thus closing

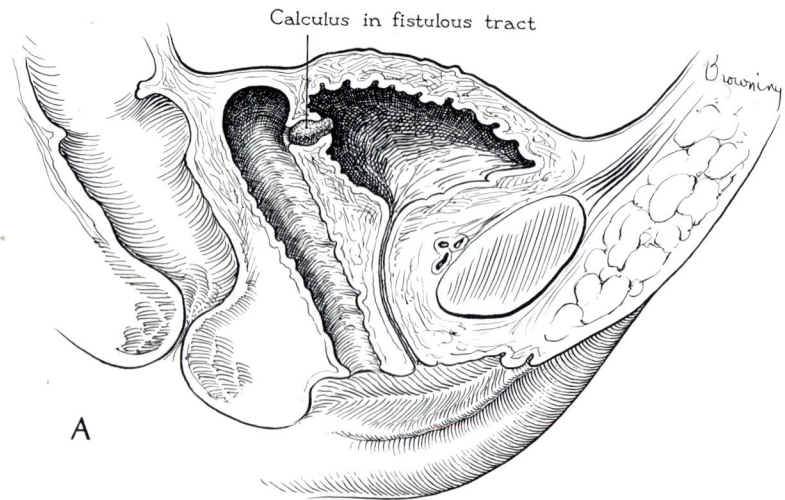

Fig. 28-18. (A) Demonstrating fistula following total abdominal hysterectomy. Six attempts had been made at closure. Calculus apparently had formed about a bit of foreign material left at previous operation.

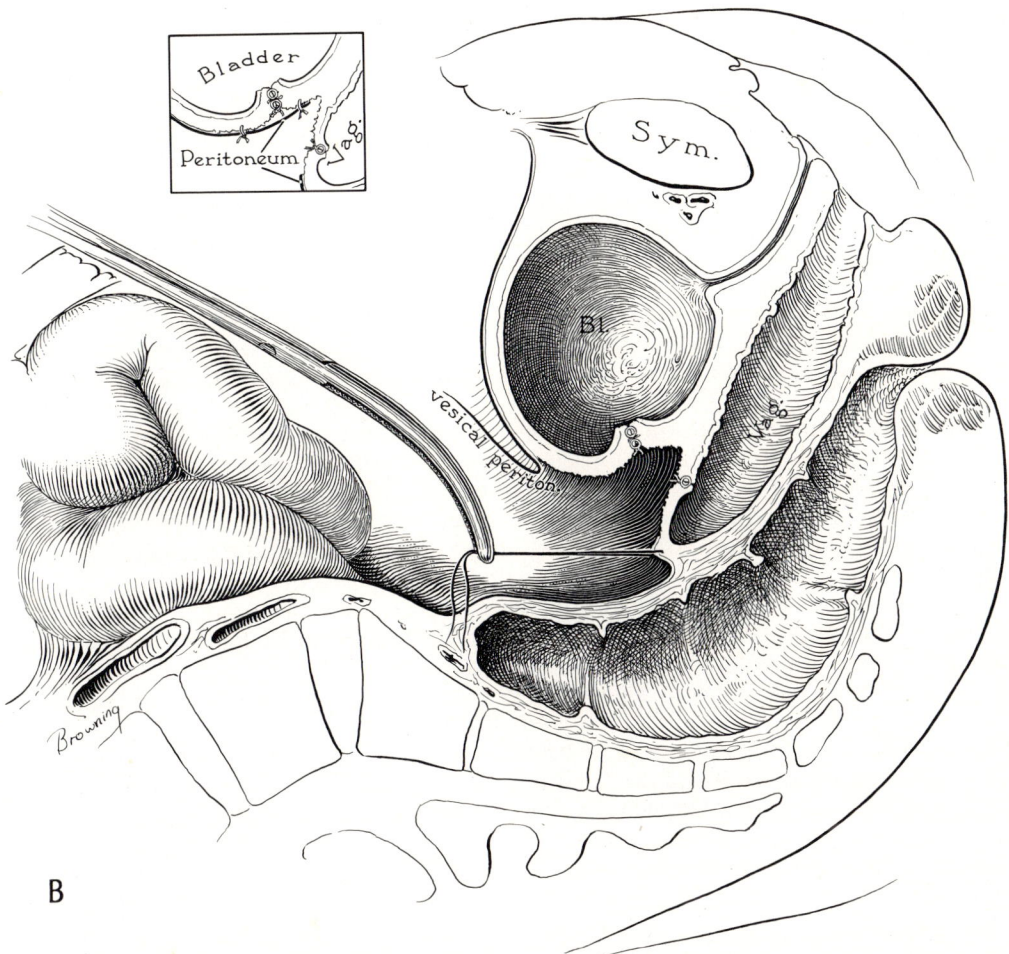

Fig. 28-18. (B) Demonstrating fistula following total abdominal hysterectomy. Intra-abdominal closure of vesicovaginal fistula. A flap of peritoneum has been dissected free. The bladder and the vagina have been separated and closed separately. Inset shows double closure of bladder wall with peritoneum sutured over the suture line. The vagina is closed with a single layer of sutures.

the bladder and the vagina, the peritoneal flap is brought down and sutured to the bladder wall so that the suture line is covered. (See inset in Fig. 28-18 B.) A drain is placed in the cul-de-sac and out through the lower portion of the midline incision. It is considered not to be serious if a vesico-abdominal fistula should develop, since such a fistula usually closes spontaneously. A retention catheter is inserted in the bladder through the urethra and left in place for 12 days.

URINARY DIVERSION

CHOICE OF TECHNIC

It is not wise to select one method of urinary diversion to be used under all conditions. Although consideration is given to this subject under the heading of vesicovaginal fistulas, urinary diversion today is used more frequently in radical surgery for cervical cancer. It can be said at the outset that cutaneous ureterostomy is unsatisfactory and should be used only in case of dire emergency when it may unhappily be resorted to as a temporary expedient. Aside from the disadvantage of the collection of urine on the abdomen, it is very difficult to keep the ends of the ureters from constricting. We have also concluded that when the urine is to be diverted for a benign condition, such as a hopeless vesicovaginal fistula, the isolated loop conduit is superior to sigmoid implantation. We prefer to implant the ureters into the ileum by the direct mucosa-to-mucosa technic. This same technic is our choice when radical pelvic surgery is done for malignancy when we believe that the patient has an excellent chance of cure of the malignancy. Even when there is some hydroureter and hydronephrosis, successful implantations may be made into the ileal conduit with frequent improvement of the kidney condition. Figure 28-19 A shows the normal unilateral upper tract of a patient who had a previous nephrectomy for tuberculosis and later developed a vesicovaginal fistula, on which many unsuccessful attempts had been made at repair. Ultimately, scar tissue constricted the terminal portion of the ureter completely. Figure 28-19 B shows the hydronephrotic kidney at this time. A pyelostomy on the anuric patient was done. As a lifesaving measure an implantation was made into an ileal loop. Figure 28-19 C shows the condition of the upper tract a year later when the patient was restored to perfect health clinically. We have had other cases in which ureterosigmoid anastomoses were causing destruction of kidney function, and reimplantation into an ileal loop resulted in restoration of kidney function (Fig. 28-20).

In spite of the failure in many cases of sigmoidal implantation, we believe that it does have a place in pelvic surgery. In anterior exenteration operations it becomes obvious in certain cases in the course of the operation that the chances of cure are almost nil. It would be folly to subject such an individual to the extensive operation of the isolated ileal loop. A sigmoidal implantation will often serve the purpose of urinary diversion until the patient dies of cancer. Also, she will have the advantage of continence. There are occasional cases of recurrent cervical cancer with involvement of the urethra and the bladder with urinary incontinence. If the patient is in otherwise generally good condition, we have, on occasion, given temporary relief by implantation into the sigmoid.

Furthermore, occasionally at the operating table a segment of the lower ureter may be removed purposely or accidentally in connection with the removal of a malignant ovarian tumor or even a benign ovarian tumor or a huge fibroid. Ureteroureteral anastomosis or implantation into the bladder may be impossible. Under such circumstances a ureterosigmoidal anastomosis may be indicated.

Hence the pelvic surgeon may be required to use one procedure or another, and often he must make a decision rapidly. Therefore we will illustrate here the modified Coffey technic, the Cordonnier-Leadbetter technic, and the isolated ileal conduit.

TRANSPLANTATION OF URETERS INTO THE SIGMOID

Occasionally, large vesicovaginal fistulas are encountered which defy all attempts at surgical closure. These cases fall into two groups. First, there are the obstetric fistulas in which the base of the bladder and the urethra, including the sphincter region, are destroyed. Although the bladder defect may be closed and a urethra made, the formation of a working sphincter may be impossible. Such reconstructed urethras do not yield well to the artificial sphincter action of the Goebell-Stoeckel procedure. Second, the large fistulas resulting from irradiation of advanced cervical cancer may be impossible to close because of the size of the defect, the inelasticity of the dense scar tissue, and inadequacy of the blood supply of the tissue surrounding the fistula.

Fortunately, fistulas of these types are rare, but it is well for the surgeon to have some procedure in his armamentarium to offer these unfortunate women.

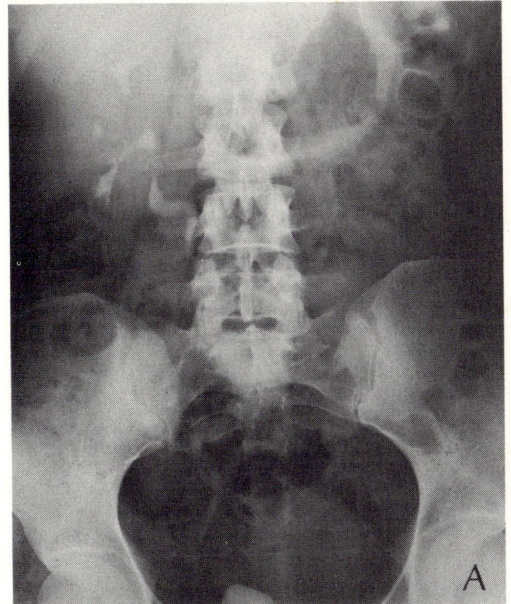
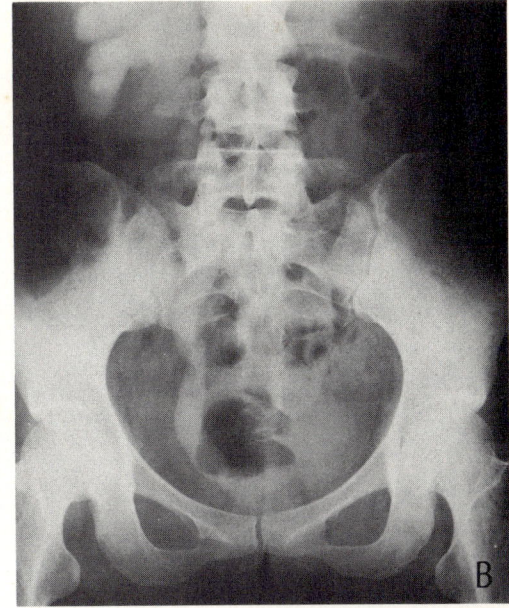
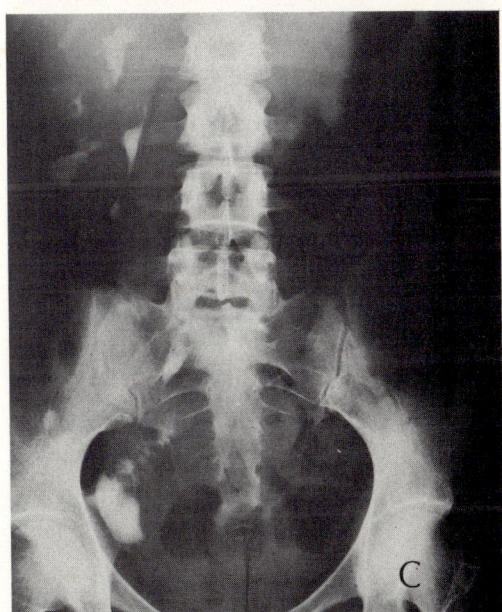

Fig. 28-19. (A) Single kidney in woman with incurable vesicovaginal fistula. (B) After complete obstruction of lower end of ureter due to scar tissue following attempts at repair of fistula. (C) Following nephrostomy and 3 weeks after implantation of ureter into ileal loop. Note complete restoration to normal of the kidney pelvis and the calyces.

Diversion of the urinary stream to the bowel by uretero-intestinal anastomosis is the only possible solution to this difficult problem.

The history of the development of the modern technic for implanting the ureters into the bowel is one of the most fascinating of American surgery. Urologists, gynecologists, and general surgeons have contributed to our present-day knowledge of the subject, which has evolved out of much experimental and clinical work. Complications due to soiling the peritoneal cavity have been almost completely overcome due to bowel preparation with antibiotics as described in Chapter 2 on preoperative care. However, hydronephrosis, renal infection, and re-

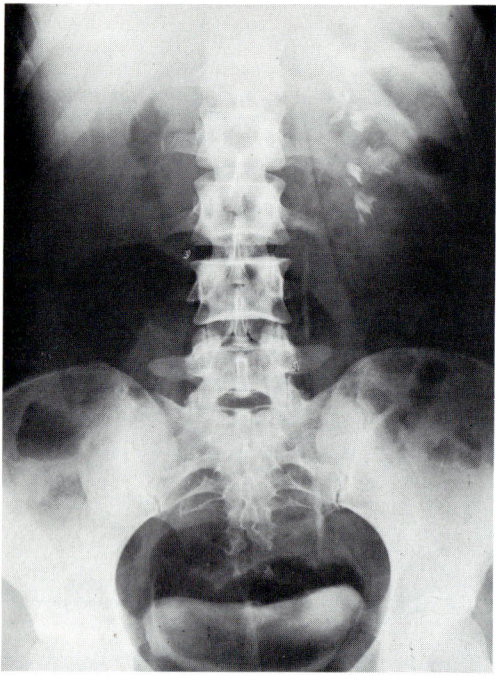
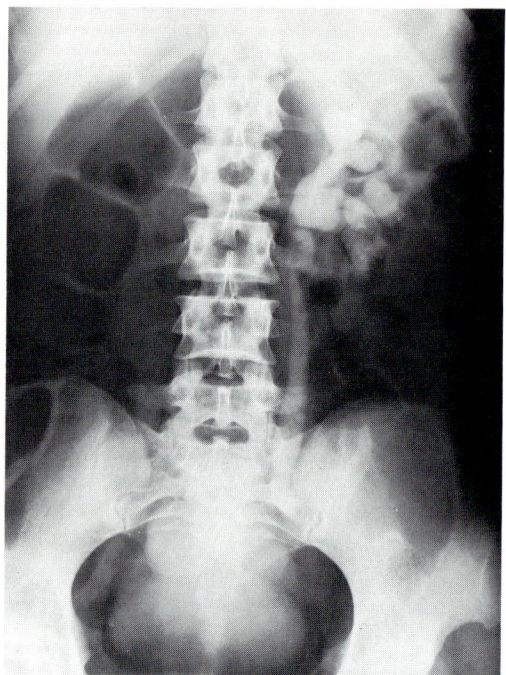
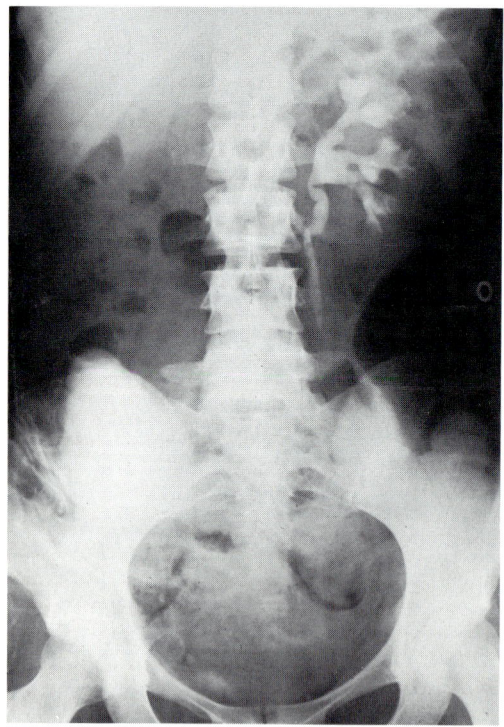

FIG. 28-20. (*Top, left*) Normal pyelogram of unilateral kidney. The patient was incontinent following resection of the vesical neck. (*Top, right*) Hydronephrosis developed several months after implantation of the ureter into the sigmoid, and the patient showed clinical and chemical evidence of retention of urinary products. (*Bottom*) Immediately after the pyelogram shown at *top, right*, was taken, the ureter was removed from the sigmoid and implanted into the ileal loop. This pyelogram illustrates return to normal contour of calyces 20 days after implantation.

absorption of urinary waste products still occur. We have patients upon whom sigmoidal implantations were done as long as 20 years ago who are in apparent good health. Even with these good clinical results, the pyelograms are mostly far from normal. Other patients have died within a few years or less of renal insufficiency. In general, we believe that the implantation of the ureters into the bowel, regardless of the technic employed, is apt to shorten the life of the individual.

As early as 1894 Maydl attempted to utilize the valve-like action at the ureterovesical orifices by transplanting, intraperitoneally, the entire vesical trigone with the intact ureters into the bowel. This method has been entirely abandoned, because it is not applicable to most of the conditions for which the implantation is done, such as carcinoma of the bladder and large vesicovaginal fistulas. Maydl's technic was modified and improved by Peters, who performed the same type of operation extraperitoneally for exstrophy of the bladder and thus eliminated the danger of peritonitis.

In 1898 Franklin Martin worked on the problem with experimental animals, with the hope of developing a radical operation for carcinoma of the cervix, excising the bladder with the uterus. He transplanted both ureters through a single opening in the sigmoid or the rectum. He was the first to use rubber catheters in the ureters, and he attempted to create a valve at the ureterosigmoidal anastomosis. It is probable that Martin actually created more of a sphincter than a valve, the distinction being that a sphincter retards emptying of the ureter, whereas a valve permits emptying but prevents backflow. Martin finally gave up his experimental attempts because the animals all developed renal infection and hydronephrosis.

Thus Coffey was unable to find in the 240 articles in the literature up to 1909 a single instance in which a true ureterointestinal valve had been constructed. The mortality was high up to this time, approximately 55 per cent. Coffey began his animal and clinical experimental work in 1909, and it extended over 2 decades. In 1911 he reported his first experimental attempts at valve formation by burying the ureter for a short distance in the musculature of the bowel, before inserting it into the lumen. The ureter was drawn into the bowel through an opening in the mucosa by means of an anchoring suture, which was made to enter the bowel lumen through the opening and emerged about a centimeter below. This is now known as the Coffey I technic.

Coffey's second method, published in 1925, was also a submucosal transplantation, but he utilized renal catheters in the ureters, which were withdrawn down into the rectum by gauze that had been previously packed in the rectum. This technic has the advantage of permitting drainage of the urine through the catheters until postoperative edema has subsided. Thus both ureters may be transplanted at one operative procedure with relative safety. Coffey's third method, published in 1930, consisted of implantation of the ureter in the submucosa of the bowel with the end of the ureter tied off but not entering the lumen. A silk or linen transfixion suture was placed through the ureteral wall near its end and into the intestinal lumen. When this ligature sloughed out, a uretero-intestinal fistula was established. Obviously, only one ureter can be transplanted at a time by this method.

In 1933 Higgins modified Coffey's transfixion suture technic and left the ureters intact, connected with the bladder. His transfixion suture penetrated the ureteral wall and the bowel wall, finally being sewed to a rectal tube which is pulled out 4 days later. Following this, the urine passes freely per rectum, and the amount passed into the bladder can be seen to decrease gradually under cystoscopic observation. Nine days after the first operation the bladder is excised for carcinoma, and the lower ends of the ureters are tied off with silk sutures.

The same year Winsbury-White also implanted the intact ureters submucosally. At the second stage of his operation the ureters are divided three fourths of an inch below their egress from the submucosal channel, at which point a longitudinal incision into the bowel is made. The ends of the ureters are inserted into this opening and fixed in place with an anchoring suture.

In 1942 Jewett described a new method

of ureteral transplantation in 2 stages for cancer of the bladder. The method consisted of burying the intact ureters in the submucosa of the sigmoid at the first stage. At the second stage an opening is cut through the ureteral and intestinal walls with a specially constructed electrode, inserted through the ureteral stump. For the first few years following the development of this technic Jewett was rather optimistic concerning the results. However, with the passage of time, his optimism has given way to pessimism on the basis of the long-term effect on kidney function.

In 1950 Cordonnier described a method of ureterosigmoid anastomosis by suturing ureteral mucosa to that of the sigmoid. Nesbit refined the technic. Later, Leadbetter, Weyrauch, and Young combined the submucosal tunnel principle of Coffey with direct mucosal anastomosis. An analysis of their cases showed that hydronephrosis was less common than after any other type of ureterosigmoid anastomosis, and that hyperchloremic acidosis did not occur in the presence of a postoperatively normal upper urinary tract.

Finally, Bricker in 1950 devised a method of using an isolated ileal loop for implantation of the ureters. It has the disadvantage of requiring the patient to use a bag upon the abdomen for the collection of the urine, but it has the great advantage of very nearly eliminating the danger of recurrent pyelonephritis and hyperchloremic acidosis. This advantage is based on the fact that the isolated loop acts simply as a conduit and does not permit reabsorption of urinary waste products, and, provided that a good ureterosigmoid anastomosis is done, it does not result in hydronephrosis.

Technic: Modified Coffey II Method

Coffey gave his patients castor oil for 2 nights preceding the operation and copious bowel irrigations the night before and early in the morning of operation. The use of Sulfasuxidine has done away with the necessity of these procedures. The patient is given 12 gm. of Sulfasuxidine per day in divided doses for 5 days preceding the operation. Early on the morning of operation she is given an ordinary saline enema followed by an instillation of neomycin.

The patient is given a small induction dose of Pentothal Sodium on arrival at the operating room. She is held in the knee-chest posture by 2 assistants, and a sterile sigmoidoscope is passed up the bowel for about 12 inches. A sterile gauze roll is used to pack the sigmoid and the rectum as the sigmoidoscope is withdrawn. Several inches of gauze are permitted to protrude from the anus, and a clamp is placed on it, so that later it may be identified easily between the patient's thighs when the operator desires it to be withdrawn. Recently, we have substituted a sterile rectal tube for the gauze because it is manipulated more easily at the laparotomy. It always should be inserted through the proctoscope in order to be certain that it is passed to the desired length up the sigmoid and not curled up in the rectum.

The patient is placed on the operating table in the Trendelenburg position, and a midline incision is made from umbilicus to symphysis. The omentum and the bowel are packed carefully into the upper abdominal cavity. Rather deep anesthesia is required to do this satisfactorily. It is our custom to change to ether anesthesia after the patient had been changed from the knee-chest to the Trendelenburg posture. The posterior parietal peritoneum is opened longitudinally over the ureter, beginning at a point just below the pelvic brim, and the ureter is visualized. A tape is placed around the ureter for identification. It is dissected from its bed with blunt dissection, down to a point near its insertion into the bladder, so that as much ureter as possible may be available for implantation into the bowel without tension. Sufficient ureter should be freed to permit easy implantation into the sigmoid, but it should not be dissected free from its bed unnecessarily high so that its blood supply will be disturbed as little as possible. With the ureter freed, it is doubly clamped near the bladder, and the distal end is ligated with No. 1 chromic catgut.

A large catheter with open end is prepared previously with a tightly fitting rubber cuff about 10 cm. from its tip end, and a suture of double medium silk is sewn through the other end of the catheter as shown in Figure 28-21 A. The prepared catheter is inserted into the upper segment of the ureter until the cuff just enters the end of the ureter. The catheter is fixed firmly in the ureter by tying with No. 1 chromic catgut just above and below the rubber cuff (Fig. 28-21 B). If a bilateral implantation is to be done, these procedures are repeated on the opposite side.

An incision, approximately 3 cm. long, is then made through the longitudinal muscle fibers of one of the taenia of the sigmoid. Care should be taken that this does not perforate the bowel lumen. If the implantation cannot be made readily at the site of the taenia, the incision is made obliquely through the circular muscular coat. A very small puncture through the bowel mucosa is made at the lower end of the gutter (Fig. 28-21 C). Thus the gauze packing or the rectal tube is exposed, and the free end of the catheter is sutured into it (Fig. 28-21 D). If a bilateral implantation is to be done, this procedure is repeated on the opposite side. An assistant then withdraws the gauze or the rectal tube from the sigmoid under the direction of the operator. Thus, the lower ends of the ureters are drawn into the lumen of the bowel. The portions of the ureters in which the rubber cuffs lie should be drawn well into the lumen of the bowel to permit them to slough away. The lower ends of the ureters are then buried in the gutter in the bowel wall, with No. 000 chromic catgut on an atraumatic needle. The first and the last stitches pass through the periureteral tissue (Fig. 28-21 E). This suture line may be reinforced with a second one, using a continuous Lembert suture. The wounds in the posterior parietal peritoneum are closed with a continuous suture of fine catgut. Sulfanilamide powder is sprinkled over the operative regions, and the abdomen is closed without drainage.

The catheters are watched carefully to make certain that they drain freely. If there is stoppage, a few cubic centimeters of sterile saline may be injected to relieve it. This should not be done by a nurse, but only by an experienced house officer who understands the danger of overdistention of the ureter. On about the 10th day gentle traction is made on one of the catheters. If it gives readily, it is removed; if not, traction is made daily until it slips out easily. If a bilateral implantation has been done, 2 or 3 days are permitted to elapse before the second catheter is removed.

TECHNIC: CORDONNIER-LEADBETTER URETEROSIGMOID ANASTOMOSIS

This technic of ureteral implantation may be used for implantation into the sigmoid.

The bowel is prepared as described in the chapter on preoperative care. The patient is put in the Trendelenburg position, and the small bowel is packed off. If either ureter is dilated, the dilated one is approached first so that it may be divided and allowed to drain while the opposite side is worked on. This allows for contraction of a dilated ureteral musculature with decrease in circumference and consequent easier transplantation.

The usual procedure is to expose the left ureter through a small incision in the peritoneum below the proximal sigmoid at the pelvic brim. It is divided, and the proximal end of the distal stump is ligated. The proximal ureter is freed from its bed to a point behind the mesentery of the sigmoid through which a small transverse incision is made. The end of the ureter is pulled through the mesentery, the operator being sure that there is no angulation.

The site chosen for the anastomosis is at the beginning of the sigmoid as it becomes mobile. The anastomosis is performed through a slightly obliquely placed incision in the anterior taenia. The ureter is carefully measured for proper length without tension, the inferior lip of the cut end is slit for a dis-

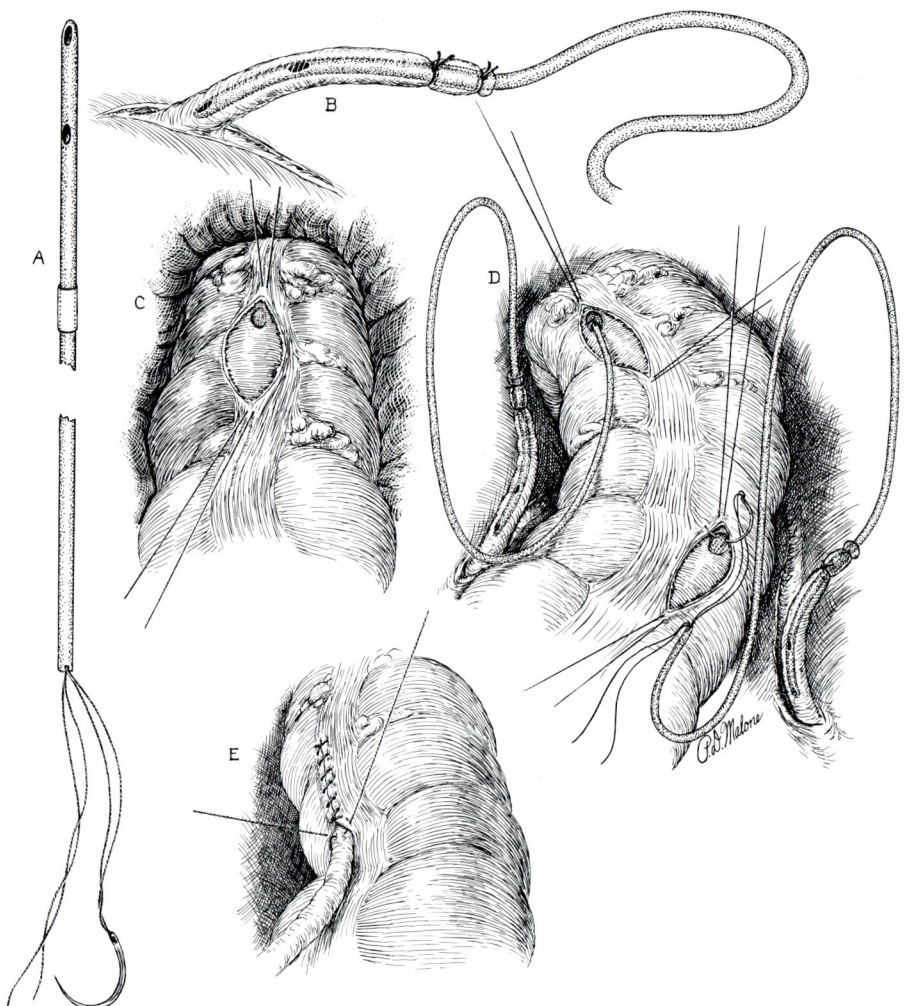

Fig. 28-21. Implantation of ureter into bowel: Coffey II technic. (A) No. 9 catheter shod with a cuff of small rubber tubing. A silk thread has been attached to end of the catheter, and the needle is left in place for subsequent suture to gauze. (B) The ureter has been cut and freed for a distance from its retroperitoneal bed. The tip end of the catheter has been threaded for a distance up the ureter and tied in place about the rubber cuff. (C) An incision has been made through the longitudinal bowel musculature and a small opening made over gauze into the bowel lumen. (D) The ends of the catheters are sutured to the gauze preparatory to withdrawal of the gauze. Thus the ureters are pulled into the vowel lumen. (E) The ureter has been buried in the bowel musculature. The final stitch is taken through the ureter to fix it to the bowel. Fine catgut with atraumatic needle is used for the continuous suture. Silk is used for the final fixation suture.

tance of 5 to 7 mm., and the sharp edges of the ureter are trimmed to leave an oval elliptical ureteral os which will be considerably larger than a cross section of the transversely cut ureter.

Then the trough in the bowel is made by incising the anterior taenia for a distance of 2.5 to 3 cm. diagonally toward the point where the ureter will emerge from the retroperitoneum. The incision in the bowel is carried down to the mucosa as shown in Figure 28-22 A. A small circular opening is made into the mucosa at the distal end of the trough (Fig. 28-22 B). A direct anastomosis is made between the prepared end of the ureter and the bowel mucosa. No. 5-0 chromic catgut is used to make a watertight anastomosis (Fig. 28-22 B). The muscular tissues along the trough are loosely sutured together over the ureter as shown in Figure 28-22 C. Retroperitonealization of the area of anastomosis and fixation of the bowel is accomplished by suturing the superior peritoneal edge of the incision in the mesentery of the sigmoid over the site of the anastomosis. Fine silk is used for this (Fig. 28-22 D).

The right ureter is implanted with the same technic at the point in the sigmoid where it can be accomplished without tension. Sutures are placed to secure the sigmoid to the posterior peritoneum to relieve any tension on the anastomosis.

A long soft-rubber tube with several perforations is placed in the rectum and strapped in place, which is frequently irrigated with saline solution to maintain free drainage. The rectal tube is removed on the 5th postoperative day.

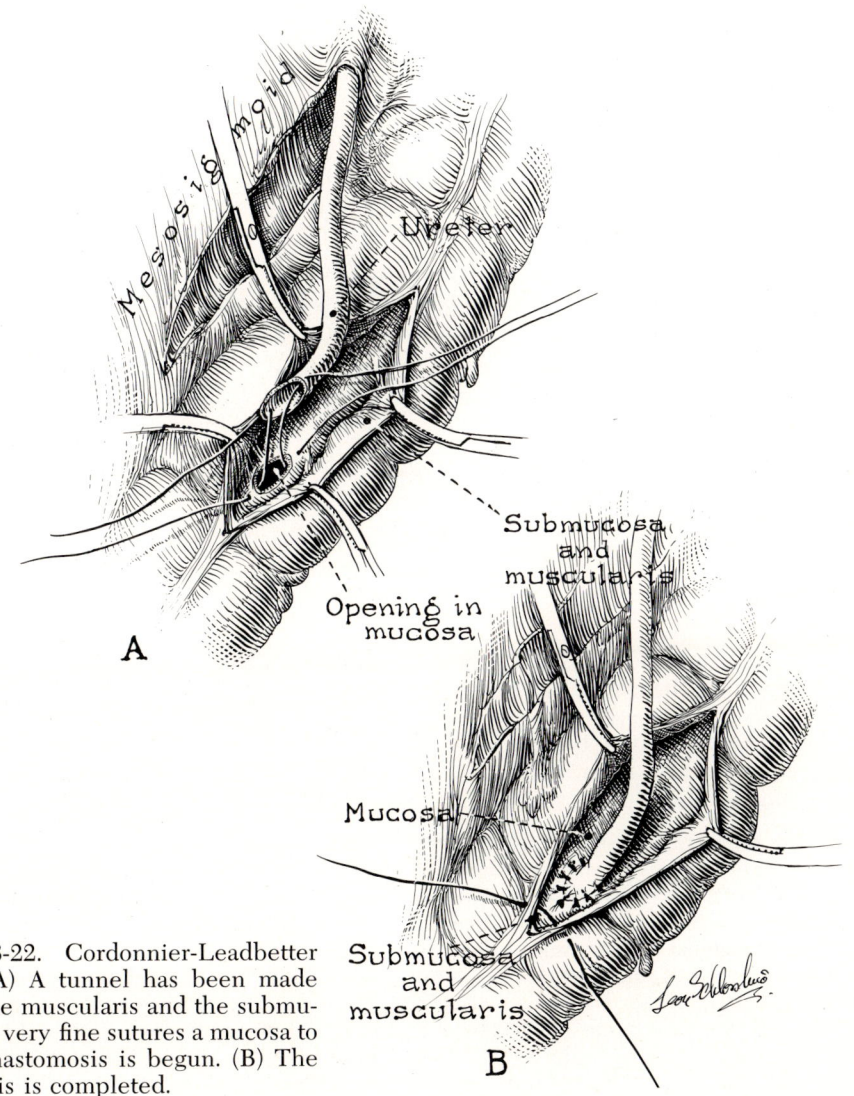

FIG. 28-22. Cordonnier-Leadbetter technic. (A) A tunnel has been made through the muscularis and the submucosa; with very fine sutures a mucosa to mucosa anastomosis is begun. (B) The anastomosis is completed.

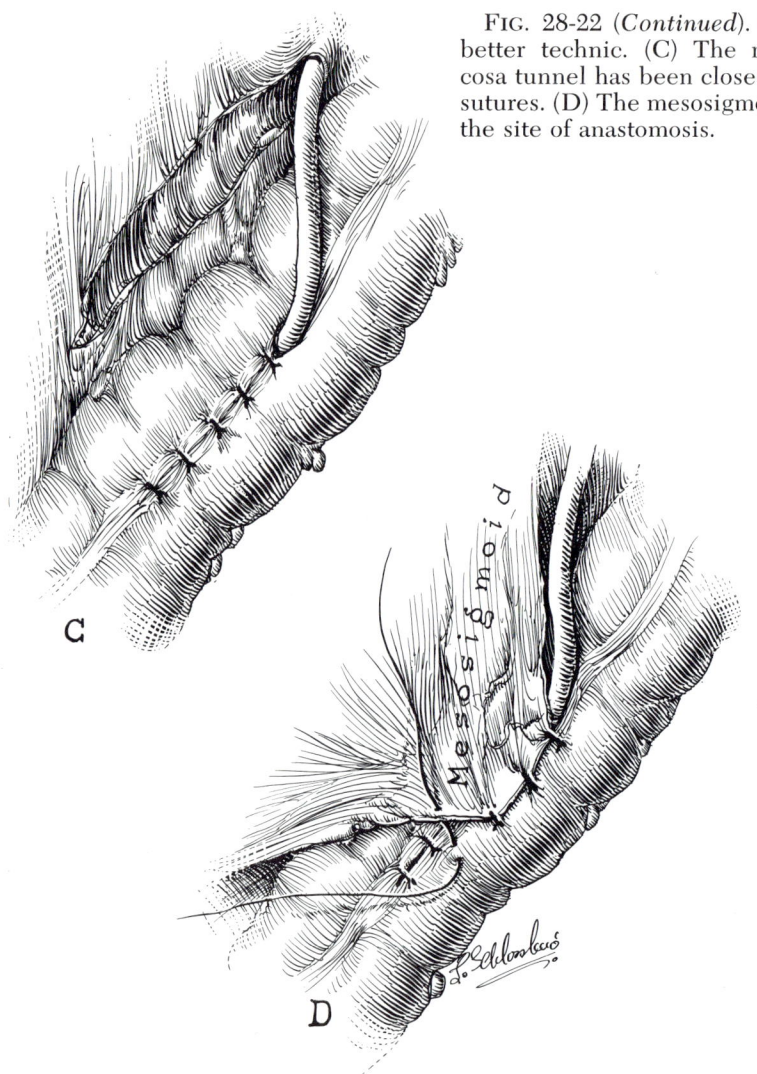

Fig. 28-22 (*Continued*). Cordonnier-Leadbetter technic. (C) The muscularis-submucosa tunnel has been closed with interrupted sutures. (D) The mesosigmoid is sutured over the site of anastomosis.

Technic: Bricker's Ileal Loop Bladder Substitution

Bricker has described the technic of the ileal loop bladder substitution operation as follows:

A 6 to 8 inch segment of ileum is isolated with its blood supply carefully preserved. The distal end of this segment is usually located about 6 inches from the ileocecal junction. An end-to-end anastomosis of the remaining ileum is done with two rows of fine interrupted cotton or silk. The proximal end of the isolated segment is closed, the ureters are anastomosed to it, and the distal end is brought out through an accessory incision to the right of the umbilicus. Great care is used for the ureterointestinal anastomosis, a meticulous end-to-side, mucosa-to-mucosa, two-layer anastomosis with fine interrupted, nonabsorbable sutures being done. No ureteral catheters or anastomotic splints are used. We no longer close the right lateral gutter since we have decided that the danger of intestinal obstruction from herniation through the large aperture is negligible. On the other hand, we now are careful to tack the left ureter to the undersurface of the mesentery in order to reduce the hazard of intestinal obstruction. It is considered of importance to make sure that the bowel segment is decompressed in the early postoperative period. This is accomplished by inserting a catheter into the segment

Transplantation of Ureters Into the Sigmoid

Fig. 28-23. The intestinal segment is isolated from the terminal ileum about 4 to 6 inches from the ileocecal junction. A segment of 4 to 6 inches is necessary. The rent in the mesentery of the small intestine is carefully repaired. An end-to-end anastomosis is made of the ileum. (From E. Bricker)

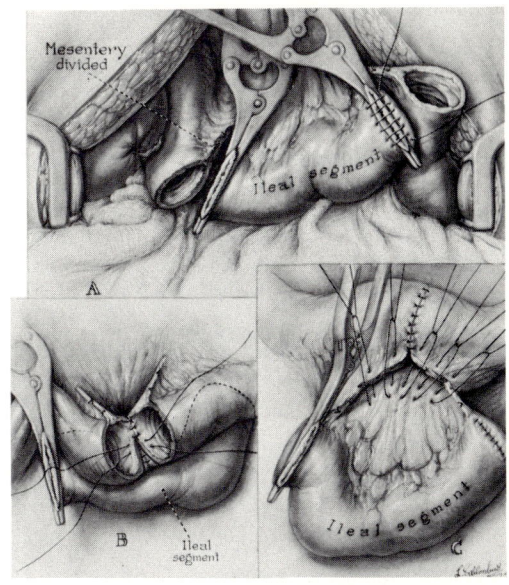

Fig. 28-23 (*Continued*). (*Right*) The ureters are sectioned 2 to 3 cm. below the level of the iliac arteries and freed sufficiently for the implantation, being careful not to strip them of their blood supply.

(*Bottom*) The side-to-end anastomosis between the ureters and the segment of ileum is completed, mucosa to mucosa, using the finest of catgut and reinforcing the anastomosis with fine silk. (From E. Bricker)

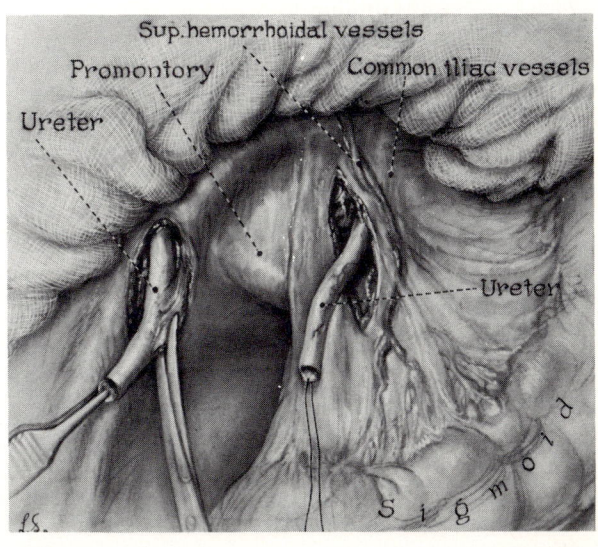

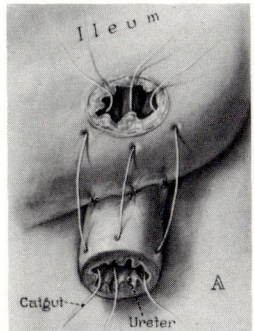 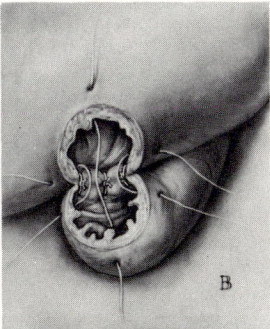 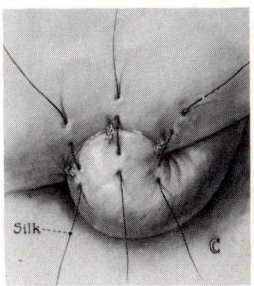 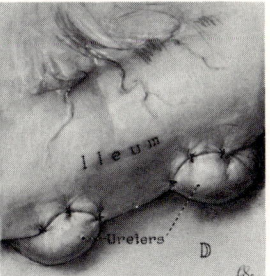

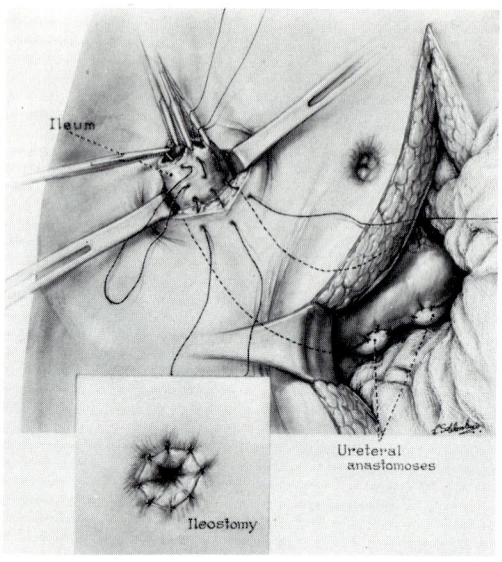

FIG. 28-23 (*Continued*). The ileostomy is completed by suturing it to the edge of the skin of a small incision in the right lower quadrant. (From E. Bricker)

through the abdominal stoma, the mucosa of which is carefully sutured to the edge of the skin incision for primary healing. This catheter is removed on the third or fourth postoperative day, and a Rutzen bag is applied to the stoma. In those few patients for whom bladder substitutes have been made as palliative procedures without pelvic evisceration, a rubber-dam drain had been inserted into the cul-de-sac in case there should be a leak of urine from one of the anastomoses. In the cases of pelvic evisceration the perineal drain is considered adequate to take care of this contingency. (Fig. 28-23)

BIBLIOGRAPHY

Babcock, W. Wagner: The operative treatment of vesicovaginal and related fistulae. Southern Surgeon, 8:34, 1939.

Bricker, E. M., and Eisman, B.: Bladder reconstruction from cecum and ascending colon following resection of pelvic viscera. Amer. Surg., *132*:77, 1950.

Clark, B. G., and Leadbetter, W. F.: Ureterosigmoidostomy: collective review of results in 2897 reported cases. J. Urol., 73:999, 1955.

Coffey, Robert C.: Physiological implantation of the severed ureter or common bile duct into the intestine. J.A.M.A., 56:397, 1911.

———: Transplantation of the ureters into the large intestine. Surg. Gynec. Obstet., 47:593, 1928

———: Transplantation of the ureters. Ann. Surg., *91*:908, 1930.

Cordonnier, J. J.: Ureterosigmoid anastomosis. J. Urol., 63:276, 1950.

Cordonnier, J. J., and Lage, W. T.: An evaluation of ureterosigmoid anastomosis by mucosa to mucosa method after two and one-half years' experience. J. Urol., 66:565, 1951.

Counseller, Virgil S.: Surgical and postoperative treatment of large vesicovaginal and rectovaginal fistulae, Surg. Gynec. Obstet., 74:738, 1942.

Danforth, W. C.: Transperitoneal approach in the management of inaccessible vesicovaginal fistulas. Amer. J. Obstet. Gynec., 39:690, 1940.

Everett, H. S., and Mattingly, R. F.: Urinary tract injuries resulting from pelvic surgery. Amer. J. Obstet. Gynec., 71:502, 1956.

Falk, H. C., and Orkin, L. A.: Nonsurgical closure of vesicovaginal fistulas. Obstet. Gynec., 9:538, 1957.

Falk, H. C., and Tancer, M. L.: Loss of urethra. Report of three cases. Obstet. Gynec., 9:458, 1957.

Graham, John B.: Painful syndrome of postradiation urinary-vaginal fistula. Surg. Gynec. Obstet., *124*:1260, 1967.

Higgins, Charles C.: Aseptic uretero-intestinal anastomosis. Amer. J. Surg., 22:207, 1933.

———: Transplantation of the ureters into the rectosigmoid. J. Urol., 37:90, 1937.

Hinman, Frank: The technic and late results of uretero-intestinal implantation and cystectomy for cancer of the bladder. Seventh Congress of the International Society of Urology, p. 464, 1939.

Holden, Frederick C.: Partial colpocleisis as an approach to vesicovaginal fistula following total hysterectomy. Amer. J. Obstet. Gynec., *44*:880, 1942.

Hunner, Guy L.: Personal communication.

Hyman, Richard M.: Coagulation therapy for small vesicovaginal fistulas. Clin. Obstet. Gynec., 8(2):465, 1968.

Jewett, H. J.: New method of ureteral transplantation for cancer of bladder: Report of 15 clinical cases. J. Urol., *48*:489, 1942.

———: Uretero-intestinal anastomosis in two stages for cancer of the bladder: Modification of original technic: Report of 33 cases. J. Urol., *52*:536, 1944.

Jobert de Lamballe: Traité des fistules, etc., Paris, 1892.

Kelly, Howard A.: The treatment of large vesicovaginal fistulae. Bull. Johns Hopkins Hosp., 7:29, 1896.

———: Operative Gynecology. New York, Appleton, 1898.

———: The history of the vesicovaginal fistula: An address. Trans. Amer. Gynec. Soc., 37:3, 1912.

Kloman, E. H.: Vesicovaginal fistula. Southern Med. J., *34*:271, 1941.

Latzko, William: Behandlung hochsitzender Blasen- und Mastdarmscheidenfisteln nach Uterusextirpation mit hohem Scheidenverschluss. Zbl. Gynäk., *38*:906, 1914.

———: Postoperative vesicovaginal fistulas. Amer. J. Surg., 58:211, 1942.

Mackenrodt, A.: Die operative Heilung der Harnleiterfisteln. Ein geheilter Fall von Harnleiter—Gebärmutterfistel. Zbl. Gynäk., *18*:1026, 1894.

Mahfouz, N.: Atlas of Obstetrical and Gynecological Museum. vol. 2, p. 580. London, John Skerrett.

Martin, F. H.: Implantation of ureters in rectum: A method having for its object the making of subsequent infection of the ureters and kidneys impossible. J.A.M.A., 32:159, 1899.

Miller, Norman F.: The surgical treatment and postoperative care of vesicovaginal fistula. Amer. J. Obstet. Gynec., *44*:873, 1942.

Pettit, A. V.: Vesicovaginal fistula. Western J. Surg., *51*:89, 1943.

Pfaneuf, L. E.: Vesicovaginal fistula management—end results. Amer. J. Obstet. Gynec., *31*:316, 1936.

Schuchardt, Karl: Über die paravaginale Methode der Extirpation uteri und ihre Enderfolge beim Uteruskrebs. Monatsschr. Geburtsch. Gynäk., *13*:744, 1901.

Sims, J. Marion: On the treatment of vesicovaginal fistula. Amer. J. Med. Sci., *23*:59, 1852.

Taussig, F. J.: Treatment of postoperative and postradiation vesicovaginal fistula. Urol. Cut. Rev., *47*:3, 1943.

von Dittel, L.: Abdominale Blasenscheidenfistel-Operation. Wien klin. Wchr., 6:449, 1893.

Winsbury-White, H. P.: A new method of implanting the ureters into the bowel. Proc. Roy. Soc. Med., *26*:1214, 1933.

29

Relaxed Vaginal Outlet, Rectocele, and Enterocele

ANATOMIC CONSIDERATIONS

Before considering the surgical repair of perineal lacerations, rectocele, and enterocele, attention should be directed to the anatomy of the vagina and the pelvic floor. The pelvic floor is formed chiefly by the levator ani muscles, aided posteriorly by the coccygeus muscles. The levator muscles form a broad muscular diaphragm which orginates in front from the posterior surface of the superior ramus of the pubis lateral to the symphysis; behind, from the inner surface of the spine of the ischium; and between these 2 points, from the obturator fascia. The muscle fibers extended posteromedially, inserting into the sides of the vagina and the rectum and into the midline of the perineum, between the vagina and the rectum. Posterior to the rectum, fibers that have passed laterally to the vagina and the rectum insert into a median raphe between the rectum and the coccyx, and finally the most posterior fibers insert into the coccyx.

Superficial to the floor formed by the levators is the urogenital diaphragm (triangular ligament). This is composed of 2 layers of fascia and covers the triangular area between the ischial tuberosities and the symphysis pubis. Lying between the layers of the trigone are the sphincter urethrae and the deep transversus perinei muscles. Superficial to the triangular ligament, and hence superficial to the levator muscles, lie the superficial transversus perinei muscles and the bulbocavernosus muscles. The former muscles arise from the ischial tuberosities and are inserted in the midline of the perineum, just posterior to the vagina. The bulbocavernosus muscles arise from the midline of the perineum, just posterior to the vagina, and pass forward along either side of the vagina to be inserted into the clitoris. The vagina, then, forms an opening between the 2 levator muscles and in the urogenital diaphragm. The bulbocavernosus muscles may be considered as the superficial vaginal constrictors; and the levator muscles, the deep constrictors.

All of these muscles are covered with fascia; hence it is the fascia, not the muscular tissue, that is visible when the dissection is carried out in doing a perineal repair.

The vagina is a musculomembranous tubal structure, reaching from the cervix to the vulva. The orifice has the smallest caliber; above this, the vagina is relatively roomy. The mucous membrane lining is covered with stratified squamous epithelium, which is thin before puberty and after the menopause. During the menstrual life of the woman it is much thicker and is thrown up into rugae. Beneath the epithelium there is fibromuscular tissue, and outside of this the perivaginal portion of the endopelvic fascia. Anteriorly, this fascia extends from the symphysis beneath the bladder and is inserted in the anterior surface of the cervix at about the level of the internal os. This is the pubovesicocervical fascia that is utilized in cystocele repair. Posteriorly, there is also an extension of endopelvic fascia which is less sturdy than the anterior fascia, but it is utilized in rectocele repair.

Posteriorly, the upper part of the vagina lies in proximity to the cul-de-sac of Douglas. In the average normal case this is not more than the upper fourth of the vagina, but in some women the cul-de-sac is congenitally much deeper. Occasionally, this peritoneal sac may dissect deeply down into the rectovaginal space and form a peritoneal pouch in which intestines lie.

Below the level of the cul-de-sac, the vagina is in close apposition to the anterior rectal wall for about half the length of the vagina. In this midportion the vagina is separated from the rectum by only a thin layer of fascia which forms the rectovaginal septum. This middle half of the posterior vaginal wall is most susceptible to rectocele formation. In the lower fourth the vagina and the rectum diverge and ultimately are separated by the perineal body. This body is formed by the union of the levator ani muscles, and superficial to them the union of the deep and the superficial transversus perinei muscles. These structures, covered with fat and skin, constitute the perineal body.

The effect of the descent of the child's head upon these structures is one of stretching and often tearing. Stretching of the vagina thins the fascia in the midportion of the vagina. The ischemia caused by prolonged pressure of the child's head in this region also weakens the rectovaginal septum. Subsequent heavy work, straining at stool, future pregnancies, and all activities which increase the intra-abdominal pressure eventually may produce herniation of the rectum into the vagina.

When the child's head reaches the outlet, there is stretching of the structures mentioned above which make up the perineal body. In most cases some laceration of the mucosa of the fourchette takes place. In those cases in which the tear continues backward, the posterior portion of the urogenital trigone with the superficial and deep transversus perinei muscles are torn apart. Then the levator muscles which lie in close apposition to each other in the midline are separated, and, when the tear is complete, it extends through the sphincter ani muscle and even up the rectal wall. Thus the perineal body may be destroyed completely, or the damaged perineum may consist eventually of only thin and weak connective tissue.

The thinning of the rectovaginal septum in the region of the upper vagina may also be a factor in the development of enterocele. This is particularly true when there is a congenitally deep cul-de-sac. All activity which increases intra-abdominal pressure will cause the peritoneal sac to dissect deeper and deeper into the potential space between the rectum and the vagina, where the fascia has already been thinned out and weakened.

SYMPTOMS OF RELAXED VAGINAL OUTLET AND RECTOCELE

First, it is important to stress the point that relaxed vaginal outlet and rectocele may be entirely asymptomatic and require no treatment. Simple relaxation of the outlet is much more apt to be asymptomatic than rectocele. Often, relaxed outlet is a contributing factor in producing a feeling of lack of support when there is an associated descensus of the uterus. The question of which condition contributes more to the symptoms is rather academic because it is well to correct both conditions when surgery is done. Also, when relaxed outlet, with or without rectocele, exists with asymptomatic cystocele, it is our custom to repair the posterior vagina and the perineum when the cystocele is repaired.

However, the rectocele itself may give rise to very definite symptoms that require relief. With a large rectocele the protruding mass may be annoying, particularly when the woman is walking. The patient may be troubled also by a collection of feces in the rectocele pouch, and pressure may be required on the mass through the vagina in order to effect an evacuation of the bowels. Frequently, hemorrhoids are associated with the relaxed condition and may contribute to the general perineal discomfort. In all such cases the hemorrhoids should be removed when the relaxed outlet and/or the rectocele are repaired.

Not uncommonly a patient attributes lack of satisfactory sex relations to the relaxed condition of the perineum. The complaint may originate from herself or her husband. This may be dependent upon the condition of the vaginal outlet and may be a legitimate reason for perineorrhaphy. However, in our experience the lack of satisfactory sex relations often is not due to the local condition. It is frequently evidence of marital incompatibility and, even more often, the natural result of increasing age of both husband and wife. One always should evaluate the whole marital picture before promising improvement from plastic vaginal surgery.

REPAIR OF RELAXED VAGINAL OUTLET AND RECTOCELE

As the gynecologist ages, his practice to a great degree grows older with him. Thus he learns that one of the commonest complaints in women over 50 is dyspareunia. With the withdrawal of estrogen the vaginal mucosa becomes thin and sensitive, and there is contracture of the outlet of varying degree. This accounts for dyspareunia, particularly in nulliparous woman and those upon whom perineal repair has been done. The gynecologist is apt to see some of his own repairs of several years before and wish that he had not done them. One should always bear in mind the effect of estrogen withdrawal when planning his repair.

First, it should be made clear that the repair of the relaxed vaginal outlet and the repair of the rectocele are two distinct operative procedures. They are frequently done together, but perineal repair is often done when rectocele is not present. Rarely, a rectocele may be present and require repair in a woman whose outlet is not relaxed. It should be stressed that in performing perineal surgery one does not see the muscles described above. They are ensheathed in fascia, and it is not wise to dissect the fascia from the muscles because the firmest union is obtained by the healing of fascia to fascia.

One should not attempt plastic surgery on the posterior vagina with a preconceived idea of the exact type of operation that one will do. Only after the posterior flap of vaginal mucosa has been dissected up, and the size and the position of the rectocele and the presence or the absence of enterocele have been determined, can one make a final decision as to what type of operation is required. A few of our standard procedures are described here, but it is understood that variations in technic must be made to fit individual cases.

TECHNIC: THE MOST CONSERVATIVE PERINEAL REPAIR

There are some women who have no rectocele and not too much relaxation but have symptoms which may be at least partially attributable to separation of the levators. One is particularly apt to encounter cases of this type when performing vaginal hysterectomy and/or cystocele repair when the major symptomatology is dependent upon the primary condition for which the operation is done. Support of the perineum can often be adequately provided by bringing the levators together with minimal narrowing of the outlet as shown in Figure 29-1.

A curved transverse incision is made posteriorly at the mucocutaneous junction, and the fascial sheath of the levators is exposed. A single suture is used to approximate the levators; or, if more narrowing of the outlet is desired, a second suture is used (Fig. 29-1 A). Without excising any mucosa, the flap is sutured transversely with a subcuticular stitch (Fig. 29-1 B).

TECHNIC: SIMPLE PERINEAL REPAIR FOR RELAXED VAGINAL OUTLET WITHOUT RECTOCELE

The ultimate size of the vaginal orifice is determined by placing mucosa clips

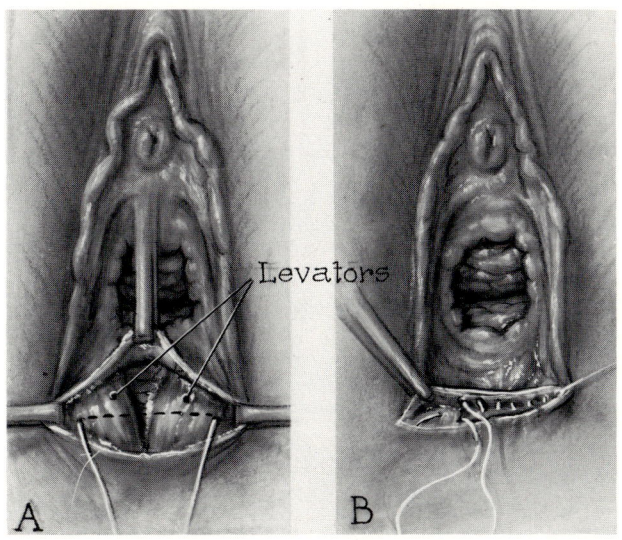

Fig. 29-1. Most conservative type of repair with minimum narrowing of introitus. (A, *left*) A single stitch is used to reunite the levators. (B, *right*) The mucosal flap is sutured to the perineal skin transversely with a subcuticular stitch of fine catgut.

on the labia minora on either side of the outlet and approximating them in the midline. These should be adjusted so that the final opening will admit 2 fingers easily. In performing a repair one always should bear in mind postmenopausal shrinkage which ultimately will further contract the orifice to some degree.

A curved transverse incision is then made posteriorly at the mucocutaneous junction, connecting the 2 mucosa clips (Fig. 29-2 A).

The posterior vaginal wall is dissected upward by blunt and sharp dissection (Fig. 29-2 B). The operation about to be described is for simple perineal relaxation, without rectocele; hence the dissection is carried high enough only to expose the fascia covering the levator muscles to permit placing of the levator sutures. The flap of mucosa is excised by transverse incision as indicated by the dotted line in Figure 29-2 B.

Next, a small inverted V-shaped piece of mucosa is excised in the midline as in Figure 29-2 C. This prevents pouting of excessive mucosa in the center of the posterior vaginal wall when the vaginal incision is closed.

Interrupted sutures of No. 0 chromic catgut are taken through the levator muscles (Fig. 29-2 D). No attempt is made to expose the muscle fibers themselves before taking these sutures. The muscles are covered with fascia, and bold stitches are taken laterally to include a liberal amount of the muscle in each bite. The number of stitches taken in the levator muscles varies, depending upon the degree of relaxation and the tightness of the closure desired. In the average case 3 stitches are taken.

Starting at the top of the inverted-V incision, the vaginal incision is closed in the midline, using a continuous lock stitch of No. 0 chromic catgut. When the levator region is reached, the muscles are approximated by tying the previously placed sutures (Fig. 29-2 E).

This mucosal suture is continued down over the perineum subcuticularly in the midline (Fig. 29-2 E). A small cutting needle is well adapted for this suturing.

Figure 29-2 F shows the completed operation. In this instance it had been done very conservatively, leaving a rather large outlet.

Technic: Repair of Relaxed Vaginal Outlet and Moderate-Sized Rectocele

The degree of closure of the relaxed outlet is determined by grasping the mucocutaneous border on either side of the outlet with mucosa clips and drawing them together. The final opening should admit 2 fingers easily An incision is

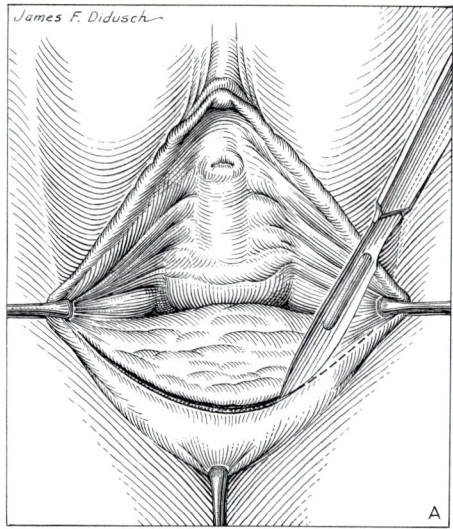
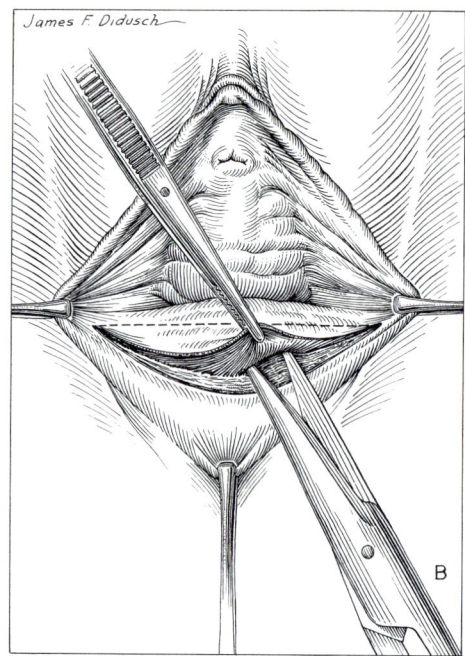
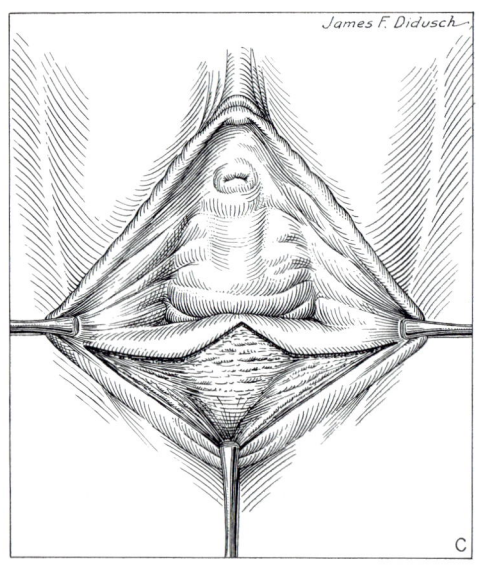

FIG. 29-2. Simple perineal repair. (A) An incision is made at the mucocutaneous border. (B) The flap of the mucosa is being dissected free. The dotted line indicates the line of excision of the flap. (C) The flap and in addition a small inverted V-shaped piece of mucosa have been excised.

made along the mucocutaneous border, posteriorly, connecting the 2 clamps (Fig. 29-3 A).

A posterior flap of vaginal mucosa is dissected up by sharp and blunt dissection (Fig. 29-3 B). When this dissection has been carried up to the level of the clips, the triangular mucosal flap is excised as indicated by the dotted line in Figure 29-3 C.

A second triangular flap of mucosa is dissected free and excised, with the apex at a point above the summit of the rectocele (Fig. 29-3 D). Thus the rectocele and the fascia of the rectovaginal septum are exposed.

Interrupted sutures of No. 0 chromic catgut are taken deeply through the levator muscles (Fig. 29-3 E). If the dissection is rather bloody, these levator sutures

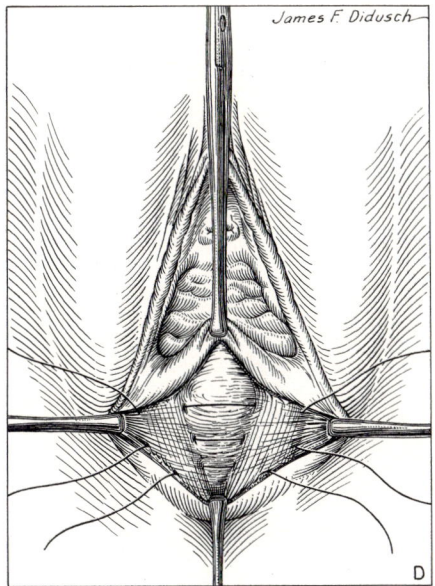

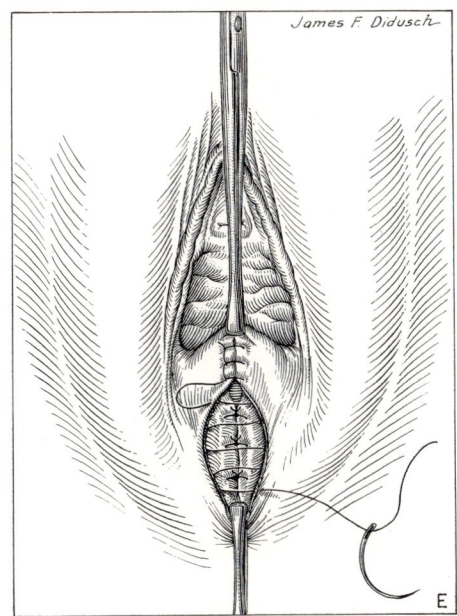

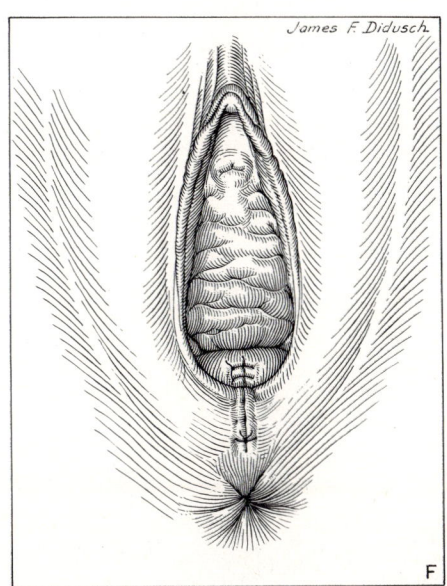

Fig. 29-2 (*Continued*). Simple perineal repair. (D) Three interrupted sutures of No. 0 chromic catgut have been placed in the levator ani muscles. (E) The levator muscles have been approximated. The mucosa has been closed with a lock stitch of No. 0 chromic catgut, and perineal skin is being approximated with a subcuticular stitch. (F) Operation completed.

may be placed before excising the mucosal flaps in order to reduce the operating time after the complete dissection and thus conserve blood. Hence we sometimes place them directly after dissecting free the first triangular flap, before the flap is excised.

The fascia of the rectovaginal septum is then dissected from the vaginal mucosa and approximated over the rectocele, using as many mattress sutures of No. 0 chromic catgut as are necessary to cover completely the bulging rectal wall (Fig. 29-3 E). In Figure 29-3 F these sutures have been tied. In some instances with a small rectocele, the perirectal fascia is approximated with 1 or 2 concentric purse strings instead of these mattress sutures. At this stage of the operation the mucosal closure is started, beginning at

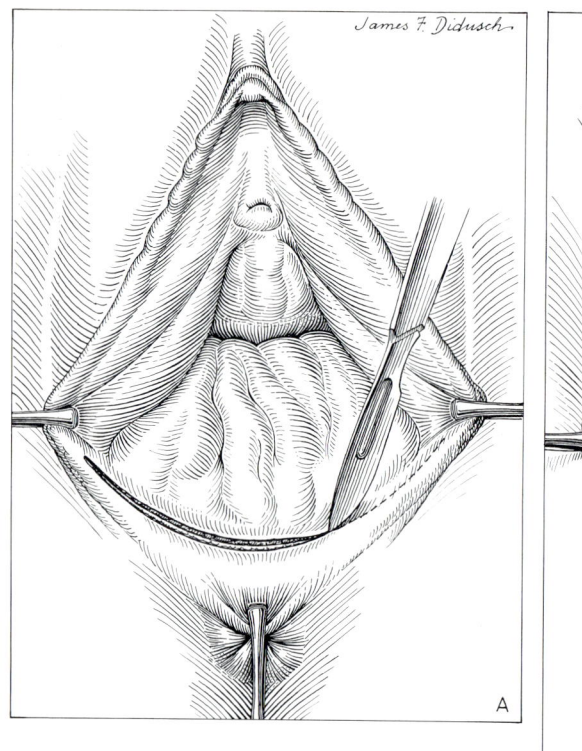
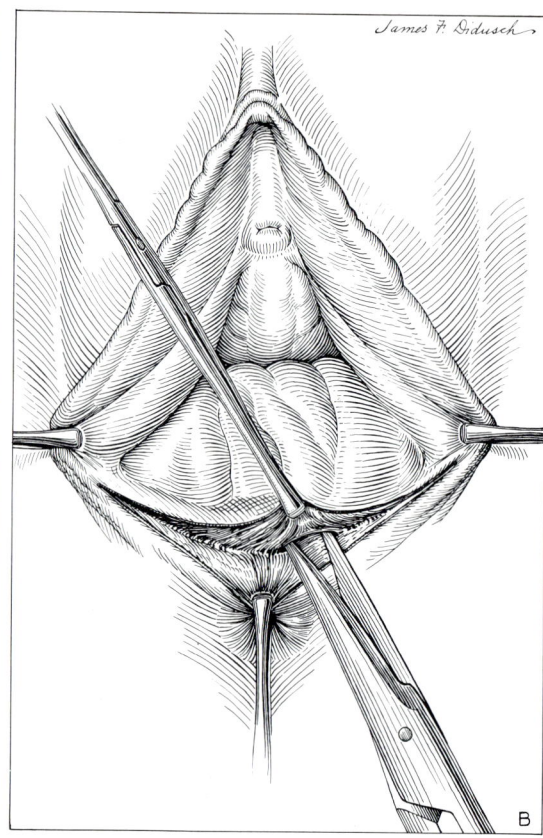
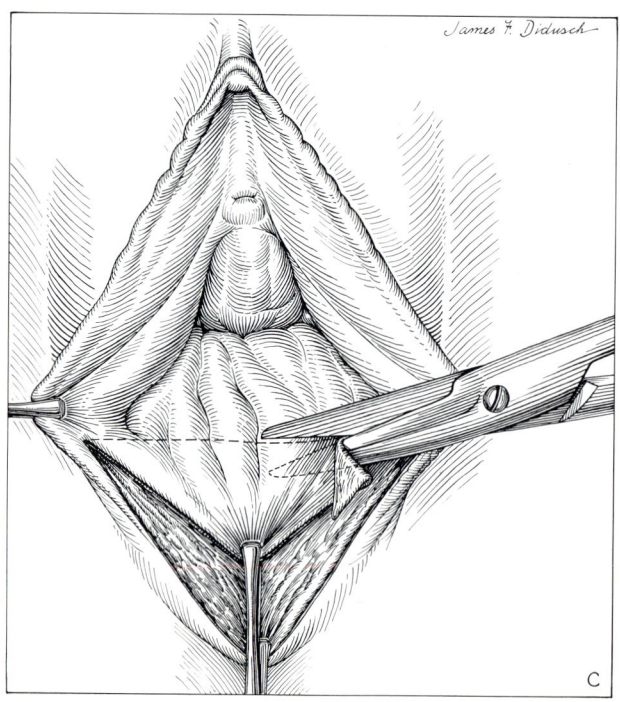

Fig. 29-3. Repair of medium-sized rectocele. (A) An incision made at the mucocutaneous border. (B) The posterior flap is being dissected free by sharp dissection. (C) The triangular flap of the mucosa is being excised.

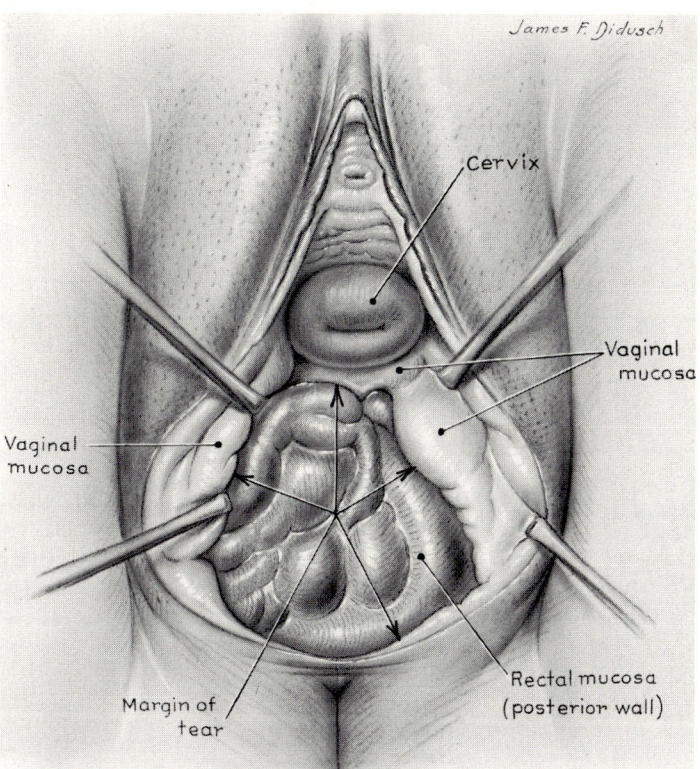

Fig. 30-2. Rectovaginal tear extending from the perineum almost to the cervix.

stools; in others the band of scar tissue that bridges the gap between the sphincter ends gives sufficient sphincter action to permit control of feces when the stool is of normal consistency and moderately good control of flatus, while in some cases the tear extends well up the rectum so that feces and gas escape at all times (Fig. 30-2). Not uncommonly a complete tear is discovered during a pelvic examination incidental to some other pelvic complaint, and frequently we are struck by the lack of complaint of incontinence. Upon direct questioning, such women will often reply that they have no difficulty in their naturally constipated state; only after cathartics are they really annoyed by the lack of a sphincter.

TREATMENT

An attempt at repair should be made at the time of delivery. If this fails and the patient is left incontinent, we believe that at least 6 months should elapse before an attempt at repair is made. This gives the tissues sufficient time to return to normal, the operation will be easier to perform, and, in our experience, the chances of success are enhanced.

Two general types of operation are used in the repair of complete lacerations: (1) *the layer method;* and (2) *the flap method as first described by Warren.* Slight modifications in both of these methods have been made from time to time by various gynecologists, but they are of no great significance. The only real addition to the original technic was made by Norman Miller, who, since 1931, has advocated cutting the rectal sphincter lateroposteriorly to permit the free escape of gas and thus prevent tension on the sutures. Miller calls this sphincter cutting the "paradoxical operation." We have used it several times with success and believe that it is especially important to cut the sphincter in the more difficult cases, and partic-

30

Complete Perineal Lacerations and Rectovaginal Fistulas

COMPLETE PERINEAL LACERATIONS

General Considerations

Laceration of the perineum involving the rectal sphincter and the rectovaginal septum is one of the more serious obstetric complications (Fig. 30-1). A surprising number of such cases may be repaired successfully at the time of delivery. Still a fairly large group confronts the gynecologist later, thus making the surgical problem of repairing them of major importance. Although nearly all of these injuries are the result of delivery, some rare cases may be attributed to operations for rectal fistulas or hemorrhoids, and, occasionally, a complete perineal laceration may result from falling astride some sharp object.

In 1929 when Smith and Linton reviewed the cases of complete perineal laceration treated at the Woman's Free Hospital, they found no decrease in the number of complete lacerations that had been seen yearly since the founding of the hospital in 1875. However, it is our impression that there has been a definite decrease in the number of cases of complete laceration in our clinics in the past decade. We are inclined to attribute this to better prenatal evaluation of the obstetric problem, the more careful use of the forceps, and especially to the more frequent use of episiotomy.

The classic symptoms of loss of control of feces and gas are present in the majority of the cases, but since there is a great variation in the "completeness" of "complete" perineal lacerations, there is also considerable variation in the degree of incontinence. In some instances a few sphincter fibers are left intact with satisfactory control except with loose

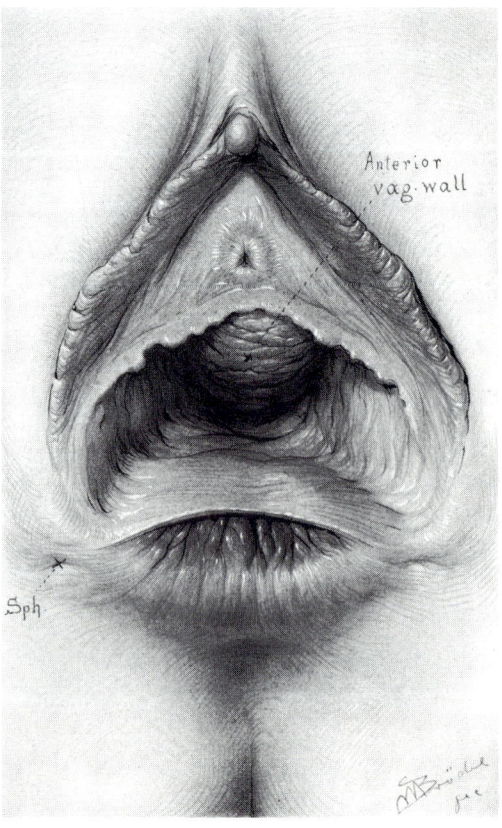

Fig. 30-1. Old 3rd-degree laceration. Note dimples on either side due to retraction of torn sphincter.

connection with vaginal hysterectomy. The subject should be considered from 4 different viewpoints, depending upon the anatomic condition present at the time of the hysterectomy.

1. The prevention of a future enterocele when the anatomy of the cul-de-sac is quite normal.
2. The prevention of a future enterocele when there is a deep cul-de-sac which could develop into a full-fledged enterocele.
3. The cure of an enterocele not associated with an appreciable rectocele.
4. The cure of an enterocele associated with a well-developed rectocele.

Many enteroceles following vaginal hysterectomy are the result of improper occlusion of the space at the top of the vagina. This space is obliterated by picking up the stumps of the uterosacral ligaments which have already been sutured at either angle of the vagina. The suture then picks up the inner surface of the posterior vaginal flap. When tied, the space at the apex of the vagina is completely obliterated. This technic is illustrated in the section on vaginal hysterectomy as a part of our routine plication of the uterosacral ligaments (Fig. 24-10).

When there is a deep cul-de-sac the excess of peritoneum can be picked up with the above stitch, and the stitch can be repeated 2 or 3 times until all of the redundant cul-de-sac serosa is plicated.

When an actual enterocele sac is present without a rectocele, it is not necessary to dissect free the entire posterior vaginal wall as shown in Figure 29-8. The sac may be dissected free through the incision existing from the vaginal hysterectomy and ligated at its neck. Then the stump of the sac is included in with the suture described above, thus obliterating the space. If there is redundant vaginal mucosa in this area a V-shaped piece may be excised.

When there is also a relaxed outlet and a rectocele requiring repair, it is best to open up the entire posterior vaginal wall and repair the enterocele as above described. After this the rectocele and the relaxed outlet are repaired as indicated.

BIBLIOGRAPHY

Baden, W. F.: Geriatric gynecology. Postgrad. Med. J., 46:241, 1969.

Goffe, J. Riddle: An operation for extreme cases of procidentia, with rectocele and cystocele. Med. Rec., 82:879, 1912.

McCall, Milton L.: Posterior culdeplasty; surgical correction of enterocele during vaginal hysterectomy; a preliminary report. Obstet. Gynec., 10:595, 1957.

Moschowitz, Alexis V.: The pathogenesis, anatomy and cure of prolapse of the rectum. Surg. Gynec. Obstet., 15:7, 1942.

Reich, W. J., Nechtow, M. J., and Keith, L.: Diagnosis and modified surgical treatment of posterior direct vaginal hernia (enterocele). Clin Obstet. Gynec., 9:1070, 1966.

Te Linde, R. W.: Prolapse of the uterus and allied conditions. Amer. J. Obstet. Gynec., 94:444, 1966.

Ward, George G.: Operative technic for repair of rectocele and injury to the pelvic floor. Surg. Gynec. Obstet., 48:399, 1929.

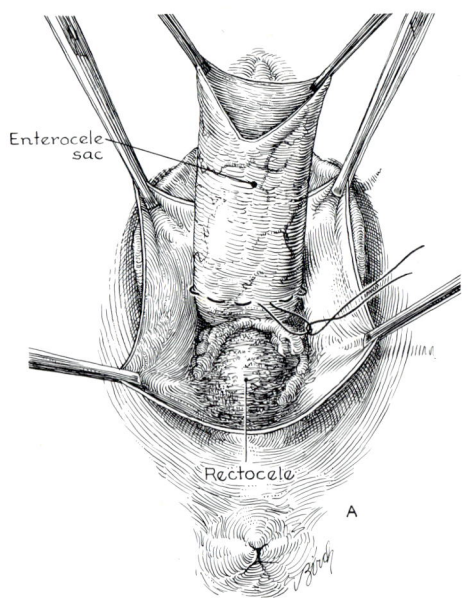

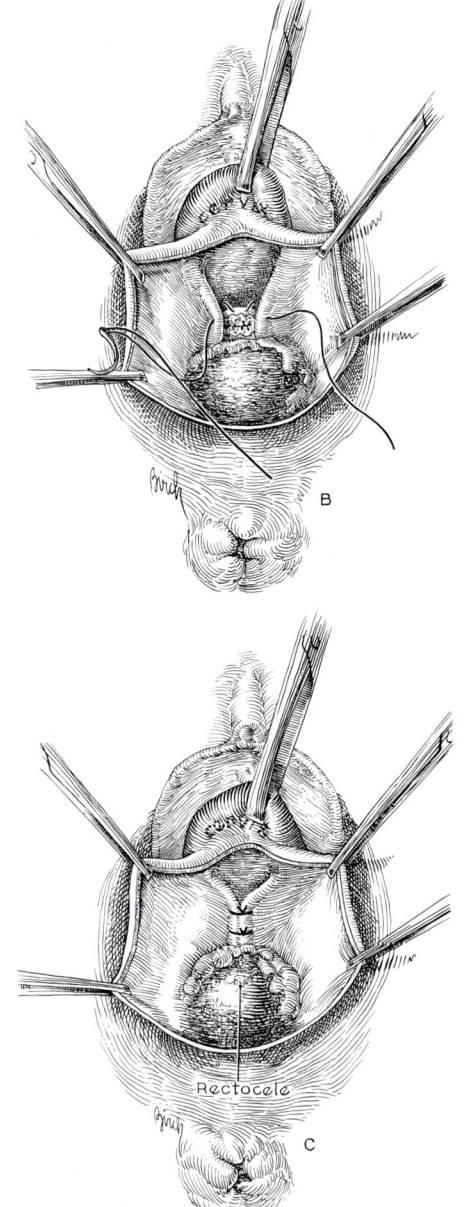

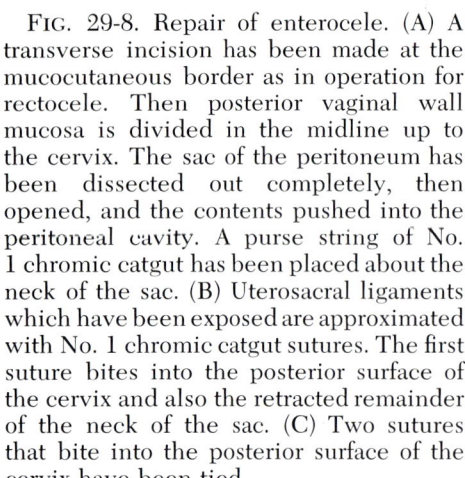

FIG. 29-8. Repair of enterocele. (A) A transverse incision has been made at the mucocutaneous border as in operation for rectocele. Then posterior vaginal wall mucosa is divided in the midline up to the cervix. The sac of the peritoneum has been dissected out completely, then opened, and the contents pushed into the peritoneal cavity. A purse string of No. 1 chromic catgut has been placed about the neck of the sac. (B) Uterosacral ligaments which have been exposed are approximated with No. 1 chromic catgut sutures. The first suture bites into the posterior surface of the cervix and also the retracted remainder of the neck of the sac. (C) Two sutures that bite into the posterior surface of the cervix have been tied.

pation, but this is not necessary if one is careful to include only the peritoneum in each bite when in the ureteral region. The number of concentric purse-string sutures depends upon the depth of the cul-de-sac, but it should be sufficient to obliterate at least the space below the level of the uterosacral ligament. Figure 29-7 shows the purse strings in place, but they have not been tied when placed, as is our usual custom; this technic has been altered here so that the method of placing them may be demonstrated.

PREVENTION AND REPAIR OF ENTEROCELE IN CONNECTION WITH VAGINAL HYSTERECTOMY

Since more and more vaginal hysterectomies are being done, it becomes important to consider enterocele repair in

be carried out equally well in connection with the Spalding-Richardson composite operation.

Technic: Repair of Enterocele

An incision is made posteriorly, at the mucocutaneous border of the vaginal outlet between lateral mucosa clips as in a posterior colporrhaphy. Inserting the curved scissors beneath the vaginal mucosa in the midline, a tunnel is made by successively opening and closing the scissors. After tunneling as far as the scissors will reach conveniently, the mucosa is cut in the midline. Then the process of tunneling and cutting is repeated until the cervix is reached. The vaginal mucosa is dissected laterally on either side, thus first exposing the rectocele, if present, and then the enterocele. The latter appears as a peritoneal pouch, much like a hernial sac, which it is in reality.

Then the sac is dissected free by blunt dissection as high as possible and then opened (Fig. 29-8 A). After making certain that the sac is free of intestines, a purse string of No. 1 chromic catgut is placed about the neck of the sac (Fig. 29-8 A). The purse string is tied, and the sac is trimmed off a little distal to the suture.

As the cervix is drawn forward, the undersurfaces of the uterosacral ligaments are visible. These ligaments are approximated in the midline with interrupted sutures of No. 1 chromic catgut, 2 or 3 of which are required. These sutures should bite into the posterior surface of the cervix and the sac (Fig 29-8 B). As they are tied, a firm new base is formed for the cul-de-sac. Figure 29-8 C shows the enterocele completely repaired. An appropriate operation is done for the cure of the rectocele, if present, and for repair of the relaxed vaginal outlet.

In 1957 McCall described an operation for enterocele which he claimed prevented shortening of the vagina. In McCall's words it was: "A posterior culdeplasty whereby the relaxed cul-de-sac of Douglas is suspended and obliterated between the uterosacral ligaments without dissection of or excision of the hernial sac." It is true that the operation described above in detail does usually shorten the vagina to some degree, but we cannot recall any complaints dependent on this. After all, most of the patients are no longer young, and the shortened vagina does not appear to be a source of annoyance.

Another method of closing a large sac is to open it through the vaginal approach and close it with a purse string, much in the manner of obliterating the cul-de-sac at laparotomy. Such a suture bites successively into the posterior surface of the cervix, a uterosacral ligament, the anterior rectal serosal surface, and finally the opposite uterosacral ligament. After tying this suture, the excessive peritoneum is excised. Then the stump of the sac may be sutured to the posterior surface of the cervix.

Technic: Repair of Enterocele from Within Abdomen (Moschowitz)

A deep cul-de-sac, a potential enterocele, may be obliterated or a well-developed enterocele may be cured by the Moschowitz operation, which was originally devised by him for cure of rectal prolapse. This procedure is used primarily in operating for other pelvic conditions which require a laparotomy.

The patient is placed in the Trendelenburg position, and the intestines are held back in the abdominal cavity by gauze. The uterus is held up and forward with a traction suture (Fig. 29-7). Beginning at the base of the sac, a purse string is taken, using medium silk or linen. This is tied, and a second is taken just above it. These sutures are placed with a small round needle, just picking up the peritoneum and biting very lightly into the musculature of the rectum. Successive purse strings are taken, and when the region of the uterosacral ligaments is reached, good firm bites are taken through the ligaments and into the posterior surface of the cervix. At the level of the uterosacral ligaments and above, care should be taken to avoid including the ureters in the sutures. The ureters may be catheterized before the operation so that they can be identified easily by pal-

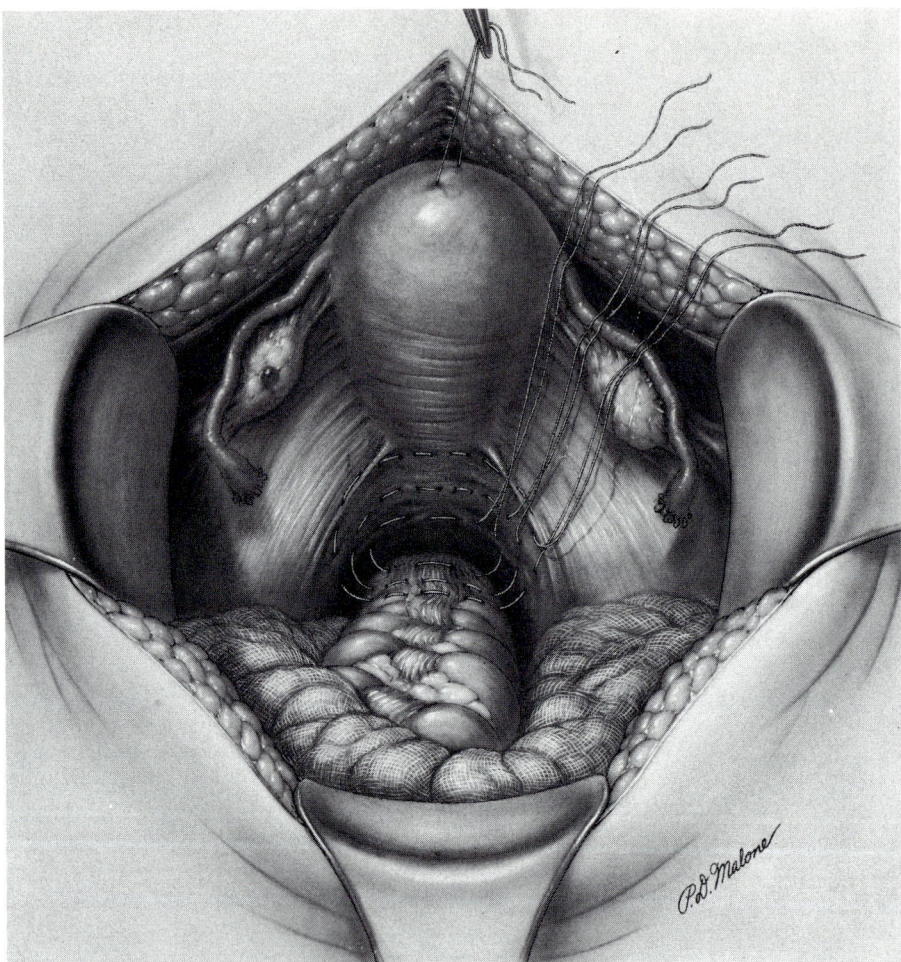

Fig. 29-7. Method of obliteration of deep cul-de-sac or enterocele, using multiple concentric purse strings.

laparotomy, the sac may be closed by a succession of concentric purse strings, starting at the bottom of the sac. This procedure, which was described by Moschowitz for cure of rectal prolapse, is shown in Figure 29-7. When the enterocele occurs as a herniation through the vaginal vault after a total vaginal hysterectomy, the sac is dissected out from below and excised; all the available ligaments are brought together and sutured to the vagina to give it support and also to secure closure of the hernial defect.

The operation to cure enterocele is often part of an extensive plastic procedure done for co-existing relaxed vaginal outlet, rectocele, cystocele, and uterine descensus of varying degrees. When total vaginal hysterectomy is done, the enterocele sac is dissected free and excised, and the neck is closed. The uterosacral ligaments are then approximated for the purpose of strengthening the floor of the cul-de-sac. A similar procedure can be carried out when the operation is combined with the interposition or Manchester operation. The appropriate time to do this may be when it is encountered on dissecting the posterior flap of mucosa free from the cervix, before amputation. In most cases, however, it is best repaired when the rectocele is repaired. These procedures can

the term "high rectocele," as this is anatomically misleading.

Failure to recognize an enterocele when it occurs along with rectocele means failure in attaining a satisfactory surgical result. Like most hernias, probably there is often a congenital factor in its formation, for enterocele has been described in nulliparous women. A congenitally deep cul-de-sac may serve as the entering wedge by which the hernia sac dissects downward in the space between the posterior vaginal wall and the anterior surface of the rectum. The most important acquired factor in promoting the formation of an enterocele is prolapse of the uterus, and, of course, childbirth is the greatest etiologic factor in prolapse. Frequently, the two conditions are combined. The descent of the uterus is apt to result in an elongation of the cul-de-sac, and the intra-abdominal pressure then carries the dissection downward. Herniation of the intestines through the uppermost part of the vagina occasionally occurs following a vaginal hysterectomy. Such a hernia may merely be the reappearance of a pre-existing enterocele which was unrecognized and hence not properly treated when the uterus was removed. On the other hand, the hernia can make its appearance through a weak point resulting from the operation. Probably the sloughing, which of necessity takes place at the distal ends of the ligaments that have been tied en masse, is responsible for lack of solid support of the newly formed upper pelvic floor.

The patient may complain of a mass protruding from the vaginal outlet on straining or standing. It usually disappears when the patient lies down. The contents of the sac are usually intestine, omentum and/or fluid. We never have observed strangulation of the intestine in these hernia sacs. The large size of the neck of the sac permits the contents to slip in and out easily. In many instances there is a history of previous operations, such as uterine suspension and perineal repair.

Recognition is the first essential factor in the cure of an enterocele. It is unfortunate that the term "high rectocele" has been applied to this condition. In the first place, it is not a rectocele; the contents of the sac are small bowel, not rectum. Second, this misnomer has induced surgeons to attempt a cure by performing a rectocele operation at an unusually high level. Often an enterocele and a rectocele occur in the same patient, although either may occur independently. When enterocele is present, without rectocele, its bulging mass may be seen protruding from a high point downward over the lower posterior vaginal wall. When rectocele and enterocele are both present, the diagnosis frequently can be made by inspection, as the division between the two is indicated more or less distinctly by a transverse furrow just above the rectocele (Fig. 29-6). A finger inserted into the rectum will demonstrate the rectocele as distinct from the bulging at a higher point that is caused by the enterocele.

After the enterocele has been recognized, the same principles of cure apply to it as to the cure of other types of hernia: isolation of the sac, disposition of the sac, and closure of the defect through which the sac leaves the pelvic floor. The technic of cure of an enterocele depends to a large extent upon the other conditions with which it is associated. When it is encountered while performing a pelvic

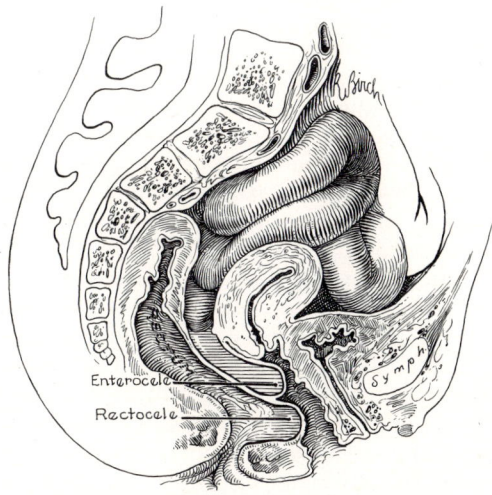

FIG. 29-6. Sagittal section, demonstrating relative position of rectocele and enterocele.

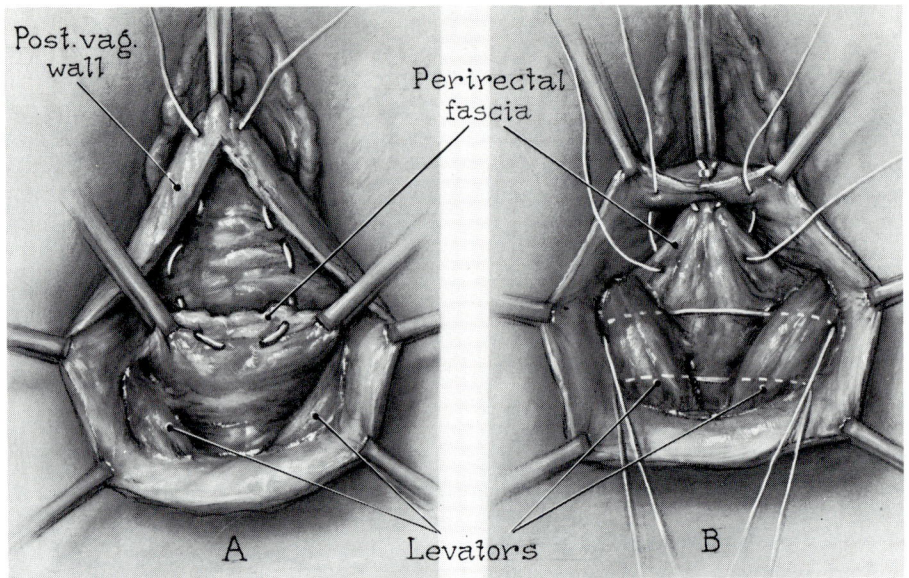

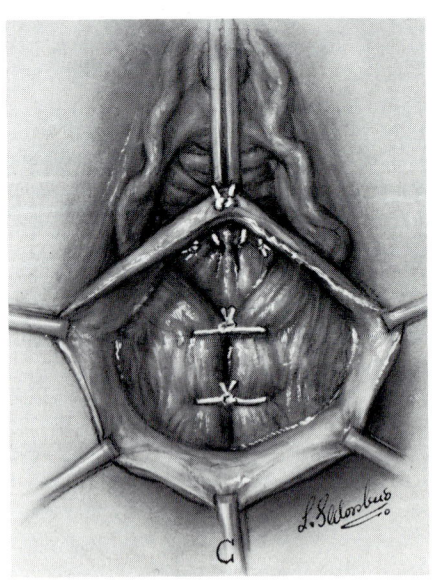

FIG. 29-5. Repair of high rectocele. (A) After dissecting out the rectocele, the well-developed rectovaginal fascia, found lower in the posterior vaginal wall, is elevated with a purse-string suture to fill in the high defect where fascia is practically nil. (B) Purse string has been tied. Lateral defects are closed with an interrupted suture on either side. (C) Levators are brought together in case outlet requires repair.

strong lower flap may be brought up and sutured to the posterior surface of the cervix and bilaterally as shown in Figure 29-5 B. This may shorten the posterior wall somewhat but not sufficiently to be of practical importance. The high rectovaginal fascia may be brought in from the sides and sutured together in the midline with interrupted sutures to reinforce this area. The remainder of the repair is done in a routine manner.

ENTEROCELE

Enterocele or herniation through the cul-de-sac of Douglas is not nearly as common as either rectocele or cystocele, but its recognition is of great surgical importance. The condition is described under various names in the literature: posterior vaginal hernia, rectovaginal hernia, cul-de-sac hernia, Douglas pouch hernia, and high rectocele. We object to

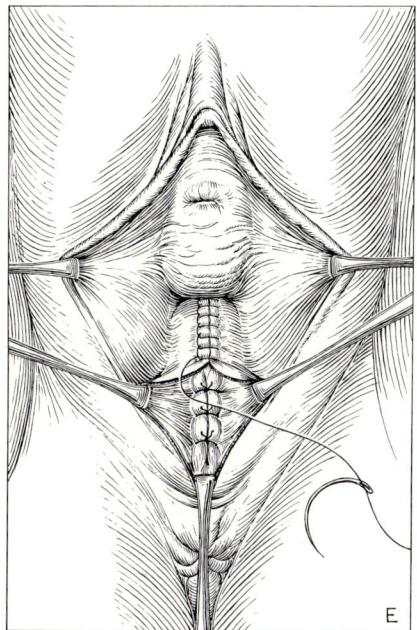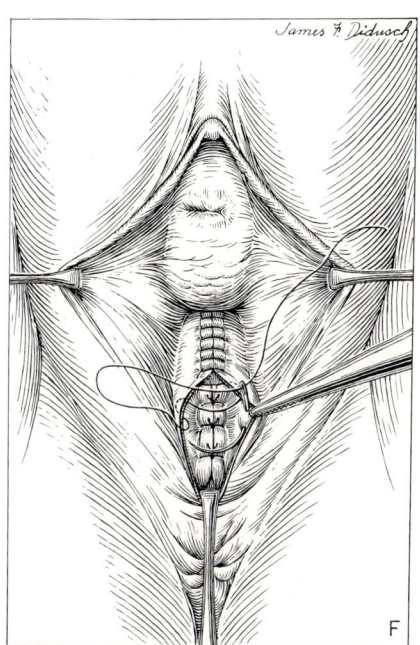

FIG. 29-4 (*Continued*). Repair of large rectocele. (E) Levator muscles have been approximated in the midline, and the mucosa is being closed with a continuous lock stitch. (F) The mucosal stitch is continued over the perineum subcuticularly.

ure 29-4 C shows 4 of such sutures tied, and 2 have been placed below but not tied. The excess of vaginal mucosa is excised as indicated by the dotted line in Figure 29-4 B.

Figure 29-4 D shows all 6 sutures tied and the fascia brought together completely over the rectum. Three interrupted sutures of No. 0 chromic catgut are placed in the levator ani muscles (Fig. 29-4 D).

Before tying the levator sutures, the closure of the vaginal mucosa incision is begun at the apex and carried down with a continuous lock stitch of No. 0 chromic catgut. When the closure is carried down to the point shown in Figure 29-4 E, the levator sutures are tied. From that point on, the continuous suture is carried down over the perineum subcuticularly as shown in Figure 29-4 F.

Technic: Repair of High Rectocele

Failure to obtain a perfect restoration of the posterior vaginal wall is not infrequently the result of neglecting to recognize weakness in the upper posterior vaginal wall. The operator may excuse himself from carrying his dissection high enough, believing that there is insufficient bulging to justify further dissection. One must remember that the upper portion of the rectovaginal fascia is normally the weakest, and all too often the patient returns years later with bulging high in the posterior vagina. The differentiation between high rectocele and enterocele is discussed in the section on enterocele. Such a differentiation may be difficult or even impossible until the entire posterior wall is dissected up to the cervix.

A useful method of utilizing the stronger lower fascia to reinforce the upper weak area is shown in Figure 29-5. After the posterior vaginal mucosal flap has been dissected completely free, the lower fascia will be visible with a frayed edge as shown in Figure 29-5 A. Above this level there may be practically nothing but areolar tissue up to the cervix, separating the rectum from the vagina. The

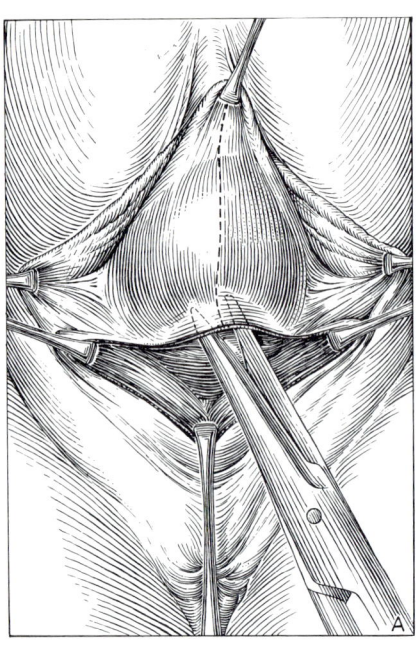 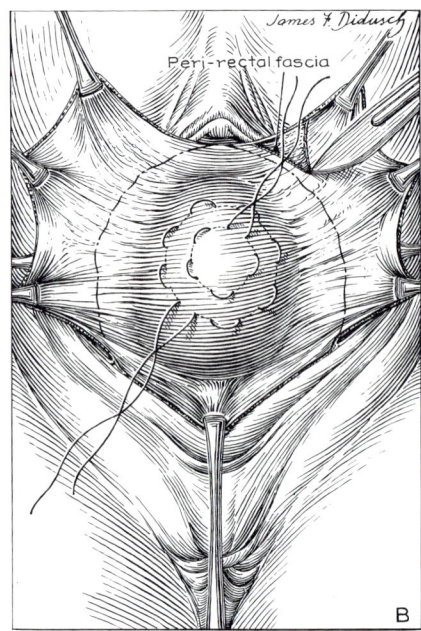
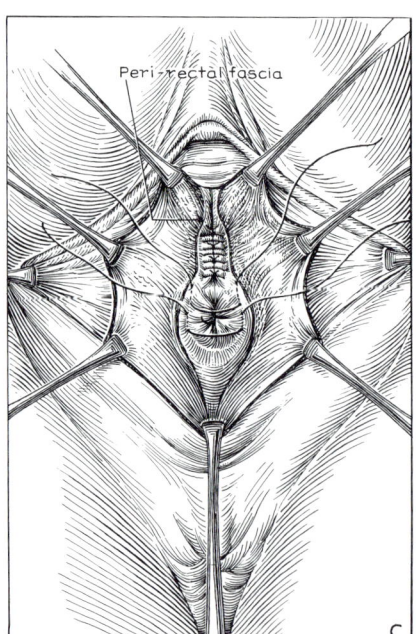 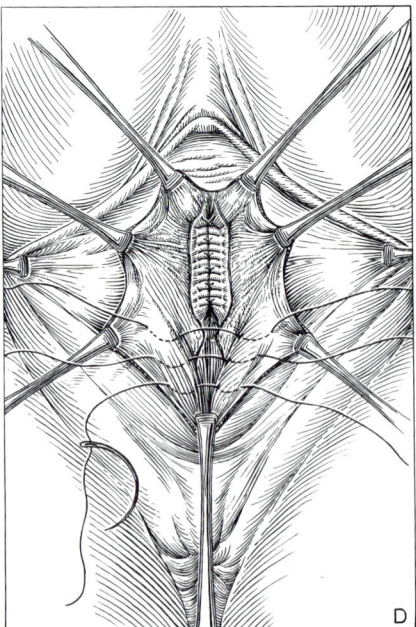

FIG. 29-4. Repair of large rectocele. (A) transverse incision has been made at the posterior mucocutaneous border. The mucosa is dissected free in the midline by alternately opening and closing Mayo scissors. The mucosal flap is divided as indicated by the dotted line. (B) Two concentric purse strings have been placed. The line of excision of the excessive mucosa is indicated by a dotted line, and the beginning of the fascial dissection with the scalpel is shown. (C) Both purse strings have been tied, and perirectal fascia is being approximated in the midline with interrupted mattress sutures. (D) Three interrupted catgut sutures have been placed deeply through the levator muscles.

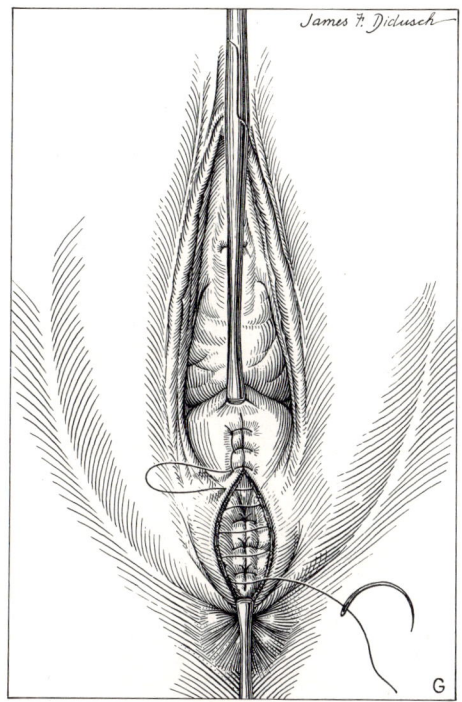 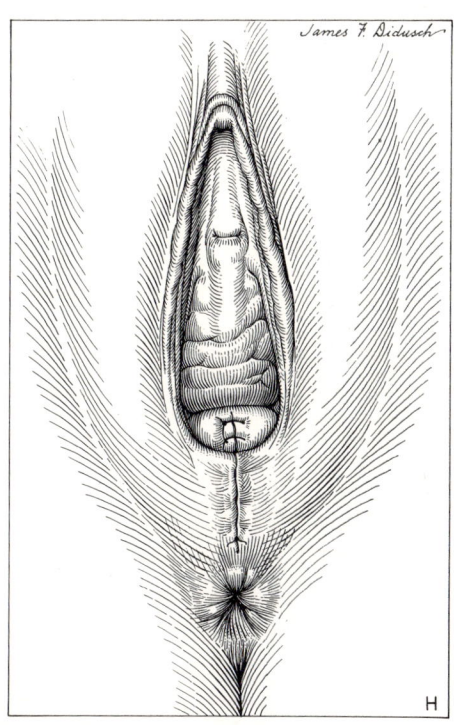

FIG. 29-3 (*Continued*). Repair of medium-sized rectocele. (G) Levator sutures have been tied, and the mucosa incision closed in the midline. This suture is carried down over the perineum subcuticularly. (H) Completed operation.

the apex of the upper triangle (Fig. 29-3 G). This is done with a continuous lock suture of No. 0 chromic catgut.

The levator sutures are tied when the continuous suture approaches the perineal region. Then the continuous suture is continued down over the perineum as a subcuticular stitch, using a small curved cutting needle (Fig. 29-3 G).

Figure 29-3 H shows the completed operation.

TECHNIC: REPAIR OF LARGE RECTOCELE

An incision is made at the posterior mucocutaneous border, and a more or less triangular piece of mucosa is excised as in an ordinary perineal repair. In Figure 29-4 A this procedure has already been carried out. The scissors are inserted in the midline beneath the mucosa, and by alternately opening and closing the scissors a tunnel is made up to a point well above the apex of the rectocele. This tunnel lies between the perirectal fascia and the rectal wall, which is often covered with some fat. After this tunnel has been completed, the mucosa and the fascia are cut in the midline as indicated in Figure 29-4 A. These 2 layers are dissected from the rectum laterally.

Concentric purse-string sutures of No. 0 chromic catgut are placed in the bulging anterior rectal wall. Very superficial bites are taken in the tissue to avoid perforation of the bowel wall. Sometimes 1 purse-string suture suffices, and again 2 or 3 are necessary to invert the bulging rectal wall (Fig. 29-4 B). Using the scalpel, the perirectal fascia is freed from the vaginal mucosa (Fig. 29-4 B). After starting the dissection with the scalpel, often the separation of the fascia from the mucosa can be carried out best with gauze over the gloved finger.

The perirectal fascia is then approximated in the midline over the rectum, using interrupted mattress sutures of No. 0 chromic catgut. These mattress sutures are placed from above downward. Fig-

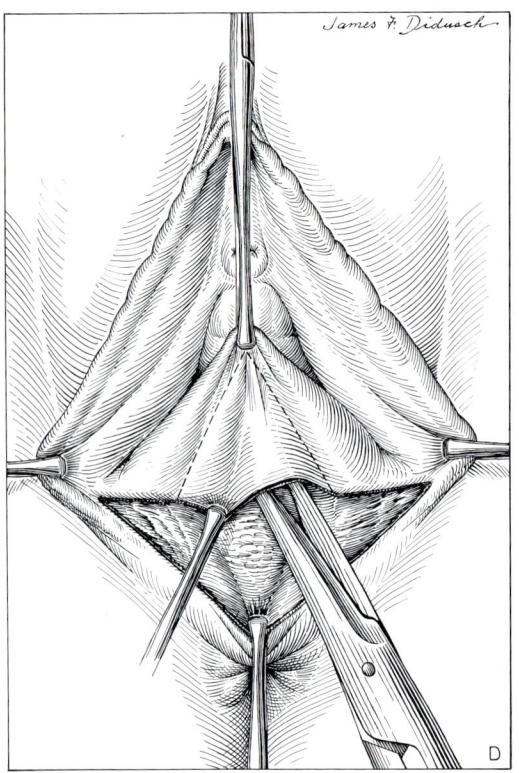
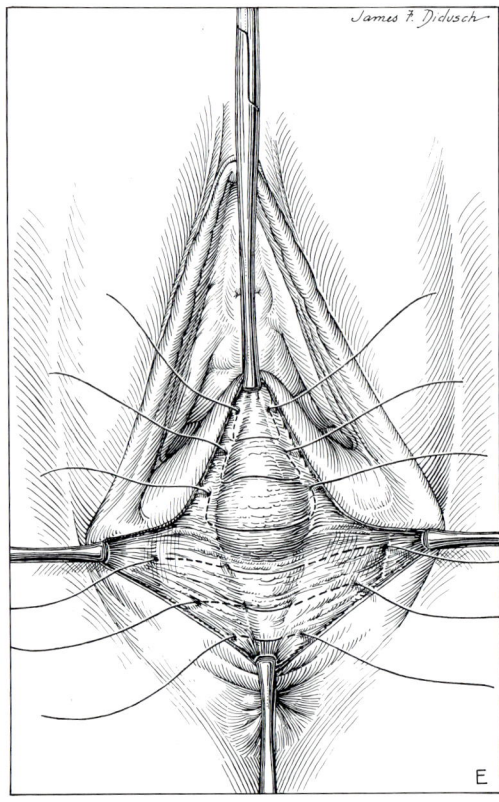
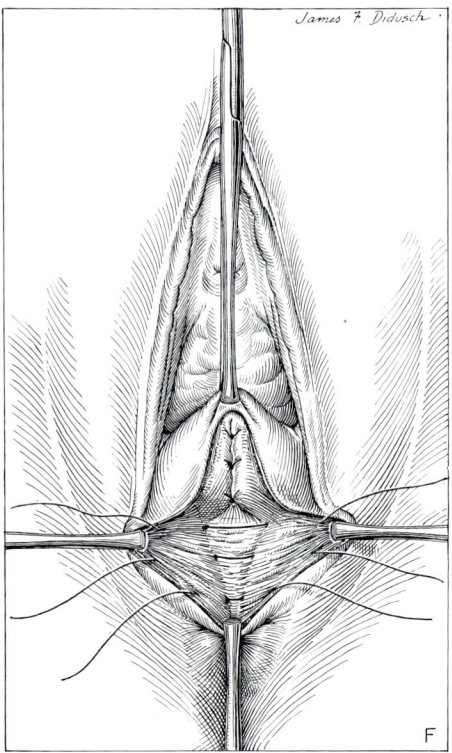

FIG. 29-3 (*Continued*). Repair of medium-sized rectocele. (D) An inverted V-shaped incision is marked out by a scalpel as indicated by the dotted line. This flap is dissected free and is excised. (E) Three deep sutures have been placed in the levators. Three mattress sutures have been placed in the perirectal fascia. (F) The fascia sutures have been tied, thus approximating fascia over rectum.

ularly in those in which previous unsuccessful attempts at repair have been made.

It is our opinion that the Warren apron or flap method is the greatest single contribution to the cure of complete perineal laceration, and for this reason Warren's own description and his original portrayal of the method of dissecting the flap are reproduced here:

The flap is formed by dissecting the "butterfly" from within outward, preserving the materials just mentioned in one continuous mass, the pedicle being formed by the entire free margin of the septum, a hinge on which the flap is swung over so as to exclude the rectum from view. The dissection will be performed with greater ease and nicety if the knife is used, and should be made chiefly from the sides in the manner indicated. In reflecting the central portion it is important to avoid "buttonholing"; for this purpose it is well to keep the septum between the thumb and forefinger of the left hand, liberating the flap by gentle strokes of the knife to and fro, while the tissues are made tense by traction on the flap with the forceps in the hands of an assistant. The dissection should stop just short of the free margin so as to leave it intact, otherwise the pedicle of the flap would be severed; on the sides the dissection is carried out sufficiently far to expose the ends of the ruptured sphincter muscle.*

It is obvious upon reviewing the results recorded in the literature that excellent results may be obtained by the layer method as well as by the flap method:

Smith and Linton. From the Woman's Free Hospital by the *layer method:*

Cured................ 89.3 per cent
Failed................ 1.8 per cent
Relieved.............. 8.9 per cent

Phaneuf. Operation by the *layer method:*

Satisfactory .... 87 per cent
Reoperation upon the remaining 13 per cent increased the satisfactory results to 97.8 per cent.

---
*Warren, J. Collins: A new method of operation for the relief of rupture of the perineum through the sphincter and rectum. Trans. Amer. Gynec. Soc., 72:324, 1882.

Campbell. From University of Wisconsin Medical School, *flap method:*

Successful .... 95 per cent

Miller and Brown report from the University of Michigan, dividing the cases done by the *Warren flap method* into two groups: those done before 1931 and those after 1931. In the latter group the sphincter was cut in most instances.

	BEFORE 1931	AFTER 1931
Function restored	71%	87%
Function improved	15%	8%
Failure	10%	5%
Unknown	5%	None

In considering the end results, the effect of future deliveries upon the reconstructed perineum should be considered. We always have taught that deliveries after a successful 3rd-degree perineal repair should be made by cesarean section. Smith and Linton's followup study on this point substantiates this viewpoint; they found that of those patients who had future vaginal deliveries, 21.2 per cent had a complete and 12.1 per cent a partial recurrence.

It is obvious from the above statistics that good results may be obtained by either of the two methods when the operations are performed properly by competent surgeons. The use of fine catgut and the avoidance of undue tension are essential, regardless of which method is used. In our clinic we are inclined to the Warren flap technic and use it in most cases, unless the tear up the anterior rectal wall is too long. In such cases a turned-down flap sufficiently long to cover the defect and protrude beyond the perineum would, of necessity, be so long that its blood supply might be imperiled, and there would exist the danger of sloughing. In such cases we suture the anterior rectal wall and close by the layer method.

During the past few years we have had remarkably good success in our surgical results with the use of Sulfasuxidine (succinylsulfathiazole), both preoperatively and postoperatively. Before the expected date of operation the patient

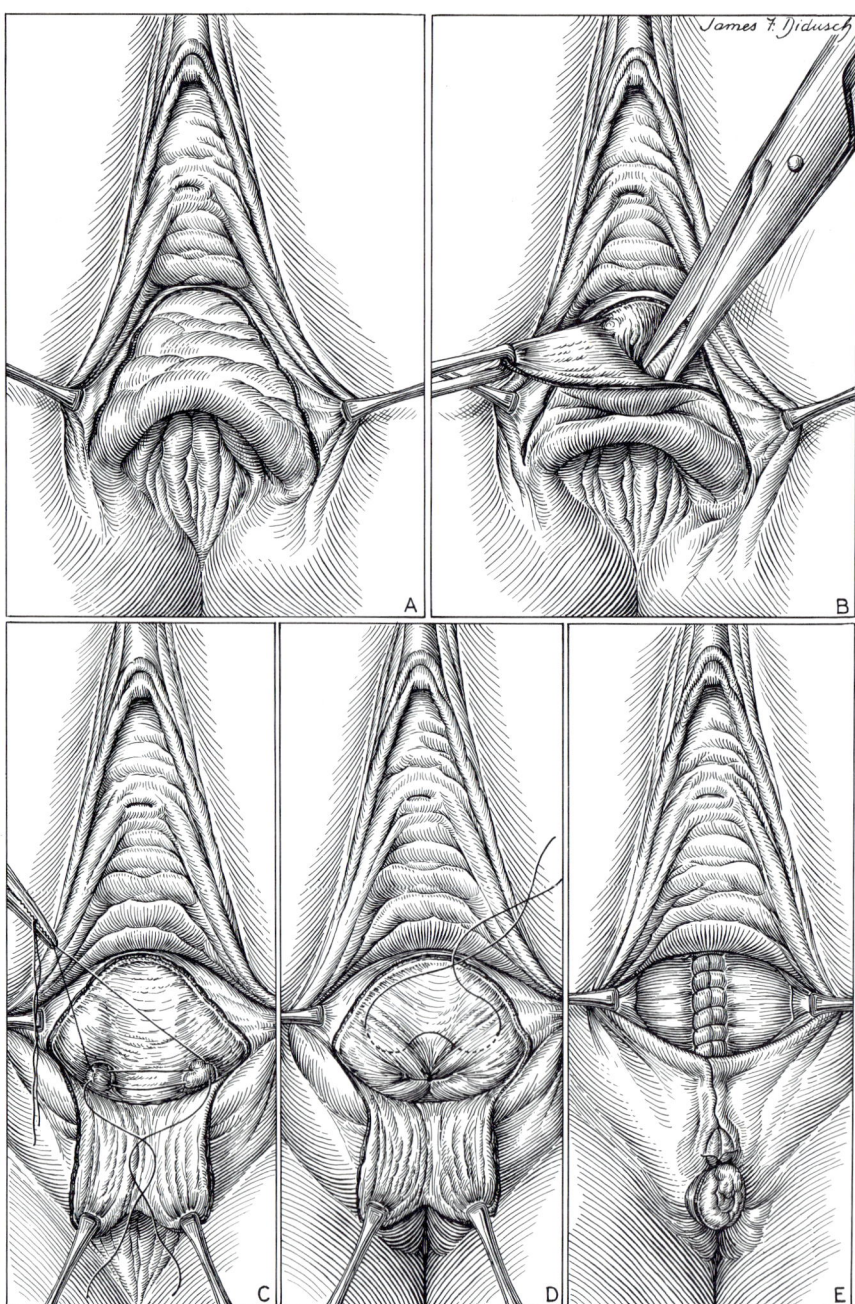

Fig. 30-3. Warren flap operation for 3rd-degree tear. (A) Indicating line of incision, outlining flap of vaginal mucosa. (B) The flap is being dissected free and turned back. (C) The flap is retracted downward. The ends of the sphincter have been delivered and are being sutured with interrupted sutures of medium silk. (D) The sphincter ends have been united and are buried by suturing the levator muscles together in the midline with No. 0 chromic catgut. (E) The vaginal incision has been closed with a continuous lock stitch that is continued subcuticularly over the perineum. The flap is thus rolled up. If too redundant, it may be trimmed off at a later time.

is given 24 Sulfasuxidine tablets (0.5 gm.) daily in divided doses. This produces a mild laxative effect, and the patient usually has 2 or 3 soft stools daily. If this regimen is carried out, the patient need not be placed on a liquid diet preoperatively. She is merely advised to eat rather lightly for a few days before operation. With this regimen the *Escherichia coli* content of the stool is reduced to almost nil, and per primum healing is the rule. A few hours before the scheduled time of operation the rectum is irrigated with sterile saline solution until the irrigating fluid returns clear. Then the rectum is instilled with 250 cc. of 1 per cent neomycin solution. As soon as the patient's stomach is settled after operation, again she is given 12 gm. of Sulfasuxidine daily and placed on a light diet. About the 3rd postoperative day the bowels usually begin to move, and she continues to have a few soft stools per day. The drug is continued for about 2 weeks after operation. During this time the patient is permitted to eat solid food, avoiding a diet with great residue.

Technic: Warren Flap Operation for 3rd-Degree Tear

An inverted V-shaped incision is made in the posterior vaginal mucosa, outlining the flap which is to be turned down. The lower ends of the incision should be just lateral to the dimples caused by retracted sphincter ends (Fig. 30-3 A).

The flap of mucosa is dissected free from above downward (Fig. 30-3 B). This should be done with care, to avoid injury to bowel wall, and the dissection should stop short of the margin of the vaginal and the rectal mucosa. If this margin should be perforated, the advantage of the flap technic would be nullified. If the flap has been demarcated properly, the areas overlying the sphincter ends will have been denuded.

Using Halsted clamps, the sphincter ends are fished for and delivered. They are sutured together with 2 or 3 interrupted sutures of medium silk (Fig. 30-3 C). It is well at this point for the operator to put a second glove on the left hand and insert a finger into the rectum to test the sphincter tone. If the operator is not satisfied with the sphincter tone, a further attempt should be made to find and approximate more sphincter fibers. The second glove is removed, and the sterile part of the operation continues as the turned-down flap, which is grasped with 2 mucosa clips, is allowed to hang down over the rectum.

The levator ani muscles are brought together with interrupted sutures of No. 0 chromic catgut (Fig. 30-3 D). These muscles re-enforce the sphincter fibers and build up the perineum. Then closure is carried out as in an ordinary perineal repair. The end of the mucosal flap eventually protrudes somewhat puckered by the approximated muscles above it (Fig. 30-3 E). It should not be trimmed flush with the perineum at this time, for it may retract to some degree. If the protrusion is annoying, it may be trimmed off later under local anesthesia. At the conclusion of the operation the sphincter is cut as shown in Figure 30-4 F.

Technic: Layer Method of Repair of Complete Perineal Laceration

An incision is made at the junction of the posterior vaginal wall and the rectal mucosa. An inverted V-shaped incision is made in the posterior vaginal wall, and the vaginal mucosa is removed (Fig. 30-4 A). The size of this V depends upon the redundancy of the vaginal mucosa. It should extend sufficiently far laterally at its base to denude the regions in which the sphincter ends are to be picked up. The ends of the sphincters are grasped with Halsted clamps (Fig. 30-4 B). The tips of the clamps are plunged down on either side to pick up the sphincter ends. The position of the sphincter ends can be estimated from the position of dimples in the skin caused by retraction of the ends of the sphincter (Fig. 30-4 A). It is difficult from inspection of the tissue caught in the clamps to judge whether or not one actually has grasped the sphincters. To test this the 2 tips of the clamps containing the tissue are brought together in the midline, and the sphincter action is tested by inserting a finger in the rectum. To do this an extra glove is

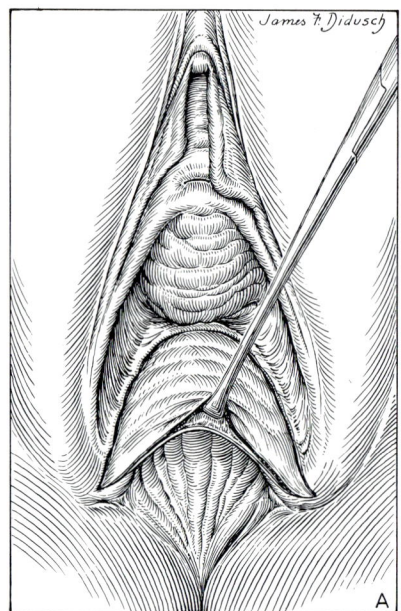

FIG. 30-4. Operation for 3rd-degree perineal laceration, layer method. (A) A transverse incision at the junction of the vaginal and the rectal mucosa has been made. An inverted V-shaped piece of mucosa is removed from the posterior vaginal wall. The size of this depends upon the redundancy of the mucosa.

put on temporarily. Two interrupted sutures of Pagenstecher linen or medium silk are placed in the sphincter ends, but they are not tied at this time.

The rent in the rectum is closed, using a continuous suture of No. 0 chromic catgut. The suture (Fig. 30-4 C) is made by taking small parallel bites along the edge of the rent, being careful to include in each stitch a good bite of rectal wall, but not to perforate the mucosa. As this suture is drawn tight, the edge is inverted into the lumen of the bowel. If there is sufficient tissue so that it can be done without tension, a second suture line is desirable.

The sphincter ends are then united by tying the 2 interrupted nonabsorbable sutures. One or more deep interrupted sutures are taken into the levator muscles (Fig. 30-4 D). These sutures are tied, thus restoring the perineum and re-enforcing the sphincter sutures. The vaginal mucosa is then closed with a continuous lock stitch of No. 0 chromic catgut, which is continued over the perineum subcuticularly (Fig. 30-4 E).

The rectal sphincter may then be cut at 5 o'clock. In the more difficult cases, and particularly those in which previous operations have failed, we make this a rule and never have experienced incontinence as a result of it (Fig. 30-4 F).

RECTOVAGINAL FISTULAS

CAUSES AND SYMPTOMS

Rectovaginal fistulas result from a number of causes. Those due to any single cause are not many, but taken together they are sufficiently frequent to demand considerable attention from the operating gynecologist. Many occur as the result of unsuccessful attempts at repair of 3rd-degree tears when a bridge of tissue or the complete sphincter heals in the anterior sphincter region, while the repair above the sphincter breaks down. There results a low rectovaginal fistula of variable size (Fig. 30-5). Small and even moderate-sized fistulas can form as a result of injury done to the rectum at the time that a perineal operation is performed. In the better clinics this practically never occurs, but such cases are encountered from less adequately trained surgeons. Even more rarely, injury to the rectum or the sigmoid takes place in the course of a total hysterectomy, and in such instances a fistula forms at the very top of the vagina. High rectovaginal fistulas result from irradiation of cervical cancer. These may be due to radium burns of normal tissue or to the destruction of carcinomatous tissue that has invaded the rectovaginal septum. We have observed sloughing of practically the entire rectal and posterior vaginal wall as the result of irradiation.

Perirectal abscesses, when opened spontaneously or surgically, may result in fistulas that open into the vagina. Attempted unsuccessful repairs of such fistulas can result in other fistulas with more scar tissue.

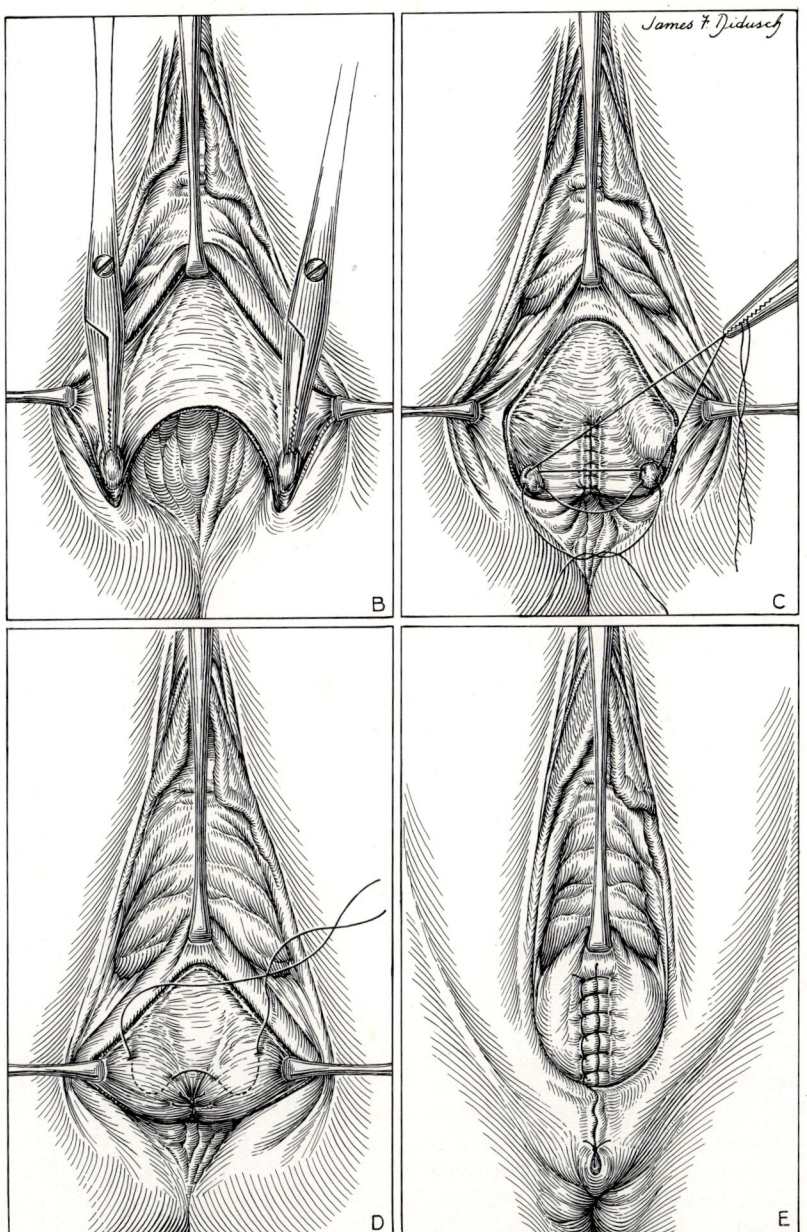

Fig. 30-4 (*Continued*). Operation for 3rd-degree perineal laceration. (B) The vaginal flap has been removed. The ends of the sphincter muscles have been delivered with Halsted clamps. (C) The rent in the rectal wall has been closed with a double layer of continuous No. 0 chromic catgut, inverting the edges into bowel lumen. (D) After approximating the silk sphincter sutures shown in C, the levators are brought together with deep interrupted sutures of No. 0 chromic catgut. (E) The vaginal incision is closed with a continuous lock stitch of No. 0 chromic catgut which is continued down subcuticularly to approximate the perineal skin.

Small rectovaginal fistulas may be entirely asymptomatic. A slight leakage of gas and seepage of feces may not be detected in the vaginal discharge. When the fistulas are slightly larger, the escape of gas may be the only complaint, or

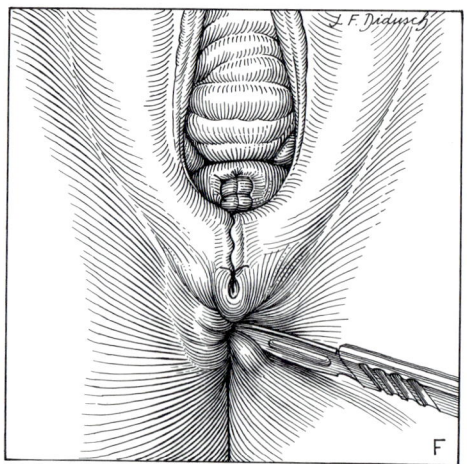

Fig. 30-4. (*Continued*). Operation for 3rd-degree perineal laceration. (F) Sphincter ani is cut at about 5 o'clock.

there may be the complaint of a slight fecal odor in the vaginal discharge. When the fistulas are large, the entire bowel content is evacuated through the vagina. Naturally, this is an extremely annoying condition, but, as in women with 3rd-degree lacerations, voluntary constipation may reduce the amount of leakage. In our experience, relatively good control of feces by constipation is attained more often with 3rd-degree lacerations than with rectovaginal fistulas.

Diagnosis and Treatment

The diagnosis of rectovaginal fistula is usually very simple. By merely spreading the labia the condition may be disclosed, or a duckbill speculum usually can be rotated so as to show a higher fistula. The opening in the vagina may be filled with feces, or if the bowel has been emptied recently, the dark rectal mucosa may be seen at the fistulous opening, in contrast with the pink vaginal mucous membrane. It may be exceedingly difficult to locate the opening in the rectum and the vagina when the fistulas are small. The location of both orifices is essential to the cure. A small probe may find its way through the fistula from the vaginal side and the tip be felt on rectal examination. If difficulty is experienced in following the fistulous tract at operation, injection with methylene blue may aid. The small fistula, resulting from rupture of an abscess, is most apt to be troublesome in following. These postabscess fistulas may open between the anal sphincter fibers, and cutting of the fibers to lay open the fistulous tract is essential to cure.

Regardless of the type of operation to be done, it is apparent that healing is enhanced by reducing the colon bacillus content of the stool. For that purpose the patient is placed on a daily dose of 12 gm. of Sulfasuxidine for 5 days preceding the operation. A few hours before operation she is given rectal irrigations with sterile saline until the fluid returns clear, and then the rectum is instilled with 250 cc. of 1 per cent neomycin solution. After postoperative nausea ceases, the Sulfasuxidine treatment is resumed; the postoperative routine is the same as that following repair of a 3rd-degree tear.

The surgical cure of a rectovaginal fistula may be exceedingly simple or quite complicated. Small fistulas may be closed by 2 or more purse strings as shown in Figure 30-6.

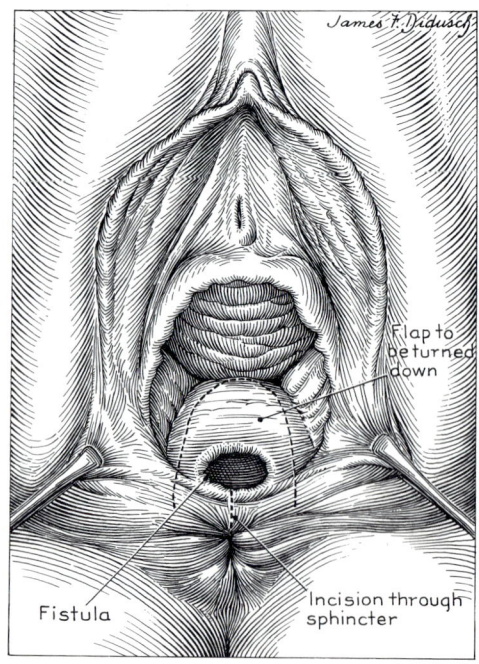

Fig. 30-5. Low rectovaginal fistula is converted into complete tear by cutting sphincter. Inverted U-shaped dotted line outlines proposed flap to be turned down.

It is desirable to approximate broad surface to broad surface for healing, regardless of the exact technic of closure. A more-or-less standard technic for closure of a typical fistula in a layer-for-layer manner is shown in Figure 30-7. When the fistula is fairly large and lies just above the sphincter or the perineal bridge, usually it is wise to cut the bridge, thus converting the fistula into a 3rd-degree tear (Fig. 30-5). The 3rd-degree tear is then repaired by the flap method as shown in Figure 30-3.

Except in the simplest fistulas, we routinely practice the cutting of the sphincter at about 5 o'clock, at the conclusion of the operation, as described by Miller (Fig. 30-3 F). If this is done, there is no pressure from the accumulation of gas in the rectum. This procedure, combined with the use of Sulfasuxidine medication preoperatively and postoperatively, has noticeably increased our successes.

Very large and difficult fistulas often require more than the routine operation. We refer particularly to fistulas that occur after irradiation and to those that, because of previous surgical attempts, have an excess of scar tissue. In such cases it is often essential to divert the feces from the field of operation by first performing a sigmoidostomy. We have found a modified Mikulicz procedure to be the best type of colostomy for this purpose (Fig. 30-9). The bowel is completely transected to ensure perfect diversion of feces, and subsequent closure is simple. Finally, the rare rectovaginal or sigmoidovaginal fistulas resulting from bowel injury at the time of total hysterectomy and lying at the apex of the vagina may require transabdominal closure. Recently we have closed such a fistula vaginally, using a technic similiar to that described by Latzko for vesicovaginal fistulas following total hysterectomy. This technic is illustrated in Figure 30-8.

Technic: Closure of Small Rectovaginal Fistula

A small circular incision is made in the vagina, encircling the fistulous opening (Fig. 30-6 A).

With small pointed-tip scissors the vaginal mucosa is dissected free for a distance sufficient to mobilize the bowel wall in order to permit closure of the opening in the bowel by 2 or 3 purse-string sutures without tension (Fig. 30-6 B). The first purse string is placed about the opening, a few millimeters from the edge, using No. 0 chromic catgut (Fig. 30-6 C). Care should be exercised not to permit perforation through the bowel mucosa in placing this suture. The edges of the fistula are inverted into the lumen of the bowel as the purse string is tied. A 2nd purse string is placed about the 1st (Fig. 30-6 D). If it can be done without tension, a 3rd purse string may be placed around the 2nd (Fig. 30-6 E). The perirectal fascia is then approximated in the midline, using a continuous suture of No. 0 chromic catgut (Fig. 30-6 F). The vaginal mucosa is excised, if redundant, and is closed with a continuous lock stitch of No. 0 chromic catgut (Fig. 30-6 G). If the fistula is closed easily, the sphincter is not cut, but if the fistula is closed with difficulty and especially if previous unsuccessful attempts have been made, the rectal sphincter may be cut as indicated in Figure 30-4 F.

Technic: Closure of Larger Rectovaginal Fistula

An incision is made around the fistulous opening through the vaginal mucous membrane, as indicated by the dotted line in Figure 30-7 A.

The vaginal mucous membrane is dissected back far enough to permit mobilization of the bowel for closure (Fig. 30-7 B). Since the opening into the bowel is too large to be closed by a purse string, it is closed by a series of mattress sutures, as indicated in Figure 30-7. The bites in the tissue are taken parallel with the edges of the fistula but do not enter the lumen of the bowel. No. 0 chromic catgut is most suitable for these stitches. The closure can also be made with a continuous suture, inverting the edges into the bowel lumen as shown in Figure 30-7 B.

After the 1st layer of stitches is tied, it is reinforced by a 2nd layer placed in the

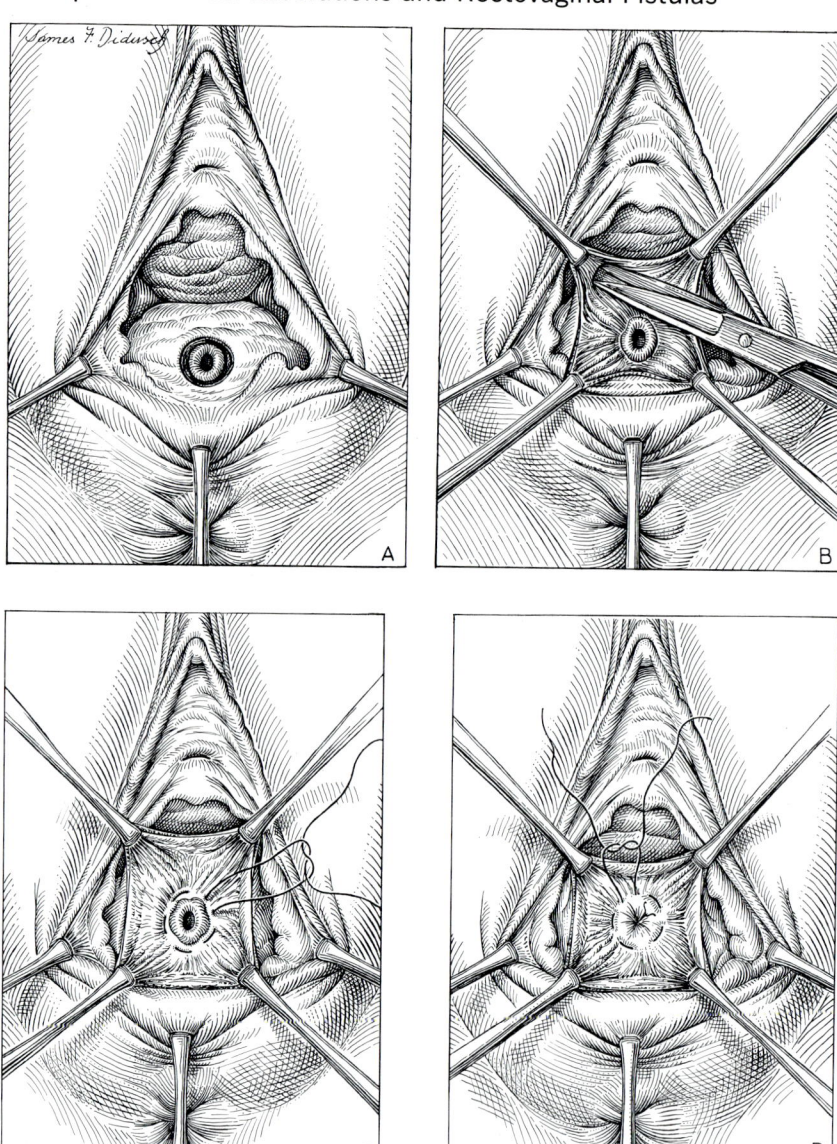

Fig. 30-6. Repair of small rectovaginal fistula. (A) A circular incision through the vaginal mucosa is made about the fistulous opening. (B) Flaps of vaginal mucosa are dissected free for about 2 cm. from the margin of the fistulous opening. (C) A purse-string suture of No. 0 chromic catgut is placed about fistulous opening. (D) The first purse string has been tied, inverting the fistulous opening. The second purse string has been placed and is about to be tied.

same way but taking somewhat coarser bites (Fig. 30-7 C). These mattress sutures should be approximated gently and snugly, but not tight enough to strangulate the tissues. In this manner broad surfaces are brought together for healing.

After the 2nd layer of stitches has been tied, the edges of the vaginal mucosa are trimmed off, and the mucosal incision is closed with a continuous suture of No. 0 chromic catgut. This suture everts the edges of the mucosa and approximates broad new surfaces for healing. When this mucosal suture is taken, bits of the

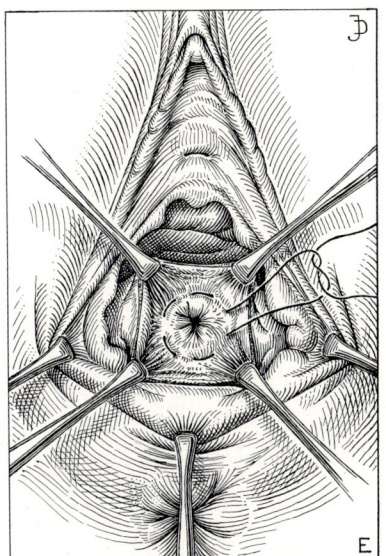
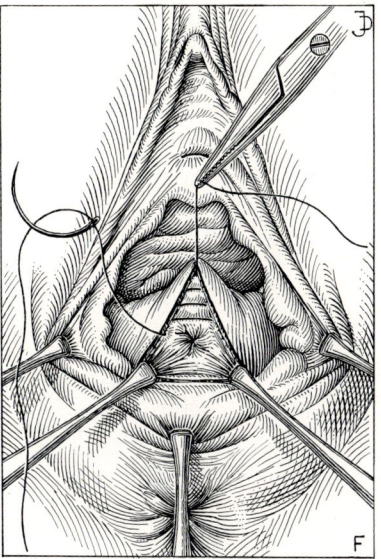
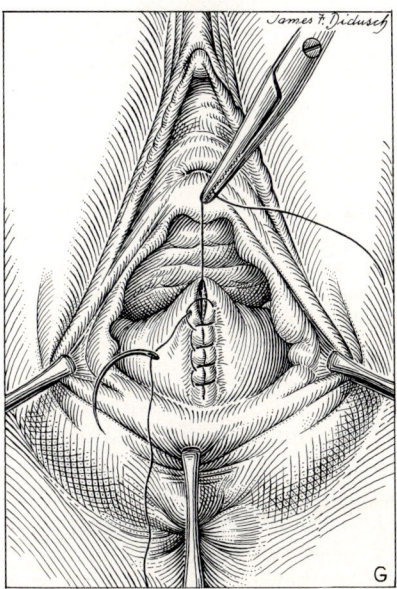

FIG. 30-6 (*Continued*). Repair of small rectovaginal fistula. (E) The second purse string has been tied, and a third has been placed. (F) Submucosal tissues are approximated with a continuous suture of No. 0 chromic catgut. (G) The mucosa is closed with a continuous lock stitch of No. 0 chromic catgut.

subjacent tissue are picked up with each bite, thus closing all potential dead space (Fig. 30-7 D).

In the large fistulas it is our custom to sever the anal sphincter, as indicated in Figure 30-4 F, to permit the free passage of gas and to prevent pressure on the operative incision.

Latzko Technic: Closure of Large Rectovaginal Fistula

The Latzko technic of using both the anterior and the posterior vaginal walls in the closure of vesicovaginal fistulas following total hysterectomy has a restricted use in the closure of selected rectovaginal fistulas. We have encountered a few large rectovaginal fistulas following hysterectomy for cervical carcinoma. These have occurred mostly in cases in which irradiation was first used, followed by a Wertheim type of hysterectomy. In such cases the interference with the blood supply by the surgery added to the already depleted blood supply resulting from irradiation is sufficient to

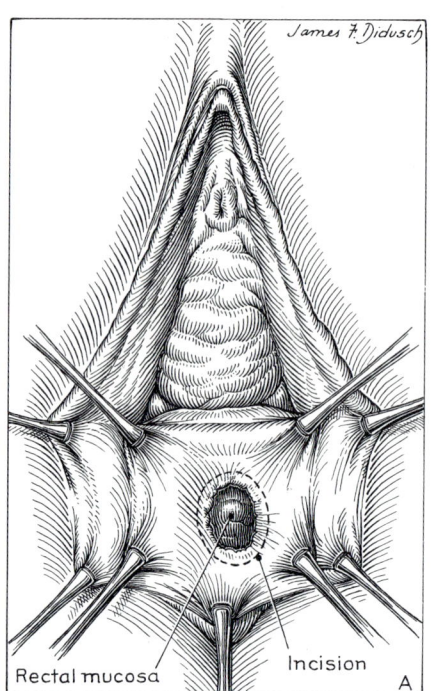 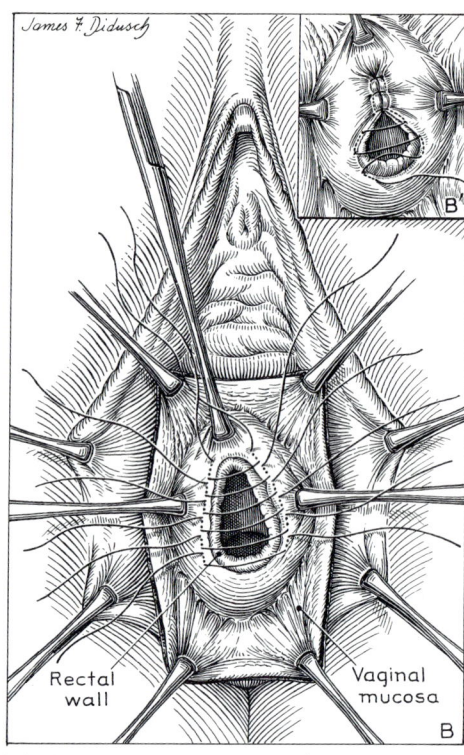

Fig. 30-7. Repair of rectovaginal fistula. (A) Shows the opening of the fistula in the posterior vaginal wall exposed and the incision indicated by a dotted line. (B) A broad flap of vaginal mucosa has been dissected away from the margin of the fistula. Interrupted mattress sutures have been placed about the margin of the fistula. When these sutures are tied, the fistulous opening will be inverted. B' shows the closure with a continuous suture.

cause sloughing of the rectal and the vaginal walls; consequently, fistula develops. Such a fistula may be large and surrounded by indurated, fibrosed tissue with poor blood supply. In that case the chance of cure by ordinary methods is poor. A sufficient area around the fistula must be denuded to approximate broad surfaces and also to approximate tissue which is well vascularized.

Figure 30-8 A shows incisions about the fistula. The area to be denuded includes both the anterior and the posterior vaginal walls. Figure 30-8 B shows the mucosa being removed; Figure 30-8 C, the 1st line of closure; the edges are inverted into the bowel lumen, using No. 0 chromic catgut. Figure 30-8 D shows the 1st suture line closed and the 2nd being placed; these sutures are of the mattress type, the bite of the needle being taken parallel with the suture line. Finally, the mucosal edges are brought together with mattress sutures of silver wire. These sutures are left in place for 2 weeks. For their removal, the patient is anesthetized with Pentothal Sodium.

Technic: Modified Mikulicz Sigmoidostomy for Diversion of Feces, in Repairing Difficult Rectovaginal Fistulas

A lower-left rectus incision is made, and the sigmoid is delivered. If the mesosigmoid is very short, the bowel may be mobilized by cutting the peritoneum as it is reflected from the bowel to the parietal wall. The sigmoid need only be brought up enough so that a small knuckle will be above the level of the skin.

A tape is placed through the meso-

Rectovaginal Fistulas 653

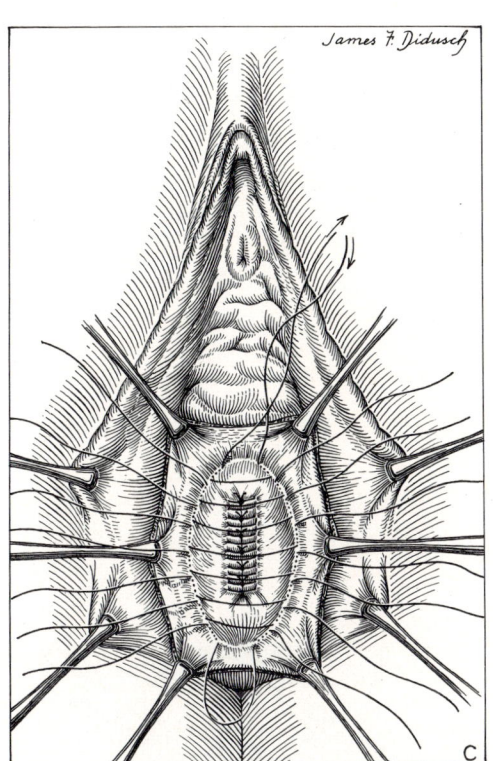 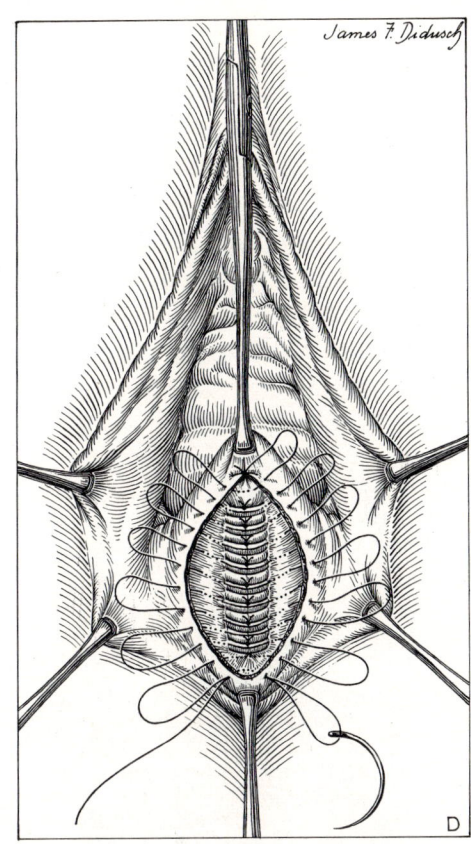

FIG. 30-7 (*Continued*). Repair of rectovaginal fistula. (C) Interrupted mattress sutures have been placed in the perirectal tissues. When tied, these sutures will invert the first row of sutures and approximate broad surface to broad surface for healing. (D) The mucosa is closed with a continuous mattress suture which picks up the subjacent tissue, thus obliterating dead space and everting the mucosal edges.

sigmoid, as indicated in Figure 30-9 A. This tape is left in place to act as a guide when the bowel is transected at a later time.

The antimesenteric surfaces of the bowel are sutured together with 2 parallel lines of interrupted sutures of fine silk, as shown in Figure 30-9 B.

The bowel is sutured to the parietal peritoneum with interrupted fine silk sutures (Fig. 30-9 C), and the wound is closed in a layer-for-layer manner (Fig. 30-9 D).

The bowel is anchored to the skin with a few interrupted silk sutures.

Forty-eight hours later the bowel is completely transected with the cautery, releasing the tape as the bowel is cut through. Only by complete transection can one be certain of perfect diversion of the feces.

About 10 days after opening the bowel, the fistula is repaired. In the 10-day interval the lower segment of bowel is irrigated daily with saline, both ways, to make certain that it is as free as possible of residual feces and mucus. A few hours before operation it is instilled with 250 cc. of 1 per cent neomycin.

About 6 weeks should be allowed for the repair of the fistula to heal firmly. Then the colostomy is closed.

This same method of fecal diversion may be used before repair of 3rd-degree tears when they appear to be especially difficult. This is very rarely necessary, but occasionally one sees cases in which several previous unsuccessful attempts

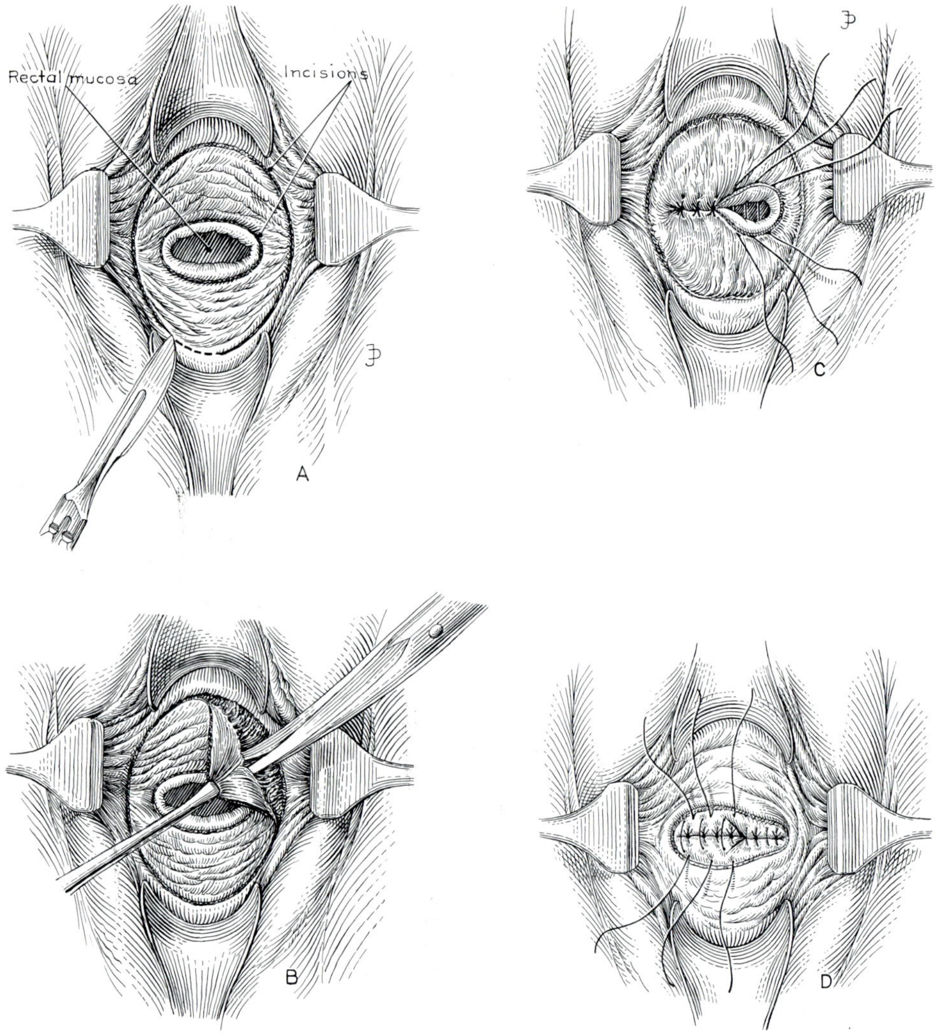

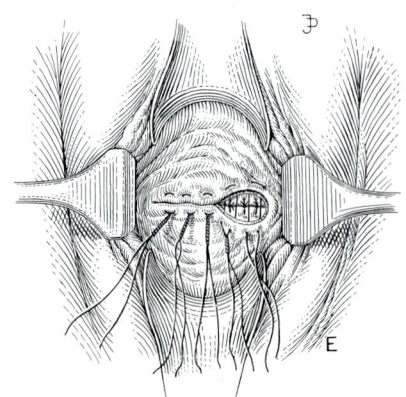

Fig. 30-8. Closure of large rectovaginal fistula by Latzko technic. (A) Demonstrating incisions. (B) Demonstrating excision of mucosa from anterior and posterior vaginal walls. (C) The 1st line of sutures is placed, inverting the edge into the rectal lumen. (D) The 1st line of sutures has been placed and tied. The 2nd line of sutures is being placed. Note mattress-type stitch used. (E) Mattress sutures of wire, forming the 3rd suture line.

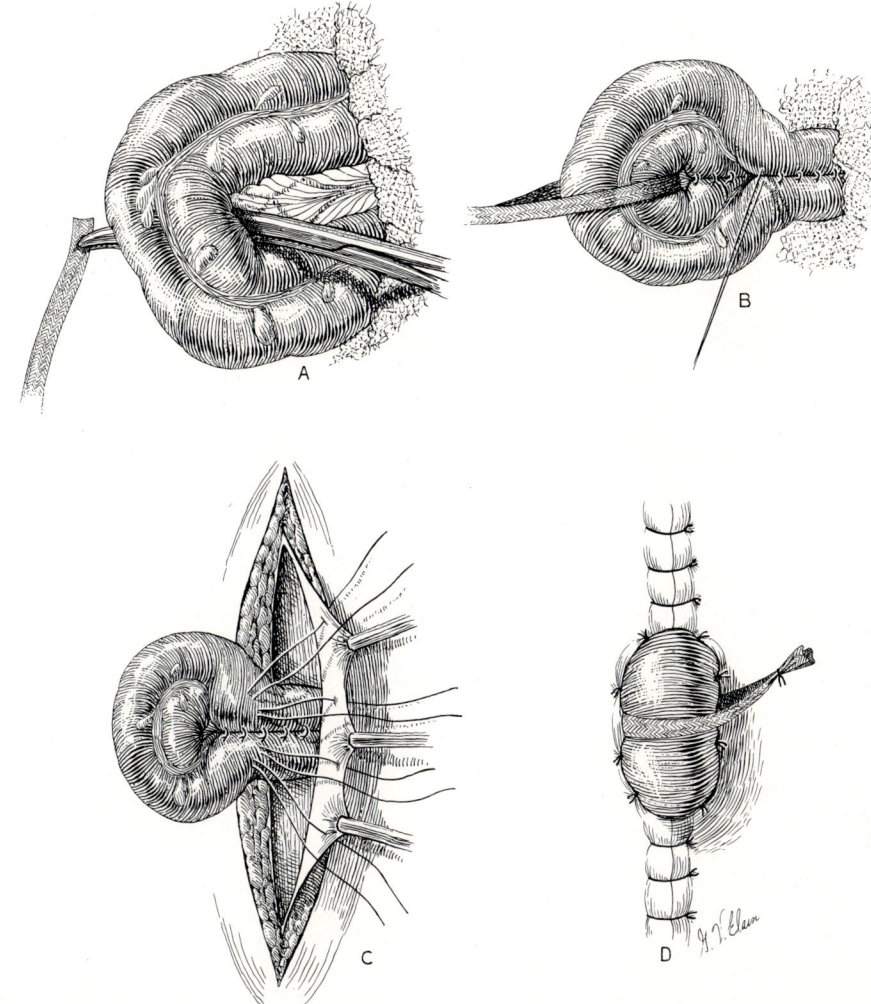

Fig. 30-9. Method of sigmoidostomy by Mikulicz principle preparatory to complete transection of bowel for diverting feces in preparation for repair of difficult rectovaginal fistula. (A) The sigmoid has been delivered, and tape has been inserted through the mesosigmoid. (B) The 1st row of interrupted silk sutures has been placed. The 2nd row is being placed. (C) The bowel wall is being anchored to the peritoneum with interrupted silk sutures. (D) The bowel wall is tacked to the skin edge with interrupted silk sutures. The tape is left in place for orientation in severing the bowel later.

have resulted in an excess of scar tissue. In making the final all-out attack on such a surgical problem, fecal diversion greatly enhances the chances of success.

CONGENITAL RECTOVAGINAL FISTULAS

Congenital communication of the rectum with the vagina is, fortunately, a rare condition. The communication may be small, or the full lumen of the bowel may open into the vagina. When the opening is small, the condition may be life-endangering, and a colostomy may be necessary for medical reasons. When the opening is the full width of the bowel lumen, complete incontinence may be present, but it is remarkable how little incontinence exists in some cases. Some of the patients control their bowels so well that surgery would scarcely be justi-

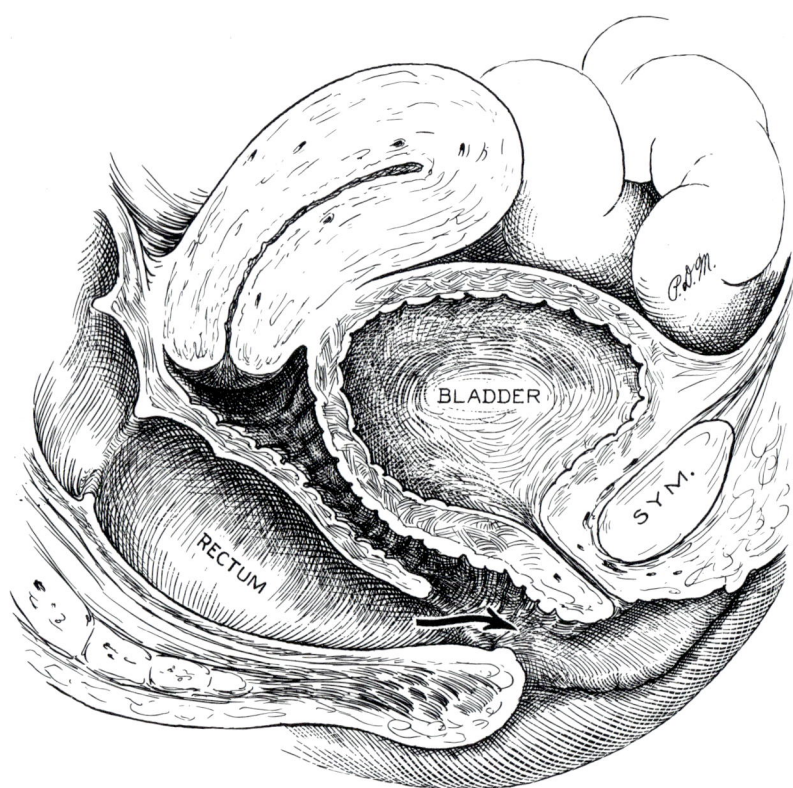

Fig. 30-10. Sagittal section showing congenital opening of rectum into vaginal vestibule.

fied for the correction of the condition were it not for the disadvantage of the fistula at coitus. The vaginal opening may occur at any level in the vagina from the posterior fornix to the fourchette. Fortunately for the repair, the majority open in the lowermost part (Fig. 30-10).

An understanding of this congenital developmental defect is best obtained by a consideration of the embryology of the parts. According to Harkin,

the allantois expands to form the primitive bladder, then courses anteriorly to open on the ventral surface of the embryo. The hindgut is at the level of and posterior to the primitive bladder. Caudad to this region the minute continuation and extremity of the intestinal tract is known as the tail gut. As early as the third week, the bladder and hindgut empty into a common cavity called the cloacal membrane. In the six-weeks' embryo the urogenital groove is beginning to grow downward, and by the seventh week the urogenital and intestinal system have been partitioned by this groove. The coacal membrane is then divided into urogenital and anal membranes respectively, and by the eighth week the urogenital membrane breaks down to establish an external opening. In the region of the future anus an invagination develops which is known as the proctodeum. Normally, the anal membrane ruptures during the eighth week to establish continuity between the proctodeum and the anus. Any failure of the anal membrane to break down results in an imperforate anus.

It is apparent that any arrest in the downward groove, which should separate the intestinal tract from the urinary system, will result in residual communicating fistulas.*

The anal sphincters are derived from mesenchyme and therefore are independent in their development from the ectodermal and entodermal origins of the

---

* Harkin, Dwight E.: Congenital malformation of the rectum and anus. Surgery, 11:423, 1942.

anus and the rectum. Harkin believes that most, if not all, of these patients are equipped with anal sphincters. This is a point of great surgical interest and may account for the perfect sphincteric action obtained when the rectum is brought down into its correct place. However, the presence of true rectal sphincter fibers is difficult to prove, for it seems probable that the closely approximated levator ani muscles might give quite adequate fecal control when the rectum is transplanted between them.

TREATMENT

The time of the treatment is important. It is probable that many pediatric surgeons would disagree with us on the time at which correction of this condition should be undertaken. From our experience we would strongly favor waiting until the child has reached puberty before attempting the operation. Before that time the parts are so small and the vaginal mucosa so delicate that dissection is difficult, and the operation is apt to be doomed to failure. A second operation is always done with greater difficulty due to scar tissue resulting from the first.

The treatment consists of bringing the rectum down to the normal anal region and closing the opening in the vagina. It is best to defer operation until after puberty to permit the vagina to enlarge enough to allow intravaginal work. The operation described here was done on a 15-year-old Negro child. The procedure originally carried out for this condition was described by Rizzoli, who made an incision from the fistula through the vagina and the perineum to the position where the anus was to be transplanted. The bowel was brought down into the new position, and the vaginal and perineal wound was closed. The operation described here was done by E. H. Richardson, Jr., and the author, who believe it to be the logical method of dealing with the condition. It has the obvious advantage over Rizzoli's operation in that nothing is done to interfere with the sphincter action of the closely approximated levator ani muscles or of the sphincter ani, if such is present, as believed by Harkin. The result in the case herewith described was excellent, including perfect sphincter action. On investigating the literature in the course of writing this book, the senior author found that Stone had described this same operation in 1936 and reported 3 cases operated on successfully. Stone gave medication to tie up the bowels for from 7 to 10 days after the operation. This is no longer necessary and, in fact, is undesirable. We place the patient on a daily dose of 12 gm. of Sulfasuxidine for 5 days preoperatively. On the morning of operation the bowel is irrigated with saline solution until it returns clear. Then 250 cc. of 1 per cent neomycin solution is instilled into the bowel. We begin Sulfasuxidine again as soon as postoperative nausea ceases and continue it for about 2 weeks. As a rule, a spontaneous bowel movement occurs on the 3rd or the 4th postoperative day, and the patient has 2 or 3 soft movements daily as long as she is on the drug.

Technic: Operation for Formation of Anus for Correction of Congenital Opening of Rectum into Vaginal Vestibule

Figure 30-11 A shows the congenital condition as it exists. The rectum opens into the vaginal vestibule and is without any sphincter musculature. The rectum and the vagina are separated by a thin septum above the congenital opening. The perineum is solid, formed by the union of the levator ani muscles in the midline. Figure 30-11 A shows the circular line of incision about the rectal opening.

The rectum is mobilized for a sufficient distance to permit it to be drawn down to its normal site (Fig. 30-11 B).

A transverse incision is made in the perineal region through the skin and the fat in the position of the normal anus (Fig. 30-11 C).

A midline incision of about 1 inch is made between the levator muscles and is stretched open by a Kelly clamp (Fig. 30-11 D). The edge of the rectal mucosa is grasped with Allis clips, and the rectum is withdrawn through the new open-

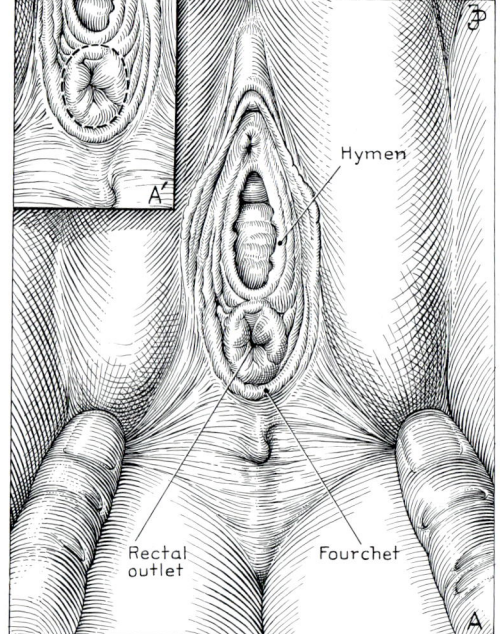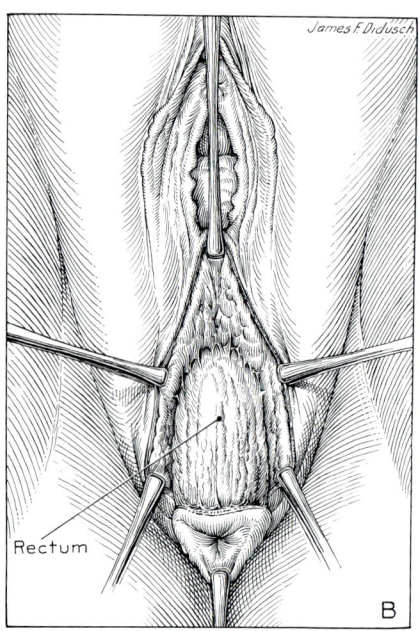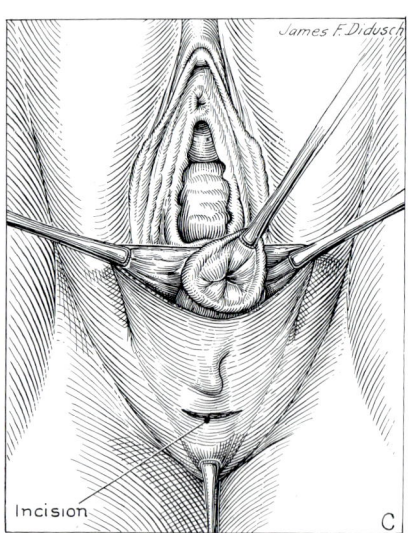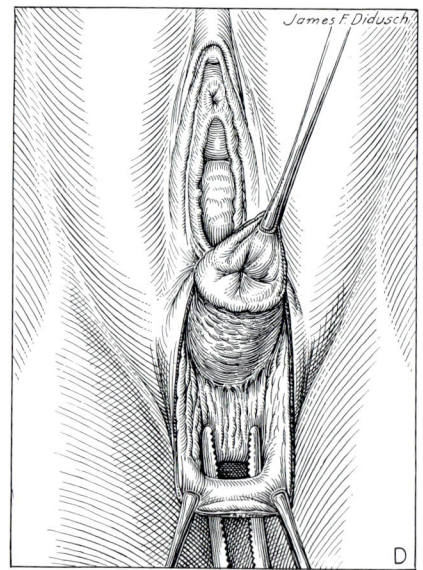

Fig. 30-11. Operation for congenital opening of the rectum into the vagina. (A) Preoperative condition. (A') Inset indicates line of incision. (B) After encircling the rectum it is mobilized for a distance sufficient to permit it to be delivered through the new opening. (C) A transverse incision is made for the anal opening. (D) After the levator ani muscles are separated in the midline, a Kelly clamp is inserted for withdrawal of the rectum.

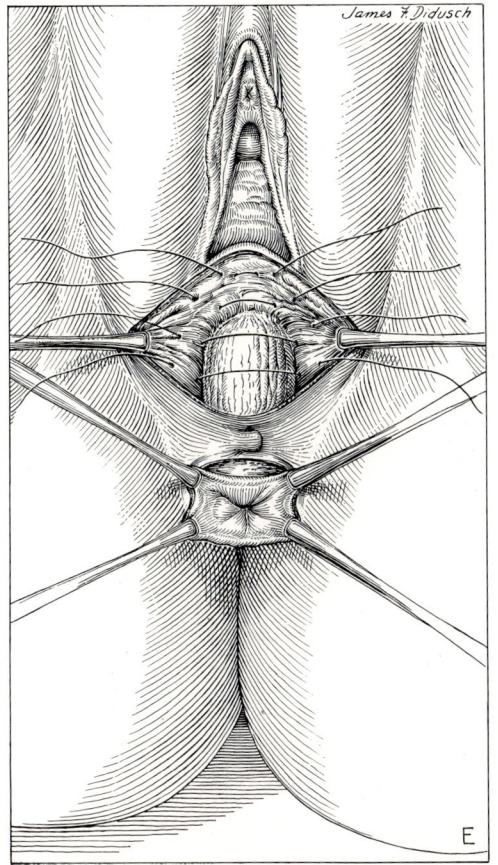
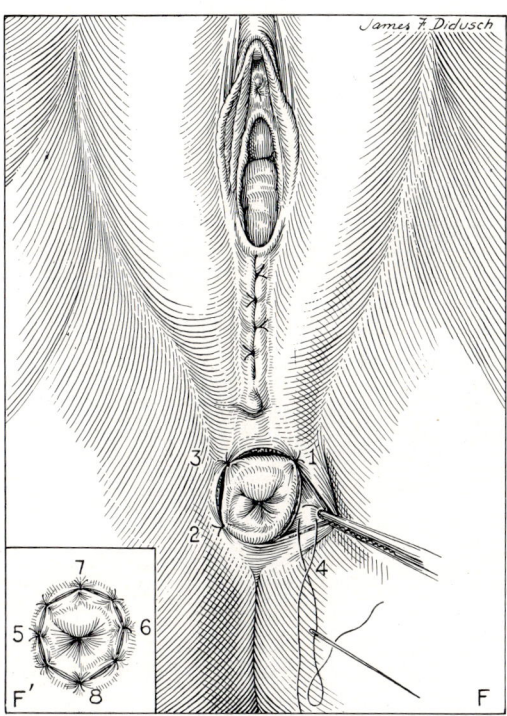

FIG. 30-11 (*Continued*). Operation for congenital opening of the rectum into the vagina. (E) After the rectum is withdrawn through the anal opening, the tissues are brought together over the anterior rectal wall by interrupted No. 0 chromic catgut sutures. (F) The incision in the vaginal vestibule and the perineum has been closed. The margins of the rectum are sutured to the skin margins to form a new anus. (F′) Suturing is complete.

ing (Fig. 30-11 E). This should be possible without tension if the rectum has been mobilized properly, but the rectum should not be mobilized any higher than necessary to minimize interference with its blood supply.

As the rectum is held in its new position by means of mucosa clips, the vaginal vestibule wound is closed, first with interrupted sutures of No. 0 chromic catgut approximating the deeper tissues (Fig. 30-11 E), then with similar sutures approximating the mucosa.

Finally, the rectal mucosa is sutured to the skin edges of the newly formed anus with interrupted sutures of fine silk (Fig. 30-11 F). The patient of whom these drawings were made had perfect sphincter action following the above procedure, and the anal region is scarcely distinguishable from a normal one.

Rizzoli Operation

Since the first edition of this book we have had a failure with the operation described above, owing to retraction of the anus and re-establishing of a rectovaginal fistula. Therefore we later performed a preliminary transverse colostomy. After cleaning out the distal loop of colon by daily irrigations for approximately 10 days, we performed the Rizzoli operation as shown in Figure 30-12. In the presence

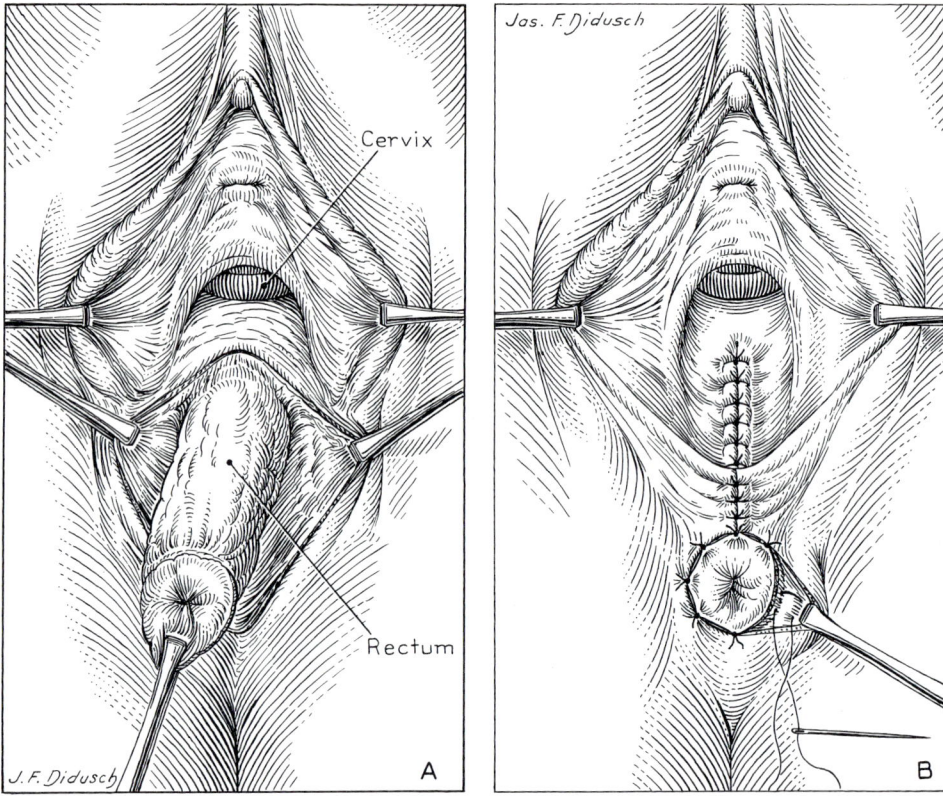

FIG. 30-12. Rizzoli operation for congenital rectovaginal fistula. (A) The incision has been carried through the perineum, and the anus has been dissected free. (B) The anal margin has been sutured to the skin, and the perineal incision has been closed.

of scar tissue from the previous operation we were able to get better exposure by cutting down through the perineum, and thus we could dissect the anus and the rectum with ease up to the peritoneal reflexion. It is our belief that the first type of operation described in this chapter may be done with frequent success, but if there is difficulty in freeing the anus and the rectum sufficiently to bring the anus down to the perineal opening without tension, cutting of the perineum as suggested by Rizzoli may facilitate the freeing of the bowel. Also, when previous surgery has been done, resulting in scar tissue, the Rizzoli type of operation may be done to advantage. Although either type of operation will often be successful with preoperative bowel sterilization without colostomy, when a previous unsuccessful operation has been done, preliminary colostomy is advisable.

BIBLIOGRAPHY

Bodenhammer, W.: A Practical Treatise on the Etiology, Pathology and Treatment of the Congenital Malformations of the Rectum and Anus. Baltimore, S. S. & William Wood, 1860.

———: Some facts and observations relative to the congenital malformations of the rectum and anus and to the operation of colotomy in such cases. New York J. Med., 49:562, 1889.

Campbell, R. E.: A report on a series of complete tears of the perineum with extension up the posterior vaginal wall, repaired by the vaginal flap method. Amer. J. Obstet. Gynec., 41:403, 1941.

Cave, H. W.: Vaginal anus with report of a case—Operation, Cured. Virginia Med. Month., 52:342, 1925.

David, V. C.: The treatment of congenital openings of the rectum into the vagina—atresia ani vaginalis. Surgery, 1:163, 1937.

Harkin D. E.: Congenital malformation of the rectum and anus. Surgery, 11:422, 1942.

Miller, N. F., and Brown, W.: The surgical treatment of complete perineal tears in the female. Amer. J. Obstet. Gynec., 34:196, 1937.

Phaneuf, L. E.: Complete lacerations of the perineum and their surgical treatment. Amer. J. Obstet. Gynec., 17:475, 1929.

———: Complete laceration of the perineum and rectovaginal fistula. Amer. J. Obstet. Gynec., 36:899, 1938.

———: Complete laceration of the perineum and rectovaginal fistulas—management and end results. Amer. J. Obstet. Gynec., 36:899, 1938.

Rizzoli, F.: Memorie dell' Accademia delle Scienze dell' Institute di Bologna, 1857.

Smith, G. van S., and Linton, J. R.: Complete laceration of the perineum: A report of 291 cases seen between 1876 and 1928 at the Free Hospital for Women, Brookline, Mass. Surg. Gynec. Obstet., 40:702, 1929.

Stone, H. B.: Imperforate anus with rectovaginal cloaca. Ann. Surg., 104:651, 1936.

Warren, J. C.: A new method of operation for the relief of rupture of the perineum through the sphincter and rectum. Trans. Amer. Gynec. Soc., 72:322, 1882.

PART FOUR

Treatment of Pelvic Tumors — Benign and Malignant

31

Surgical Conditions of the Vulva

FIBROMA AND FIBROMYOMA OF THE VULVA

Fibroma and fibromyoma of the vulva are rare but occur more frequently than any other benign tumors of this region (Fig. 31-1). There are three sources of origin: the fibrous tissue of the vulva, the extraperitoneal portion of the round ligament, and the intrapelvic connective tissue. The tumors arising from the connective tissue of the vulva are apt to be fibromas, and hyaline degeneration is common in them. The tumors arising from the round ligament contain more smooth muscle and usually feel firmer. Those arising from the intrapelvic connective tissue present at the vulva as the growth extends downward have been known to reach enormous size.

Symptoms arise as a result of the size and the weight of these tumors. The patient may complain of difficulty in walking, sitting, coitus, and urination. Over a fifth of those reported by Leonard from the laboratory at Johns Hopkins Hospital were said to have undergone sarcomatous degeneration, but our more recent experience does not bear out such a high percentage of malignant change.

The treatment is surgical excision. Figure 31-2 A shows a typical large fibroma, arising from the right labium majus. It was connected by a very large pedicle, which encroached on the base of the right labium minus, so that the removal of the labium with the tumor was necessary. The large defect caused by such an excision is closed with interrupted sutures of No. 00 chromic catgut, and the skin incision was closed with a lock stitch of fine silk (Fig. 31-2 C).

LIPOMA OF THE VULVA

In spite of the fact that the labia majora are composed chiefly of fat, lipoma of the vulva is very rare. Lipomatous tumors are sessile when small, but because of their position they may become pedunculated when they reach considerable size. The soft consistency of the fat frequently suggests that they are cystic, and the possibility of hernia must be considered. As in lipomata elsewhere, the lobulation gives one the cue to their real nature. The smaller lipomata are quite asymptomatic. When they become larger, they may interfere with walking, sitting, coitus, or urination. A few enormous vulval lipomas have been reported in the literature—the largest by Lovelace, who reported a 44-pound tumor that extended as far as the patient's knees.

The treatment of lipoma of the vulva is excision. Small sessile tumors are easily enucleated. When large tumors are attached by small pedicles, excision may also be simple, but large tumors that are sessile or attached by large pedicles may present surgical problems of considerable difficulty. The electrosurgical knife is a great aid and saves much operating time. Surgical excision is similar to the technic demonstrated for removal of a fibroma but is frequently more difficult to dissect because of indistinct tissue planes.

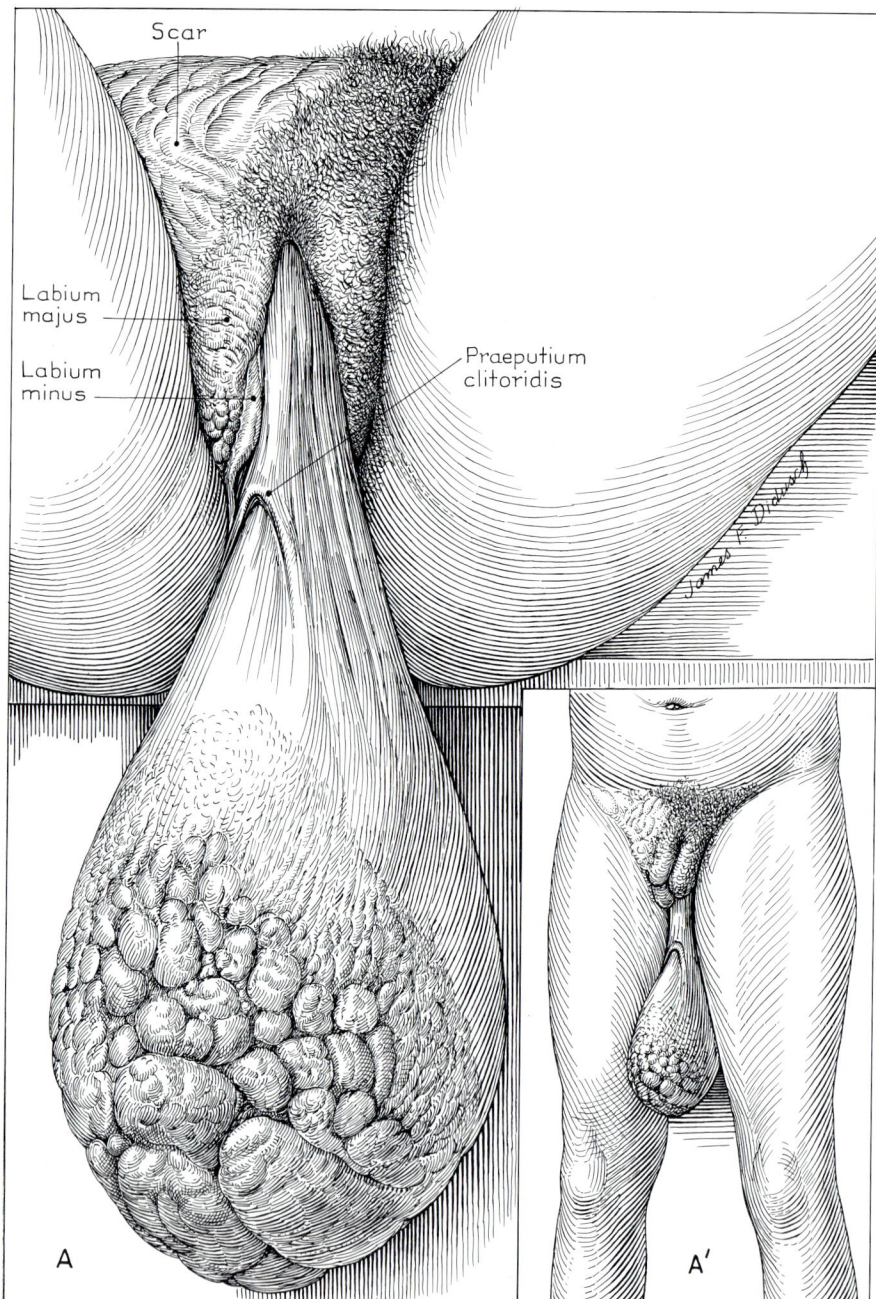

Fig. 31-1. Large fibroma of the vulva.

HIDRADENOMA (SWEAT-GLAND TUMOR) OF THE VULVA

This rare benign tumor of the vulva was first described by Schickele in 1902. Approximately 120 have been reported since that time. It is of importance to the gynecologic surgeon because it is often mistakenly diagnosed as malignant and treated unnecessairly radically. The possibility of error in microscopic diagnosis is understandable, since the adenomatous pattern of the growth may have a proliferative appearance; if the pathol-

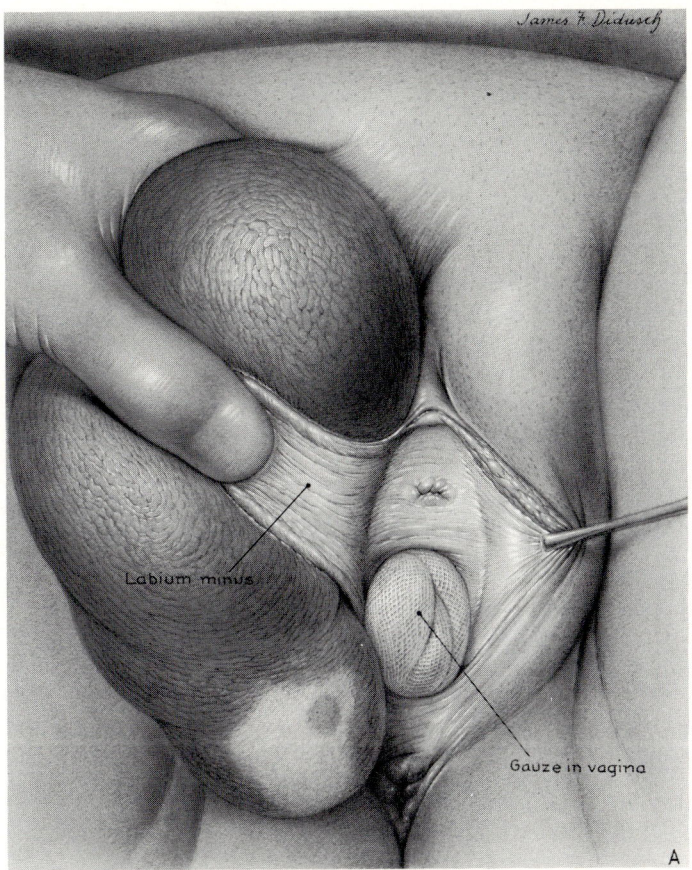

Fig. 31-2. Partial vulvectomy for benign lesion. (A) A large fibroma arising from the right labium majus, to be removed by partial vulvectomy.

ogist lacks definite clinical follow-up knowledge of such cases, he might easily consider the tumor to be malignant.

Novak and Stevenson have carefully studied 14 hidradenomas from our laboratory. They have noted considerable variation in the microscopic picture. The usual pattern is of the adenomatous type, with the glands closely packed and varying greatly in size (Fig. 31-3). The epithelial lining of the glands may be single, but in many tumors the glands are lined by an inner layer of short columnar or cuboidal cells, and beneath this layer is another layer of cells, closely packed with small dark nuclei. In many of the tumors there is a great tendency to epithelial proliferation, and the gland lumina are filled with epithelial plaques, similar to those found in the cervix, due to epidermidization. Obviously, tumors of this type may be considered malignant if the pathologist is without clinical knowledge of the course of the disease.

The practical question from the point of view of the operating gynecologist is whether or not the lesion is malignant, and a consideration of the evidence is worthwhile. Novak and Stevenson have made a critical review of the cases found in the literature, many of which were reported as malignant. It is obvious that most of the cases which have been considered malignant have been judged purely on histologic grounds. In fact, in only one case did Novak and Stevenson conclude that there was indisputable evidence of adenocarcinoma. In that case the left labium majus, on which the tumor grew, was widely excised, together with

668   Surgical Conditions of the Vulva

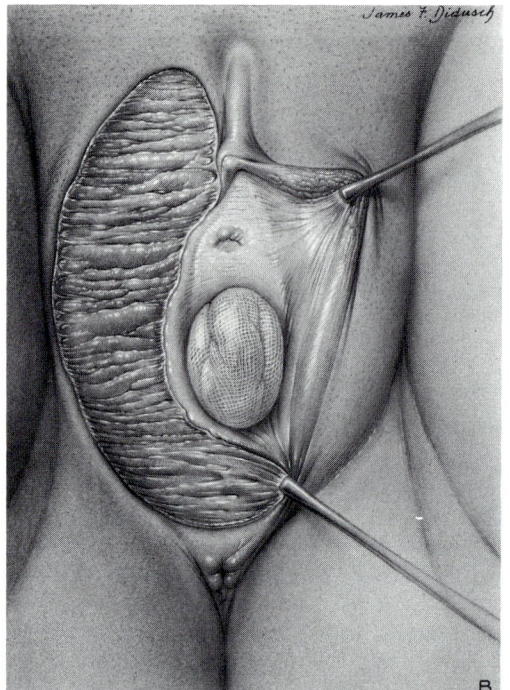
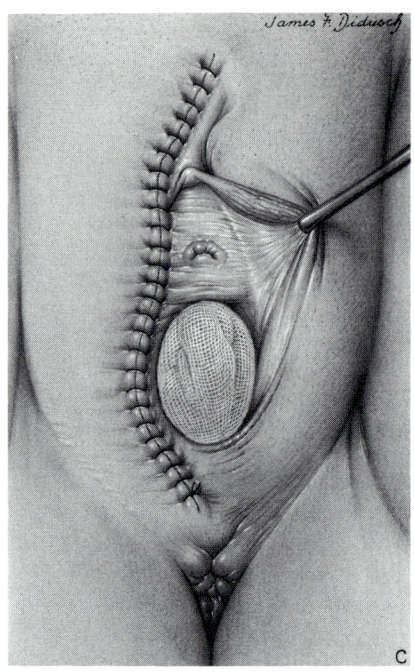

Fig. 31-2 (*Continued*). Partial vulvectomy for benign lesion. (B) Partial vulvectomy has been performed, leaving fatty base. (C) The subcuticular fat has been approximated with interrupted sutures of fine catgut. The skin is closed with a continuous suture of fine silk.

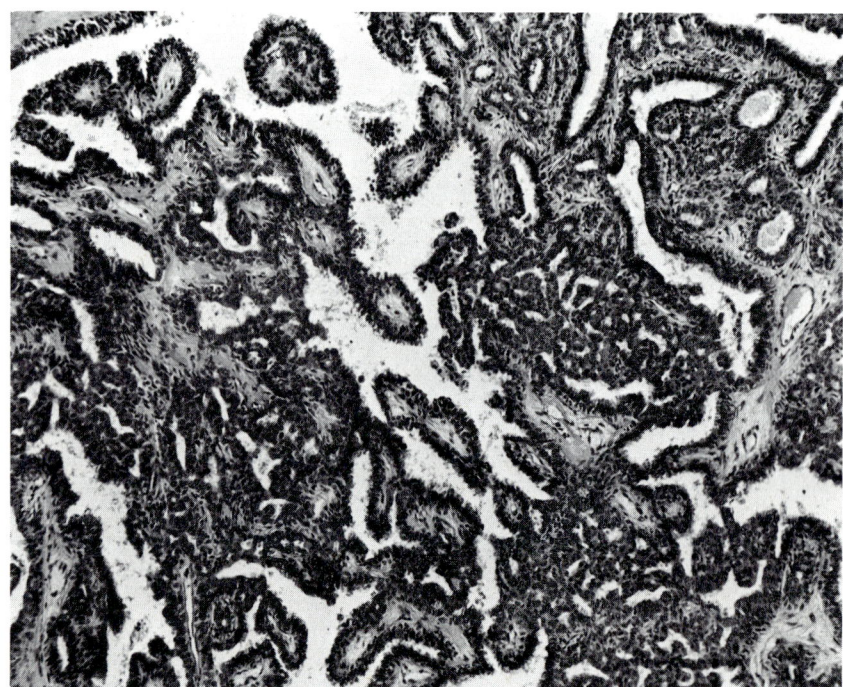

Fig. 31-3. Low-power magnification section of hidradenoma of the vulva.

the left inguinal glands. The glands showed definite metastases, but the patient was well 2 years after the operation. However, in considering the question of malignancy of these tumors, it is only fair to say that occasionally adenocarcinoma of the vulva is encountered in which it is quite impossible to ascertain the origin, and a sweat-gland origin is possible but not certain. Two such tumors in our laboratory were described by Novak and Stevenson in connection with 14 undoubtedly being hidradenomas.

Clinically, the tumors are small, usually not over a centimeter in diameter (Fig. 31-4). They are sessile and are covered with normal skin. Their consistency may be firm or as soft as a sebaceous cyst, with which they are often confused. The majority are found on the labia majora, but they also occur on the perineum, the labia minora, the vaginal vestibule, and on the perilabial skin. A small superficial granular area is often seen on the surface, and in some instances reddish-brown pulpy exudate may be expressed. There is no discomfort from the growth, and many hidradenomas are discovered incidentally on routine pelvic examination.

The treatment consists of complete local excision. Recurrences have been noted from incomplete excision, but excision of the local recurrences has resulted in cure. The important thing is to have the excised tumor examined by a competent gynecologic pathologist so that its true nature is recognized, thus avoiding an unnecessary mutilating operation.

PAPILLOMATA OF THE VULVA

Papillomata of the vulva are of two types. The ordinary papilloma of the skin may occur on the labia majora or the mons veneris. It is covered with normal-looking skin, is usually attached by a small pedicle, and does not become ulcerated.

Condylomata acuminata represent the other type. They characteristically occur on the vulva, the perianal skin, and some-

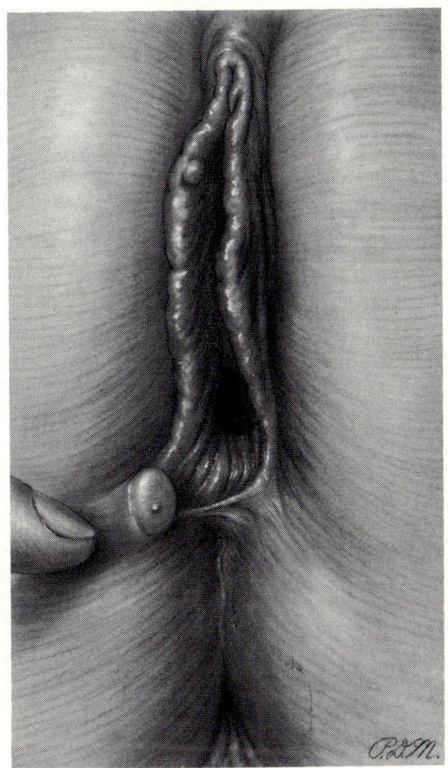

Fig. 31-4. Hidradenoma of the vulva.

times in the vagina. They have been designated as venereal warts, but actually they are not a venereal disease. It is true that they are often present in women with chronic gonorrheal cervicitis, but any vaginal discharge favors their growth. However, we have seen them in women with no abnormal vaginal discharge, in whom there is no suggestion of previous neisserian infection, who are very clean in their habits. Nonetheless, there is no doubt that excessive moisture favors their growth. Recent evidence identifies a virus which thrives in a moist environment as the etiologic agent. They vary in size from small excrescences of 1 or 2 mm. in diameter to massive conglomerations of papillomata as large as a cauliflower (Fig. 31-5). Histologically, condylomata acuminata differ from the ordinary papillomata. The latter are covered with normal-appearing epithelium over a tree-like connective-tissue core. Condylomata acuminata are covered with markedly hypertrophied,

670 Surgical Conditions of the Vulva

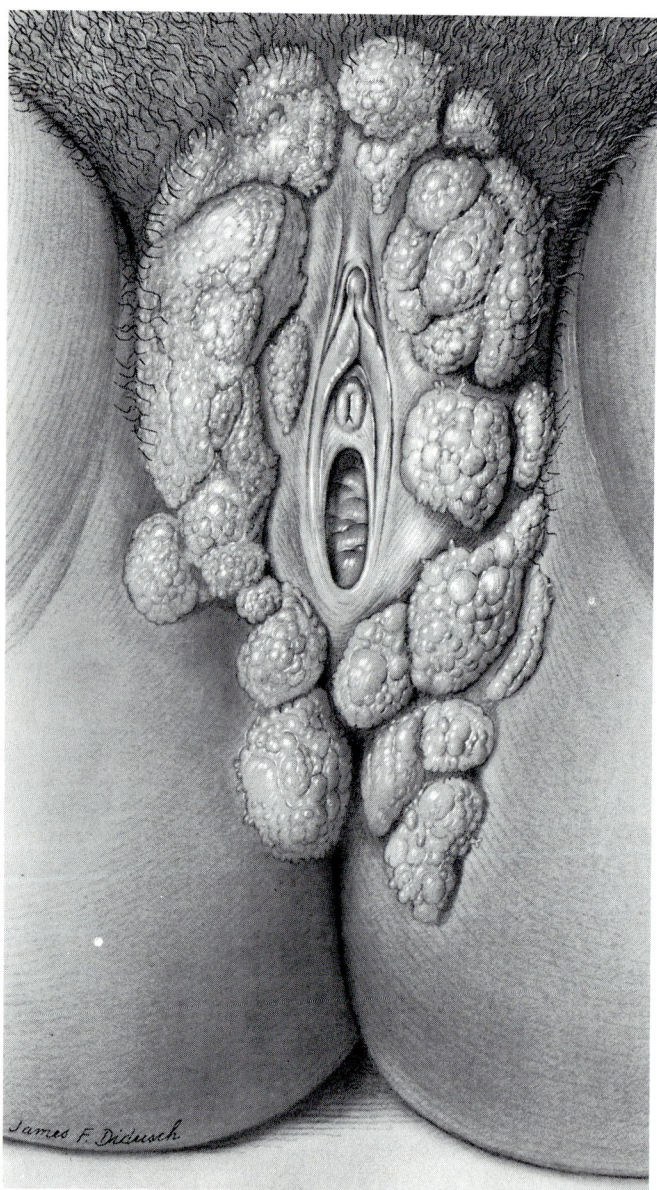

FIG. 31-5. Multiple large condylomata acuminata.

stratified squamous epithelium, with marked cornification. There is always a marked infiltration of the epithelium and subjacent connective tissue with lymphocytes, plasma cells, and polymorphonuclear leukocytes.

The treatment of the smaller lesions is very simple. Broad-spectrum antibiotics are used to clear the secondary infection. Weekly applications of a 25 per cent solution of podophyllin in benzoin are quite effective in removing small lesions. To avoid chemical burns, care must be taken to allow the solution to dry thoroughly before permitting other areas of the vulva, perineum, or vagina to come into contact with this cauterizing agent. Effective eradication of smaller lesions by local application of sulfa cream has been reported, but this is quite time-consuming and is better utilized as an adjunct to more definitive therapy. Each lesion may be completely destroyed by fulguration. The massive growths may require excision with the electrosurgical knife. They should not be excised during pregnancy, when they often grow rapidly due to estrogen stimulation. Spontaneous regression, and even disappearance, often occurs after pregnancy, and the increased vascularity during pregnancy makes the excision of massive condylomata dangerous. Massive growths may necessitate delivery by cesarean section. To prevent recurrence of the condylomata, vaginal discharge, if present, should be cleared up.

CYSTS OF THE VULVA

Bartholin's-Gland Cysts

Cysts of Bartholin's glands are common, and by far the commonest cysts occurring in the vulval region. They are nonneoplastic and result from retention of glandular secretions due to blockage somewhere in the duct system. The commonest cause of this obstruction is gonococcal infection. However, such obstruction does occur rarely in virginal women and occasionally in parous women who never have had a neisserian infection. It is probable that the Bartholin's duct may become obstructed by the healing of obstetric tears or abrasions. The contents of most of the cysts are clear mucoid material, but hemorrhage may occur in them and darken the fluid. More commonly the cyst contents become secondarily infected, usually with the colon bacillus, forming a pseudoabscess with an epithelial-lined wall, with many or few layers, depending on the part of the duct that forms the cyst. If the cyst wall is formed by a terminal duct or acinus, the lining is of cuboidal epithelium. If the wall is lined by epithelium of the duct system nearer the surface, it is of the transitional or squamous type. The epithelium may be flattened by pressure or even entirely destroyed.

Most small Bartholin's cysts are incidental findings at routine pelvic examinations. They are quite asymptomatic, unless infected. The larger cysts may also give rise to no symptoms, even when they have attained considerable size. Discomfort at coitus, sitting, or walking is the usual complaint when the cyst does become symptomatic.

Technic: Excision of Bartholin's-Gland Cyst

In the removal of Bartholin's-gland cysts it is our custom to make an elliptical incision in the mucosa which is distended over the cyst (Fig. 31-6 A). We believe that an incision on the mucosal side is preferable to one through the skin, because if the incision is made through the skin, it is often difficult to dissect the cyst wall from the very thin and delicate mucosa without incision or tearing it.

If an opening is accidentally made through the mucosa, a buttonhole-like opening is apt to persist. If, on the other hand, the incision is made on the mucosal side, usually no difficulty is encountered in dissecting the cyst from the inner surface of the skin.

Since cyst formation is usually preceded by inflammation, the cyst wall is adherent and cannot be shelled out easily with blunt dissection. The blunt-pointed Mayo scissors serve admirably for sharp dissection of the cyst wall from its bed (Fig. 31-6 B, C, and D). Often when the cyst is large, it will have developed posteriorly, close to the rectum. This should be borne in mind in dissecting the cyst free. If danger seems to be imminent, the assistant may insert his finger in the rectum, but this is rarely necessary. Complete removal of the gland tissue adherent to the cyst wall is essential, for if some is left, the residual glandular tissue may form another cyst. In making the dissection, the noncystic portion of the gland usually can be detected easily by palpation. It feels quite indurated in contrast with the surrounding soft tissues. Occasionally, we deliberately open the cyst and dissect the wall from the surrounding tissue. At times this procedure is extremely convenient.

Directly beneath the Bartholin cyst is the vestibular bulb, which is composed of anastomosing venous channels. Care must be taken to avoid bleeding when

672 Surgical Conditions of the Vulva

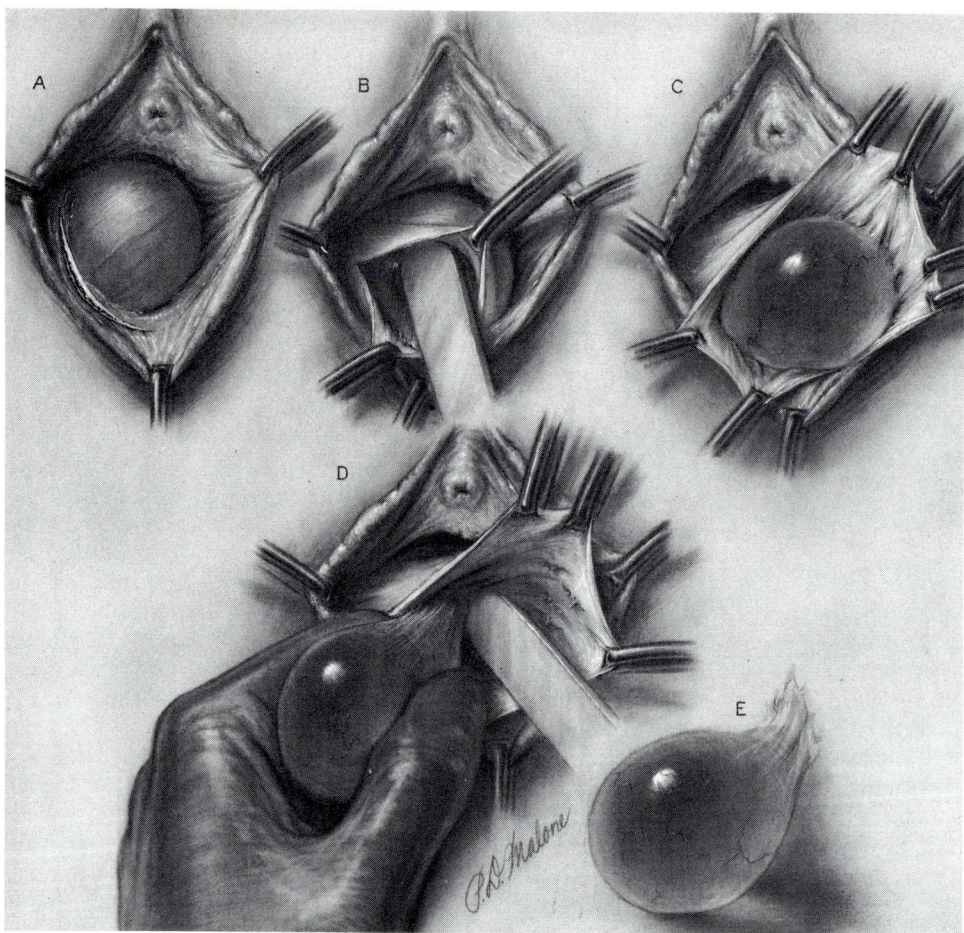

FIG. 31-6. Excision of Bartholin's-gland cyst. (A) An incision is made in the mucosa over the cyst. (B) Dissection is begun, using the handle of the scalpel. (C) Dissection has been continued by sharp and blunt dissection. (D) Dissection is almost complete. (E) Shows intact cyst after removal.

dissecting the gland from its attachment to the vascular bulb. Finally, to ensure permanent hemostasis, the entire cavity must be obliterated by approximating the walls with fine chromic catgut. The final approximation of the mucosa is accomplished best by a continuous submucosal suture of No. 0 chromic catgut. Bleeding from this area is the usual cause of a postoperative hematoma of the labia which may dissect up over the mons pubis and onto the abdominal wall beneath Scarpa's fascia. Bed rest, ice packs, and a pressure dressing to the vulva is the primary treatment of this complication, whereas attempts to ligate the venous bleeding points are futile. The blood will usually reabsorb with adequate time, but it is sometimes necessary to evacuate the blood and drain.

Technic: Marsupialization of Bartholin's-Gland Cyst

In recent years, permanent drainage of a Bartholin's-gland cyst by marsupialization of the cyst wall has become an established method of treatment. Since the cyst wall is composed primarily of the duct of the gland, effort has been made to preserve the secretory function of the gland for vaginal lubrication rather than to excise the gland with the cyst. It

Cysts of the Vulva

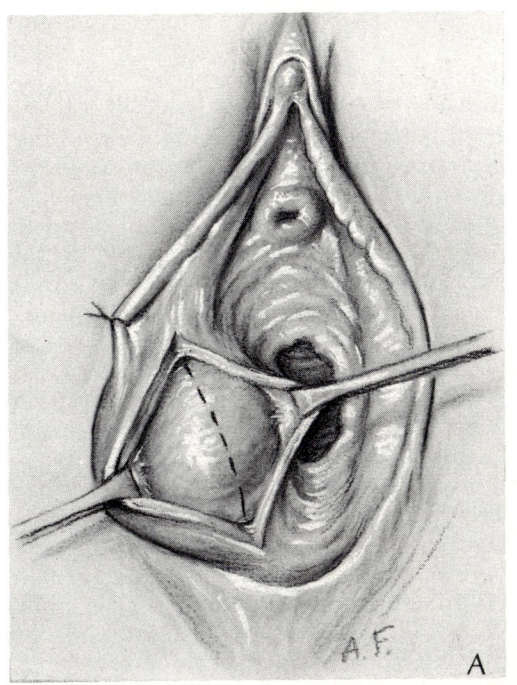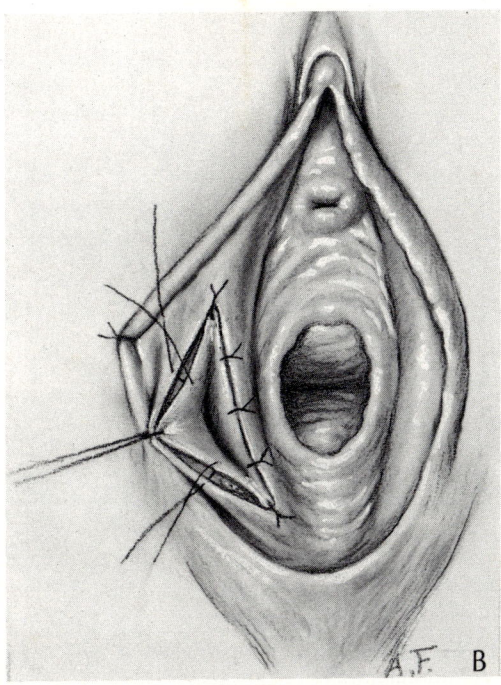

FIG. 31-7. (A) Incision for marsupialization. (B) Marsupialization. (Tancer, M. L., Rosenberg, M., and Fernandez, D.: Cysts of the vulvovaginal (Bartholin's) gland. Obstet. Gynec., 7:609, 1956)

is certainly a less involved technical procedure and eliminates many of the complications resulting from excision of the cyst.

The procedure may be performed under local, regional, or general anesthesia. Briefly, a vertical incision is made in the vagina mucosa over the center of the cyst outside the hymenal ring. The incision is made as wide as possible to enhance patency of the stoma postoperatively. After opening the cyst wall and draining it of its contents, the lining of the cyst is everted and sutured to the vaginal mucosa with interrupted sutures of No. 00 chromic catgut (Fig. 31-7). If desired, a portion of the cyst wall may be excised, although this appears to offer little assurance that the stoma will remain patent. Drains and packs are not necessary, and the patient's postoperative care includes daily sitz baths after the 3rd or 4th postoperative day.

An adverse sequella of this procedure is a 10 to 15 per cent recurrence rate which is the result of closure and secondary fibrosis of the vaginal orifice following marsupialization. Recurrence of cyst and abscess formation can also occur. According to Matthews excision of an area of skin over the lesion and packing the cavity at the time of the procedure has not prevented the stoma from closure. In deciding whether to marsupialize or excise a Bartholin gland cyst, one must balance these adverse sequellae against the possibility of dryness of the vagina following excision. In our opinion this is more of a theoretical than a practical objection, for having excised hundreds of Bartholin gland cysts, we have had no complaints.

OTHER CYSTS

Sebaceous cysts are also common (Fig. 31-8), but they do not often cause symptoms unless they become infected. Small cysts, 3 to 5 mm. in diameter, are common; they constitute incidental findings on routine pelvic examination. They rarely reach a diameter of 1 cm. When uninfected, they are usually entirely

674 Surgical Conditions of the Vulva

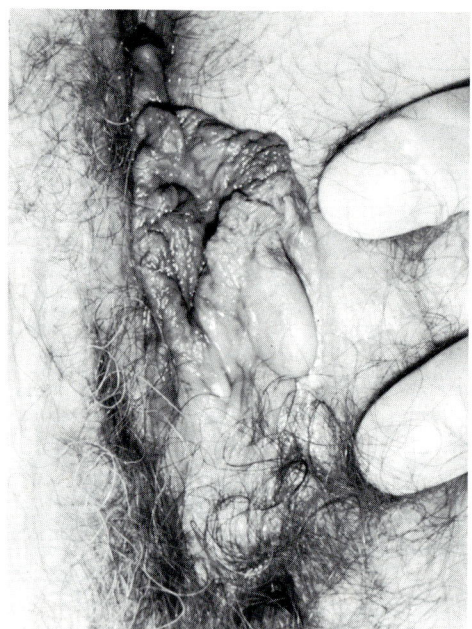

FIG. 31-8. Showing sebaceous cyst on labia majora.

asymptomatic, or else the patient may have noticed a small nodule for which she wishes an explanation. Usually they are brought to the patient's attention when they become infected and tender. They occur most often on the labia and especially on the inner surfaces. The yellowish color imparted to them by their sebaceous contents makes them readily recognizable. The cysts rarely become large enough to require removal. More commonly, the smaller ones require incision when infected. Hot compresses of salt solution or sitz baths, following incision, usually give the patient comfort promptly. They very seldom require removal after incision.

Cysts arising from the terminal portions of the wolffian ducts occasionally occur in the region of the hymen, the clitoris, or the labia minora. They are usually thin-walled and translucent (Fig. 31-9). Since they arise near the junction of the wolffian duct and the skin, they may be lined with columnar or stratified squamous epithelium or a combination of both. They are always benign, and excision is required only if they annoy the patient, but such occasions occur only infrequently.

KRAUROSIS OF THE VULVA

The term *kraurosis* was first used by Breisky in 1885. Since then it has been employed loosely and indefinitely in the literature, and one is left in utter confusion as to the exact pathologic entity designated by the term. It has been confused particularly with leukoplakia, for in the later stages of leukoplakia extreme shrinkage often occurs. Kraurosis literally means shrinkage, and in this text it will be used to indicate exactly that.

The histologic picture of kraurosis is that of an atrophic process. The changes in the mucosa and the skin are similar to those seen in senile atrophy of the skin. There is a uniform atrophy of the various layers of the epidermis, with flattening of the rete ridges and merging of the elastic and connective tissue in the cutis. Woodruff states that it is impossible to differentiate kraurosis microscopically from lichens sclerosis and from senile atrophy, and should not be attempted, as they represent the same clinical entity.

Following the cessation of ovarian activity, with a resultant withdrawal of the estrogenic hormone, there is a normal physiologic shrinkage of the vulva and the vagina. Great variation occurs in the degree of shrinkage within physiologic limits. In rare instances the shrinkage is

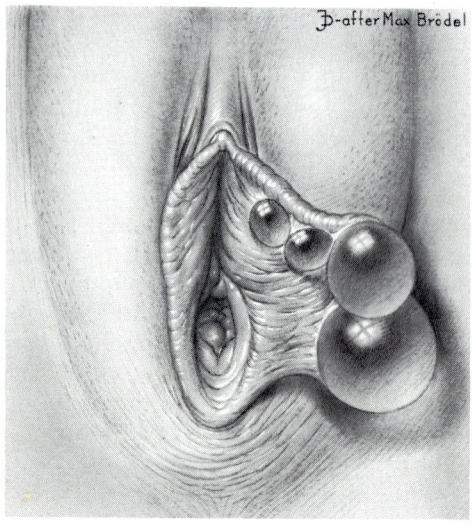

FIG. 31-9. Cysts of labium minus.

excessive, and the atrophic changes of the vulva and the vaginal orifice cause extreme contraction, so that marital relations are impossible. We believe that the term *kraurosis* should be applied to this excessive and pathologic degree of postmenopausal change. As the atrophic postmenopausal vaginal mucosa is subject to abrasions and ensuing infection, so the atrophic skin of the vulva is easily broken, and crevices form through which infection readily enters. The parts become edematous, reddened, and indurated as the result of chronic inflammation. The mucosa of the parts becomes smooth, shining, and dry, and the folds of mucous membrane and skin become flattened. Often the labia minora disappear completely. The infected skin and mucosa may itch, but often kraurosis vulvae is entirely asymptomatic.

This form of simple kraurosis usually demands no treatment. When it occurs in postmenopausal women who are relatively young and in whom there is still a desire for sexual intercourse, plastic enlargement of the vaginal outlet is occasionally indicated. A healing ointment, such as that of zinc oxide or dienestrol cream, can be used to heal the abrasions, and this usually brings relief from the irritation.

In addition to this simple kraurosis there often results, as a late stage of leukoplakia, a marked vulval shrinkage. This is discussed under the section dealing with leukoplakia.

LEUKOPLAKIA OF THE VULVA

The term *leukoplakia* or *leukoplakic vulvitis* has been confused in the literature and has been used to designate both true leukoplakia and also simple kraurosis, which has not true leukoplakia's characteristic—whitish, parchment-like changes in the skin. In this text we shall use the term *leukoplakia* to include only those cases in which gross whitish changes are visible in the skin. Histologically, they are characterized by the changes described below.

In order to define more clearly the nature of the lesion, the histopathology as described by Taussig follows:

In the early stage we find extensive subepithelial leukocytic infiltration with pronounced elongation of the epithelial papillae (acanthosis) and beginning thickening of the keratin layer. In the beginning, nuclear elements are still present to some degree in this keratin layer, and the term parakeratosis has been applied to this stage in distinction from the later hyperkeratosis where only thickly packed keratin fibers are found. In the course of a few months or a year, if the pruritus has been pronounced, there is noted a marked increase in the thickness of the eleidin layer and in the quantity of eleidin deposited in these cells. Since this substance stains very deeply with hematoxylin, this layer often appears as a thick black band beneath the keratin. The epithelial layer in this early hyperplastic stage is as a rule from four to six times thicker than in the normal individual. In the connective tissue there is considerable hyperemia and marked round-cell infiltration. Only toward the conclusion of this stage do we notice increasing connective tissue formation with some sclerosis.

The late atrophic stage is not an abrupt change. There are gradations between it and the hyperplastic stage so that areas midway between the two are commonly found. Yet the lesions of this late stage are so characteristic and different from the early stage that it seems histologically almost like two diseases. As we approach the late stage we observe increasing hyperkeratosis, pronounced eleidin but lessened acanthosis. The papillae become much flatter and shorter, even though the total thickness of the epithelial layer is still twice that of the normal. There is also diminished round-cell infiltration and increasing sclerosis of the dermis.

The typical late atrophic stage is a very distinctive picture.... The epithelial layer in these cases consists of a considerable layer of hyperkeratosis, beneath which is found a thin layer of eleidin cells, and then, with papillae absent, a flat strip of pavement cells that may or may not be covered by a single layer of basement epithelium. In many areas the border of this pavement epithelium appears frayed out and irregular without any sharp distinction from the connective tissue beneath. Even more marked are the changes in the dermis. The round-cell infiltration is in more-or-less circumscribed lymph zones, much less marked than in the early cases, with plentiful plasma and mast cells scattered through the connective tissue. This connective tissue in many areas directly beneath the epithelial layer undergoes a peculiar collagenous change, forming patches of glairy tissue containing only a few normal cells. . . . I never failed to note some diminution in the amount of elastic tissue between the epithelial papillae of the skin and directly beneath the basement membrane.*

The etiology remains obscure although many factors have been implicated, including infection, trauma, nutritional effects, and hormonal changes.

Clinical Characteristics

Leukoplakia vulvae is a disease of the menopausal years or beyond. The average age in Taussig's group was 49 years. In three quarters of the total number of patients the menses had ceased, and in the remaining quarter there was clincal evidence of some ovarian dysfunction. Although the cause of leukoplakic vulvitis is not known, there can be little doubt that a deficiency of estrogenic hormone predisposes to its development. In spite of this general statement, however, we have seen a rare case in a young individual with normal ovarian function (insofar as it can be determined by the menstrual history).

The presenting symptom is in almost all instances pruritus, and in most cases this symptom has existed for a period of many months or even for years. The patient may describe the vulval sensation as a feeling of rawness or burning, especially if scratching has caused minute ulcerations. In the later stages of the disease when the vaginal orifice has contracted, dyspareunia may become a major complaint. Remissions occur, but the history in most cases suggests a steady progression of the disease.

Grossly, the vulva may be generally and symmetrically involved (Fig. 31-10), or there may be localized patches of leukoplakia which are most often on the inner aspects of the labia majora or in the region of the prepuce. The generalized type of lesion is the more common, but the degree of leukoplakia is not always uniform over the entire area. The preputial folds above and the perineal region below are often the most severely involved. The dull whitened areas are usually thick and parchment-like in appearance, and small crevices are common. In the advanced atrophic stage the changes in the subepithelial connective tissue produce contractions so that the labial and the preputial folds are obliterated, and the vaginal orifice is markedly narrowed. This end picture may be properly designated as leukoplakic kraurosis, but not simply as "kraurosis" (Plate 1).

Leukoplakia of the vulva is one of the few conditions in the human body that can be definitely considered as a precancerous lesion. Many reports indicate that leukoplakic lesions may eventually become malignant, as frequently as 20 to 25 per cent, although statistics are inconsistent on this point.

In contrast, however, more than 50 per cent of vulvar carcinoma demonstrates coexisting leukoplakia. We have had occasion to observe a few cases of vulval leukoplakia over a number of years which were not operated upon because of various reasons. Under our observation ulcerations developed which on biopsy showed epidermoid cancer. Approaching the question from the aspect of the fully developed cancer, Smith and Graves found that in 21 vulvas removed for cancer there were 16 in which leukoplakia was present elsewhere on the vulva. Figure 31-11 shows an early cancer on a leukoplakic vulva of long standing. Plate 1 shows a similar picture of advanced leukoplakia with beginning cancer.

Treatment

Since there appears to be such a direct association between estrogen deficiency and leukoplakia, one naturally turns to endocrine therapy, but supplying estrogens has been disappointing. More recent reports, however, from Williams, Richardson, and Hathcock confirm their earlier studies of the beneficial effect of

---

* Taussig, F. J.: Leukoplakic vulvitis and cancer of the vulva (etiology, histopathology, treatment, five-year results). Trans. Amer. Gynec. Soc., 54: 60, 1929.

PLATE 1

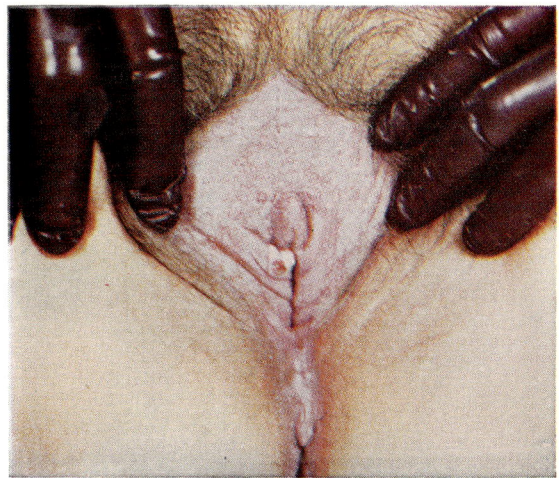

Marked leukoplakia of long standing. Carcinoma has developed just below the clitoris on the atrophic labium minus.

PLATE 2

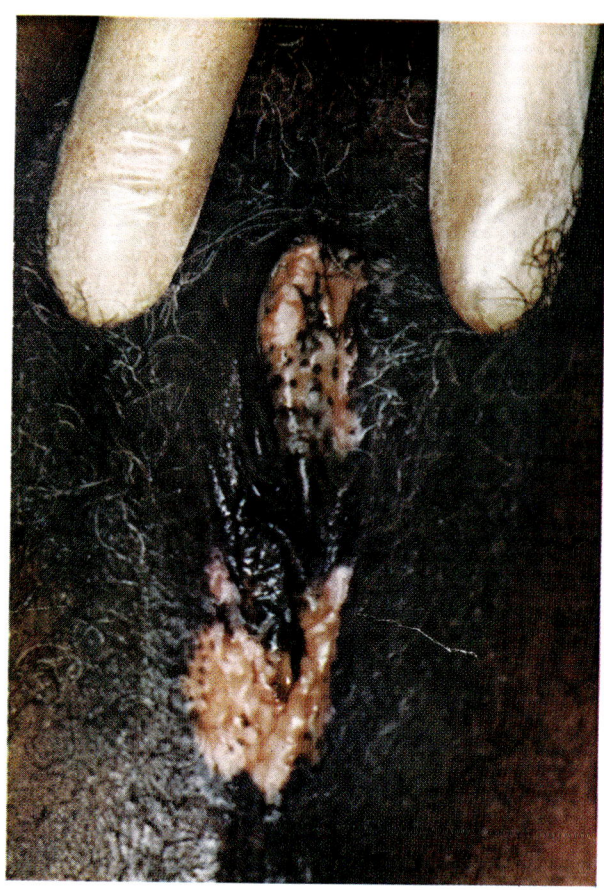

Gross appearance of carcinoma in situ of vulva with multicentric foci of raised pinkish white areas of the vulvar skin involving the labia minora, perineal body, prepuce of the clitoris, and inner aspect of labia majora.

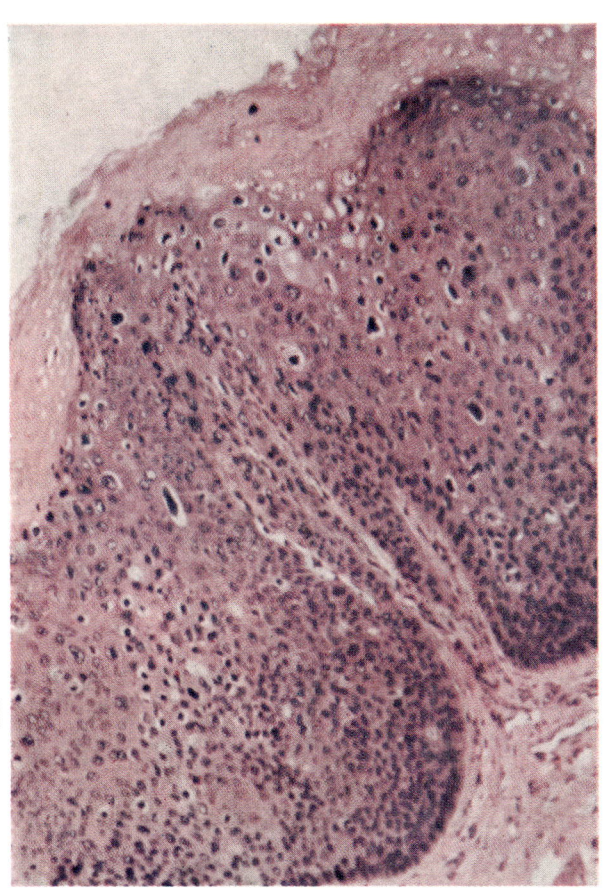

PLATE 3

Microscopic changes of carcinoma in situ of vulva showing the surface epithelium with hyperkeratosis and full-thickness alteration of the squamous epithelium, containing cells of varying size, shape, and nuclear content, as well as Bowenoid (clear cell) changes and corps ronds formation.

PLATE 4

Invasive carcinoma of vulva with replacement of the labia minora and clitoris and extension of the lesion into the vaginal introitus and periurethral area.

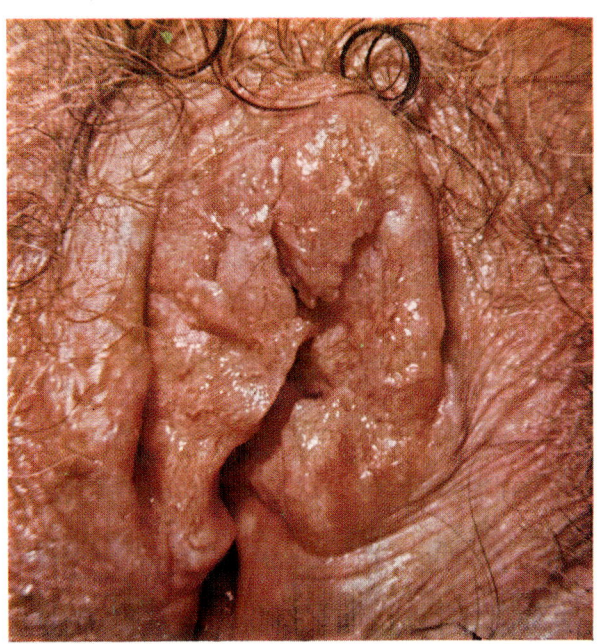

PLATE 5

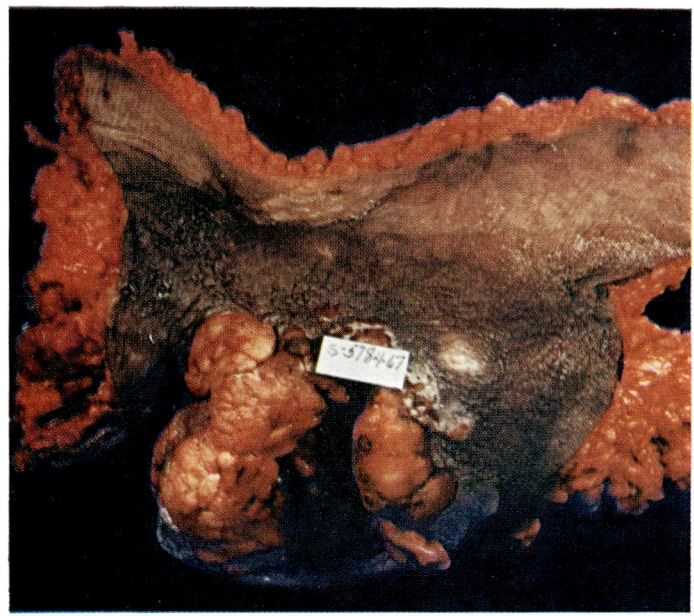

Radical vulvectomy showing complete specimen after en bloc dissection.

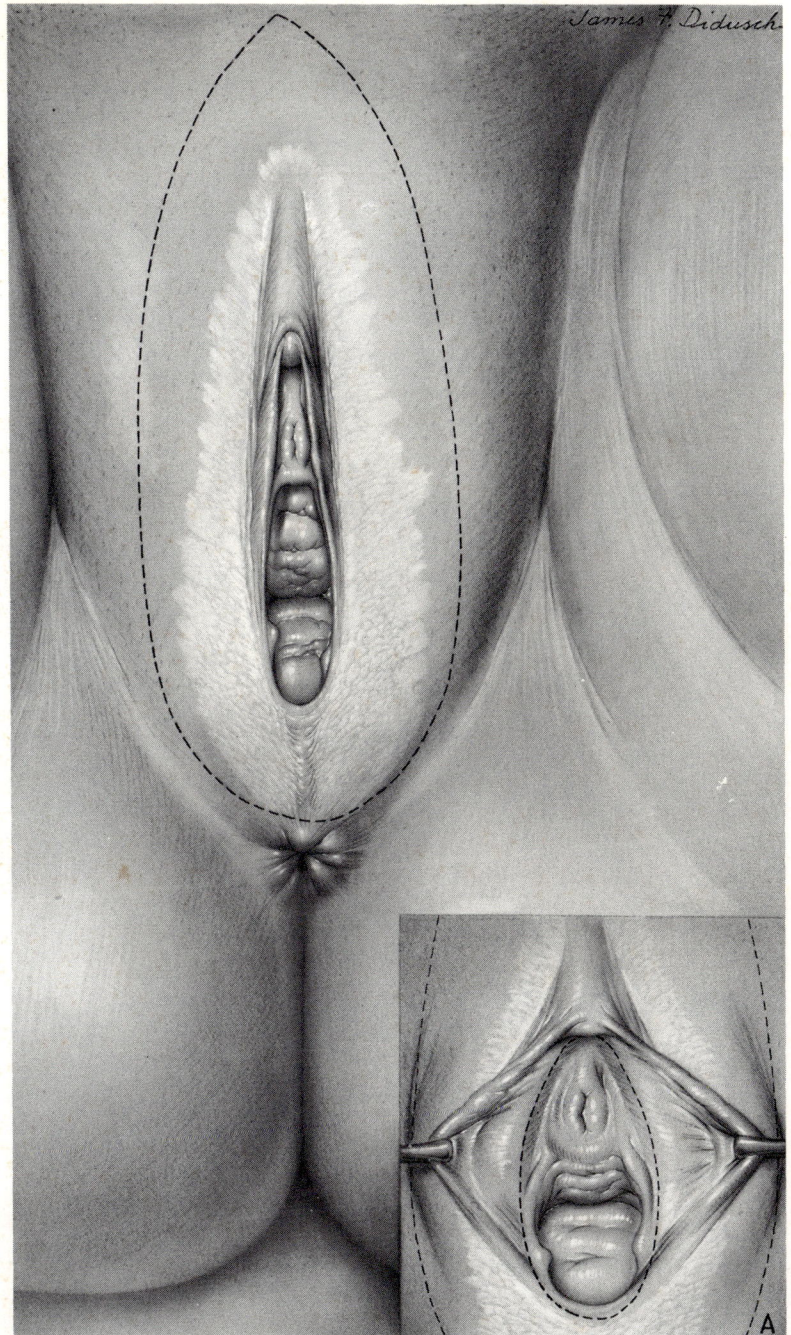

Fig. 31-10. Conservative vulvectomy for leukoplakia of the vulva. The large oval incision demarcates the outer incision. Inset A shows the inner incision.

topical testosterone for the relief of symptoms and improvement of the epithelium in dystrophic diseases of the vulva, including leukoplakia. Their treatment, using 50 mg. of testosterone per cc. of white petrolatum, recommends the use of approximately 10 mg. of testosterone daily, which is rubbed into the vulva after bathing. Their results are difficult to discount, as half of their cases were ob-

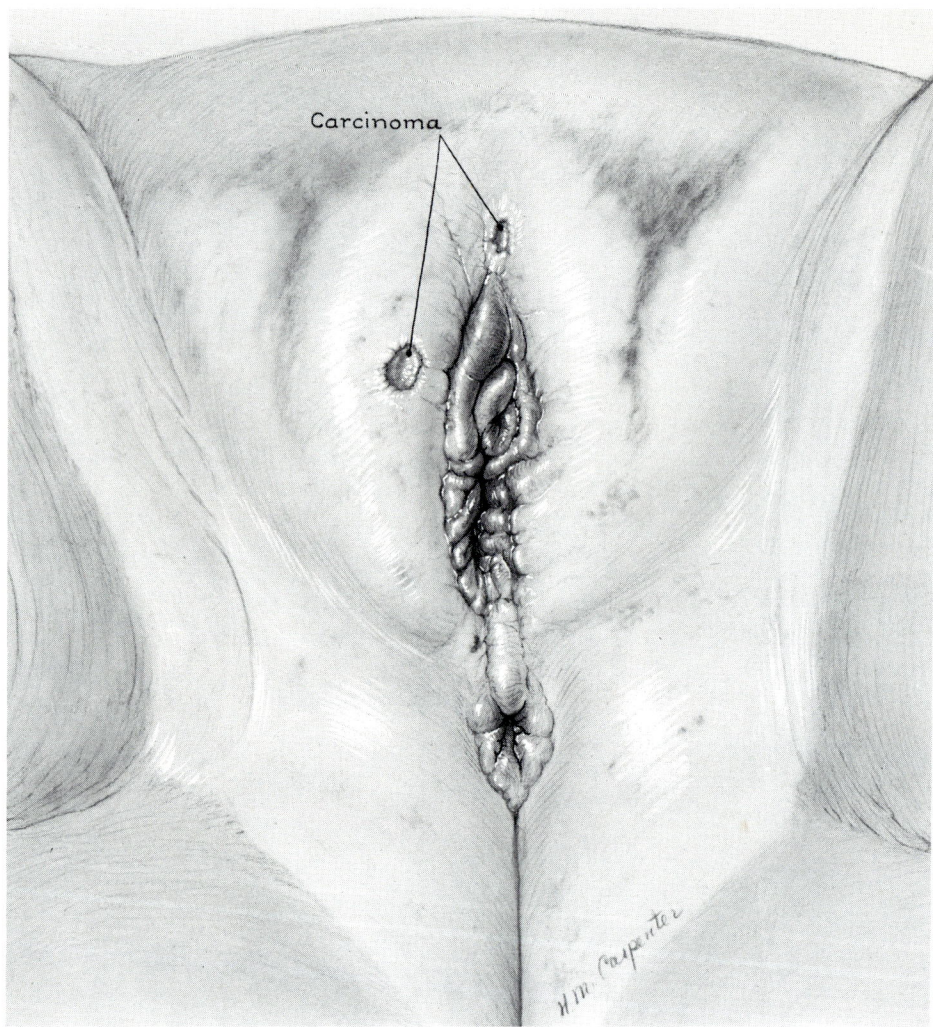

Fig. 31-11. Long-standing and extensive leukoplakia in which carcinoma has eventually developed.

served from 8 to 15 years or more. While there was 100 per cent relief of symptoms of prutitis, these symptoms generally returned if therapy was discontinued. Of their 56 cases, of which only 26 were primarily cases of leukoplakia, they have not observed vulvar malignancy to date, and they reported rebiopsy in 49 of the 56 patients so treated. Not only were all patients relieved of dyspareunia, but there was a definite surge in libido, and thickening of the vulvar epitheleum.

In spite of this report, our own experience has led us to believe that in the generalized form of the disease, a vulvectomy is indicated. Most of the cases a gynecologist sees have been treated conservatively for a long period of time and have not responded.

When the disease is quite localized to a definite area, local excision of this area is acceptable treatment, with the clear understanding that the etiologic stimulus is not focal but generalized and recurrence must be anticipated. This fact is one of the major criticisms of the use of vulvectomy for this senile vulvar disease, since the recurrence of both symptoms and skin changes at the surgical margins are quite common and require additional medical or local surgical treatment. If, however, conservative treatment is used in place of vulvectomy, it is important to make certain by means of multiple biopsies that coexistent malignancy is not present.

Technic: Conservative Vulvectomy for Leukoplakia

Conservative vulvectomy is done partially or completely for leukoplakia, carcinoma in situ, and benign tumors. The operation described here is a typical one for leukoplakia which involves all of the inner aspects of the labia majora and extends back to, but does not encircle, the anus. An elliptical incision is made about the vulva as indicated in Figure 31-10. It is well to have a fair margin about the leukoplakic skin, but in the case illustrated it was necessary to cut close to the leukoplakic area near the rectum. This incision is best made with the cutting current of the electrosurgical instrument, the bleeding vessels being clamped and coagulated from time to time.

After the outer incision is completed, an inner incision is made in the zone of the carunculae myrtiformes (Fig. 31-10). The two incisions are continued through the vulval fat until they meet, thus excising the vulva. The superficial muscles of the urogenital diaphragm, including the bulbocavernosis and transverse perineal muscles, are not excised with this procedure; only the skin and subcutaneous fat are included in the dissection. In instances in which the perianal region is involved, Taussig has advised leaving a bridge of anal skin on either side about 1.5 cm. in width. In addition, the posterior vaginal mucosa may be dissected free from the underlying rectovaginal fascia, and the mucosal flap everted over the perineal body to the denuded area of the pararectal skin (Fig. 31-12).

After complete hemostasis, the subcutaneous tissues are approximated with interrupted sutures of No. 00 chromic catgut. The skin is approximated with a subcuticular continuous suture of No. 00 chromic catgut by use of a small cutting needle.

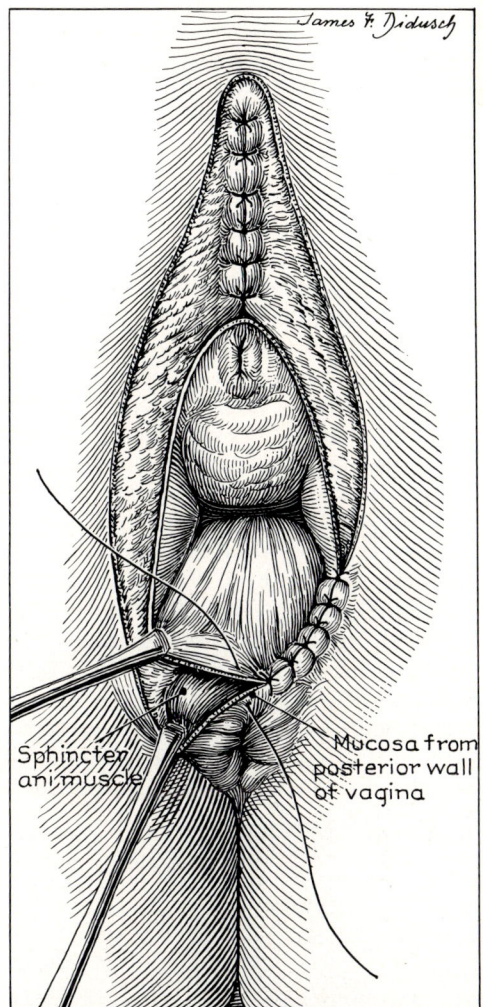

Fig. 31-12. Demonstrating the method of covering perineum by utilizing a flap of mucosa which has been dissected from the posterior vagina.

An indwelling Foley catheter is usually left in the urethra for 10 or 12 days postoperatively, although more recently in our clinic the use of suprapubic bladder drainage with a polyethylene tube has proven to have a distinct advantage in cases of simple vulvectomy.

PAGET'S DISEASE OF THE VULVA

This epithelial lesion has been the subject of controversy since the original report of the entity by Sir James Paget in 1874 as a disease of the breast. Paget's original report makes reference to a similar entity of the glans penis but does not describe the lesion. The disease was documented in the male by Crocker in 1899, involving the penis, scrotum, and pubic regions. The first reported case of Paget's disease of the vulva was made by Dubreuilh in 1901, and during the past three quarters of a century fewer than 100 cases have been reported.

At present there are two hypotheses regarding the pathogenesis. Woodruff considers vulvar Paget's disease to be of epithelial origin, arising from the embryonal stratum germinativum from which the apocrine system is developed. Consequently anaplasia may develop in both the surface epithelium and the adjoining adnexa either concomitantly or separately. In contrast, Weiner, and more recently Dockerty and Pratt as well as Koss and others, support the thesis that Paget's cells migrate into the skin from an underlying apocrine gland carcinoma. Koss feels that Paget's disease is an intraepithelial spread of adenocarcinoma of the adjacent ducts. An underlying apo-

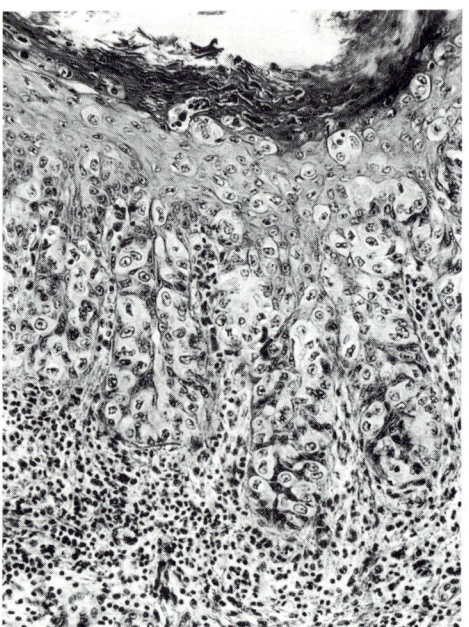

FIG. 31-14. Paget's disease of the vulva. Note the large clear apocrine cells.

crine adenocarcinoma is demonstrable in anogenital Paget's disease in 30 to 50 per cent of the cases, as reported by Helwig and Graham.

Grossly, the lesion involves the labia, usually unilaterally, and often extends to the clitoris, the perineum, and the buttock. The labia are red and edematous, and the lesion itself is brilliant red with small whitish islands of epithelium scattered throughout (Fig. 31-13). Microscopically, most of the epithelium is thickened and distorted by masses of large clear cells with pale finely granular cytoplasm (Fig. 31-14). The nuclei vary in size and chromatin content. Degeneration and vacuolization are prominent. Mitoses are present but vary considerably in number in different cases. These large clear cells are also seen diffusely scattered throughout the ducts of the sweat glands and the root sheaths of the hair follicles. In some areas masses of these cells seem to form a definite adenomatous tumor not unlike the comedocarcinoma of the breast.

The clinical picture is that of a slowly progressive disease. The usual story is one of vulvar irritation and of pruritis

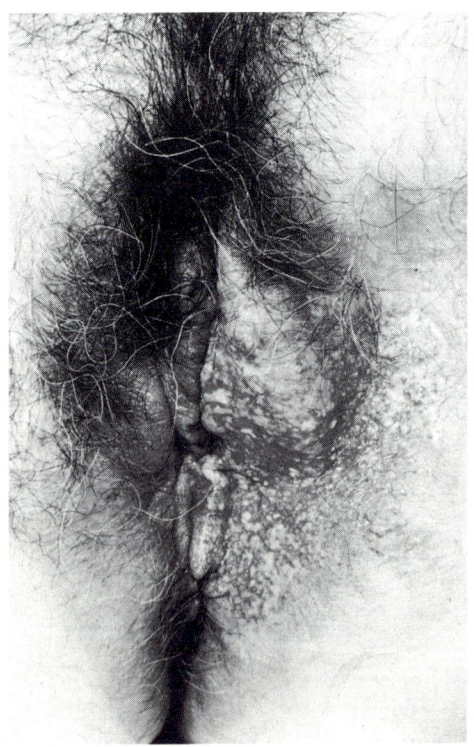

FIG. 31-13. Paget's disease of the vulva.

which has existed for months and frequently years. Ointments and often x-ray therapy have usually been tried with little or no success. The disease should be looked upon as a type of intra-epithelial malignancy which may remain as such for many years. That metastasis may eventually take place in some cases has been proved by Weiner as well as Woodruff and Richardson, and others. In fact, in one case of Richardson's, the outcome was fatal, and the autopsy showed involvement of the uterus, the tubes, and the inguinal and the retroperitoneal lymph glands.

Treatment should consist of a simple vulvectomy, but because of the possible extension of the disease into the underlying apocrine sweat glands, it may be preferential to remove the superficial muscles of the perineum, including the bulbocavernosis and transverse perinei muscles. The important aspect of this procedure is obtaining a wide tumor-free margin, both along the surface and in depth. Due to the fact that many of these lesions are multicentric in origin, it is inadvisable to perform less than a total simple vulvectomy.

The relationship of vulvar Paget's disease to adenocarcinoma of the apocrine glands is frequently misinterpreted for the lesion involving the perianal area. While many authors consider Paget's disease of the vulva to be associated with adenocarcinoma of the sweat glands in 30 to 50 per cent of the cases, this statement needs clarification. Vulvar Paget's disease appears to be less frequently associated with extensive adenocarcinoma of the apocrine glands than that form of extramammary Paget's disease that involves the perianal region. Nonetheless, the prognosis must be considered less favorable than that of other varieties of intra-epithelial carcinoma of the vulva.

CARCINOMA IN SITU OF THE VULVA

The importance of recognizing carcinoma of the vulva in its preinvasive stage needs scarcely to be emphasized to the readers of this work who are quite familiar with the high mortality of invasive vulval cancer. Although the vulva is an area which is easily studied by biopsy, there are distressingly large numbers of women with vulval cancer who come to gynecologists after long periods of delay. The reluctance of some elderly patients to submit to an embarrassing examination and the habit of many physicians to prescribe ointments for vulva irritation are undoubtedly responsible for much of this delay.

Historical Consideration. Bowen described the first two cases of intra-epithelial carcinoma of the skin in 1912. Both cases occurred in moles. Since then many cases have been reported on the vulva, although it is still a rare disease. Several of the reported lesions have been adjacent to invasive neoplasms, and others have developed invasive cancer after treatment. For example, Gardner et al. in 1953 described 8 cases, only 2 of which were without invasive cancer, and these 2 subsequently developed invasive lesions 7 and 11 years after the initial therapy. There have been enough of such cases to establish the relationship between these curable lesions and invasive cancer.

In 1958 Woodruff and Hildebrandt studied 14 cases from the Johns Hopkins Gynecological Pathology Laboratory, which represented all the cases recorded since the inception of the laboratory more than 60 years before. However, all but 3 occurred in the last 20 years, probably an indication of an increasing alertness in the detection of the condition by patient, practicing physician, and pathologist. During the same 20-year period, 58 cases of invasive vulval cancer were seen in one clinic. The average age of the women with the preinvasive lesion was 53, which is, as expected, several years younger than the average age of invasive vulval cancer.

Symptoms. Symptomatology varies, but in about half of Woodruff's cases the presenting symptom was itching and/or irritation. Some of the patients complained of a "growth," soreness, or pain. One of his cases was found on routine examination.

Gross and Microscopic Pathology. There is a great variation in the gross appearance of the lesions. They are described by the examiners in our histories as "punched out," "raised and whitened areas," "leukoplakic areas," "pinkish white and raised," "firm white and glistening," "white, shiny and moist" and "granular" (Plate 2).

Microscopically, the lesions vary from one type to another with some cases demonstrating the classic changes of Bowen's disease with areas of focal stratification while in other areas there is full-thickness change of the epithelium. The abnormal cells may completely replace the normal stratification or may be scattered throughout the residual maturing layers. These changes include the size, shape, and chromatin content of the various nuclei, with interruption of the normal maturation process and the presence of corps ronds ("fried egg" cells with central hyperchromatic nucleus and broad, pale, cytoplasmic border). The surface epithelium may show hyperkeratonization and rete peg formation. Other areas show the typical full-thickness epithelial change similar to carcinoma in situ of the cervix, with complete loss of stratification and cells which show individual anaplastic change (Plate 3). There is no breakthrough in the underlying dermis, but round cell infiltration is present.

Diagnosis

The diagnosis can be made only by biopsy, and multiple biopsies are required, for the lesion is frequently multicentric in origin. Since the occurrence of carcinoma in situ of the cervix is frequently associated with this disease, rountine Papanicolaou smears or cervical biopsies should be taken in every case in which there is a suspicion of vulvar carcinoma.

Treatment

Simple vulvectomy with a wide margin of normal skin is the treatment of choice. Multiple foci of squamous cell carcinoma of the vulva were reported in 20 per cent of the cases by Green, and 26 per cent of the cases in Gosling's experience. Basal cell carcinoma of the vulva, composed of hyperchromatic basal cells, is usually in situ and is well recognized for its multicentric origin. Carcinoma of the vulva is well known to be associated with other primary neoplasms, especially of the genital tract. At the Mayo Clinic, in a group of 137 patients with vulvar carcinoma, 12.3 per cent of the patients had second primaries in either the vagina or the cervix. There is inescapable evidence that the carcinogenic influence on the lower genital tract may involve the vulva, the vagina, and the cervix, either at the same time or at different intervals.

While an occasional case may require individual consideration and local excision rather than complete vulvectomy, it is important to recognize the possibility of a recurrent lesion which may go unrecognized and become invasive. Of all the in situ lesions of the vulva, perhaps the basal cell carcinoma is the least aggressive, as discussed later in this chapter. However, there have been many cases reported in which metastatic disease has occurred in the inguinal lymph nodes, but the invasive character of the primary disease was missed at the time of original surgery for in situ disease.

INVASIVE CARCINOMA OF THE VULVA

Carcinoma of the vulva is one of the less commonly occurring malignancies of the genital tract (Plate 4), with a reported incidence of 3 to 4 per cent of all gynecologic tumors. For the most part, it is a disease of advanced years; the average age of incidence is 60. However, in the M. D. Anderson series of 254 patients, approximately 27 per cent were between 20 and 50 years of age. In addition, in the West Indies it is reported to be preceded by granulomatous disease in 45 per cent of the cases, where it is also found at a much earlier age. In the M. D. Anderson series, 60.2 per cent had invasive squamous carcinoma, while the remainder of the cancer was distributed as follows:

	CASES
Melanoma	19
Bartholin gland	14
Sarcoma	5
Basal cell	2
Carcinoma in situ	29
Paget's disease	7
Urethra	25

SYMPTOMS AND DIAGNOSIS

The most frequent symptom is pruritis. Since leukoplakia precedes the development of cancer in approximately half of the patients, frequently the pruritis has been present for months and even for years before the appearance of the carcinoma. The cancer is often painful, and, when advanced, the pain may be extreme. Sometimes the appearance of a lump or an ulcer first draws the patient's attention to the vulval region. When the cancer breaks down, the ulceration weeps a bloody discharge. One of the presenting symptoms may be a burning on urination; this is due to irritation of the ulcerated area. When a patient complains of any or all of these symptoms, diagnosis usually gives little difficulty after inspection of the vulva. A nodule or raised ulceration, often on an old leukoplakic background, is a characteristic picture, but lymphopathia, tuberculosis, and other ulcerative lesions may simulate carcinoma. In all cases a biopsy should be taken before proceeding with therapy.

The most frequent question asked about the diagnosis of carcinoma of the vulva is: On what portion of the diffusely abnormal vulvar skin does one take the biopsy? Recognizing that invasive carcinoma is frequently associated with leukoplakia and other dystrophic vulvar epithelial lesions, the concern of the clinician that he may possibly miss the area of malignancy is a serious one.

Recently Collins reported on the use of 1 per cent toluidine blue solution as a method of staining the abnormal epithelium. After painting the vulva with toluidine blue, the stain is allowed to remain for 2 or 3 minutes and then removed with a decolorizing solution of 1 per cent aqueous acetic acid. The abnormal epithelium retains the stain and identifies the suspicious areas for biopsy.

In 242 vulvar cases in which this stain was utilized, the diagnosis of invasive cancer was accurately determined in 14 cases with no false negative occurrences. It was even effective in detecting recurrent tumor in previous vulvectomy cases. As expected, this stain is rapidly absorbed by all types of benign atypical epithelium, similar to the way in which Schiller stain is absorbed as a test for cancer of the vagina and cervix. Consequently, false positive results occurred in 16 per cent of Collins' cases. Our own experience has been less successful in diagnosing proven cancer with this stain. It has not proven to be useful in our hands in diagnosing the earliest in situ lesions, which are the most troublesome to detect clinically.

The disease is usually relatively slow in growing. In spite of this and the fact that the growth is on the exterior of the body, patients often present themselves with very advanced lesions. The reasons for delay are several. Since the disease occurs so frequently in elderly women in whom false modesty is common, patients are often reluctant to consult a physician. Salves and other home remedies are often used until time demonstrates their futility.

TREATMENT

Since the turn of the 20th century, views have differed on the extent and type of surgical procedure advisable for the treatment of carcinoma of the vulva. However, there is now agreement that wide excision of the entire vulva and dissection of the inguinal and femoral lymph nodes (Basset operation) is the minimum procedure required for the cure of this disease. The basis for recommending a lymphadenectomy of the groin stems from the original work of Sappey (1874), who was the first anatomist to demonstrate that the lymphatic drainage of the vulva flows to the inguinal and femoral nodes en route to the iliac and para-aortic lymph vessels.

The earliest reports on the use of groin

dissection in vulvar cancer came from Europe in 1895, when various individuals, including Ruprecht, Schauta, and Kustner, as well as Mauclaire (1903), advocated bilateral groin lymphadenectomy in patients with carcinoma of vulva. In the treatment of malignant melanomas, Pringle (1908) must be given credit for originally recommending a monobloc excision of the tumor together with its lymphatic bed. In 1912 Basset recommended the monobloc excision of both groin lymphatics for the primary treatment of carcinoma of the clitoris in a study of 147 cases of this disease. Taussig's report in 1931 was responsible for developing this technic in the United States, and Way has perhaps the widest experience in the diagnosis and surgical treatment of vulvar carcinoma of anyone in the British Isles.

The current use of bilateral extraperitoneal pelvic lymphadenectomy in conjunction with radical vulvectomy and groin dissection was initially suggested by Kehrer in 1918. His approach was through two independent, low oblique incisions for each iliac fossa. Stoeckel a few years before had recommended the same surgical approach but advocated preliminary exploratory laparotomy to determine the extent of the intrapelvic and abdominal spread. If the aortic lymph nodes and abdominal viscera were not involved, he performed a pelvic lymphadenectomy, followed by a bilateral groin dissection and vulvectomy. It is of interest to note that recently Williams and Butcher have revived this approach for the pelvic lymphadenectomy.

The recent study of Parry-Jones in defining the lymphatic drainage of the vulva added further information to the previous work of Way on the inguinal and femoral lymph drainage of the vulva. By the injection of Patent Blue dye and colloidal iron subcutaneously into the vulva, he demonstrated that there is no lateral spread of the vulvar lymphatics onto the thigh, but that the lateral spread of the dye was arrested in all cases at the labiocrural fold. Only from the perineum were the lymphatics demonstrated to skirt the vulva on the adjacent thigh rather than to travel along the labia majora (Fig. 31-15). In addition, the lymphatics on the medial side of the labia minora were demonstrated to drain toward the urethral orifice, suggesting that tumor in this area may spread directly to the lymphatics of the outer urethra. Parry-Jones' contribution was particularly significant in calling attention to the probable deep lymphatic pathway from the vulva to the internal iliac lymph chain, which is more commonly seen with lesions that approach the outer portion of the vagina and communicate with the internal pudendal lymphatics.

Operability

The operability of patients with vulvar carcinoma is rarely limited by the extent of the lesion or the presence of metastasis to the lymph nodes of the groin. Rather, the operability is now based primarily on the criteria of whether or not the patient is a surgical candidate, as evaluated by cardiovascular-pulmonary-renal reserve. McKelvey, however, considers that nearly all patients (93% of his series) are candidates for surgery, as he utilizes local anesthesia for the entire operative procedure, thereby avoiding the complications of a general anesthesia.

The correctness of the attitude that lymph gland metastases are no contraindication to radical surgery is reflected in Taussig's statistics on his results from the Basset operation. In the group with metastatic cancer to regional nodes, there was a 5-year cure rate of 52.6 per cent, which was only 11 per cent lower than the cure rate without metastases. The ability to predict metastatic spread of vulvar carcinoma to the inguinal and femoral lymph nodes preoperatively has been unsuccessful in more than 50 per cent of the cases, according to Berven, because the presence of lymph node enlargement from infection cannot be accurately differentiated from tumor. In 43 patients with no clinical evidence of glandular involvement, Way found 17 (39%) to show carcinoma histologically. While lymphography has been useful to alert the clinician to the presence of "sus-

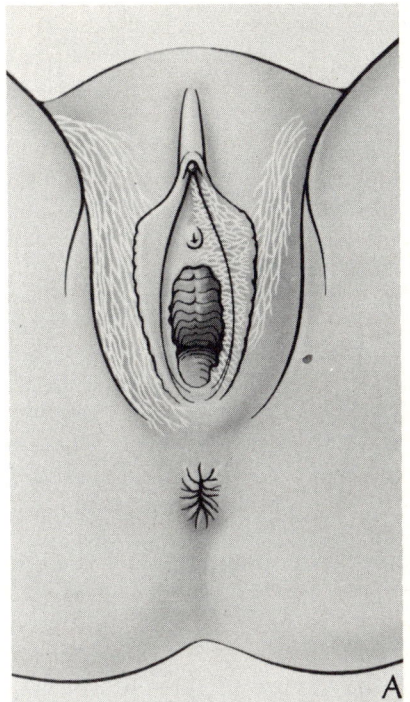 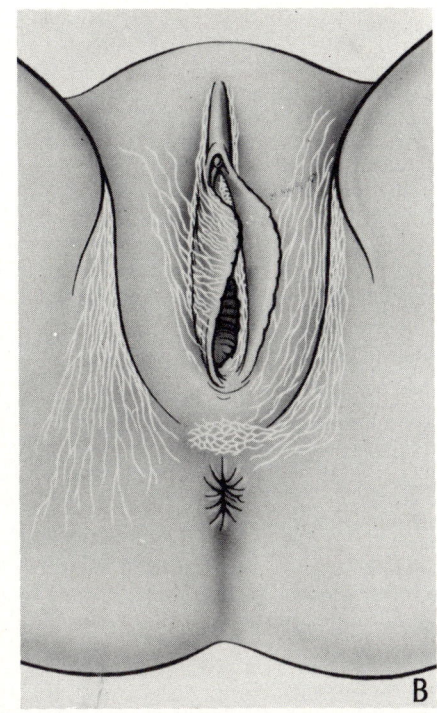

Fig. 31-15. (A) Lymphatic drainage of vulva demonstrating the discreet margin of lymphatic channels of the labia majora at the labiocrural fold. Periurethral and labia minora (medial surface) lymphatics may communicate with drainage of outer vagina. (B) Lymphatic drainage of inner aspect of thigh, and perineal body of superficial inguinal and femoral nodes. (Parry-Jones, E.: Lymphatics of the vulva. J. Obstet. Gynaec Brit. Comm., 70:751, 1963)

picious" nodes, as demonstrated by defects in the radiographic architecture of the femoral, inguinal, iliac, and para-aortic lymph nodes, this technic has not proven sufficiently accurate to serve as a reliable guide to the surgeon on the presence or absence of distant metastases. In general, the presence of tumor must be confirmed histologically, since there are many artifacts that alter the architecture of the lymph node, mainly those of inflammation, scarring, and failure to fill afferent lymphatics. The major benefit of lymphography in the treatment of vulvar carcinoma is in the radiographic demonstration of the completeness of the lymph node dissection at the time of surgery.

Technic: Operation for Carcinoma of the Vulva With Radical Node Dissection

The surgical treatment for carcinoma of the vulva consists of a 1-stage en bloc dissection of the inguinal and femoral lymphatic chain and a total vulvectomy with wide margins. The groin incision extends in an arcuate fashion to each anterior iliac crest and includes the adjacent skin and underlying fat and lymphatic channels which lie directly over the inguinal ligament and mons pubis. Figure 31-17 A demonstrates the outline of the superior and inferior incisions, which includes the area of primary lymphatic drainage from the vulva and mons pubis to the inguinal and femoral lymphatics. While Way and Marshall include additional skin over the region of the fossa ovale and inner thigh (Fig. 31-16), our primary healing rate has been much improved by the present groin incision without right-angle extensions. It is important to remove the overlying skin and subcutaneous fat, which includes both Camper's and Scarpa's fascia, in order to remove the

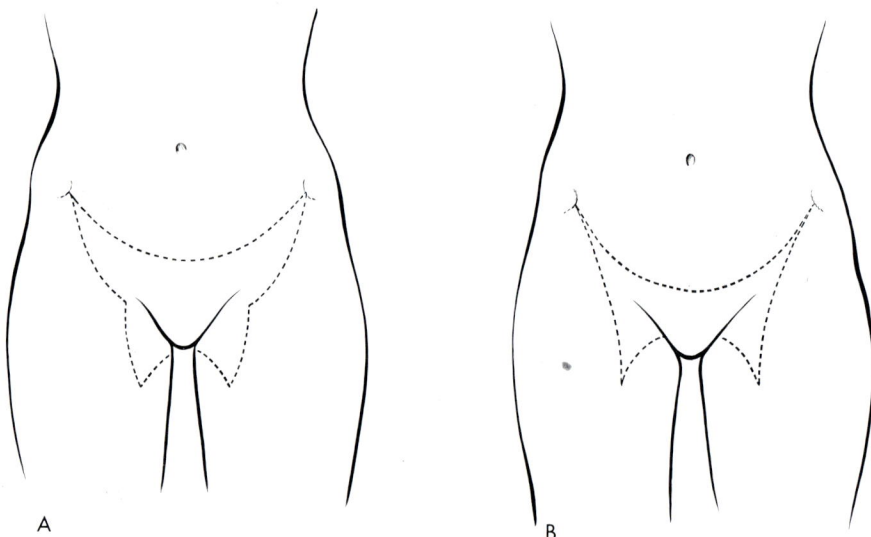

FIG. 31-16. (A) Skin incision of Way including area of fossa ovale and inner thigh. (B) Skin incision of Marshall and Parry-Jones removing less tissue and including area of femoral nodes without skin of inner thigh.

superficial lymphatic channels and to avoid necrosis of devitalized skin from the dissection. The vulvar incision depends on the location and the extent of the vulvar lesion. Contrary to Sappey's original description of the vulvar lymphatics, Parry-Jones has demonstrated that the lymphatics of the vulva drain through the labia majora and do not leave the vulva during their course to the inguinal and femoral nodes. Only from the perineum do the lymphatics skirt the vulva and pass onto the inner thigh rather than travel up the labia majora. Our incision, therefore, is confined to the labiocrural folds except when the tumor involves the perineum or extends laterally into the crural fold. As shown in Figure 31-17 B, the gross lesion is in the region of the clitoris while the extensive leuoplakia is confined to the boundaries of the labia majora. It is important to remove all of the leukoplakic lesion in the dissection and to have a wide skin margin (at least 2 cm.) from the tumor. As shown in Figure 31-17 C, the boundaries of the incision are marked on the skin, with the upper incision extending 1 or 2 cm. above the inguinal ligament and approximately 2 cm. above the symphysis pubis. This is particularly important for vulvar lesions in the region of the clitoris, where the lymphatics of the mons are frequently involved. The groin dissection is accomplished with two teams, which has reduced the operating time of this portion of the procedure by more than 50 per cent. The inferior incision extends to the fascia lata, while the superior incision removes all the lymphatic and areolar tissue down to the external oblique and anterior rectus fascia from the lateral aspect of Poupart's ligament to the region of the mons pubis (Fig. 31-18 A).

Figure 31-18 B demonstrates the technic of incising the femoral sheath at the medial margin of the sartorius muscle. This landmark is identified by palpation of the femoral artery and making the incision lateral to the artery adjacent to the femoral nerve. The artery is thoroughly cleaned of its fascial sheath, and care is taken to identify and ligate the external pudendal artery, which serves to identify the entrance of the saphenous vein into the fossa ovale as a major tributary of the femoral vein. The proximal end of the saphenous vein is transfixed and doubly ligated as demonstrated in Figure 31-18 C, and the femoral sheath is dissected medially as an en bloc procedure. Later the saphenous vein is

Invasive Carcinoma of the Vulva 687

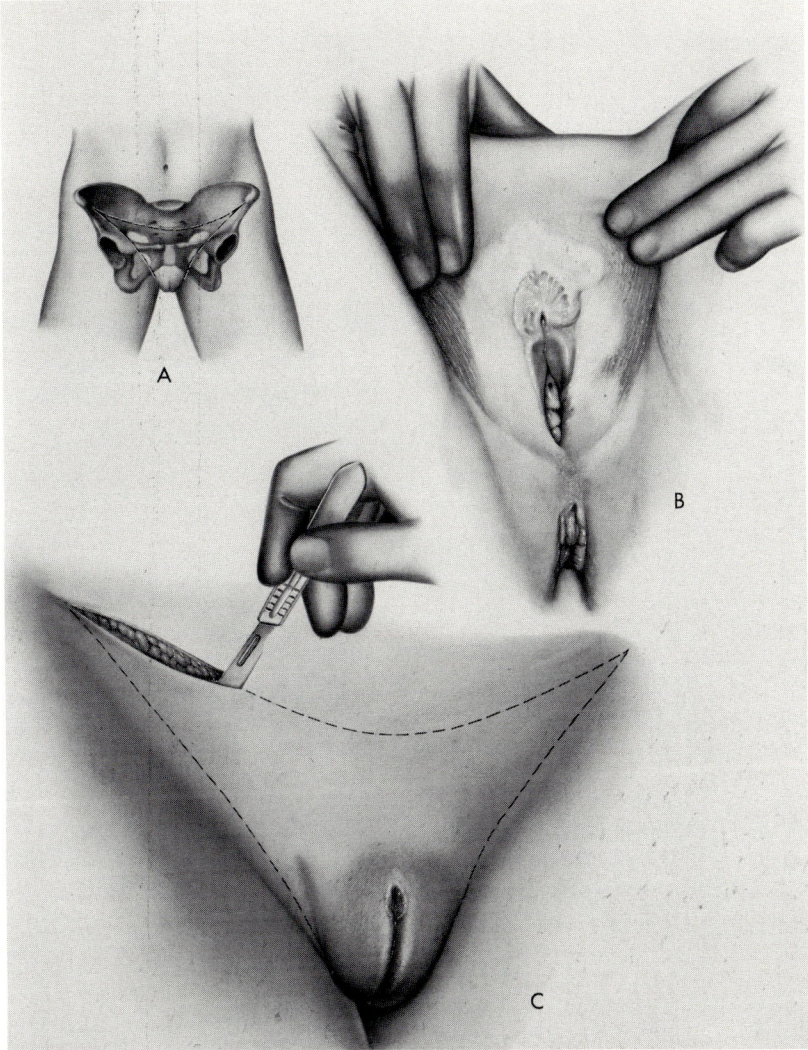

Fig. 31-17. (A) Outline of groin and vulvar incision overlying the area of primary lymphatic drainage of the vulva to the femoral and inguinal lymphatics. (B) Ulcerated carcinoma of clitoris with adjacent leukoplakia of labia majora. (C) Crescent-shaped incision above inguinal ligament extending above symphysis pubis to anterior iliac spine bilaterally.

again excised and ligated as the dissection continues toward the inner thigh and mons pubis.

Figure 31-19 A demonstrates the dissection of the deep femoral lymph chain surrounding the artery, vein, and femoral canal. Particular effort is made to identify and remove Cloquet's node or the node of Rosenmüller, which is the sentinel node beneath Poupart's ligament. This gland filters the lymphatic channels entering the femoral canal. If this node is negative for metastatic tumor on frozen section, we are in complete agreement with Taussig's opinion on the inadvisability of doing a deep extraperitoneal gland dissection of the iliac, obturator, and hypogastric nodes. Way has shown that if the superficial nodes are negative for tumor, 3 per cent of the cases or less will have metastases to the deep pelvic nodes. The increased morbidity, blood

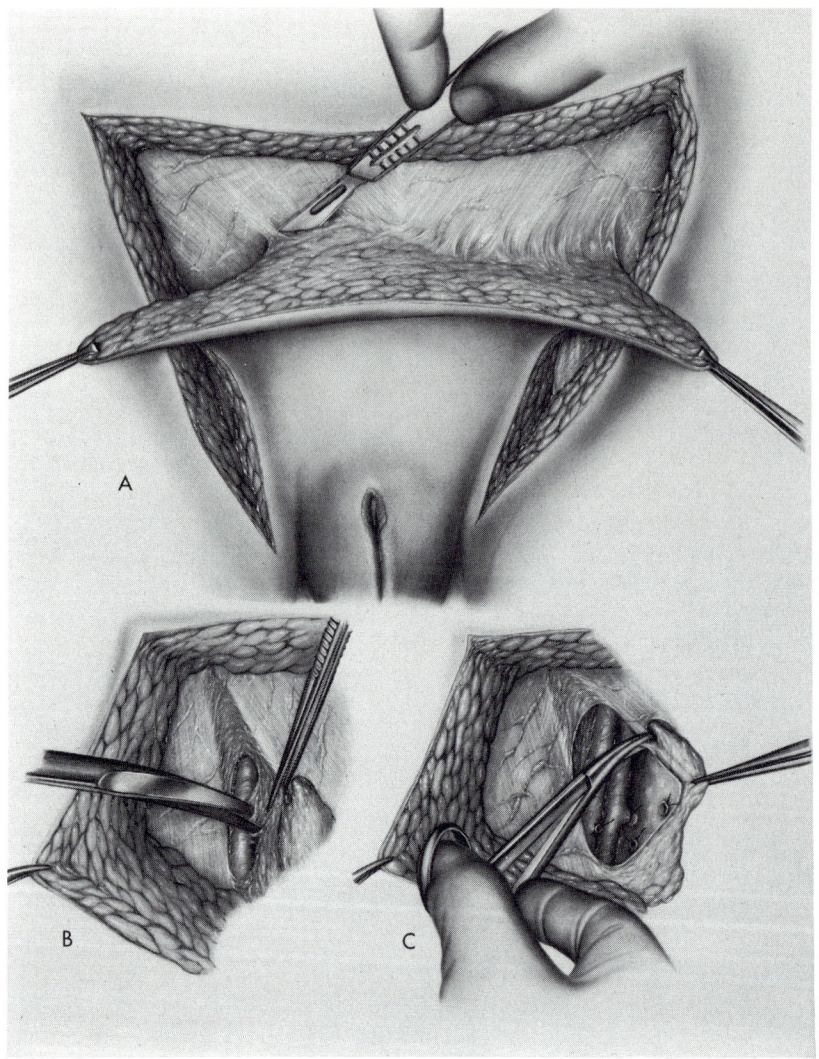

FIG. 31-18. (A) En bloc dissection of the groin lymphatics with attached skin and subcutaneous fat to the region of the mons pubis. (B) Opening of femoral sheath along medial border of sartorius muscle. Femoral artery is cleaned of adherent fascia. Inguinal lymphatics are seen entering external inguinal ring. (C) Dissection of femoral sheath medially following ligation of the saphenous vein and external pudendal artery. Superficial inguinal lymph chain is seen entering inguinal canal.

loss, and operating time associated with the extraperitoneal lymph node dissection is not justified unless Cloquet's node or adjacent femoral or inguinal nodes contain metastatic tumor. When such metastases are present, a cure rate of 18 per cent (Way) encourages one to perform the deep node dissection.

As demonstrated in Figure 31-19 B, the deep inguinal chain is dissected by opening the inguinal canal from the external inguinal ring. The internal ring is identified by the round ligament as it passes into the canal from the peritoneal cavity. The round ligament is excised, and the deep inguinal lymphatic tissue is removed.

When indicated, the deep nodes are approached through the abdominal wall by extending the inguinal canal incision.

Invasive Carcinoma of the Vulva 689

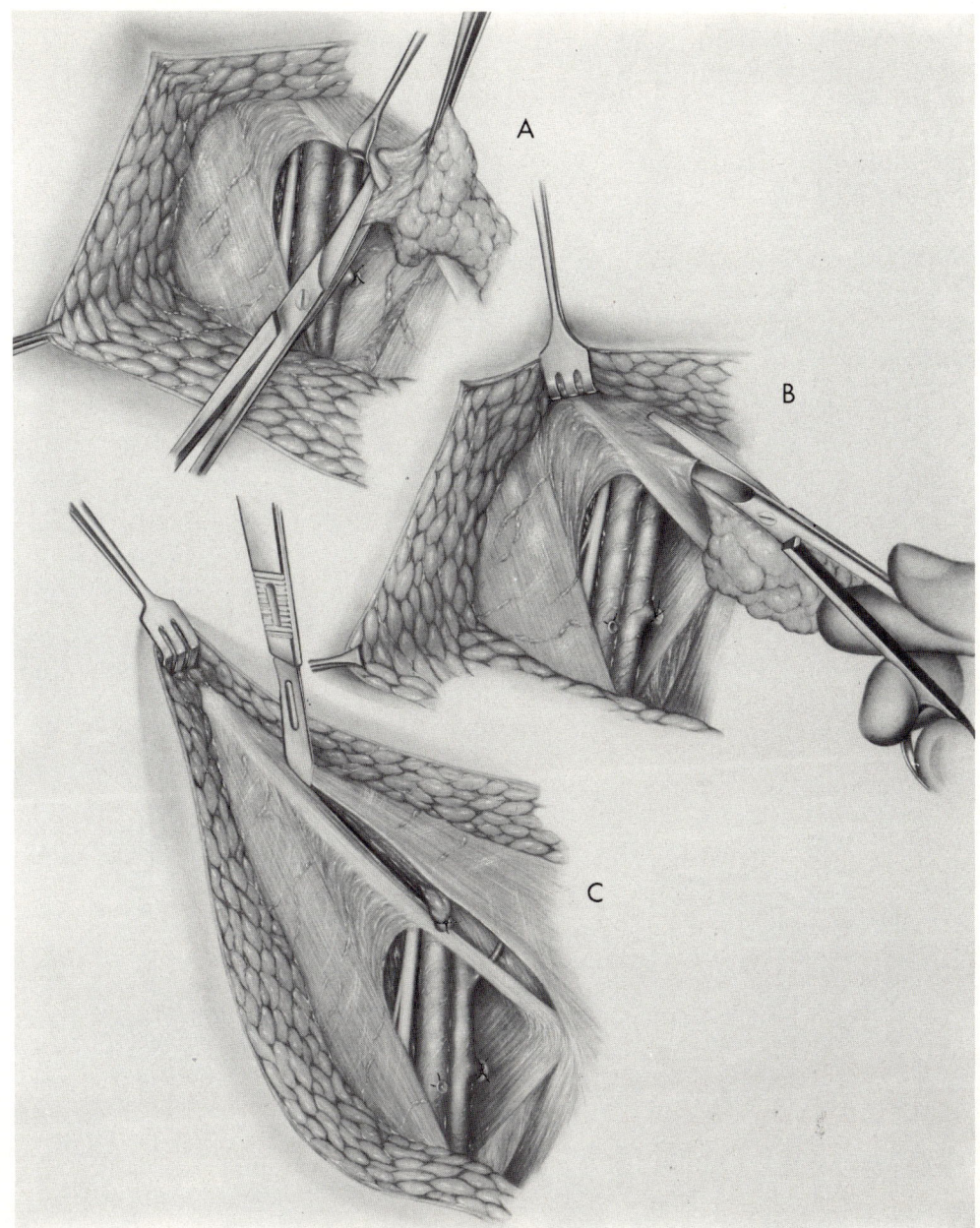

FIG. 31-19. (A) Dissection of femoral canal and Cloquet's node. The femoral triangle, including artery, vein, and nerve, is completely dissected. Inguinal ligament is elevated for dissection of deep femoral lymphatics from femoral canal. (B) Opening inguinal canal for dissection of deep inguinal lymph chain. Scissors placed in external inguinal ring to open roof of canal. (C) Incision of external oblique muscle from inguinal canal for extraperitoneal node dissection. Round ligament protudes from internal inquinal ring. Inferior epigastric vein arises from external iliac vein above medial border of inguinal ligament.

Figure 31-19 C demonstrates opening the external oblique muscle 2 cm. above Poupart's ligament, which can be extended as far laterally as necessary. The incision is continued through the internal oblique and transversalis muscles,

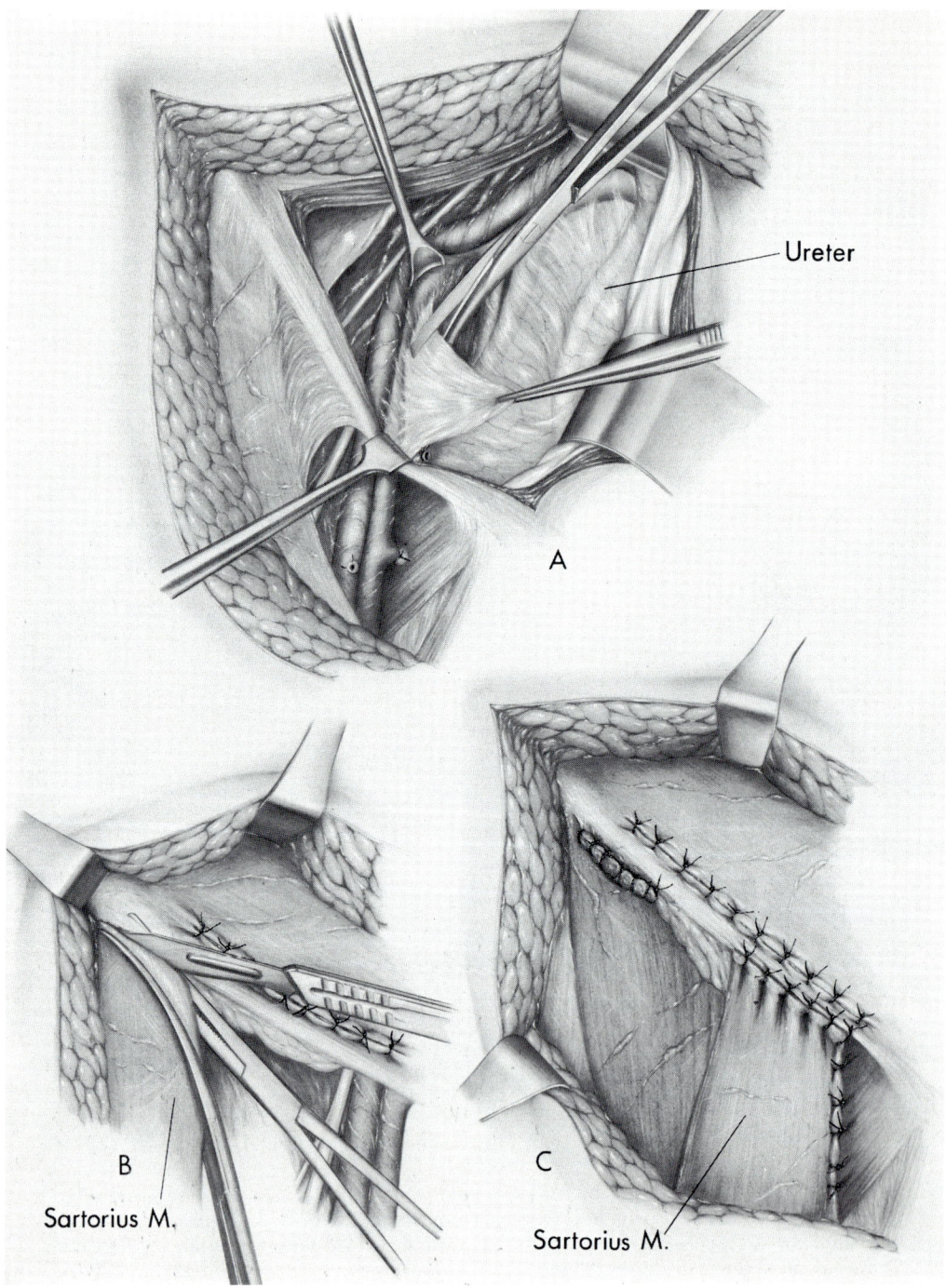

Fig. 31-20. (A) Extraperitoneal pelvic lymphadenectomy. Dissection includes external iliac, common iliac, hypogastric, and obturator lymph nodes. Ureter is reflected medially, attached to parietal peritoneum. (B) Excision of proximal portion of sartorius muscle at origin from anterosuperior iliac spine. (C) Transposed sartorius muscle over femoral vessels with suture of muscles to medial border of inguinal ligament and pectineus muscle. Abdominal musculature is closed following extraperitoneal pelvic lymphadenectomy.

and the iliac vessels are demonstrated by retracting the peritoneum medially.

Figure 31-20 A shows the extraperitoneal lymphadenectomy, which includes the external iliac, common iliac, and hypogastric vessels. The obturator space is thoroughly cleaned, as discussed in the radical Wertheim hysterectomy. The inferior epigastric artery and vein should be ligated at their origin from the external iliac vessels just inside Poupart's ligament as they course upward to supply the abdominal wall. An anomalous obturator artery and vein may arise from the external iliac vessels and enter the obturator fossa along the lateral pelvic wall. As demonstrated in Figure 31-20 A, the ureter is displaced medially with the parietal perineum to avoid injury. It is easily identified as it enters the pelvis at the bifurcation of the common iliac vessels. While it is important to clean meticulously the deep lymphatic channels along the pelvic vessels, it is essential to avoid trauma to the vessel walls by skeletization. It is best to leave a loose layer of adventitia attached to the vessel wall rather than to risk injury, thrombosis, and bleeding from the vessel. The retroperitoneal space is drained only when venous bleeding is troublesome, and there is concern for hematoma formation. The external oblique, internal oblique, and transversalis muscles are closed in a 2-layer fashion with obliteration of the inguinal canal by the second suture layer.

An important step in this procedure was innovated by Baronofsky in 1948 and popularized by Way. This includes transposing the sartorius muscle over the femoral neurovascular trunk to protect the femoral vessels from postoperative infection, thrombophlebitis, and possible hemorrhage. As shown in Figure 31-20 B, the origin of the sartorius muscle is excised from the anterior superior iliac spine and adjacent inguinal ligament and is sutured to the medial border of the inguinal ligament with interrupted silk sutures. The medial border of the sartorius muscle is sutured to the pectineus fascia to avoid collection of serum and exudate in the femoral space (Fig. 31-20 C). Large French rubber catheters (No. 18) are sutured in place above the inguinal ligament for suction drainage postoperatively. The inguinal incision is then approximated by mobilizing the upper and lower skin flaps sufficiently to permit closure without tension, as demonstrated in Figure 31-21 A. The groin specimen is wrapped in a sterile towel, and the patient is placed in the lithotomy position.

The vulvar incision, as shown in Figure 31-21 B, is continued along the labiocrural folds and includes the perineal skin above the anus. Dissection is continued along the periosteum of the symphysis (Fig. 31-21 A), and the underlying fascia and deep musculature of the urogenital diaphragm (Fig. 31-21 B). Most of the bulbocavernosus and transverse perinei muscles are removed in the vulvar dissection. At this point it is important to identify and ligate the internal pudendal vessels (Fig. 31-21 C) which provide the major blood supply to the vulva. These vessels can be identified as they emerge from Alcock's canal at approximately 4 and 8 o'clock in the dissection.

The vaginal incision is made just above the external urethral meatus and circumscribes the introitus just outside the carunculae hymenales (Fig. 31-22 A). The posterior vaginal wall mucosa is undermined for 3 to 4 cm. to form a mucosal flap for anastomosis to the perianal skin to avoid tension on the suture line. The vulva is removed after carefully ligating the blood supply to the clitoris, which can be troublesome if these vessels retract beneath the inferior pubic ligament (Fig. 31-22 A). In the event that there is tumor on the medial aspect of the labia minora near the urethra, based on Parry-Jones' demonstration of the lymphatic drainage from this area to the periurethral region, it is advisable to excise the outer third of the urethra. The outer urethra distal to the urogenital diaphragm can be removed without concern of producing urinary incontinence unless there is a prominent cystourethrocele. In such cases plication of the urethrovesical angle is necessary.

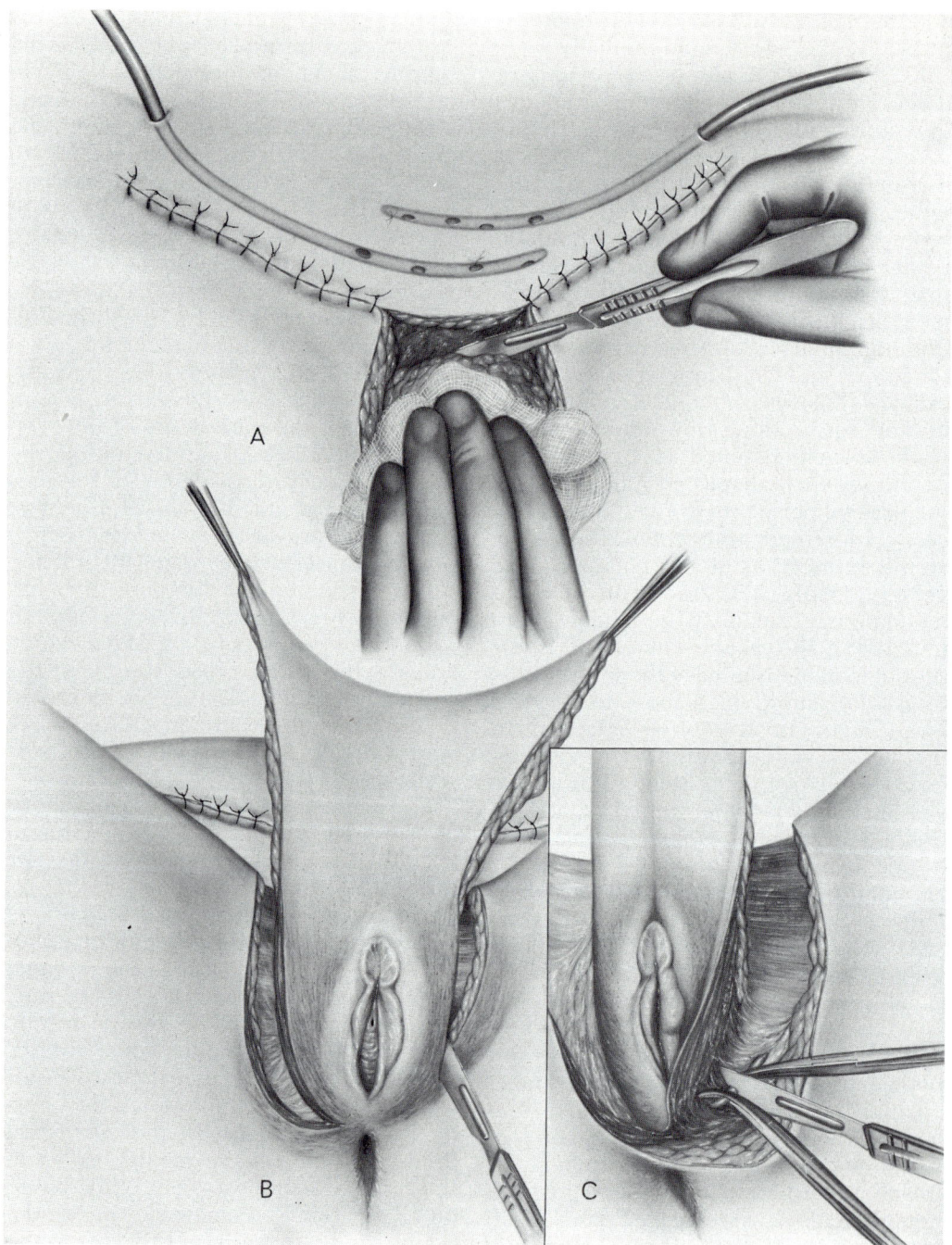

FIG. 31-21. (A) Closure of skin margins over groin with rubber catheter drains sutured beneath skin flap. (B) Vulvar incision along labiocrural fold with dissection to deep musculature of urogenital diaphragm. (C) Clamping and incision of internal pudendal vessels at posterior lateral margin of vulvar incision.

Closure of the vulvar incision (Fig. 31-22 B) is accomplished by undermining the thigh skin flaps and the outer vaginal mucosa. In the event the outer urethra has been removed, care must be taken in approximating the skin near the excised

Invasive Carcinoma of the Vulva   693

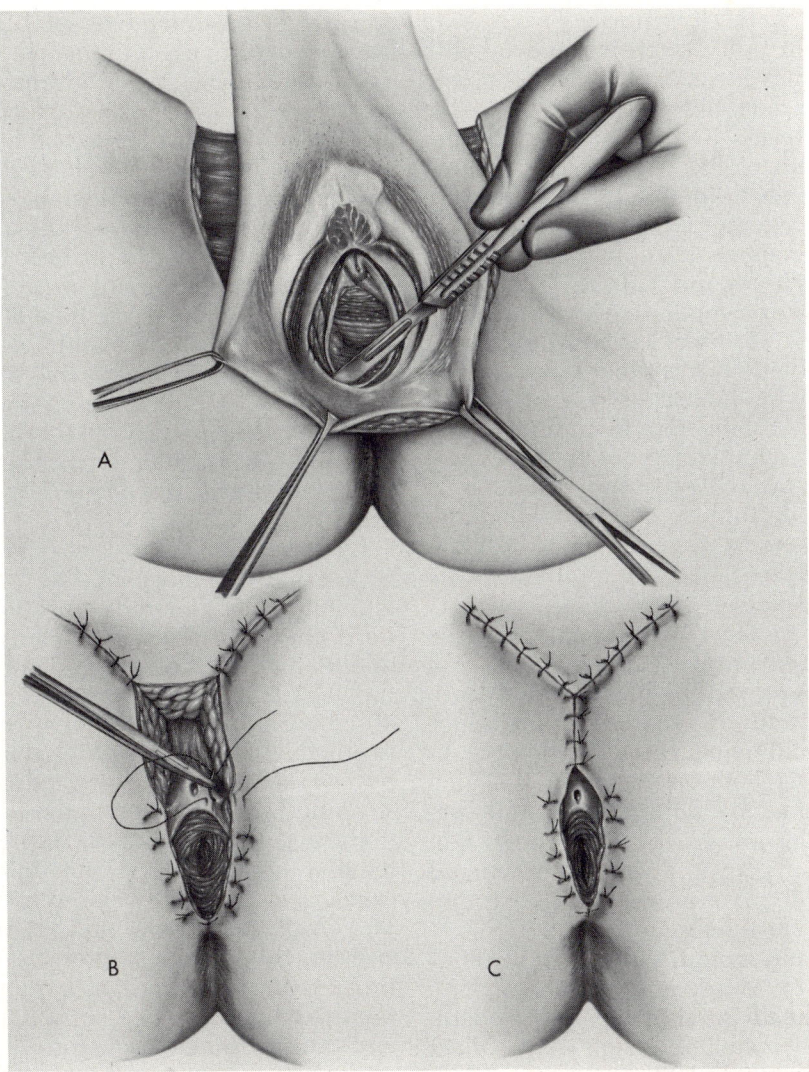

FIG. 31-22. (A) Vaginal incision made just above the meatus and circumscribing the introitus. (B) Closure of undermined vaginal mucosa to thigh skin flaps. (C) Complete closure of vaginal suprapubic and inguinal incision with horizontal mattress sutures.

urethra. Retraction of the urethra beneath the vulvar suture line can be avoided by anchoring the periurethral fascia to the subcutaneous fat of the lateral skin margins. The vaginal mucosa is sutured to the mobilized skin flaps of the thigh with horizontal mattress sutures, bringing broad surface to broad surface (Fig. 31-22 C). It is important, if at all possible, to avoid tension on the skin margins. Extensive mobilization of the vaginal mucosa is occasionally required.

Plate 5 shows the complete specimen after block dissection.

COMPLICATIONS

Necrosis and Infection of Skin Flaps. This is a universal problem and varies in frequency from 40 to 100 per cent of the reported series. The more extensive the dissection, the more frequent is the skin necrosis. This results from ischemia of the skin margins and secondary infection. The incision utilized in this technic avoids leaving large areas of devitalized skin, which is removed with the operative specimen. Nonetheless, partial or complete breakdown of the incision occurs in approximately 50 per cent of our cases. Way advises fixation of the legs, with the thighs flexed and the legs tied together for 1 week or more, in order to remove tension from the skin margins. He reports that this technic has reduced the postoperative hospitalization by as much as 3 weeks. His method has not been widely accepted, however, because of the increased risk of venous stasis and thromboembolic complications. Adequate mobilization of full-thickness skin margins with the subcutaneous fat and blood supply attached, together with suction drainage beneath the flaps, has greatly reduced this problem of incision breakdown.

Efforts to clear the infection of the glands preoperatively with the use of antibiotics as well as postoperative antibiotics has also decreased the incidence of wound infection. If the incision breaks down, it is better to shorten the total healing time by débridement and secondary closure or split thickness skin graft rather than to await the prolonged hospitalization required for the wound slowly to close by granulation.

Serum and Lymph Collection. Copious amounts of serum and lymph are collected beneath the skin flaps in the operative site. Suction drainage may collect as much as 300 to 500 cc. a day, depending on the amount of adipose tissue of the groin and the degree of secondary infection following the operation. However, meticulous ligation of the margins of the lymphatic dissection will significantly reduce the amount of this drainage. The large rubber drainage catheters are connected to low Gomco suction and left in place as long as there is drainage beneath the skin flaps. As a rule, these catheters may be first advanced on the 5th day and removed within the 1st postoperative week.

Postoperative Hemorrhage and Retroperitoneal Hematoma. While hemorrhage from infection and necrosis of the denuded femoral vessels was formerly a serious postoperative problem, this has been virtually eliminated with the transposition of the sartorius muscle over the femoral vessels, which is now fairly routine. Retroperitoneal hematoma formation from deep pelvic gland dissection remains a problem and may frequently point into the cul de sac, where drainage can be accomplished. If venous bleeding from obturator or pelvic floor veins is a problem at the time of surgery, retroperitoneal drains should be inserted to avoid a pelvic hematoma. Thrombophlebitis and emboli from the pelvic veins as a complication of hematoma formation is an added risk to this procedure and requires vigorous antibiotic therapy.

Lymphedema. Transient lymphedema is a usual sequence of this procedure although it is generally only temporary until there is re-establishment of secondary lymphatic drainage channels from the leg. However, approximately 30 to 40 per cent of our cases have significant residual lymphedema, which is improved by the continuous use of fitted elastic stockings and elevation of the legs.

Hernia. Postoperative inguinal and femoral hernias may occur unless both canals are specifically closed at the completion of the femoral and inguinal dissection. Silk suture is preferable in approximating the inferior border of the inguinal ligament to Cooper's ligament and the pectineus fascia for obliteration of the femoral canal. It is considered inadvisable to transsect the inguinal ligament for the deep pelvic node dissection as postoperative hernias frequently result from poor healing and secondary infection of the inguinal region.

Mortality and Cure Rate

Mortality. There is still a significant mortality from this procedure mainly due to the uncontrollable problem of pulmonary emboli from the pelvic and leg veins. In addition, as a result of generalized cardiovascular disease in this elderly age group, myocardial infarctions and cerebral vascular accidents are admitted complications of this type of radical pelvic surgery. Way acknowledges a hospital mortality of 19 per cent in a recent follow-up report of late results of extended radical vulvectomy. McKelvey reports a primary mortality of only 5.1 per cent, which is lower than that of other series and is probably due to his use of local anesthesia for the entire dissection.

The prophylactic use of anticoagulants has not decreased the incidence of postoperative pulmonary emboli nor improved the mortality rate, but it will increase the morbidity from postoperative bleeding. In preference to prophylactic anticoagulation, we have recently employed the use of clinical dextran (dextran 70), 500 cc. daily for 2 days *before* and 5 days *after* surgery, in an effort to prevent RBC and platelet sludging. Thrombophlebitis and pulmonary emboli have been decreased mainly by early ambulation, decrease in cellulitis of the wound, and exercise of the lower extremities.

Cure Rate. The determining factor in the cure of this disease is related directly to the presence of metastases to regional lymph nodes at the time of operation. In a long-term follow-up of 69 patients for more than 10 years, Way reports a 5-year survival of 70 per cent in the absence of lymph node involvement, while the cure rate decreases to 47 per cent with lymph node metastases. When there was metastasis to the deep pelvic nodes, a survival rate of 18 per cent, although a discouraging figure, justifies continued efforts for cure of the disease by deep node dissection.

Collins, in a report on the 5-year survival of 94 patients with cancer of the vulva, relates the prognosis to both the size of the lesion and the positive lymph nodes. With lesions *less* than 3 cm. with *negative* nodes, the 5-year cure rate is 90 per cent. At the other end of the scale, where the lesion is *greater* than 3 cm. in size with *positive* lymph nodes, the 5-year survival is 18 per cent. When the gross lesion is greater than 3 cm. in longest diameter, the chance of node involvement is 50 per cent, whereas if the lesion is less than 3 cm. in diameter, the chance of node involvement is 20 per cent. For all cases with negative nodes, Collins' 5-year cure rate is 76 per cent, whereas those with positive nodes had a 5-year cure rate of 20 per cent. Lymph node involvement at the time of operation in Way's series was 42 per cent, and the cure rate did not correlate well with the size of the tumor. Green reports a 5-year survival of 88 per cent with *negative* nodes and 41 per cent with *positive* nodes in 54 patients treated for carcinoma of the vulva.

Radical vulvectomy and bilateral inguinal and femoral lymphadenectomy was performed in McKelvey's clinic in 113 (93.5%) of 124 patients who had no previous definitive therapy, with a 54 per cent absolute 5-year cure rate. The overall operative mortality was 5.1 per cent. Lymph nodes were involved in 29 per cent of the patients. Only 25 per cent of the patients with lymph node metastases were cured whereas a 5-year survival of 68.2 per cent was achieved in patients with no disease in regional lymph nodes.

In a recent report by Rutledge, Smith, and Franklin from M. D. Anderson Hospital, 127 treated patients were evaluated for survival after radical vulvectomy and lymphadenectomy. Of 49 patients with negative superficial groin dissection, none died of recurrent malignancy. Thirty-one patients had positive nodes, of whom 42 per cent survived free of disease.

BASAL CELL CARCINOMA OF THE VULVA

Basal cell carcinoma of the vulva differs from other forms of vulvar cancer both in treatment and prognosis. Although the tumor occurs infrequently, representing 2 to 3 per cent of all vulvar malignancies, in general it is a slow-growing lesion which rarely metastasizes except in its unusual form, the basosquamous variety. Figure 31-23 shows the gross lesion with its characteristic, slightly elevated, rolled edge surrounding a superficial ulcer, commonly called "rodent ulcer" when appearing on other parts of the skin. Figure 31-24 shows the microscopic picture with the deeply stained basal cells extending into the stroma from the overlying epithelium. While giving the histologic appearance of invasion, these cells maintain continuity with the overlying epithelium and, with the exception of the squamous cell variety, rarely metastasize.

Such tumors are quite radiosensitive, but the vulva is a difficult area to treat because of the irritation of the adjacent tissues, including the vagina, urethra, and anus. While simple vulvectomy has been recommended by Marcus and others, who found the origin of the lesion to be multicentric, local excision is considered adequate therapy by many gynecologists. Schueller from Roswell Park estimates that 95 per cent are curable by a wide local excision. Our own limited experience corroborates this opinion. If a squamous cell component is present, it has been our policy to treat such lesions as squamous cell vulvar carcinoma with radical vulvectomy and lymphadenectomy. Local recurrences of basal cell lesions may be repeatedly excised with an excellent chance of cure. This may be explained more by the problem of multicentric origin of basal cell carcinoma, as stressed by Marcus, than by failure to remove the primary lesion adequately. For this reason some authors favor a simple vulvectomy for all types of intraepithelial carcinomas of the vulva.

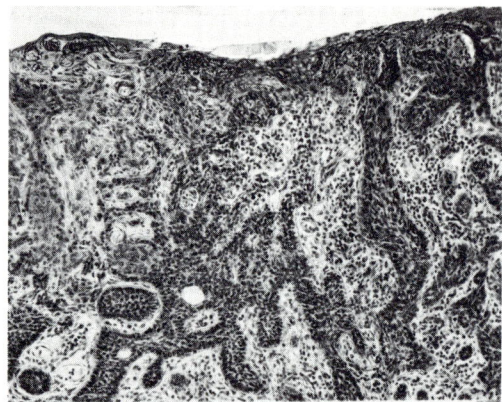

FIG. 31-24. Low-power view of a section of a basal cell carcinoma of the vulva.

UNUSUAL MALIGNANCIES OF THE VULVOURETHRAL REGION

Melanoma of the Vulva

Malignant melanoma is one of the more uncommon lesions of the lower genital tract and represents about 3 to 5 per cent of primary malignant lesions of the vulva. Similarly, the vulva is one of the more unusual locations for this malignancy, accounting for approximately 3 per cent of melanomas in women (Booher and McPeak, 1965). They are thought to arise from the junctional nevus, and their growth is known to be stimulated by the hormones of pregnancy. It is important, therefore, to recognize any change in color or size of nevi on the external genitalia and vagina, and, wherever noted, to perform immediately an excisional biopsy. It is important to avoid biopsy of the margin of a melanoma because of the possibility of disseminating tumor cells in the underlying tissue.

Pack has recently reported 41 patients with histologically proved melanoma of

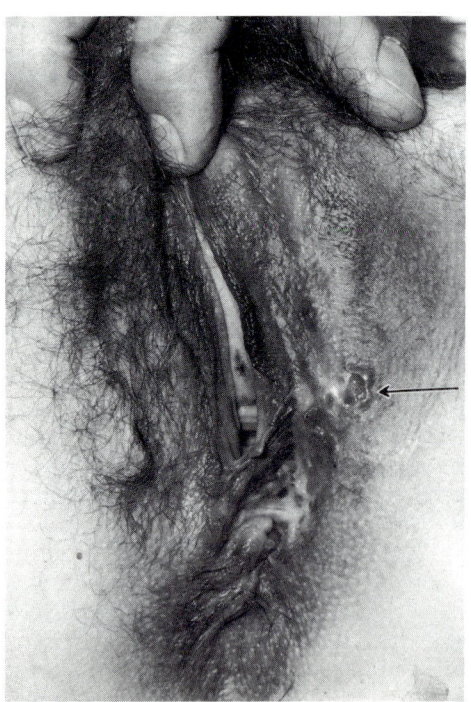

FIG. 31-23. Basal cell carcinoma of the vulva. Note the elevated edge of the localized lesion.

the vulva and 3 patients with melanoma of the vagina and compared their clinical course with 58 patients with epidermoid carcinoma of the vulva seen in the same period. A majority of the primary melanomas were located on the labia minora and mucosa of the vulva, whereas the majority of the epidermoid carcinomas were located on the labia majora. There is agreement that the treatment of choice is radical vulvectomy and groin dissection, although the prognosis is poor when metastases have occurred to the regional nodes. The incidence of metastasis to nodes in melanomas is not accurately reported but is known to be much higher than that of squamous carcinoma. Das Gupta and D'Urso reported a 34.7 per cent incidence of positive regional nodes in 26 cases of melanoma of the vulva and vagina. Only 26 per cent of the patients with metastatic disease survived. With extension of the disease to the vagina, the disease is generally fatal as a result of the rapid spread of the tumor to the deep pelvic nodes by the vaginal lymph chain. While an extraperitoneal lymph node dissection of the deep pelvic nodes is generally recommended for this disease, it is usually more informative than beneficial since few cases have been cured in which the disease has reached the internal lymphatics of the pelvis. Factors which adversely affect the prognosis of this disease include: (1) the size of the lesion, (2) metastases to regional lymph nodes with frequent bilateral involvement, (3) extension to the vagina, and (4) occurrence of the disease in pregnancy. While White and associates, in a series of 71 patients, reported a 73 per cent 5-year survival in 30 pregnant patients, this fortuitous result occurred where early lesions had been treated before there was spread of the disease. Melanomas in pregnancy are known to pass the placental barrier and metastasize to the fetus as 4 known cases were recently reported from the literature by Hormann and Lemtis.

CARCINOMA OF BARTHOLIN'S GLAND

Carcinoma of Bartholin's gland is one of the more uncommon malignancies occurring in the female genital tract and represents 3 to 4 per cent of all vulvar malignancies. This tumor is almost always unilateral, although Lewis (1956) has described 1 case of bilateral Bartholin's-gland carcinoma.

Klob reported the first case of Bartholin's-gland tumor in 1864, and to date over the next century there have been more than 150 new cases reported in the world literature. By 1951 Wharton and Everett could find only 2 cases of carcinoma of Bartholin's gland that had been treated at the Johns Hopkins Hospital. Undoubtedly, the 150 cases mentioned above do not represent all the cases of Bartholin's-gland carcinoma as individual cases are infrequently reported.

The neoplasm is sometimes first noticed as a small, firm, and painless nodule in the position of the Bartholin's gland. Initially it is well-circumscribed, but as the growth extends, it infiltrates the surrounding tissue so that its origin may be difficult to determine from the gross appearance of the lesion. As the tumor increases in size, it may become painful, and often this brings the patient to seek medical advice. The tumor frequently undergoes necrosis, so that the mass may feel fluctuant and may be confused with a benign cyst. One of the best points of differential diagnosis is the age of the patient. The majority of these carcinomas occur between the ages of 40 and 55 years, whereas most cysts and abscesses make their appearance in younger women. However, since the chances of a Bartholin lesion are so overwhelmingly in favor of inflammation or a retention cyst, a great proportion of these neoplasms are excised or incised with the belief that they are not neoplastic. Only when the tumor is found at operation to be solid is its true nature recognized.

Histologically, there are two types of Bartholin's-gland carcinoma. The majority of the tumors are adenocarcinoma, but several epidermoid cancers have been described. The glandular histology corresponds to that of the cuboidal cells which line the acini, and the superficial ducts near the surface are lined with stratified squamous epithelium. The ducts lying between the acini and the superficial squamous-lined ducts are lined by a transitional type of epithelium.

It is often difficult to be certain that a vulvar neoplasm arises primarily in Bartholin's gland. Honan has enumerated four criteria which must be satisfied if the Bartholin's-gland origin is to be established with certainty: (1) typical vulvar location, (2) position deep in the labium, (3) connection with the gland duct, and (4) the presence of intact gland tissue. If, in addition to the above, the skin is intact over the growth, one can be certain of the Bartholin's-gland origin. Obviously, in advanced cases all of the above criteria cannot be fulfilled.

Extension to the inguinal glands occurs early, and in some cases the femoral glands are also involved. Because of its location deep in the vulva, metastases to the deep lymphatics of the pelvis, including the hypogastric and obturator nodes, are a frequent occurrence. By the time the tumor is recognized clinically, the prognosis is unfavorable, chiefly because early diagnosis is infrequent.

Accurate 5-year survival rates are unavailable, for such statistics are fragmentary in the literature. The prognosis also relates to the histology of the lesion as the squamous tumors may remain localized for longer periods of time and metastasize less frequently, whereas the adenocarcinomas appear more virulent. The relationship of the size of the tumor and the spread to regional lymph nodes has a prognostic significance similar to that of other malignancies of the vulva. From the present survey, a 20 to 30 per cent survival rate would appear to be the most optimistic figure currently available.

The treatment is surgical and consists of a radical vulvectomy and groin dissection (Basset operation) similar to the other types of treatment of carcinoma of the vulva. Supervoltage irradiation therapy may be given, but the results are poor when used alone. The addition of irradiation to the groin and vulvar regions following radical surgery may be beneficial in cases in which the surgical procedure did not encompass the entire disease.

BIBLIOGRAPHY

Barclay, D. L., Collins, C. G., and Macey, H. B., Jr.: Cancer of the Bartholin gland; a review and report of eight cases. Obstet. Gynec., 24:329, 1964.

Basset, A.: Traitement chirurgical opératoire de l'epithelioma primitif du clitoris. Rev. de chir., 46:546, 1912.

Berven, E.: The treatment of cancer of the vulva—Symposium. Brit. J. Radiol., 22: 498, 1949.

Booher, R. H., and McPeak, C. J.: Melanoma. In Nealon, T. F. (ed.): Management of the Patient With Cancer. p. 333. Philadelphia, W. B. Saunders, 1965.

Breisky [ed., Zeitschrift für Heilkunde, Prag.]: Ueber Kraurosis vulvae, eine wenig beachtete Form von Hautatrophie am Pudendum muliebre. Z. Heilk., 6:69, 1885.

Collins, C. G.: Cancer of the vulva. In Marcus, C. C., and Marcus, S. L. (eds.): Advances in Obstetrics and Gynecology. p. 603. Baltimore, Williams & Wilkins, 1967.

Crocker, H. R.: Paget's disease, affecting the scrotum and penis. Trans. Path. Soc. London, 40:187, 1889.

Das Gupta, T., and D'Urso, J.: Melanoma of female genitalia. Surg. Gynec. Obstet., 119:1074, 1964.

Dockerty, M. B., and Pratt, J. H.: Extra-mammary Paget's disease. Cancer, 5:1161, 1952.

Dubreuilh, W.: Paget's disease of the vulva. Brit. J. Derm., 13:407, 1901.

Gardiner, J.: Modified technique of inguinal lymphadenectomy. Obstet. Gynec., 28: 147, 1966.

Gardiner, S. H., Stout, F. E., Arbogast, J. L., and Huber, C. D.: Intraepithelial carcinoma of the vulva. Amer. J. Obstet. Gynec., 65: 515, 1953.

Gosling, J. R. G., Abell, M. R., Drolette, B. M., and Loughrin, T. D.: Infiltrative squamous cell (epidermoid) carcinoma of vulva. Cancer, 14:330, 1961.

Green, T. H., Jr.: Radical vulvectomy. Clin. Obstet. Gynec., 8:642, 1965.

Green, T. H., Jr., Ulfelder, H., and Meigs, J. V.: Epidermoid carcinoma of the vulva;

analysis of 238 cases. I. Etiology and diagnosis. Amer. J. Obstet. Gynec., 75:834, 1958.

Helwig, E. B., and Graham, J. H.: Anogenital Paget's disease. Cancer, 16:387, 1963.

Helwig, E. B.: Cited by Koss, L. G., Ladinsky, S. and Bockunier, A., Jr. In Paget's disease of the vulva. Obstet. Gynec., 31:513, 1968.

Honan, J. H.: Ueber die Carcinome der Glandulae Bartholini, inaugural dissertation. Berlin, 1897.

Hormann, G., and Lemtis, H.: The question of diaplacental metastasis of malignant blastomas in the mother. Z. Geburtsh. Gynaek., 164:1, 1965.

House, T. E., and Hester, L. L., Jr.: Radical vulvectomy for carcinoma of the vulva. Obstet. Gynec., 31:739, 1968.

Hovnanian, A. P.: The evaluation and present status of pelvi-inguinal lymphatic excision. Surg. Gynec. Obstet., 124:851, 1967.

Johnsson, J. E.: Radiation treatment of vulvar cancer. Geriatrics, 19:447, 1964.

Kehrer, E.: Soll das Volvakarzinom operiert oder bestrahlt werden? Geburtsh. Franuenh., 48:346, 1918.

Kelly, H. A.: Operative Gynecology. New York, Appleton, 1898.

Koss, L. G., Ladinsky, S., and Bockunier, A., Jr.: Paget's disease of the vulva. Obstet. Gynec., 31:513, 1968.

Leonard, V. N.: Fibroid tumors of the vulva: a report of 12 cases and a digest of the literature on this subject. Bull. Johns Hopkins Hosp., 28:373, 1917.

Lewis, T. L. T.: Progress in Clinical Obstetrics and Gynecology. London, J. & A. Churchill, 1956.

Lovelace, W. R.: Fibrolipoma of left labium majus. J.A.M.A., 80:375, 1923.

Marcus, S. L.: Basal cell and basal-squamous cell carcinomas of the vulva. Amer. J. Obstet. Gynec., 79:461, 1960.

Marshall, C. M.: The newer gynecology; some of its surgical and anatomical implications. Amer. J. Obstet. Gynec., 65:773, 1953.

Masterson, J. G., and Goss, A. S.: Carcinoma of the Bartholin gland. Review of the literature and report of a new case in an elderly patient treated by radical operation. Amer. J. Obstet. Gynec., 69:1323, 1955.

Matthews, D.: Marsupialization in the treatment of Bartholin's cyst and abscesses. J. Obstet. Gynaec. Brit. Comm., 73:1010, 1966.

Mauclaire, P.: Évidement lympatique bilatéral et néoplastic en bloc pour les cancers du pénis et du clitoris. Tribune Méd. Par., 36:277, 1903.

McKelvey, J.: Malignant tumors of the vulva. In Pack, G. T., and Ariel, I. M. (eds.): Treatment of Cancer and Allied Diseases. vol. 6, p. 69. New York, Paul B. Hoeber, 1962.

McKelvey, J. L., and Adcock, L. L.: Surgical cure of carcinoma of the vulva—relation to stage of tumor. Obstet. Gynec., 26:455, 1965.

Novak, E., and Stevenson, R. R.: Sweat gland tumors of the vulva, benign (hidradenoma) and malignant (adenocarcinoma). Amer. J. Obstet. Gynec., 50:641, 1945.

Novak, E. R., and Woodruff, J. D.: Gynecologic and Obstetric Pathology. ed. 6. Philadelphia, W. B. Saunders, 1967.

Pack, G. T., and Oropeza, R.: A comparative study of melanomas and epidermoid carcinomas of the vulva; a review of 44 melanomas and 58 epidermoid carcinomas (1930-1965). Rev. Surg., 24:305, 1967.

Paget, J.: Disease of the mammary areola, preceding cancer of the mammary gland. St. Bartholomew's Hospital Rep., 10:87, 1874.

Parry-Jones, E.: Lymphatics of the vulva. J. Obstet. Gynaec. Brit. Comm., 70:751, 1963.

Pringle, J. H.: A method of operation in cases of melanotic tumors of the skin. Edinburgh Med. J., 23:496, 1908.

Purola, E., and Widholm, O.: Primary carcinoma of the Bartholin's gland. Report on two cases. Acta Obstet. Gynec. Scand., 45:205, 1966.

Rutledge, F. N.: Cancer of vulva and vagina. Clin. Obstet. Gynec., 8:1051, 1965.

Rutledge, F. N., Smith, J., and Franklin, E.: Experience with the treatment of carcinoma of the vulva. Presented at 80th Annual Meeting of Amer. Assoc. of Obstetricians and Gynecologists, Hot Springs, Va., September 1969.

Sackett, N. B.: Carcinoma primary in Bartholin's gland—five year survivals after radical surgery. Amer. J. Obstet. Gynec., 91:1149, 1965.

Schueller, E. F.: Basal cell cancer of the vulva. Amer. J. Obstet. Gynec., 93:199, 1965.

Smith, G. Van S., and Graves, W. P.: Kraurosis vulvae. J.A.M.A., 92:1244, 1929.

Stoeckel, W.: Wie lassen sich die dauerresultate bei der Operation des Vulvakarzinoms verbessern? Zbl. Gynaek., 36:1102, 1912.

Tancer, M. L.: Bartholin's cysts paraurethral lesions. Clin. Obstet. Gynec., 8:982, 1965.

Taussig, F. J.: Leukoplakic vulvitis and cancer of the vulva (etiology, histopathology, treatment, five-year results). Trans. Amer. Gynec. Soc., 54:60, 1929.

———: Diseases of the Vulva. p. 141. New York, Appleton-Century-Crofts, 1931.

Way, S.: The anatomy of the lymphatic drainage of the vulva and its influence on the radical operation for carcinoma. Ann. Roy. Coll. Surg. Eng., 3:187, 1948.

———: Malignant Disease of the Female Genital Tract. Philadelphia, Blakiston, 1951.

———: Late results of extended radical vulvectomy for carcinoma of the vulva. J. Obstet. Gynaec. Brit. Comm., 73:594, 1966.

Weiner, H. A.: Paget's disease of the skin and its relation to carcinoma of apocrine sweat glands. Amer. J. Cancer, 31:373, 1937.

Wharton, L. R., Jr., and Everett, H. S.: Primary malignant Bartholin gland tumors. Obstet. Gynec. Survey, 6:1, 1951.

Wight, O. B.: Melanoma of the labia. Western J. Surg., 39:98, 1931.

Williams, G. A., Richardson, A. C., and Hathcock, E. W.: Topical testosterone in dystrophic diseases of vulva. Amer. J. Obstet. Gynec., 96:21, 1966.

Williams, K., and Butcher, H. R., Jr.: A technic for inguinal and iliac lymphadenectomy. Amer. Surgeon, 27:55, 1961.

Woodruff, J. D., and Hildebrandt, E. A.: Carcinoma in situ of the vulva. Obstet. Gynec., 12:414, 1958.

Woodruff, J. D., and Richardson, E. H., Jr.: Malignant vulvar Paget's disease. Obstet. Gynec., 10:10, 1957.

32

The Epidemiology of Cancer of the Cervix

The past quarter of a century has witnessed a number of interesting paradoxes in the diagnosis and treatment of cervical cancer. Following Papanicolaou and Traut's classic presentation of "The Diagnosis of Uterine Cancer by the Vaginal Smear" in 1943, the detection of cervical cancer in its earliest presymptomatic phase has reversed the previous clinical finding of 70 per cent invasive cancer with spread beyond the confines of the cervix to the present-day status in which 70 per cent or more of the cervical disease is detected as in situ, or early invasive (Stage 1 A) lesions. At the same time the radiotherapeutic approach to cervical cancer has accelerated from the conventional 250-400 KV beam to the present megavoltage unit including 2 MeV cobalt 60, 6 MeV linear accelerator, and 25 MeV betatron. While the supervoltage therapy units afford greater versatility and deeper penetration in treatment, recent reports from the M. D. Anderson Hospital (1967) show very little difference in survival rates when compared with orthovoltage, stage for stage. Instead, the improvement in cervical cancer cure is better related to the aggressive efforts of early detection by mass screening programs. As recently reviewed by Constable and Truskett, the increased detection of Stage I and II lesions at the expense of Stage III and IV lesions accounts for the overall improvement in survival rates.

When the overall 5-year survival figures are compared between poorly

TABLE 32-1. CANCER OF THE CERVIX: COMPARISON OF STAGE I DISTRIBUTION, STAGE I 5-YEAR SURVIVAL, AND OVERALL 5-YEAR SURVIVAL WITH EFFECTIVENESS OF SCREENING PROGRAM*

AREA	PER CENT OF ALL PATIENTS ALLOCATED TO STAGE I	STAGE I 5-YEAR SURVIVAL	OVERALL 5-YEAR SURVIVAL
		Percentages	
Great Britain	14.3 to 41.0	68.9	40.6
Poorly screened U.S.A.	17.9 to 47.9	72.9	48.5
Well-screened U.S.A.	42.4 to 56.5	82.3	61.9

* Constable, W. C., and Truskett, I. D.: Relationship of cytological screening facilities and cure rate in cancer of the cervix. Brit. J. Radiol., 40:691, 1967.

TABLE 32-2. CANCER OF THE CERVIX: POORLY SCREENED AREAS*

CENTER	FEMALE POPULATION OVER 20 YEARS SCREENED IN STATE ANNUALLY	PATIENTS ALLOCATED TO STAGE I	STAGE I 5-YEAR SURVIVAL	OVERALL 5-YEAR SURVIVAL
	Percentages			
Boston	13	30.7	75.9	50.0
New Orleans	11	21.7	75.6	44.4
Royal Marsden	—	29.4	73.1	43.8
Manchester	—	14.3	68.7	42.1

* Constable, W. C., and Truskett, I. D.: Ibid.

screened and well-screened areas of the United States and Great Britain, it is clear that there is a 21.3 per cent greater overall survival in the well-screened centers (61.9% against 40.6%).

It is equally clear that in centers where less than 14 per cent of the adult female population (over the age of 20) is screened annually (designated "poorly screened"), the overall cure rates are similarly poor in both the United States and England.

In contrast, the well-screened centers in the United States, where 18 per cent or more of the adult female population is screened annually, demonstrate an increased number of early Stage I cases and a resultant overall improvement in the 5-year cure rate.

The M. D. Anderson Hospital demonstrates a variance in the generalized trend toward an increase in the detection of Stage I lesions. Instead, this hospital has a smaller percentage of Stage I cases but an increase in the number of cases allotted to Stage III. However, as discussed later, its survival rates, stage by stage, are excellent and demonstrate the beneficial effect of a major interest of this hospital in the treatment of this disease.

PRESYMPTOMATIC DIAGNOSIS

Additional data concerning the effectiveness of cytologic screening is obtained from the screening program in British Columbia, which has been continued since 1949. The program developed gradually until 1966, at which time approximately 1 out of 5 adult women was screened annually. By the end of 1966, 75 per cent of all women over the age of 20 had been screened at least

TABLE 32-3. CANCER OF THE CERVIX: WELL-SCREENED AREAS*

CENTER	FEMALE POPULATION OVER 20 YEARS SCREENED IN STATE ANNUALLY	PATIENTS ALLOCATED TO STAGE I	STAGE I 5-YEAR SURVIVAL	OVERALL 5-YEAR SURVIVAL
	Percentages			
Los Angeles	19	42.4	85.7	63.6
Seattle	26	53.7	73.8	59.9
San Francisco	19	56.5	80.7	65.3
M. D. Anderson	18	13.9	92.7	63.2
New Haven	18	44.1	78.7	57.6

* Constable, W. C., and Truskett, I. D.: Ibid.

once. This data, as reported by Fidler, Boyes, and Worth (1968), documents a decreased rate of invasive cancer of the cervix of more than 50 per cent between 1955 and 1966: the incidence of invasive carcinoma dropped from a rate of 28.4 per 100,000 female population to the present rate of 13.6. This decline is due to the detection and elimination of a large number of patients with carcinoma in situ and premalignant lesions. This fact is supported by the observation of a rate of clinical cancer in 4.8 per 100,000 women screened as contrasted with a rate of 28.6 in the unscreened population.

In the British Columbia population, the ultimate effect of the screening program in the reduction of the overall mortality rate of the disease has only recently become evident. Unfortunately, mortality data is often inaccurate. Consequently, this group has refined the death figures by obtaining clinical and pathological information on all patients in the province who had the diagnosis of carcinoma of the cervix or carcinoma of the genital tract included on the death certificate. By so doing, many of the deaths unrelated to carcinoma have been excluded, and a refined mortality rate is more meaningful and shows a definite decline in recent years from 11.8 per 100,000 population (1958) to 7.8 per 100,000 (1966). This and other data previously presented support the thesis that in situ carcinoma of the cervix is a precursor of invasive carcinoma, and that its removal from a population will result in a significant lowering of the morbidity and mortality of this disease.

In the State of New York, where an expanding cervical cancer screening program has been in existence since 1955, an increasingly higher rate of in situ cases has been detected (45.8% of all cervical cancer in upstate New York in 1963). The incidence rate of invasive cancer has steadily decreased, as has the mortality rate from this disease. Factors other than early diagnosis have obviously influenced this mortality rate for New York State, as the sharp decline began in 1945, 10 years before the onset of the state screening program, and the slope of the curve has been uninfluenced by the impact of the population screening program. The American Cancer Society reports that during the 33-year interval between 1931 and 1963, 520,000 deaths occurred in the United States from cancer of the uterus. Had the 1933 death rate from cancer of the uterus prevailed, there would have been approximately 715,000 deaths from this disease. Thus approximately 200,000 women may have been saved from death from uterine cancer, a result which is attributable primarily to the effect of the cytologic screening programs in this country.

In comparing the average cost of screening a patient for cervical cancer with the average cost of treatment for this disease, some amazing comparisons are evident. In the State of New York, the average cost of screening is $4.00 per head, with a case finding load of 4 per 1,000 patients screened. This cost amounts to approximately $1,000 per detected case. The total cost of investigation and treatment of a patient with early carcinoma of the cervix, according to Clark (1960), is $1,611.80. The cost of investigating and treating late stage cases is $2,536.92 per person. The average cost of treating a patient in New York State who does not survive is more than $33,000. The cost of diagnosing and treating a patient with an early case of cervical cancer is reduced 30 times as compared with the cost of treating a patient with a late stage of the disease, in which the patient will not survive even with our best efforts.

A number of population studies in the United States and Canada provide sufficient data for a fairly accurate evaluation of the pathogenesis of cervical cancer. Studies in British Columbia and Memphis reveal that the prevalence rate for carcinoma in situ is centered between the ages of 30 and 45. The incidence rate, as determined from the second and subsequent rescreenings, demonstrates a much earlier occurrence of carcinoma in situ between the ages of 20 and 29. It seems apparent that carcinoma in situ may remain dormant for 10 years or more in a presymptomatic state prior to invasion.

The cumulative evidence from the Aberdeen, Scotland, screening program, which includes 56,000 women, indicates a progression from carcinoma in situ through a microinvasive stage before overt clinical cancer occurs. Macgregor states that this may take as long as 20 years. In this study the highest incidence of positive smears was found from 10 to 19 years after first coitus, and the highest incidence of clinical cancer was 30 to 39 years after marriage. When preclinical microinvasive cancer was found, it required an average of 4.1 years to reach the point at which symptoms lead to diagnosis.

In a mass population screening program in Washington County, Maryland, initiated in 1963, Davis and Jones have utilized the irrigation vaginal smear technic. Cell material collected by women themselves provided cytologic examinations from over 61,000 women. Following a screening program of women between the ages of 30 and 45, the invasive cervical cancers now appear primarily from the unscreened population. In the 5 years since the program was initiated, only 3 invasive cancers were observed per 10,000 women at risk after detection and treatment of the preinvasive disease. In the unscreened population, the risk of invasive cancer was 80 per 10,000 women at risk, or 27 times greater than that in the screened population. The magnitude of this difference in rates of invasive cancer is so great that there can be no doubt of the effectiveness of the cancer control program.

In view of the convincing evidence of the effectiveness of cervical cancer screening programs for the early detection of carcinoma of the cervix, it is regrettable that no more than 20 per cent of the adult female population receives annual cytologic examinations. Even more regrettable is the fact that a large portion of this figure includes patients receiving regular annual examinations who are in a high socioeconomic category, where this disease is least frequent. How, then, can we anticipate screening the entire female adult population, which currently includes 61 million women, in order to control cervical cancer effectively? It has been estimated that to achieve this mammoth task, it would require the full-time professional services of every member of the American College of Obstetricians and Gynecologists 6 hours and 30 minutes each day of the year to do Papanicolaou smears and pelvic examinations. Obviously, the task cannot be achieved by our present medical manpower. There are several alternatives, however, which are immediately available and could be effectively implemented:

1. Nonprofessional, technical personnel, either technicians or nurses, could be trained for the purpose of obtaining the Papanicolaou smear as a mass population screening program. Mobile health units, which currently include minature chest x-rays and immunizations, could serve as a means of obtaining a Papanicolaou smear.

2. The irrigation vaginal smear, self-obtained by the patient, which has been effectively documented by Davis and Jones in Maryland to be an accurate screening method, is an additional method of mass population screening for cervical cancer. In addition to Davis and Jones, Mattingly, Boyd, and Frable have recently confirmed the effectiveness of this technic. A major objection to this method is the fear that the patient will obtain a false sense of security concerning the status of the remaining pelvic organs. This can be at least partially overcome by including, with the irrigation material, literature telling the woman just what the smear will do and what it will not do. One of the supporting features of the irrigation smear is the requirement that the patient must obtain the cytology report from her gynecologist or family physician.

3. Approximately 8 million adult females are admitted annually to hospitals in the United States for a variety of medical and surgical conditions. It is obvious that this group represents a large segment of the female population who would have a unique opportunity to obtain a Papanicolaou smear by a physician, nurse, or technician. At present less than

15 per cent of all adult females receive a pelvic examination and Papanicolaou smear as a part of the admission physical examination. The enactment of hospital rules to require a cytologic examination of all females admitted to a hospital, similar to the requirement for a routine chest x-ray, would provide the impetus necessary for the total control of cervical cancer.

ETIOLOGY

An increasing body of evidence identifies the sexual act as a major etiologic factor in the pathogenesis of cervical cancer. Since the classic report of Gagnon in 1950, which reviewed the death certificates of 13,000 nuns in French Quebec with no reported case of cervical cancer, the role of coitus, circumcision, human smegma, age of marriage, and age of first coitus have been intensively investigated as etiologic factors of this disease.

Convincing evidence is now available that identifies the act of coitus and prolonged exposure to coitus by marriage earlier than the age of 20 as significant factors in the future development of cervical cancer. In addition, multiple marriages and multiple sexual consorts have been shown statistically to be related to cervical cancer. The significance of coitus is further documented by Nix in a recent retrospective study of hospital records and autopsies of 100,000 Catholic nuns, among whom there was only 1 death due to squamous cell cancer of the cervix in a 93-year-old nun, and 7 cases of endometrial cancer were detected. Of 1,000 nuns who received the irrigation smear and pelvic examination as a part of a routine health examination, there has been no case of cervical cancer detected. Celibacy would therefore seem to protect the female from cervical cancer, a virtue which would probably not sell well on this basis alone.

Christopherson and Parker present evidence in a studied population of 38,939 women that 38.6 percent of this group married before the age of 20, and this high risk group accounted for 61 per cent of the detected cases of invasive cancer and 57 per cent of in situ disease. The 6.8 per cent of women who never married accounted for only 1.5 per cent of the cases of invasive cancer. The first pregnancy occurred before the age of 20 in 25 per cent of the cases, and these cases accounted for 48 per cent of all of the invasive cervical cancer. Over 64 per cent of patients with invasive cervical cancer began sexual activity in their teens.

Rotkin, from the Kaiser Foundation Hospital, has recently reviewed the association of adolescent coitus and cervical cancer. He concludes his survey of 416 cervical cancer patients and matched controls with the following formula:

For women who have experienced at least one coital act, where coitus began during adolescence, where there was more than one marriage and/or coital mate, who are derived from a non-Caucasian population and are of non-Jewish origin, risk is greatest. For prevention on population levels, educational programs may not be impossible. It is well known that the adolescent girl generally benefits little in any sense by sexual exposure and that early coital as well as marital beginnings are disadvantageous for her from many points of view.

Such evidence concerning the venereal origin of cervical cancer is difficult to refute. While recent evidence produced by Masters and Johnson demonstrates the fact that the coital act does not produce trauma to the ectocervix, the sexual experience, by some chemical means or another, does seem to have a carcinogenic influence. Data is inadequate at the present time on women who have continually utilized the vaginal diaphragm for family planning purposes, which would protect the cervix from semen and the coital act; such data might provide additional information on this subject.

The fact that cervical cancer is extremely rare among Jewish women is thought to result from both genetic and hygienic factors. The hypothesis is that this is due to circumcision of the male, but in the Arab population, among whom circumcision is also a religious ritual, cervical cancer is as common as in the non-Jewish population throughout the world. The Moslems of India, where circumcision is practiced at a later age than among the Jews, have a decreased incidence as compared with the Hindus, whose men are not circumcised. The Fijians, who practice circumcision, have a decreased rate of cervical cancer as compared to Indians, who do not practice circumcision. Cervical cancer is also uncommon among the Parsees of India, who do not practice circumcision, but who keep their genitalia scrupulously clean. The evidence for and against circumcision is thus inconclusive at this time.

BIBLIOGRAPHY

Bryans, F. E., Boyes, D. A., Boyd, J. R., and Fidler, H. K.: The cytology program in British Columbia. III. Management of preclinical carcinoma of the cervix. Canad. Med. Assoc. J., 90:62, 1964.

Bryans, F. E., Boyes, D. A., and Fidler, H. K.: The influence of cytological screening programs upon the incidence of invasive squamous cell carcinoma of the cervix in British Columbia. Amer. J. Obstet. Gynec., 88: 898, 1964.

Christopherson W. M., and Parker J. E.: Relation of cervical cancer to early marriage and childbearing. New Eng. J. Med., 273: 235, 1965.

Clark, R. L.: Introduction. In Carcinoma of the Uterine Cervix, Endometrium and Ovary. Fifth Annual Clinical Conference on Cancer, 1960, at the University of Texas M. D. Anderson Hospital and Tumor Institute, Houston, Texas. p. 9. Chicago, Year Book Medical Publishers [1962].

Constable, W. C., and Truskett, I. D.: Relationship of cytological screening facilities and cure rate in cancer of the cervix. Brit. J. Radiol. 40:691, 1967.

Davis, H. J.: Personal communication.

Davis, H. J., and Jones, H. W., Jr.: Population screening for cancer of the cervix with the irrigation smear. Amer. J. Obstet. Gynec., 96:605, 1966.

Dorn, H. F., and Cutler, S. J.: Morbidity from cancer in the United States. PHS Publ. No. 590 (Public Health Monogr. No. 56). Washington, D.C., Government Printing Office, 1959.

Dunn, J. E., Jr.: The presymptomatic diagnosis of cancer with special reference to cervical cancer. Proc. Roy. Soc. Med., 59:1198, 1966.

Dunn, J. E., Jr., and Martin, P. L.: Morphogenesis of cervical cancer. Findings from San Diego County Cytology Registry. Cancer, 20:1899, 1967.

Friedell, G. H., Hertig, A. T., and Younge, P. A.: Carcinoma in Situ of the Uterine Cervix. Study of 235 Cases in the Free Hospital for Women. Springfield, Ill., Charles C Thomas, 1960.

Fidler, H. K., Boyes, D. A., and Worth, A. J.: Cervical cancer detection in British Columbia. J. Obstet. Gynaec. Brit. Comm., 75:392, 1968.

Gagnon, F.: Contribution to study of etiology and prevention of cancer of cervix of uterus. Amer. J. Obstet. Gynec., 60:516, 1950.

Gray, L. A.: Dysplasia, Carcinoma in Situ and Micro-Invasive Carcinoma of the Cervix Uteri. Springfield, Ill., Charles C Thomas, 1964.

Greene, H. J., Oppenheim, A., and Olswang, A. Results of routine Papanicolaou smears in two venereal disease clinics in New York City. Acta Cytol., 9:319, 1965.

Haenszel, W.: Cancer mortality among the foreign born in the United States. J. Nat. Cancer Inst., 26:37, 1961.

Haenszel, W., and Hillhouse, M.: Uterine cancer morbidity in New York City and its relation to the pattern of regional variation within the United States. J. Nat. Cancer Inst., 22:1157, 1959.

Horn, D., and Watanabe, G.: Report on a national survey of cytologic facilities. CA, 15:161, 1965.

Kennaway, E. L.: Racial and social incidence of cancer of the uterus. Brit. J. Cancer, 2:177, 1948.

Kmet, J., Damjanovski, L., Stucin, M., Bonta, S., and Cakmakov, A.: Circumcision and carcinoma colli uteri in Macedonia, Yugoslavia. Brit. J. Cancer, 17:391, 1963.

Kottmeier, H.-L. (ed.): Annual Report on the Results of Treatment in Carcinoma of the Uterus and Vagina. vol. 13. Stockholm, published under the patronage of the International Federation of Gynecology and Obstetrics; sponsored by American Cancer Society, et al., 1963.

Lemon, F. R., Walden, R. T., and Woods, R.

W.: Cancer of the lung and mouth in Seventh-Day Adventists. Cancer, 17:486, 1964.

Levin, M. L., Haenzel, W., Carroll, B. E., Gerhardt, P. R., Handy, V. H., and Ingraham, S. C.: Cancer incidence in urban and rural areas of New York State. J. Nat. Cancer Inst., 24:1243, 1960.

Martin, C. E.: Marital and coital factors in cervical cancer. Amer. J. Public Health, 57:803, 1967.

Masters, W. H., and Johnson, V. E.: Human Sexual Response. Boston, Little, Brown & Co., 1966.

Mattingly, R. F., Boyd, A., and Frable, W. J.: Vaginal irrigation smear: a positive method of cancer control. Obstet. Gynec., 29:463, 1967.

Macgregor, J. E.: Cervical cancer, the beginning of the end? Lancet, 2:1296, 1967.

Naguib, S. M., Lundin, F. E., Jr., and Davis, H. J.: Epidemiologic factors related to cervical cancer detected by a screening program in Washington County, Maryland. Obstet. Gynec., 28:451, 1966.

Nix, J. T.: Personal communication.

Pemberton, F. A., and Smith, G. Van S.: The early diagnosis and prevention of carcinoma of the cervix. Amer. J. Obstet. Gynec., 17:165, 1929.

Pereyra, A. J.: The relationship of sexual activity to cervical cancer. Obstet. Gynec., 17:154, 1961.

Reagan, J. W., and Wentz, W. B.: Genesis of carcinoma of the uterine cervix. Clin. Obstet. Gynec., 10:883, 1967.

Røjel, J.: The interrelation between uterine cancer and syphilis. Acta Path. Microbiol. Scand. (Suppl.) 97:3, 1953.

Rotkin, I. D.: Adolescent coitus and cervical cancer: associations of related events and increased risk. Cancer Res., 27:603, 1967.

Slate, T. A., and Merritt, J. W.: Discussion. In Symposium on Cervical Lesions. Acta Cytol., 6:185, 1962.

Wynder, E. L., Cornfield, J., Schroff, P. D., and Doraiswami, K. R.: A study of environmental factors in carcinoma of the cervix. Amer. J. Obstet. Gynec., 68:1016, 1954.

Wynder, E. L., Lemon, F. E., and Bross, I. J.: Cancer and coronary artery disease among Seventh-Day Adventists. Cancer, 12:1016, 1959.

33

Carcinoma in Situ of the Cervix

Three fundamental questions regarding carcinoma in situ require answers. When the correct answers to these questions are at hand, much progress will have been made in the prevention of invasive cervical cancer. These questions are:
1. What is carcinoma in situ?
2. What is the relation between carcinoma in situ and invasive cervical cancer?
3. How should the condition be treated?

The answers to the third question should be based on sound histologic and clinical evidence and a correlation of the first two answers.

THE MICROSCOPIC PICTURE

The first question—what is carcinoma in situ?—will be answered briefly, and then the microscopic evidence to support this definition will be presented. *Carcinoma in situ* is a term that should be applied to a microscopic picture of the surface cervical epithelium in which the individual cells through the full thickness of the epithelial layer have the same characteristics as those of invasive cancer.

As a point of departure, the microscopic picture of the normal cervical epithelium should be reviewed. Figure 33-1 is a typical section. Upon the basement membrane, immediately adjacent to the fibromuscular stroma of the cervix, is a layer of fat spindle cells, the nuclei of which are oval and take a deep hematoxylin stain. The cytoplasm of these cells also stains lightly with hematoxylin. Just superficial to these cells there usually is a layer or two of cells which stain lightly basophilic. As one progresses toward the surface, the cells become polyhedral. The nuclei still stain with hematoxylin, but the cytoplasm takes a light eosin stain. Still more superficially the cells become flattened, and although the nuclei stain with hematoxylin, the cytoplasm stains rather deeply pink. The most superficial cells are completely flattened and keratinized. In short, there is a gradual transition in form and staining qualities between the perpendicular basal spindle cells and the horizontally flattened superficial cells.

In carcinoma in situ there is a complete

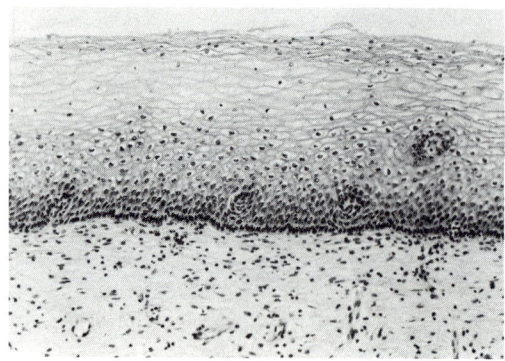

FIG. 33-1. Normal cervical epithelium. Note the stratification from deepest layer of basal cells to superficial flattened spinal cells.

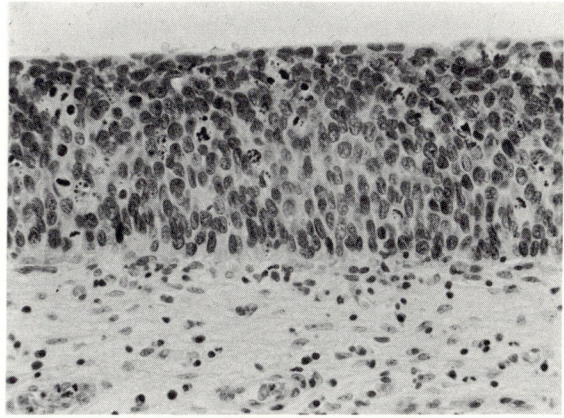

FIG. 33-2. Showing complete loss of stratification and distribution of atypical cells and mitotic figures through full thickness of epithelium.

absence of this stratification. The individual cells vary in size and shape, and the nuclei, which are also variable in form, tend to be larger in relation to the cells than those of the normal cells. Many of the nuclei stain heavily with hematoxylin, and mitotic figures are frequent. This microscopic picture, if seen in the depth of the cervix or in a metastatic position, would mean cancer to the eye of any pathologist. Figures 33-2 to 33-4 illustrate typical examples.

The transition between carcinoma in situ and normal cervical epithelium is often abrupt. The line of demarcation may be perpendicular, as in Figure 33-5, or oblique, as in Figure 33-6. On the other hand, the transition between the normal epithelial cells and the abnormal may be gradual, but when the entire thickness of the surface epithelium is composed of the cells that are abnormal, the ultimate picture is that of intra-epithelial carcinoma.

There is another microscopic picture in which the hyperactive cells are limited to the deeper portions of the surface epithelium. We have chosen to call this picture "basal cell hyperactivity." All degrees of this abnormal cellular activity are found. Figure 33-7, for example, shows only hyperactive-looking cells in the basal layers, whereas the upper layers of cells retain their normal char-

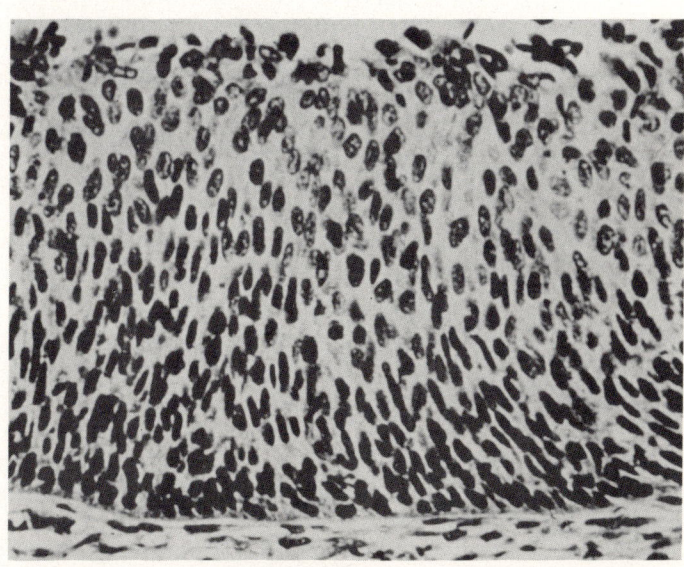

FIG. 33-3. Carcinoma in situ (high-power view).

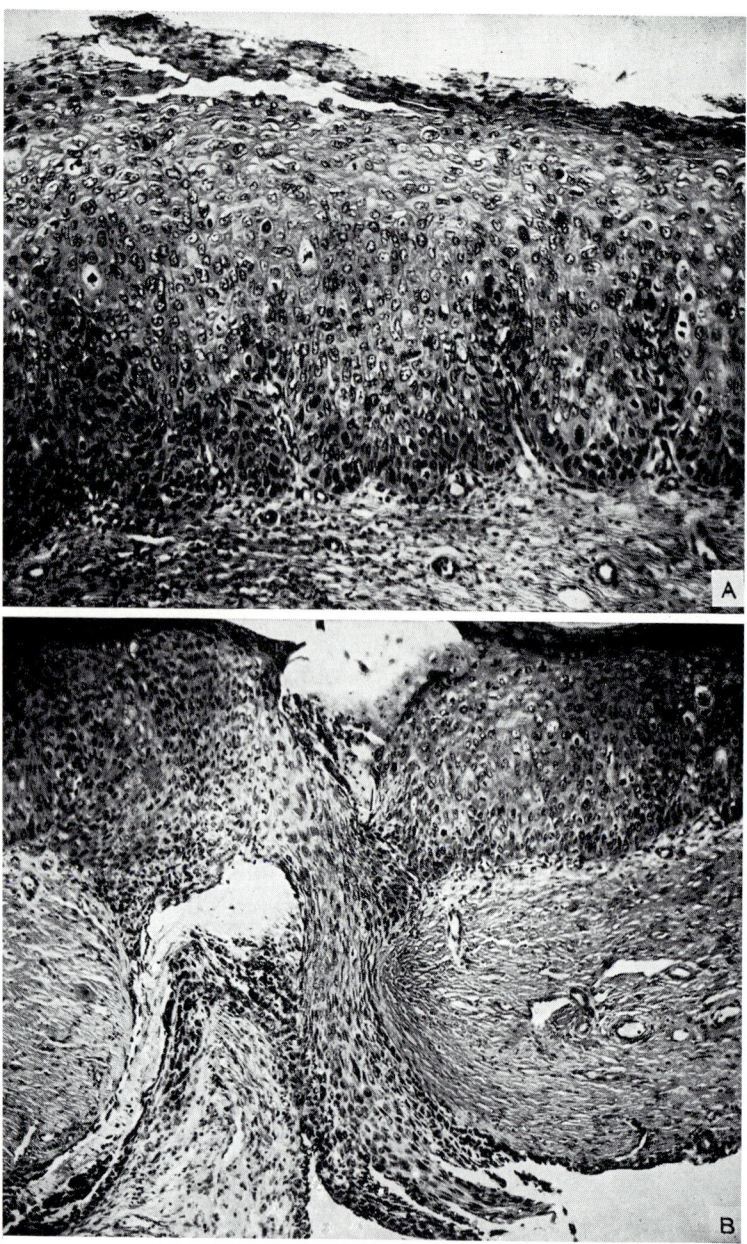

Fig. 33-4. (A) Carcinoma in situ. (B) Section from the same case, showing surface cancer growing into lumen of the gland.

acter and stratification. Figure 33-8 shows a much higher degree of involvement of the epithelium with hyperactive cells, and the transition from abnormal to normal cells is gradual, but the more superficial cells appear to be perfectly benign. Since there are all degrees of involvement of the surface epithelium with hyperactive cells, naturally there will arise differences of opinion about its significance.

The microscopic description of carcinoma in situ would not be complete without calling attention to a lesion which sometimes is confused with it. We refer to epidermidization or squamous cell

The Microscopic Picture 711

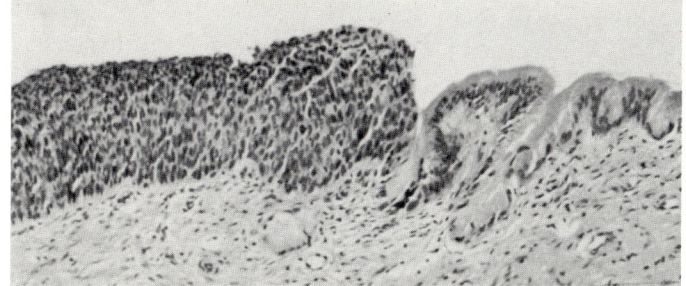

FIG. 33-5. Showing definite perpendicular line between abnormal (*left*) and normal epithelium (*right*).

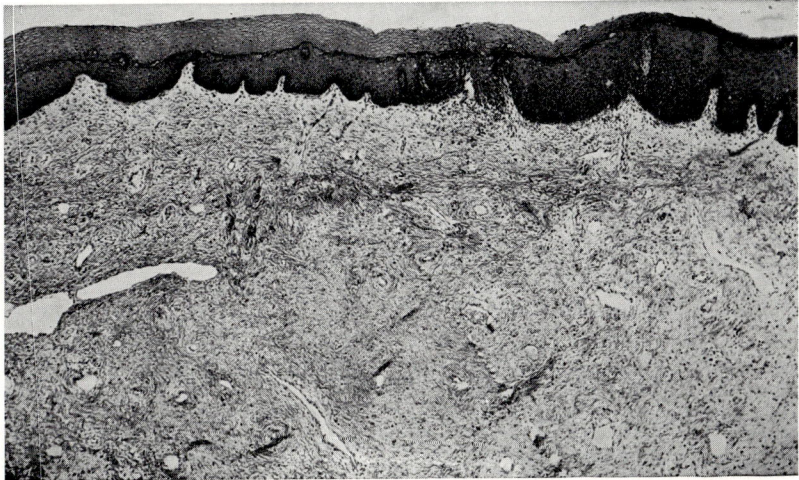

FIG. 33-6. Oblique line of demarcation between carcinoma in situ on the right and normal epithelium superficially on the left.

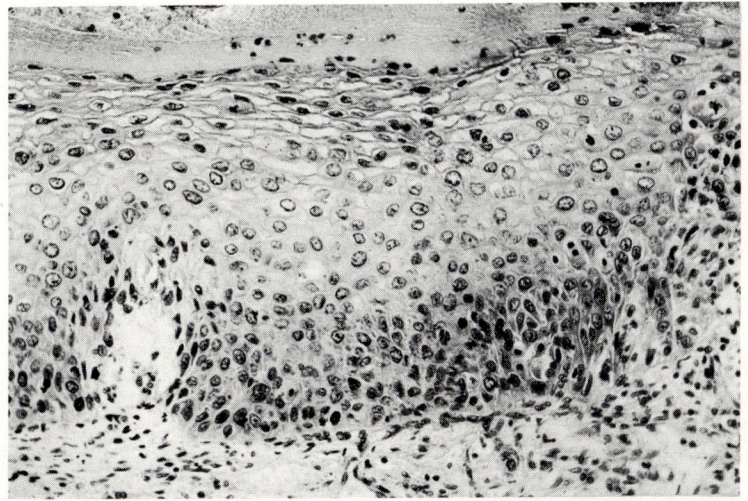

FIG. 33-7. Slight basal cell hyperactivity of cervical epithelium.

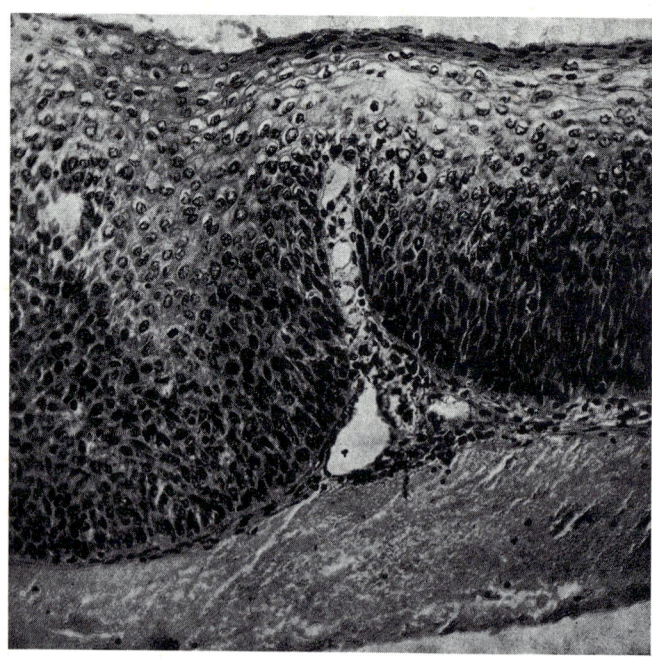

FIG. 33-8. Moderate basal cell hyperactivity or dysplasia of cervical epithelium.

metaplasia. This condition is found in many chronically infected cervices and especially in cervical polyps. Replacing the columnar epithelium on the surface and in the depths of the glands is multi-layered squamous-like epithelium. Often the cells are vacuolated and otherwise atypical but do not contain the hyperchromatic nuclear changes and mitoses seen in intra-epithelial cancer. Although greatly distorted, some semblance of stratification of the atypical cells remains.

The description is best made by photomicrographs, such as Figures 33-9 and 33-10. Replacement of all of the columnar epithelium of glands is not uncommon, and the picture may be suggestive of invasion; but careful examination under high-power magnification of the individual cells will show them to be of a benign character. The final differentiation, as in all malignancy, is made by clinical follow-up of women showing this condition. The authors have done this

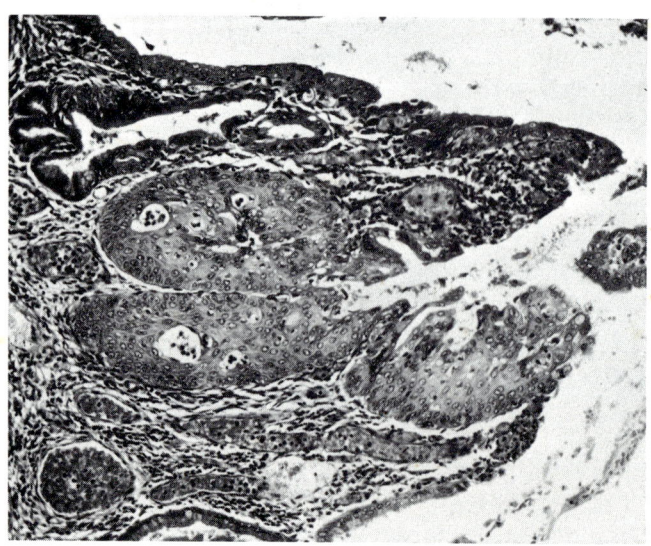

FIG. 33-9. Epidermidization displacing cervical glands well into cervix.

PLATES 6 to 8

PLATE 6

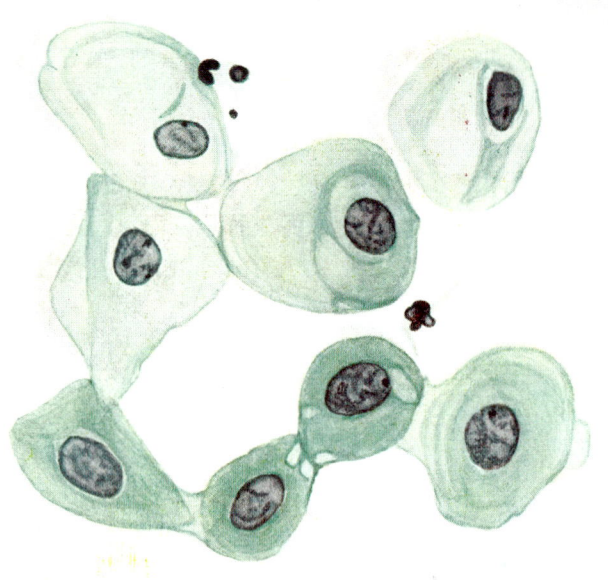

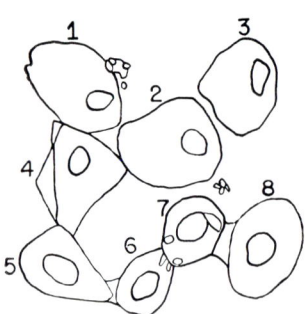

KEY TO BASAL CELL PLATE

1. Outer layer basal, vesicular nucleus, thin transparent cytoplasm.

2. Outer layer basal, finely granular nucleus, unevenness in density of cytoplasm.

3. Outer layer basal, degenerate, partially pyknotic nucleus, perinuclear vacuole.

4. Early precornified cell, showing square shape and folding of transparent cytoplasm.

5. Outer layer basal, oval nucleus, cellular form slightly elongated.

6 and 7. Inner layer basals, dense cytoplasm showing beginning of vacuolization, round vesicular nuclei.

8. Outer layer basal, with central nucleus containing finely divided chromatin. (Graham, Ruth M.: The Cytologic Diagnosis of Cancer. ed. 2. Philadelphia, W. B. Saunders, 1963)

PLATE 7

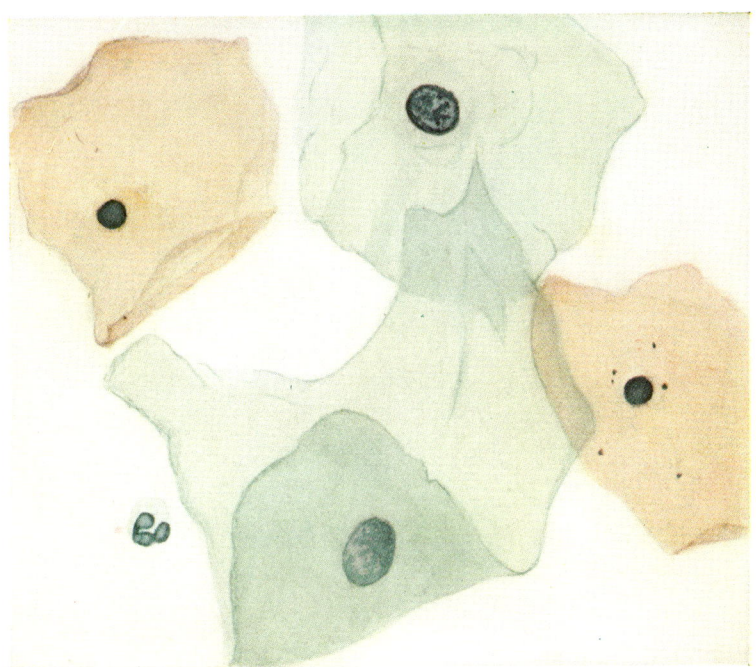

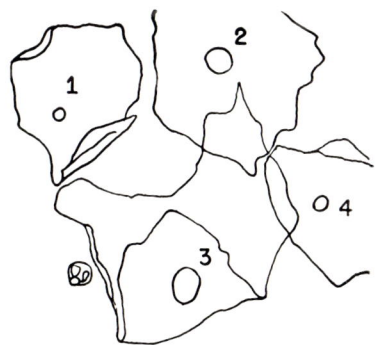

KEY TO CORNIFIED AND PRECORNIFIED
CELL PLATE

1. Flat cornified cell with pyknotic nucleus and fairly even cellular border.

2. Precornified cell showing wrinkled, transparent cytoplasm and a vesicular nucleus.

3. Precornified cell with large amount of folded transparent cytoplasm and bland nucleus.

4. Cornified cell with small dense nucleus, irregular cytoplasm with granules, and evidence of a perinuclear vacuole. (Graham, Ruth M.: *Ibid.*)

PLATE 8

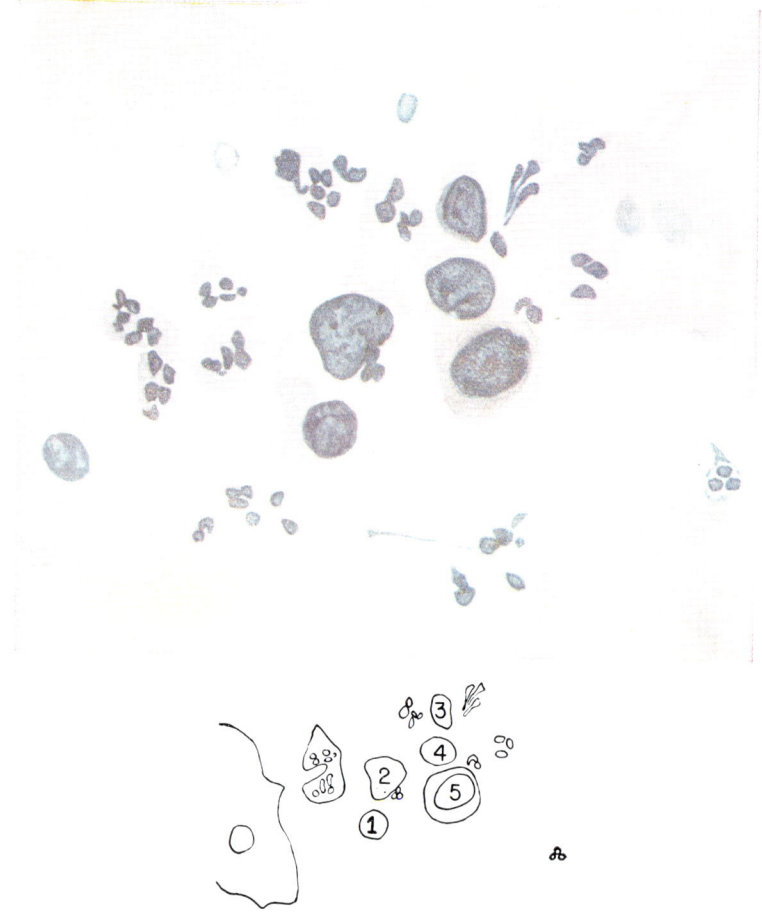

KEY TO SQUAMOUS CELL CANCER PLATE

1. Round, undifferentiated malignant cell with a clear nuclear border, strands of chromatin and no visible cytoplasm.
2. Large, triangular-shaped undifferentiated cell showing prominent clumps of chromatin and a sharp nuclear border.
3. Undifferentiated cell with two obvious clumps of chromatin. This nucleus is smaller than the rest. There is no cytoplasm.
4. Slightly irregular, but definite nuclear border. Coarse clumps of chromatin and no cytoplasm.
5. Undifferentiated cell with a dense hyperchromatic nucleus and a small amount of cytoplasm with an indistinct cell border. The rest of the field contains cornified and precornified cells and leukocytes. (Graham, Ruth M.: *Ibid.*)

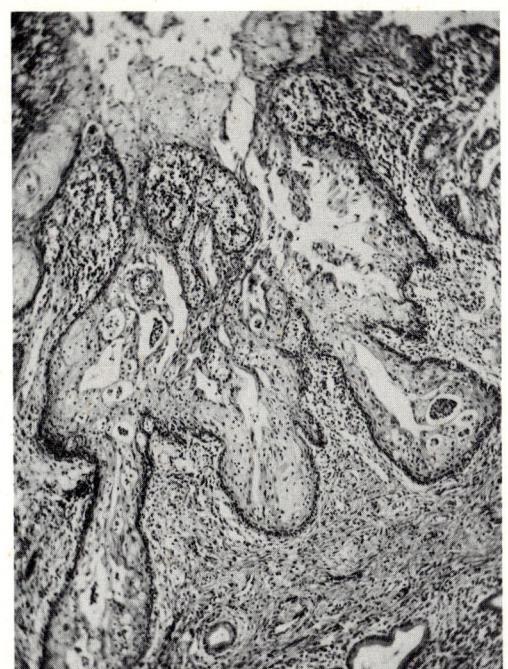

FIG. 33-10. Nonmalignant cervical lesion. Although cancer-like in appearance, it is benign epidermidization.

over several years and have found no evidence that these lesions eventuate in malignancy. Uncertain pathologists have straddled their decision by calling such lesions precancerous, but there is no evidence that they bear any relation to cancer.

The above descriptions represent our conception of the microscopic picture of carcinoma in situ and other conditions related to or confused with it. The histologic conception of intra-epithelial cancer means nothing unless its relation to true cervical cancer can be proved. Hence we shall attempt to answer our second question on the relation of carcinoma in situ to invasive cervical cancer.

THE RELATION OF DYSPLASIA TO CARCINOMA IN SITU

Advances in the field of cytopathology have produced impressive correlations between the morphologic changes of the desquamated cell from the cervix and that observed by biopsy and conization. Although it is not within the scope of this volume to be concerned with the details of cytology, Plates 6, 7, and 8 give an excellent idea of typical cervical cytology patterns, Plates 6 and 7 showing normal cells and Plate 8 showing malignant squamous cells.

Many new cytologic definitions have arisen in the past decade; one of the most frequent in relation to cervical cancer is that of dysplasia. Dysplasia has a number of interpretations which vary from such terms as "borderline lesion," "precancerous metaplasia," and "atypical epithelial hyperplasia" to "basal cell hyperactivity." Previous studies by Galvin, Jones, and Te Linde attempted to correlate the relationship between basal cell hyperactivity and carcinoma in situ. Their study, as have many other studies, demonstrated that the more severe the dysplasia, the more frequent is the finding of carcinoma in situ (Fig. 33-11). Other retrospective and prospective studies of cervical dysplasia indicate a varied outcome of the dysplastic epithelium (Fig. 33-12). Of the "borderline lesions" described by Koss, only 40 per cent progressed to carcinoma in situ, whereas 38 per cent disappeared. Stern and Neely reported progression of dysplasia to carcinoma in situ in 12 per cent of their cases, whereas 40 per cent regressed to normal and 49 per cent persisted as dysplasia. In all of these studies, however, there is criticism of the requirement for repeated cervical biopsies, which may interfere in the progress of the lesion or remove a small focus completely. Certainly, conization of the cervix destroys any prospective experiment to determine the outcome of early epithelial lesions. Reagan, however, takes an opposite view and states that women with dysplasia of the cervical epithelium are no more likely to develop carcinoma in situ or invasive carcinoma than are those without dysplasia. He considers the outcome of dysplasia to be unpredictable. In a recent discussion on the genesis of carcinoma, Reagan reports on 1,261 cases of dysplasia occurring primarily in the premenopausal woman. Only in the presence of estrogen

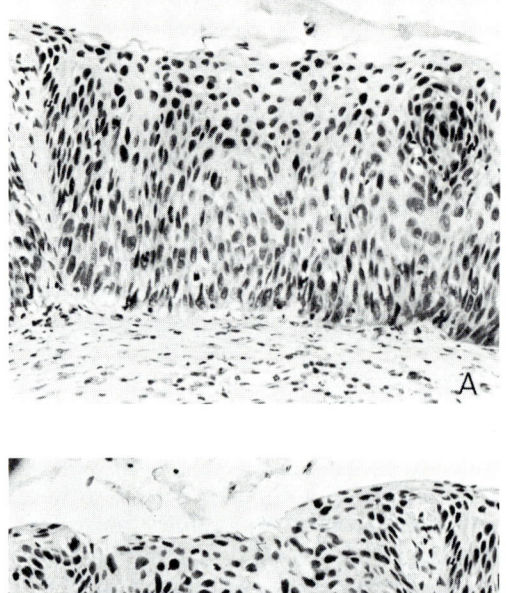

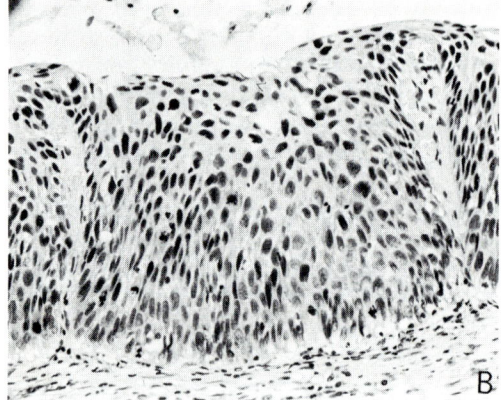

Fig. 33-11. (A and B) Severe dysplasia of cervix with epithelial changes extending through most of the surface epithelium but lack of full-thickness change for diagnosis of carcinoma in situ.

quently found to have carcinoma in situ, and 0.9 per cent were ultimately proven to have invasive squamous cell carcinoma. In an effort to eliminate the possible effects of biopsy, an additional 120 women with dysplasia were followed only by cytology studies. In this group, 60 per cent of the women had dysplastic lesions that regressed, 38.3 per cent had lesions that persisted, whereas 1.7 per cent of the women were ultimately found to have carcinoma in situ. Reagan's study showed no relation between the severity of the dysplasia and its potential development of carcinoma in situ.

In contrast to the above statistics, Richart followed 750 patients with abnormal smears and repeated cytologic

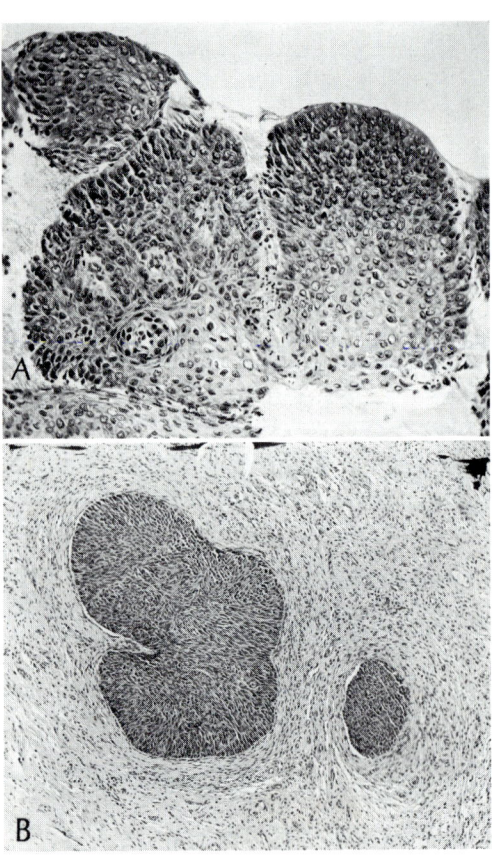

Fig. 33-12. Relation of basal cell hyperactivity to invasive carcinoma. (A) Original biopsy, showing carcinoma in situ. (B) Section from tissue obtained by conization 1 week later, showing microscopically invasive carcinoma.

is such a lesion found in the postmenopausal female, suggesting that estrogen may be a factor in the development of this lesion. In evaluating the topography of the uterine cervix for the location of dysplastic epithelium, Reagan defines a band-like zone encircling the cervical canal at the squamocolumnar junction. This area was found to overlap the distribution of carcinoma in situ, which is slightly higher in the endocervical canal.

His study included 221 women with follow-up histology, of whom 48.9 per cent were subsequently found to have no residual dysplasia, and 43.9 per cent had lesions that persisted as dysplasia, whereas only 6.3 per cent were subse-

examination and colpomicroscopy, which avoided the criticism of biopsy studies. His work suggests that approximately 30 per cent of all patients with cervical dysplasia progress to carcinoma in situ within 2 years.

The question may be critically posed, therefore: What is the true significance of the cytologic diagnosis of cervical dysplasia? Regardless of the conflicting reports in the literature, it is our interpretation that cervical dysplasia should serve as a "red flag" to the clinician, making him acutely aware of cellular atypia. Whether due to infection, trauma, intra-uterine contraceptives, or other causes, it should be investigated. The importance of follow-up studies of atypical cervical epithelium cannot be overstressed. Repeated cytologic studies with multiple cervical biopsies, utilizing the Schiller iodine stain, are essential. In the event that the suspicious cytology persists on repeated examination, and there is histologic evidence of dysplasia from cervical biopsies, more intensive studies of the cervix with colposcopy and directed biopsy or conization of the cervix are required.

THE RELATION OF CARCINOMA IN SITU TO INVASIVE CANCER

The first portrayal of carcinoma in situ in the world literature is in Cullen's volume *Cancer of the Uterus,* published in 1900. It is designated as a case of early cervical cancer. On the basis of the cytologic changes Cullen assumed that it was cancer, although there was no invasion of the subjacent tissues. In 1910 Isador Rubin described and pictured 2 cases, microscopically identical with Cullen's, and labeled them "incipient carcinoma." In 1912 Schottländer and Kermauner described the same microscopic picture in the surface epithelium surrounding advanced cervical cancer (Figs. 33-13 and 33-14). This has been observed repeatedly since then, extending about the periphery of the invasive growth. Schottländer and Kermauner considered this to be a method of extention of the growth.

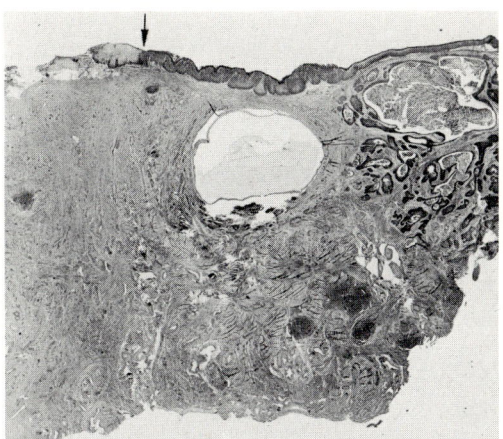

FIG. 33-13. Low-power section of entire lip of cervix. The dark surface epithelium on the right is carcinoma in situ. The bit of epithelium on the left is normal (arrow). Deep in the section on the right is extensive glandular involvement and true microscopic invasion. Grossly this cervix appeared to be normal.

To Schiller belongs the credit for the original thought that cancer of the cervix might begin as a surface lesion, remaining on the surface for a considerable time before eventually invading the stroma. He presented some clinical evidence to support his view that this surface lesion was actually early cancer. Such evidence consisted of reported deaths following recurrence after total hysterectomy for lesions which were thought to be in situ.

Since 1950 several workers, notably Younge, Pund, Blumberg, Galvin, and the senior author, have made histologic studies in an attempt to answer the question regarding the relationship of carcinoma in situ to invasive cancer. There is general agreement among these workers that carcinoma in situ is often a precursor of the invasive lesion, but there is some disagreement as to the microscopic interpretation of "invasion." Galvin and the senior author undertook a histologic study on cervices that had been removed following a biopsy diagnosis of carcinoma in situ. The removed cervices were cut up completely in blocks, and many sections were made of each block in a search for microscopic

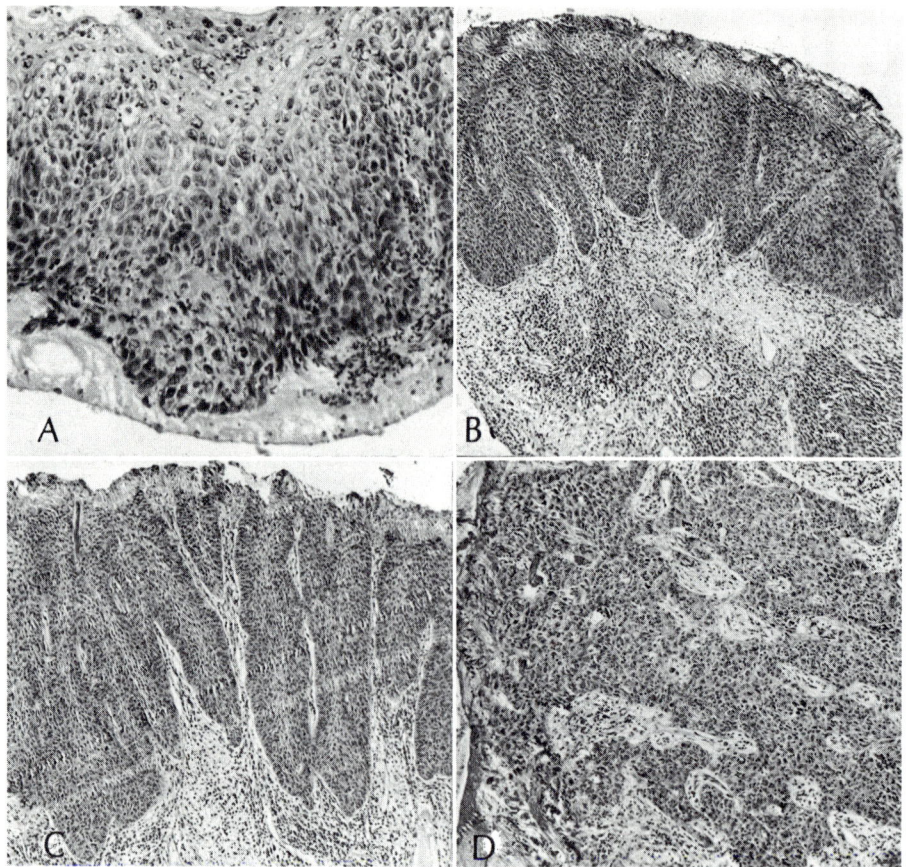

Fig. 33-14. Demonstration of progression from carcinoma in situ to invasive cancer. (A) Carcinoma in situ as found in biopsy. ×200. (B) Carcinoma in situ as found in removed cervix. ×100. (C) Early invasive cancer adjacent to B. (D) Advanced microscopic invasive cancer adjacent to C.

invasive cancer. In a total of 108 cases, there were 72 in which atypical cells which appeared to be malignant were found beneath the surface epithelium. Many were within gland lumina, but in some instances they were definitely within the stroma. Glandular involvement is not true invasion; nor is it equivalent to the filling of the gland with benign cells, as is seen so frequently in epidermidization (Fig. 33-9). In epidermidization, growth stops when the gland lumen is full. In carcinoma in situ this is not the case. Figure 33-15, for example, shows masses of malignant epithelial cells beneath the surface epithelium, which is also malignant. In approximately the center of the field is a gland which is filled with malignant cells, with destruction of almost all of the columnar epithelium. A bit of columnar epithelium remains, sufficient to show that this plug of cancer cells is "glandular involvement."

Pathologists differ in their opinion on where glandular involvement stops and invasion begins, but in the authors' opinion invasion occurs when the mass of tissue exceeds the reasonable limits of a gland. Also, it appears from our studies that unquestionable stromal invasion follows glandular involvement. Figure 33-13 demonstrates the close relationship between glandular and stromal invasion. In some cases unquestionable stromal invasion seems to proceed directly from the surface epithelium, as in Figure 33-14.

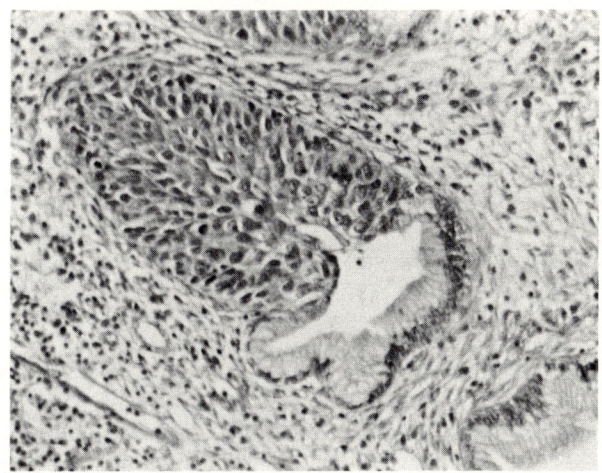

FIG. 33-15. Carcinoma in situ with glandular involvement showing neoplastic epithelium "snowplowing" beneath glandular epithelium and filling of the gland lumen.

From the above cited work it is evident that the finding of carcinoma in situ in a biopsy many indicate three possibilities as regards the condition of the entire cervix:

1. That the biopsy was taken from the periphery of an advanced cervical cancer, as described by Schottländer and Kermauner.
2. That the carcinoma in situ is limited to the surface epithelium.
3. That microscopic glandular involvement or true stomal invasion is present.

It is obvious that in order to know the true status of the cervix, one must leave no stone unturned in getting all possible data. Needless to say, the cervix should be carefully inspected and palpated, and all suspicious tissue biopsied for study. This may reveal a truly invasive lesion. If this is not found, the cervix should be studied thoroughly by colposcopy or conized as described under technic in Chapter 20. A curettage of the uterine cavity should be done after the cone is taken. The cone should be cut into multiple blocks, and many sections taken from each block. It is only by meticulous examination of these sections that one can learn the true condition of the cervix. This fact is best exemplified by a recent study of Burghardt from Graz, where cases with 15 routine sections taken from a conization specimen were restudied by taking 80 additional sections from the coned cervix. In the restudied cases there was a 22 per cent error found in the original diagnosis. Even with these precautions there will be occasional failures to learn the extent of the lesion. For example, in one instance the lesion which was intra-epithelial on the cervix extended the entire length of the uterine cavity and became invasive at the fundus. Such a case is, of course, most unusual, but it does illustrate the necessity of complete investigation.

It appears that little, if any, more information on the relation of carcinoma in situ to invasive cervical cancer can be gained by simple histologic study. Therefore we must turn to clinical studies to see what evidence can be found. Such studies began with the evidence presented by Schiller when he reported 1 recurrence after 5 years and 2 recurrences before the lapse of 5 years following hysterectomy for this lesion. Galvin and the senior author reported 1 death following irradiation for what appeared to be carcinona in situ. The death occurred 6 months after treatment, and necropsy showed metastatic cancer. However, conization was not performed routinely in these earlier studies. There are more than 40 cases in the literature of clinically advanced cancer in which a review in retrospect of previous biopsies showed intra-epithelial cancer. One may object to this type of evidence on the theory that it is coincidental. A recent review of our cases reported by Galvin,

Jones, and the senior author would seem to refute this objection. These investigators examined the hospital records of the 723 cases of cervical cancer treated in our therapy clinic for the years 1940 to 1950 inclusive. It was found that 13 of them had had previous cervical biopsies from 1 to 17 years before. Three of these 13 cases were International Stage 0, and the remaining were Stage I to Stage III. The paraffin blocks of the biopsies were still available and were sectioned serially. Of these 13 cases, 11 showed intra-epithelial cancer in the sections thus obtained. In the 12th case there was marked basal cell hyperactivity, and in the 13th case no surface epithelium could be found in the sections. These findings would indicate that invasive cervical cancer is preceded by noninvasive cancer in a high percentage of the cases.

It would seem that there often is a latent period of several years during which the intra-epithelial cancer exists before becoming truly invasive. As evidence of this is the fact that the average age of women with intra-epithelial cancer is about 10 years less than that of women presenting themselves with invasive cancer. In Galvin and the senior author's series the average age of the women with intra-epithelial cancer was 37.1 years; in Pund's series, 36.6 years; and in Younge's series, 38 years. The average age of women with clinical cancer is 48 years. The longest reported interim between the biopsy showing carcinoma in situ and invasive cancer was 17 years, as reported by Galvin, Jones, and the senior author.

The study of Peterson of Copenhagen throws further light on this question. He kept under observation 127 patients without treatment who had been diagnosed by biopsy as having carcinoma in situ. All were followed for at least 3 years; 104 (82%) for at least 5 years; and 38 (30%) for a minimum of 10 years. After 1 year's follow-up 4 per cent of the untreated patients had developed manifest carcinoma of the cervix; at the end of 3 years, 11 per cent; at the end of 5 years, 22 per cent; and at the end of 9 years, 33 per cent. At the time of his report 34 of the 127 patients had developed cancer. In 10 the disease was still microscopic; in 17, in Stage I; in 4, in Stage II; in 2, in Stage II, and in 1, in Stage IV. A similar report from Copenhagen by Lange revealed that 24 per cent of 100 patients developed invasive carcinoma while under observation.

From the evidence presented by Galvin and the senior author and that of Peterson, it is evident that invasive cervical cancer is often preceded by carcinoma in situ. This is not equivalent to saying that carcinoma in situ invariably becomes invasive. In fact, it is quite obvious that some women will die of intercurrent disease before the development of the invasive disease. In fact, 8 of Peterson's patients died of other causes within 10 years after the diagnosis of preinvasive cancer had been made.

Naturally, the question arises: Does intra-epithelial carcinoma *invariably* become invasive? Galvin, Jones, and the senior author have reported 3 such cases with intervals of 6, 4, and 3 years. However, since these studies were conducted primarily by biopsy, it is possible that the invasive lesion was present at the time of the original biopsy.

The best evidence to date concerning the frequency of invasion of carcinoma in situ is indirect and comes from population screening programs. During the 20-year interval from 1942 to 1961, there has been a gradual but steady decline in the mortality from carcinoma of the cervix in British Columbia (Boyes), where approximately 75 per cent of the adult female population has been screened. This has resulted in a decline of clinical invasive carcinoma of about 50 per cent. From these and other data there is suggestive evidence that approximately 50 per cent of all cases of carcinoma in situ will become invasive if untreated.

With the passage of time, since the publication of the third edition of this book, we have accumulated further evidence regarding the relationship of carcinoma in situ and invasive cancer in the form of recurrences following hysterectomy. Among 690 cases treated by the modified Wertheim hysterectomy or total hysterectomy in our clinic since 1944, we have had 7 recurrences (1%). In 3 of these the lesion recurred as an invasive lesion, and in 4 as an in situ lesion. These recurrences present further evidence of the true malignant nature of this disease.

The above facts may leave the clinical gynecologist somewhat confused as to the course to be taken when a diagnosis of carcinoma in situ is made by biopsy or suspected from a positive smear taken from a relatively normal-looking cervix. Today most cases are discovered as the result of a positive or suspicious cervical smear. First, the cervix should be biopsied. We do this instead of proceeding directly with conization, because invasive cervical cancer may be discovered, making conization unnecessary. Conization is a simple surgical procedure, but it is not entirely innocuous with reference to subsequent treatment by hysterectomy or irradiation. Younge has been a strong advocate of cervical biopsy with a sharp, square-jawed biopsy punch and endocervical curettage with a narrow, sharp curette. His recent report (Griffiths and Younge) from the Boston Hospital for Women includes his total experience since initiating this program in 1936. In 248 patients with biopsy-diagnosed carcinoma in situ and microinvasive cancer, the incidence of unsuspected invasive cancer is 0.4 per cent (1 patient), which is an achievement difficult to contest.

One should remember in biopsying the cervix that the pathologist can judge only from the tissue under his microscope. Therefore a random biopsy means very little from a relatively normal-looking cervix. Directed biopsy of a suspect lesion by colposcopic visualization of the cervix is the most accurate method of studying the abnormal cervix. If this is not available, several biopsy specimens should be taken around the circumference of the squamocolumnar junction after meticulous inspection of the cervix *before* and *after* staining with Gram's iodine solution (Schiller test). In addition, 2 or 3 bites should be taken from within the cervical canal. This may be impossible with the nulliparous cervix and in the contracted postmenopausal cervix, and this difficulty is a shortcoming of biopsying versus conization.

If the biopsy specimens show invasive cancer, the case is classified as Stage I and treated with irradiation or surgery. If the biopsy shows carcinoma in situ or no malignancy, a conization should be done promptly. Sections of the cone will usually reveal the site and the extent of the lesion. If nothing is found, the patient should be followed with further smears. If they remain permanently negative, one may dismiss the thought of malignancy; but if they persist as positive, further cervical tissue should be removed by biopsy and curettage until the lesion is located.

The question arises whether a persistently positive smear ever justifies a hysterectomy in the absence of positive evidence by biopsy or curettage. We have emphasized that histologic evidence should be had before treatment. This is important for two reasons: (1) The smear may be falsely positive. (2) It is important to know as exactly as possible the location and the extent of the lesion. It should be emphasized that a positive smear never constitutes an emergency, and ample time may be taken for a thorough investigation. However, even after thorough and repeated investigations, nothing may be located, and there comes a point when the emotional trauma of the patient must be considered. We have on a rare occasion performed a hysterectomy under such circumstances after prolonged observation. In spite of the most meticulous examination of the removed uterus, no malignancy may be found. Nevertheless, we believe that the hysterectomy was justified in this case, but such cases are extremely rare if all measures are taken to locate the source of the malignant cells seen in the smear.

DIAGNOSIS

Today most cases of carcinoma in situ are discovered by evidence found in the routine use of the Papanicolaou smear for all adult females over the age of 20. At Johns Hopkins Hospital from 1940–44 only 26 per cent of cervical carcinomas were found in the in situ or Stage I classification, whereas by 1960–61 this statistic had risen to 69 per cent. At Marquette-Milwaukee County General Hospital, 20 per cent of all cases of carcinoma of the cervix were detected as Stage 0 or Stage I from 1940–49, whereas during the 6-year period from 1960 through 1965, 74 per cent of all cases were detected as in situ or Stage I lesions (Fig. 33-16).

Although the Papanicolaou smear has made the greatest contribution to date of any available clinical tool for the early detection and control of cervical cancer, it cannot be regarded as infallible. Too frequently, clinicians rely completely on the report of a single cytologic smear examination as evidence of the absence of genital cancer, even though the patient may continue to have symptoms. We simply do not know the true false-negative rate of the Papanicolaou smear, and the only authoritative information on this point comes from mass population screening programs, in which repeat

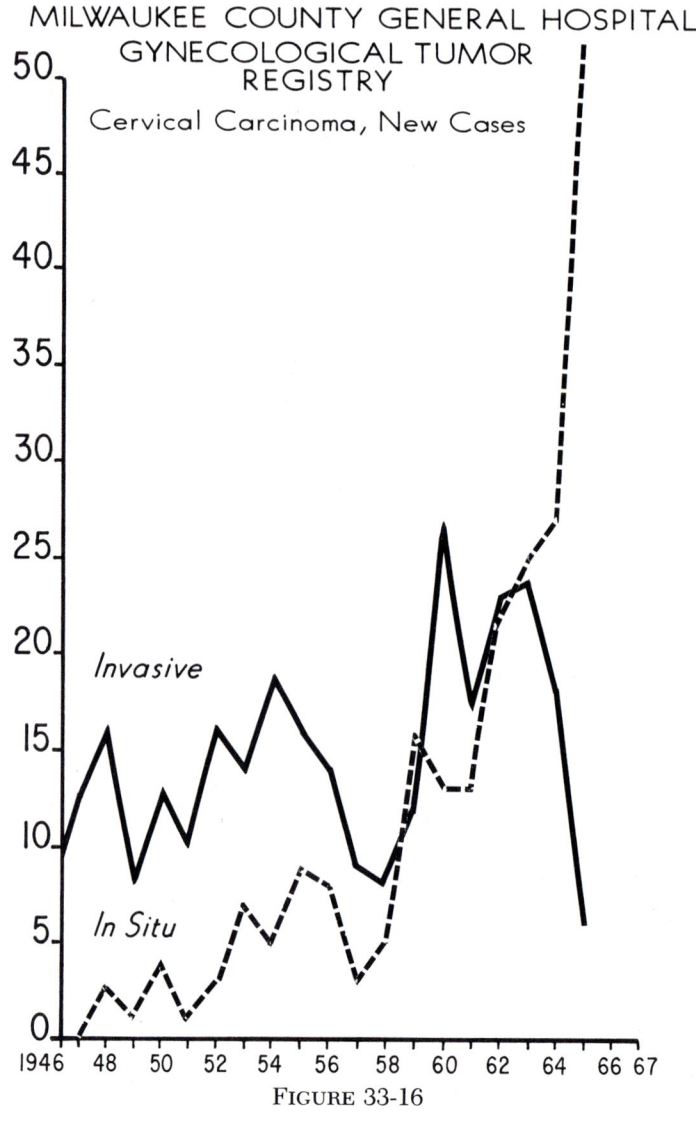

FIGURE 33-16

cytologic examinations on an annual basis demonstrate an error in the original smear in more than 15 per cent of the cases. A recent report from M. D. Anderson Hospital by Singleton, Grant, and Rutledge reveals a 21.1 per cent false-negative rate for the initial Papanicolaou smear where cervical biopsy revealed carcinoma in situ. In addition, 19.7 per cent of the cases with negative Papanicolaou reports in 518 patients later proved to have Stage I carcinoma by cervical biopsy.

The false-negative rate, however, cannot be directed only to the cytology laboratory, but the accuracy of cancer screening must be a shared responsibility between the clinician and the cytopathologist. An inadequate cell sample is the most common cause of incorrect cytologic diagnoses, and, in general, the Papanicolaou study is no better than the clinician who takes the smear. Unless the smear includes a full sample of cells from the posterior fornix, as well as a complete circumferential scrape of the squamocolumnar junction, it is impossible for the cytopathologist to give an accurate interpretation. Therefore any suspicious cervical lesion should have not only a Papanicolaou smear but an adequate cervical biopsy immediately at the time of observation.

The cervical biopsy is frequently obtained by outlining the abnormal cervical epithelium with the Schiller iodine stain. Biopsies should include a complete circumferential sample with no less than 4 to 6 generous biopsies. Even this, however, is not always adequate for complete evaluation of the cervix, and many reports have criticized the adequacy of the cervical biopsy alone in establishing a diagnosis of the presence or absence of cervical cancer.

Singleton, Grant, and Rutledge reported that cervical biopsy alone failed to detect carcinoma in situ in 13.2 per cent of the cases in which further conization detected the disease, while 14.3 per cent of the Stage I carcinomas were incorrectly diagnosed by biopsy alone and were later diagnosed by conization. Silbar and Woodruff in the Hopkins Gynecological Pathology Laboratory recently reported on the evaluation of the biopsy, cone, and hysterectomy sequence for carcinoma in situ and revealed a false-negative rate of the initial Papanicolaou smear of 18.2 per cent of 110 patients. In their entire study of 124 patients, only 75.8 per cent of their cases of carcinoma in situ were diagnosed on the initial biopsy. Only 1 case, however, was entirely negative, whereas the remainder showed some degree of cellular atypia.

Continued atypical or suspicious Papanicolaou smears, in the absence of histologic evidence of cancer, require further study by colposcopy with directed biopsy or full evaluation of the cervix by conization. The recent use of colposcopy in demonstrating areas of dysplasia as the cause of suspicious cytology has greatly reduced the frequency of conization of the cervix. It is lamentable that cervical biopsy is frequently bypassed in the presence of an abnormal smear in preference for immediate conization. Since biopsy will detect 85 to 90 per cent of invasive lesions of the cervix, only a small group of patients with early *invasive* carcinoma require conization.

Conization is not an innocuous procedure, and unless it is performed by a competent and experienced person, there can be serious complications such as serious hemorrhage, requiring transfusion in 5 to 10 per cent of the cases; perforation of the uterus; pelvic cellulitis, and injury to the rectum and bladder. The latter complications are usually in cases in which there is extreme atrophy with obliterated vaginal fornices. The recent use of a weak solution of Neo-synephrine (1:200,000) has greatly reduced the incidence of hemorrhage and provides adequate time for the surgeon to perform a cold-knife conization of the cervical canal to the region of the internal os, while including a 2-cm. margin of the ectocervix. The confines of the lesion should be identified prior to the cone with Schiller's stain. No attempt should be made to dilate the cervix prior to the cone, and only gentle sounding of endocervix and uterine cavity to identify the direction of the canal is considered advisable to avoid removing the fragile cervical epithelium prior to the cone. If the cone has been adequate, a differential curettage will add little to endometrial curettage alone, but if there is suspicion of an endocervical or endometrial lesion, a differential curettage can be accomplished prior to placing Sturmdorf sutures in the anterior and posterior lip of the cervix. Many clinics have recommended the use of frozen-section evaluation of the cone specimen in order that the operative procedure may be carried out immediately upon receiving the report from the pathologist.

The use of the cone-cryostat procedure has been in vogue for many years at the Mayo Clinic and is now receiving more widespread use in recent years. Clinical experience with the conization-hysterectomy sequence has shown that the morbidity rate is lowest when the hysterectomy is performed either immediately or within 48 hours of the conization; otherwise the hysterectomy should be deferred for a period of 6 weeks postconization. The most frequent complication of postconization-hysterectomy is pelvic cellulitis and hematoma formation resulting from the spread of bacteria in the paracervical lymphatics and tissue friability.

COLPOSCOPY*

Although colposcopy was developed by Hinselmann in 1925, and the method is a standard procedure in most European clinics, it has gained acceptance in the United States only within the past decade. The earlier evolution of cytology in this country and the lack of personnel skilled in the use of the colposcope have tended to delay its wider utilization.

Basically, the colposcope provides a magnified inspection of the squamocolumnar juncture or transformation zone of cervical epithelium. This is the area of histologic epidermidization in which the advancing edge of squamous epithelium gradually replaces the original columnar epithelium (showing ectopy or eversion), visible on the ectocervix in 85 per cent of premenopausal women.

Cervical neoplasia is first manifest in the transformation zone, and once the clone of abnormal cells has expanded to replace a few millimeters of the original columnar epithelium, the neoplastic tissue, penetrating between the original columnar capillary loops, produces characteristic vascular patterns, e.g. punctation, mosaicism, or an atypical transformation zone. In addition, localized exuberant growth of the neoplastic epithelium may produce zones of whitish or grayish-white appearance (leukoplakia). The use of green filters, Schiller's solution, and 2 per cent acetic acid provide additional information.

Colposcopy has proven of definite value in managing cases of atypical or positive cytology by making possible an independent evaluation of the severity and extent of the lesion, and by improving the precision of biopsies for histologic appraisal. Adequate colposcopic inspection, combined with directed biopsies, permits sampling of the "heart" of the lesion and more precise exclusion of significant invasion. Of the 152 invasive carcinomas of the cervix treated at the Johns Hopkins Hospital from 1963 through 1967, only 7 cases of microinvasion were discovered by conization which had been previously unsuspected by colposcopy and biopsy. Only 2 cases of frank invasive carcinoma were discovered primarily by conization: in one case colposcopy was omitted, and in the second case conization was recommended because of colposcopically suspected invasion despite biopsy reports of lesser severity. Thus, over 99 per cent of significant invasive carcinoma has been diagnosed by appropriate biopsies.

The procedure is obviously of little value in that small fraction of cases with high endocervical localization, which is therefore inaccessible to inspection

---

* The section on Colposcopy was written by Dr. Hugh J. Davis, Assistant Professor of Gyn-Obstetrics, International Health, and Population and Family Health, and Gynecologist-Obstetrician in the Department of Gynecology and Obstetrics, School of Medicine, Johns Hopkins University.

PLATE 9

PLATE 9

Colposcopic findings in cervical neoplasia.

(A) Case 2. Low-power view of anterior lip showing multiple gland openings and islands of columnar epithelium in transformation zone. Very delicate mosaicism is present, compatible with atypia in metaplasia.

(B) Case 4. Low-power view of anterior lip of cervix showing a portion of atypical transformation zone characterized by ground-glass appearance. There was contact bleeding on procurement of material from this area.

(C) Case 5. Low-power view of left anterior lip of cervix showing an agar-strip marker between focal zone of neoplasia and squamous epithelium. Punctation in lesion cannot be appreciated at this magnification. Macular lesions due to trichomonas are seen on portio.

(D) Case 5. Low-power view of right anterior lip of cervix showing a sharp-bordered focal lesion with punctation. Area between India ink tattoo marks was sampled for histology.

(E) Case 6. Low-power view of anterior lip of cervix showing a pattern of punctation with some areas of mosaicism compatible with Stage O carcinoma. Distinct border between this lesion and normal squamous epithelium is not seen in this view.

(F) Case 6. High-power view of cervix showing details of pattern of punctation and mosaicism in focal lesion. Tattoo marks delineate zone from which biopsy was obtained.

(G) Case 7. Low-power view of cervix showing a sharp-bordered, slightly raised focal lesion occupying half of anterior lip. Elevated mosaic pattern can be seen in upper part of lesion.

(H) Case 7. High-power view of edge of lesion at external os demonstrating detail of markedly atypical vessels compatible with invasive carcinoma. Branching of vessels is distinctly abnormal. (Jones, H. W., Jr., Katayama, K. P., Stafl, A., and Davis, H. J.: Chromosomes of cervical atypia, carcinoma in situ, and epidermoid carcinoma of the cervix. Obstet. Gynec., 30:795, 1967)

PLATE 9

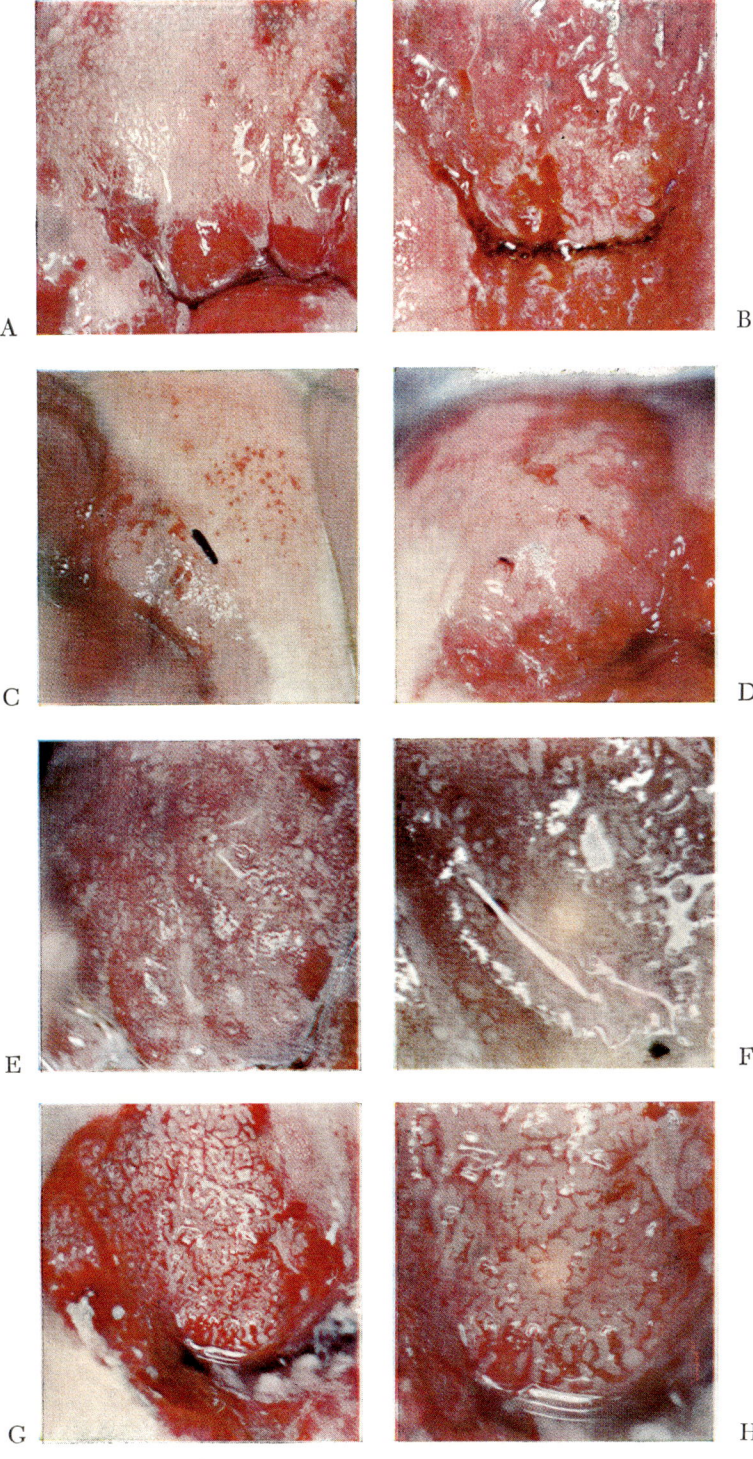

and biopsy. But if used judiciously, with careful weighing of cytologic and histologic patterns, colposcopy is a most useful adjunct in the management of cervical neoplasia.

TREATMENT

The standard treatment of carcinoma in situ has been a rather radical removal of the uterus, including an ample vaginal cuff. In patients over 40 we remove the adnexa, but in younger women ovaries are conserved since there is no hazard with the preinvasive disease. Prior to the routine use of conization of the cervix for evaluation of possible early stromal invasion, our surgical procedure for carcinoma in situ included dissection of the paracervical tissue medial to the lower ureter. This extensive procedure, which is best performed with ureteral catheterization, may no longer be considered essential for well-defined carcinoma in situ, following conization. Recent experience has shown that this surface disease can be adequately managed by a simple hysterectomy with removal of a 3-cm. vaginal cuff or more if the Schiller stain shows more vaginal involvement.

In cases in which there is adequate uterine descensus and vaginal relaxation, a vaginal hysterectomy with removal of an adequate mucosal cuff may be performed. The wider hysterectomy demonstrated in this chapter, however, is considered most useful in those cases of Stage I A carcinoma of the cervix in which there is early microinvasion that does not require a lymphadenectomy. As a matter of fact, the original development of the modified Wertheim hysterectomy was specifically designed for those cases in which prior to surgery early stromal invasion may have been unrecognized by means of cervical biopsy alone. If microinvasion has been ruled out by conization, the wider operation is not necessary. The importance of an adequate vaginal cuff is an essential part of this operation, in order to avoid recurrence of the disease in the upper vagina, which may result from extension from the in situ lesion of the cervix or the multicentric origin of the in situ disease. Topek, who has recently reviewed the recurrence rate of carcinoma in situ, records 48 reported cases of in situ recurrence in the vaginal cuff or invasive carcinoma from 2,614 patients treated for carcinoma in situ. This incidence of 1.65 per cent recurrence in the vaginal vault, which does not include all of the cases that have occurred, probably represents the approximate frequency, namely, 2 per cent.

In recent years interest in the conservative treatment of carcinoma in situ by therapeutic conization of the cervix has grown. Perhaps the largest experience in the use of conization for the treatment of carcinoma in situ has been that of Krieger at the Cleveland Clinic. Krieger's most recent experience includes 433 patients treated for carcinoma in situ during the period 1950 through 1966. His premise is that there is no truly definitive treatment for this disease, and that conization, which is necessary for diagnosis, also constitutes sufficient treatment in the majority of cases. Krieger bases the need for hysterectomy on those cases in which follow-up cytology reveals persistently abnormal cells. In his study, 314 cases were treated with conization alone, whereas an additional 100 had either a hysterectomy or its equivalent. Unfortunately, 20 patients (6.5%) treated only with conization were lost to follow-up. This occurred in a socioeconomic group which was considered highly responsible. In addition, 2 patients died of cervical carcinoma 5 and 6 years postconization who refused follow-up care. The Cleveland Clinic technic of "radical" conization utilizes a Heyman cautery cone attachment for conization of the endocervix following conization. Apparently there is minimal bleeding and only 5½ per cent incidence of postoperative stenosis. In a total group of 414 patients who underwent conization, 20 patients were lost to follow-up study, while 36 of the remaining 394 cases had persistent or progressive cervical disease. Hence conization failed in primary treatment of carcinoma in situ of the cervix in 9.1 per cent of the 394 patients. Yet one cannot ignore the 20 patients lost to follow-up and the 2 cases of death from progressive cancer who refused follow-up care. A similar conservative report by McLaren from England shows that conservative treatment of 151 patients with conization was considered adequate in 82 per cent of the cases, and that follow-up observation is being continued. However, a 10 per cent loss of patients to follow-up is a similar criticism of this study.

Because there is nearly 100 per cent cure of this disease if treated by hysterectomy initially, conization should be considered only for those patients who are genuinely interested in future childbearing, and in whom there is assurance of reliability for continued follow-up care.

Many studies demonstrate residual carcinoma in situ in the hysterectomy specimen following conization, varying in incidence from 21 to 47 per cent. Silbar and Woodruff found residual carcinoma in situ in 21.7 per cent of the postconization-hysterectomy specimens, while Singleton, Grant, and Rutledge found 37 per cent carcinoma in situ. An even higher percentage is found in patients during pregnancy. It is obvious, therefore, that hysterectomy for carcinoma in situ with removal of an adequate vaginal cuff remains the most acceptable primary method of treatment of this disease in most cases.

TREATMENT OF RECURRENCES

There is a reported incidence of approximately 2 per cent recurrence of carcinoma in situ in the vaginal vault (Topek). Our own experience at Johns Hopkins Hospital since 1944 includes 690 cases treated either by a modified Wertheim hysterectomy or by a simple total hysterectomy. We have had 7 vault recurrences to date (1%), 3 of which have recurred as an invasive lesion (although conization was not done routinely in earlier years). Several other reported cases have developed invasive cancer following treatment for carcinoma in situ. Some of these might have been avoided if a Schiller test or colposcopic examination of the cervix and upper vagina had been performed on all cases preoperatively to ascertain the extent of the lesion. If the recurrence is in the form of invasive cancer, it should be treated as indicated in Chapter 34. If the recurrent lesion is still in situ, the lesion may be treated with equal success with either partial vaginectomy or irradiation. We have used both methods, and all of our cases are living and well to date. Our personal preference is for partial vaginectomy, but if the patient strongly desires a more adequate vagina, we have used irradiation. The use of vaginal ovoids to the vaginal vault is a most satisfactory method of treatment. Invasive carcinoma should be treated by both radium and external irradiation therapy. If the in situ recurrence is sufficiently extensive to require complete vaginectomy, it is best started from below as shown in Figure 33-17.

MICROINVASIVE CARCINOMA

Since the last edition of this textbook, the International Classification of carcinoma of the cervix has been modified to include a separate clinical classification of early Stage I lesions. As adopted at the Congress of the International Federation of Gynecology and Obstetrics in September 1961 in Vienna and effective January 1962, Stage I carcinoma has been officially subdivided into Stage I A and I B. As outlined previously, Stage I A includes early stromal invasion (preclinical carcinoma), or microinvasive carcinoma. This substage of the International Classification is further defined thus:

... a case should be allotted to Stage I A only following microscopic diagnosis of the *earliest* stromal invasion performed before planned treatment. Stage I A represents that group of cases of carcinoma of the cervix which can only be diagnosed microscopically following biopsy. They have often formerly been called microcarcinoma. In the remainder of Stage I cases a clinical diagnosis will be possible.

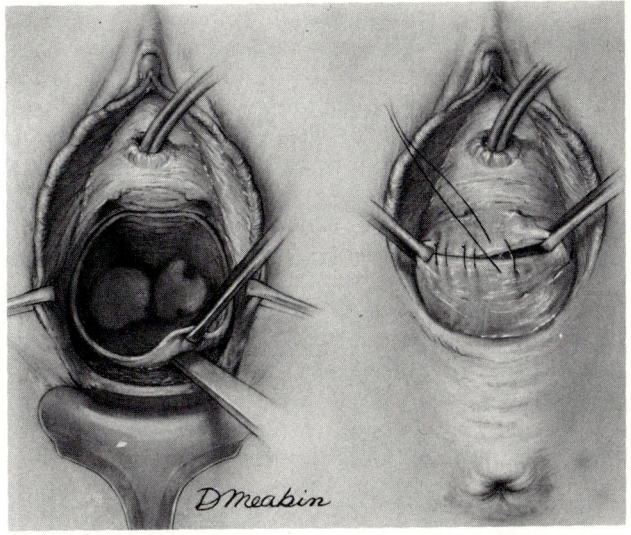

FIG. 33-17. Recurrent carcinoma in situ shown by Schiller's test. In order to be certain of complete removal, the vagina is circumcised and dissected free as far as feasible before completing the vaginectomy abdominally.

The main issue in establishing a uniform classification of Stage I carcinoma concerns both the method of treatment and the comparability of reported cure rates. The currently accepted definition of Stage I A carcinoma includes those lesions in which there is microscopic evidence of invasion of the superficial stroma of 5 mm. or less in depth, and in which there is no evidence of microlymphatic involvement. Such microscopic lesions have a cure rate which approaches that of carcinoma in situ and therefore should be identified separately from the more advanced Stage I lesions.

The diagnosis therefore requires adequate tissue and serial sections. A cone is essential in studying this lesion and reports based on cervical biopsy alone are subject to criticism (Fig. 33-18). Short of definite invasion, pathologists still disagree about the significance of various changes that can affect the epithelium.

In a recent review of 20 cases of microinvasive carcinoma of the cervix diagnosed at Milwaukee County General Hospital during the years 1945–65, utilizing the criteria of a maximal depth of penetration of 5 mm., Mattingly and Borkowf could accept only 7 of these 20 cases (35%) as truly representative of microinvasive carcinoma. The remaining 65 per cent of the cases demonstrated either carcinoma in situ or frank invasive tumor. Morton has recently studied this disease, which he has termed "incipient carcinoma of the cervix." He divides these superficial epidermoid lesions into seven categories ranging from carcinoma in situ in the surface epithelium through the more advanced state of carcinoma in situ

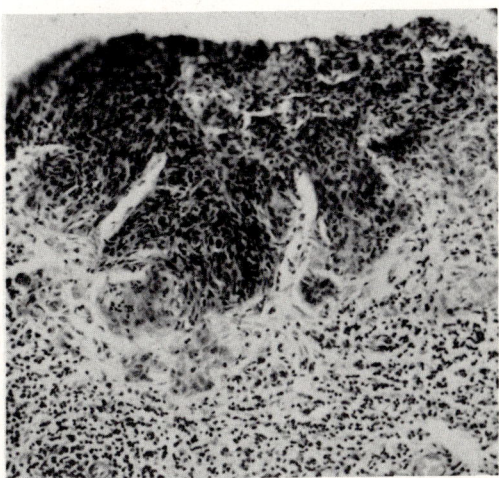

FIG. 33-18. Microinvasive carcinoma of the cervix showing breakthrough of the basement membrane with isolated nests of tumor cells located in the underlying stroma, with a 5-mm. margin of the surface epithelium.

with lymphatic emboli. Other studies, including those by Frick (1963) and by Przybora (1965), are in agreement that unless there are emboli in the lymphatic channels, microinvasive carcinoma (Stage I A) should be treated more conservatively than frank invasive Stage I B carcinoma of the cervix. The 5-mm. depth limit was chosen arbitrarily, based on reports that such cervical lesions showed no lymphatic involvement after radical operation with lymph node dissection. It is particularly important to differentiate accurately those cases of microinvasive Stage I A carcinoma from Stage I B because the latter group has an incidence of positive lymph nodes in 10 to 17 per cent of the cases.

TREATMENT

In the absence of microlymphatic involvement, Stage I A lesions can be adequately treated by a simple total hysterectomy with a wide (3-cm.) vaginal cuff, similar to that for carcinoma in situ. For a more adequate surgical procedure in which the parametrium is dissected out to the ureters, we feel that the modified Wertheim hysterectomy, described in this chapter, is preferable for early invasive, Stage I A lesions. In the event that the patient is not a good surgical risk, such Stage I A lesions may be effectively treated by intracavitary irradiation alone. In these cases, 2 intracavitary radium insertions, 14 days apart, with a total dose of 8,000–10,000 mg./hr., depending on age and physical status, is considered adequate treatment. External therapy is not indicated in such lesions as there have been only rare instances in which positive lymph nodes have been found. In such lesions, adequate study of the cone specimen should reveal evidence of microlymphatic spread. With intracavitary radiation therapy, Kottmeier reports a 97 per cent 5-year cure in 133 cases of microinvasive carcinoma. Vaginal hysterectomy is not preferred in this disease since abdominal exploration is important in the complete evaluation of the pelvic organs and lymph nodes at the time of surgery, although the Schauta radical vaginal hysterectomy has been used extensively in European clinics with excellent cure rates (Navratil).

Microinvasive, Stage I A carcinoma of the cervix with microlymphatic emboli in the adjacent stroma is best treated with either a full complement of intracavitary and external irradiation or by primary radical hysterectomy and pelvic lymphadenectomy. It is in such cases that lymph node metastases have been detected with early lesions of the cervix.

TECHNIC: MODIFIED WERTHEIM HYSTERECTOMY FOR MICROINVASIVE (STAGE I A) CERVICAL CARCINOMA

Before being anesthetized, the patient is cytoscoped and both ureters are catheterized with No. 7 catheters. Before the laparotomy the vagina and the cervix should be painted or sprayed with iodine solution. The Schiller test is useful in determining the extent of the surface involved by the lesion.

The patient is then placed on the operating table and anesthetized. The vagina is cleaned up with soap, water, and alcohol. Then it is swabbed out with Scott's solution, and a dry sterile sponge is placed in the vagina to absorb secretions that may be massaged from the uterus on manipulation at operation. This sponge is removed just before the vagina is opened. The abdomen is prepared according to routine and draped for an infraumbilical midline incision, and the table is put in a marked Trendelenburg position.

A midline incision is made, extending from umbilicus to symphysis. If it is necessary for proper exposure of the pelvic organs to carry the incision above the umbilicus, it should be done, but such procedure is seldom required. The intestines are packed back with moist gauze packs. It is well to spend a little time and do this quite thoroughly in order not to be annoyed during the course of the operation by loops of intestine getting into the operative field. The pelvis is explored manually to make certain that there has been no extension of the growth beyond the uterus. Since one is dealing with microscopic cancer of the cervix, such an extension is very unlikely, but it is well to carry out this precaution on the rare chance that the cervical lesion was misjudged.

The round ligament on one side is clamped, cut, and ligated at least 1 cm. from the uterine cornu. The infundibulopelvic ligament is then clamped, cut, and doubly ligated well out toward the pelvic wall. In doing this one should be certain that the ureter is not included in the suture ligature—a likelihood that is not great, although it can occur. The ureters that have been catheterized are easily palpable, and there is no difficulty in avoiding them.

This procedure is repeated on the opposite side, or, if the adnexa are to be conserved on one side, the clamps and the ligatures are placed accordingly.

The bladder peritoneum is cut at its reflexion onto the anterior surface of the uterus, as in the ordinary hysterectomy. This cut is made so as to join the openings in the anterior leaves of the broad ligaments resulting from cutting the round ligaments. The bladder is then dissected down from its attachment to the cervix. To prevent unnecessary bleeding, the freeing of the bladder from the vagina to the point ultimately required should not be done at this stage. Up to this point the operation does not differ from an ordinary hysterectomy.

The peritoneum forming the posterior leaf of each broad ligament is then cut downward parallel with the side of the uterus, and the structures in the bases of the broad ligaments are exposed. The catheterized ureters should then be easily palpable and located to permit double ligation of the uterine vessels as far laterally as possible (Fig. 33-19 A). The uterine end of the vessels should also be ligated to free the operative field of clamps. This procedure of ligation of the uterine vessels can be carried out without freeing the ureters from their beds, and thus any injury to their blood supply is avoided.

After the uterine vessels have been ligated bilaterally in this way, another bite of paracervical tissue is made with Ochsner clamps on both sides 1 or 2 cm. from the side of the cervix, care again being taken to avoid the ureters. This clamped tissue which constitutes the bases of the broad ligaments is then cut and ligated. This tissue is ligated by a suture placed just beyond the tip of the clamp and tied as the clamp is slowly released. In some instances it is necessary to take a second bite of tissue parallel and lateral with the cervix below the first.

Next, the uterosacral ligaments are clamped at a point at least 1 cm. from the cervix. They are ligated on the uterine side and cut between the clamps and the ligatures, as shown in Figure 33-19 B.

The bladder is now dissected farther down, freeing it from the pubovesicocervical fascia which covers the vagina. This fascia is easily recognized by its longitudinal fibers. The lateral paravaginal tissue is next clamped, cut, and ligated on either side of the vagina, taking successive bites with Ochsner clamps until a point is reached where the vagina can be cut across well below the cervix.

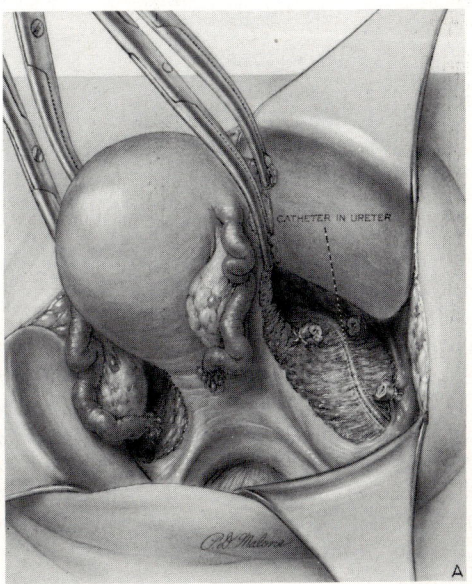

FIG. 33-19. Radical hysterectomy for microinvasive carcinoma. (A) Round ligaments and infundibulopelvic ligaments have been cut and ligated as in the usual hysterectomy. The broad ligament has been opened widely, exposing the ureter which has been catheterized. The right uterine vessels have been ligated lateral to the catheter.

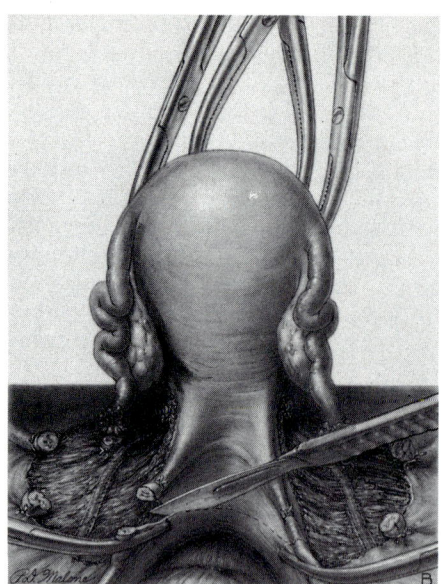

FIG. 33-19 (*Continued*). Radical hysterectomy for microinvasive carcinoma. (B) Uterosacral ligaments have been clamped and ligated and are being cut. The peritoneum between the two ligaments is cut as indicated by the dotted line.

In carrying this lateral clamping, cutting, and ligating down to this point it is necessary from time to time to dissect the bladder down still farther to avoid catching it in the clamps. Sometimes bleeding is encountered from both the bladder and the fascia in making this dissection. It is well to clamp and ligate these vessels as they are encountered in order to keep the field as dry as possible.

When the vagina has been freed sufficiently far down to permit amputation with a good cuff of vagina on the cervix, the lateral portions of the vagina, covered with the pubovesicocervical fascia, are clamped for a short distance with Ochsner clamps (Fig. 33-19 C). As the vagina is cut across, an assistant grasps the anterior and the posterior vaginal walls with straight Ochsner clamps as necessary to control bleeding.

The vagina is closed with figure-of-eight sutures of chromic catgut (Fig. 33-19 D). The vagina is suspended by bringing in the round and the uterosacral ligaments and suturing them to the cut edge of the vagina. Because the uterine vessels have been ligated so far laterally in this operation, no attempt is made to bring in these vessels with the basal broad ligament tissue attached to them, as is done in the conservative hysterectomy.

The pelvis is peritonized by suturing the bladder peritoneum to the posterior surface of the vagina and closing the broad ligaments by suturing the anterior and the posterior leaves together with a continuous suture of No. 000 chromic catgut. The infundibulopelvic stumps are inverted beneath folds of peritoneum (Fig. 33-19 E).

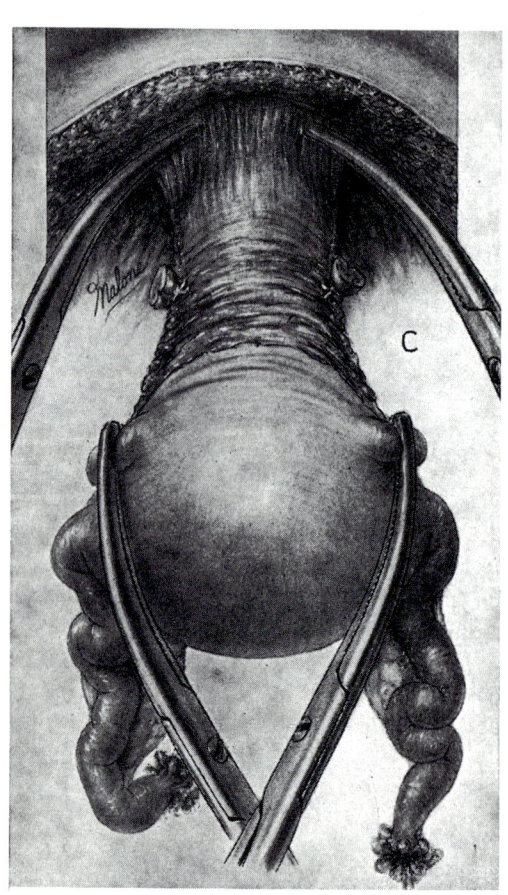

FIG. 33-19 (*Continued*). Radical hysterectomy for microinvasive carcinoma. (C) The bladder has been dissected down from the pubocervical fascia, well below the tip of the cervix. The pubocervical fascia and the vaginal wall are grasped on both sides with curved Ochsner clamps.

Microinvasive Carcinoma 729

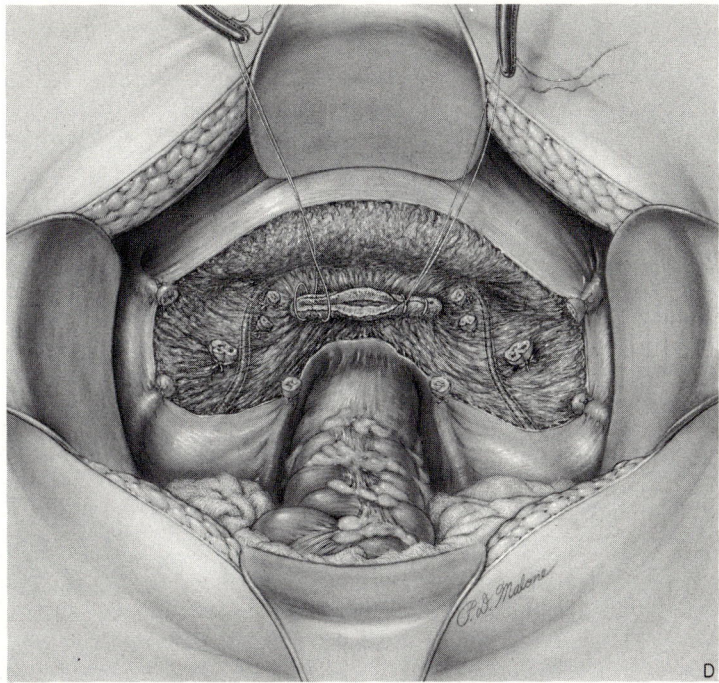

FIG. 33-19 (*Continued*). Radical hysterectomy for microinvasive carcinoma. (D) The uterus has been removed, and the vagina is being closed with figure-of-eight sutures of chromic catgut. Note the ligated uterine vessels and the ligatures about the vessels of paracervical and paravaginal tissues.

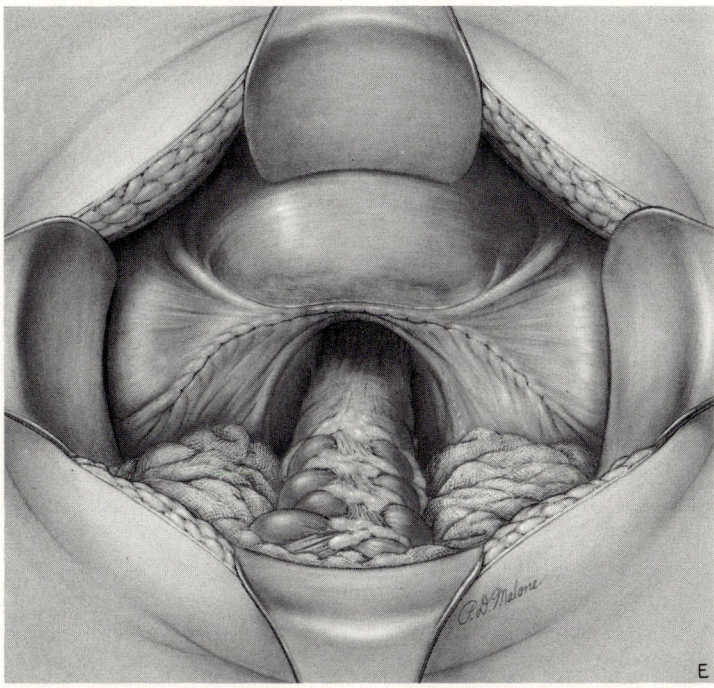

FIG. 33-19 (*Continued*). (E) Pelvis is completely peritonized after vagina is closed without drainage.

BIBLIOGRAPHY

Ashley, D. J. B.: Biological status of carcinoma in situ of uterine cervix. J. Obstet. Gynaec. Brit. Comm., 73:372, 1966.

Boyes, D. A.: The British Columbia screening program. Obstet. Gynec. Surv., 24:1005, 1969.

Burghardt, E.: Die Diagnostische Konisation der Portio Vaginalis Uteri. Geburtsch. Frauenheilk., 23:1, 1963.

Frick, H. C., Janovski, N. A., Gusberg, S. B., and Taylor, H. C.: Early invasive carcinoma of the cervix. Amer. J. Obstet. Gynec., 85:926, 1963.

Frost J. J.: Gynecologic and obstetric cytopathology. In Novak, E. R., and Woodruff, J. D.: Novak's Gynecologic and Obstetric Pathology. ed. 6, p. 575. Philadelphia, W. B. Saunders, 1967.

Galvin, G. A., Jones, H. W., and Te Linde, R. W.: Significance of basel-cell hyperactivity in cervical biopsies. Amer. J. Obstet. Gynec., 70:808, 1955.

Galvin, G. A., and Te Linde, R. W.: The present-day status of noninvasive cervical carcinoma. Amer. J. Obstet. Gynec., 57:15, 1949.

———: The minimal histological changes in biopsies to justify a diagnosis of cervical cancer. Amer. J. Obstet. Gynec., 48:774, 1944.

Govan, A. D. T., Haines, R. M., Langley, F. A., Taylor, C. W., and Woodcock, A. S.: Changes in the epithelium of the cervix uteri. A study by the panel of pathologists engaged in the survey of carcinoma in situ carried out by the Royal College of Obstetricians and Gynaecologists. J. Obstet. Gynaec. Brit. Comm., 73:883, 1966.

Graham, Ruth [M.]: Carcinoma in Situ of the Cervix: The Cytologic Method in Diagnosis and Study. Monographs on Surgery. p. 64, New York, Nelson, 1951.

———: The Cytologic Diagnosis of Cancer. ed. 2. Philadelphia, W. B. Saunders, 1963.

Gray, L. A.: Dysplasia, Carcinoma in Situ, Micro-Invasive Carcinoma of the Cervix Uteri. Springfield, Ill., Charles C Thomas, 1964.

Griffiths, C. T., and Younge, P. A.: The clinical diagnosis of early cervical cancer. Obstet. Gynec. Surv., 24:967, 1969.

Hirst, J. C., and Brown, M. L.: The diagnosis of very early carcinoma of the uterine cervix during pregnancy. Amer. J. Obstet. Gynec., 64:1296, 1952.

Kottmeier, H.-L. (ed.): Annual Report on the Results of Treatment in Carcinoma of the Uterus and Vagina. Published under the patronage of the International Federation of Gynecology and Obstetrics. vol. 14, collated 1966. Stockholm, Norstedt & Söner, 1967.

Krieger, J. S.: Graded treatment for in-situ carcinoma of uterine cervix. Amer. J. Obstet. Gynec., 101(2):171, 1968.

Lange, P.: Clinical and Histological Studies on Cervical Carcinoma; Precancerous, Early Metastasis, and Tubular Structures in the Lymph Nodes. p. 40. Copenhagen, Munksgaard, 1960.

Margulis, R. R., Ely, C. W., and Ladd, J. E.: Diagnosis and mangement of Stage IA (micro-invasive) carcinoma of the cervix. Obstet. Gynec., 29:529, 1967.

Mattingly, R. F., and Borkowf, H. I.: Unpublished data.

Morton, D. P.: Incipient carcinoma of the cervix. Amer. J. Obstet. Gynec., 90:64, 1964.

Navratil, E.: Radical vaginal hysterectomy (Schanta-Amveich operation). Clin. Obstet. Gynec., 8:676, 1965.

Peckham, B. M., and Greene, R. R.: Follow-up on cervical epithelial abnormalities. Amer. J. Obstet. Gynec., 74:804, 1957.

Peterson, O.: Spontaneous course of cervical precancerous conditions. Amer. J. Obstet. Gynec., 72:1063, 1956.

Przybora, L. A.: Incipient invasion of cervical cancer: morphological aspects of carcinogenesis in 74 cases. Gynaecologia, 160: 69, 1965.

Pund, E. R., and Blumberg, J. M.: Cancer in Situ (Preinvasive) of the Cervix Uteri. Monographs on Surgery. p. 42. New York, Nelson, 1951.

Richart, R. M.: Natural history of cervical intraepithelial neoplasm. Clin. Obstet. Gynec., 10:748, 1967.

Schottländer, J., and Kermauner, F.: Zur Kenntnis des Uteruskarzinoms. Berlin, Karger, 1912.

Singleton, W. P., Grant, D., and Rutledge, F.: To cone or not to cone. Obstet. Gynec., 31:430, 1968.

Stern, E., and Neely, O. M.: Carcinoma and dysplasia of the cervix. Acta Cytol., 7:357, 1963.

Te Linde, R. W.: The relation of "intra-epithelial carcinoma" to invasive cancer of the cervix. In Progress in Gynecology. p. 349. New York, Grune & Stratton, 1946.

———: Carcinoma in Situ of the Cervix. Monographs on Surgery. p. 5. New York, Nelson, 1951.

Te Linde, R. W., and Galvin, G. A.: The minimal histological changes in biopsies to justify a diagnosis of cervical cancer. Amer. J. Obstet. Gynec., *48*:774, 1944.

Topek, N. Y.: Surgical treatment of carcinoma in-situ of cervix. Clin. Obstet. Gynec., *10*:853, 1967.

34

Invasive Carcinoma of the Cervix

CLASSIFICATION

INTERNATIONAL CLASSIFICATION

In 1937 the Health Organization of the League of Nations adopted a gross classification of cervical cancer which has been in general use abroad and in most of the clinics in the United States. In 1950 this classification was simplified and modified to include preinvasive (in situ) cancer. No alteration of the basic principle of the League of Nations classification was made, but the appearance of preinvasive cancer on the clinical horizon made it necessary to add another stage, which was designated Stage 0. New recommendations for the clinical classification of carcinoma of the cervix were adopted at the Congress of the International Federation of Gynecology and Obstetrics in September 1961 in Vienna and were enacted, effective January 1, 1962. The following description includes the redefined International Classification:

PREINVASIVE CARCINOMA OF THE CERVIX

Stage 0. Carcinoma in situ, intra-epithelial carcinoma.

INVASIVE CARCINOMA OF THE CERVIX

Stage I. Carcinoma strictly confined to the cervix (extension to the corpus should be disregarded).

  Stage I A. Cases of early stromal invasion (preclinical carcinoma).

  Stage I B. All other cases of Stage I with the disease confined to the cervix.

Stage II. The carcinoma extends beyond the cervix but has not extended on to the pelvic wall.

The carcinoma involves the vagina, but not the lower third.

Subgrouping of Stage II cases into II A (no parametrial involvement) and II B (parametrial involvement) is recommended.

Stage III A. The tumor involves the lower third of the vagina.

Stage III B. The carcinoma has extended on to the pelvic wall. On rectal examination there is no cancer-free space between the tumor and the pelvic wall.

Stage IV. The carcinoma has extended beyond the true pelvis or has involved the mucosa of the bladder or rectum.

Stages II, III, and IV are essentially unchanged from the 1950 classification; the major revision is in the redefinition of Stage I, and a statement from the official definition further defines Stage I A (see the introductory paragraph under Microinvasive Carcinoma in Chapter 33).

MICROSCOPIC CLASSIFICATIONS

Several attempts have been made to classify carcinoma of the cervix histologically and to relate the histology to the choice of therapy. Much of this work is only of historical interest, but the student of cervical cancer should be familiar with it. The gross classification described above remains the most useful and practical guide to therapy, and is illustrated in Figure 34-1.

In 1923 Martzloff made a histologic

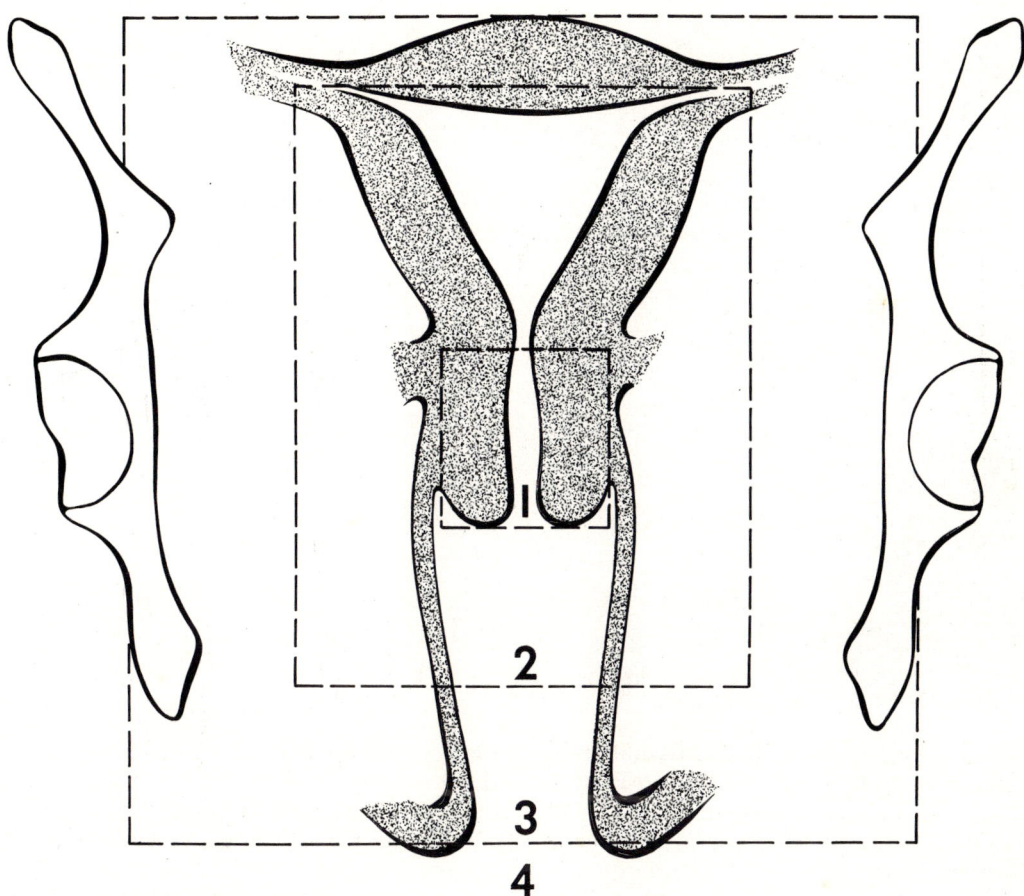

FIG. 34-1. Clinical staging of carcinoma of the cervix.
Stage 1: The tumor is strictly confined to the cervix.
Stage 2: The tumor extends beyond the cervix but has not reached the pelvic wall; involves the vagina but not the lower third.
Stage 3: The tumor extends on to the pelvic wall or involves the lower third of the vagina.
Stage 4: The tumor has extended beyond the true pelvis or has involved the mucosa of the bladder or rectum.

and clinical study of carcinoma of the cervix based on the material in the gynecologic pathology laboratory of the Johns Hopkins Hospital. He found that epidermoid cancer of the cervix could be divided into 3 morphologic groups, dependent upon the predominant cell type. He designated these groups as spinal cell, transition cell, and fat spindle cell cancer. In the spinal cell type of cancer the predominating cells resemble those polyhedral cells of the upper part of the stratum mucosum of ordinary cervical epithelium. Epithelial pearl formation occurs in some but not in all growths of this type (Fig. 34-2). The predominating cell of the transitional cell cancers resembles those of the intermediate zone of cervical epithelium situated between the spinal layer above and the basal layer below. These cells are closely packed and have round nuclei that are separated from each other by cytoplasm deeper in staining properties and less in quantity than in the spinal cells (Fig. 34-3). The fat spindle-like cell type of cancer resembles the basal cells in the stratum germinativum of the cervical epithelium.

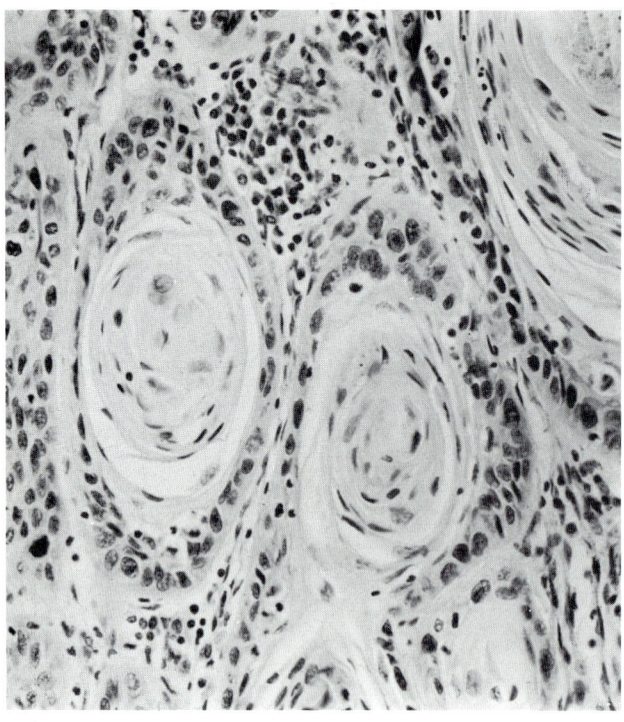

FIG. 34-2. Epidermoid carcinoma of the cervix. High-power view of spinal cell type.

These cells have dark hematoxylin-staining nuclei with scanty eosin-staining cytoplasm (Fig. 34-4).

On studying the operative results, Martzloff, judging by the percentage of clinical operative cures, showed that the spinal cell type of cancer was the least malignant; the fat spindle cell type was the most malignant; and the transitional cell type occupied an intermediate position. From the radiologic point of view, it appears that the reverse is true: spinal cell cancer is the least radiosensitive; the fat spindle cell type is the most sensitive

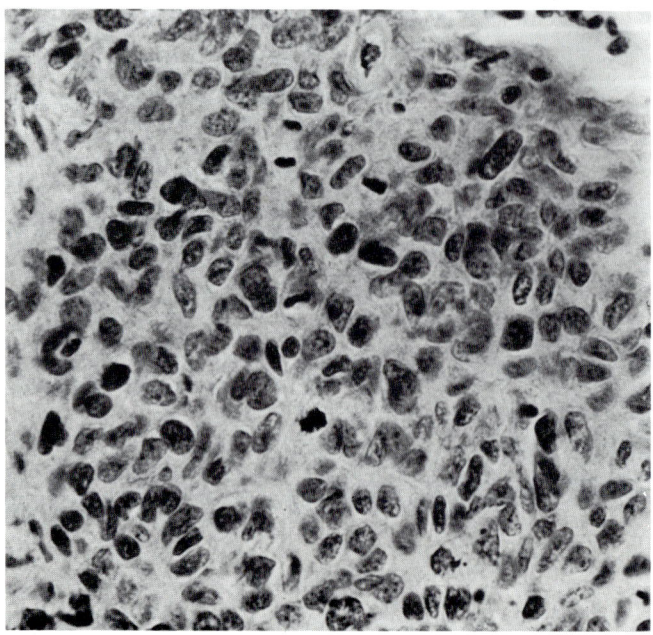

FIG. 34-3. Epidermoid carcinoma of the cervix. Transitional cell type.

FIG. 34-4. Epidermoid carcinoma of the cervix. Fat spindle or basal cell type.

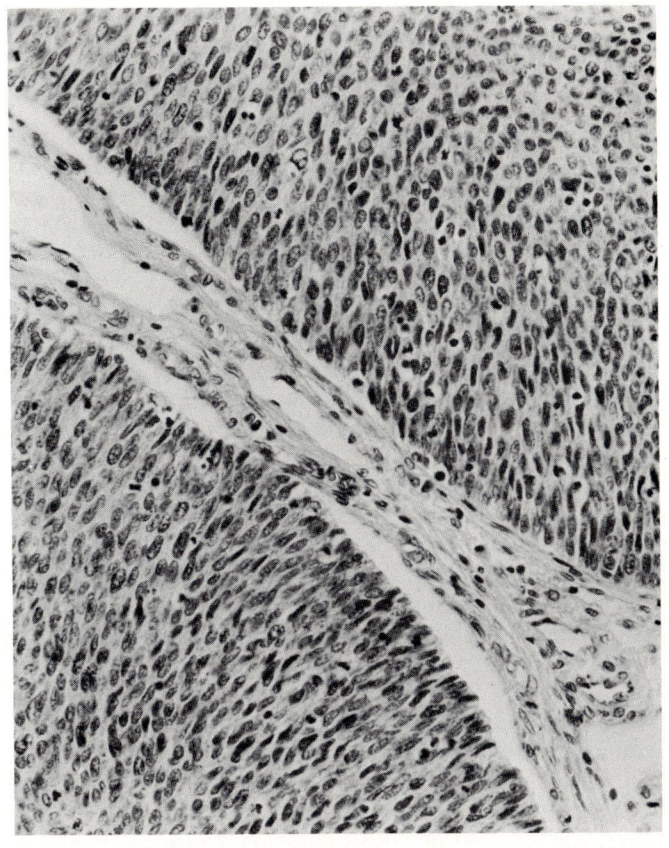

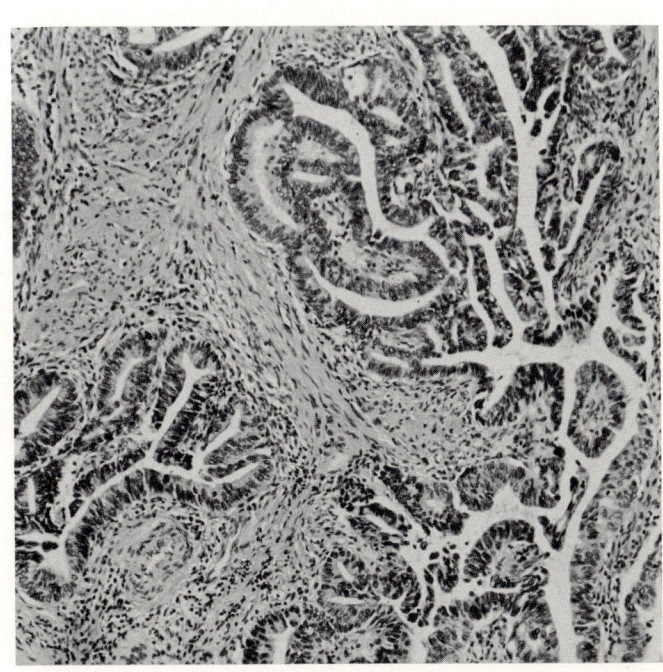

FIG. 34-5. Adenocarcinoma of the cervix.

to irradiation, while the transitional cell type of cancer occupies an intermediate position in its radiosensitivity. Adenocarcinoma of the cervix (Fig. 34-5) was intermediate in its degree of malignancy between the spinal cell and the transitional cell type.

The Martzloff classification is similar to that of Broders', which uses the numerical grades 1 through 4. The designation of a grade is based on percentage of immature cells in the tumor. Therefore Broders' Grade 1 classification would be that tumor that has the greatest percentage of well-differentiated tumor cells, while Grade 4 would be the most undifferentiated type of tumor, or that derived from the fat, spindle, or basal cell type.

A classification by Wentz and Reagan is based on both the cytologic and histologic pattern of the predominant cell and includes: Group 1, keratinizing carcinoma; Group 2, large cell nonkeratinizing carcinoma; and Group 3, small cell cancer. These groups are similar to Martzloff's spinal, transitional, and spindle cell types, respectively. Survival in a composite group of 420 patients from Wentz's series revealed the large cell nonkeratinizing type (transitional cell type) to have the most favorable outcome in radiation treatment. However, Martzloff was unable to make a definite correlation of clinical response based on histology alone as his material demonstrated that about one third of the 70 cases failed to indicate correctly the predominating cancer cell on biopsy when compared with the surgical specimen. There has been no histopathologic correlation of clinical response with adenocarcinoma of the cervix, which comprises 3½ to 5 per cent of the cervical neoplasms in this clinic.

Clinical experience in the treatment of this disease refutes the oft-quoted law of Bergonie and Tribondeau, which identifies the immature or undifferentiated cell as being the most radiosensitive. Instead, these tumors would seem to be autonomous in their response and unpredictable from a histologic pattern alone.

THE DIAGNOSIS

In this section the diagnosis of *gross* lesions only is to be considered. Diagnosis of the macroscopically invisible lesions is considered in Chapter 33, Carcinoma in Situ of the Cervix. The *gross* lesion may often be suspected and *almost* diagnosed from simple palpation of the cervix. To the palpating fingers the carcinomatous growth may be friable, as is usually the case with the everting type of growth. It may have a stony hard but smooth feeling when the growth develops beneath normal mucosa. The lesion may take the form of a punched-out ulcer, or the cervix may feel quite normal when a relatively extensive lesion exists in the cervical canal.

To inspection, the friable lesion appears like a roughened, granular, bleeding surface which may be sloughing, infected, and foul-smelling. The ulcerative lesion may appear like a fairly clean punched-out ulcer, or there may be a crater-like excavation with a necrotic base. Rarely, a growth starting in the cervical canal may protrude from the external os much like a benign polyp. The stony hard cervix that is the site of an extensive growth beneath relatively normal mucosa may not appear very abnormal, even when the growth is quite advanced. The inverting type of growth may extend well into the musculature of the cervix without changing the appearance of the vaginal portion of the cervix as viewed through the speculum. The important point is that every suspicious-feeling cervix should be inspected through a speculum with good visualization, and that every cervix should be visualized when there has been abnormal bleeding, even though it feels entirely normal to palpation.

After inspection of the cervical lesion, it always should be smeared and biopsied. The most "typical" appearing lesion may not prove to be carcinoma. We have seen tuberculous lesions of the cervix as well as other granulomas which could not be distinguished grossly from cancer. Furthermore, the diagnosis must be verified microscopically to permit the case to be included in the 5-year salvage reports.

Biopsy of the cervix can be done in several different ways. There is no better method of making satisfactory biopsies than to excise wedge-shaped pieces of tissue with a scalpel, including the surface and some of the subjacent tissue. There are numerous biopsy instruments on the market, but we have found the Gaylor and the Younge forceps to be of great value in taking biopsies in the office, the out-patient department, and the operating room (Fig. 34-6). Conization of the cervix seldom is necessary when a gross lesion is present. It is done routinely in our clinic in evaluating microscopic cervical cancer, and the reader is referred to Chapter 33, Carcinoma in Situ of the Cervix. However, curettage of the cervical canal is frequently done in the presence of gross cervical cancer to determine the extension of the lesion up the canal. The information thus obtained is of value in planning the irradiation therapy.

CHOICE OF TREATMENT

Opinion among gynecologists has not yet crystallized on the best method of treating carcinoma of the cervix. This statement, which was made in the first edition of this book, still is equally true at the time of this revision. In general, in the United States and Canada, radical hysterectomy with lymph node dissection was abandoned in the 1920's in favor of irradiation. After using irradiation for many years in many clinics, much has been accomplished in the successful treatment of the disease. Its shortcomings and complications have also became apparent. Because of these, radical surgery in the form of modifications of the Wertheim operation was renewed by Meigs in 1939 at the Massachusetts General Hospital and by others. Over a period of several years Taussig resected the pelvic lymph nodes, leaving the uterus in situ and treating the cervix with radium. Some clinics have combined the Wertheim type of operation with preoperative or postoperative irradiation. In England, Victor Bonney, throughout his long professional life, persisted in using the radical abdominal hysterectomy in a form slightly modified from that originally described by Wertheim. As will be noted later in this chapter, Bonney's pupils and successors have greatly narrowed their indications for surgery. On the contininent of Europe, the radical abdominal hysterectomy, irradiation, and the radical vaginal extirpation of the uterus and the parametria, as described by Schauta, have all been and still are being practiced in some clinics. The greatest advocate of the radical vaginal approach currently is Navratil of Austria, van Bouwdijk-Bastiaanse of Amsterdam having advocated it strongly until his death a few years ago.

Since Martzloff's study in 1923, many attempts have ben made to determine the radiosensitivity of cancer cells with the hope of ascertaining which tumors would respond best by irradiation and which by surgery, but the studies have

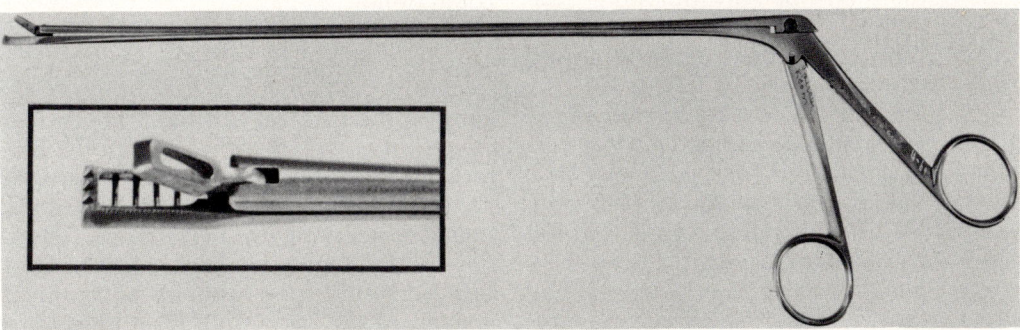

FIG. 34-6. Younge square-jawed biopsy forceps.

not been very helpful. Ruth Graham has presented evidence to show that the response of a tumor to irradiation depends principally upon the response of the nonmalignant cells rather than upon the malignant cells themselves. Her evidence, called radiation response (RR), was obtained from studying vaginal smears of irradiated cases, but has not proven clinically useful as her data has not been reproducible by other clinics.

Gusberg and Herman recently have reported on continued studies on the cytomorphologic response of the tumor cells to a test dose of external irradiation. In addition, they compare their findings with the histologic evidence of lymphatic involvement on pretest cervical biopsy as well as the clinical observation of the tumor response. Their data demonstrate that patients with good RST (radiosensitivity testing) have a higher survival rate when treated with irradiation than patients with poor RST. Their method of applying a test dose of 400 r by cobalt 60 or Betatron for 3 days, and observing the cytologic changes in the tumor cells 1 week later, is similar to that in previous studies of Glucksmann and Spear 25 years ago. This work confirms the well-known triad of factors involved in the response of tumors, namely, virulence of the tumor, radiosensitivity of the neoplastic cell, and the quality of treatment. In recognition of the importance of each factor, the search continues for the key to the unanswered question: Which tumor will respond best to which modality of treatment, surgery or irradiation? Current investigation on tritiated thymidine labeling of tumors as a more accurate method of documenting the mitotic activity of a cell cycle may prove to be a clinical method of determining tumor radiosensitivity.

The presence of persistent fever in patients under treatment for cervical carcinoma has an ominous prognosis. In a recent report from the Mayo Clinic by Van Herik, the incidence of sustained fever increased in direct proportion to the advancement of the disease. The fact that in the majority of cases no etiologic factor can be found for the presence of fever suggests a thermogenic influence of advance tumor which is related to tissue breakdown and metastases. Since concurrent pelvic inflammatory disease can exist with cervical carcinoma, it is particularly important to document this diagnosis because of the adverse effect the presence of infection can have on irradiation. Certainly, intracavitary radium should not be applied until the pelvic inflammatory disease has been completely suppressed with proper antibiotic therapy; if necessary, in rare instances laparotomy and surgical removal of the adnexa may be required prior to treatment. Death from uncontrolled pelvic inflammatory disease following irradiation therapy was a serious clinical problem prior to the availability of effective antibiotics. In the presence of urinary tract obstruction with cervical cancer, the possibility of pyelonephritis must be evaluated as well as the more frequent occurrence of pyometra. The later diagnosis is important since intracavitary radium should not be used in the presence of pyometra. The prognosis worsens as the course of fever is prolonged. In the Mayo Clinic series, patients with fever for more than 7 days had a 5-year survival of only 25.8 per cent as compared with an overall 5-year survival rate of 41.2 per cent where fever was present for less than 7 days.

Since the first edition of this book, a school of ultraradical surgeons has appeared on the clinical scene who are performing more or less complete pelvic exenterations for advanced and recurrent cervical cancer. In Chapter 35 the various methods and results are considered in some detail.

Operative Results

In order to obtain a fair opinion regarding the surgical treatment of cervical cancer, it is well to view some of the historical milestones. The surgical approach to treatment of carcinoma of the cervix had its inception in 1879, when Theodore McGraw strongly urged total hysterectomy in treatment of cervical cancer. At the same time Freund in Germany developed a technic for total hysterectomy, although this procedure included an operative mortality of 50 per cent. Six years later, in 1895, Reis demonstrated in autopsy material the technic of lymph gland removal with part of the broad ligament at the time of total hysterectomy. The earliest record of radical surgery in this country was made in 1895 by J. G. Clark, who, while a resident gynecologist at Johns Hopkins Hospital, reported two cases of a more radical hysterectomy for carcinoma of the uterus. Clark catheterized the ureters with bougies in order to obtain a better dissection of the broad ligament at the lateral pelvic wall and to facilitate ligation of the uterine vessels at their origin, as well as to enable removal of a large portion of the vagina without injuring the ureter. In 1898 Wertheim of Vienna developed the philosophy of routine removal of pelvic lymph nodes and total hysterectomy for the treatment of cervical cancer. Wertheim reported his first series of 270 cases in 1905 and elaborated further on his experience with 500 cases in 1911. Due to the high surgical mortality rate and urinary and bowel complications initially, the treatment for cervical cancer was gradually replaced by radium and deep x-ray therapy in the United States from 1920–40.

Experience with radical hysterectomy and pelvic lymphadenectomy in this country was renewed in 1939 by the late J. V. Meigs, who was dissatisfied with the results of irradiation therapy. Although this procedure has become known as the radical Wertheim hysterectomy, Meigs's operation routinely removed all of the pelvic lymph nodes whereas Wertheim performed only a selective lymphadenectomy in which only the enlarged and palpable lymph nodes were removed. In Meigs's report of 344 cases of primary invasive carcinoma of the cervix, which was a highly selected group, there was a 5-year cure of 75 per cent of Stage I cases and 54 per cent of Stage II cases in 193 patients eligible for 5-year follow-up. Meigs's original operative fistula rate was 9 per cent (45 patients), although one third of the patients who developed fistula had received previous irradiation.

Ureteral complications continue to be a serious problem, as reported by Green in 1962. A 12.5 per cent ureteral complication rate, including 8.5 per cent ureterovaginal fistula and 4 per cent ureteral stricture, has been reportedly improved by continuous bladder drainage for 6 weeks postoperatively and by suspension of the ureter off the pelvic floor, with suture of the distal ureter to the obliterated portion of the hypogastric artery. We have recently initiated the technic of wrapping the denuded ureter with the adjacent parietal peritoneum, as described by Ohkawa. Both procedures are aimed at protecting the lower ureters from the usual pelvic cellulitis that occurs in the operative site, which is thought to produce ureteral scarring and fistulae. In general, the frequency of urinary tract fistulas is markedly increased when surgery is performed for radioresistant cervical carcinoma. The current incidence of urinary tract fistula is summarized in Table 34-1.

Masterson's recent unselected series of 180 radical hysterectomies and lymph node dissection performed during the period 1950–64 for primary cervical cancer revealed a 5-year cure rate in 150 patients of 87 per cent in Stage I and 63 per cent in Stage II. There was a 10 per cent incidence of positive lymph nodes in Stage I and 20 per cent in Stage II. The total incidence of fistula was 5 per cent, which was reduced from 12 per cent in an earlier report. Parker reports a corrected 5-year survival in Stage I disease as 84 per cent, with a high fistula rate. However, the 10- to 22-year survival rate in Stage II lesions with positive nodes is practically nil (4%).

The radical vaginal hysterectomy (Schauta-Amreich operation) has been used primarily in Europe but has had only limited use in this country, primarily by McCall. Navratil of Graz, Austria, has recently reported on a series of 426 cases of epidermoid carcinoma of the cervix operated on from 1952 through 1958. He reports a 5-year survival of 88 per cent, 56.6 per cent, and 66.6 per cent for Stages I, II, and III, respectively, with an overall cure of 79.1 per cent. Where no

TABLE 34-1. INCIDENCE OF URINARY TRACT FISTULA AFTER RADICAL HYSTERECTOMY

SOURCE	DATE OF REPORT	TYPE OF FISTULA, %	
		Ureterovaginal	Vesicovaginal
Welch, Pratt and Symmonds	1961	5.0	3.0
Green	1962	8.5	2.2
Sweeny and Douglas	1962	10.0	1.0
Louros	1964	2.0	2.0
Foley and Fetherston (MCGH)*	1965	11.0	5.0
Calame and Nelson	1967	13.4	
Masterson	1967	4.4	0.6
Parker, Wilbanks, Yowell and Carter	1967	12.0	7.0

* Milwaukee County General Hospital.

preoperation radiation was given, the 5-year cure rate was 87.4 per cent in Stage I cases and 59.2 per cent in Stage II cases. A low incidence (2.2%) of operative injury to the bladder, ureters, and rectum was reported in the 724 operations, with only 2 injuries to the ureter (0.2%). The incidence of postoperative fistula was extremely low, only 1.2 per cent. Ingiulla reports an incidence of ureterovaginal fistula in 871 patients operated by the Schauta technic to be only 1.95 per cent, and most of these were in Stage II and Stage III lesions. Vesicovaginal fistulas occurred in the same group of patients in 2.8 per cent and were principally found in Stage II lesions. Rectal fistulas occurring in this group of 871 cervical cases were very low (1.6%).

Although the previous discussion has been focused primarily on squamous cell carcinoma of the cervix, the identical conclusion can be drawn for adenocarcinoma of the cervix. As reported by Rutledge et al., Cuccia et al., Decker et al., and others, in adequate-sized series, the cure rate for adenocarcinoma is identical, whether treated by primary surgery or primary irradiation. The general belief expressed in the literature that radiation therapy may not be as effective for adenocarcinoma as for squamous cell carcinoma, as well as the fact that this tumor of endocervical origin may have a more rapid parametrial spread, has encouraged the primary surgical treatment of this disease. At the present time, however, current statistics are not convincing for significant improvement in the cure rate by surgery in preference to irradiation, but surgery is followed by a much higher complication rate.

The therapeutic debate during the past 25 years concerning primary treatment of cervical cancer would seem to be fairly well resolved at the present time. It seems evident that the cure rate for both modalities of treatment is relatively the same, stage for stage. The decision regarding the use of primary surgery versus irradiation therapy remains one of personal preference and is related to the experience and competence of the pelvic surgeon. The following conclusions can be drawn from a survey of the world literature on this subject:

1. The 5-year cure rate for Stage I and Stage II epidermoid carcinoma of the cervix is comparable by both primary surgery or irradiation therapy. For Stage I lesions, the cure rate varies between 85 and 89 per cent.

2. There is a significantly higher complication rate with radical surgery, with an overall fistula rate varying between 10 and 12 per cent. With experience and specific precautions, this figure should be no more than 3 to 5 per cent.

3. In the young patient with an early cervical lesion, in whom conservation

of the ovaries is desired, primary radical surgery is particularly useful. The treatment of cervical cancer should be individualized to fit the particular case. Patients with surgical contraindications should not be subjected to radical surgery for the treatment of this disease.

4. At the same time, irradiation therapy cannot be claimed as a panacea as there are specific tumors that are radioresistant in spite of more than adequate supervoltage irradiation dosage. It is generally believed, however, that lateral pelvic wall recurrence of this disease is more commonly related to inadequate tumorcidal dosage than to radioresistant disease.

Our Current Views on Treatment

After considering the results of treatment with surgery and irradiation, it is probable that the reader is left with a certain amount of confusion about the best therapy for this disease. The authors, after attempting to evaluate the pros and cons with an unbiased mind, have arrived at certain conclusions regarding the treatment of cervical cancer of Stages I, II, III, and IV. Carcinoma in situ is considered in Chapter 33, and the treatment of recurrent cancer is considered separately.

From the previous discussion on the operative and irradiation results, one can only conclude the following facts: The incidence of fistulas resulting from surgery is greater than that of this same group when treated by irradiation; most of the fistulas resulting from irradiation occur in the advanced cases in which life expectancy is generally limited. This must be considered a point against surgery.

We believe that, in general, carcinoma of the cervix, Stage I, had best be treated with irradiation, as outlined in this chapter, except in selected cancer treatment centers in this country and abroad where vast surgical experience and skills have been achieved. Perhaps one of the greatest sins of many gynecologists in the country is to attempt the radical hysterectomy with lymph gland dissection and slight the completeness of the operation because of technical difficulties. Whenever a surgeon contemplates surgery for cervical cancer, he would do well to consult his conscience and ask himself whether or not he is capable of doing the complete and extensive surgery required to equal or better the patient's chance of cure offered her by irradiation. Unless he is performing this type of surgery regularly in a well-staffed medical center with trained assistants, he should not subject the patient to such untoward risks.

Irradiation Results

At the change of the century, when the approach toward radical surgery was being explored in Europe, two important radiologic discoveries occurred about the same time. Roentgen's discovery of the x-ray in 1895 and the discovery of radium by Pierre and Marie Curie in 1898 were key factors in the later use of radium and deep x-ray for the treatment of malignant disease. Although the first report of the use of radium in the treatment of carcinoma of the cervix appeared in 1903 by Margaret Cleaves, it was not until the pure element was first prepared in 1910 by Madame Curie at the Sorbonne in Paris that this radioactive element became widely used in European and American medical centers.

Several different methods of radium therapy were developed including the Stockholm technic (Radiumhemmet), the Paris technic (Curie Foundation), and the Manchester technic in England. The Stockholm radium technic consisted of high-intensity irradiation repeated 2 or 3 times in 3 weeks, while the Paris technic included low-intensity irradiation delivered continuously over 1 week. The Manchester technic was developed from the Paris school and gave low hourly dosage rates with at least 2 insertions. From 1920–40 radium therapy virtually replaced the surgical treatment of carcinoma of the cervix in the United States, and at the present time remains the most common form of therapy internationally. With the establishment of the roentgen as a defined unit of radiation exposure (Stockholm, 1921), radiation dosage be-

TABLE 34-2. SURVIVAL RATES FOR RADIOTHERAPY PATIENTS*

Stage	5-Year Survival Rate† (%)		10-Year Survival Rate† (%)	
	Kilovoltage	Megavoltage	Kilovoltage	Megavoltage
SQUAMOUS CELL CARCINOMA IN AN INTACT UTERUS‡				
I	90.5	91.5	87.0	90.0
II$_A$	81.5	83.5	78.5	79.0
II$_B$	60.0	66.5	51.0	57.0
III$_A$	41.5	45.0	39.0	39.5
III$_B$	31.0	36.0	21.5	30.0
IV	5.0	14.0	5.0	14.0
Total	62.5		57.0	
CANCERS OF CERVICAL STUMP§				
I	86.0	97.0	86.0	97.0
II$_A$	64.0	93.0	64.0	89.0
II$_B$	64.0	67.0	57.0	67.0
III$_A$	40.0	61.0	40.0	61.0
III$_B$	40.0	32.0	40.0	32.0
IV	0		0	
Total	68.5		66.5	

* Fletcher, G. H., and Rutledge, F. N.: Overall results in radiotherapy for carcinoma of the cervix. Clin. Obstet. Gynec., 10(4):960, 1967.
† Kilovoltage—September 1948–September 1954. Megavoltage—September 1954–December 1963.
‡ Patients dying from intercurrent disease are excluded. Percentages are of a total of 2,200 patients.
§ Percentages are of a total of 189 patients.

came a measure of the voltage of the x-ray unit. With the recent utilization of high-energy nuclear radiation sources, ranging between 3 million electron volts (cobalt 60) and 25 MeV (Betatron), irradiation therapy has achieved new vistas in the treatment of pelvic cancer. The combination of intracavitary radium and supervoltage external irradiation combines the advantage of the high surface irradiation from the radium (gamma) source in the center of the pelvis with effective treatment of the lateral pelvic wall by augmenting the radium dose with the deeply penetrating megavoltage ray.

A recent report from the M. D. Anderson Hospital by Fletcher and Rutledge is evidence of the success which can be achieved by this modality at the present time. Their series of 2,200 patients, treated between September 1948 and the end of December 1963, included the use of the 22 MeV Betatron, which became available in September 1954. Consequently, the last 6 years of their treatment program utilizing megavoltage can be compared with the results of their earlier treatment with orthovoltage.

Their figures do not support the statement that there is significantly better irradiation control of the disease in the megavoltage series. Apparently, more patients died in the megavoltage series from distant metastasis presumably outside the pelvis at the time of therapy. Five-year survical of 62.5 per cent and a 10-year survival of 57 per cent by both kilovoltage and megavoltage are indeed evidence of meticulous and laudable therapy and perhaps better than any other surgical or radiotherapeutic clinic in this country. Cervical stump carcinomas were also effectively controlled with irradiation, with a somewhat better 5-year survival of 68.5 per cent as compared with cases involving the intact uterus. The cure rate of adenocarcinoma of the cervix was found to be comparable,

TABLE 34-3. RESULTS OF TREATMENT PROGRAM AT THE UNIVERSITY OF MINNESOTA, 1935–55*

	5-YEAR	10-YEAR
Stage I	81.3%	66.8%
Stage II	60.0%	50.0%
Stage III	35.0%	28.0%
Stage IV	3.4%	—
Overall 5-year	58.8%	
Overall 10-year	47.5%	

* Makowski, E. L., McKelvey, J. L., Flight, G. W., Stenstrom, K. W., and Mosser, D. G.: Results of radiation therapy of carcinoma of cervix. J.A.M.A., 182:637, 1962.

stage for stage, whether treated with irradiation therapy alone or in combination with radiation plus surgery. The latter method included a simple total hysterectomy for removal of the parent tumor in the endocervix but did not include a lymph node dissection.

Makowski, McKelvey and co-workers report a 20-year treatment program at the University of Minnesota from 1935–55 with a total of 1,200 cases. Their series included three major types of irradiation:
   1939–42...240 Kv (orthovoltage)
   1942–53...400 Kv (orthovoltage)
   1953–55...alternating 400 Kv and cobalt 60 teletherapy

Although this material admittedly included some cases of carcinoma in situ in the Stage I category, the 5- and 10-year results for more advanced diseases are commendable.

In comparing figures with the data from 124 institutions of 26 countries in the *Annual Report,* volume 14, edited by Kottmeier and collated in 1966, one can observe the favorable results of current treatment programs by irradiation.

As has been emphasized repeatedly in this text, one of the major improvements in the cure of cervical carcinoma has been the progressive increase of early cases in all series throughout the world as a direct result of cervical cancer screening programs.

Complications, Morbidity, and Mortality of Irradiation Therapy. The biologic effect of ionizing irradiation produces an interruption of the biochemical and metabolic processes of the human cell, which causes mitotic inhibition or reproductive failure of the cell and finally cell death. Lethally irradiated cells may show no visible damage initially, but eventually they degenerate owing to their inability to undergo continued cell division. Other cells will undergo an immediate interruption of viability, with rapid cellular death ensuing. Successful irradiation treatment, therefore, is a delicate balance between the normal tissue tolerance of the reproductive tract and adjacent organs and the tumorcidal dosage required for permanent arrest of the tumor cell. Irradiation complications

TABLE 34-4. OVERALL RELATIVE APPARENT 5-YEAR RECOVERY RATE*

	108 COLLABORATORS REPORTING IN BOTH VOLUME 13 AND VOLUME 14	ALL COLLABORATORS
Vol. 13 (1953–57)	48.5	48.5
Vol. 14 (1956–60)	50.1	50.4

* Kottmeier, H.-L. (ed.): Annual Report on the Results of Treatment in Carcinoma of the Uterus and Vagina. Stockholm, vol. 13, 1963; vol. 14, collated 1966, published, 1967.

TABLE 34-5. COMPARISON OF THE 5-YEAR RESULTS OBTAINED BY 108 INSTITUTIONS COLLABORATING IN BOTH VOLUME 13 AND VOLUME 14*

	VOLUME 13 (1953–57)		VOLUME 14 (1956–60)	
	Relative Apparent 5-Year Recovery Rate	Proportion of Cases in the Different Stages (Per Cent)	Relative Apparent 5-Year Recovery Rate	Proportion of Cases in the Different Stages (Per Cent)
Stage I	74.8	24.7	75.8	25.5
Stage II	52.9	37.9	54.4	37.8
Stage III	30.1	31.7	31.4	31.1
Stage IV	8.0	5.7	8.6	5.6
	48.5		50.1	

* Kottmeier, H.-L. (ed.): *Ibid.*

occur when the ionization tolerance of the nonmalignant cell is exceeded. Consequently, the bladder and rectum are constantly threatened with the hazard of receiving excessive irradiation during the course of treatment of the cervical malignancy. Tissue tolerance depends not only on the dose but also on the amount of tissue irradiated. The current direction of irradiation therapy is in the use of megavoltage machines due to the deep penetrability of the emitted ray (80% depth dose at 10 cm.) and the feasibility of whole pelvis irradiation in preference to the conventional split field technic. With such radiobiologic advantages of the supervoltage unit, the superficial skin is no longer a barrier to the depth dose of irradiation. Unfortunately, the effective penetrability of the megavoltage ray is a double-edged sword and is currently producing a series of untoward reactions to adjacent pelvic structures.

As recently reported by Kottmeier, the complication rate is directly related to the dosage received by the bladder and the rectum. The glandular mucosa of the bowel is unfortunately more radiosensitive than the transitional epithelium of the bladder, and serious rectal injuries occurred at the Radiumhemmet with the Stockholm technic when more than 6,000 r was given to the rectum. When the rectum received more than 8,000 r, serious injuries occurred in 26.1 per cent. While local measures of hydrocortisone enemas and analgesic rectal suppositories may be helpful, the radiobiologic effect of ischemic endarteritis is progressive and irreversible. Rectal dosage of greater than 6,000 r produce a high incidence of rectal stricture and frequently require permanent colostomy. McLennan, McLennan, and Bagshaw report frequent rectal complications with the linear accelerator (6 MeV), which have not been reduced in recent years by rotational therapy. Of equal concern to these investigators is the fact that the predicted overall survival of cases treated with megavoltage between 1961 and 1965 is only 54 ± 9.6 per cent, which is lower than their previous experience.

Bladder injuries are less frequent, and usually the symptoms are more delayed. In Kottmeier's report 1.4 per cent had serious bladder injuries with irradiation therapy. Bladder injuries of all types, including fistulas, occurred in 31.2 per cent of the cases in which irradiation dosages to the bladder wall exceeded 6,000 rads. His fistula rate was 0.8 per cent for all cases. Ureteral obstruction likewise may occur from radiation fibrosis but usually occurs as a result of recurrent pelvic tumor.

As the combined irradiation dosage of both intracavitary radium and supervoltage external therapy increases above 6,000 rads to the lateral pelvic wall, one can expect an increased incidence of pelvic cellulitis, ureteral and rectal strictures, and fistula formation. Greiss found 55 per cent complications of various degrees of severity when the combined midpelvic dose exceeded 7,000 rads. In order to preserve the integrity of the bladder and rectal wall, meticulous monitoring of the irradiation dosage to the rectovaginal and vesicovaginal septa is of major importance in the treatment of cervical cancer. As discussed in Dosimetry of Irradiation Therapy, the use of a scintillation probe counter in the bladder and rectum at the time of radium application is essential for accurate documentation of the exact dosage to the bowel and bladder wall. This instrument records the number of roentgens per hour which the bladder and rectal mucosa receives during the radium treatment. The combined irradiation dosage from external therapy and intracavitary radiation should not exceed 5,000 to 6,000 rads to these structures.

Aseptic necrosis and spontaneous fracture of the head of the femur may also occur. This is most frequently noted with rotational therapy or the use of lateral treatment portals. McKelvey's report includes 13 patients (1.1%) with aseptic necrosis of the femur which was directly related to the use of lateral portals. This complication occurs more frequently with orthovoltage, in which the absorption capacity of bone is greater than with megavoltage.

While death from radiation has been reported in the past, this is an uncommon complication of modern radiotherapy. In the past, most of the deaths resulting from irradiation therapy occurred in patients with pelvic inflammatory disease when irradiation ignited the disease, and it became generalized and uncontrollable. Modern antibiotic therapy, however, and the more liberal use of primary surgery for such cases has virtually eliminated deaths from infection as a complication of radiation therapy.

TECHNIC OF IRRADIATION

The subject of irradiation treatment for carcinoma of the cervix has become so complex in the past decade that it is impossible to present a complete treatise on the subject in this textbook; instead, the reader is referred to numerous texts on the subject. The present review includes a general statement of the principles of current treatment and some standard technics. In the treatment of cervical carcinoma full advantage is taken of the combined treatment with high-dosage, controlled gamma irradiation from intracavitary radium and the high-voltage x-ray beam for lateral pelvic wall treatment.

In general, most radium treatment programs have evolved as modifications of the Stockholm, Paris, or Manchester technics. Intracavitary radium therapy is based on the physics of the inverse square law, which simply states that a dose rate from a point source is inversely proportional to the square of the distance from the source of the radiation. Therefore, the dose rate of radium for an area that is twice the distance away from a defined source would be only one fourth the dose rate of the original area. The depth dose, however, from this point source of irradiation is increased as the treating distance is increased. The proportional dose to the vaginal mucosa, to the paracervical area, and to the immediate broad ligament is more favorable as the diameter of the vaginal colpostat increases.

Prior to initiation of therapy, it is essential that the patient have complete evaluation of the contiguous organs, namely, the rectum and urinary tract, to make certain that there is no involvement of these organs by the tumor. Consequently, in addition to a thorough general physical examination, including complete cardiopulmonary evaluation with chest x-ray for possible metastatic disease, a proctosigmoidoscopy and barium enema are essential to make certain that the rectal mucosa and rectal wall are not involved in extension of the cervical tumor.

The urinary tract is evaluated routinely by intravenous pyelogram and water cystoscopy with direct visualization of the urethra and bladder mucosa. The importance of documenting the status of the bladder and upper urinary tract has been repeatedly demonstrated by studies that show the prognostic influence of ureteral obstruction from lateral spread of the cervical carcinoma (Everett, 1939). In Everett's original study, patients with Stage III carcinoma of the cervix having ureteral obstruction showed poor response to irradiation therapy, while 75 per cent of Stage III patients with no obstructive uropathy survived for 5 years. This suggests that parametrial induration may not necessarily be related only to tumor, but may be due to an associated inflammatory process which responds under therapy. In 1956 a review of the problem regarding the urinary tract as it relates to the prognosis of cervical cancer was conducted by Burns, Everett, and Brack which confirmed the original experience at Hopkins. Where the pretreatment pyelograms were normal, the 5-year survival rate was 70.3 per cent as compared to a 5-year survival of 22.4 per cent for those pretreatment pyelograms showing hydronephrosis. Schewe reported similar results in 102 cases of carcinoma of the cervix, in which 54 per cent of the patients demonstrating abnormal excretory urograms were dead within 1 year following therapy. It is important to view the bladder for the possibility of bullous edema, which suggests lymphatic obstruction in the bladder wall. However, in order to classify the lesion clinically as Stage IV, evidence of disease in the bladder must be proven by biopsy. The same requirement is true for rectal lesions, which may be purely inflammatory rather than tumor.

Radiation therapy for invasive cancer of the cervix at Marquette School of Medicine consists of a fairly standard combination of external pelvic irradiation and intracavitary radium. The objective of our technic is to deliver a total, combined dose of approximately 10,000 r to Point A (paracervical triangle) and 6,000 r to classical Point B (the lateral parametrium). For purposes of brevity, the treatment policy in management of carcinoma of the cervix is outlined below.

Stage I:

I A: Two intracavitary radium insertions 10 to 14 days apart with a total dose of 8,000 to 10,000 mg. hours, depending on the age and physical status of the patient.

I B: If the lesion is fungating or exophytic, 2,000 r whole pelvic irradiation, with the dose calculated at midplane. This is followed by 2 intracavitary radium insertions at 2-week intervals for a total of 8,000 mg. hours. With the midline shielded (5-cm. lead bar), 2,000 r additional is added to the parametrium (15 cm. × 15 cm. anterior and posterior portals).

I B: Alternate Plan for nonexophytic lesions: 8,000 to 10,000 mg. hours of radium in 2 insertions, 14 days apart, with no precedent external irradiation. This is followed by 3,000 to 4,000 r to the parametrium with midline structures shielded.

Stage II:

II A: 2,000 r whole pelvis irradiation followed (at 2 weeks) by 8,000 mg. hours of intracavitary radium in 2 insertions, 14 days apart; 2,000 r additional to parametrial structures with midline structures shielded by lead bar.

II B: May be treated as II A; *or* 4,000 r whole pelvis in 4 weeks followed by 5,500 to 6,500 mg. hours of radium in 2 insertions (14 days apart). The total radium dose is influenced by the rectal dose per scintillation probe.

Stage III:

III A: 4,000 r whole pelvis in 4 weeks (Betatron), followed by 5,500 to 6,500 mg. hours of radium in 2 insertions; *or* 6,000 r to entire pelvis in 6 weeks (Betatron) without shielding, followed by 2,000 to 3,000 mg. hours of radium in 1 insertion. Dosage is influenced by rectal dose rate per probe. The intracavitary increment may be omitted if general status is poor.

III B: 6,000 r whole pelvis in 6 weeks without shielding, followed by 2,000 to 3,000 mg. hours of radium in 1 insertion.

Stage IV: 6,000 to 7,000 r whole pelvis (Betatron) in 6 to 8 weeks per tolerance and general physical status; *or* same as stage III B.

The 25 MeV Betatron is employed in our clinic for external irradiation and the dose rate is 1,000 r per week calculated at depth. The Manchester system of fitted rubber ovoids and plastic tandems is employed where possible.

Treatment is initiated with either external irradiation or intracavitary radium. It has been our policy to initiate treatment of the more advanced lesions (Stages II, III, and IV) with external irradiation by opposing anterior and posterior pelvic fields (15 × 15 cm.) until a midpelvic depth dose of 2,000 r has been attained. At this point, intracavitary radium therapy is started. By means of suturing an intrauterine tandem to the cervix (Fig. 34-7), approximately 3,500 r is delivered to point A, utilizing 20 mg., 10 mg., and 10 mg. radium sources in the uterine cavity and cervical canal. Silverstone spring colpostats or Manchester ovoids are used for the vaginal application of radium with a dose of approximately 2,500 r being delivered to Point A with a 20-mg. radium source in each colpostat. The bladder and rectum are probed at the time of application, utilizing a sterile rubber sheath to cover the probe. The maximum dosage is recorded in roentgen per hour and should not exceed 50 r/hr. Because of the normal anatomical depth of the posterior vaginal wall, the rectum is probed approximately 10 to 12 cm. before reaching the area of the posterior fornix and the location of the vaginal colpostat. The bladder is probed for approximately 6 to 8 cm. from the urethral meatus, before reaching the area of the colpostats in the anterior fornix, where the maximum irradiation to the bladder involves the area of the trigone.

IRRADIATION THERAPY

From this radium system utilizing 2 applications at 2-week intervals, approxi-

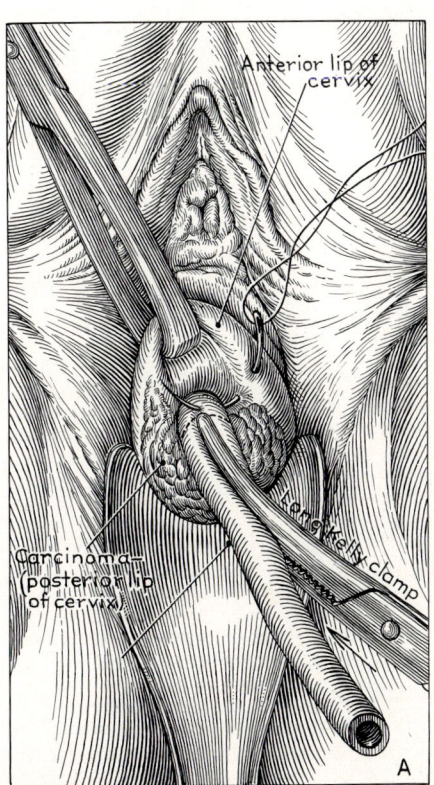 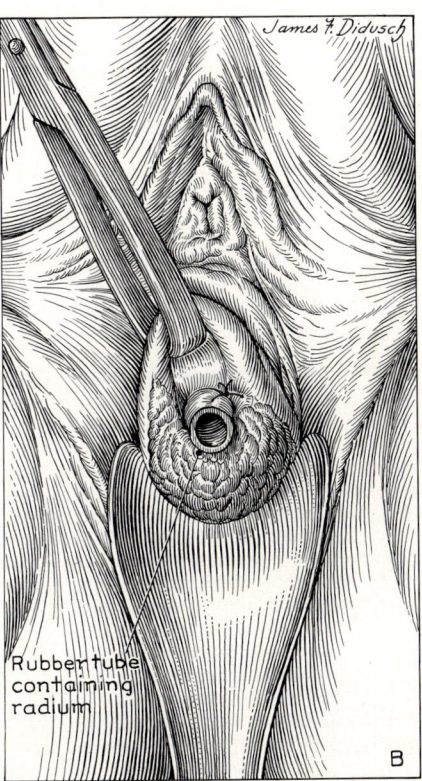

FIG. 34-7. Method of placing radium. (A) Tube with radium inserted into cervical canal. (B) Tube sutured to cervix and cut flush with cervix.

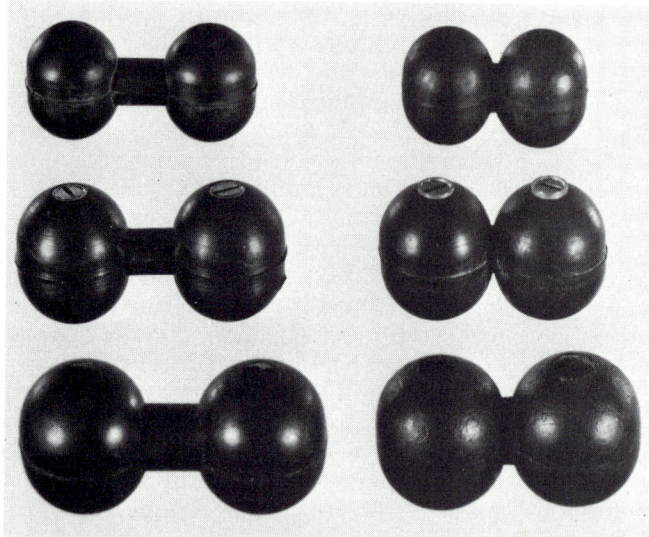

FIG. 34-8. Vaginal ovoids of various sizes with fixed separator of different distances.

mately 6,000 gamma r are delivered to point A and 1,500 to 2,000 gamma r to point B (Figs. 34-7 and 34-8). External irradiation completes the treatment by a split field technic, using a 5-cm. median lead shield over the pubic and sacral areas. Four ports are thus produced, and an initial 2,000 r is delivered to the midpelvis at Point B. Thus over a period of 6 weeks a total of 4,000 r is delivered to Point B by means of external pelvic irradiation. With advanced lesions (Stage II B, III, and IV), this technic is reversed with the initial use of external irradiation to approximately 2,000 r midpelvic dosage in an effort to shrink the tumor mass, improve the inflammatory reaction, and provide a more effective radium application.

The following anatomic and physical principles of intracavitary radium therapy are employed:

1. There must be multiple insertions.
2. Tandem must reach the top of the fundus.
3. Use ovoids of as large a diameter as the vaginal vault allows.
4. Ovoids must be carefully positioned in each fornix with adaption to the existent anatomical situation.
5. The radium system must not slip downward.
6. The relative proportion of uterine and vaginal radium is determined by the type of disease.

The following maximum radium dosages are used in our radiation program:

1. 10,000 to 11,000 mg./hr. if no external irradiation is used.
2. 10,000 mg./hr. if parametrial treatment is to be given.
3. 8,000 to 9,000 mg./hr. if prior therapy of 2,000 r has been given to the whole pelvis.
4. 5,500 to 6,500 mg./hr. if prior therapy of 4,000 r has been given to the whole pelvis.
5. 4,000 to 5,000 mg./hr. if prior therapy of 6,000 r has been given to the whole pelvis.
6. 3,000 mg./hr. if prior therapy of 7,000 r has been given to the whole pelvis.

The importance of all methods of combined intracavitary radium and external irradiation therapy is to achieve a tumoricidal dose of ionizing irradiation of approximately 6,000 r to the midplane of the pelvis; this plane is equidistant between the symphysis pubis and the sacrum and presumably includes the broad ligament and the lymphatics from the uterus to the lateral pelvic wall. This dose range is effective for both squamous cell carcinoma and adenocarcinoma of the cervix. Irradiation dosages in excess of 6,000 r, as previously stated, are associated with progressive and serious complications of the bowel and urinary tract.

One of the advantages of the initial use of intracavitary radium is the opportunity to stage the tumor under anesthesia at the beginning of the treatment program. In the event that one is dealing with an advanced lesion (Stage II or more), or if one wishes to confirm the stage of the disease before initiating therapy, there should be no hesitancy in examining the patient under anesthesia, and at the same time performing a D and C and fractional curettage of the endocervical and endometrial cavity as basic information for defining the limits of the cervical cancer.

DOSIMETRY OF IRRADIATION THERAPY

In order to evaluate effectively the results of irradiation therapy in the treatment of cervical carcinoma, it is important to have an accurate method of documenting irradiation dosages to the tumor-bearing areas of the pelvis. Todd and Meredith designated Points A and B as reference points in the pelvis, in which Point A was originally located 2 cm. above the lateral fornix and 2 cm. lateral to the cervical canal, and Point B was 3 cm. lateral to Point A. Ten years later, Paterson redefined Point A as 2 cm. up from the external cervical os and 2 cm. lateral from the cervical canal. Theoretically, Point A is superimposed on the paracervical area at the junction of the crossing of the uterine artery with the ureter. Recently, Nathanson has shown by direct anatomical placement of microdosimetry units that Point A is not a specific anatomical point; that is, it is not located precisely at the crossing of the ureter by the uterine artery. However, as crude as both points may be, they serve as radiologic points of reference for dosimetry studies.

A plane passing through the internal os and the center of the vaginal colpostats bisects the lower uterine segment and the paracervical areas. This plane is chosen for the isodose curve calculation, which is a standard method of evaluating the amount of radiation per hour to be given to various points emanating from the central radium source. In our understanding of irradiation therapy, it is important to recognize from the beginning that the rad is the internationally accepted unit of an absorbed radiation dose. In practice, this is frequently confused with the term *roentgen*, which in reality is only a unit of radiation exposure. The roentgen (r), often incorrectly used to indicate dosage, is a unit which indicates the ability of a proton beam to produce ionization in the air, and should be used only for the unit of radiation exposure rather than the unit of absorbed radiation in the tissue. There is a difference in dosage if measurements are reported in rads instead of roentgens. Actually, rads = roentgens $\times$ f, in which the value of "f" depends on the material being irradiated and the energy of the irradiation. Tabulated values of "f" are available for various energies and materials.

In monitoring the amount of irradiation delivered to the tissue, sensitive ionizing chambers, including materials that scintillate and other radiation-sensitive elements, have been utilized at the tip of small-diameter, long-stem instruments which are known as dose rate probe detectors. The amount of ionization is recorded on a read-out meter and may be recorded for high radiation levels as roentgens per hour (Fig. 34-9). Such instruments have proven uniquely valuable in assessing the amount of irradiation to the bladder and rectal wall at the time of radium application. A probe of this kind is used in conjunction with the application of radium to make certain that the total amount of irradiation delivered by radium does not exceed the normal tissue tolerance of the rectovaginal and vesicovaginal septum. In general, the combined radiation dosage to the bladder and rectal wall should not exceed 5,000 to 6,000 roentgens. By observing the read-out meter for the

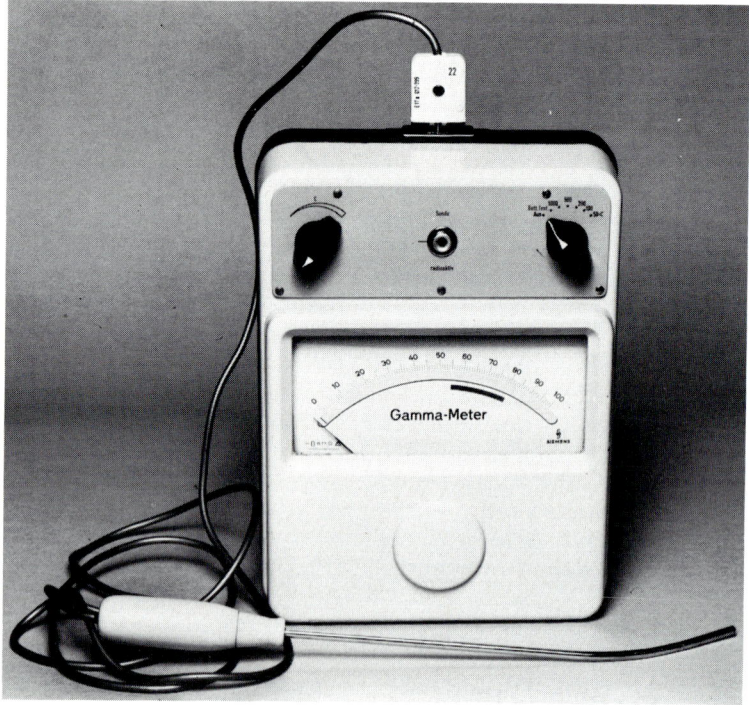

Fig. 34-9. Dosimeter with dose rate probe detector containing sensitive ionizing chamber in tip.

amount of radiation to the rectal mucosa at the time of radium application, one can multiply the reading of roentgens per hour by the number of hours that the radium is to be left in place to determine the amount of radiation given to the rectal wall by that application. If the radium is to be repeated, one must assume a similar amount for the next application. In addition, it is important to include the amount of unshielded midline irradiation produced by deep x-ray therapy as an additive component to the rectal and vesical wall in calculating the total bladder and rectal dosage. In general, probe dosimetry measurements to the rectal and vesical wall should not exceed a rate of more than 50 roentgens per hour, and it is preferable to keep the irradiation between 30 and 40 roentgens per hour. In the event this limit is exceeded, the colpostat should be removed and reapplied with repacking of the bladder and rectal wall away from the radium source.

RADICAL WERTHEIM HYSTERECTOMY

Preparation

It is advisable to emphasize three important requirements for patients undergoing radical surgery: adequate hydration, adequate blood volume, and adequate bowel preparation.

It is advisable to have the bowel prepared with antibacterial therapy as well as mechanical cleansing. The use of Neothalidine, 15 ml. every 4 hours for 24 to 48 hours preoperatively, and enemas until clear fluid is returned prior to surgery, with the last enema of 1 per cent neomycin solution, will adequately prepare the bowel for any operative procedure. This is particularly important if a radical Wertheim hysterectomy is being considered for radioresistant carcinoma, for which the operative procedure may be more extensive. The fact that radical surgery in the treatment of radioresistant cancer is occasionally associated with bowel injury is an additional indication for adequate bowel preparation. It is preferable to give only a liquid diet on the day prior to surgery to promote complete emptying of the intestinal tract with the bowel preparation. During the many preoperative studies which require the fasting state, there is a tendency toward dehydration, which is also exaggerated by multiple enemas and diarrhea produced by the bowel preparation. To provide an adequate tissue hydration preoperatively, 2 liters of 5 per cent glucose and normal saline is given on the day prior to surgery, and additional fluid is given until the urinary specific gravity is within the normal range (1.010-1.015). Blood volume studies, which are essential in evaluating red cell mass and plasma volume, are used as baselines for blood replacement postoperatively. Preoperative transfusion is required until a hematocrit of 40 per cent or greater is achieved. The placement of a central venous catheter is an additional preoperative procedure which is considered essential for proper monitoring of the patient's intravascular compartment and cardiac reserve during and after the operation. This is inserted in the subclavian or external jugular vein, as described in Chapter 4. In order to maintain patency of the tube, it may be used for intravenous fluid replacement when it is not being utilized for periodic monitoring of the central venous pressure. Only if bowel resection is definitely planned preoperatively is a long intestinal tube (Cantor tube) positioned in the ileum on the day prior to surgery.

Baseline electrolyte studies, serum protein with A/G ratio, urea nitrogen, and baseline liver function studies are a part of the normal laboratory evaluation of the patient.

TECHNIC: RADICAL WERTHEIM HYSTERECTOMY

Following proper abdominal and vaginal preparation, an indwelling catheter is placed in the bladder to keep it decompressed throughout the operative procedure. An adhesive plastic skin drape (Vi-drape) is of assistance during prolonged operative surgery in protecting the incision from bacterial contamination. A low midline periumbilical incision, extending approximately 3 cm. above the umbilicus, is required for adequate exposure. The incision is protected by moist gauze beneath self-retaining retractors. In any prolonged operative procedure it is advisable to release the mechanical retractors and the tension on the walls of the incision after 2 hours in order to improve the circulation through rectus muscles, which become ischemic under prolonged retraction.

Abdominal and Pelvic Exploration

If this type of radical hysterectomy is to be successful, it is important to evaluate meticulously the parietal and visceral surfaces of the peritoneal cavity, as well as the para-aortic lymph nodes, for the possibility of metastatic tumor already beyond the limits of cure by this procedure. The liver surface, diaphragm, omentum, mesentery, and bowel are thoroughly examined, and the kidneys are palpated retroperitoneally for possible gross abnormalities. Of paramount importance is an adequate evaluation of the para-aortic lymph chain. This is meticulously palpated from the region of the bifurcation of the aorta to the celiac plexus. Although gross metastatic disease is easily palpable, it is important to provide histologic proof of the absence of metastatic disease by routinely sampling lymph nodes from the lower portion of the aorta and vena cava adjacent to the bifurcation. If these nodes are grossly normal and are proven to be histologically benign on frozen-section study, it can be assumed with relative certainty that metastasis does not occur higher up the lymphatic chain. This point is emphasized, due to the fact that occasionally the most benign and innocuous-appearing soft lymph node will contain histologic evidence of embolic tumor. Patients who have undergone radical pelvic surgery, and later develop recurrence in the upper abdomen, are those patients in whom disease was unrecognized in the lymphatic chain above the pelvic brim at the time of surgery.

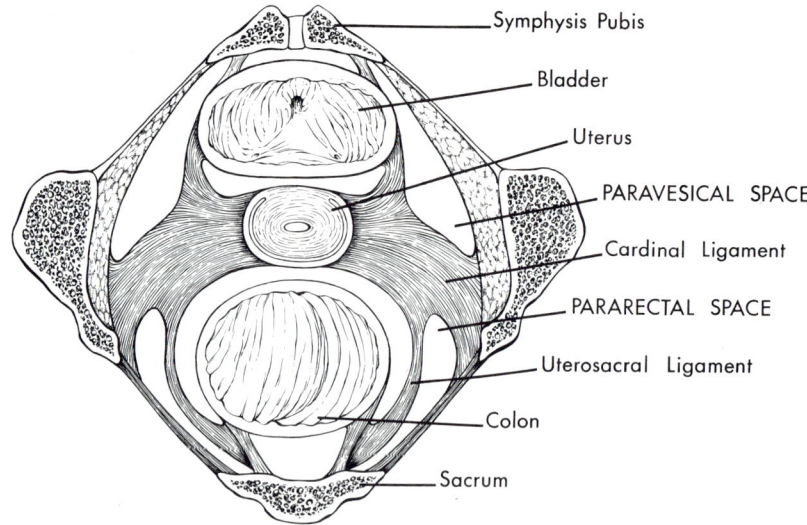

FIG. 34-10. Cross section of pelvis showing paravesical space and pararectal space. The base of the broad ligament (cardinal ligament) extends to the lateral pelvic wall and contains the major lymphatics draining the cervix.

Accurate evaluation of the extent of tumor in the pelvis proper can be accomplished easily and rapidly by opening the paravesical and pararectal spaces (Fig. 34-10), which provides an opportunity for thorough exploration of the intervening base of the broad ligament. As this is the direct pathway of lateral extension of cervical cancer in the pelvis, this tissue must be carefully examined for tumor and its relationship to the adjacent pelvic floor and lateral pelvic wall. This procedure is easily accomplished by ligating the round ligament and infundibulopelvic ligaments close to the lateral pelvic wall, and opening the anterior leaf of the broad ligament (Fig. 34-11). The index finger can be inserted easily into the paravesical space, which is developed bluntly until the fascia of the levator muscle is identified (Fig. 34-12). The posterior peritoneal leaf is opened next (Fig. 34-13 A), and the pararectal space is developed bluntly by initiating a plane with the finger between the cardinal ligament anteriorly and the uterosacral ligament posteriorly. This space is gently developed until the pelvic floor is completely visible. While the paravesical space is relatively avascular, the pararectal space must be carefully dissected due to the anastomotic channels of the hypogastric vein, which courses freely across the pelvic floor and broad ligament in this area. The major branches of the hypogastric artery are lateral to the pararectal fossa and are not damaged in this step of the operation. The ureter is left attached to the pelvic peritoneum and is medial to the paravesical and pararectal fossae. As demonstrated in Figure 34-13 B, the intervening tissue between these two planes constitutes the base of the broad ligament, which is attached to the lateral pelvic wall in the region of the obturator fossa. If one can be certain that there is no gross evidence of tumor invading the fascia of the levator muscles of the pelvic floor, or the fascia at the lateral pelvic wall, including the obturator muscle and the fascial sheath of the external iliac vessels, the case is considered operable, and attention is now turned to the pelvic lymphadenectomy.

Pelvic Lymphadenectomy

Skeletonization of the lymphatic tissue along the iliac vessels begins in the region of the bifurcation of the aorta. The opening of the posterior peritoneal leaf of the broad ligament must be extended to

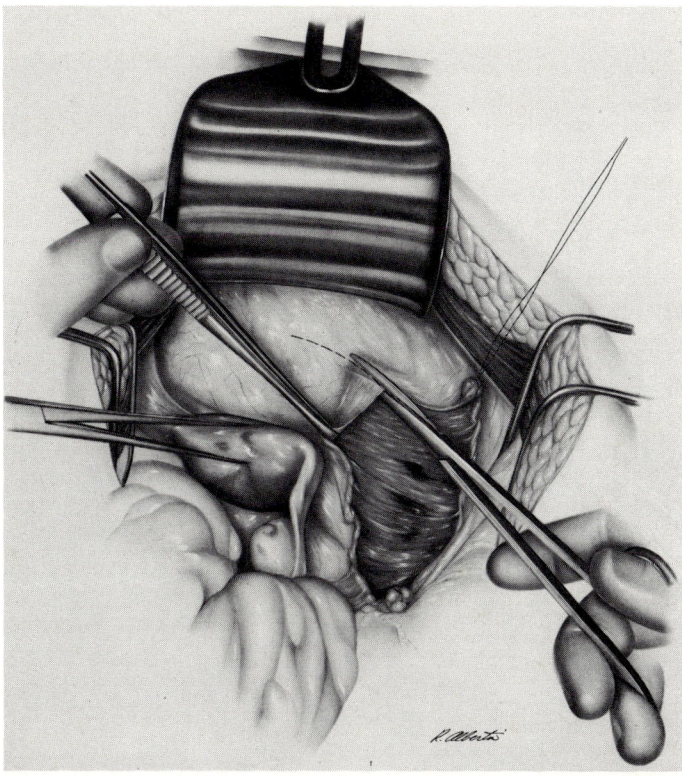

FIG. 34-11. Opening the anterior leaf of the broad ligament after ligating the round ligament and infundibulopelvic ligament.

the area of the pelvic brim, where the ureter is easily identified as it enters the pelvis at the bifurcation of the common iliac artery into the external and hypogastric vessels. On the right side, the ureter is generally in close relation to the common iliac bifurcation, while on the left side the ureter enters the pelvis 1 to 2 cm. lateral to the bifurcation of the left common iliac artery and at this point is related more directly to the left external iliac artery and vein. In dissecting the presacral area in the angle of the bifurcation of the aorta, care must be taken to avoid bleeding from the middle sacral vessels, as well as the proximal part of the external iliac vein, which course through this retroperitoneal space. It is best to ligate the middle sacral vessels as they are identified, but if traumatized, positive pressure will usually control the venous bleeding. The lymphatic tissue is removed by sharp dissection with the points of the Mitzenbaum scissors upwards, while special care is directed toward avoiding trauma to the ureter (Fig. 34-14). The ureter is reflected medially during the dissection of the common iliac vessels and left attached to the parietal peritoneum in order to maintain its blood supply.

It is important to remove the fascial sheath of the iliac vessels, but in order to avoid trauma to the intima or wall of the vessels, particularly the veins, one should not attempt to skeletonize the pelvic vessels to the point of producing a "naked," pearl-white, vascular tree. If there is tumor in the adventitia of the vessel wall, the patient will likely not be cured by this procedure, and consequently such compulsive efforts produce far more complications than benefits. It is important to rotate the vessels medially and laterally with a vein retractor during the dissection of the common and external iliac trunks in order to obtain the lymphatic tissue behind the vessels

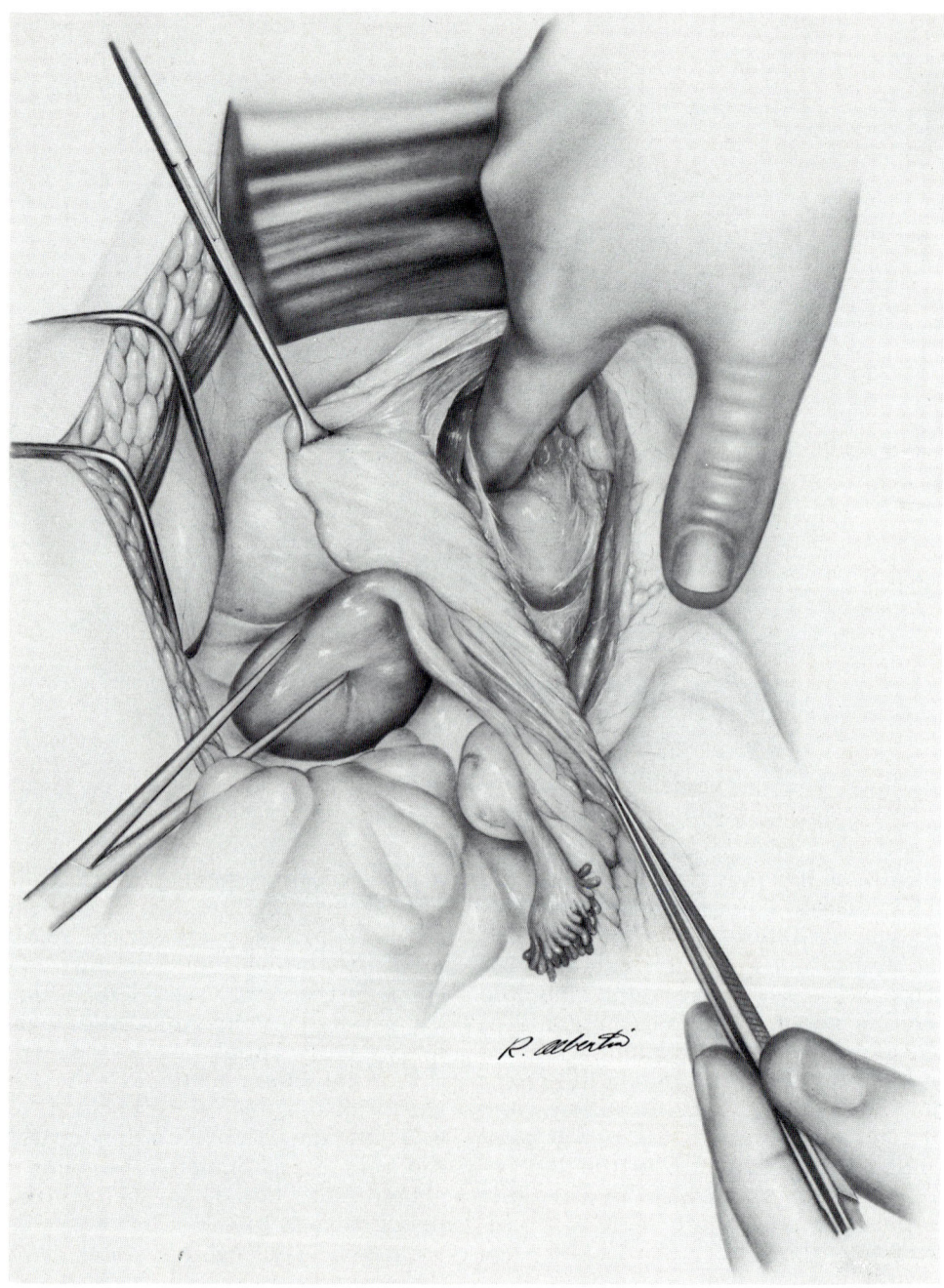

FIG. 34-12. Development of paravesical space to region of pelvic floor.

along the psoas muscle. The genitofemoral nerve which is seen lateral to the external iliac vessels should be preserved, as damage to this peripheral nerve will produce postoperative discomfort in the region of the groin and medial aspect of the thigh.

The external iliac vessels are carefully dissected until they are seen to pass beneath the inguinal ligament. At this

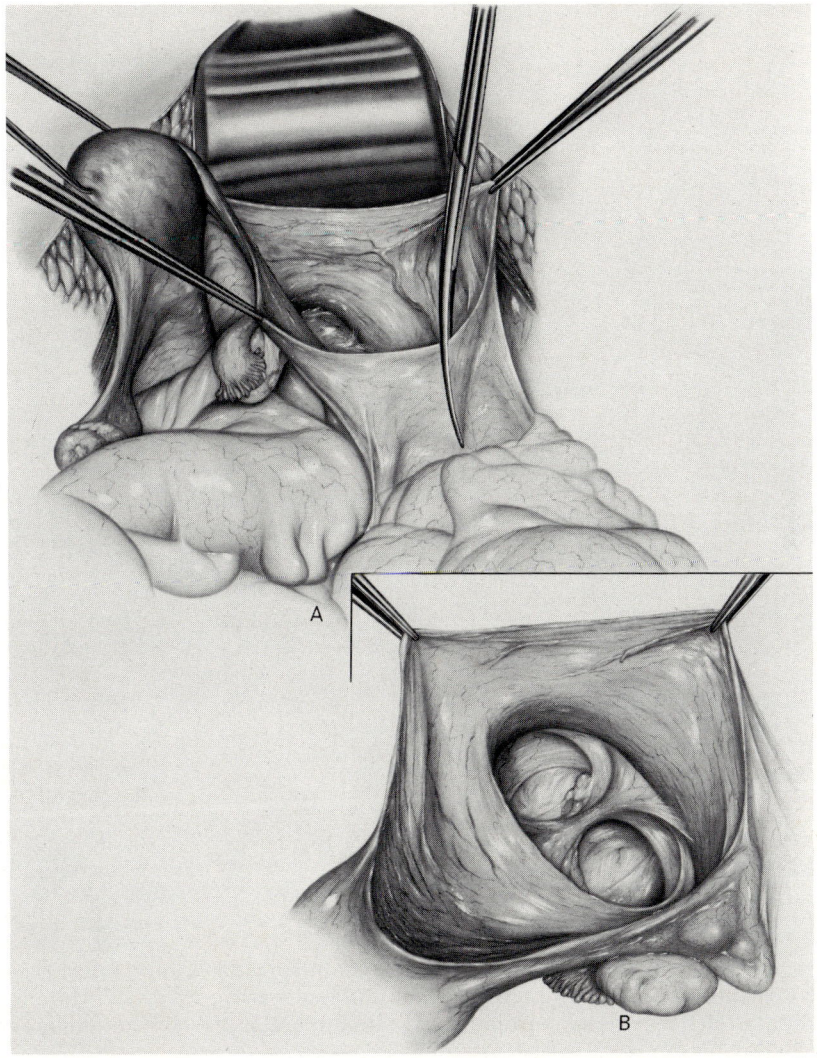

FIG. 34-13. (A) Opening the posterior leaf of the broad ligament for development of the pararectal fossa. (B) Paravesical and pararectal fossae with intervening base of broad ligament attached to pelvic floor and lateral pelvic wall.

point care must be taken to avoid injury to the inferior epigastric artery and vein which come from the anterior and medial side of the iliac vessels and run along the anterior peritoneum into the lower abdominal wall. One must also be cognizant of the anomalous obturator artery and vein which frequently arise from the lower portion of the external iliac vessels and course down over the pelvic sidewall into the obturator space. If accidentally traumatized, they should be ligated at their point of origin from the artery or vein. In order to avoid bleeding in the obturator space, these vessels are frequently ligated, regardless of their origin, as they course through the obturator space.

The obturator space is entered by reflecting the external iliac vessels medially and freeing the areola tissue that lies directly beneath these vessels at the lateral pelvic wall (Fig. 34-15). Once the space has been entered and the adjacent tissue cleaned from the external iliac vessels, these vessels are now gently

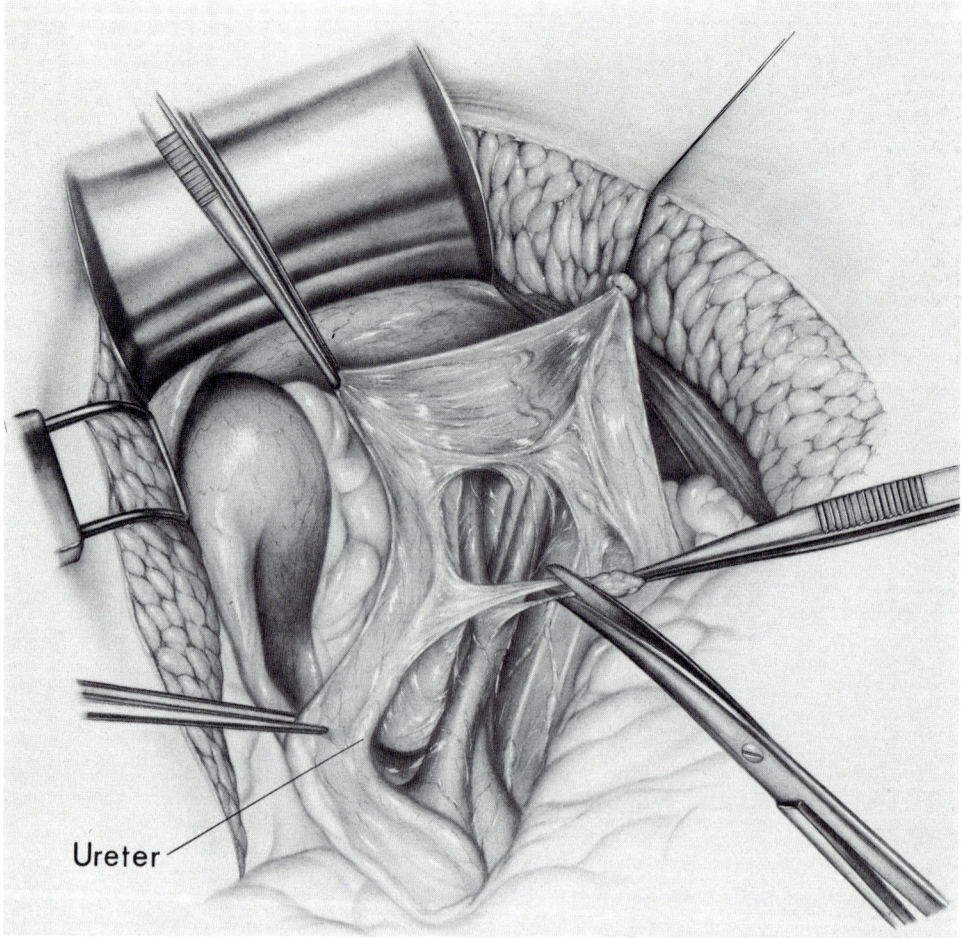

Fig. 34-14. Pelvic lymphadenectomy with dissection of right common iliac vessels and their branches, including the external iliac and hypogastric artery and vein. Note attachment of ureter to parietal peritoneum. Genitofemoral nerve courses along psoas muscle.

retracted laterally with a vein retractor, and the obturator space is clearly exposed. The dissection is continued by removing all of the nodes below the bifurcation of the iliac vessels, including the hypogastric nodes and the nodes in the obturator fossa. A lymph node may be encountered in the angle formed by the external iliac and hypogastric arteries and must be carefully dissected out.

The obturator artery can be demonstrated along the obturator muscle at the lateral pelvic wall adjacent to the easily defined obturator nerve (Fig. 34-15). The nerve, artery, and vein course toward the obturator foramen, where they leave the pelvis. Care must be taken to avoid trauma to all of these structures, particularly the obturator veins, which have a rich anastomotic network against the lateral pelvic wall and communicate freely with the adjacent hypogastric veins. It is best to ligate routinely the obturator vessels, but in the event that trauma to the vessels should occur in this area, hemostasis is best obtained by packing the space with a hot pack and providing adequate time for a fibrin clot to occur. If excessive bleeding occurs on one side of the pelvis, dissection may continue on the opposite side in the interim after pressure packing.

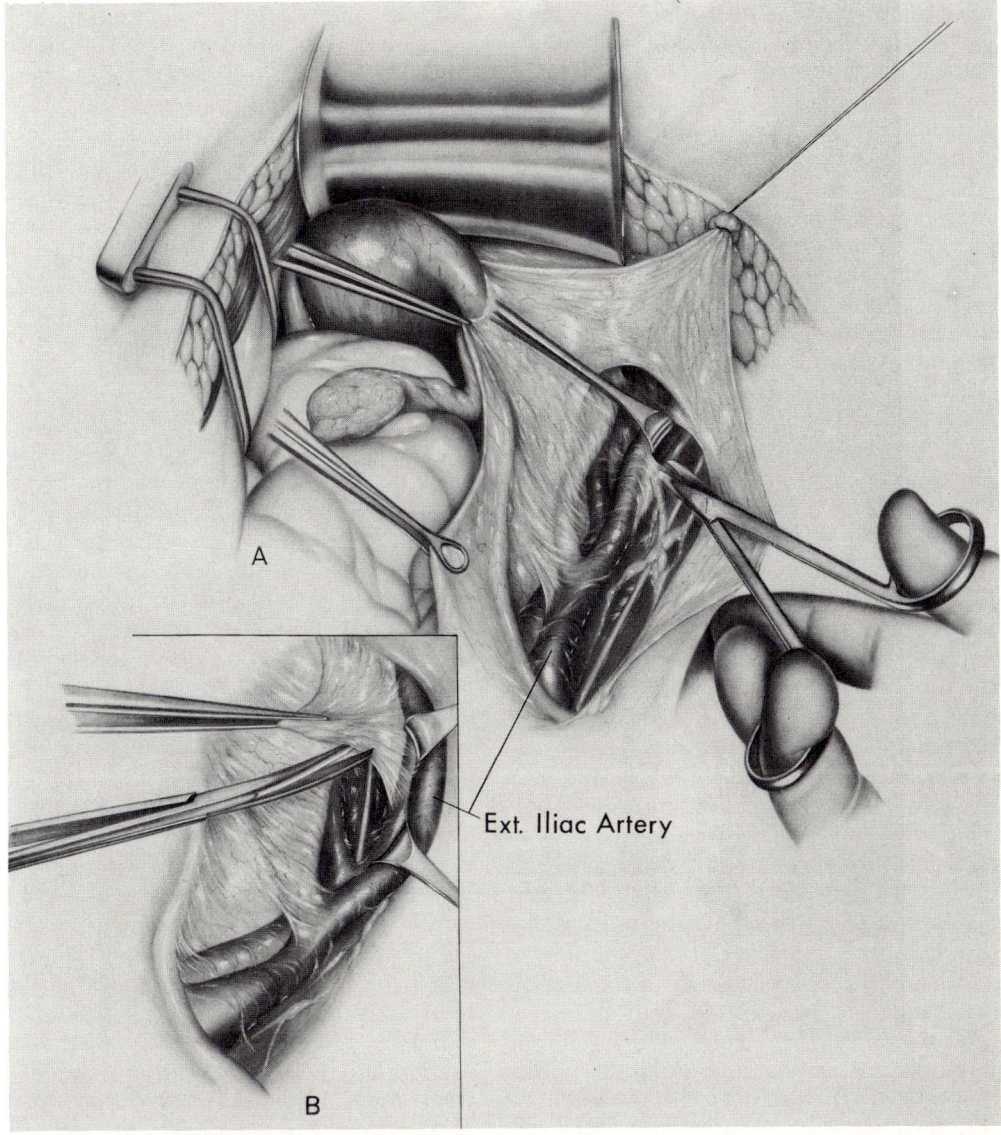

FIG. 34-15. (A) Entry into obturator space by medial reflection of external iliac vessels. (B) Dissection of obturator fossa demonstrating obturator nerve with areolar tissue attached superiorly to external iliac vessels.

The hypogastric artery is now dissected, after identification of the anterior visceral trunk, which branches into the superior vesical, uterine, inferior vesical, vaginal, and middle hemorrhoidal arteries. The anterior division of the hypogastric artery continues along the paravesical fossa to become the obliterated umbilical ligament. It can be ligated distal to the superior vesical artery.

Should the superior vesical artery be damaged, it can be ligated without serious compromise to the blood supply of the bladder. The uterine artery is ligated at its origin from the anterior branch of the hypogastric artery, and the uterine portion of the vessel remains in the broad ligament as a part of the web of paracervical fascia surrounding the ureter. The adjacent uterine veins should also be ligated in order to avoid brisk bleeding in this area. The bladder is now reflected off the lower uterine segment by incising the bladder peritoneum from its attachment to the uterus, and the fascial adhesions of the base of the bladder to the cervix and upper vagina are released by sharp-scissors dissection. The bladder is gently retracted away from the anterior wall of the vagina, and the lower portion of the ureter is identified as it courses through the fascial fibers of the base of the broad ligament. The ureter tunnels between the anterior and posterior fascial bundles of the broad ligament prior to entering the bladder. This tunnel is opened by sliding the Mitzenbaum scissors along the anterior surface of the ureter and spreading the blade as demonstrated in Figure 34-16 A. One will observe the uterine artery coursing along the fascial roof of the ureteral tunnel. As demonstrated in Figure 34-16 B, the roof of the tunnel is opened by doubly clamping and incising this tissue, which demonstrates the ureter attached to the posterior sheath of the broad ligament as though it were lying in a hammock (Fig. 34-16 C). The fascial bundles are suture-ligated for control of bleeding, and the ureter is separated from the posterior fascial leaf of the broad ligament by sharp dissection.

Adson clamps are useful in dissecting the tunnel of the ureter, which is frequently called the "web." These clamps have long handles and delicate points that make them useful in this area, where trauma to the adjacent ureter and bladder is to be avoided. After dissecting the anterior and posterior leaf of the ureteral tunnel, the ureter itself is free from its fascial attachment and is consequently devoid of direct blood supply in this area for approximately 5 to 6 cm. before it is re-attached to the parietal peritoneum. Care must be taken to avoid damage to the adventitia and serosal surface of the ureter, which contains the remaining collateral circulation to the lower ureter. In the event that the blood supply to the ureter is compromised in this region, fistula formation is a serious and frequent complication. The anterior and posterior attachments of the broad ligament to the base of the bladder in this area are now clamped and ligated, a step which completely separates the broad ligament from its attachment to the base of the bladder. Bleeding is frequently troublesome in this region, but can be greatly diminished by clamping and ligating the fascia in this area rather than by sharp dissection. The bladder base contains a rich plexus of vesical veins which should be avoided if at all possible.

Deep Pelvic Dissection

The base of the broad ligament (the cardinal ligament) may now be excised from its attachment at the lateral pelvic wall. A Wertheim clamp is placed as far laterally as possible, with one jaw in the paravesical space and the other jaw in the pararectal space (Fig. 34-17 A). Dissection can be carried down to the pelvic floor with complete freedom from injury to the bladder, ureter, and hypogastric vessels. Should serious bleeding occur in the region of the pelvic floor from the hypogastric veins, hemostatic control is best obtained by firm packing of the pelvis with a hot pack and alternating the dissection to the opposite side of the pelvis. Figure 34-17 demonstrates the lateral fibers of the cardinal ligament, which blend with the fascia of the obturator muscle. Note the presence of the obturator nerve at this point of the dissection and the excised cardinal ligament, with the dissection extending to the pelvic floor (Fig. 34-17 B).

The uterus is retracted sharply forward, and the uterosacral ligaments are placed on stretch. The peritoneal reflection from the cul-de-sac of Douglas is now excised, removing the peritoneum as it reflects from the anterior surface of the rectum well away from its attachment to the lower uterine segment. Care must be taken not to injure the lower ureters as they course just lateral to the uterosacral ligament in this area (Fig. 34-18 A). The areolar tissue between the vaginal wall and the rectum is separated by both blunt and sharp dissection (Fig. 34-17 B). This step develops the posterior reflec-

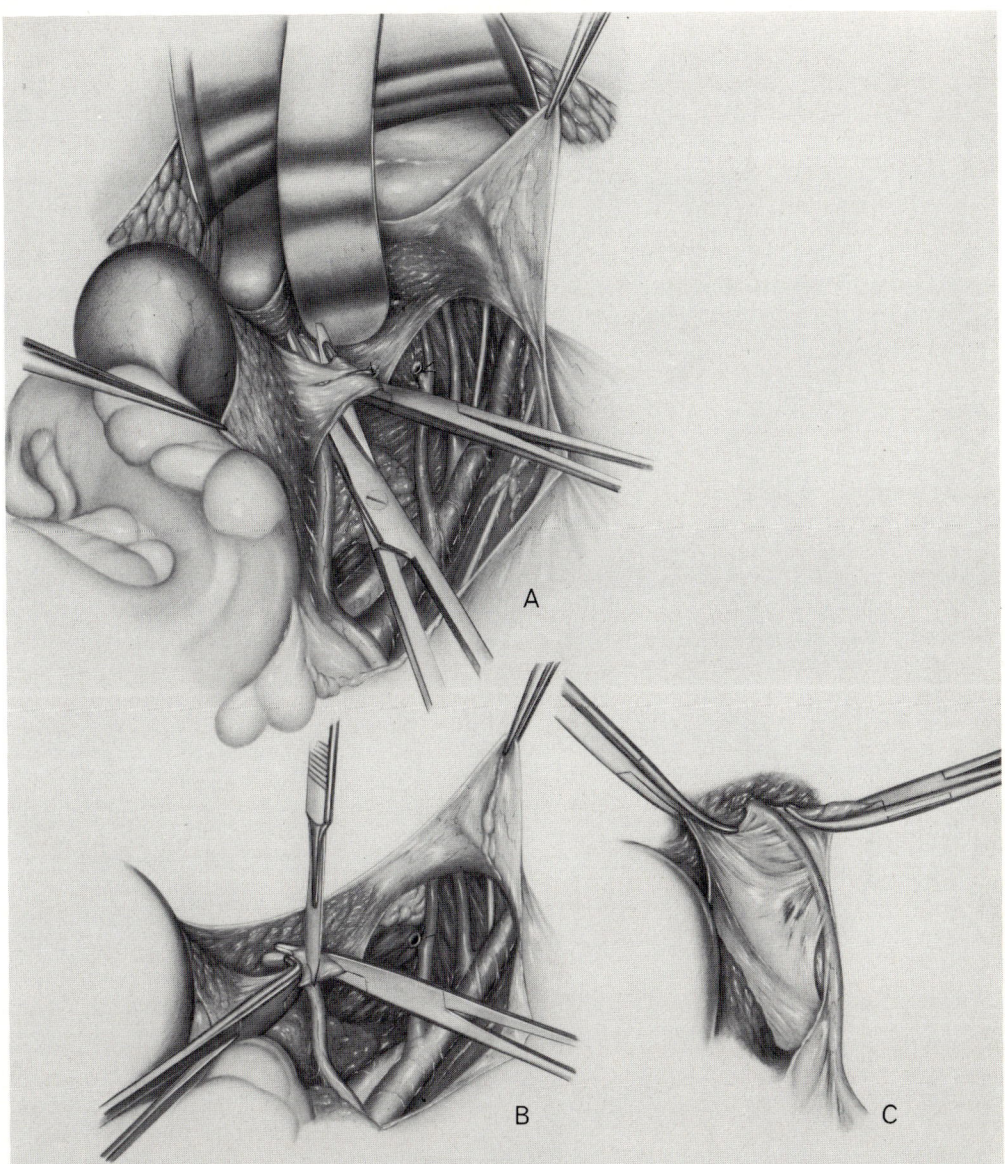

FIG. 34-16. (A) Mitzenbaum scissors inserted above the ureter in the "web" or ureteral tunnel of the broad ligament. Note ligated uterine artery in anterior fascial sheath of tunnel. (B) Roof of tunnel is opened between clamps, with ureter attached to posterior sheath (C).

tion of the pelvic fascia around the lateral wall of the rectum and includes the more superficial uterosacral ligaments. The entire fascial bundle is identified as the "rectal stalk." The rectal stalk is clamped as far posteriorly as possible, taking special care to avoid the ureter, which is retracted laterally, and the rectum, which is posterior (Fig. 34-18 C).

Continuation of this plane of dissection develops the paravaginal fascia, which is clamped, excised, and ligated adjacent to the posterior surface of the inferior ramus of the pubis. The bladder and lower ureters are gently reflected away from the operating field (Fig. 34-19 A). This procedure routinely removes the upper 4 or 5 cm. of the vagina

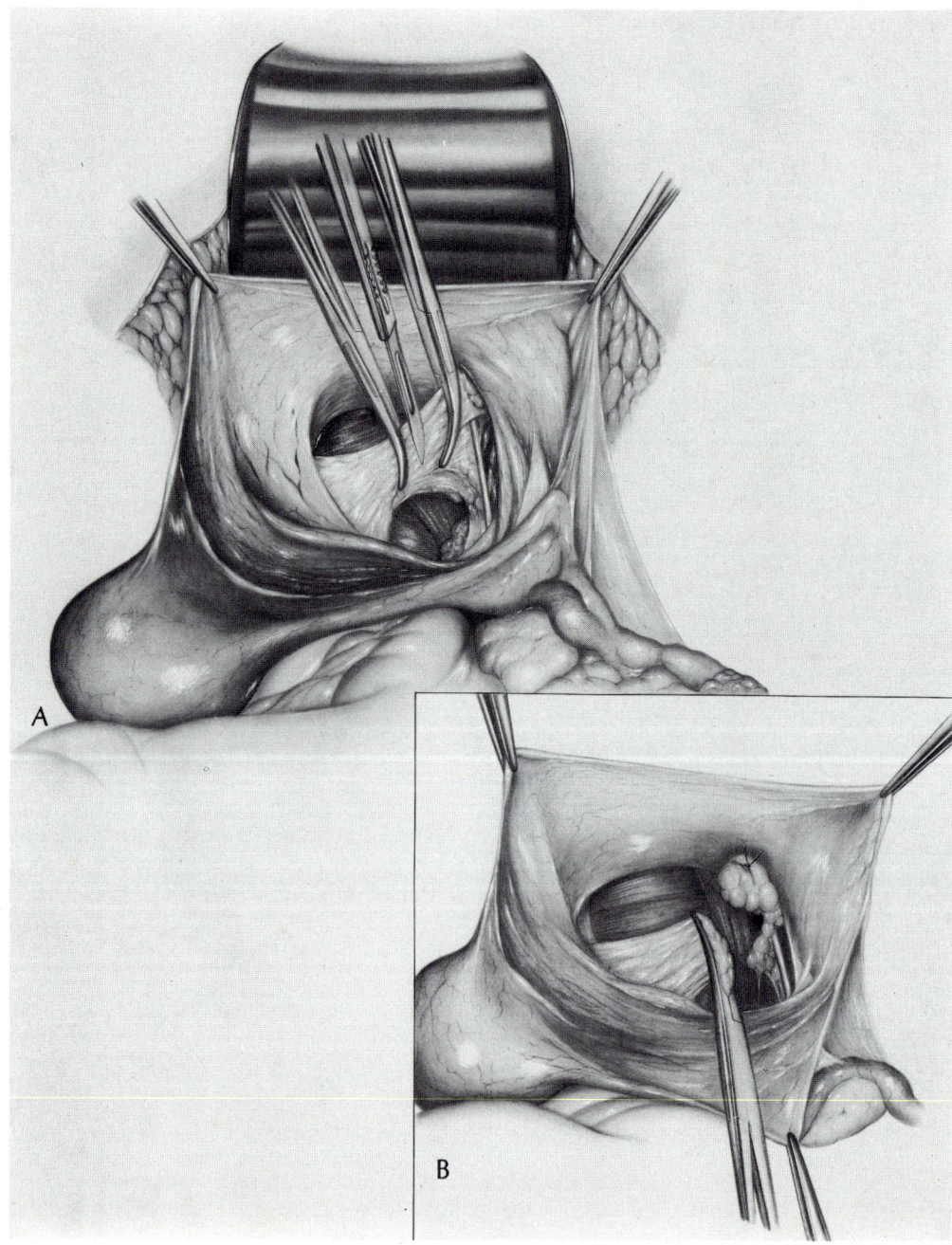

FIG. 34-17. (A) Clamping and incision of lateral portion of cardinal ligament adjacent to the lateral pelvic wall. (B) Excised ligament showing pelvic floor and levator muscles. Dissected obturator nerve is seen in obturator space.

and requires gentle dissection of the bladder and rectum from their attachments to the adjacent vaginal fascia. Care must be taken to avoid injury to the bladder and rectum at this point of the operation, as it is easy to traumatize these organs by compromising their blood supply or developing the plane of dissection too close to their muscular wall. Therefore the fascial planes must

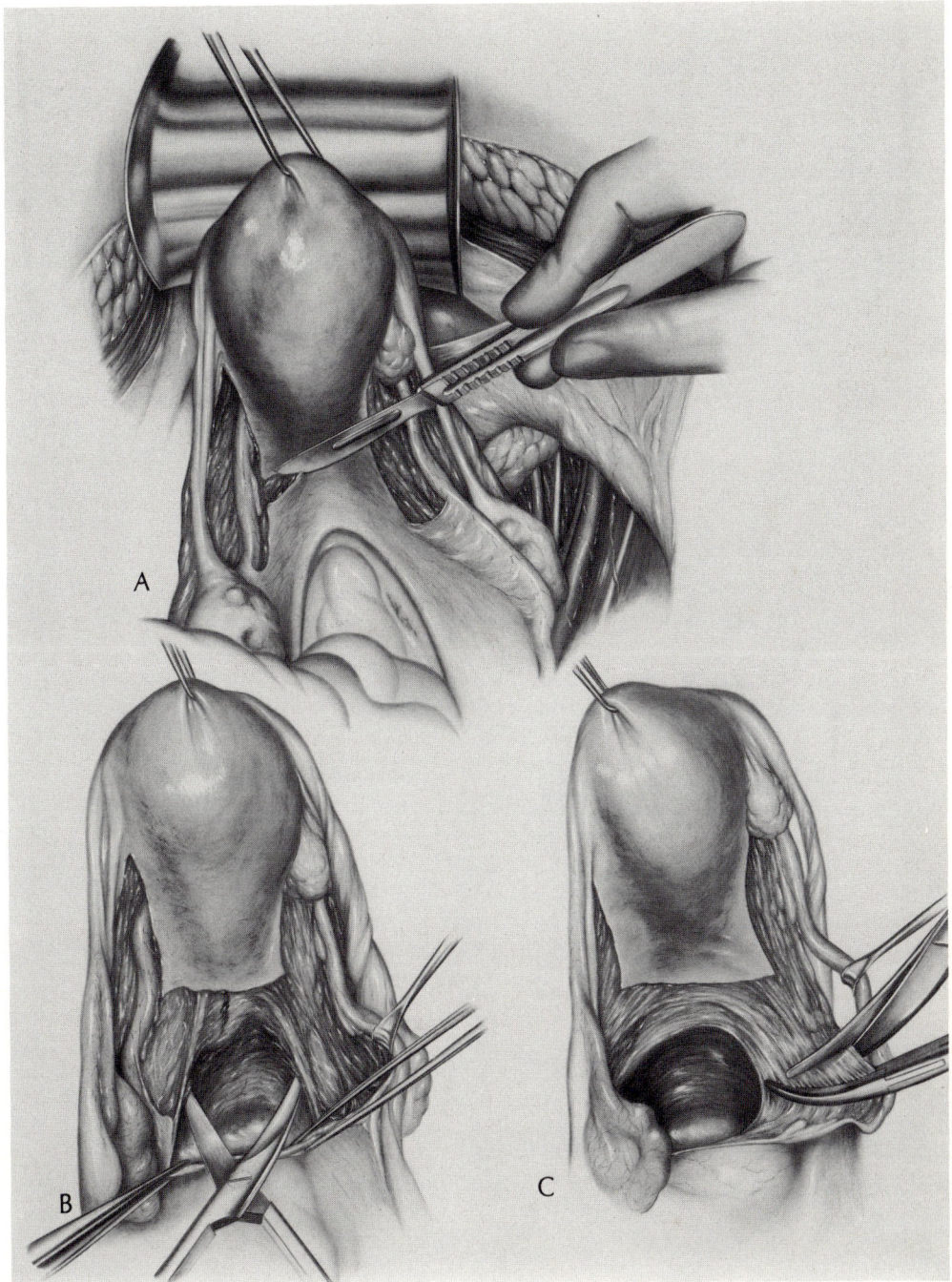

FIG. 34-18. (A) Cutting the cul-de-sac peritoneum as it reflects onto the rectum. Ureters course laterally devoid of peritoneum. (B) Dissection of the rectovaginal septum with development of rectal stalks (uterosacral ligaments) laterally. (C) Clamping of the rectal stalks, which includes the uterosacral ligament. Ureter is gently retracted to avoid trauma.

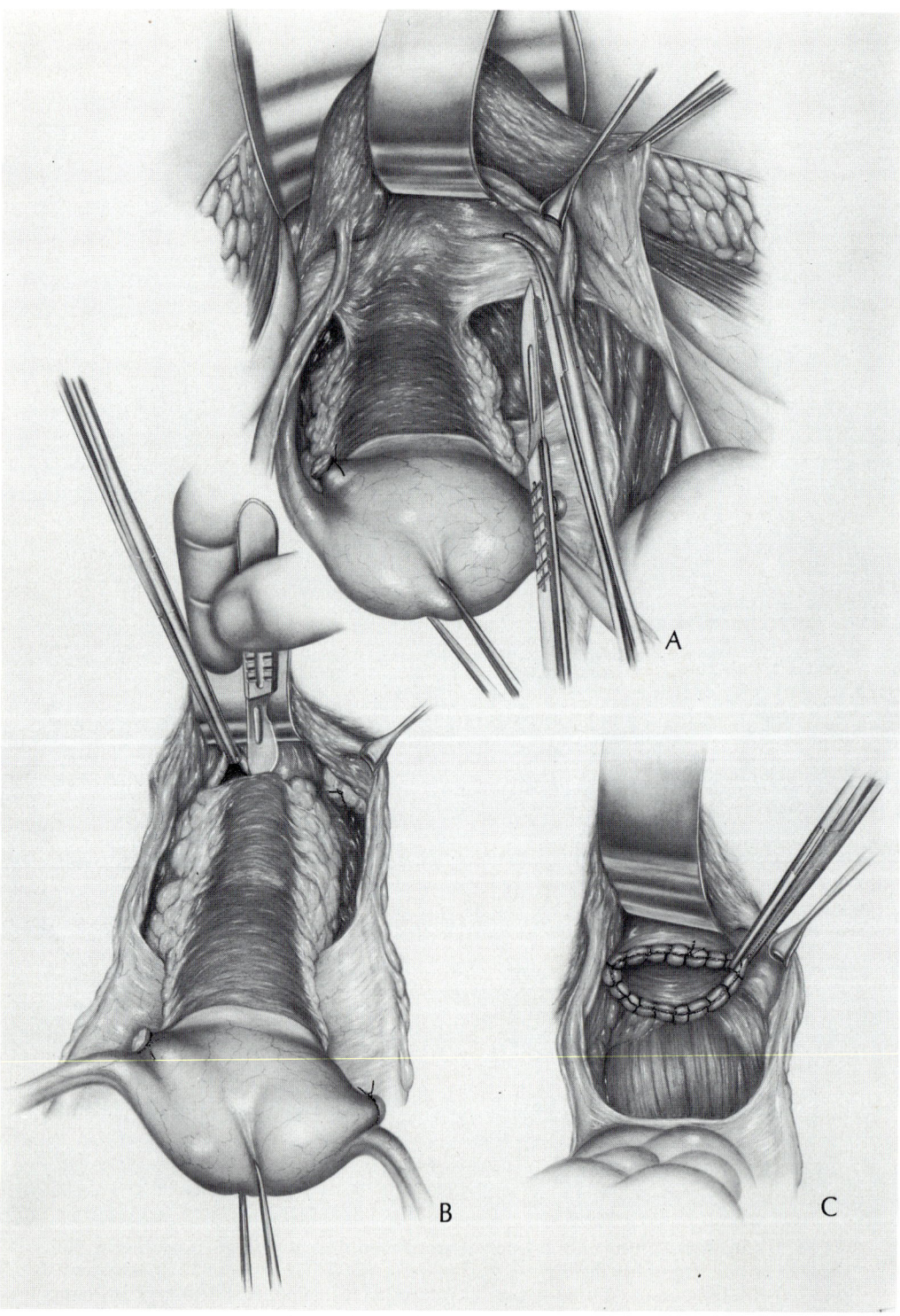

FIG. 34-19. (A) Dissection of bladder from vagina and excising the paravaginal fascia from the lateral pelvic wall. Lower ureter is retracted from operating field. (B) Opening of vagina and securing lower vaginal cuff. Upper half of vagina is included with surgical specimen. (C) Open vaginal cuff with continuous locking suture for hemostasis. Ureters are seen laterally and denuded rectum posteriorly.

be developed by sharp dissection rather than attempting to displace the bladder and rectum forcibly by the blunt end of a poorly protected sponge forceps. The specimen is removed, preferably by the closed technic, but to obtain a larger vaginal cuff, the vagina is partially opened, as shown in Figure 34-19 B, prior to applying long, right-angle clamps to the surgical specimen to avoid spillage of the tumor cells into the pelvis. Hemostasis is controlled by a continuous locking suture of No. 1 chromic catgut, and the vagina is left open to obtain adequate pelvic drainage. Figure 34-19 C illustrates the open vaginal vault, the adjacent ureters, and the base of the bladder with the underlying rectal wall devoid of peritoneum. No additional effort is made to support the remaining vagina as all of the fascial support of the pelvic organs has been removed. The remaining vagina is well supported by its attachments to the lateral pelvic wall and urogenital diaphragm.

Two cigarette drains are placed on either side of the denuded pelvic floor and brought out through the vagina. In addition, drainage from the obturator fossa and lateral pelvic wall can be enhanced by the use of large, straight French rubber catheters placed along each lateral pelvic wall beneath the peritoneum and brought out through stab wounds in the lower quadrant bilaterally. Additional holes are cut into the catheter to provide adequate drainage for the collected blood, lymph, and lymph exudate in the pelvis. These rubber catheters are connected to a low-pressure Gomco suction apparatus postoperatively and are most beneficial in preventing lymphocyst formation. Lymphocyst formation as a complication of radical Wertheim hysterectomy occurs in reportedly 2 to 5 per cent of the cases.

Management of the denuded pelvic ureters remains a controversial subject. Most gynecologists prefer to leave them in their retroperitoneal position to develop a collateral circulation from the longitudinal surface vessels of the ureter and from the lateral pelvic wall. Green believes that anchoring the serosa of the ureter to the umbilical ligament has reduced the incidence of ureteral complications in his experience by elevating the ureters away from the pelvic cellulitis that develops postoperatively. Excessive elevation of the ureters, however, has produced kinking with obstruction and fistula formation in some of our own cases. We have recently initiated the technic of wrapping the exposed segment of the pelvic ureter with the adjacent parietal pelvic peritoneum, as described by Ohkawa. While our experience with this procedure is limited, we are impressed with the anatomic result of loosely wrapping the ureter in peritoneum, which provides protection from the postoperative pelvic cellulitis and a capillary source for a collateral blood supply.

The pelvis is peritonized with a continuous running stitch of No. 000 chromic catgut, beginning in the region of the infundibulopelvic ligament on each side of the pelvis and approximating the parietal and visceral peritoneum to the midpoint of the vagina. This will completely extraperitonealize the denuded pelvis from the peritoneal cavity. An additional step in peritonizing the pelvis is frequently utilized to provide additional protection to the denuded bladder base. This includes suturing the free edge of the bladder peritoneum to the anterior cuff of the vagina prior to placing the continuous fine suture which approximates the bladder peritoneum to the peritoneal reflection from the cul-de-sac and rectum. In essence, this provides an extra peritoneal layer of tissue between the base of the bladder and the raw pelvis and is an added method of decreasing vesicovaginal fistulae. This technic avoids the use of abdominal packing as advocated by Brunschwig and Masterson, for we find no difficulty in obtaining sufficient peritoneum for complete closure of the pelvis.

In the event of persistent bleeding from the pelvic floor veins which is not controlled at the time of completion of the operative procedure, one should have no hesitancy in leaving a gauze pack firmly placed in the pelvis prior to closure of the pelvic peritoneum, with the free end brought out through the vaginal vault. The pack can then be advanced in 48 hours and removed in 72 hours without concern for continued bleeding. The vaginal drains are advanced on the 3rd postoperative day and removed on the 5th postoperative day if drainage has subsided. In the event that there is copious vaginal drainage, the drains are left in place until this subsides. The lower quadrant drains are likewise advanced on the 4th or the 5th day and removed as soon as the lymph drainage from the pelvis subsides. If all the lymphatic channels have been ligated at the margins of the dissection, there should be minimal leakage of lymph into the pelvis following this procedure. In general, lymphocyst formation is much more common where previous irradiation has not been given, and where the lymphatic channels remain patent.

COMPLICATIONS OF RADICAL HYSTERECTOMY

While many of the complications from the radical Wertheim hysterectomy have been discussed previously with the method of treatment of cervical cancer, it is important to review briefly the major factors which contribute directly to the serious problems that can result from this operative procedure.

1. *Experience of the operator:* the morbidity, mortality, and complication rates are inversely proportional to the experience of the surgeon. The greater the experience of the pelvic surgeon with radical pelvic surgery, the fewer are the complications. Hendriksen has shown that the casual operator frequently performs inadequate surgery, and that the morbidity and survival rates reflect this. In a review of 88 cases of early cervical carcinoma, he found that where the operative procedure had been inadequate, the 5-year survival was only 44 per cent as opposed to an expected 75 to 85 per cent.

2. *Previous irradiation:* experience with the combination of irradiation followed by radical surgery clearly demonstrates that the incidence of fistulae after radical surgery is, in general, double the rate of that occurring in nonirradiated patients. In 46 cases of radical Wertheim hysterectomy *following irradiation* at Johns Hopkins Hospital between the years 1949 and 1960, there was a 15 per cent incidence of ureterovaginal fistula; 7 per cent vesicovaginal fistula; and 7 per cent rectovaginal fistula, for a total fistula rate of 29 per cent. Similar experience has been reported by Welch, Pratt, and Symmonds, and many others.

3. *Obesity, pelvic inflammatory disease, endometriosis, and metabolic disease* (diabetes in particular) when present, have a much higher rate of complications and untoward results because of the influence of these factors on healing, thromboembolism and the remaining vascularity of the pelvis.

4. *Thrombophlebitis and lower extremity complications*: the hazard of postoperative thrombophlebitis is markedly increased where there has been trauma to the wall of the large veins during the pelvic dissection. Accumulation of thromboplastin on the intima of the vein is one of the earliest responses of vein trauma. Such effects frequently result from overenthusiastic stripping of the adventitia of the vessels, and prolonged kinking and retraction of a major vessel during the operative procedure. The prophylactic use of anticoagulants has not been a practical solution to this problem because of increased bleeding during the procedure and postoperatively. The use of clinical dextran is known to decrease blood viscosity and reportedly prevents venous thrombosis in vascular surgery. Its disadvantages, however, are its interference in crossmatching with prolonged use and its known interference with coagulation factors. Nonetheless, when injury has occurred to a pelvic vein, the use of dextran might be considered a wiser immediate choice than anticoagulation. Currently, we are using clinical dextran (70) for 2 days preceding radical surgery (500 cc./day) and for 3 to 5 days postoperatively, in an effort to decrease the incidence of this complication.

5. *Urinary tract complications*: this subject has been previously discussed in detail. The incidence of vesicovaginal fistula varies from 3 to 7 per cent in re-

ported series, and there is a greater hazard to the ureter, with a reported incidence of ureterovaginal fistula varying between 2 and 13 per cent. The major contributory factors to these problems are the experience of the operator and previous irradiation. Urinary tract fistulas usually present clinically between the 5th and 14th postoperative day, and are heralded by the presence of unexplained fever, tachycardia, lower quadrant and flank pain, and leukocytosis. Repair of a ureterovaginal fistula, following radical Wertheim hysterectomy, should be deferred for a minimum of 8 to 12 weeks. In the interim, should there be progressive hydronephrosis and calyectasis, a temporary nephrostomy or ureterostomy is far preferable to too early an attempt at repair. Reimplantation of the ureter into the bladder is by far the preferred method of treatment for such ureteral fistulae and may require the use of a bladder flap to accomplish successfully the anastomosis to a shortened pelvic ureter. Vesicovaginal fistulas should always be deferred for a minimum of 6 months prior to repair, and one should be certain that there is no recurrence of malignancy before attempting repair. Due to the frequent occurrence of the defect high on the bladder wall from ischemic necrosis of the bladder base, it is sometimes necessary to repair such fistulas by both the vaginal and the abdominal route. We have routinely used the Latzko procedure for such repairs, and except where the fistula resulted from radical surgery following full irradiation, this procedure has proven successful in over 85 per cent of the cases.

ADENOCARCINOMA

There are two distinct types of adenocarcinoma of the cervix which bear separate consideration:

1. That which originates only in the endocervix as determined by careful fractional curretage.
2. That which is shown to be present in both the endocervix and the endometrium where the histologic origin of the adenocarcinoma is indistinct, called Corpus et Collum. This lesion is discussed in Chapter 36.

The most effective method of treating adenocarcinoma originating in the endocervix has been a subject of confusion in the literature. Primary surgery has been advocated by many on the basis that adenocarcinoma is considered to be less sensitive to radiation, as are other glandular-secreting tumors. Adenocarcinoma of the endometrium is frequently cited as being less sensitive than squamous carcinoma. In addition, endocervical tumors may extend into the endometrial cavity, where their cure would be less assured by irradiation alone. These and other personal preferences have initiated interest in treating such lesions by primary radical surgery or a combination of preoperative irradiation followed by either simple total hysterectomy or radical Wertheim hysterectomy and lymphadenectomy. Comparative studies, however, simply do not support the clinical impression that the more extensive therapy for adenocarcinoma of the cervix is more effective in curing the disease than irradiation alone, when compared stage for stage. Furthermore, recent reports by Cuccia *et al*, and Rutledge *et al*, clearly demonstrate the fact that the cure rates of adenocarcinoma of the cervix by current methods of irradiation therapy are similar, if not identical, to those of squamous cell carcinoma.

Dose response curves of irradiation are markedly affected by the concentration of oxygen in the tissue. Any biological deficit which would reduce the oxygen concentration at the cellular level would render the tumor cell less radiosensitive because it could undergo rapid repair. For maximum tumor response, it is important, therefore, that anemia and a decreased circulating blood volume be corrected prior to the initiation of irradiation therapy.

CARCINOMA OF CERVIX IN PREGNANCY

The coexistence of carcinoma of the cervix in pregnancy is relatively rare, occurring in approximately 0.5 per cent of all pregnancies, and has been detected more frequently during the past decade as a result of the routine use of cytologic vaginal smears. This figure varies somewhat because some reports include the first 12 to 18 months postpartum. It is logical to include invasive carcinoma detected during the first postpartum year as part of the pregnancy statistics, for the time interval required for the development of invasive cancer would probably include the period of the previous pregnancy.

To look at the disease in another way, approximately 1½ to 2½ per cent of all cases of carcinoma of the cervix occur during pregnancy, the majority being carcinoma in situ. Carcinoma in situ has approximately the same occurrence in both the pregnant and the nonpregnant state. Since the peak incidence of carcinoma in situ occurs during the peak age of childbearing, the coexistence of both entities is not surprising. The well-known etiologic factors of cervical cancer make obstetric patients a high-risk group for the detection of early carcinoma. Regrettably, Papanicolaou smears are still used routinely in less than 50 per cent of asymptomatic pregnant patients, according to Hofmeister and Barbo. Fear of biopsying the pregnant cervix is a common factor in the delay in diagnosing cancer of the cervix during pregnancy.

Diagnosis

Since 75 to 80 per cent of patients with carcinoma of the cervix in pregnancy have no specific gross abnormalities, diagnosis in pregnancy must be made by the routine use of the Papanicolaou smear. It is our feeling that pregnancy does not alter the cytologic interpretation of the Papanicolaou smear and should be a guide to further evaluation of the cervix in cases with suspicious or positive reports. While there is a hesitancy to biopsy the cervix during pregnancy because of bleeding, this should not dissuade the physician from his responsibility to biopsy the cervix when indicated by either a gross lesion or abnormal cytology.

The recent use of colposcopy with directed biopsies has reduced the problem of blood loss to some extent because the entire circumference of the cervix need not be sampled as one would do after examination with the naked eye. In addition, colposcopy has reportedly reduced the use of conization to about one tenth of its previous use without this technic. It is our belief, however, that conization of the cervix, even in the pregnant patient, is still the preferential method to rule out micro- or macroinvasion. The recent use of a weak solution of Neo-Synephrine (1:200,000) has greatly diminished the amount of blood loss from conization in pregnancy. A maximum of 20 cc. is used throughout the procedure, and while this may elevate the systemic blood pressure slightly, this effect is quite transient and is not detrimental to placental circulation. The use of vasopressors, plus the routine ligation of the descending branch of the uterine artery, has removed all serious restrictions from conization of the cervix during pregnancy. This procedure should be undertaken regardless of the duration of pregnancy, and should include at least three quarters of the endocervical canal. As one approaches a full-term pregnancy, there is added risk to premature labor and rupture of the membrane from an extensive cone, but the risk of vaginal delivery through a cervix with invasive carcinoma poses an even greater hazard to the patient. In the event that labor should occur following recent conization in a term pregnancy, cesarean section would be advisable rather than risking the possibility of cervical trauma and hemorrhage.

Treatment

In considering treatment, several factors should be taken into consideration: (1) the effect of pregnancy on the carcinoma, (2) the effect of carcinoma on the pregnancy, (3) the effect of carcinoma on the method of delivery, and (4) the stage of the pregnancy when the carcinoma is detected.

Current statistics have clarified the

earlier statements that carcinoma of the cervix is aggravated by pregnancy. When evaluated, stage for stage, the cure rates are identical to those of the nonpregnant state except for those cases treated at term and postpartum. Bosch and Marcial have shown an improvement in the survival rate in cases treated in the first two trimesters of pregnancy as compared to that of cases treated in the third trimester and postpartum period, which is attributed by most authors to the detrimental effect of cervical dilatation and vaginal delivery. Similar results have been reported by Schmitz, Smith, and Isaacs. Most authors have considered vaginal delivery to be contraindicated in patients with invasive carcinoma of the cervix associated with pregnancy, an opinion in which we concur.

Prem, Makowski and McKelvey take a conservative view concerning patients in the third trimester and permit them to progress to 35 or 36 weeks of pregnancy before initiating treatment. This seems to be a reasonable viewpoint. There appears to be no difference in results for Stage I lesions regardless of the deliberate delay in treatment during the third trimester of pregnancy. It seems apparent, therefore, that the prognosis of carcinoma of the cervix in pregnancy is related primarily to the stage of the disease rather than to the stage of pregnancy. This statement is certainly true in the treatment of carcinoma in situ in pregnancy. Once the lesion has been histologically proven by biopsy and conization to be an intraepithelial lesion, the patient should be permitted to deliver vaginally and treatment of the disease should be deferred for 3 to 6 months postpartum, at which time a simple hysterectomy with a wide cuff is performed.

When invasive cervical cancer is detected during the first trimester of pregnancy, treatment should be initiated immediately with complete disregard for the fetus. When the invasive disease is detected during the second trimester or before the 7th month (28th week), it is still our opinion that treatment should not be delayed. However, when invasive cervical cancer is detected in the third trimester, particularly between the 28th and 32nd week, there is precedent for delaying treatment until the 34th to 36th week, when the fetus would have an improved chance of survival. In series similar to McKelvey's, the delay in treatment, particularly for Stage II lesions, is defensible statistically, but the physician must be certain of the stage of the disease and must present this questionable decision to the patient and her family, since the facts are far from clear in this matter. Certainly no gynecologist would be criticized for immediate treatment of the disease, but he must be willing to accept the fact that the disease may progress if he chooses to delay. The choice of therapy remains debatable, as has been brought out in the discussion for this disease in the nonpregnant state. Whether one would choose primary surgery or irradiation would depend on the stage of the disease, the stage of pregnancy, the age of patient, and her general medical health. In a young patient where there is interest in conserving ovarian function, there is considerable interest in the use of a radical Wertheim hysterectomy and pelvic lymphadenectomy for Stage I carcinoma. This has particular merit during the 2nd and 3rd trimesters of pregnancy in those cases in which abdominal delivery would be required to avoid cervical dilatation and vaginal delivery. The complication rate, however, is much higher than the same operative procedure in a nonpregnant state, with an increase in blood loss, operating time, and general morbidity. Nonetheless, surgery has the advantage of avoiding premature castration and other side-effects of irradiation, as well as the added knowledge of the exact location and extent of the disease. Irradiation therapy, however, is more uniformly used, has fewer complications, and has equal therapeutic effect, stage for stage. The irradiation treatment is identical to that in the nonpregnant state, with the exception that it is usually initiated with external therapy and that hysterotomy is required for the treatment of lesions occurring beyond the first trimester of pregnancy.

BIBLIOGRAPHY

Bonney, V.: The results of 55 cases of Wertheim's operation for carcinoma of the cervix. J. Obstet. Gynaec. Brit. Emp., 48: 421, 1941.

———: Wertheim's operation in retrospect. Lancet, 1:637, 1949.

Bickenbach, W.: Surgical treatment or irradiation for treatment of cervical carcinoma. Med. College of Virginia Quarterly, 3(1): 35, 1967.

Broders, A. C.: Grading of carcinoma. Minnesota Med., 8:726, 1925.

Brunschwig, A.: The surgical treatment of cancer of the cervix. Stage I & II. Amer. J. Roentgen., 102:147, 1968.

———: The surgical treatment of cancer of the cervix uteri (A radical operation for cancer of the cervix). Bull. N.Y. Acad. Med., 24: 672, 1948.

———: Radical vaginal operation (Schauta) for carcinoma of the cervix. Amer. J. Obstet. Gynec., 66:153, 1953.

Burns, B. C., Jr., Everett H. S., and Brack, C. B.: Value of urologic study in the management of carcinoma of the cervix. Amer. J. Obstet. Gynec., 80:997, 1960.

Calame, R. J., and Nelson, J. H., Jr.: Ureterovaginal fistula as a complication of radical pelvic surgery. Arch. Surg., 94:876, 1967.

Calame R. J., and Wallach, R. C.: An analysis of complications of the radiologic treatment of carcinoma of the cervix. Surg. Gynec. Obstet., 125:39, 1967.

Corscaden, J. A., Kasabach, H. H., and Lenz, M.: Intestinal injuries after radium and roentgen treatment of carcinoma of the cervix. Amer. J. Roentgen., 39:871, 1938.

Cosbie, W. G.: The contribution of radiotherapy to the modern treatment of female pelvic cancer. J. Obstet. Gynaec. Brit. Emp., 66:843, 1959.

Cullen, T. S.: Cancer of the Uterus. Philadelphia, W. B. Saunders, 1900.

Decker, D. G., and Smith, R. A.: Sequential radiation therapy and surgery for Stage I and Stage II cancer of the cervix. Amer. J. Roentgen., 102:152, 1968.

Diehl, W. K., and Hundley, J. M., Jr.: Urinary tract changes in cervical carcinoma. Surg. Gynec. Obstet., 87:705, 1948.

Everett, H. S.: The effect of carcinoma of the cervix and its treatment upon the urinary tract. Amer. J. Obstet. Gynec., 38:889, 1939.

Everett, H. S., Brack, C. B., and Farber, G. J.: Further studies on the effect of irradiation therapy for carcinoma of the cervix upon the urinary tract. Amer. J. Obstet. Gynec., 58:908, 1949.

Fletcher, G. H., and Rutledge, F. N.: Overall results in radiotherapy for carcinoma of the cervix. Clin. Obstet. Gynec., 10:958, 1967.

Foley, D. V., and Fetherston, W. C.: Complications of radical pelvic surgery. Clin. Obstet. Gynec., 8:771, 1965.

Friedell, G. H., and Graham, J. B.: Regional lymph node involvement in small carcinoma of the cervix. Surg. Gynec. Obstet., 108:513, 1959.

Freund, W. A.: Method of complete removal of the uterus. Amer. J. Obstet. Gynec., 7: 200, 1879.

Green, T. H., Jr.: Urologic complications of Wertheim hysterectomy—incidence, etiology, management and prevention. Obstet. Gynec., 20:293, 1962.

Glucksmann, A.: In Way, S.: Malignant Diseases of the Female Genital Tract. p. 83. Philadelphia, Blakiston, 1951.

Greiss, F. C., Blake, D. D., and Lock, F. R.: Complications of intensive radiation therapy for cervical carcinoma. Obstet. Gynec., 18:417, 1961.

Gusberg, S. B., and Herman, G. G.: Radiosensitivity and virulence factors in cervical cancer. Amer. J. Obstet. Gynec., 100:627, 1968.

Henriksen, E.: The lymphatic spread of carcinoma of the cervix and body of the uterus. Amer. J. Obstet. Gynec., 58:924, 1949.

Hinselmann, H.: Zur Kenntnis der präancerösen Veränderungen der Portio. Zbl. Gynaek., 51:901, 1927.

Inguilla, W., and Cosmi, E. V.: Vesical, ureteral and rectal fistulas following operation for carcinoma of the cervix—study of 1,000 consecutive cases. Amer. J. Obstet. Gynec., 99:1078, 1967.

Kottmeier, H.-L. (ed.): Annual Report on the Results of Treatment in Carcinoma of the Uterus and Vagina. Published under the patronage of the International Federation of Gynecology and Obstetrics. vol. 13, Stockholm, 1963; vol. 14, collated 1966. Stockholm, Norstedt & Söner, 1967.

———: Complications of radiotherapy of carcinoma of the cervix. In Marcus, S. L., and Marcus, C. C. (eds.): Advances in Obstetrics and Gynecology. vol. 1, p. 633. Baltimore, Williams & Wilkins, 1967.

Liu, W., and Meigs, J. V.: Radical hysterectomy and pelvic lymphadenectomy. Amer. J. Obstet. Gynec., 69:1, 1955.

Louros, N. C.: Suggestions and technique

for what should be considered radical hysterectomy in carcinoma of the cervix. Amer. J. Obstet. Gynec., 89:432, 1964.

Macgregor, J. E.: Cervical cancer; the beginning of the end? Lancet, 2:1296, 1967.

McGraw, T. A.: Cases of operations for cancer of the womb. Mich. Med. News, 2:98, 1879.

McLennan, C. E., McLennan, M. T., and Bagshaw, M. A.: Linear accelerator in treatment of cervical cancer—a decade of experience. Amer. J. Obstet. Gynec., 98:675, 1967.

Makowski, E. L., McKelvey J. L., Flight G. W., Stenstrom, K. W., and Mosser, D. G.: Results of radiation therapy of carcinoma of the cervix. J.A.M.A., 182:627, 1962.

Martzloff, K. H.: Carcinoma of the cervix uteri: a pathological and clinical study with particular reference to the relative malignancy of the neoplastic process as indicated by the predominant type of cancer cell. Bull. Johns Hopkins Hosp., 34:141, 1923.

——: Epidermoid carcinoma of cervix uteri; histologic study to determine resemblance between biopsy specimens and parent tumor obtained by radical panhysterectomy. Amer. J. Obstet. Gynec., 16:578, 1928.

Masterson, J. G.: Radical surgery in early carcinoma of cervix. Amer. J. Obstet. Gynec., 87:601, 1963.

Meigs, J. V.: Carcinoma of the cervix—the Wertheim operation. Surg. Gynec. Obstet., 78:195, 1944.

——: The Wertheim operation for carcinoma of the cervix. Amer. J. Obstet. Gynec., 49:542, 1945.

Nathanson, B. N., Liegner, L. M., Rudolph, J. D., and Hodara, M.: Dose verification studies in radium therapy of carcinoma of the cervix. Amer. J. Obstet. Gynec., 97:808, 1967.

Navratil, E.: Vaginal Surgery of Cervical Carcinoma. Proc. A.C.S. Mtng. Munich, Springer-Verlag, 1968.

Nebel, W., Singleton, H. M., and Swanton, M. C.: Cold knife conization of the cervix uteri. Surg. Gynec. Obstet., 125:780, 1967.

Ohkawa, K.: Personal communication.

Parker, R. T., Wilbanks, G. D., Yowell, R. K., and Carter, F. B.: Radical hysterectomy and pelvic lymphadenectomy with and without preoperative radio-therapy for cervical cancer. Report of 265 patients followed 10 to 22 years. Amer. J. Obstet. Gynec., 99:933, 1967.

Paterson, R.: Treatment of Malignant Disease by Radium and X-ray: Being a Practice of Radiology. p. 622. Baltimore, Williams & Wilkins, 1948.

Paunier, J. P., Declos L., and Fletcher, G. H.: Causes, time of death, and sites of failure in squamous cell carcinoma of the uterine cervix on intact uterus. Radiology, 88:555, 1967.

Peham, H. V., and Amreich, J.: Operative Gynecology. Philadelphia, J. B. Lippincott, 1934.

Read, C. D.: The role of surgery in the treatment of carcinoma of the cervix. Amer. J. Obstet. Gynec., 56:1021, 1948.

Rutledge, F. N., Gutierrez, A. G., and Fletcher, G. H.: Management of Stage I and II adenocarcinomas of the uterine cervix on intact uterus. Amer. J. Roentgen., 102:161, 1968.

Schauta, F.: Die Operation des Gebärmutterkrebes mittels des Schuchardt'schen Paravaginalschnittes. Montasschr. Geburtsh. u. Gynäk., 15:133, 1902.

Schewe, E. J., and Sala, J. M.: Bilateral ureteral obstruction complicating the treatment of carcinoma of the cervix. Amer. J. Roentgen, 81:125, 1959.

Schiller, W.: Untersuchungen zur Enststehung der Geschwulste; Collumcarcinom des Uterus. Virchow's Arch. Path. Anat., 263:279, 1927.

——: Early diagnosis of carcinoma of the cervix. Surg. Gynec. Obstet., 56:210, 1933.

Sweeny, W. J., and Douglas, R. G.: Treatment of carcinoma of the cervix with combined radiation and extensive surgery. Amer. J. Obstet. Gynec., 84:981, 1962.

Stoeckel, W.: Die vaginale Radikaloperation des Collum-Carcinoms. Zbl. Gynäk., 52:39, 1928.

Taussig, F. J.: Iliac lymphadenectomy for Group II cancer of the cervix. Amer. J. Obstet. Gynec., 45:733, 1943.

Tod, M. C., and Meredith, W. J.: Dosage system for use in treatment of cancer of the uterine cervix. Brit. J. Radiol., 11:809, 1938.

Thompson, J. D., and Brack, C. B.: Radical surgery for radioresistant cervical cancer. Obstet. Gynec., 9:676, 1957.

Van Bouwdijk-Bastiaanse, M. A.: Vaginal hysterectomy, with special regard to use in cancer. Nederl. T. geneesk., 93:2132, 1949.

Van Herik, M.: Fever as a complication of radiation therapy for carcinoma of the cervix. Amer. J. Roentgen., 93:104, 1965.

Ward, G. G.: The treatment of carcinoma of the cervix complicated by pregnancy. J. Mt. Sinai Hosp., 14:674, 1947.

Welch, J. S., Pratt, J. H., and Symmonds, R. E.: Wertheim hysterectomy for squamous cell carcinoma of the uterine cervix. Amer. J. Obstet. Gynec., 81:978, 1961.

Wentz, W. B., and Lewis G. C., Jr.: Correlations of histologic morphology and survival in cervical cancer following irradiation therapy. Obstet. Gynec., 26:228, 1965.

Wentz, W. B., and Reagan, J. W.: Survival in cervical cancer with respect to cell type. Cancer, 12:384, 1959.

Wertheim, E.: Discussion on the diagnosis of treatment of carcinoma of the uterus. Brit. Med. J., 2:689, 1905.

———: Die erweiterte abdominale Operation bei Carcinoma Colli Uteri (Auf Grund von 500 Fällen). Berlin, Urban, 1911.

———: Zur Frage der Radikaloperation beim Uteruskrebs. Arch. Gynäk., 61:627, 1900.

Adenocarcinoma

Cuccia, C. A., Bloedorn, F. G., and Onal, M.: Treatment of primary adenocarcinoma of the cervix. Amer. J. Roentgen., 99:371, 1967.

Rutledge F. N., Gutierrez, A. G., and Fletcher, G. H.: Management of Stage I and II adenocarcinomas of the uterine cervix on intact uterus. Amer. J. Roentgen., 102:161, 1968.

Carcinoma of Cervix in Pregnancy

Bosch, A., and Marcial, V. A.: Carcinoma of the uterine cervix associated with pregnancy. Amer. J. Roentgen., 96:92, 1966.

Greene, R. R., and Peckham, B. M.: Preinvasive cancer of the cervix in pregnancy. Amer. J. Obstet. Gynec., 75:551, 1958.

Henriksen, E.: Basic problems in the management of early carcinoma of the cervix uteri. Amer. J. Surg., 102:304, 1961.

Hofmeister, F. J., and Barbo, D. M.: Cancer detection in private gynecologic practice; a concluding study. Obstet. Gynec., 23:386, 1964.

Kinch, R. A.: Factors affecting the prognosis of cancer of the cervix in pregnancy. Amer. J. Obstet. Gynec., 82:45, 1961.

Mikuta, J. J., Enterline, H. T., and Braun, T. E., Jr. Carcinoma in-situ of the cervix associated with pregnancy. J.A.M.A., 204:763, 1968.

Peckham, B., Greene, R. R., Chung, J. T., Bayly, M. A., and Benaron, H. B.: Epithelial abnormalities of the cervix during pregnancy. Amer. J. Obstet. Gynec., 67:21, 1954.

Prem, K. A., Makowski, E. L., and McKelvey, J. L.: Carcinoma of the cervix with pregnancy. Amer. J. Obstet. Gynec., 95:99, 1966.

Schmitz, H. E., Smith, C. J., and Isaacs, J. H.: Cancer of the cervix and cancer complicating pregnancy. Trans. New England Obstet. Gynec. Soc., 11:167, 1957.

Stander, R. W., and Lein, J. N.: Carcinoma of cervix and pregnancy. Amer. J. Obstet. Gynec., 79:164, 1960.

35

Pelvic Exenteration

INDICATIONS

General knowledge of the life history of a particular disease is one of the most valuable clinical tools available in assessing the proper method of therapy. The predictable pathway of spread of cervical carcinoma has made this disease the target of both irradiation and surgery as the primary treatment of choice. The fact that this disease has a protracted growth period localized to the cervix and immediate paracervical tissues, later spreading to the lateral pelvic wall lymph nodes, makes this tumor most accessible for the *en bloc* treatment, either by irradiation or surgical methods. While this therapeutic debate has been active since the initial surgical reports of Freunc, Reis, Wertheim, Bonney, Meigs, and others, the introduction of the pelvic exenteration by Brunschwig (1948) provided the initial "ultraradical" surgical approach for advanced and radioresistant cervical cancer.

The initial 10-year experience with such procedures was associated with a high morbidity and mortality rate, but was a direct reflection of the initial selection of patients who had a more advanced disease than the operative procedure could encompass. This resulted in the development of strict guidelines regarding the precise indications and contraindications of these procedures. At the present time less than 40 per cent of all patients explored for radioresistant cervical cancer are candidates for the *en bloc* exenteration. This fact suggests that the tumor is usually cured centrally with an extremely high midline roentgen dosage provided by an intracervical and contracervical radium source, as well as the additional benefit of supervoltage external irradiation. The residual cervical cancer is most frequently attached to the lateral pelvic wall, which limits the use of this surgical procedure.

Following complete irradiation therapy, the surgeon has neither the acute vision nor the discerning touch to determine accurately the presence or absence of microscopic foci of tumor in adjacent tissues surrounding the cervix. Perez-Mesa and Spjut have shown by pathological study of exenteration specimens that the bladder and rectum are commonly involved with tumor, 61 per cent and 44 per cent, respectively, even though there is infrequent evidence of disease in the mucosal surface. As advocated by Brunschwig, Bricker, Schmitz, Parsons, and others, when the surgeon is faced with an unresponsive tumor at the "court of last appeal," the most successful surgical procedure has proven to be the most radical. Not only must one consider the probability of extension of the malignancy to contiguous organs, such as rectum and bladder, but such organs can no longer be considered normal even if uninvolved in the neoplastic process. The vascular effects of irradiation therapy result in an obliterative endarteritis and progressive ischemia of the pelvic viscera. When one adds the final insult of skeletonization of the remaining blood supply of the pelvis by a radical hysterectomy alone, a serious complication rate of 20 to 30 per cent of the lower bowel and urinary tract must be expected. In an effort to avoid such morbidity, as well as to provide the maximum opportunity for complete eradication of the disease, a total pelvic exenteration, which usually includes bladder, uterus, vagina, and rectum, as well as pelvic lymphadenectomy, has become the most effective procedure in operable cases of recurrent cervical cancer.

However, it is very important that the pelvic surgeon be flexible in his surgical approach toward such cases and maintain an open-minded policy regarding the type of radical procedure to be utilized. Occasionally the fascial planes and tissues are pliable and will dissect easily to permit a Wertheim operation. If such a procedure is not possible, either an anterior pelvic exenteration or a total pelvic exenteration should be utilized. A posterior exenteration has been associated with an unacceptably high urinary tract fistula rate, which has eliminated its use for this disease.

As Related to Stage of the Disease

Radioresistant Stage I cervical carcinoma provides the most ideal group of patients for some type of radical surgery. The more advanced the recurrent tumor, the more difficult is the *en bloc* removal of the disease. Consequently, Stage II cervical lesions will have a decreased survival rate and should be considered only where there is surgical assurance that the tumor can be encompassed with the pelvic dissection. If tumor is adherent to the fascia of the pelvic musculature or found to be invading the fascial sheath of the iliac vessels, the exenterative procedure should be abandoned. Parsons has no living case of 5 years or more, in which pelvic exenteration for radioresistant cervical carcinoma revealed positive pelvic lymph nodes. Ingersoll and Ulfelder have only 1 patient living 5 years or longer with positive pelvic nodes who was treated with a pelvic exenteration for radioresistant carcinoma of the cervix.

There has been sporadic interest in utilizing the total pelvic evisceration as a primary procedure for the rare Stage IV cervical malignancy that has spread in the anteroposterior direction, involving bladder and/or rectum. The use of irradiation in such cases will assuredly produce fistulae which remain uncorrectable, following necrosis and slough of the tumor. It is important to stress, however, that there is no justification for pelvic evisceration as a solely palliative procedure. The morbidity, mortality, and complication rates are too high to warrant such extensive surgery when it enforces the patient to spend the first 6 months of the remaining year of her life recovering and being rehabilitated from the surgical procedure and the last 6 months dying from the persistent tumor.

Carcinoma of the endometrium is not considered an ideal disease for the *en bloc* dissection because of the rapidity of extrapelvic spread by the hematogenous and lymphatic routes. However, Brunschwig has reported a 28 per cent 5-year survival following radical surgery where the disease was confined to the pelvis. There has been no significant success with radical surgery for ovarian carcinoma.

CONTRAINDICATIONS

The main contraindications to radical pelvic surgery are time-honored and are a reliable index of far-advanced disease:

1. *Sciatic nerve pain*, usually unilateral, as evidence of encroachment of tumor on the perineural sheath of the sciatic nerve plexuses.

2. *Progressive leg edema*, indicating lymphatic obstruction of the external iliac lymphatic channels. While irradiation therapy, particularly supervoltage, may produce lymphatic obstruction, it is necessary to demonstrate that the edema is not the result of metastatic tumor. In establishing the etiology of the obstruction, a lymphangiogram is frequently helpful but not diagnostic.

3. *Obstructive uropathy*, with either unilateral or bilateral hydronephrosis, is one of the most sensitive barometers of advancing cervical carcinoma. As shown by Cox et al., unilateral hydronephrosis is associated with only 40 per cent resectability of the recurrent malignancy, while bilateral obstruction connotates nonsectability in more than 88 per cent of the cases. This prognosis was documented by Everett in 1939 and confirmed more recently by Burns and Brack. In our clinic this prediction is referred to as Everett's law.

4. *Extrapelvic metastasis* in paraaortic nodes or abdominal viscera, as demonstrated at the time of exploration. A lymphogram or venogram may be beneficial in evaluating possible metastatic disease, which usually requires surgical verification.

5. *Obesity*, although not an absolute contraindication, should be strongly considered in the final evaluation of surgical risk of the patient, for the complication rate varies directly with the weight of the patient.

While these guidelines are valuable in the selection of the ideal candidate for radical pelvic surgery, they are by no means diagnostic of inoperability. Even an adequate evaluation of the pelvis under anesthesia cannot be used to define the operability of a given case, since the tissue response of high-voltage irradiation is frequently indistinguishable from that of invasive tumor. Therefore, unless there is clinical evidence of metastases to bone or extrapelvic organs, *the final decision regarding resectability of this disease must be made by meticulous evaluation of the pelvic viscera at the time of exploratory laparotomy.* In this sense, laparotomy is sometimes considered as the final portion of the diagnostic work-up of such patients, and should not be omitted.

OPERATIVE PROCEDURE

The procedure is initiated abdominally, but may require completion by the vaginal approach, depending on the factors of obesity, depth and configuration of the bony pelvis. A generous midline incision is used, extending well above the umbilicus for adequate exposure. A transverse incision interferes with the final placement of the urinary and fecal ostia in both lower quadrants. Protection of the free edges of the incised abdominal wall with moist abdominal gauze will avoid ischemia and improve healing of the incision following prolonged retraction.

Exploration of the abdominal viscera, particularly the liver surface, followed by meticulous evaluation of the paraaortic lymph nodes for evidence of extrapelvic metastases, is the most important single step in the critical decision of the operability of the patient. At the present time there is no accepted indication for a total pelvic exenteration for palliative therapy in the presence of extrapelvic metastatic disease. Pelvic lymph node metastases contraindicate an exenteration only when there is invasion of the adjacent vessel or fascia of the pelvic wall. Palpation of the parametrial tissues for evidence of tumor usually requires direct examination by opening the anterior and posterior leaves of the broad ligament for final evaluation of the extent of spread of the disease. For the technic of evaluating the paravesical and pararectal spaces, the reader is referred to Figures 34-10 to 34-12 of Chapter 34, Invasive Carcinoma of the Cervix.

We are in complete agreement with Cox et al. that the resectability of radioresistant carcinoma must be determined at the operating table and not solely by pelvic examination. A "frozen pelvis" following irradiation may well be the resultant effect of the therapy alone and not an indication of inoperability. Because of the magnitude of the operation and the social repugnance to a pelvic exenteration, this procedure should not be performed in the absence of a histologic diagnosis of residual tumor.

It is important to understand that the operation is *completely reversible* at this point and can be discontinued if tumor is not identified or cannot be completely encompassed by the operative procedure. As demonstrated in Chapter 34 (Figs.

34-10 to 34-12), the index finger is used to explore the avascular paravesical and pararectal spaces after ligating and excising the ovarian vessels at the pelvic brim and the round ligament near the lateral pelvic wall. By careful finger dissection along the lateral pelvic wall, one can determine the resectability of the broad ligament, paravesical and pararectal tissues without disturbing the arcade of pelvic blood vessels. Exploration is continued gently into the obturator fossa by retracting the uterus and parametrium to the opposite side of the pelvis. Indurated and suspicious areas are biopsied, particularly where there is question of tumor extending to the fascia of the levator ani or obturator muscle. If tumor is confirmed by frozen section and adherent to the fascia or pelvic vessels, the disease is considered too advanced for surgical cure, and the operation is discontinued following closure of the broad ligament.

If the disease is resectable by the above criteria, the dissection of the pelvic contents begins by extending the peritoneal reflection of the broad ligament and incising the peritoneum around the entire pelvis just below the pelvic brim (Fig. 35-1). Note that a peritoneal flap is left attached to the ureter for preservation of its blood supply and utilization later in the urinary diversion. In excising the ureters in the lower pelvis, all the tumor-free portion of the pelvic ureter that is available is utilized. The pelvic peritoneum is incised along the mesosigmoid to the margin of the sigmoid musculature prior to dividing the terminal sigmoid colon at the junction of the rectosigmoid. Care must be taken to avoid injury to the middle sacral artery and vein, which enter the pelvis along the sacral promontory.

URINARY DIVERSION

Although most exenteration procedures defer the urinary diversion until the end of the operation, the present technic is

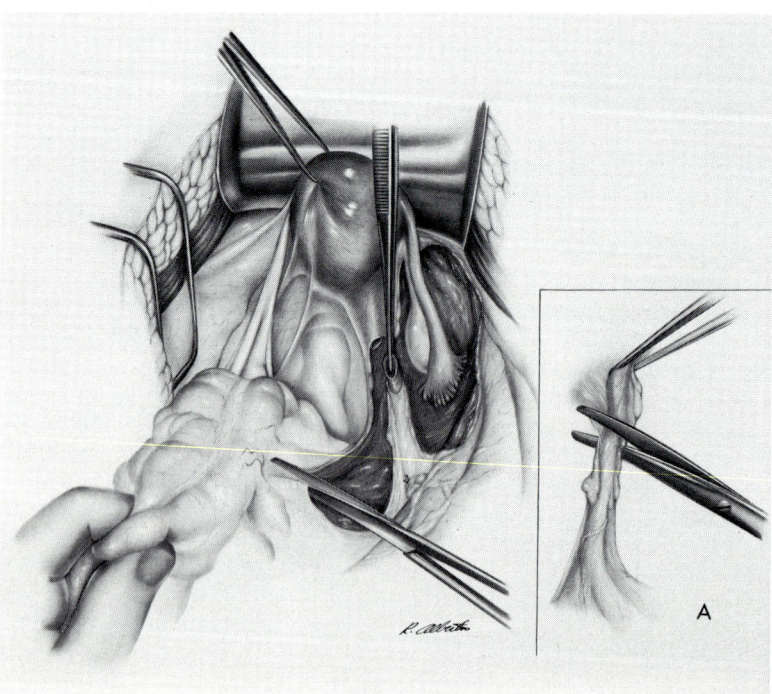

FIG. 35-1. Exenteration showing transection of ureter and incision of peritoneum below pelvic brim and along sigmoid mesentery. (Insert A) Showing cutting of ureter, which remains attached to the pelvic peritoneum.

focused around the early diversion for the following reasons:

1. Critical and meticulous evaluation of the abdomen and pelvis has indicated that the disease is surgically resectable.

2. The *en bloc* dissection is technically easier and more rapid with the ureters free from the specimen and the rectum detached from the sigmoid colon.

3. The urinary diversion is the most delicate and time-consuming step in the entire procedure. This is accomplished more efficiently when the surgeon is more alert and refreshed at the beginning of the operation than when he is compromised by fatigue and by the precarious condition of the patient at the later part of the dissection.

4. Early diversion provides an excellent opportunity for the surgeon to evaluate the competence of the ureterointestinal anastomosis while the remainder of the pelvic dissection is completed.

The sigmoid colon has proven to be an ideal segment of bowel for the urinary conduit, although the isolated terminal ileal segment, as developed by Bricker, has been the most frequently used method of urinary diversion. However, the mobility of the sigmoid mesentery permits easy diversion of the sigmoid ostia to the right lower quadrant and avoids an end-to-end small bowel anastomosis, which decreases the total operative time significantly. The advantages of rapid urinary runoff, augmented by the peristaltic action of the large bowel without the complication of hyperchloremic acidosis, are similar assets of the isolated ileal segment. The placement of the ostia in the abdominal wall is deferred until later in the operation in order to avoid trauma to the bowel and ureters during the remainder of the procedure.

Approximately 15 to 18 cm. of the sigmoid colon is carefully selected for the conduit, with particular attention given to an area which includes a rich arcade of blood vessels from the inferior mesenteric artery (Fig. 35-2). The final length of the bowel segment is determined by the thickness of the abdominal wall, in order to provide sufficient bowel for the intra-abdominal segment without placing undue tension on the ureteral anastomosis. In some instances this may include approximately 6 to 8 cm. of intra-abdominal bowel. In the event that additional large bowel is needed to construct a urinary conduit of adequate length and to fashion a colostomy, the descending colon can be easily mobilized by carefully excising the attachment of the splenic flexure to the parietal peritoneum. In preparing the conduit, care must be exercised to avoid damage to the anastomotic arcade of inferior mesenteric and superior hemorrhoidal vessels. Following division of the proximal and distal ends of the sigmoid segment, the proximal end is closed with a continuous inverting suture of fine chromic catgut (3-0) as an initial layer, followed by interrupted Lembert sutures of fine silk (3-0). The angles of the bowel must be well inverted to ensure against leakage of urine from the ureteral transplant. The rectosigmoid portion of the remaining pelvic bowel, which is attached to the pelvic tumor mass, is closed with a continuous inverting suture to prevent soilage of the operating field during the remainder of the dissection.

Anastomosis of the ureters to the antimesenteric wall of the isolated sigmoid conduit utilizes the mucosa-to-mucosa technic of Leadbetter (Fig. 35-3). Each ureter is positioned for final anastomosis so that the attached peritoneal flap remains on its anterior exposed surface after the ureter is turned back over the mesosigmoid and removed completely from the pelvis. This is accomplished following complete mobilization of the pelvic ureter by rotating the ureter so as to bring the retroperitoneal portion of the ureter along the inferior surface of the sigmoid pouch and mesentery, permitting the ureter to remain covered by its peritoneal flap at all times. The adventitia of the ureter is anchored posteriorly to the serosa of the sigmoid with three fine silk sutures (5-0), beginning in the middle of the ureter initially and followed by sutures at each edge of the ureter (Fig. 35-3 A and B). These initial

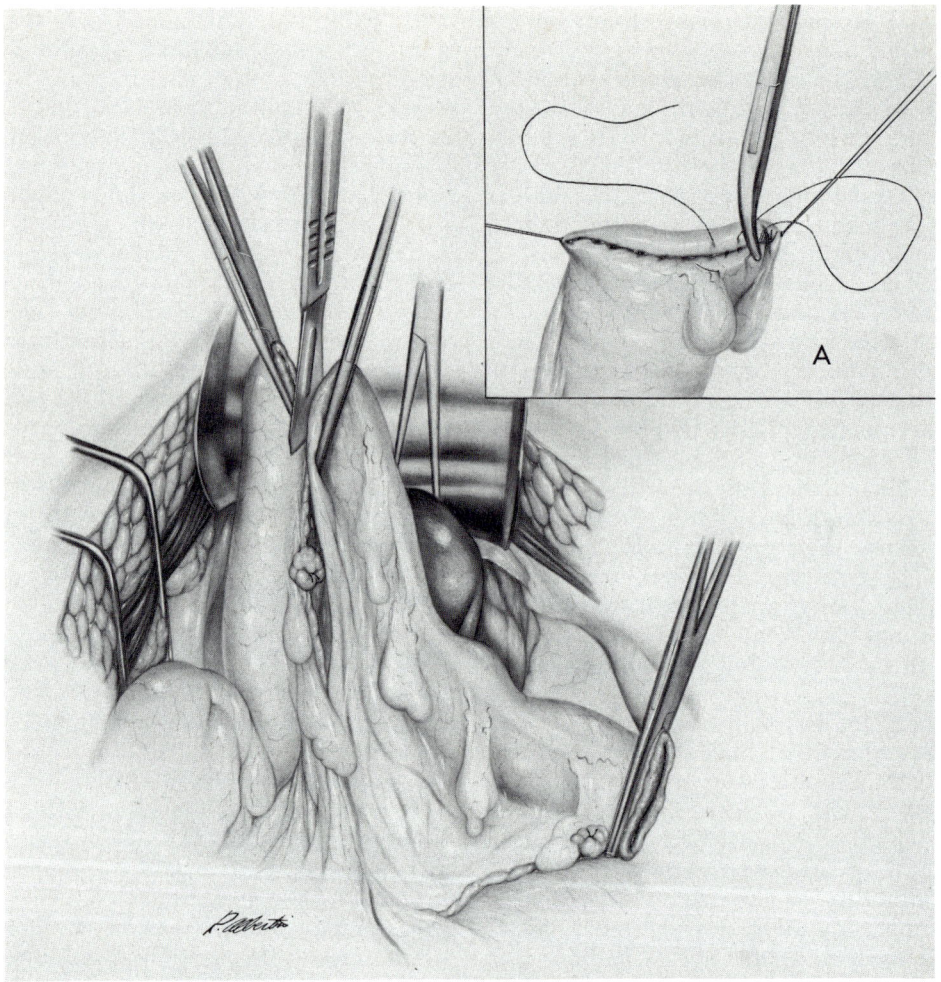

Fig. 35-2. Section of sigmoid has been excised. (Insert A) Showing two-layer closure of one end of sigmoid segment.

sutures are placed approximately 1 cm. from the excised end of the ureter and provide the main support to the mucosal anastomosis. The location for anastomosis of the left ureter is chosen to avoid encroachment on the closed end of the colon and should be at least 3 to 4 cm. from the bowel suture line. The right ureter should be implanted in such a position that it falls most naturally upon reflection from the pelvis, but should be separated from the opposite ureter by at least 4 to 5 cm. The anastomoses appear closer together in Figure 35-3 E for illustrative purposes only.

A small longitudinal incision is made through the muscularis of the bowel along the position and length of the ureteral orifice. In order to avoid the natural tendency of excessive enlargement of the orifice in the bowel mucosa, 2 empty round needles or skin hooks are used to anchor and elevate the mucosa for easy entry into the bowel lumen, as well as to secure the mucosal edge until the first mucosa-to-mucosa suture is placed (Fig. 35-3 C). In suturing the full-thickness wall of the ureter to the mucosa of the bowel, the middle suture is placed first, followed by the 2 angle sutures and utilizing 4-0 chromic catgut material. In recent cases we have used Silastic

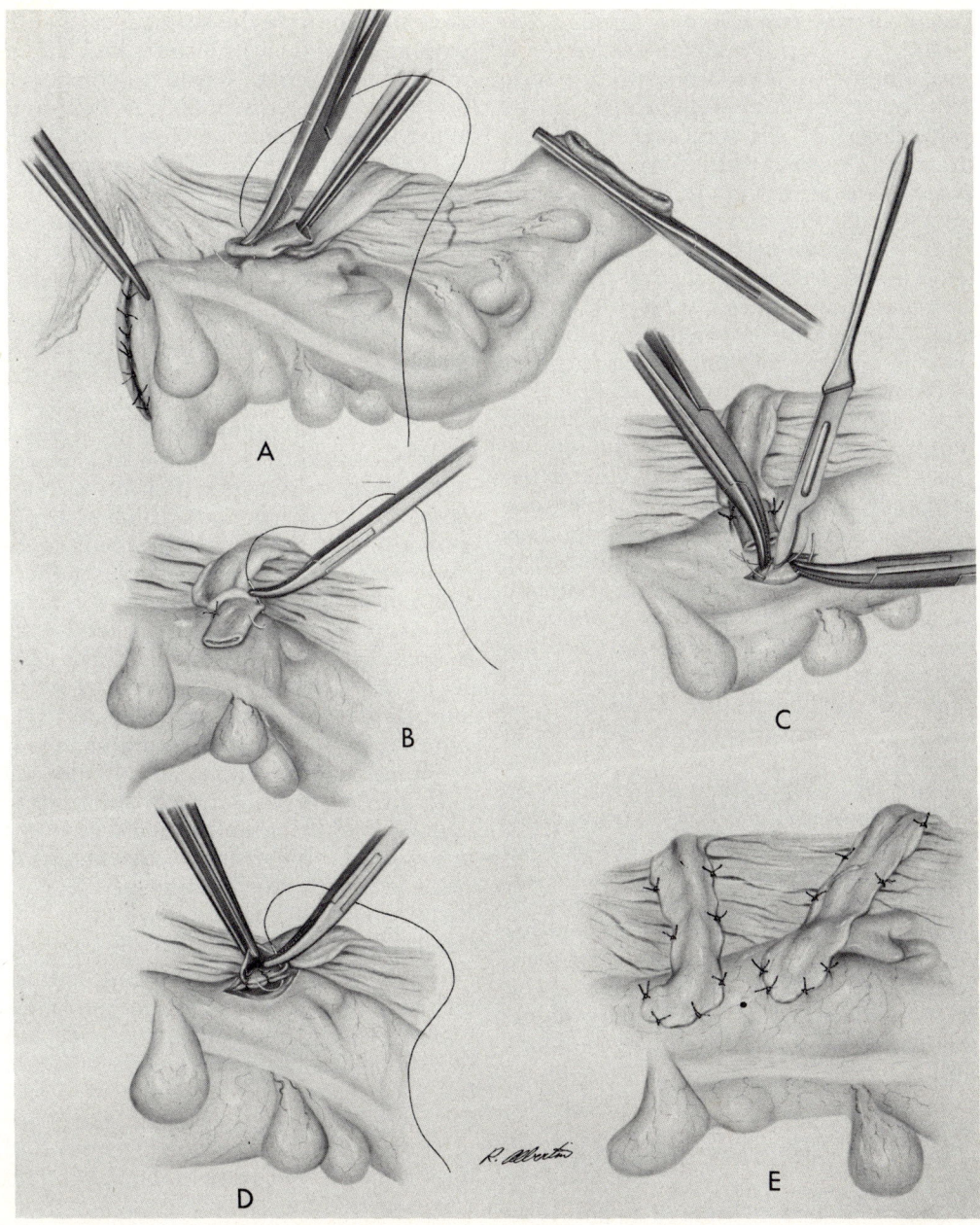

FIG. 35-3. Showing mucosa-to-mucosa anastomosis of ureter to sigmoid conduit. Note that the peritoneum attached to ureters may be used to extraperitonize the two-layer ureteral anastomosis.

tubing (ID*.078 or .062) as ureteral splints to enhance the healing process of the uretero-intestinal anastomosis. As advocated by Rutledge and Burns, this

---

* Internal diameter.

malleable splint is most useful for previously irradiated tissues, where leakage of the ureter is a common complication. One end of the silastic tubing is inserted up the ureter to the renal pelvis, and the opposite end is directed through the lumen of the conduit out through the ostia. The anterior wall of the ureter is than anastomosed in 2 or 3 locations to the bowel mucosa, depending on the redundancy of the mucosal ostia. No attempt is made to produce a leakproof anastomosis at this point, as the second, supporting layer of fine silk serosal sutures will reinforce the anastomosis and seal the orifice. The peritoneal flap of the ureter is now sutured with silk to the serosa of the bowel over the anastomotic site, and to the mesentery, in order to extraperitonize the ureter completely. This will ensure an adequate blood supply, as well as reinforce the anastomosis and prevent displacement of the ureters by movement of the abdominal viscera. The blind end and midportion of the conduit are securely sutured to the posterior peritoneum of the abdomen to make certain that the urinary bladder remains stationary and does not fall into the pelvis, where it might be involved in the resultant cellulitis from the procedure and place tension on the ureteral anastomosis.

The ureteral Silastic catheters are removed in approximately 14 days and are irrigated with 1 per cent neomycin solution only if there is evidence of diminished drainage from either catheter. In general, it has been our experience that the outcome of the exenterative procedure is reflected in the outcome of the urinary diversion. If the urinary diversion goes well, the entire operation goes well.

PELVIC LYMPHADENECTOMY

Attention can be directed to the lymphadenectomy, as the previous peritoneal reflection has uncovered the bifurcation of the aorta and vena cava. During the sharp dissection of the pelvic vessels, it is advisable to avoid traumatizing the vessel wall, which produces reaction of the intima of the vessel and enhances the possibility of postoperative emboli. We no longer advocate stripping the vessels until they are pearl-white and devoid of all adventitia, as it is evident that this does not improve the surgical cure of the patient. As shown in Figure 35-4, a filmy residue of areolar tissue is considered optimum. The dissection is continued along the external iliac vessels until they pass beneath Poupart's ligament and into the femoral canal. Care must be taken to avoid injury to the inferior epigastric and anomalous obturator vessels at the lower end of the iliac vessels.

The hypogastric vessels are clamped and double ligated with silk (Fig. 35-4 A). If one prefers to excise the hypograstric vessels as a part of the *en bloc* dissection, it is important to spend the valuable time necessary to ligate the branches of the hypogastric artery and vein at this point in the dissection, which will prevent difficult deep pelvic bleeding and excessive blood loss at a later point in the operation. The posterior branches are easily demonstrated by reflecting the hypogastric vessels forward (Fig. 35-4 B) so that the iliolumbar, lateral sacral, and gluteal vessels may be ligated. The internal pudendal and obturator vessels are encountered next, and finally the anterior trunk containing the uterine, vaginal, middle hemorrhoidal, and vesical arteries. The hypogastric vessels may be included with the ligation of the pararectal stalks, if desired, which is discussed later.

Particular care must be taken with the adjacent network of anastomosed veins, which, when traumatized, retract into the sacral foramina and pelvic musculature. It is usually more beneficial to pack the area temporarily, when necessary, until the venous bleeding is controlled, if there is any difficulty in identifying the origin of the vein.

Continuation of the lymph node dissection into the obturator fossa (Fig. 35-5) is facilitated by previous ligation of the blood supply of the pelvis and by elevation of the external iliac vessels with a vein retractor. The obturator nerve and obturator muscle are thoroughly cleaned by sharp dissection. The distal ends of the obturator vessels are ligated (Fig. 35-5 A) prior to their exit through the obturator foramen. Attention is

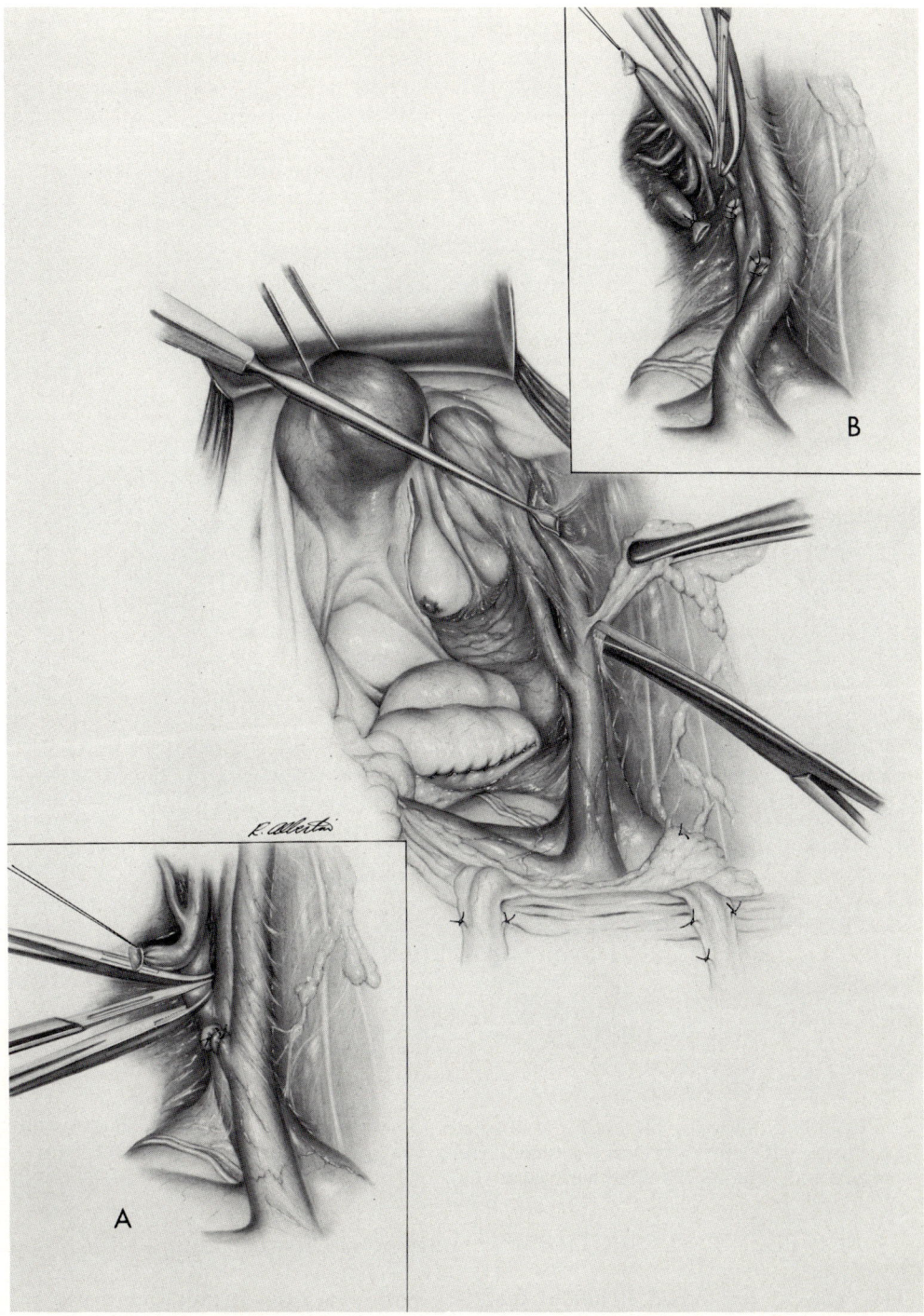

FIG. 35-4. Showing lymphatic dissection along external iliac vessels with clamping (A) and excision (B) of hypogastric vessels.

directed to the occasional anomalous obturator vessels which enter the distal portion of the fossa from the external iliac vessels. The upper portions of the sciatic nerve roots are visible at this time and must not be traumatized.

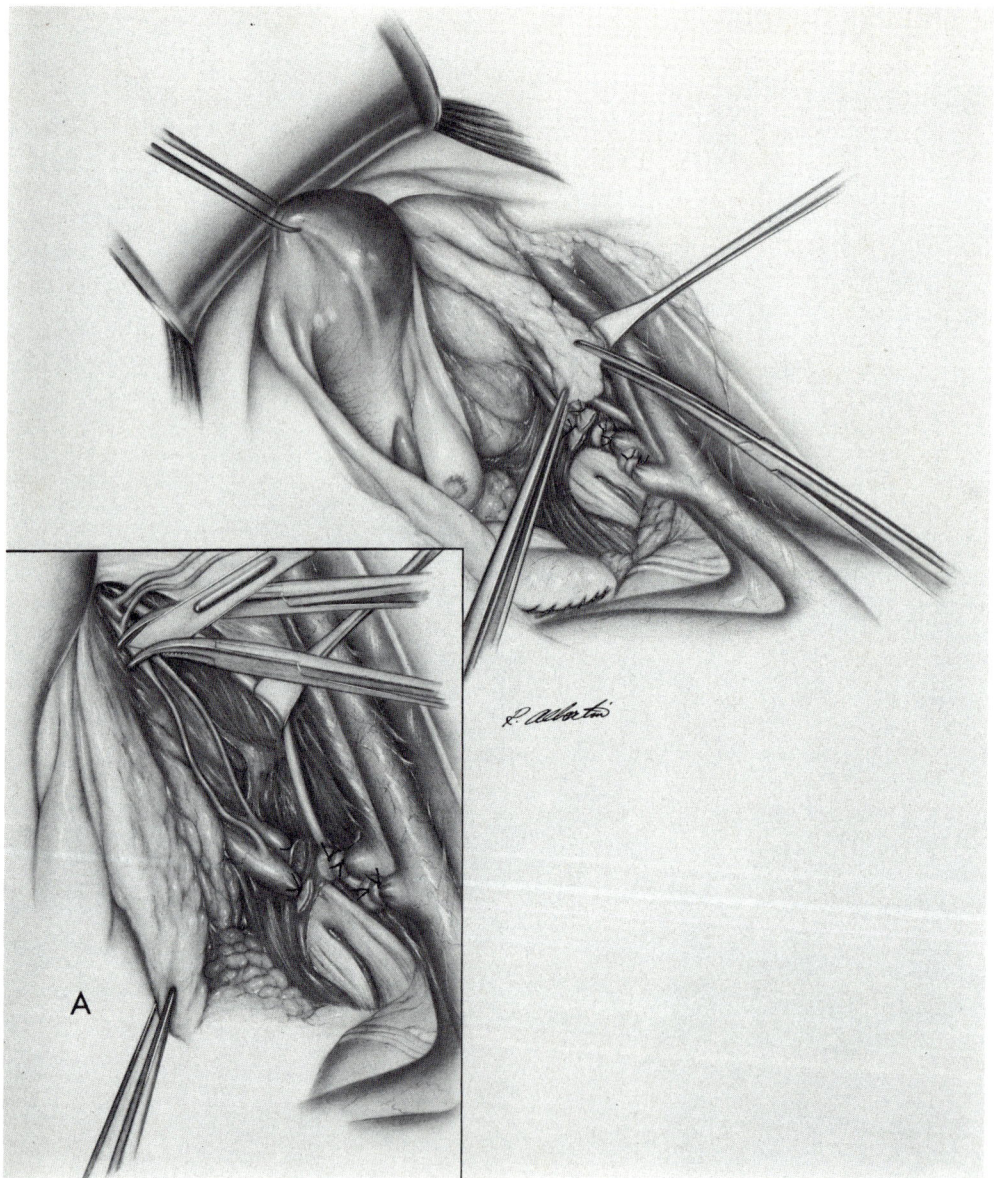

FIG. 35-5. Showing dissection of obturator fossa. (Insert A) Shows cleaned obturator fossa with obturator nerve retracted from underlying obturator muscle. Obturator artery and vein are clamped and cut as they enter obturator foramen.

DEEP PELVIC DISSECTION

The base of the broad ligament (cardinal ligament) is now excised at the lateral pelvic wall by placing one jaw of the Wertheim clamp in the paravesical space and in the pararectal space, respectively, which will free most of the parametrium down to the levator muscles and pelvic floor, as illustrated in Figure 34-17.

With the major pelvic vessels previously ligated, the rectum may be dissected bluntly from the anterior surface of the sacrum by strong forward traction of the rectum and uterus and insertion of the hand behind the rectum (Fig. 35-6). The pararectal stalks blend with

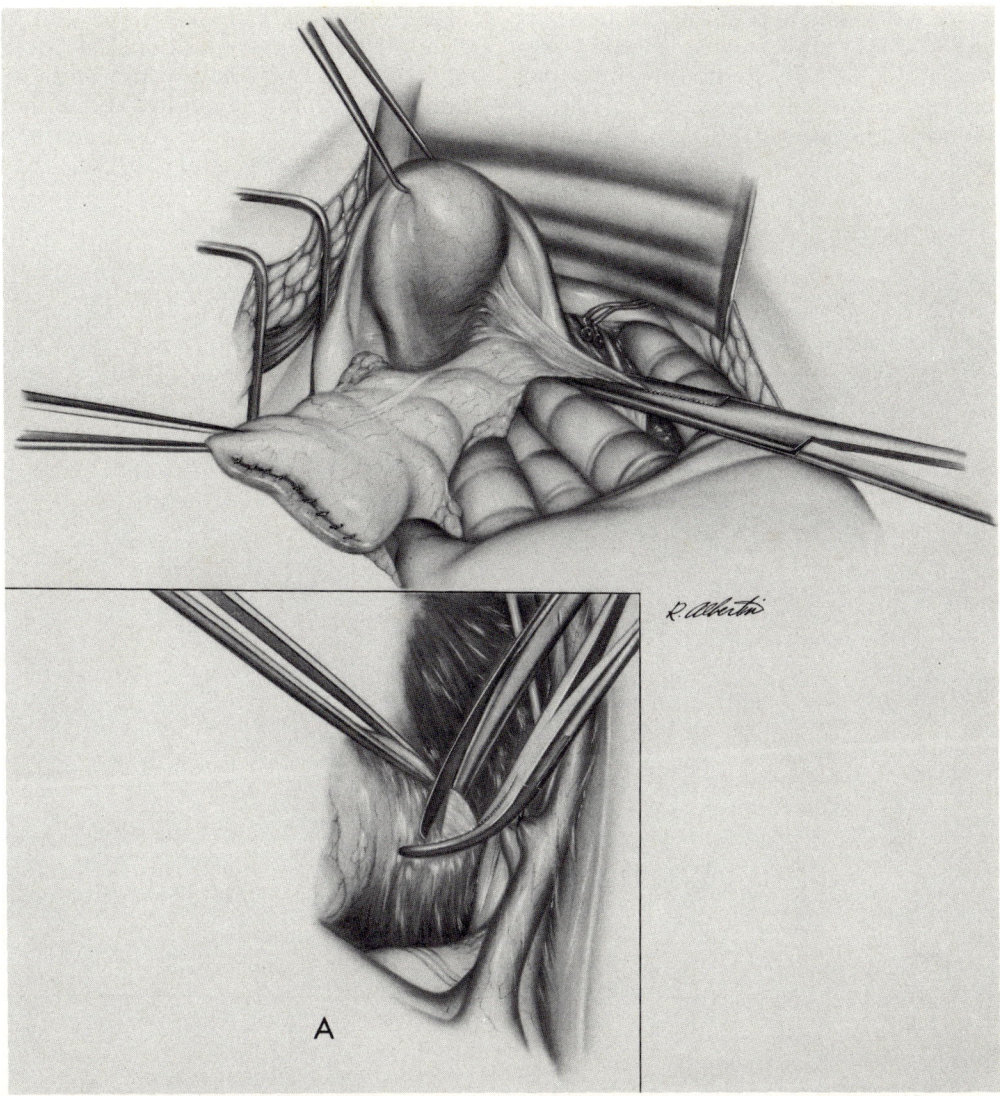

FIG. 35-6. Showing dissection of rectum from anterior surface of sacrum. (Insert A) Showing use of Wertheim clamp in excising pararectal tissue close to pelvic wall.

the lateral parametrial lymphatic tissue and anchor the rectum and uterus to the posterolateral pelvic wall. Large Wertheim clamps are utilized to ligate this tissue as close to the pelvic wall and underlying sciatic nerve roots as possible (Fig. 35-6 A). In the event that the hypogastric vessels have not been excised prior to this time, they are included in the successive pararectal sutures that completely free the specimen from the lateral pelvic wall.

The bladder and urethra are dissected from their subpubic attachments by both sharp and blunt dissection. Care is taken to preserve every available centimeter of bladder peritoneum, which will be utilized later in the construction of a peritoneal hammock to close the pelvic inlet from the abdominal cavity. The entire surgical specimen is retracted cephalad to facilitate the subpubic and paravaginal dissection. To complete the deep pelvic dissection, the rectum is retracted for-

782 Pelvic Exenteration

ward, and the adherent areolar tissue is excised from the lower sacrum and coccyx (Fig. 35-7). Brisk bleeding may occur from the anterior sacral plexus of veins and is best controlled by a pressure pack.

The entire *en bloc* procedure can be accomplished by the abdominal route, but it is frequently easier and more expedient to use the combined abdominal-perineal approach. The separate perineal dissection is particularly useful in a

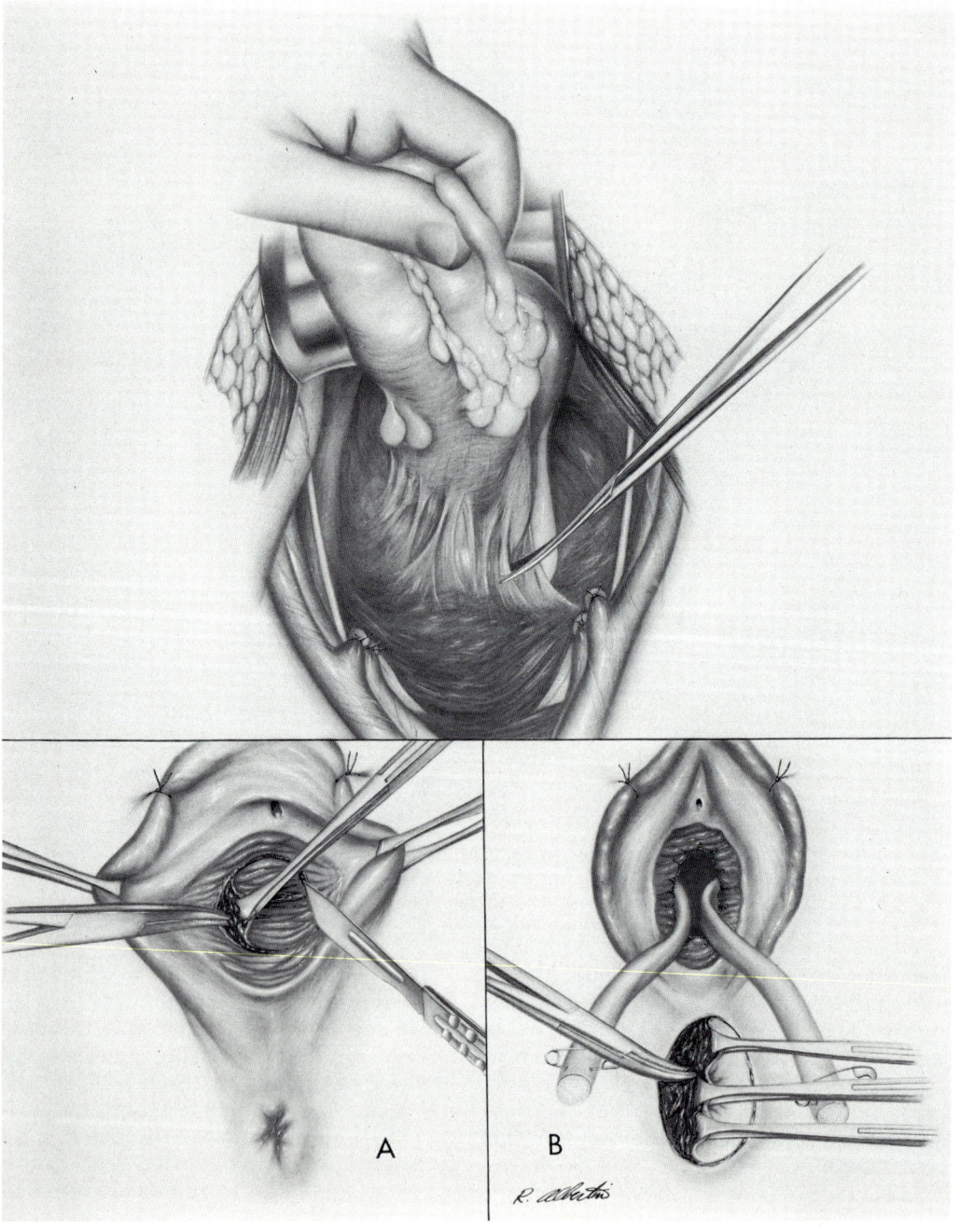

FIG. 35-7. Showing completion of dissection of sigmoid from lower sacrum. (Inserts A, B) Showing vaginal and anal dissection from below by a second team.

young patient when an effort is made to preserve the outer one third of the vagina. While one surgical team is completing the deep pelvic dissection, another team incises the outer one third of the vagina (Fig. 35-7 A) and ligates the vaginal vessels bilaterally. The outer third of the urethra is transected, and the paraurethral vessels are secured. The paravaginal tissues are dissected medially, the adjacent fascia and the areolar tissue being removed until the levator ani muscles are visible. At this point the vaginal dissection should communicate with the pelvic cavity, which completely frees the specimen except for the anal attachment. In preserving the outer rectovaginal fascia, the anus is circumscribed and closed by a continuous inverting suture to prevent soiling of the pelvic cavity with fecal material, and the inferior hemorrhoidal vessels are ligated (Fig. 35-7 B). Separation of the rectum from the lateral fibers of the puborectalis portion of the levator, followed by sharp-scissor dissection of the rectovaginal and parasacral fascia, will free the rectum. The entire surgical specimen is removed through the abdominal incision. The anal space is obliterated by approximation of the puborectalis muscles, and the skin is closed with a subcuticular suture. A continuous, locking chromic catgut suture is placed along the excised vaginal mucosa for hemostasis, and two cigarette drains are inserted into the pelvis (Fig. 35-8).

CLOSURE OF THE PELVIC PERITONEUM

The pelvis is now devoid of all structures except the levator and obturator muscles, the obturator nerve coursing across the obturator fossa, and the roots of the sciatic nerve. The vaginal drains are placed on either side of the pelvis and anchored with catgut sutures, while gauze packs are used against the raw pelvis only in the event that there is persistent venous oozing at the time of closure. These are brought out through the vagina, advanced on the 3rd postoperation day, and removed on the 5th day. The drains remain in place until the perineal drainage has subsided and are usually removed on the 7th to 10th postoperative day.

This procedure emphasizes the importance of closing off the raw pelvis from the abdominal cavity. While some authorities believe this to be unnecessary, this additional step has greatly decreased the incidence of postoperative intestinal obstruction. In addition, the usual pelvic cellulitis is excluded from the peritoneal cavity, and peritonitis is greatly diminished. The preserved bladder peritoneum is used along with the parietal peritoneum from the anterior abdominal wall to close the pelvis completely from the abdominal cavity along the pelvic brim, the anterior peritoneum being approximated to the residual posterior peritoneum. One must avoid tension on the posterior peritoneum adjacent to the ureters, which might jeopardize the ureteral anastomosis. The effect of this peritoneal closure is to create a peritoneal hammock across the pelvic inlet, which will gradually stretch as the small bowel settles into the pelvis, creating a peritoneal barrier between the serosa of the bowel and the raw pelvis (Fig. 35-8). If there is insufficient peritoneum for adequate coverage of the entire pelvis, the omentum may be utilized for this purpose. This may be accomplished as a pedicle graft by leaving a small portion of the omentum attached to its blood supply and reflecting the free, excised portion into the pelvis and suturing the free edges to the pelvic peritoneum. We have frequently excised the entire omentum and sutured it in the pelvis as a free omental graft which quickly regains a parasitic blood supply.

The sigmoid urinary conduit is brought through the lower abdominal wall in the right lower quadrant, midway between the umbilicus and the anterior superior iliac spine. The sites for the urinary and fecal ostia are marked on the abdomen with methylene blue prior to draping the patient. Regardless of where the urinary ostium is placed, it is important to have a flat surface for attach-

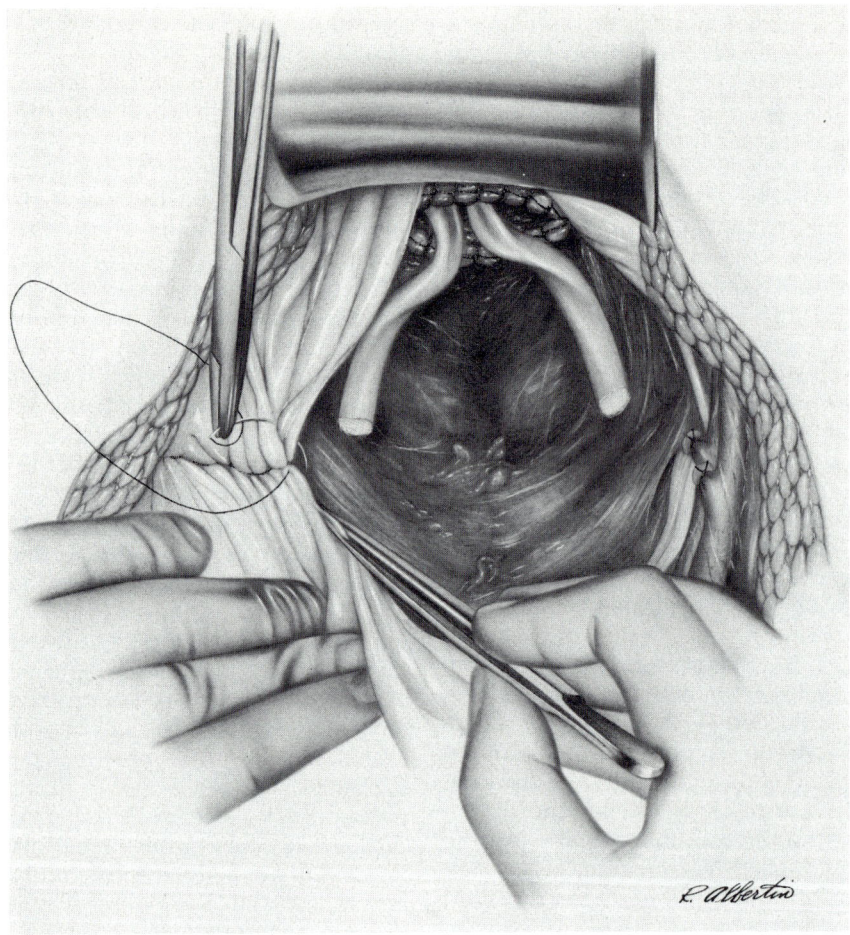

FIG. 35-8. Showing drainage of denuded pelvis and closure of peritoneum.

ment of the prosthesis. The sigmoid colostomy site is marked in the left infraumbilical area, so that the inferior pole of the fecal ostia is on a horizontal line with the level of the superior pole of the urinary ostia. The abdominal wall is prepared by excising an ovoid tunnel, 3 cm. in diameter, through its entire thickness—skin, subcutaneous fat, external oblique fascia, and muscle. This is important in creating an unobstructed free flow of urine from the conduit. The serosa of the bowel is anchored to the fascia and subcutaneous fat of the abdominal wall, and the bowel musosa is everted so as to create a raised "rosebud" stoma projecting from the abdominal wall, which is completely covered with bowel mucosa. This will greatly reduce the occurrence of stricture of the urinary ostia.

The fecal stream is diverted to the left abdominal wall in similar manner, the upper portion of the sigmoid colon being brought to the skin just lateral and slightly inferior to the umbilicus. Both ostia cannot be placed along the same plane of the lower abdomen because of interference from the urinary prosthesis belt. The colostomy bud should be placed below the beltline for cosmetic purposes. It is important to suture the serosa of both the urinary conduit and the sigmoid colostomy to the lateral parietal peritoneum. This will avoid leaving peritoneal pockets for possible herniation and obstruction of bowel. Stay sutures are utilized in closing the incision, as such patients are excellent candidates for impaired healing and evisceration.

ANTERIOR PELVIC EXENTERATION

A similar operative technic is utilized in the anterior pelvic exenteration where the rectum is found to be free of disease at the time of exploration and dissects easily from the vagina. In leaving the rectum intact in such cases and removing the remainder of the pelvic organs (uterus, vagina, and bladder), one must accept the possibility of residual tumor in small lymphatic channels in the rectal wall as well as the risk of compromising the blood supply of the rectum during the operative procedure.

In such cases the identical operative procedure is performed as that described for total exenteration, with the exception that the terminal ileum is used for the urinary conduit. This procedure, as introduced by Bricker, utilizes a mucosa-to-mucosa anastomosis of the ureter to the ileum following double-layer closure of the blind end of the ileal pouch.

The pelvic lymph node dissection is similar to that described in the total exenteration, although the hypogastric vessels are usually not sacrificed in this procedure. An effort is made to maintain a blood supply to the middle and inferior hemorrhoidal vessels, while the anterior division of the hypogastric artery is ligated and removed with the specimen. Dissection of the parametrium is achieved by development of the paravesical and pararectal spaces including all the paracervical tissues to the lateral pelvic wall.

The uterosacral ligaments are ligated as far posteriorly as possible after separation of the rectum from the rectovaginal fascia by both sharp and blunt dissection. Removal of the bladder and vagina is accomplished, as previously described, with preservation of as much of the bladder peritoneum as possible. The major problem at this point is the control of bleeding from the paravesical plexus of veins at the base of the bladder. If bleeding is excessive, packing usually is more effective in producing hemostasis, during which time the dissection is continued on the opposite side. Peritonealization and drainage through the vagina are accomplished as previously described, and the ileal conduit is brought through the low abdominal wall, midway between the umbilicus and the anterior superior iliac spine on the right side. The serosa of the conduit is carefully sutured to the posterior abdominal peritoneum above the pelvic brim to avoid displacement of the conduit and tension on the ureteral anastomosis.

As previously mentioned, this procedure is currently being replaced by total pelvic exenteration for recurrent cervical carcinoma. It is frequently indicated in vulvar, vaginal, or urethral carcinoma where the disease has involved the anterior vaginal wall.

COMPLICATIONS

The major complications following exenterative procedures are related primarily to the urinary tract and bowel. The problem of urinary tract fistulas at the site of the uretero-intestinal anastomosis continues to plague the pelvic surgeon and occurs most frequently following megavoltage pelvic irradiation. Occasionally the wall of the urinary conduit will become involved in an area of pelvic cellulitis with subsequent fistula formation. Surgical correction of such fistulas should be delayed for at least 3 months until the inflammatory reaction of the conduit and adjacent fistulous tract has subsided. In the event that stenosis of the ureter should occur with resultant diminished renal function as demonstrated by serial intravenous pyelograms, an earlier repair is necessary.

Intestinal obstruction continues to be a serious problem, particularly in those cases in which adequate peritonization of the pelvis is not accomplished, accounting for the most frequent serious complication (11%) in Bricker's vast experience with 207 exenterations for postirradiation carcinoma of the cervix. In those cases in which intestinal obstruction occurred, 6 out of 26 patients (25%) died postoperatively. Bowel fistula or obstruction occurred in 14 per cent of 118 exenterations at the Mayo Clinic, and other series report an incidence of 12 to 20 per cent for similar bowel complications. Bowel complications have not been a clinical problem in our own clinic, primarily because the sigmoid colon is used for the urinary conduit, and a bowel anastomosis is not required. Pelvic cellulitis, a frequent occurrence following such procedures, is caused by contamination of the pelvis with intestinal flora at the time of surgery and the continuous drainage of lymph and serum into the raw open pelvic floor.

Septicemia and death resulting from resistant bacteria are serious complications of this procedure, and intensive antibiotc therapy is frequently required.

Thromboembolic disease is always a hazard in such prolonged operative procedures, particularly with trauma to the pelvic veins from the pelvic dissection. Prophylactic anticoagulation is impractical in such procedures because of the hazard of postoperative hemorrhage from many small pelvic veins which are not individually ligated.

The operative mortality from pelvic exenteration for recurrent carcinoma of the cervix has improved in the past decade and is currently 8 per cent in Milwaukee and other clinics. In Brunschwig's extensive experience in total exenteration, including 217 patients, a surgical mortality rate of 17 per cent reflects the original use of this procedure for palliative treatment in poor-risk patients rather than its current use for surgical cure. An idea of the operative mortality and 5-year survivals in various clinics can be obtained by examining Table 35-1.

CURE RATE

The combined world experience in pelvic exenteration is less than 2,000 cases. In all the reported series, the average 5-year cure rate is 20 to 25 per cent (Symmonds, Pratt, and Welch). Undoubtedly this cure rate will remain unchanged until there is uniform adherence to the specific indications and

Table 35-1. Patients Treated for Advanced Pelvic Cancer by Exenteration of the Pelvic Organs Reported in the Past 10 Years*

First Author	Institution	Number of Patients Treated	Number of Operative Deaths	Number Surviving 5 Years
Dargent, M. (1957)	Lyon, France	83	26	13
Douglas, R. (1957)	New York Hospital	23	1	5
Smith, R. (1963)	National Cancer Institute	71	6	11
Parsons, L. (1964)	Boston	112	24	24
Rutledge, F. (1965)	M. D. Anderson	108	18	31
Brunschwig, A. (1965)	Memorial Hospital	535	86	108
Bricker, E. M.	St. Louis	153	15	53
Total		1,085	176 (16%)	265 (24%)

* Kiselow, M., Butcher, H. R., Jr., and Bricker, E. M.: Results of the radical surgical treatment of advanced pelvic cancer: 15 year survey, Ann. Surg., 166:428, 1967.

contraindications for this procedure. As long as pelvic surgeons experiment with such cases in the vague hope that the disease will be completely removed instead of having a clear understanding of the limits of success of such procedures, the cure rate will remain unchanged.

SUMMARY

1. In patients with radioresistant carcinoma of the cervix, where the recurrent disease is confined to the cervix, the immediate adjacent parametrium, or has spread in an anteroposterior direction, the surgical procedure of choice is an *en bloc* pelvic exenteration and lymphadenectomy.

2. Due to the frequence of fistulae, an anterior pelvic exenteration is an occasionally acceptable procedure for radioresistant disease. The posterior exenteration has been largely abandoned in postirradiated cervical carcinoma because of the high incidence of urinary and rectal fistulae.

3. At the "court of last appeal," the clinical absence of gross tumor in the bladder or rectum should not deter the pelvic surgeon from a total exenteration since the surgical specimen commonly demonstrates residual tumor in the wall of adjacent viscera. The irradiated, ischemic bladder and rectum cannot be considered normal tissue and should be included in the pathologic specimen to ensure adequate tumor margins.

4. The total pelvic exenteration should not be performed in the absence of histologically proven recurrent carcinoma; nor should it be undertaken when such disease has spread beyond the pelvis. This operation has no place in palliative therapy and should be utilized only when the pelvic tumor is considered anatomically resectable and where one would anticipate complete surgical control of the disease.

5. It is impossible to predict accurately the operability of recurrent cervical carcinoma following full irradiation therapy and resultant pelvic scarring. A more liberal use of laparotomy for final evaluation of the extent of tumor spread provides a more realistic and definitive approach toward the use of radical surgery for an otherwise lethal disease.

6. The *en bloc* dissection provides an effective, logical method of control of radioresistant cervical carcinoma, and its acceptance by well-informed patients is excellent. Its success or failure in arresting the disease is a reflection of the proper selection of the surgical candidate by the pelvic surgeon. Consequently, the most important step in this procedure is to make certain by multiple frozen section biopsies that the disease is confined to the pelvis and completely free from pelvic musculature *prior* to beginning the exenteration. Utilization of the avascular paravesical and pararectal anatomical spaces is the key to the accurate evaluation of the location and extent of the neoplastic disease.

BIBLIOGRAPHY

Berkeley, C., and Bonney, V.: The radical abdominal operation for carcinoma of the cervix uteri. Brit. Med. J., 2:445, 1916.

Bricker, E. M.: The technique of ileal segment bladder substitution. *In* Meigs, J. B. (ed.): Progress in Gynecology. Vol. III. New York, Grune & Stratton, 1957.

Bricker, E. M., and Modlin, J.: The role of pelvic evisceration. Surgery, 30:76, 1951.

Bricker, E. M., Butcher H. R., Jr., Lawler, W. H., Jr., and McAfee, C. A.: Surgical treatment of advanced and recurrent cancer of the pelvic viscera. Ann. Surg., 152:388, 1960.

Brunschwig, A.: Complete excision of the pelvic viscera for advanced carcinoma. Cancer, 1:177, 1948.

———: Surgical treatment of recurrent endometrial cancer. Obstet. Gynec., 18:272, 1961.

———: What are indications and results of pelvic exenteration? J.A.M.A., 194:274, 1965.

———: Surgical treatment of carcinoma of the

cervix, recurrent after irradiation or combination of irradiation and surgery. Amer. J. Roentgen., 99:365, 1967.

Burns, B. C., Jr., and Brack, C. B.: Prognostic factors in radioresistant cervical carcinoma. Obstet. Gynec., 16:1, 1960.

Cox, E. F., Ketchum, A. S., Villa Sant, U., and Mumford, R. S.: Patient evaluation for pelvic exenteration. Amer. Surg., 30:574, 1964.

Crisp, W. E., Davis, C. E., and Snow, D. L.: Preservation of vaginal function following radical pelvic surgery. Arch. Surg., 81:632, 1960.

Dargent, M., Mayer, M., and Colon, J.: Limits and indications for pelvic exenteration in advanced phases of gynecologic cancers. C. R. Soc. Franc. Gynec., 27:293, 1957.

Douglas, R. G., and Sweeney, W. J.: Exenteration operations in treatment of advanced pelvic cancer. Amer. J. Obstet. Gynec., 73:1169, 1957.

Everett, H. S.: The effect of carcinoma of the cervix uteri and its treatment upon the urinary tract. Amer. J. Obstet. Gynec., 38:889, 1939.

Freund, W. A.: Eine neue Methode der Exstirpation des ganzen Uterus. Samml. klin. Vort., No. 133 (Gynäk., No. 41:911) Leipzig, 1878.

Gary, R. K., Sala, J. M., and Spratt, J. S.: The detection and treatment of postirradiationally recidivated cancers of the cervix uteri. Radiology, 83:208, 1964.

Green, T. H., Jr., Meigs, J. V., Ulfelder, H., and Curtin, R. R.: Urologic complications of radical Wertheim hysterectomy; incidence, etiology, management and prevention. Obstet. Gynec., 20:293, 1962.

Henriksen, E.: The lymphatic spread of carcinoma of the cerivix and the body of the uterus. Amer. J. Obstet. Gynec., 58:924, 1949.

——: Distribution of metastases in Stage I carcinoma of the cervix; a study of 66 autopsied cases. Amer. J. Obstet. Gynec., 80:919, 1960.

Ingersoll, F. M., and Ulfelder, H.: Pelvic exenteration for carcinoma of the cervix. New Eng. J. Med., 274:648, 1966.

Kiselow, M., Butcher, H. R., Jr., and Bricker, E. M.: Results of the radical surgical treatment of advanced pelvic cancer: a 15-year survey. Ann. Surg., 166:428, 1967.

Leadbetter, W. F.: Consideration of problems incident to performance or ureteroenterostomy: report of a technique. J. Urol., 65:818, 1951.

Mattingly, R. F.: Surgery in the aging female. Clin. Obstet. Gynec., 7:573, 1964.

Meigs, J. V.: Radical hysterectomy with bilateral pelvic lymph node dissections. Report of 100 cases operated on 5 years or more. Amer. J. Obstet. Gynec., 62:854, 1951.

Mikuta, J. J.: Pelvic exenteration in carcinoma of the cervix, a review of the literature. Amer. J. Med. Sci., 236:797, 1958.

Parsons, L.: Pelvic exenteration. Clin. Obstet. Gynec., 2:1151, 1959.

Parsons, L., and Bell, J. W.: An evaluation of pelvic exenteration operation. Cancer, 3:205, 1950.

Parsons, L., and Friedell, G. J.: Radical surgical treatment of cancer of cervix. Proc. Nat. Cancer Conf., 5:241, 1964.

Parsons, L., and Sommers, S. C.: Gynecology. Philadelphia, W. B. Saunders, 1962.

Perez-Mesa, C., and Spjut, H. J.: Persistent postirradiation carcinoma of cervix uteri. Arch. Path., 75:462, 1963.

Ries, E.: Eine neue operationsmethode des uteruscarcinoms. Z. Geburtsh. Gynäk., 32:266, 1895.

Rutledge, F. N., and Burns, B. C., Jr.: Pelvic exenteration. Amer. J. Obstet. Gynec., 91:692, 1965.

Schmitz, R. L., Schmitz, H. E., Smith, C. J., and Molitor, J. J.: Details of pelvic exenteration evolved during an experience with 75 cases. Amer. J. Obstet. Gynec., 80:43, 1960.

Smith, R. R., Ketchum, A. S., and Thomas, L. B.: Carcinoma of the uterine cervix: experience with radical surgery. Cancer, 16:1105, 1963.

Symmonds, R. E., Pratt, J. H., and Welch, J. S.: Exenterative operations. Amer. J. Obstet. Gynec., 101:66, 1968.

Ulfelder, H.: Extended radical surgery for recurrent and advanced cervical cancer. Clin. Obstet. Gynec., 10:940, 1967.

Wertheim, E.: Die erweiterte abdominale Operation die Carcinoma colli uteri (auf grund von 500 fallen). Berlin, Urban und Schwarzenberg, 1911.

——: The extended abdominal operation for carcinoma uteri. Translated by H. Grad. Amer. J. Obstet. Gynec., 66:169, 1912.

36

Carcinoma of the Corpus Uteri

GENERAL CONSIDERATIONS

The apparent increase in the incidence of carcinoma of the uterine fundus during the past two decades is related to several factors. During this recent interval, the incidence of cervix cancer has decreased in the United States as a direct result of mass population screening programs. While the earlier comparison of carcinoma of the cervix to endometrial carcinoma was historically recorded as 8:1, present statistics have dropped this ratio to a reported 4:1 and in some clinics 1:1 (Novak and Villa Santa). The current ratio in our own clinic is approximately 4.7:1. Although well-controlled studies are lacking, it is the experience of many clinicians that cancer of the endometrium is more frequent among middle and upper income groups, as reported by Graham, as well as Boutselis (58% occurring in private patients) and Corscaden (57% in private patients). Consequently, the ratio of these two diseases may depend on the type of patient admitted to a specific clinic. In addition, the life expectancy for the female has increased during the past quarter century to the present rate of age 72, which includes a larger group of females in the age category for endometrial carcinoma. More specifically, medical data for uterine cancer has become more accurate in defining the death rate from fundal carcinoma separate from carcinoma of the cervix.

The average age of women at diagnosis of endometrial carcinoma varies between 55 and 60 in most reported large series. In our own clinic, the average age of this disease is 56, as reported by Pentecost and Brack. This corresponds with the average age of 56.9 as reported by Davis in 525 patients, and age 57 as summarized from several reports by Morton. Endometrial carcinoma infrequently occurs in younger women under the age of 40, varying between 2 and 5 per cent. Peterson's recent report of 650 cases of endometrial carcinoma included 5 per cent occurring under the age of 40 at the time of diagnosis. Of this group, 81 per cent gave a long history of amenorrhea or other menstrual irregularities for several years prior to the diagnosis, suggesting an associated endocrine dysfunction. Kempson and Pokorny recently studied the pathology in 22 such patients at Barnes Hospital, where the adenocarcinoma occurred in young women under the age of 40, among a larger group of 1,280 cases over the age of 40. On restudy of the histology of each case, they found that 7 of these young cases represented only endometrial hyperplasia. These authors share our view that the better prognosis in young women may be related to atypical endometrial hyperplasia being overdiagnosed and treated as adenocarcinoma.

Many investigators have noted that late menopause is one of the menstrual traits found in patients who eventually develop corpus cancer. Way noted a 5-year delay for endometrial cancer patients as compared to a control group. In a statistical review by Wynder and his associates, 13 per cent of the patients in these cancer cases underwent menopause at the age of 55 or over, as compared to 5 per cent in the control group. Although 75 to 85 per cent of such patients with endometrial carcinoma are postmenopausal, Barter *et al.* noted that only 15.9 per cent of the patients in their group were reportedly having menstrual periods, and that many of these were actually menopausal.

HISTOPATHOLOGY IN RELATION TO PROGNOSIS

Histologic Grading

The prognosis for endometrial carcinoma is governed primarily by two factors: (1) the histologic grading of the tumor and (2) the extend of the lesion at the time of diagnosis and treatment. This histologic grading system was developed by Broders in 1932, with frank adenocarcinomas divided into four groups morphologically, based on the degree of cellular differentiation. This grading system correlates consistently with the 5-year survival rate. Mahle was one of the early investigators who applied Broders' classification to his series of 186 cases of corpus carcinoma at the Mayo Clinic, and demonstrated that a definite relationship exists between the histologic pattern of the tumor and the surgical end-result. A recent report by Roman, Beck, and LaTour clearly correlates the 5-year results in 266 cases of endometrial carcinoma ranging from 86.8 per cent (Grade 1) to 45.8 per cent (Grade 4).

Broders' Classification. Grade 1 (Fig. 36-1) is characterized by a frank adenocarcinoma with irrefutable neoplastic change as evidenced by an increase in the number of glands and back-to-back crowding, as well as alterations in the epithelial cells lining the gland that are typical of neoplasia. This group includes those tumors in which 100 to 75 per cent of the adenomatous tumor is well-dif-

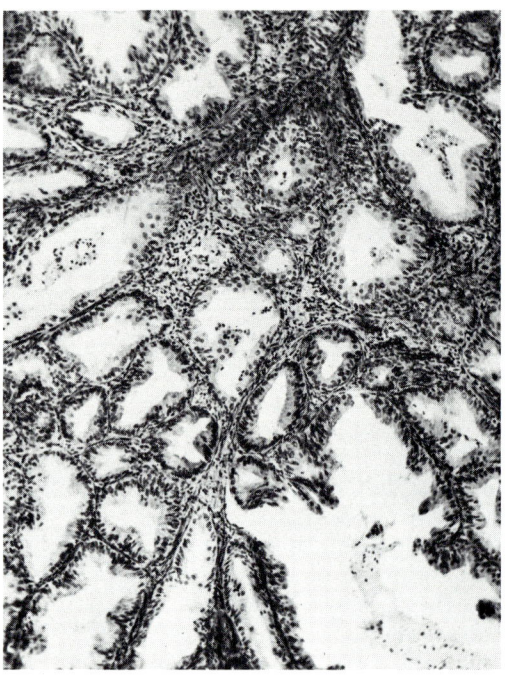

Fig. 36-1. Well-differentiated adenocarcinoma (Grade 1).

ferentiated with a distinctly identifiable gland pattern.

Grade 2 (Fig. 36-2). The proportion of differentiated epithelial cells lining the gland structures is approximately 75 to 50 per cent, while 25 to 50 per cent of the tumor is undifferentiated.

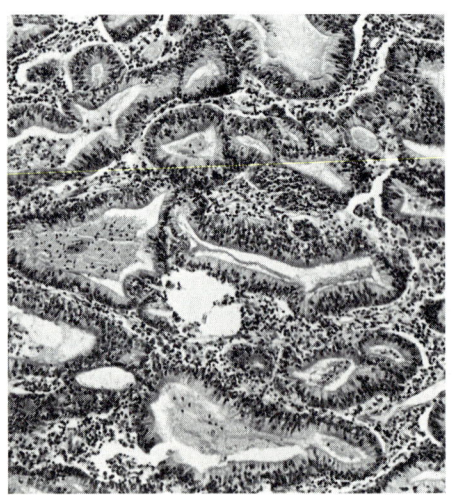

Fig. 36-2. Adenocarcinoma with minimal undifferentiation (Grade 2).

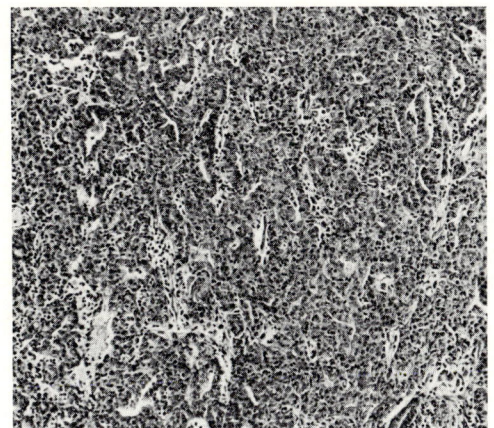

Fig. 36-3. Adenocarcinoma with marked undifferentiation (Grade 3).

GRADE 3 (Fig. 36-3). Fifty to 25 per cent of the glandular pattern remains well-differentiated, while 50 to 75 per cent of the tumor shows an undifferentiated pattern.

GRADE 4 (Fig. 36-4). This is clinically the most malignant of all types and includes those lesions with 25 to 0 per cent differentiated cells, while 75 to 100 per cent of the tumor is composed of a highly undifferentiated histologic pattern.

In 1932 Broders reintroduced the term *carcinoma in situ*, which was originally suggested by Rubin in 1918. In 1949 Hertig and Sommers made an extensive study of the genesis of endometrial cancer and described the histologic changes of carcinoma in situ, a pathologic entity which has had various interpretations by pathologists and clinicians since that time. Hertig's classification included endometrial glands composed of large cells with abundant clear eosinophilic cytoplasm. The nuclei were described as pale with fine granular chromatin arranged in irregular palisades and having a slightly irregular nuclear membrane. Although there is some cellular disorientation and disparity in the size and stratification of nuclei, the staining quality is generally uniform. While there is moderate crowding of the affected glands, there is no back-to-back arrangement or invasion of the endometrial stroma by the glandular elements. There is marked reduplication of the gland lumina and infolding of glands, but external budding of the glands is not a part of this microscopic picture. If any invasion of either the stroma or myometrium is present, the carcinoma is no longer regarded as *in situ*. Although Hertig and co-workers concluded that this microscopic change was not capable of regression spontaneously, recent ex-

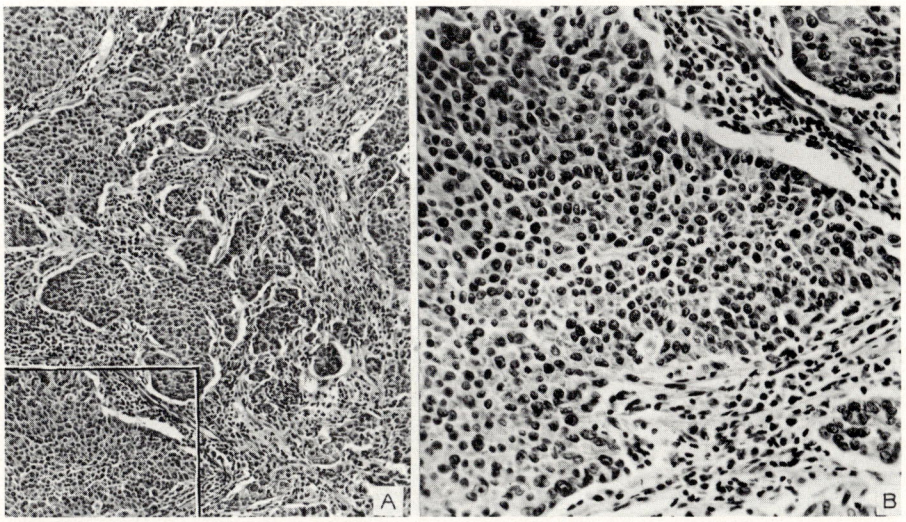

FIG. 36-4. (A) Adenocarcinoma with highly anaplastic cells showing almost complete undifferentiation (Grade 4). (B) Shows enlarged section indicated by lines in A.

perience with this lesion at Marquette has demonstrated complete reversal of this histologic picture by the continuous treatment with progesterone (Delalutin or Provera) for 3 to 6 months. Consequently, the entity remains debatable as a form of clinical carcinoma and should not be included in the general discussion and management of invasive adenocarcinoma of the endometrium.

A separate classification of adenoma malignum was described by Ewing and in general conforms to the Grade 1 well-differentiated adenocarcinoma described above. In order to avoid confusion by a plurality of terms, this classification should probably be abandoned for a more standardized histologic classification.

Histologic Types

The major histologic type of carcinoma of the uterine fundus is one of adenocarcinoma. The occurrence of islands of squamous epithelium (acanthosis) with endometrial carcinoma, commonly referred to as adenoacanthoma, occurs in approximately 15 per cent of the cases of fundal carcinoma. This lesion varies in reported incidence from less than 1 per cent (Scheffey et al., 1943) to 43.7 per cent (Tweeddale et al., 1964). Baggish and Woodruff have demonstrated squamous metaplasia almost uniformly in benign endometrium during the menstruating phase of the cycle and conclude that the origin of this cell stems from the duopotential cell lying between the glandular epithelium and the basement membrane. While estrogen administered to a variety of experimental animals has been observed to produce squamous metaplasia of the endometrium, the prolonged use of progesterone in high dosages for recurrent endometrial carcinoma has been repeatedly observed at Marquette and by other investigators to produce this same metaplastic pattern in the endometrium. Novak and Nalley, in reviewing the experience with adenoacanthoma at the Johns Hopkins Clinic in 1957, found this lesion to be associated with well-differentiated adenocarcinoma and therefore with an excellent cure rate. However, recent reports from Woodington et al., and from Charles, as well as Gusberg and Yannopoulos, show that adenoacanthoma has no bearing on the cure rate of the disease. Rather, the prognosis of such cases is dependent on the histologic grade of the glandular elements of the tumor and the clinical extent of the disease. The acanthosis is rarely malignant but has been found in metastatic lesions.

Primary squamous cell carcinoma of the body of the uterus has been reported infrequently since the criteria of this lesion were outlined by Fluhmann in 1928. For such lesions to be acceptable, it must be clearly established that (1) there is no co-existing adenocarcinoma, (2) there is no connection between the tumor and the squamous epithelium of the cervix, and (3) the absence of a primary growth in the cervix has been confirmed conclusively. Baggish and Woodruff have reviewed the literature on this subject and report a total of 13 acceptable cases of primary squamous cell carcinoma of the endometrium to date. Although the follow-up of these cases has been inadequate, the prognosis appears to be poor. All such cases occurring at Hopkins have died within 5 years.

The relationship of endometrial hyperplasia to endometrial cancer has been the subject of increasing debate for many years. The problem has been studied morphologically in three main ways: (1) study of prior endometrial biopsies in patients who have developed carcinoma; (2) prospective study of patients with various hyperplastic or atypical endometrial patterns, and (3) examination of the noncancerous endometrium in patients with definite endometrial carcinoma. Historically, study of prior biopsies was initiated in 1932 by Taylor, who reported 5 patients who ultimately developed adenocarcinoma and who had hyperplasia diagnosed in previous biopsies.

In 1949 Hertig and Sommers reviewed previous endometrial biopsy material from 32 patients who ultimately developed endometrial carcinoma from 1 to 23 years later following a previous dilatation and curettage. They were able to demonstrate progressive atypical hyperplastic changes in the endometrium as the time approached closer to the time when the adenocarcinoma was diagnosed. They described carcinoma in situ of the endometrium as a histologically separate lesion from adenomatous hyperplasia. Hertig concluded that once the carcinoma in situ had occurred, it was incapable of regression, and reported 6 cases of invasive cancer that developed from 1 to 11 years later. In 1947 Gusberg called attention to a pattern of adenomatous hyperplasia of the endometrium which he believed bore a constant relation to prolonged estrogen stimulation in both benign and malignant tissue. In a more recent report on 191 patients with adenomatous hyperplasia, Gusberg and Kaplan found coexistent adenocarcinoma in 20 per cent of 91 patients treated by hysterectomy, while an additional 13 per cent had borderline lesions. In 1953 Te Linde, Jones, and Galvin reported on the difficulty encountered at Johns Hopkins in identifying the glandular pattern of atypical endometrial hyperplasia separate from frank adenocarcinoma. In 11 of 13 cases of this series, the operative specimen revealed undoubted endometrial cancer. Copenhaver has studied our recent experience at the Johns Hopkins Hospital with 23 patients who were followed pathologically after having atypical hyperplasia in the preoperative curettings. Eight patients were found to have invasive cancer at the time of hysterectomy.

While benign cystic hyperplasia is rarely followed by adenocarcinoma, Corscaden, Fertig, and Gusberg conclude that a patient with premenopausal hyperplasia still has a tenfold greater chance of developing adenocarcinoma after the menopause than does the patient who has never had endometrial hyperplasia. Endometrial polyps are rarely malignant in themselves (less than 1%), but a patient with a benign endometrial polyp over the age of 45, according to Armenia, is reported to have a ninefold increased risk of developing adenocarcinoma. In studies in which noncancerous endometrium was present with endometrial carcinoma, Gray and Barnes in a study of 109 patients found endometrial hyperplasia in 56, atypical hyperplasia in 50, and endometrial polyps in 46, distributed among a total of 72 patients (66%). In an earlier report Novak and Yui found endometrial hyperplasia present in 39 per cent of 104 patients with endometrial carcinoma similar to that shown in Figure 36-5.

ASSOCIATED CLINICAL CONDITIONS

The clinical triad of *diabetes mellitus*, *obesity*, and *hypertension* is repeatedly included in most reports on this subject, not only as associated clinical features of such patients but also in reference to possible underlying endocrinologic factors responsible for the pathophysiology

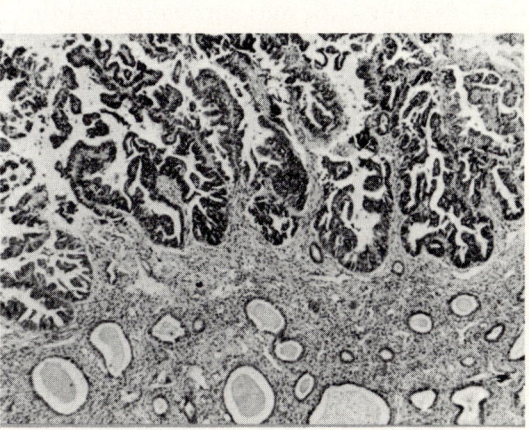

Fig. 36-5. Adenocarcinoma in the corpus and endometrial hyperplasia.

of these clinical diseases, including endometrial adenocarcinoma.

Obesity. Kottmeier reported that 29 per cent of his series of Swedish patients weighed more than 180 pounds, and an additional 7 per cent weighed over 220 pounds. Twenty patients (63%) of Peterson's series weighed more than 200 pounds, while a total of 81 per cent of this group were grossly overweight, weighing more than 150 pounds. The correlation of both obesity and tallness by Wynder and his group suggests the possibility of pituitary growth hormone dysfunction. However, to date, accurate growth hormone assays are not available for a critical evaluation of this factor.

Diabetes Mellitus. Dunn and co-workers have reviewed the reported frequency of *altered carbohydrate metabolism* among patients with endometrial carcinoma, which varies from 1.3 to 22 per cent. Regrettably, the data is inconclusive on this subject, since most of the previous reports were from poorly evaluated, retrospective surveys of hospital records with very few laboratory studies available for critical evaluation of this disease. In addition, few studies have taken into account other factors that influence glucose tolerance, such as age, parity, obesity, family history, and the like. This controlled study by Dunn and co-workers, using an oral glucose tolerance test, and a recent, well-executed prospective study by Frazier, utilizing an intravenous glucose tolerance test, are two noteworthy reports which are available for serious consideration. When corrected for both age and weight, both studies failed to show a significant increase in abnormal glucose tolerance in the carcinoma groups. Dunn reviewed the data of 25 investigators regarding the correlation of diabetes and endometrial carcinoma, and by combining the observations of 6,157 women with endometrial carcinoma, he found an average of 7.25 per cent to be diabetic. Interestingly, this figure is consistent with the findings of the National Health Survey of 1960–62 of the general population, which demonstrated that 9 per cent of women, aged 55 to 64, had blood glucose levels in excess of 200 mg./100 ml. 1 hour after a glucose load. Additional studies of this type are necessary for final confirmation of this metabolic problem in order to confirm conclusively or permanently to lay to rest this clinical relationship.

Hypertension. The relationship of hypertension to the problem of endometrial carcinoma is one of equal controversy. Current reports include an association of hypertension in endometrial cancer patients, varying in frequency from one third to three quarters of the patients studied. However, when blood pressure findings are correlated with weight, there is no statistical difference noted by Wynder or by Dunn between patients with endometrial carcinoma and the control groups. Many retrospective studies have linked other clinical entities with this disease, including a reported increased incidence of spontaneous abortion and increased intensity and length of menstrual flow, as well as premenstrual breast swelling. Such related factors were only suggestive in Wynder's epidemiologic study rather than conclusive. In well-controlled studies, the underlying basis for these associated clinical distrubances appear to be related primarily to *obesity* than to pathologic changes in any of the endocrine systems.

Multiple primary malignancies were present in 11 per cent of Lynch and co-workers' study in which the most frequent combinations of endometrial carcinoma occurred with carcinoma of the ovary, breast, and cervix.

SYMPTOMS

The most common symptoms include some form of abnormal bleeding in approximately 80 per cent of patients who have the diagnosis of adenocarcinoma of the endometrium established. In our clinic, endometrial carcinoma is second only to cervical cancer as an etiologic cause of postmenopausal bleeding. Vaginal discharge may precede postmenopausal bleeding by several months, although the discharge frequently is blood-tinged before frank bleeding occurs. Pelvic pain may occur, but is usually associated with advanced cancer, or occasionally cramps may result from pyometra. Healy and Brown found that 66 per cent of the patients complaining of pain eventually died of endometrial cancer, and in nearly half of these cases the initial examination revealed no evidence of extension of carcinoma beyond the uterus.

DIAGNOSIS

It is important to bear in mind the possibility of corpus carcinoma in every woman over the age of 40 with abnormal menstrual bleeding or postmenopausal bleeding. This clincal diagnosis should be considered even when this bleeding is slight or when it appears for the first time. On the basis that 15 to 20 per cent of such cases occur prior to the menopause, a dilatation and curettage should be performed on any patient with abnormal bleeding in the perimenopausal age group. In addition, approximately 5 per cent of the disease occurs in younger women under the age of 40 and requires, with persistent symptoms, a thorough histologic evaluation of the endometrium. Abnormal uterine bleeding must be investigated even in the presence of postmenopausal vaginitis, cervical polyps, fibroids, and, more currently, with the popular use of progesterones for family planning, as well as estrogen for menopausal symptoms. At the time of curettage a large amount of friable material may be obtained, but care must be taken in assuming this to be carcinoma. Endometrial hyperplasia frequently mimics the gross appearance of carcinoma and may be indistinguishable. On the other hand, we have repeatedly found endometrial cancer to be present on microscopic examination when no grossly visible endometrium suggesting cancer was present in the blood obtained at curettage.

Although other methods are available for establishing the diagnosis of endometrial carcinoma, we consider dilatation and curettage or endometrial biopsy to be the only definitive methods whereby the histopathology of the endometrial tissue may be observed. Reports vary in the literature regarding the efficacy of cytologic examinations of vaginal or cervical smears. In general, endometrial carcinoma is detected in no more than 60 per cent of all reported cases. In some clinics the success rate is far less. The most accurate method is endometrial biopsy, which establishes the diagnosis in 90 to 95 per cent of the cases. As reported by Reagan and Ng, aspiration of the endometrium has yielded up to 90 percent positive diagnosis in well-controlled series. When cervicovaginal smears are used routinely, along with endometrial aspiration smears, the accuracy rate of such combined methods of cytologic screening is approximately 85 per cent. Hofmeister utilizes the endometrial biopsy as a routine office procedure for endometrial evaluation, and in approximately 18,000 examinations, he has detected endometrial carcinoma in 0.7 per cent of all patients examined. This incidence is similar to that of carcinoma of the cervix in certain clinics, and demonstrates the effectiveness of this diagnostic tool, particularly in asymptomatic women. In addition, endometrial lavage and the use of the endometrial brush are other effective methods in the detection of abnormal endometrial cytology. Frost obtains excellent results in the detection of endometrial carcinoma with the use of the combined cervicovaginal fast smears. With the current liberal use of estrogen and progesterones in the perimenopausal age group for pregnancy protection and menopausal symptoms, the physician must be particularly alert to the camouflaged symptoms of endometrial carcinoma in patients using steroid hormones. Regardless of the possibility that symptoms of abnormal bleeding may be related to the use of these hormones, the physician is obligated to investigate the cause of any abnormal bleeding with the Papanicolaou smear, endometrial biopsy, and other technics. If the diagnosis remains unanswered, a dilatation and curettage are absolutely required.

The one contraindication to curettage which we do observe is pyometra. If, on cervical dilatation, pus is encountered coming from the uterine cavity, the cervical canal is well dilated, and nothing more is done. The patient is treated vigorously with antibiotics for 10 days, following which the cervix is dilated again and curettage performed. If pus is obtained again, an endometrial biopsy may be gently obtained without great risk of infection in the patient who is well protected with antibiotics. A thorough curettage should be deferred, however, until the intra-uterine drainage and infection cease. Not only is there a risk of producing pelvic cellulitis, but the uterine wall is usually softened and friable with pyometra, and uterine perforation may result. If such a complication should inadvertently occur, it may be necessary to do a hysterectomy to avoid seeding the peritoneal cavity with bacteria or tumor. At this point the patient is seriously compromised, both from the standpoint of potential peritonitis as well as the spread of malignant cells in the pelvis.

Similarly, we do not schedule patients for operation as having "curettage, possible hysterectomy." The inference in such a posting is that in case an abundance of suspicious looking endometrium is obtained at curettage, a hysterectomy will be done immediately. We insist on microscopic examination of the tissue before deciding on definitive therapy. Either a frozen section diagnosis with the use of a cryostat is necessary or a transient delay of surgery is required until permanent sections of the histology are prepared. Any female who has sufficient symptoms to warrant a dilatation and curettage should have a more accurate diagnosis than one based on what the naked eye can perceive, before a final decision is made concerning the type of treatment appropriate for the disease, either benign or malignant.

CLINICAL STAGING AND FACTORS INFLUENCING PROGNOSIS

Of all malignancies of the female reproductive tract, carcinoma of the endometrium has experienced the greatest variety of proposed clinical classifications, as well as the greatest delay in acceptance of an International Classification. Prior to 1961, the International Classification was based on two factors: (1) tumor confined to the uterus, and (2) the general physical health and operability of the patient.

The International Classification of 1950, which includes most of the current statistics, is as follows:

Stage I: Cases with operable disease, i.e., disease confined to the uterus.

  Group 1: Cases suitable for surgical treatment.

  Group 2: Cases with the disease confined to the uterus but bad operative risks.

Stage II: Cases in which the growth has spread outside the uterus.

Unfortunately, this classification does not include those cases with spread of the disease to the endocervix.

The International Classification was revised in 1961 by the Cancer Committee of the International Federation of Obstetrics and Gynecology. This pretreatment classification has been adopted by the American College of Obstetricians and Gynecologists, and is the current method of staging in use:

Stage I: The carcinoma is confined to the corpus.

Stage II: The carcinoma has involved the corpus and the cervix.

Stage III: The carcinoma has extended outside the uterus but not outside the true pelvis.

Stage IV: The carcinoma has extended outside the true pelvis or has obviously involved the mucosa of the bladder or rectum.

Although this classification is a definite improvement over the former one, and should be universally adopted in reporting carcinoma of the endometrium, it has many clinical objections. First, it continues to concentrate most of the operative cases in Stage I by failing to differentiate uterine size, and it therefore provides an unequal distribution of this disease. Second, Stage II (with cervix involvement) will have a lower cure rate in some series than Stage III (outside the uterus but not outside the pelvis), as reported by Gusberg. Of particular concern is the fact that this classification does not include a histologic differentiation of the tumor, which bears directly on the prognosis of this disease.

Although there have been many attempts to improve the clinical staging of this disease, one of the most acceptable classifications to date has been proposed recently by **Gusberg**, as follows:

Stage I: Normal size uterus.
  a: Differentiated.
  b: Anaplastic.
Stage II: Enlarged uterus.
  a: Differentiated.
  b: Anaplastic.
Stage III: Cervix involvement.
Stage IV: Contiguous organs or distant metastases.

This proposal clearly separates uterine size, tumor anaplasia, and endocervical involvement, all of which relate to the cure rate of this tumor. Additional factors affecting prognosis include not only the size of the uterus but the depth of invasion of tumor into the uterine wall. As reported by Carmichael from Saskatchewan, gross myometrial invasion reduces the 5-year survival rate to 65 per cent and correlates with lymph node and hematogenous spread.

Lymph Node Involvement. The incidence of lymph node involvement by endometrial carcinoma is derived from reported series in which radical surgery was the primary method of treatment. The incidence varies between 10 and 40 per cent although it must be recognized that these figures are from patients selected according to age and operative risk and may not reflect the true incidence of lymph node spread. Liu and Meigs record an incidence of 23 per cent in their general series but noted involvement of the lymph nodes in 7 of 14 cases in which the tumor extended to the cervix. Roberts (1961), in a selected series of cases from Chelsea Hospital for Women (London), found 5 patients with positive nodes (23%) among 22 cases of Stage I endometrial cancer. Davis reported 13 per cent with positive nodes in 151 cases from the New York Hospital. A more recent report, however, by Rickford from St. Thomas' Hospital and the Chelsea Hospital for Women (London) is of interest as he performed Wertheim hysterectomy on *all* cases during the past 10 years without selection for operability, unless there was gross general peritoneal spread at operation. In a series of 50 patients so treated, positive nodes were found on 5 occasions (10%). The incidence was only 5 per cent in Stage I disease where the tumor was confined to the uterus. When the disease had spread to the cervix, the nodes were involved 4 times as frequently (22%).

In view of such a low incidence of lymphatic spread in Stage I carcinoma of the endometrium, there is general agreement that a Wertheim hysterectomy is not indicated unless there is spread of the disease to the cervix.

TREATMENT AND EVALUATION OF TREATMENT

The two major factors that weigh heavily on the success of any form of treatment of endometrial cancer include (1) the extent of the disease at the time of initiating treatment, including intrauterine and extra-uterine spread, and (2) the histologic differentiation of the tumor. To compare accurately results achieved in clinics throughout the world, it is essential that the data be based on comparable groups of patients. To date, the International Classification of this disease does not provide such accuracy, and therefore the reported survival rates, comparing the various methods of treatment, are most unsatisfactory and confusing to the reader.

There are **three general methods of treatment** of endometrial carcinoma:

1. Surgery alone, including a total hysterectomy and bilateral salpingo-oophorectomy.
2. Irradiation alone, usually combining external irradiation and intracavitary radium.
3. Irradiation, either preoperative or postoperative, and surgery including external irradiation, or intracavitary radium followed by surgery.

"Which is better? How can we know?" These are legitimate questions which

Miller and other students of this disease have asked since the addition of irradiation to the armamentarium of therapy for this tumor became popular. The debate concerning the value of supplemental irradiation in the surgical treatment of carcinoma of the endometrium stems from the early reports of Cullen in 1900, who noted the possibility of surgical implantation of endometrial carcinoma during either vaginal or abdominal hysterectomy. In 1926 Ward suggested the use of 100 mg. of radium inserted into the uterus for a period of 24 hours, followed by a hysterectomy 6 weeks later. However, due to the high surgical mortality rate from the associated medical complications of this disease, there was reluctance to perform surgery in certain clinics abroad during the early part of the present century. Prior to 1930, Heyman devised a single intra-uterine radium tandem containing 35 to 45 mg. of radium elements. Unfortunately, this single tube of radium (Fig. 36-6) proved effective only for a narrow uterine cavity, whereas the large irregular uterus failed to receive a homogeneous dose of irradiation.

In 1934 Heyman developed the so-

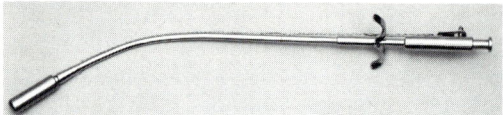

FIG. 36-7. Heyman screen applicator. The capsule at the tip contains the radium which is released after being inserted.

called "packing" method, in which the uterine cavity was packed with multiple small radium capsules containing 8 or 10 mg. of radium elements until the large uterine cavity was filled completely. This produced closer proximity of the radium to the tumor and provided a uniform distribution of the irradiation dose. The radium applicator shown in Figure 36-7 is still in use in most clinics today which prefer preoperative radium treatment. After 1930 and following the reduction of the primary surgical mortality in the treatment of this disease, the combined treatment of preoperative radium followed by total hysterectomy became the treatment of choice in many clinics, including our own, despite the fact that the Radiumhemmet in Stockholm reported excellent results with radium therapy alone.

The combination of preoperative irradiation plus surgical treatment has, in our view, the following advantages:

1. Irreversible damage or necrobiosis of the tumor, to prevent dissemination or implantation at the time of subsequent surgery.

2. Production of sclerosis and obliteration of lymphatics in the uterine wall and broad ligament, to prevent tumor dissemination.

3. Decreased incidence of vaginal recurrence and lessened incidence of latent distant metastases.

Despite the controversy regarding the improvement in cure rate with preoperative irradiation, there is tangible evidence that preoperative intra-uterine and/or vaginal irradiation does decrease the incidence of vaginal recurrences, particularly where there has been uterine enlargement by the tumor. A number of recent reports lend support to this fact, as outlined in Table 36-1.

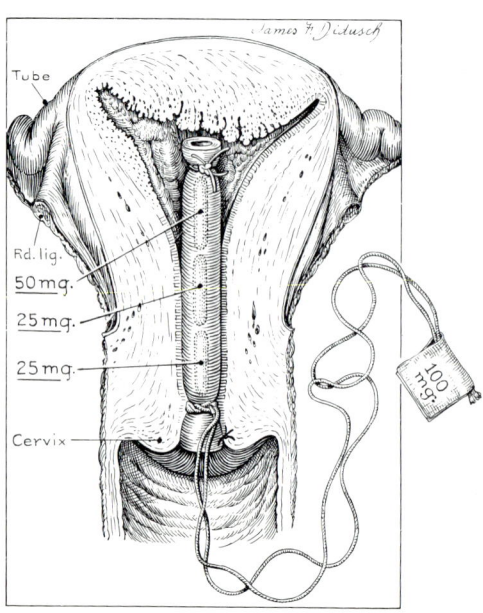

FIG. 36-6. Application of radium for carcinoma of corpus uteri.

TABLE 36-1. REPORTED RESULTS OF RADIUM APPLICATIONS

AUTHORS	SITE OF RADIUM APPLICATION	VAGINAL RECURRENCE (PER CENT)	
		Without Irradiation	With Irradiation
Boutselis et al.	Intra-uterine and vagina	15	1.8
Chau (M. D. Anderson Hospital)	Intra-uterine and vagina	25.4	2.1
Gusberg and Yannopoulos	Intra-uterine and vagina	15	1.8
Hill	Intra-uterine and vagina	7.7	1.2
Price et al.	Intra-uterine	14	3.6
Sweeney and Davis	Vagina	9.7	3.4
Wall et al.	Intra-uterine and vagina	10	4

Overall cure rates for endometrial carcinoma reveal very little difference in the method of treatment when data is compared from the *Annual Report* (vol. 14; H.-L. Kottmeier, editor).

Most investigators today agree that total hysterectomy, with bilateral salpingo-oophorectomy and removal of an adequate vaginal cuff, is the preferential treatment where possible. The addition of preoperative or postoperative irradiation remains a matter of individual philosophy of therapy. Morton has recently collated the results of treatment according to the various methods available and reports very little difference in 5- and 10-year recovery rates, as shown in Tables 36-2 and 36-3.

TABLE 36-2. RESULTS OF TREATMENT OF ENDOMETRIAL CANCER, *All Stages (1948–1957)**

PRIMARY TREATMENT	ALL CASES TREATED	NO. OF SURVIVORS	APPARENT 5-YEAR RECOVERY RATE (%)
Predominantly radiation	3,025	2,031	60.5
Exclusively radiation	2,687	1,533	57.6
Predominantly surgery†	5,161	3,257	63.1
Preoperative radiation and surgery	2,421	1,480	61.1

* Morton, D. G.: Carcinoma of the endometrium. Amer. J. Obstet. Gynec., 95:358, 1966. Figures were as of June 1966.
† One clinic, surgery only.

TABLE 36-3. THE 5- AND 10-YEAR RESULTS OF TREATMENT OF ENDOMETRIAL CANCER—38 CLINICS, 8,119 CASES OF *Stage I, Group 1* (1948–1957)*

PRIMARY TREATMENT	APPARENT 5-YEAR RECOVERY RATE (%)	APPARENT 10-YEAR RECOVERY RATE (%)
Predominantly radiation	81	70.3
Exclusively radiation	77.1	51.6
Predominantly surgery†	74.1	58.7
Preoperative radiation and surgery	74.5	60.2

* Morton, D. G.: *Ibid.*
† One clinic, surgery only.

Current data collated by Kottmeier in the 14th volume of the *Annual Report* compares the 5-year survival rates in Stage I, Group 1 cases based on the use of preoperative irradiation (Table 36-4).

There is available evidence at the present time from many clinics, including reports by Gusberg and more recently by Nolan and his associates, that there is no particular benefit from the use of preoperative irradiation with a small uterus and a well-differentiated tumor. This has been the experience in our own clinic and has been the only indication for primary surgery without the use of preoperative irradiation. Although debated by McLennan and others who favor primary surgery, Nolan's recent data suggest that preoperative irradiation improves the 5-year salvage by about 10 per cent in cases with a large uterus or undifferentiated tumor.

The vaginal route is used occasionally for the surgical treatment of this disease, but in our opinion it should be performed only in the very obese patient where the abdominal route would be extremely difficult or in certain cases associated with marked vaginal relaxation and uterine prolapse. The Mayo Clinic has recently reported the treatment of 100 cases of endometrial carcinoma by vaginal hysterectomy. This represents 15.2 per cent of the Mayo Clinic's entire series of 659 patients. This clinic has an excellent cure rate of 84 per cent after 5 years although it is admitted that the patients are selected according to the size of the uterus, the stage and grade of the lesion, and the general medical condition of the patient. Surprisingly, only 1 vaginal vault recurrence is reported even though 45 patients had cystocele, rectocele, or both repaired. That the ovaries were removed from only 57 patients is a major disadvantage to this procedure because this disease spreads to the ovary in 5 to 10 per cent of the cases. In Italy, Ingiulla

TABLE 36-4. PREOPERATIVE IRRADIATION VS. PRIMARY SURGERY IN TREATMENT OF ENDOMETRIAL CARCINOMA, *Stage I, Group 1* (1951–1960)*

PRIMARY TREATMENT	NO. CASES TREATED	APPARENT 5-YEAR RECOVERY RATE (%)
Preoperative irradiation	3,985	73.8
Primary surgery without preoperative irradiation	4,668	76.2

* Kottmeier, H.-L. (ed.): Annual Report on the Results of Treatment in Carcinoma of the Uterus and Vagina. vol. 14, collated 1966. Stockholm, Norstedt & Söner, 1967.

prefers the vaginal route for the primary surgical treatment of this disease and has treated 91 per cent of his total cases by vaginal hysterectomy. In a recent series on 140 cases, 112 underwent simple vaginal hysterectomy; 18, the Schauta-Amreich operation; and 10, abdominal hysterectomy. The operative mortality (5%) was higher than most reports of 1 to 3 per cent surgical mortality of the abdominal operation. The 5-year survival rate of 73.2 per cent is comparable to that of other clinics performing surgery by the abdominal route.

The use of the radical Wertheim hysterectomy has not proven to have significant advantage in the surgical treatment of endometrial carcinoma. The complication rate of 10 to 15 per cent and the low yield of positive pelvic lymph nodes in Stage I disease (approximately 3 to 5%) does not justify the increased morbidity and mortality associated with this procedure. The necropsy data of Beck and Latour revealed that when pelvic lymph nodes were involved, the tumor had spread out of the pelvis in 90.5 per cent of the cases. In addition, there was spread to the para-aortic lymph nodes in 13.8 per cent of the cases in which the pelvic nodes were negative.

Messinger and Jones have recently reviewed the literature regarding the prognosis of patients with endometrial cancer with positive pelvic lymph nodes including 351 patients in 6 series who were treated by radical hysterectomy and lymphadenectomy. Among 41 patients with positive nodes, only 4 patients (10%) lived 5 or more years. In the 11 cases of positive pelvic nodes treated at the Memorial James Ewing Hospital for recurrent or persistent endometrial disease, only 1 case survived 5 or more years. Although this data would not support the general philosophy of the use of the radical Wertheim hysterectomy and pelvic lymphadenectomy in Stage II lesions where the tumor had extended to the endocervix, the proponents for such treatment emphasize the increased frequency of pelvic lymph node metastases with similar spread of the disease, as in cases of carcinoma of the cervix.

PLAN OF THERAPY IN OUR CLINIC

Based on the data quoted above, as well as our own experience, which is included in the *Annual Report*, we have chosen the combined treatment of preoperative irradiation followed by total hysterectomy and bilateral salpingo-oophorectomy 4 to 6 weeks later. In general, the following plan of therapy is followed in our clinic:

Stage I. In cases in which the uterus is small and the histology of the tumor is well-differentiated (Grade I), we proceed directly to a total abdominal hysterectomy and bilateral salpingo-oophorectomy without preoperative irradiation. It must be stressed that this stage can be confirmed *only* after a thorough differential dilatation and curettage to be certain of the absence of endocervical extension. In the absence of preoperative irradiation, the cervix is usually sutured closed per vaginum with figure-of-eight sutures of chromic catgut prior to the hysterectomy.

In cases in which the uterine cavity is grossly enlarged, the uterine cavity is sounded, and the vaginal vault is measered for the proper size of vaginal ovoid forms prior to application of radium. Multiple Heyman capsules of 10 mg. radium each are used to pack the uterine cavity to capacity, while vaginal ovoids containing 20 mg. radium in each ovoid are placed in each lateral fornix, with the radium capsule directed in the anterior-posterior position. A single application of radium is given to provide approximately 5,000 mg. hours in the uterine cavity, which will deliver a depth dose of approximately 5,000 gamma r to the uterine wall approximately 1.5 to 2 cm. from the uterine cavity.

In general, our method of treatment provides a 1:1 ratio between mg. hours and gamma r, calculated at approximately 1.5 to 2 cm. from the radium source in the uterine cavity (i.e., 5,000 mg. hours of radium in the uterus will contribute approximately 5,000 gamma r at 1.5 to 2 cm. from the radium source). This technic also provides approximately 10,000 gamma r to the endometrial surface of the uterine cavity. As a general rule, the vaginal ovoid which we employ, with a 2 or 2.5 cm. diameter, provides approximately 100 gamma r/hr. surface dosage to the vaginal mucosa, utilizing 20 mg. of radium in each ovoid (100 gamma r/hr. × 50 hr. application = 5,000 gamma r surface dose). Radium location films are taken, and isodose curves are plotted by computer technic similar to the method described in the treatment of cervical carcinoma, to provide accurate dosage measurements to multiple points throughout the pelvis. A typical application of radium with 10 Heyman's capsules of 10 mg. each in the uterine cavity and vaginal ovoids containing 20 mg. each is shown in Figure 36-8.

In 4 to 6 weeks after the radium therapy, a total abdominal hysterectomy, plus bilateral salpingo-oophorectomy, is performed with removal of 2 to 3 cm. of the vaginal cuff.

Stage II. Because of spread of the tumor to the endocervix, this lesion must be treated vigorously, similar to that for carcinoma of the cervix. In such cases approximately 8,000 mg. hours of radium is given in divided doses of approximately 4,000 mg. hours each, similar to the amount of radium used in the treatment of carcinoma of the cervix. In such cases 2,000 rads whole pelvis irradiation is given initially, prior to the application of radium, utilizing the Betatron (25 MeV) without shielding by means of 15 × 15 cm. portals both anteriorly and posteriorly. If the patient is a suitable candidate, a radical Wertheim hysterectomy with pelvic lymphadenectomy is performed in 4 to 6 weeks following completion of preoperative irradiation. Patients who are not candidates for radical surgery have their full irradiation treatment completed by an additional 2,000 rads of external irradiation administered primarily to the lateral pelvic wall by shielding the midline structures.

Stage III. With carcinoma extending outside the uterus but confined to the pelvis, it may be difficult to remove all of the tumor initially by a total hysterectomy and adnexectomy. Consequently, aggressive preoperative irradiation is given, beginning with 4,000 rads, whole pelvis, external therapy by the Betatron unit (25 MeV) with 15 × 15 cm. portals anteriorly and posteriorly. Four thousand mg. hours of radium is given with Heyman's capsules in the uterine cavity, which contributes approximately 4,000 gamma r to the uterine wall at approximately 1.5 to 2 cm. depth dose. Vaginal ovoids are used at the same time to achieve a dosage of at least 5,000 gamma r to the vaginal mucosa. Usually, 25 mg. or larger radium sources are used in the ovoid to achieve this dose because of the decreased time that the intra-uterine Heyman's capsules are left in place. Four to 6 weeks later the patients is explored, and appropriate surgery is performed, which usually consists of a total abdominal hysterectomy and adnexectomy. Such cases are usually not considered candidates for radical Wertheim hysterectomy because of the advanced stage of

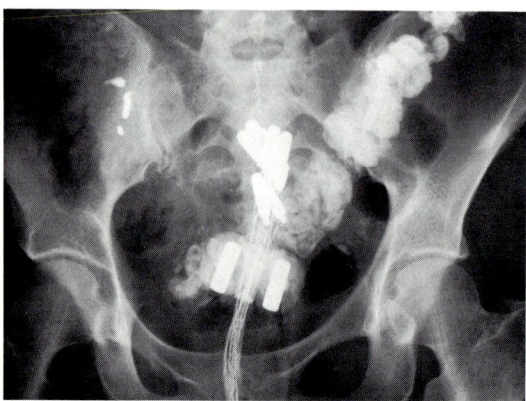

FIG. 36-8. Radium location films showing AP view of pelvis with Heyman's capsules of radium in uterine cavity and vaginal ovoids placed in the lateral vaginal fornices.

the disease. However, if the uterus and adnexa can be removed, our experience has shown a definite improvement in the cure rate by this procedure alone. More extensive surgery, including pelvic exenteration, should be reserved for the rare patient in whom the disease is confined to the pelvis and involves primarily the bladder or rectum, while the lateral parametrium and pelvic sidewalls are free of metastatic disease. In such rare cases every effort must be made to verify that the disease has not extended to the abdomen and para-aortic lymph nodes.

Stage IV. Patients in Stage IV are not surgical candidates and must be treated completely by irradiation. We prefer to treat such patients primarily with whole pelvic irradiation, using supervoltage therapy (Betatron), with delivery of 6,000 rads to the midpelvis. The abdomen is less vigorously treated and is usually encompassed with a maximum of 3,000 rads to the abdominal viscera. Additional supervoltage therapy will produce radiation nephritis and damage to liver and bowel. However, the abdominal viscera may be shielded, and 4,500 to 5,000 rads may be administered to the para-aortic lymph chain from the diaphragm to the bifurcation of the aorta by means of paravertebral portals. In addition, the patient is usually treated with chemotherapy, preferably progestogens, as discussed below.

TECHNIC: TOTAL HYSTERECTOMY FOR CARCINOMA OF THE CORPUS UTERI

A few precautions should be taken when total hysterectomy is done for endometrial carcinoma. It has been recommended that the cervix be closed with figure-of-eight chromic catgut sutures prior to laparotomy in the patient receiving primary surgery. However, with proper intracavitary and vaginal preoperative irradiation, the dissemination or implantation of viable tumor cells in the vaginal cuff at the time of surgery is considered unlikely. Most investigators believe that vaginal vault recurrence results from preoperative lymphatic emboli rather than implantation. At the M. D. Anderson Hospital, and at Johns Hopkins and Marquette, with the use of 5,000 mg. hours of intra-uterine radium preoperatively, approximately 25 to 35 per cent of the cases will show residual carcinoma in the operative specimen, although it is believed that this tumor has been biologically altered by the radiation therapy and should not implant as may be the case in the unirradiated patient. Nonetheless, many gynecologists prefer to suture the cervix prior to abdominal hysterectomy after preoperative irradiation.

When the abdomen is open, the fallopian tubes are clamped at the cornual portion of the uterus to prevent retrograde passage of carcinoma while the uterus is handled. The tubes and the ovaries are always removed regardless of the age of the patient or the early stage of the growth. Ovarian metastases from endometrial carcinoma occur in approximately 5 to 10 per cent of the cases. The total hysterectomy differs slightly from that described in this volume for benign uterine disease. The cervix is not hugged quite so closely in clamping the base of the broad ligament, and the pubocervical fascia is not stripped from the cervix and the vagina. This type of an extrafascial hysterectomy is performed in view of the fact that this fascia is rich in lymphatics, and its removal would seem to be desirable in those cases in which the corpus carcinoma is low in the uterus. As in hysterectomy for benign uterine disease, we usually close the vagina without drainage.

On rare occasions endometrial carcinoma will be discovered when the uterus is opened in the operating room, following a hysterectomy for supposedly benign uterine disease. If the cervix or the adnexa on either side has not been removed, they should be taken out before the abdomen is closed. Finally, there are those cases in which unsuspected endometrial cancer is found in the laboratory when the hysterectomy was done for a supposedly benign condition, and the adnexa were not removed. If the patient's general condition will permit, re-operation with removal of the adnexa is advisable due to the frequency of ovarian metastases with this disease. If age or the medical condition of the patient makes further surgery inadvisable, one must rely entirely on postoperative irradiation therapy.

TREATMENT OF RECURRENT ENDOMETRIAL CARCINOMA

The frequency of persistent or recurrent endometrial carcinoma is difficult to obtain from the varied reports in the literature. However, based on the relative apparent 5-year recovery rate from the 14th volume of the *Annual Report* on 14,796 patients, 62.6 per cent of this disease is cured by a variety of therapeutic technics. On the basis that approximately 7 per cent of the female population in this age group (45 to 55) will die during a 5-year period from unrelated causes, one must assume that approximately 25 to 30 per cent of all patients treated for endometrial carcinoma will have residual or recurrent disease.

In most reported series, nearly two thirds of the recurrences appear within 2 years after initial therapy (Dede, 62%; Speert, 75%; Finn, 69%; and Lindgren, 62%).

Four factors appear to relate directly to the recurrence of this disease, namely, (1) the adequacy of the primary treatment, (2) the extent of the disease at the time of treatment, (3) the degree of anaplasia of the tumor, and (4) the individual host resistance. The rapidity of recurrence of the disease following primary therapy and the degree of dedifferentiation of the tumor have an adverse effect on the longevity of the patient's life following recurrence. In contrast, well-differentiated tumors that have a long period of clinical quiescence before recurrence show the greatest response to all modalities of therapy. As reported by Dede, Plentl, and Moore, the efficiency of a combination of adequate radiotherapy and surgery is documented by their findings that 75 per cent of their series of patients with recurrent endometrial carcinoma who were initially treated by this combined technic had recurrence of the disease outside the pelvis. The fact that approximately 50 per cent of endometrial cancer recurs locally in the pelvis suggests that less than adequate treatment may have been given initially. Of the sites of pelvic recurrence, the most frequent location is that in the upper vagina, parametrium, and the uterus.

The most meaningful data on recurrent endometrial carcinoma is limited to vaginal recurrence. In the absence of preoperative irradiation, approximately 10 to 15 per cent of the cases receiving primary surgery have either persistent or recurrent disease in the vagina. The ultimate cure rate after treatment of vaginal recurrence varies widely between 10 and 50 per cent, depending on whether the recurrence represents persistent pelvic disease or an isolated implantation. In Dede, Plentl, and Moore's study, the absolute survival rate with vaginal recurrence was only 13.3 per cent, regardless of the method of treatment.

The methods available for treatment of recurrent endometrial carcinoma are varied but may be condensed into three major approaches:
1. Radiation therapy, including external therapy and/or radium.
2. Surgery, usually radical.
3. Chemotherapy.

RADIATION THERAPY

Concerning the management of recurrent disease, irradiation has been the most common treatment and includes both intravaginal radium as well as external therapy. In treating the rectovaginal or vesicovaginal septum, one must be cautious of exceeding the normal tissue tolerance of the vagina, which is approximately 8,000 rads. Irradiation therapy is obviously most effective when the recurrence is local and confined to the central portion of the pelvis.

With pelvic recurrence following preoperative radium therapy and surgery, our approach for treatment is to provide a midpelvic dose of irradiation of approximately 5,000 rads by external

(Betatron) therapy. In the treatment of recurrence following primary surgery without previous irradiation, we prefer giving 6,000 rads, whole pelvis, supervoltage irradiation, followed by the use of a small amount of additional central irradiation given by 2,000 mg. hours of radium in vaginal ovoids. The poor cure rates of 15 to 20 per cent from the Columbia-Presbyterian Hospital experience, even if the recurrent lesion is confined only to the vagina, indicates the grave prognosis of this recurrent disease. The Mayo Clinic, however, has had a much better experience, with a 50 per cent 5-year survival in 30 cases treated with irradiation.

RADICAL SURGERY

The use of radical surgery for recurrent cancer of the uterus has received only sporadic acceptance. The most recent report from Memorial Hospital by Barber and Brunschwig provides legitimate concern for this form of treatment for recurrent endometrial disease, based on their poor 5-year survival rates. Of 36 patients treated at Memorial Hospital by pelvic exenteration, either anterior or total, 5 or more years ago, 27 (75%) died within 1 year of the exenteration, and 21 patients of that group died with persistent cancer, suggesting either an inadequate surgical procedure or an ill-advised choice of treatment. While 5 patients (13.8%) lived 5 or more years, 3 of these patients died subsequently with renal complications, leaving a final cure rate of only 6 per cent. The obvious fact from these results is quite clear, namely, that the natural history of endometrial carcinoma is related to both lymphatic and hematogenous spread and does not remain confined to the pelvis for a prolonged period of time, where *en bloc* radical pelvic surgery is most beneficial. The autopsy studies of Beck and Latour, revealing para-aortic metastases in 13.8 per cent of patients in the presence of negative pelvic nodes, provide added evidence of the difficulty in proper selection of cases. The high operative mortality rate of 5 to 8 per cent in the best clinics, as well as the serious postoperative morbidity (50 to 60%) associated with this procedure, provides only a limited and highly selected place for pelvic exenteration in the treatment of recurrent endometrial cancer.

CHEMOTHERAPY

Although a wide spectrum of chemotherapeutic agents has been used for the treatment of recurrent endometrial carcinoma, there has been very little therapeutic response of such tumors to even the most cytotoxic agents. However, recent experience with the use of progestogens has demonstrated a definite role in the treatment of disseminated endometrial disease. The rationale for the use of progestogens is based on the clinical association between carcinoma of the endometrium and prolonged, unopposed estrogen stimulation of the endometrium, as previously discussed. In addition, the clinical effect of such steroids in producing degeneration of benign endometrial glands in the treatment of endometriosis provided the stimulus for Kistner and others to use this agent in early, Stage 0 lesions of the endometrium. In addition, the synthetic progestogens have been shown to inhibit carcinogenesis in the experimental animal and to cause regression of established endometrial carcinoma (rabbit). Additional support for the use of steroids in the therapy of this tumor was based on the initial success with estrogens and androgens in the management of advanced cancer of the breast and prostate.

In 1961 the initial beneficial results of 17-alpha-hydroxyprogesterone caproate (Delalutin) were reported by Kelley and Baker, showing objective remission in 6 of 21 cases with pulmonary metastasis of endometrial carcinoma lasting 9 months to 4½ years. More recently, they have noted objective remissions in 32 per cent of their patients, while Kistner has reported objective remissions obtained with progestational agents in 30 per cent of the treated cases. In general, the patients who have responded to this treatment were noted to have slowly growing tumors which were well-differentiated histologically, or only slightly undifferentiated. Anaplastic tumors have been shown to be refractory to this method of therapy by many investigators. Summation of all patients with adenocarcinoma of the endometrium with metastases treated with 17-alpha-hydroxyprogesterone caproate, as discussed by Kennedy, has shown an objective remission in 30 per cent of 596 patients. In all studies to date, pulmonary metastases respond the best, while osseous and hepatic lesions are more resistant. Recurrent tumor localized in the previously irradiated pelvis shows the poorest response and is probably related to the impairment of perfusion of the tissue by the hormone because of diminished vascularity.

A current study at Marquette, utilizing 2 gm. of 17-alpha-hydroxyprogesterone caproate weekly, has been in effect for the past 5 years. Of the 35 cases of recurrent endometrial carcinoma treated with this agent, a 25 per cent objective remission rate has been observed, the criteria for clinical response being a 50 per cent decrease in size of the tumor mass. The mean duration of the clinical response in our study has been 20 months. We have also treated 6 patients with Stage 0 adenocarcinoma of the endometrium with 17-alpha-hydroxyprogesterone caproate for 6 months, using 2 gm. of this progesterone per week in divided doses, and have had excellent results in all 6 cases. As is seen in Figures 36-9 to 36-11, the initial biopsy shows histologic evidence of Hertig's carcinoma in situ which has undergone complete histologic regression and necrobiosis of the epithelium after therapy for 3 to 6 months. Following cessation of

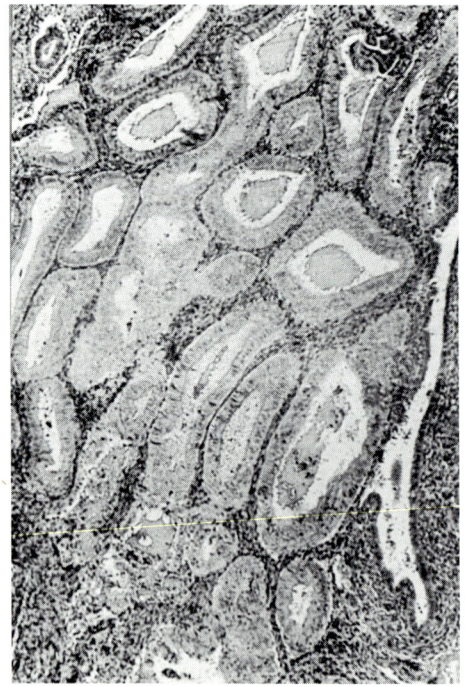

FIG. 36-9. Carcinoma in situ of the endometrium with glandular proliferation and crowding as well as nuclear hyperactivity and pseudostratification. The glandular cell cytoplasm is pale and esosinophilic-staining. Most nuclei demonstrate a fine granular chromatin pattern with frequent mitoses.

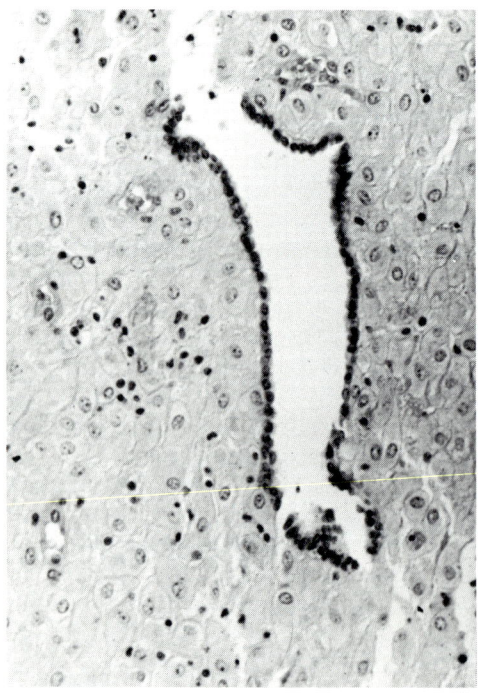

FIG. 36-10. Carcinoma in situ of endometrium treated for 6 weeks with 17-alpha-hydroxyprogesterone caproate (Delalutin), 500 mg., 3 (or 4) × weekly. Note the extensive decidual reaction of stromal cells and the exhaustive secretory change of the glandular epithelium. Epithelial cells now are low cuboidal and atrophic.

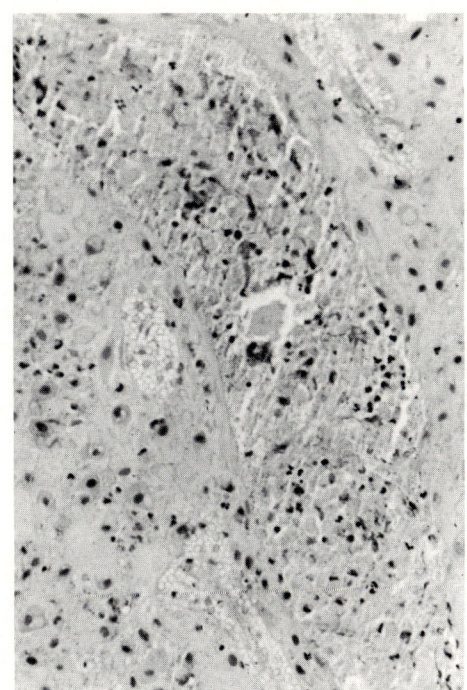

FIG. 36-11. Carcinoma in situ of the endometrium following progesterone treatment for 3 months. Note the complete necrosis of glandular epithelium with necrobiosis of stromal cells as well.

therapy at 6 months, follow-up dilatation and curettage on all cases revealed only atrophic endometrium. Kistner prefers the use of medroxyprogesterone acetate (Provera) and obtains the maximum response by the use of 400 to 1000 mg. monthly as a maintenance dose. His loading dose includes at least 3 gm. within the first 6 weeks of therapy, and, as in all studies, therapy must be continued for a minimum of 6 weeks to be considered adequate for evaluation.

Recently, Kennedy reported on the treatment of 75 patients with advanced endometrial carcinoma using either 17-alpha-hydroxyprogesterone caproate or a new progesterone, dihydroxyprogesterone acetophenide. Both drugs appear to give a similar response, with 19 or 25.3 per cent of the patients showing objective improvement. The duration of clinical response was more than 27.2 months in Kennedy's study. The duration of treatment is difficult to define but should be continued, without decreasing the dosage, as long as the patient shows evidence of clinical response.

The mechanism of action of the drug is thought to be primarily at the cellular level although there have been some reports by Varga and Henriksen suggesting that the biologic effect is mediated through suppression of luteinizing hormone (LH). However, the histologic evidence obtained by Kistner and Griffiths on direct injection of the agent into the cavity of the uterus suggests a definite local effect of the progestational agent. Currently a collaborative study among several clinics in the United States is under way to evaluate the use of progestogens as an adjuvant to the conventional treatment of endometrial carcinoma. To date, such data are too inconclusive to justify formulating conclusions regarding the prophylactic use of this agent.

BIBLIOGRAPHY

Alford, C. D., Betson, J. R., and Disonti, N.: Wertheim hysterectomy and pelvic lymphadenectomy for carcinoma of the uterine corpus. Amer. J. Obstet. Gynec., 83:1306, 1962.

Anderson, J. L. C., and Stephens, S.: Survival in carcinoma of the endometrium following pelvic node dissection. Danish Med. Bull., 11:5, 1960.

Armenia, C. S.: Sequential relationship between endometrial polyps and carcinoma of the endometrium. Obstet. Gynec., 30: 524, 1967.

Baggish, M. S., and Woodruff, J. D.: The occurrence of squamous epithelium in the endometrium. Obstet. Gynec. Survey, 22:69, 1967.

Barber, H. R. K., and Brunschwig, A.: Treatment and results of recurrent cancer of the corpus uteri in patients receiving anterior and total pelvic exenteration. CA, 22:949, 1968.

Barber, K. W., Jr., Dockerty, M. B., and Pratt, J. H.: Clinicopathologic study of surgically treated carcinoma of the endometrium with nodal metastasis. Surg. Gynec. Obstet., 115:568, 1962.

Barnett, H.: Squamous cell carcinoma of the body of the uterus. J. Clin. Path., 18:715, 1965.

Barter, R. H., Brennan, G., Newman, W., and Merrill, K. W.: The place of curettage in the diagnosis of carcinoma of the endometrium. Amer. J. Obstet. Gynec., 100:696, 1968.

Beck, R. P., and Latour, J. P. A.: Necropsy reports on 36 cases of endometrial carcinoma. Amer. J. Obstet. Gynec., 185:307, 1963.

Blaikley, J. D., Kottmeier, H.-L., Marthius, H., and Meigs, J. V.: Classification and clinical staging of carcinoma of the uterus. Amer. J. Obstet. Gynec., 75:1286, 1968.

Boutselis, J. G., Bair, J. R., Voyrs, N., and Eury, J. C.: Carcinoma of the uterine corpus—a study of 269 cases, 1947 to 1959. Amer. J. Obstet. Gynec., 85:994, 1963.

Broders, A. C.: Carcinoma in situ contrasted with benign penetrating epithelium. J.A.M.A., 99:1670, 1932.

———: The grading of carcinoma. Minnesota Med., 8:726, 1925.

Brown, J. M., Dockerty, M. D., Symmonds, R. E., and Banner, E. A.: Vaginal recurrence of endometrial carcinoma. Amer. J. Obstet. Gynec., 100:544, 1968.

Burnam, C. F.: The treatment of cancer of the body of the uterus by radiation. Ann. Surg., 93:436, 1931.

Carmichael, J. A., and Bean, H. A.: Carcinoma of the endometrium in Saskatchewan. Amer. J. Obstet. Gynec., 97:294, 1967.

Charles, D.: Endometrial adenoacanthoma. A clinicopathological study of 55 cases. CA, 18:737, 1965.

Chau, P. M.: Technique and evaluation of preoperative radium therapy in adenocarcinoma of the uterine corpus. In Carcinoma of the Uterine Cervix, Endometrium and Ovary. p. 235. Chicago, Yearbook Medical Publishers, 1962.

Copenhaver, E. H.: Atypical endometrial hyperplasia. Obstet. Gynec., 13:264, 1959.

Corscaden, J. A.: Cancer of the endometrium. In Corscaden, J. A.: Gynecologic Cancer. ed. 3, Chap. 6. Baltimore, Williams & Wilkins, 1962.

Corscaden, J. A., Fertig, J. W., and Gusberg, S. B.: Carcinoma subsequent to radiotherapeutic menopause. Amer. J. Obstet. Gynec., 51:1, 1946.

Corscaden, J. A., and Gusberg, S. B.: The background of cancer of the corpus. Amer. J. Obstet. Gynec., 53:419, 1947.

Cullen, T. S.: Cancer of the Uterus. Philadelphia. W. B. Saunders, 1900.

Davis, E. W., Jr.: Carcinoma of the corpus uteri: 525 cases seen at the New York Hospital, 1932-1961. Amer. J. Obstet. Gynec., 88:163, 1964.

Dede, J. A., Plentl, A. A., and Moore, J. G.: Recurrent endometrial carcinoma. Surg. Gynec. Obstet., 126:553, 1968.

Dobbie, B. M., Taylor, C. W., and Waterhouse, J. A. H.: A study of carcinoma of the endometrium. J. Obstet. Gynaec. Brit. Comm., 72:659, 1965.

Dunn, L. J., Merchant, J. A., Bradbury, J. T., and Stone, D. D.: Glucose tolerance and endometrial carcinoma. Arch. Intern. Med., 121:236, 1968.

Ewing, J.: Neoplastic Diseases. Philadelphia, W. B. Saunders, 1940.

Finn, W. F.: Time, site and treatment of recurrence of endometrial carcinoma. Amer. J. Obstet. Gynec., 60:773, 1950.

Fluhmann, C. F.: Squamous epithelium in the endometrium in benign and malignant conditions. Surg. Gynec. Obstet., 46:309, 1928.

Frazier, G. B.: Carbohydrate metabolism in endometrial carcinoma. J. Obstet. Gynaec. Brit. Comm., 75:1049, 1968.

Frost, J. F.: In Novak's Textbook of Gynecology. ed. 7, p. 703. Baltimore, Williams & Wilkins, 1967.

Graham, J. B.: Characteristics of women with various gynecologic cancers. Obstet. Gynec., 23:176, 1964.

Graham, J. B.: Treatment of choice in cancer of the uterine corpus. New Eng. J. Med., 254:1112, 1956.

Gray, L. A., and Barnes, M. L.: Histogenesis of endometrial carcinoma. Ann. Surg., 159:976, 1964.

Gusberg, S. B.: Precursors of corpus carcinoma: Estrogens in adenomatous hyperplasia. Amer. J. Obstet. Gynec., 54:905, 1947.

———: The problem of staging endometrial cancer. Obstet. Gynec., 28:305, 1966.

Gusberg, S. B., and Kaplan, A. L.: Precursors of corpus cancer: Adenomatous hyperplasia as Stage 0 carcinoma of the endometrium. Amer. J. Obstet. Gynec., 87:662, 1963.

Gusberg, S. B., and Yannopoulos, D.: Therapeutic decisions in corpus cancer. Amer. J. Obstet. Gynec., 88:157, 1964.

Healy, W. P., and Brown, R. L.: Experience with surgical and radiation therapy in carcinoma of the corpus uteri. Amer. J. Obstet. Gynec., 38:1, 1939.

Hendriksen, E.: Lymphatic spread of carci-

37

Sarcoma of the Uterus

Sarcoma of the uterus is the most lethal of all tumors of the uterus and has been recognized as a pathologic entity since 1860, when the first recorded case was presented by C. Meyer to the Berlin Obstetrical Society. It is a relatively rare condition. Novak and Anderson reported an incidence of 3.1 per cent of uterine malignancies in the gynecologic pathologic laboratory at the Johns Hopkins Hospital over a 25-year period. Kimbrough reported an almost identical incidence of 3.2 per cent. The disease most frequently occurs in middle life, the greatest incidence being in the fifth decade. On the other hand, sarcoma botryoids usually occur in infants, while endometrial sarcoma often occurs in the elderly. The symptomatology is not distinctive. Bleeding or blood-tinged discharge is the usual presenting symptom, but when the sarcomatous change occurs in the depths of a myoma, there may be no bleeding or abnormal discharge.

Sarcoma of the uterus may have its origin in one of four sites and, according to its origin, presents a variety of clinical pictures:

1. *Sarcomatous change in myoma.* This is the largest group, although the incidence of malignant change in fibroids is very low.

2. *Sarcoma of the endometrium.* The incidence of this type of uterine sarcoma is next to that of sarcomatous change in myoma but still must be considered a rare disease. Carcinosarcoma (mixed mesodermal tumor) arising from the endometrium will be considered separately in this chapter.

3. *Sarcoma arising in the musculofibrous wall of the uterus.* This rare tumor appears in some instances to arise from the musculofibrous coat of the blood vessels as judged by the perivascular arrangement of the sarcoma cells. In the majority of these cases it is scarcely possible to identify the exact origin of the neoplasm when it finally gets into the hands of the pathologist as separate from those tumors arising in a myoma.

4. *Sarcoma of the cervix* may be grapelike, forming the so-called sarcoma botryoids, or may be ulcerative, being grossly indistinguishable from carcinoma.

To the surgeon a very important point is concerned with the recognition of sarcoma at the operating table, for the recognition of the lesion may dictate radical surgery rather than a more conservative procedure. Sarcomatous change in myomas may be obvious at the operating table, but often the malignant change is confined to the central portion of a perfectly normal-appearing large fibroid. As the sarcomatous growth continues, the outer surface of the myoma is invaded and changes in appearance. Instead of the smooth, glistening fibrous capsule, the surface becomes dull and more irregular, suggesting that malignant tissue growing from within has penetrated the pre-existing capsule. The neoplastic tissue soon invades surrounding structures and becomes adherent.

Independent nodules in the omentum, the lymph glands, and the liver may clearly indicate metastatic sarcomatous growths. The consistency of the sarcomatous growth is usually softer than that of the average fibroid, but, as every experienced operator knows, benign fibroids can be remarkably soft. If in doubt, the tumor should be cut by an assistant in the operating room after removal. Instead of the firm, glistening cut surface and the whorl-like appearance of the fibrous tissue in the ordinary fibroid, the surface of the sarcoma may have a homogeneous, raw pork-like appearance. In some instances the malignant tumor may have become necrotic, and broken-down friable areas replace the solid tissue. If one scrapes the cut surface of a benign fibroid with a knife blade, a sharp, scraping sound is heard, and no tissue collects on the blade. Scraping of the softer sarcomatous tissue causes no sound, and pultaceous material may collect on the knife blade.

Intramural sarcoma, arising directly from the musculature or the fibrous tissue of the uterine wall, may cause a symmetrical uterine enlargement; but as the growth continues, the malignant tissue breaks through the serous surface, creating irregularities of the surface.

Endometrial sarcomas usually grow into the uterine cavity in a polypoid manner. Often they advance downward through the cervical canal and into the vagina. We have encountered a few that have practically filled the vagina. In such instances the diagnosis may be strongly suspected from the chicken-fat color of the tissue, which is very friable and easily torn through with the examining fingers.

Cervical sarcoma may present a sloughing, ulcerated appearance much like that of advanced cervical cancer. Sarcoma botryoides, which occurs more often in infants than in adults, more commonly arises in the upper vagina and secondarily involves the cervix with multiple pinkish and edematous grape-like polyps.

HISTOLOGY

Most of the bizarre cellular changes found in malignant connective tissue tumors elsewhere in the body are found in uterine sarcoma. Wide variations in cell types are frequently seen in different parts of a single tumor. Round and spindle cells are commonly found in the same tumor, and it is probable that the "round cells" are the result of cutting bundles of spindle cells transversely. Hyperchromatic nuclei are common, and mitotic figures may be rare or exceedingly frequent. Figure 37-1 shows sarcomatous change in a fibroid, and the histology is similar for sarcoma arising in the endo-

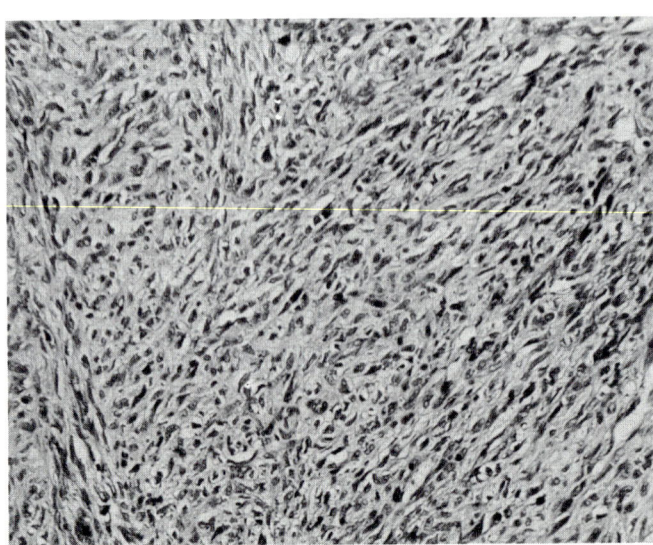

FIG. 37-1. Sarcomatous change in myoma.

metrium. Giant cells with huge, darkstaining nuclei are common in sarcoma arising in myomas. They may represent abnormal cellular activity, but equally often they appear to be the result of a degenerative process with cytoplasmic confluence of degenerating cells. In attempting to correlate the microscopic picture with clinical malignancy, it has been shown that even a great number of giant cells is not necessarily indicative of a grave prognosis. In 1920 Evans, of the Mayo Clinic, studied a large number of "malignant myomas" and made quantitative mitotic figure counts on many microscopic fields of uniform thickness. He concluded from a follow-up study of the cases that malignancy was in direct proportion to the number of mitotic figures. Novak and Anderson's study confirms that of Evans. However, we have examined microscopically metastatic sarcomatous nodules in the liver and found mitotic figures to be completely absent. The cases about which there is greatest confusion are those fibroids in which there is little or no nuclear activity but which are exceedingly cellular. The difference in the interpretation of these tumors undoubtedly accounts for the great difference in the incidence of malignancy reported in fibroids.

An incidence up to 4 per cent of sarcomatous degeneration in fibroids has been reported, but that figure is undoubtedly too high. More critical studies by Novak and Anderson, from Johns Hopkins, report an incidence of 0.7 per cent, and more recently, Montague et al., who have updated our experience at Hopkins, find the incidence to be 0.29 per cent during a 30-year period. However, it must be remembered that these calculations are based on the fibroids which reach the laboratory. Since they represent only a small proportion of the existing fibroids, the percentage of sarcomatous change in fibroids must be even smaller.

DIAGNOSIS

The preoperative diagnosis of uterine sarcoma may be easy or difficult, depending on the type. Endometrial sarcoma may be suspected when a relatively large, friable, polypoid mass presents itself through the dilated cervix into the vagina. It must be differentiated from the sloughing, submucous fibroid which is usually of firmer consistency and does not have the yellowish appearance of sarcoma. The polypoid type of sarcoma arising from the cervix may be suspected when a relatively large friable polypoid mass can be seen attached to the cervix. Removal of the polyps for biopsy will establish the diagnosis. Sarcomatous change in a fibroid may be suspected when there is evidence of rapid growth in a fibroid at any age, but when there is unquestionable postmenopausal growth in a fibroid, sarcomatous change is almost certain. If the sarcomatous change is near the uterine cavity, postmenopausal bleeding may occur, and a diagnostic curettage should be done. Finding sarcomatous tissue in the material obtained at curettage establishes the diagnosis, but the absence of sarcomatous tissue by no means rules out the possibility, as the degenerative process is often in the center of the tumor. More often, bleeding from the postmenopausal fibroid uterus indicates coincidental malignancy of the cervix or the endometrium.

TREATMENT

The treatment of uterine sarcoma is usually total abdominal hysterectomy and adnexectomy, supplemented in some instances by irradiation. However, there must be individualization, depending upon the type of sarcoma, the extent of the disease, the general condition of the patient, and whether or not the diagnosis is made preoperatively.

Let us consider first the sarcomatous fibroid or intramural sarcoma arising directly from the fibromuscular wall of the uterus. These conditions may have been diagnosed preoperatively, but it is more likely that the surgeon will be confronted with the condition after the abdomen is open. If possible, the surgeon should perform a total hysterectomy and a double salpingo-oophorectomy. An omentectomy is probably desirable whether it is grossly involved or not. The liver should be palpated, and a search should be made throughout the abdomen for lymphatic enlargement. Even if extension beyond the uterus is found, it may be advisable to perform the recommended surgery if it can be done without too great risk. This will facilitate the postoperative x-ray therapy. The extent of the growth with involvement of surrounding structures may make complete surgery impossible and, indeed, may only permit the removal of a specimen for biopsy. Following obviously incomplete surgery, deep x-ray therapy to the abdomen and the pelvis may be carried out unless the extent of the disease and the general condition of the patient are such as to make the disadvantages of irradiation outweigh the possible benefits. In case of complete surgery with sarcomatous change limited to the central portion of a large fibroid and particularly when the malignancy appears histologically to be of low grade, it is our custom not to follow the surgery with irradiation. The value of x-ray therapy is supplemental, while surgery remains the backbone of treatment.

Every surgeon who has done a large number of hysterectomies for fibroids is confronted eventually with a pathologic report of sarcoma in a fibroid uterus which he presumed to be benign at the operating table. If a subtotal hysterectomy was done or adnexa left in, the question of further surgery presents itself. We are inclined against further surgery. If the sarcoma is found high in the uterus and well away from the level of amputation, it is probable that the chances of cure are almost as good with subtotal as with the total operation. If the sarcoma is found low in the uterus, radium may be placed in the cervical stump and deep x-ray therapy given to the pelvic region. Irradiation by means of x-ray is also indicated if the adnexa have not been removed.

Sarcoma of the endometrium probably should be treated with intracavitary irradiation, followed in 3 to 4 weeks by total hysterectomy and double salpingo-oophorectomy. We never have seen an endometrial sarcoma cured with intracavitary irradiation alone. The tumor frequently melts away with irradiation but in our experience invariably recurs; hence the necessity of the hysterectomy. If the polypoid mass of sarcoma is large, extending into the vagina, the greater part of it should be curetted away before radium is applied. Because such a polypoid mass is always infected, penicillin, or a similar antibiotic, should be given when the tissue is removed and at the time of irradiation.

Sarcoma of the cervix should be diagnosed by biopsy. Irradiation in dosage comparable with that given for cervical cancer should be used, usually beginning with external irradiation and followed by intracavitary radium and vaginal colpostats. Hysterectomy with a generous vaginal cuff has been advocated following irradiation by some authors in the past, while radical Wertheim hysterectomy and pelvic node dissection provide a more complete pelvic dissection with a better chance to encompass the pelvic tumor. In cases of sarcoma botryoides involving vagina and cervix, Daniel, Koss and Brunschwig advocate pelvic exenteration in an attempt to achieve some, although few, cures of patients with this disease. Age or a generally poor medical condition may contraindicate the surgery. No one has had sufficient experience with this rare disease to justify a too-dogmatic opinion on treatment.

It is impossible to obtain any statistical data regarding prognosis in sarcoma of the uterus based on any set routine of treatment. Aaro, Symmonds and Dockerty report a 41 per cent 5-year survival for leiomyosarcoma, with surgery as the primary method of treatment. The grade and extent of the sarcoma were the most significant prognostic factors. They achieved a reduced cure rate of 32 per cent in patients with endometrial sarcoma, utilizing surgery alone. The experience at Hopkins as reported by Montague et al. was also quite favorable with primary surgery in patients treated for leiomyosarcoma. A 3-year survival of 53 per cent was observed in patients under the age of 50, while there was little success in the older age group. While Norris, Roth and Taylor refute the advantage of the combined treatment of surgery and irradiation, the experience at the M. D. Anderson Hospital (Edwards) is in support of this combined treatment. Preoperative intracavitary radium produced tumor sterilization in 10 (34.5%) of 29 patients so treated, with 15 of the 29 patients living without evidence of disease. In contrast, only 6 of 21 patients in the group that did not use preoperative radium are living. Based on our own experience and data from various clinics, the preferable current treatment for sarcoma of the uterus includes total abdominal hysterectomy and bilateral salpingo-oophorectomy, either preceded or followed by pelvic irradiation.

THE MIXED MESODERMAL TUMOR

The histogenesis of the mixed mesodermal tumor is obscure. The term *carcinosarcoma* has often been applied to these tumors in which malignant connective tissue and epithelial elements are both present (Fig. 37-2). Most gynecologic pathologists are convinced that the lesion is a real entity containing both sarcomatous and carcinomatous elements and not merely a collision of two separate tumors. Rubin has concluded from tissue culture that there are two distinct cell types. One cell type had the characteristics of carcinoma, the other of sarcoma. No intermediate cell types or evidence of transition from one form to the other was seen. The tumors often contain a variety of mesodermal elements such as striated muscle fibers and cartilage. Clinically, the tumor grows in polypoid form within the uterine cavity, often presenting into the vagina through the cervical canal. It is classically a disease that occurs in the postmenopausal period; consequently, the most common symptom is postmenopausal bleeding. The lesions usually metastasize early, quite in contrast with

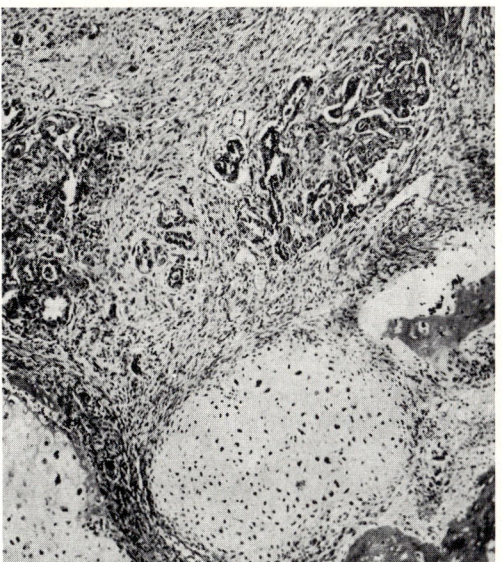

FIG. 37-2. Mixed mesodermal tumor of endometrium. Glands and stromal elements both appear to be malignant. Note cartilage, which is occasionally found in these very malignant tumors.

the usual carcinoma of the endometrium. Their great malignancy is indicated by the fact that some series are reported with no 5-year survival. For example, Sternberg, Clark, and Smith reported 21 cases from the Charity Hospital in New Orleans with no 5-year survivors — the longest survivor being 27 months after the appearance of symptoms. However, all reports are not that pessimistic. Rachmaninoff and Climie reported a 5-year survival rate of 21 per cent of 30 patients.

Because of the generally poor results of therapy, the pattern of treatment is variable. Previously it was our custom to give approximately 5,000 mg. hours of intracavitary irradiation followed by hysterectomy, but there has been considerable evidence to show that cures are little if any affected by preoperative irradiation. Intracavitary radium has proven valuable in the M. D. Anderson Hospital experience (Edwards), with 9 patients (42.9%) in a series of 21 cases living with no evidence of disease for at least 2 years. However, Rachmaninoff and Climie found no evidence in their follow-up of 30 cases that preoperative irradiation improved their results. None of their patients with residual tumor survived 5 years after hysterectomy. They concluded that the preferable treatment was to proceed as rapidly as possible with removal of the uterus and adnexa, and deep x-ray therapy was reserved for recurrent or metastatic lesions. We concur in this plan of therapy, but prefer to use supervoltage pelvic irradiation routinely following definitive surgery whenever possible in an effort to arrest the spread of the disease. When the disease is found above the pelvis, abdominal irradiation may provide added palliation.

BIBLIOGRAPHY

Aaro, L. A., Symmonds, R. E., and Dockerty, M. B.: Sarcoma of the uterus; a clinical and pathological study of 177 cases. Amer. J. Obstet. Gynec., 94:101, 1966.

Daniel, W. W., Koss, L. G., and Brunschwig, A.: Sarcoma botryoides of the vagina. Cancer, 12:74, 1959.

Edwards, C. L.: Undifferentiated tumors. In M. D. Anderson Hospital and Tumor Institute, Houston, Texas: Cancer of the Uterus and Ovary. p. 84. Chicago, Year Book Medical Publishers, 1969.

Evans, N.: Malignant myomata and related tumors of the uterus. Surg. Gynec. Obstet., 30:225, 1920.

Montague, A. C.-W., Swartz, D. P., and Woodruff, J. D.: Sarcoma arising in leiomyoma of uterus: factors influencing prognosis. Amer. J. Obstet. Gynec., 92:421, 1965.

Norris, N. J., Roth, E., and Taylor, H. B.: Mesenchymal tumors of the uterus. II. A clinical and pathological study of 31 mixed mesodermal tumors. Obstet. Gynce., 28:57, 1966.

Novak, E., and Anderson, D. F.: Sarcoma of uterus. Amer. J. Obstet. Gynec., 34:740, 1937.

Rachmaninoff, N., and Climie, A.R.W.: Mixed mesodermal tumors of the uterus. Cancer, 19:1705, 1966.

Rubin, A.: The histogenesis of carcinosarcoma (mixed mesodermal tumor) of the uterus as revealed by tissue culture studies. Amer. J. Obstet. Gynec., 77:269, 1959.

Sternberg, W. H., Clark, W. H., and Smith, R. C.: Malignant mixed Müllerian tumor (mixed mesodermal tumor of the uterus). Cancer, 7:704, 1954.

38

Adnexal Tumors

GENERAL CONSIDERATIONS

The presence of an ovarian neoplasm is an indication for laparotomy, whether or not the tumor gives rise to symptoms. The justification for this statement is the incidence of malignancy in ovarian neoplasms, which is in the neighborhood of 15 per cent. This is too high to justify a policy of waiting. The problem of ovarian neoplasms may be compared with the problem of nodules in the breast. Ovarian tumors must be regarded as potentially malignant, even though pelvic examination gives no hint of malignancy. Even at operation, with the tumor under direct inspection and palpation, one occasionally has difficulty in determining whether the tumor is benign or malignant. Clinical experience coupled with pathologic studies has demonstrated that an ovarian tumor may be benign for years and finally become malignant. Consider, as an example, the large ovarian tumor that has been responsible for noticeable abdominal enlargement for years. Suddenly there is a rapid increase in the size of the abdomen. The tumor is removed. On pathologic examination much of it is found to be typical benign cystadenoma, but other parts show signs of unmistakable carcinoma. A case such as this demonstrates that the history suggesting long duration by no means rules out present malignancy when dealing with ovarian tumors.

Because of the malignant potentialities of ovarian tumors, and because they are so often asymptomatic until the hopeless state, routine pelvic checkups at intervals of a year should be made. The possibility of ovarian neoplasm represents the second most important reason for annual examinations, the first being the more common malignancy of the cervix. In some women with familial histories of cancer, examination at 6-month intervals is desirable. Apropos of prophylaxis, the question arises as to the desirability of castration in pelvic surgery. This is discussed in some detail in the chapter on myomata, since it is usually in connection with hysterectomy for benign uterine disease that this question arises. Randall's statistics are of importance in considering this. He estimates that at the age of 40 a woman has approximately a 1 per cent chance of developing ovarian cancer during the remainder of her life. After that age the chance diminishes so that at 50 the chance is reduced to 0.9 per cent.

Aside from the possibility of malignancy, other potentialities may indicate operation, may complicate the operation, or may increase the operative risk. The commonest of these are torsion of the pedicle, infection, and rupture.

Torsion of the pedicle of an ovarian tumor is accompanied by sudden, severe pain. This may be the first symptom noted by the patient and the reason for her visit to the physician. The history of repeated episodes of pain before the final severe attack which leads to surgery suggests that patients may suffer partial twisting and spontaneous untwisting. If the torsion is not released spontaneously, the venous circulation is first interfered with, and then the arterial blood supply is cut off. The tumor becomes purple and subsequently almost black in color (Plate 10). Thromboses of the vessels of the pedicle occur, and gangrene results. A little exudate comes forth from the tumor, and the adjacent peritoneum becomes inflamed; fine fibrinous adhesions form rapidly between the tumor and the neighboring structures. The peritoneal irritation gives rise to abdominal muscle spasm; nausea and vomiting are common; and there is moderate elevation of the temperature, the pulse rate, and the leukocyte count. These signs and symptoms indicate immediate surgical intervention.

Rupture of true neoplastic ovarian cysts is a rare complication. Retention cysts and endometrial cysts more frequently rupture; each of these conditions is considered elsewhere. However, rupture of serous and mucinous cysts in the benign and the malignant forms does occur. The contents of the cysts are irritating to the peritoneum—mucin more so than serous fluid. A sterile chemical peritonitis results. Pain, nausea, vomiting, abdominal distention, and muscle spasm follow. The occurrence of these signs and symptoms, coupled with pelvic findings suggesting an ovarian cyst, indicates the advisability of immediate surgical intervention. Confirmation of intraperitoneal fluid is easily made by culdocentesis, at which time a sample may be obtained for cytologic study.

GROSS PATHOLOGY IN RELATION TO TREATMENT

One cannot consider intelligently the treatment of ovarian tumors without discussing pathology. An important difference between the well-trained gynecologic surgeon and the incompletely trained operator lies in the knowledge of pathology that the former possesses. This knowledge is particularly necessary when dealing with ovarian tumors. *The selection of the correct type or extent of surgical procedure depends more upon the operator's knowledge of gross pathology than upon anything else.* Prior to operation one can speculate on the nature of the tumor and the type of operation he expects to carry out, but the final decision cannot be made, and should not be made, until the surgeon carefully inspects the pelvis and considers the pathology of the lesion with which he must deal. The age of the patient, the number of pregnancies, the desire for children, the emotional background of the patient and her probable reaction to a surgical menopause should also be considered. However, the most important single decision concerns whether or not the growth is benign or malignant. If a needlessly radical operation is performed for a benign ovarian tumor upon a young woman, it may precipitate disagreeable menopausal symptoms as well as sterilize her unnecessarily; on the other hand, an incomplete operation for a malignant ovarian tumor practically always means recurrence and death.

Because of the importance of a knowledge of gross pathology at the operating table, the distinguishing gross characteristics of the various tumors, together with their special clinical characteristics, will be considered.

PHYSIOLOGIC (RETENTION) CYSTS OF THE OVARY

A physiologic cyst may occur in either the follicle or corpus luteum whenever there is alteration of the normal pituitary-ovarian hormonal axis, which results in the failure of either follicular or corpus luteum regression and in cyst formation. Because of their physiologic origin, these cysts usually regress with the following menstrual cycle and do not require surgery unless symptoms of acute pain warrant.

Follicular cysts vary in size from 1 to 5 or 6 cm., and in rare instances they attain a larger size. They are a product of follicular enlargement with excessive

PLATE 12

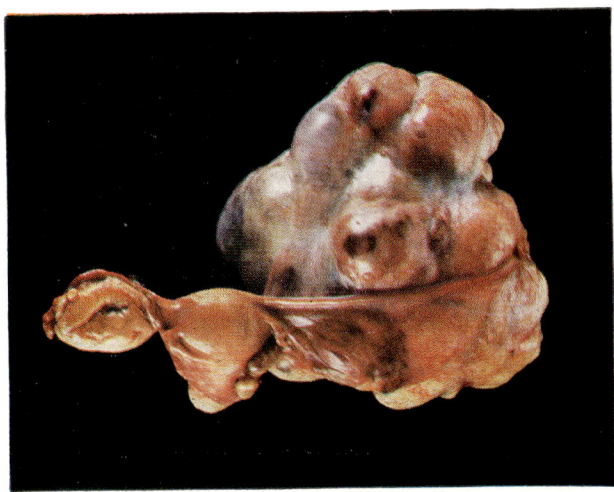

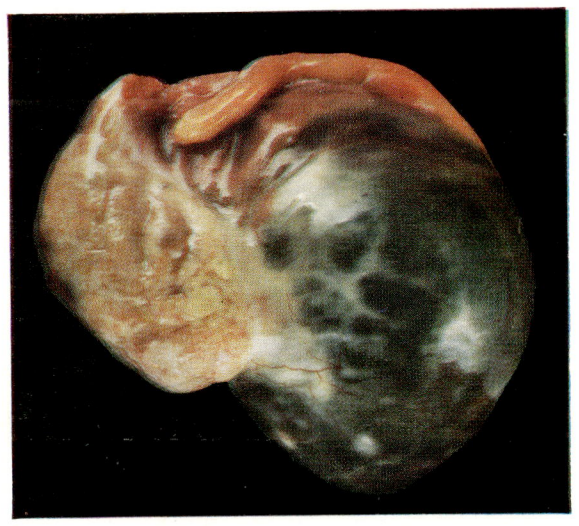

(*Top*) Granulosa cell tumor of ovary.
(*Bottom*) Parovarian cyst.

PLATE 11

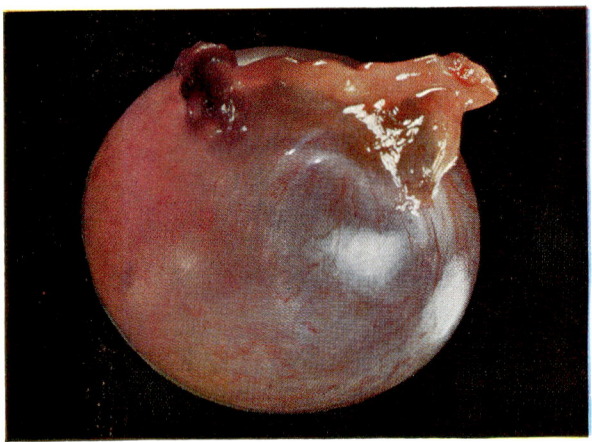

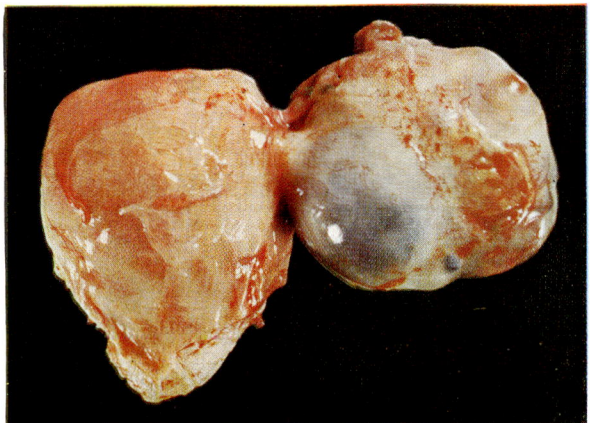

(Top) Follicular retention cyst. *(Bottom)* Cystic ovary. The enlargement is due to multiple follicular retention cysts.

PLATE 10

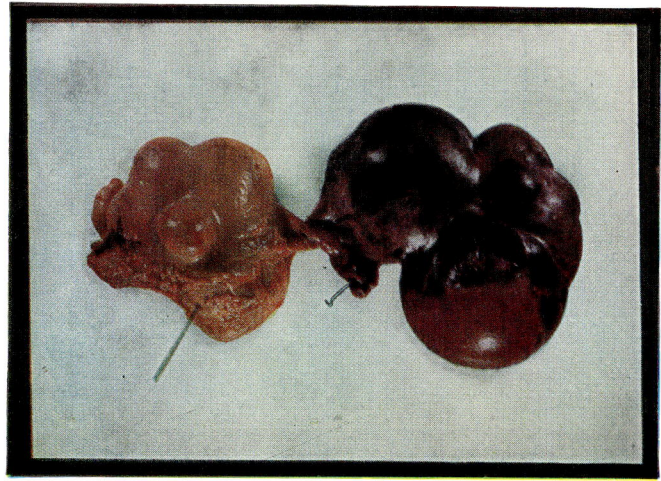

Ovarian cyst twisted with tube on pedicle.

PLATES 10 to 12

fluid formation and may be multiple or single. They are thin-walled, of a smooth consistency, and bluish white in color, and because they are retention cysts, the larger the cyst, usually the thinner is the wall (Fig. 38-1). The fluid content is straw-colored or slightly blood-tinged, rarely pure blood; if the content is pure blood, the cyst is more properly classified as a follicular hematoma. Multiple small follicular cysts may cause considerable ovarian enlargement of a semisolid nature (Plate 11). Such ovaries are usually symptomless, and operation for their removal is not justified. When such a condition is encountered at the operating table in the course of a hysterectomy, it is usually advisable to leave the ovaries in, especially in young individuals. If only one ovary is cystic and the other ovary normal, removal of the cystic ovary may be indicated. Needling such small cysts is practiced by some gynecologists. The procedure is harmless, but it is doubtful whether any permanent benefit results from it. Multiple follicular cysts in adherent ovaries after salpingectomy may be painful and require removal (Plate 11).

Large single follicular cysts may give rise to discomfort and even pain (Fig. 38-1). If one can be reasonably certain that one is dealing with this follicular type of cyst, which frequently disappears spontaneously, a period of observation is wise. Often part of the wall of the cyst is of paper thinness, and rupture on pelvic examination occasionally takes place. In the event of such an accident, the patient should be watched for possible hemorrhage, but this is rare. The patient usually becomes comfortable after a few days of abdominal soreness. The ruptured cyst may or may not re-form. Hemorrhage into a maturing follicle may cause rupture, and the evacuation of a small amount of blood into the peritoneal cavity results in pain, slight fever, and usually leukocytosis. Or, in rare instances, profuse hemorrhage may take place from this rupture. The symptoms are often confused with those of acute appendicitis or tubal pregnancy, but the differentiation is important, since

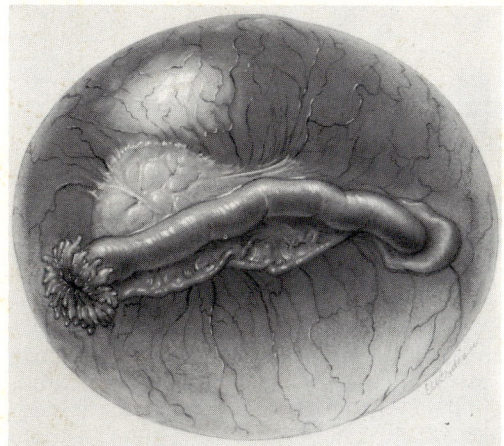

Fig. 38-1. Large follicular retention cyst.

surgery is seldom necessary for the slight hemorrhage from a follicle. The accident of follicular hemorrhage occurs most frequently at the time of ovulation, although it is by no means confined to that time.

Follicular cysts are commonly encountered incidentally at the operating table, when it is often quite possible to shell them out with the conservation of a good quantity of normal ovarian tissue. When most of the ovarian tissue is markedly thinned by the pressure of the cyst, oophorectomy is generally preferred to resection, if the patient's other ovary is normal. When the opposite ovary is absent, one may go to extremes to save a bit of ovarian tissue, and the younger the woman, the greater the effort should be at ovarian conservation. The closure of the ovarian defect and control of bleeding is best made with fine catgut, used as a lock stitch with an atraumatic needle (Fig. 38-2).

Corpus luteum cyst formation may occur following ovulation. Instead of retrogressing normally, the corpus luteum remains cystic, with an excess of fluid content. The lutein cells persist in a variable degree of preservation, and a wall of fibroblasts is deposited on the inner surface of the lutein zone. In the older cysts the lutein cells almost completely disappear, and the fibrous zone is heavy, whereas in the more recent cysts there is a zone of healthy-looking lutein cells

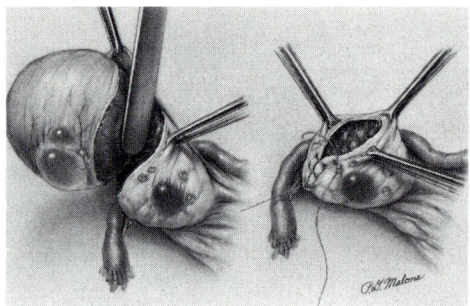

FIG. 38-2. Resection of a small cyst from an ovary. (*Left*) An incision has been made around the ovary near the junction of the cyst wall and normal ovarian tissue. The knife handle is a convenient instrument for shelling out the cyst. (*Right*) The wound in the ovary is closed with a continuous lock stitch of No. 00 chromic catgut on an atraumatic needle.

with only a little fibrous tissue within (Fig. 38-3). Often the thinner portion of the cyst wall has a yellow cast. A distinction should be made between the normally functioning cystic corpus luteum and the corpus luteum cyst that is the product of abnormal regression. The normally functioning corpus luteum contains a small amount of straw-colored or blood-tinged fluid. Occasionally this is excessive, forming a cyst, and yet the function of the corpus luteum is undisturbed. Such a functioning corpus luteum seldom attains a diameter of over 3 cm. The corpus luteum cyst sometimes attains a diameter of 5 to 6 cm. and in rare instances an even greater diameter.

The normally functioning corpus luteum may become of surgical importance because of excessive bleeding into it. The hemorrhage may cause rupture and create a clinical picture simulating appendicitis or tubal pregnancy. This accident may occur at any time following ovulation and usually is associated with coitus or strenuous activity; we have seen it during menstruation and even during early pregnancy. As in the case of the follicle, the bleeding is usually slight, and surgery is not necessary. Occasionally surgery is required because of excessive bleeding, but more often the abdomen is opened because of symptoms suggesting acute appendicitis or tubal pregnancy. The cystic lutein wall in most instances can be shelled out and the ovary saved.

The true corpus luteum cyst is commonly associated with a disturbance of or delay in menstruation, but the variation is not uniform. When the menstrual period is delayed, with discomfort in the lower abdomen, a differentiation must be made from tubal pregnancy. A period of watchful waiting for spontaneous disappearance of the cyst is usually justifiable. A peritoneoscopic examination of the abdominal cavity is frequently of value. If the cyst and discomfort of sufficient severity persist, surgery is indicated. Although enucleation of the cyst is always preferable, oophorectomy is contingent upon the condition of the rest of the ovary, the condition of the opposite ovary, and the age of the patient.

Corpus luteum cysts are not to be confused with multiple lutein cysts of the ovary occurring with hydatidiform mole and chorioepithelioma.

NEOPLASTIC CYSTS OF THE OVARY

Mucinous cystadenomas may attain an enormous size and average much larger than the serous variety (Fig. 38-4). They derive their name from their thick,

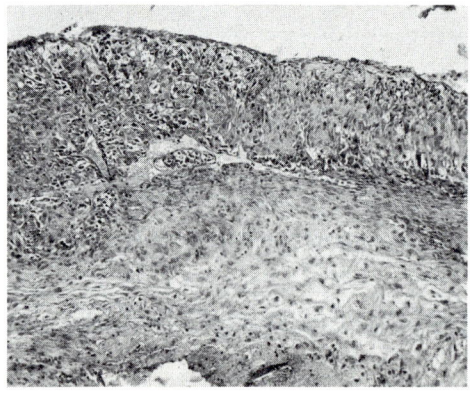

FIG. 38-3. Wall of a corpus luteum retention cyst. Lutein tissue is shown on the upper surface of the photograph.

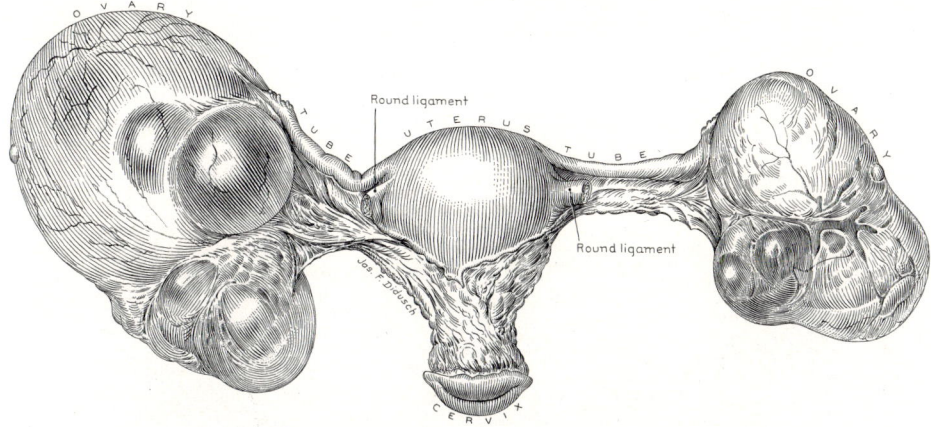

Fig. 38-4. Bilateral mucinous cystadenomas of the ovary.

viscid, mucinous contents. Although formerly called pseudomucinous cystadenomas because of a predominantly glycoprotein content, Fisher's histochemical study in 1954 showed the secretion of these tumors to be similar to the mucin from the intestinal mucosa, namely, an acid-mucopolysaccharide. This may be as thin as egg albumin, but in some instances it is gelatinous and too thick to flow. As in all cystic tumors, hemorrhage may occur in them, changing the usually almost colorless fluid to chocolate color. These tumors are multilocular or parvilocular and are composed of large, rounded cystic compartments. The walls of the tumors are of variable thickness; the thicker portions are bluish white, while the thinner portions are darker; when there is intracystic hemorrhage, they may be very dark. The thicker areas in the wall may contain innumerable small locules which constantly increase in size, and thus the tumor grows. As this process is going on within the cyst, the walls of the larger compartments become thinned by pressure, and often there is rupture of one locule into another. Papillary excrescences on the outer surface of these tumors and within the cysts are characteristics of malignant change, since these tumors are nonpapillary in their benign form. This is in contrast to the papillary appearance of the benign serous cystadenomas. However, they do occur as shown microscopically in Figure 38-5 as folds in the lining of the cyst. The tumors are commonly bilateral, so that when a unilateral tumor is encountered, the opposite ovary should be inspected carefully to make certain that it does not contain a very small cyst. Mucinous cysts become secondarily malignant in a small percentage of cases (5%, Meyer; 12%, Woodruff). Those cysts with papillary ingrowths or outgrowths are much more apt to become carcinomatous than cysts without papillary growths. The history of long-standing abdominal enlargement and the finding of areas of malignancy in an otherwise benign cystadenoma indicate that cystadenomas may persist for years as benign tumors and then become malignant. When mucinous cystadenomas are encountered in young individuals, unilateral adnexal removal is indicated, unless there is a suggestion of malignant change. After the age of 40, bilateral oophorectomy is usually advisable because of the tendency to bilaterality.

Occasionally a mucocele of the appendix is found associated with these cysts (Fig. 38-6). Pseudomyxoma peritonei may result from rupture of mucinous cysts or appendiceal mucoceles due to the transplantation of secreting cells of the tumor onto the peritoneum. Although this condition is a low-grade malignancy, it is impossible to remove completely all the myxomatous material at operation; its reaccumulation is sure to follow

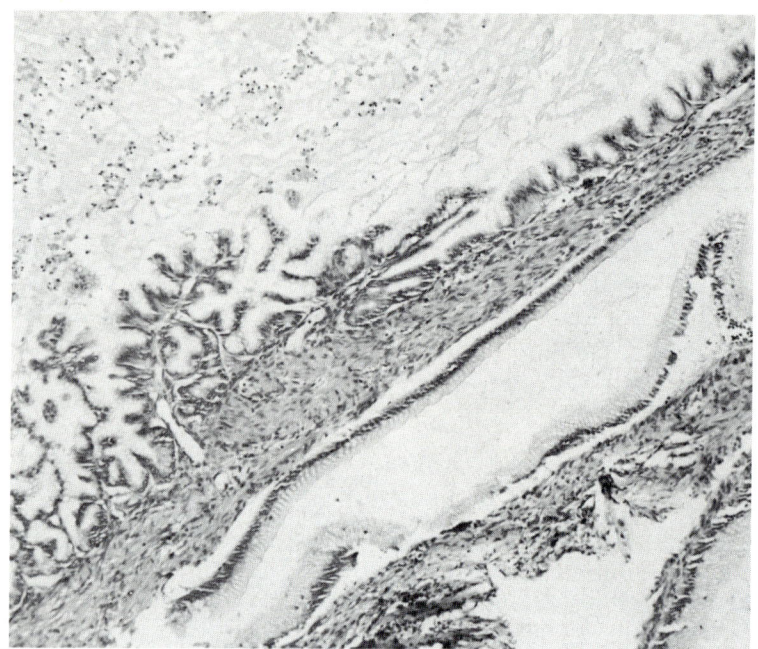

FIG. 38-5. Mucinous cystadenoma with microscopic folds in the lining epithelium.

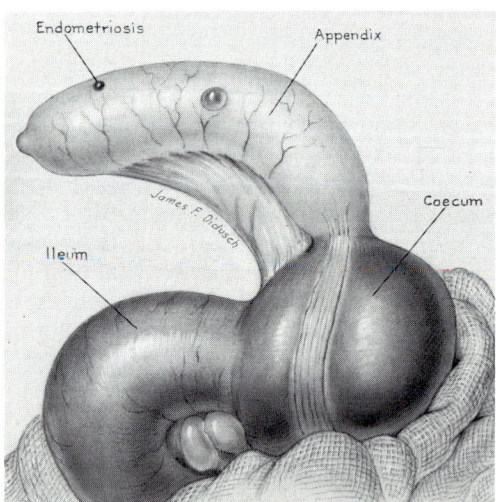

FIG. 38-6. Mucocele of the appendix.

eventually and reoperation must be done with removal of as much as possible. Death usually eventually results.

Serous cystadenomas are slightly more frequent than the mucinous variety (Fig. 38-7). They, too, may become enormous, but their average size is less than that of the mucinous cysts. They are named from the serous fluid that they contain, which is usually straw-colored; if there is hemorrhage, the fluid may be altered to the color of chocolate or coffee. These cysts are multilocular or parvilocular and appear to be composed of a conglomeration of round cystic masses. They may also give the appearance of being single large cysts which on section may have a few large compartments and many small ones in the thicker portions of the wall. Papillary excrescences are common on the exterior of the cyst wall but are even more common on the interior. They are shown grossly in Figure 38-7 and microscopically in Figure 38-8. These papillary growths frequently implant upon the serous surfaces of the abdominal viscera and may or may not produce ascites. Grossly, these implants suggest malignancy, although histologically they are graded in their malignant potential. When implants are present, a hysterectomy and a double salpingo-oophorectomy should be done, even though the other ovary appears to be normal. When the papillary serous cystadenoma is unilateral and entirely free, and no implants are found on other viscera, one should still consider doing a

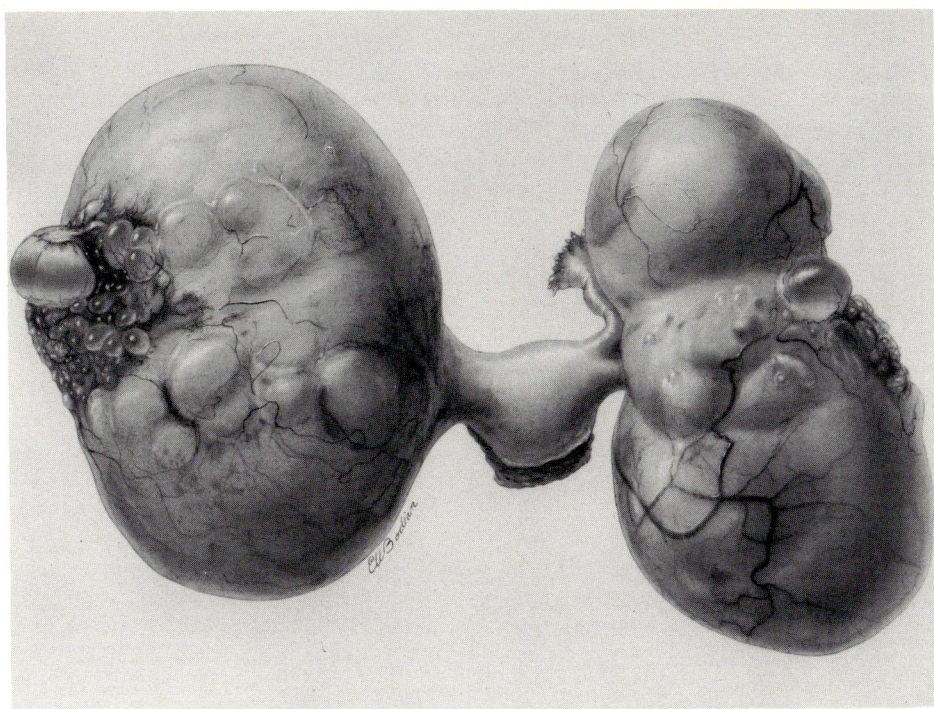

FIG. 38-7. Papillary serous cystadenomas of the ovaries.

complete operation, especially in women in their late thirties and beyond. The justification for this lies in the tendency of these tumors to become bilateral ultimately and to change to malignancy. The incidence of secondary malignant change in serous cystadenomas greatly exceeds that of the mucinous variety and

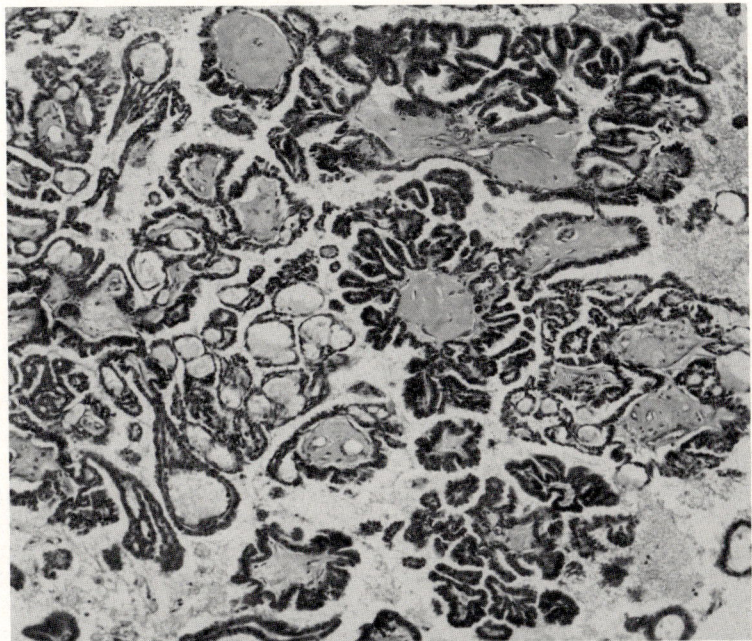

FIG. 38-8. Section of papillomata from serous cystadenoma.

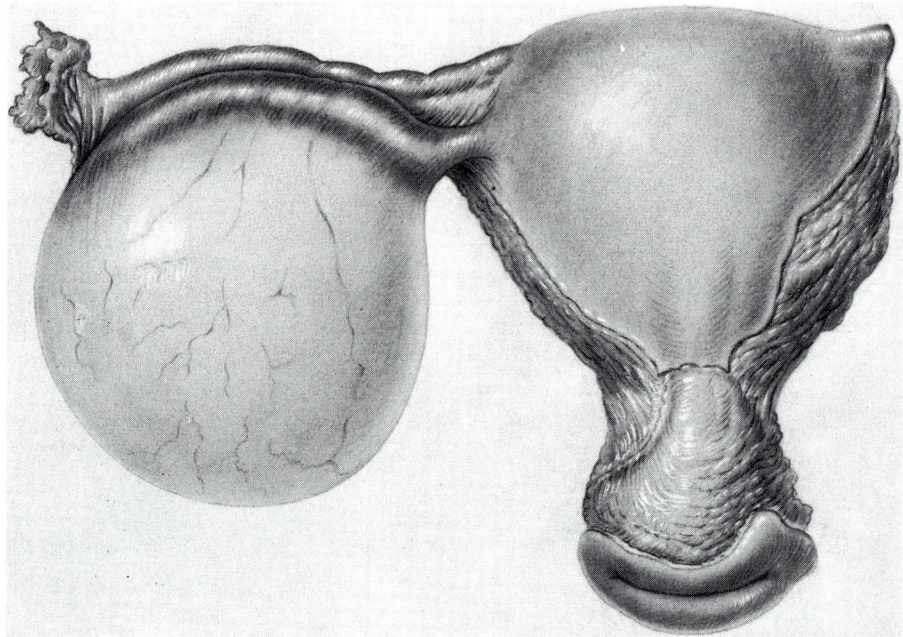

Fig. 38-9. Unilocular serous cystoma.

approximates 30 per cent in our experience.

The temptation to insert a trocar into these serous cysts should be resisted; instead, the incision should be enlarged to permit removal intact. With enormous cysts, evacuation by trocar may be unavoidable. However, before inserting the trocar the exterior of the cyst should be inspected carefully for papillary excrescences, and their presence should weigh heavily against puncture. When evacuation by trocar cannot be avoided, the area to be punctured should be protected carefully by a purse-string suture; on withdrawal, the opening in the cyst should be drawn closed quickly to avoid spilling of the contents.

Simple Serous Cystomas. Closely related to the serous cystadenomas is a unilocular cyst filled with thin fluid which is clear unless stained from intracystic hemorrhage (Fig. 38-9). Histologically, the low epithelial lining is similar to that of the serous cystadenomas, but the walls of the cyst are not formed of adenomatous tissue. They are almost always smooth-walled externally, but rarely have papillary excrescences been seen on the surface. When small, they must be distinguished from retention cysts, but their wall is usually thicker. They are quite benign and almost uniformly unilocular; unilateral ovarian removal is all that is necessary for cure, but when they occur after the menopause, a hysterectomy and a double salpingectomy should be done, if the patient's condition warrants it.

Dermoid cysts are among the commoner ovarian tumors, but they occur less frequently than the cystadenomas. Figure 38-10 shows the gross appearance of a cyst that has been opened, and Figure 38-11 shows a typical microscopic section of the wall. They range from microscopic size to very large tumors. We have seen a dermoid cyst weighing 50 pounds, but usually they are not larger than 10 to 12 cm. They are considered to arise from teratomas of the ovary, with predominance of the ectodermal component. They are cystic, their tissues are chiefly ectodermal in origin, and the incidence of malignancy is low, probably less than 1 per cent. Their rather thick walls are usually bluish white in color and very smooth; the thickness of the

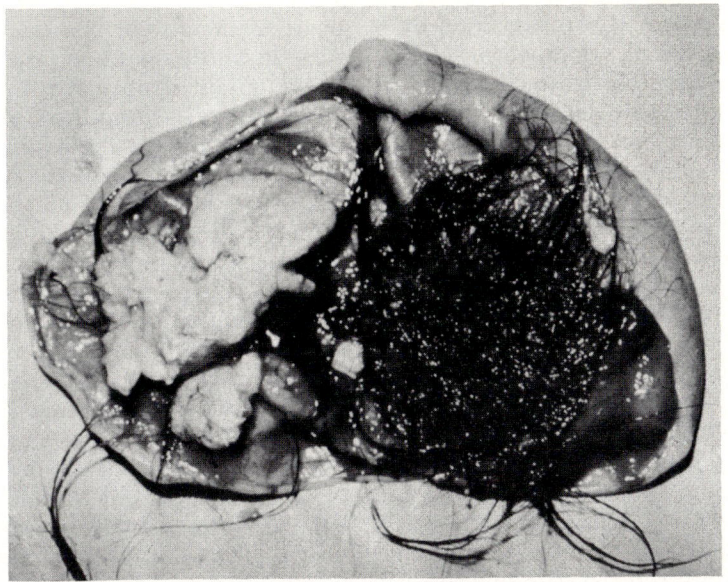

Fig. 38-10. Dermoid cyst of ovary. Cyst has been opened, and sebaceous contents and a ball of hair are pouring forth.

wall and the sebaceous contents give them a semisolid feeling, and they are heavy for their size. If the operator is uncertain of the nature of the cyst, it can be identified easily by its sebaceous and hairy contents when it is opened after removal.

Between 10 and 25 per cent of the dermoid cysts are bilateral. Because of this tendency to bilaterality, these cysts

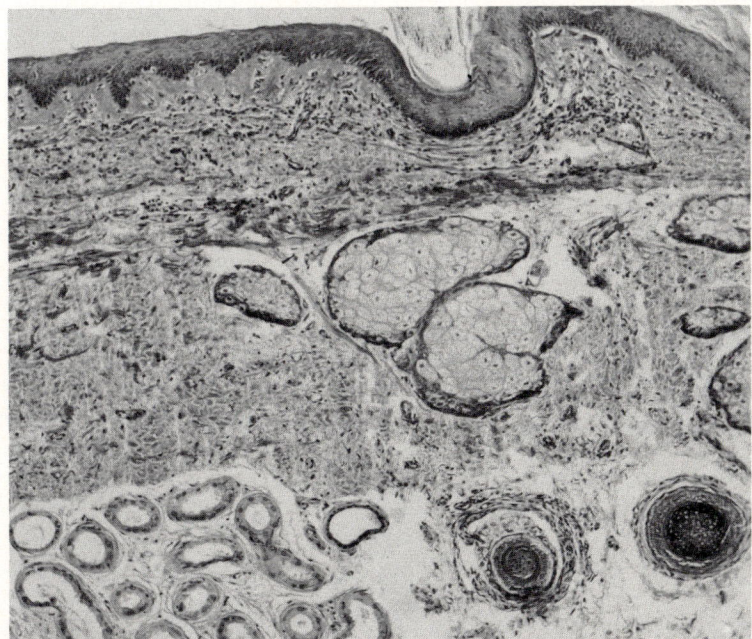

Fig. 38-11. Wall of a dermoid cyst, showing stratified squamous epithelial surface, sebaceous glands, sweat glands, and hair follicles.

often require bilateral oophorectomy and, consequently, total hysterectomy. They may come to light clinically in a patient of any age, but their occurrence in young women, and even in children, is not uncommon. When they appear at a very early age and are bilateral, they constitute one of the tragedies of gynecologic surgery. When the opposite ovary appears to be normal, it should be inspected carefully or bisected for a very small dermoid. A small suspicious cyst may be needled; if the content is oily, the diagnosis of dermoid can be made. In young women such a cyst may then be resected, if possible leaving the patient sufficient ovarian tissue to preserve the menstrual function.

Struma Ovarii. Thyroid tissue is not infrequently found in small amounts in ovarian teratomas. Von Kahlden in 1895 and Gottschalk in 1899 were the first to recognize the true nature of these tumors. Rarely, the thyroid tissue appears to outgrow all other elements, and such tumors may properly be called *struma ovarii*. Not only is the histologic picture of thyroid tissue unmistakable, but its true nature can be demonstrated by the chemical determination of its iodine content. Radioactive iodine uptake has also been demonstrated in thyroid tissue in the ovary. The ovarian struma is usually not overactive. However, cases have been reported (10%) in which overactivity of the ovarian thyroid gave rise to symptoms of hyperthyroidism. Most of these tumors are benign, but 5 to 10 per cent of struma ovarii are said to be malignant. Gonzalez-Angulo and co-workers reported 3 cases of malignant struma ovarii and found 37 cases in the literature. Malkasian recently described 3 cases, in all of which distant metastases were seen initially. However, removal of metastatic thyroid nodules, identical histologically with the original tumor, has in some instances resulted in cure.

The relation of the ovarian thyroid tissue to that of the neck is interesting. Neumann reported a case in which the struma in the neck, together with the toxic symptoms, disappeared after removal of the ovarian tumor. On the other hand, Woodruff and Markley reported a case in which the thyroid in the neck enlarged a year after the removal of the ovarian struma. In addition to total abdominal hysterectomy and bilateral salpingo-oophorectomy, malignant struma ovarii is usually treated with I^{131}.

BENIGN SOLID TUMORS OF THE OVARY

Fibromas of the ovary of sufficient size to give rise to clinical symptoms are rather uncommon. Small fibromas on the surface of the ovary occur quite frequently; and in dealing with them when they are discovered accidentally at operation, they must be considered as possible forerunners of the larger tumors. Also there is a condition which for want of a better name we have called "fibrosis ovarii," shown in Figure 38-12 and in

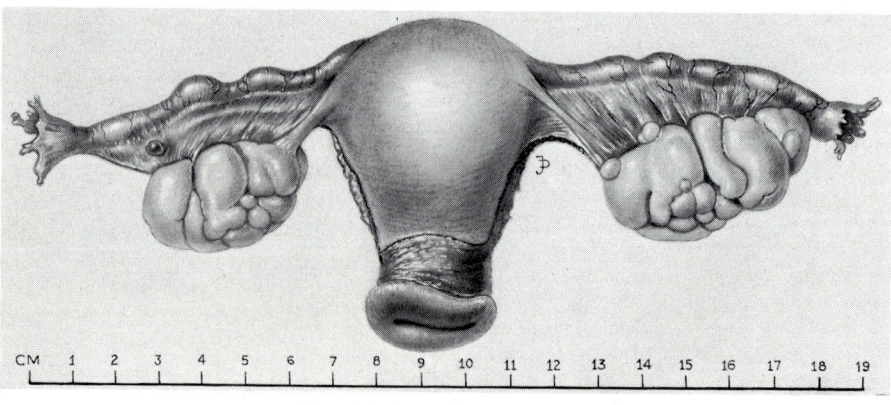

Fig. 38-12. Fibrosis ovarii.

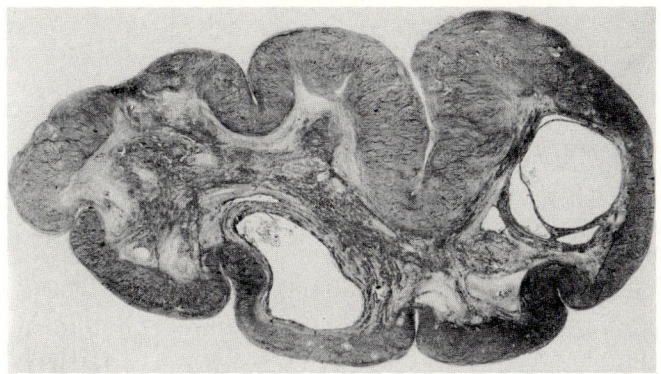

FIG. 38-13. Low-power view of a section of an entire ovary. The ovary is about twice normal size and is enveloped in the extremely thick fibrous capsule and adjacent cortical stroma as seen in this photograph.

low-power magnification in Figure 38-13. As can be seen in Figure 38-12, the ovaries are perhaps twice normal in size. The surface is markedly convoluted, and the ovaries are extremely firm. The firmness is due to great thickening of the capsule and adjacent cortical stroma, shown in Figure 38-13. The relation of this condition to fully developed fibromas is unknown, but the finding of such a condition on pelvic examination requires laparotomy to determine the nature of the enlargement. We have seen the condition occur unilaterally, but it is generally bilateral. True fibromas feel very solid and heavy; they are smooth-walled and usually more or less spherical (Fig. 38-14). Because of their weight, twisting is common.

Ascites is much more common with ovarian fibroids than with pedunculated uterine fibroids. Occasionally, abdominal ascites is accompanied by hydrothorax, giving rise to the symptom complex known as Meigs's syndrome, which is discussed later in this chapter. Fibromas are benign and usually unilateral. They are cured by simple oophorectomy, but when they occur in postmenopausal women—as they frequently do—there is no advantage in saving the opposite ovary. If the opposite ovary is to be left in, it should be inspected carefully for small surface papillary fibromas.

The Brenner tumor is the only other solid benign tumor worthy of mention; it is a rare type with gross characteristics that cannot be distinguished from those

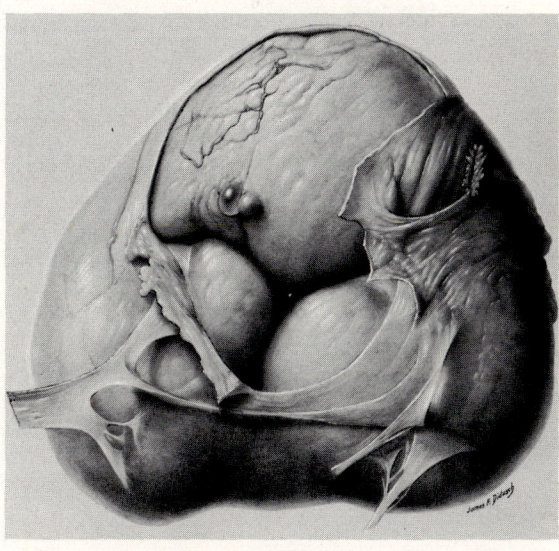

FIG. 38-14. Fibromyoma of ovary.

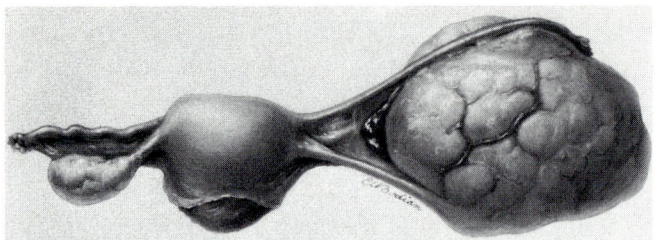

FIG. 38-15. Brenner tumor of ovary.

of the ordinary fibroma (Fig. 38-15). Microscopically, it appears like a simple fibroma through which are distributed islands of epidermoid-like cells (Fig. 38-16). The position of these deep-lying epithelial nests suggests malignancy, but under high-power magnification they do not appear malignant. Clinically, Brenner tumors are, in fact, benign and are cured by simple oophorectomy. Since they appear grossly like fibromas, most of them are removed under the assumption that they are such. When on microscopic examination epithelial elements are found deep in the fibrous growth, there is no cause for alarm, because a followup of patients from whom Brenner tumors have been removed by conservative surgery indicates that they are benign. Malignant change is primarily squamous in pattern.

MEIGS'S SYNDROME

In 1937 Meigs and Cass reported 7 cases of fibroma of the ovary associated with ascites and right hydrothorax. However, Spiegelberg was the first to report this syndrome in 1886, and Cullingworth (1879) and Tait (1891) reported similar cases. The condition is rare but important, because it points out the fact that it is possible for a solid ovarian tumor to be responsible for ascites and hydrothorax and yet be perfectly benign. Such a

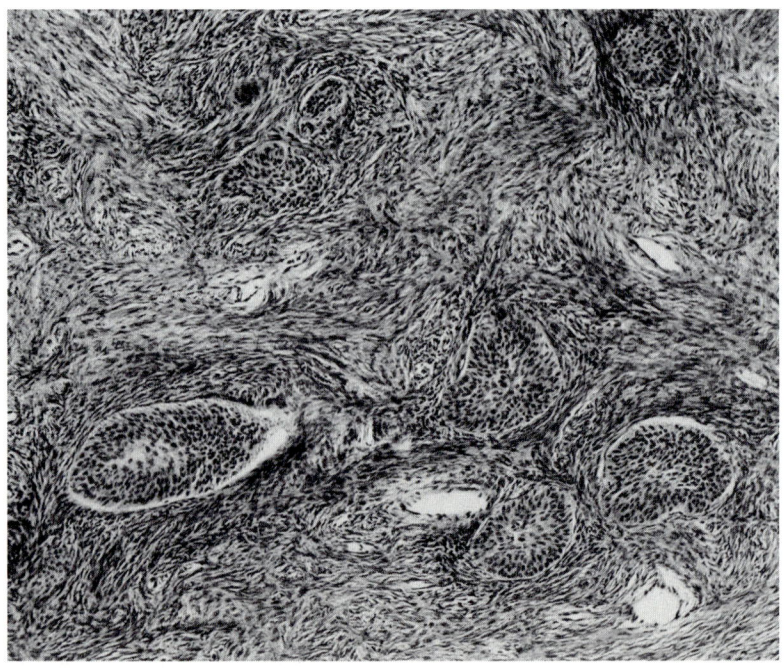

FIG. 38-16. Section of Brenner tumor. The islands of benign epithelium distinguish it from the ordinary fibroma.

symptom complex therefore calls for abdominal exploration, even though the chances are in favor of advanced malignancy. The syndrome has been defined as limited to (1) cases with fibroma, thecoma, granulosal cell tumors, and Brenner tumors; (2) ascites; (3) hydrothorax; (4) and cure after removal of the tumor. All of these tumors have one common characteristic—fibrous tissue in greater or lesser degree. Pure fibromas associated with fluid in the chest and the abdomen far outnumber the other types of tumors. It is true that some malignant ovarian tumors have been reported which were associated with ascites and clear straw-colored fluid in the chest. These should not be included in the true Meigs's syndrome, even though the cytologic examination of the chest fluid fails to reveal malignant tumor cells. The finding of undoubted malignant cells automatically rules out this syndrome.

The modus operandi of both the abdominal and the chest fluid is not clear. There is no evidence of inflammation of the serosa; pressure on lymphatics or veins does not seem likely because the fluid keeps forming even though the tumor is floating free in the ascitic fluid. Twisting of the pedicle does not seem to be the explanation, because no evidence of twisting is found at operation, and some of the tumors are large and wedged in the pelvis where twisting would be impossible. It has been suggested that these tumors by their very nature excrete fluid through their own lymphatics. Of course, this is not a real explanation but simply a hypothesis grasped at because all other explanations seem to have been excluded. The entrance of the fluid into the chest seems to be either through the diaphragmatic lymphatics or small openings in the diaphragm. The direction of flow of the fluid is from abdomen to chest, as has been proved by the introduction of India ink into the abdomen and later recovering it in the chest fluid. Ink introduced into the chest fluid will not go into the abdomen. Recently, Hodari and Hodgkinson demonstrated by lymphography that the thoracic duct and pulmonary lymphatics are involved with right hydrothorax, whereas the development of ascites occurs by another mechanism.

Since the tumors are benign, simple salpingo-oophorectomy cures the patient. The ascites and the pleural effusion promptly disappear and do not recur. If the patient is near or past the menopause, the uterus and the opposite adnexa should be removed. If the tumor is thought to be granulosal, one is confronted with the possibility of some degree of malignancy. A frozen section should be made after removing the unilateral ovary and tube. If it proves to be granulosal, the opposite adnexa and the uterus should be removed except in those cases in which future childbearing is a major concern. In such cases, bisection of the opposite ovary and meticulous evaluation of the pelvis and abdomen must assure the surgeon of the absence of residual disease.

PRIMARY SOLID CARCINOMA OF THE OVARY

Primary solid ovarian cancers present a host of microscopic patterns; classifications based upon microscopic structure are not uniform and are extremely confusing. In this work on operative gynecology we are not concerned with the details of histopathology, but with the gross characteristics of ovarian carcinomata so that they may be recognized at the operating table and treated properly. Figure 38-17 shows a solid ovarian cancer. Figure 38-18 is one of the many microscopic pictures of solid ovarian cancer. The fact that an ovarian tumor is solid should immediately cause the operator to suspect malignancy. However, the more firm the tumor, the more likely it is benign, such as the fibroma and Brenner tumor. In contrast, the semisolid tumors are more frequently malignant as their consistency is produced by areas of degeneration in proliferating tumor tissue. The surface of solid ovarian carcinomata may be perfectly smooth; more often, however, they are irregular

830 Adnexal Tumors

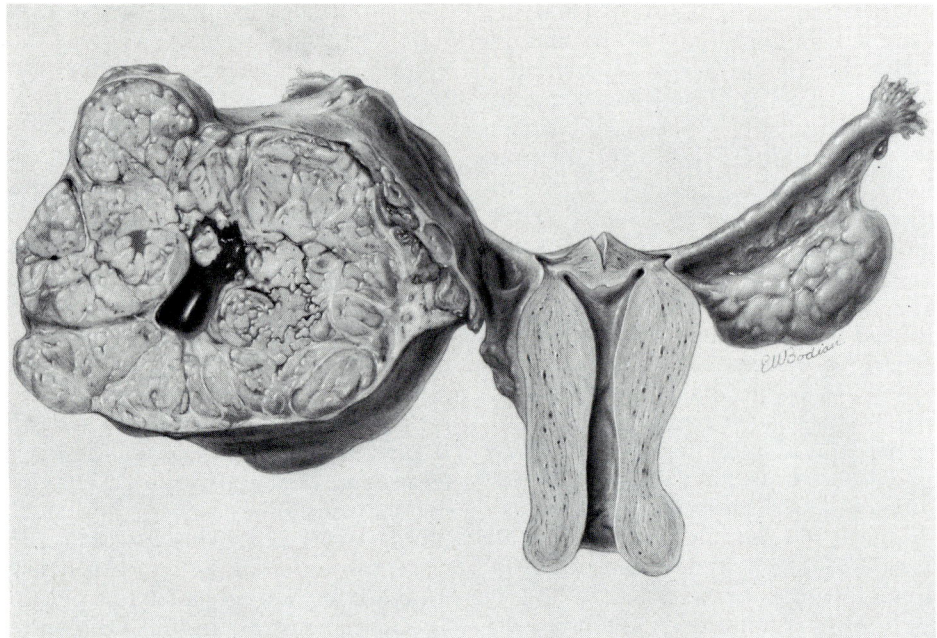

Fig. 38-17. Solid ovarian carcinoma. Although rather large, the tumor is still encapsulated.

and nodular due to outgrowths of the carcinoma through the original capsule. When in doubt about the malignant nature of a tumor, at times the decision can be made by a careful inspection of the pelvic structures for secondary growths. The omentum is a favorite place for metastases, and this fact justifies Mun-

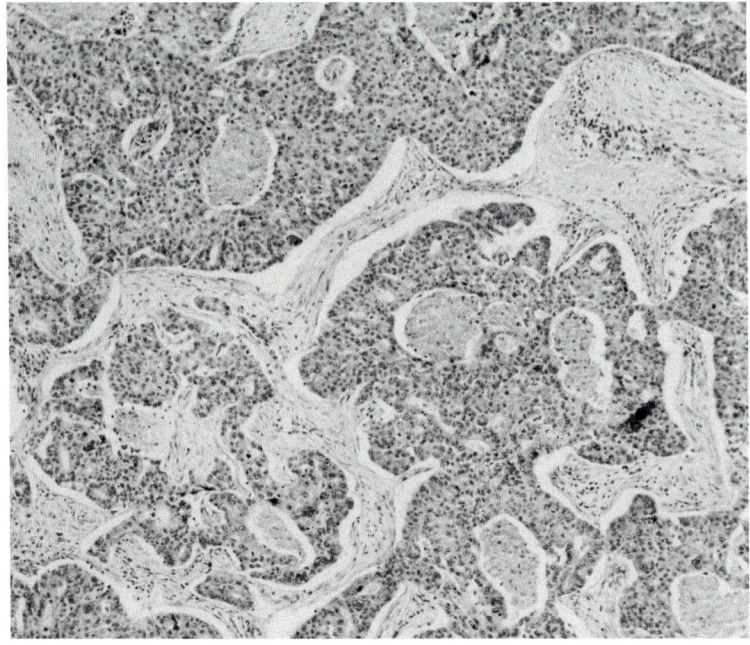

Fig. 38-18. Microscopic picture of solid ovarian carcinoma.

nell's routine removal of the omentum in all cases of ovarian carcinoma. Doubtful solid ovarian tumors should be opened in the operating room by an assistant. Although the cut surface in smaller tumors is frequently quite firm, by the time the carcinomata attain even moderate size, section usually discloses crumbling friable areas.

From the onset, solid ovarian carcinomata are often bilateral, and in advanced cases bilaterality occurred in 31 per cent of McKay and Sellers' series. Removal of both ovaries, the uterus, and omentum should be the established procedure in all solid ovarian carcinomas regardless of age, even though the opposite ovary appears to be entirely normal. We have found well-established microscopic carcinoma in the interior of the normal-appearing opposite ovary, tube, and omentum removed at operation, when the carcinoma seemed grossly to be unilateral. When feasible, a total hysterectomy is to be preferred to a subtotal.

PRIMARY CYSTIC CARCINOMA OF THE OVARY

Many cystic carcinomas of the ovary result from malignant changes in preexisting cystadenomas. As mentioned above, the incidence of malignant change in the serous cystadenomas varies between 30 and 50 per cent and is much greater than in the mucinous variety (5 to 12%). From these pathologic facts it is obvious that all cystadenomas should be considered as potentially malignant, especially those with papillomatous growths. Even though these tumors appear to be entirely benign, they should be opened in the operating room by an assistant and inspected carefully for grossly malignant areas. If the nature of the tumor is in doubt and one is considering conservative surgery, frozen sections may be made.

Clinically, the primary cystic carcinomas of the ovaries have been subdivided by Meyer into three main categories:

1. *Serous cystadenocarcinoma,* accounting for approximately 60 per cent of malignant ovarian tumors.
2. *Mucinous cystadenocarcinoma,* constituting 15 to 20 per cent of malignant ovarian tumors. Serous and mucinous tumors comprise 80 per cent or more of the malignant tumors of the ovaries.
3. *Carcinomas arising in a dermoid cyst,* usually squamous in type, which account for less than 1 per cent of malignant ovarian tumors.

An additional tumor has been added to this more traditional classification by the Cancer Committee of the International Federation of Gynecology and Obstetrics (F.I.G.O.) in 1964, which replaces the conventional list of malignant ovarian tumors with the following categorization:

1. *Serous cystomas,* benign and malignant.
2. *Mucinous cystomas,* benign and malignant.
3. *Endometrioid tumors,* benign and malignant.
4. *Unclassified tumors* (tumors which cannot be allotted to Groups 1, 2, or 3).

In addition to these carcinomata arising secondarily, there are tumors of the cystoadenomatous architecture which may be carcinomatous from the start (Ewing), all epithelial elements being unquestionably malignant (Figs. 38-19 and 38-20). In fact, the commonest malignancy of the ovary is the serous cystadenocarcinoma, 60 to 70 per cent. In some cases the tumor is almost a solid papillomatous growth with very little cystic portion. In others the cystic portion of the tumor predominates. The malignant papillomata are more friable than those of the benign cystadenomas and have a greater tendency to disseminate over the peritoneal surface. Unfortunately, they often grow painlessly, and the patient does not seek relief until abdominal enlargement is apparent.

Clinically and histologically, there seems to be every gradation of malignancy in these papillomatous tumors. On a few occasions we have observed extensive papillary implantation over the peritoneum, with extensive ascites sec-

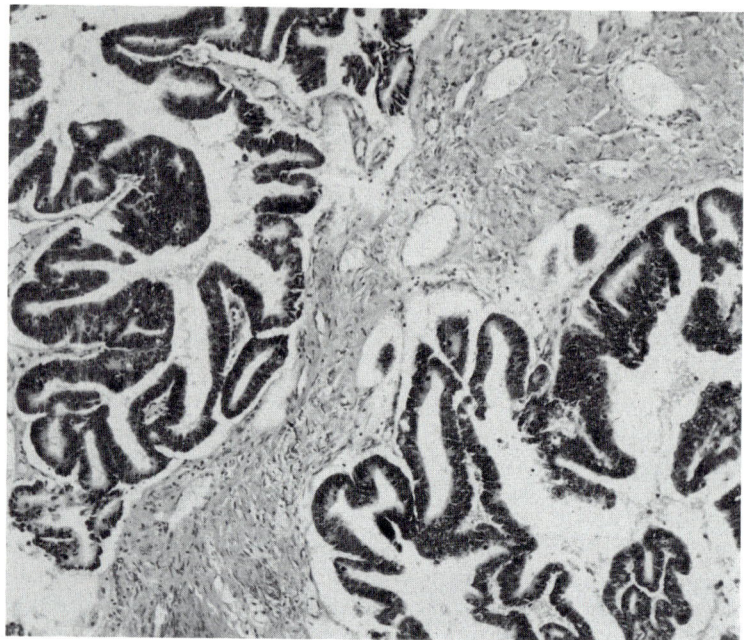

Fig. 38-19. Wall of serous cystadenocarcinoma of ovary.

ondary to papillary tumors of the ovaries, the whole picture appearing to be grossly typical of malignancy, only to find that microscopically the papillomata appeared to be surprisingly benign, and that the patient remained clincally well. Hence it is our custom to give all patients with symptoms suggesting disseminated papillary ovarian carcinoma the benefit of the doubt and to perform, if possible, a

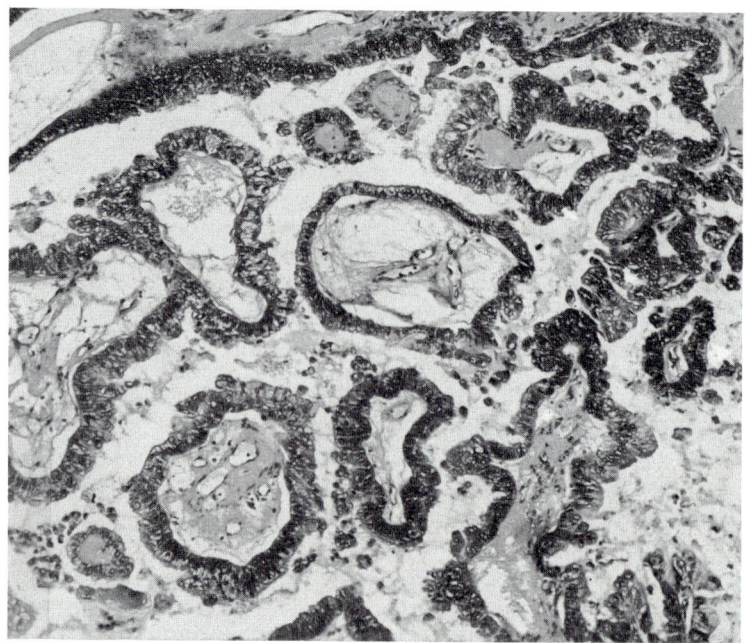

Fig. 38-20. Papillary serous cystadenocarcinoma of ovary.

complete operation with pelvic cleanout and omentectomy.

Endometrioid tumors, although a recent addition to the F.I.G.O. classification, have been discussed for many years since they were first described by Herxheimer in 1907. In 1952 Kottmeier reported that such tumors were more common than were usually recognized. In 1954 Dockerty applied the term *endometrial-like carcinoma* to a group of ovarian neoplasms. Thompson in 1957 reported 30 cases and added 70 of his own from the Ovarian Tumor Registry. Santesson has recently reviewed the experience of this tumor at the Radiumhemmet in 1,361 primary ovarian tumors, and confirms that these tumors are slow-growing and less malignant than other types of ovarian tumors. The present classification of endometrioid carcinoma is somewhat confusing and may overlap other histologic patterns. The tumor may be papillary, cystic, or solid in character, but the clinical course of the disease is primarily related to the degree of spread of the tumor at the time of its treatment.

CARCINOMA IN DERMOID CYSTS

Carcinoma in dermoid cysts is rare (1.8%) and usually occurs as the result of malignancy arising in the epidermoid elements (Peterson, 1957; Kelley and Skully, 1961). The clinical course, gross appearance of the tumor, and treatment are similar to that outlined for the other cystic carcinomas of the ovary.

METASTATIC OVARIAN CANCER

Metastatic ovarian cancer may be secondary to many primary tumors, but the most common sources are the breast, the uterus, and the gastrointestinal tract. The incidence of metastases to the ovary varies from 15 to 30 per cent. It may be impossible at the operating table to determine the origin of advanced carcinoma of the ovaries if they are involved in massive abdominal growths. The microscopic picture of the secondary cancer may reproduce that of the original growth; often, however, the histologic picture of the specimen obtained by biopsy is not sufficiently distinctive to permit one to form an opinion about its origin.

There is a special type of ovarian cancer, secondary usually to gastrointestinal neoplasm, known as the Krukenberg tumor, in which the cancer cells, regardless of their primary source, assume distinctive characteristics. Histologically, this type may appear to be more closely related to sarcoma than to carcinoma; the primary neoplasm certifies it as carcinoma. Signet-ring cells with eccentric nuclei are found in a fibrous or myxomatous stroma. Such tumors, which in the majority of cases are bilateral, are quite characteristic in their gross appearance (Fig. 38-21). They are solid and have a tendency to retain the general shape of ovaries, reproducing on a grand scale the surface convolutions seen in normal ovaries. Even when they have attained considerable size, they are apt to remain free, without attachment to surrounding structures. On gross section they appear to be fibrous or gelatinous. Surgically, the essential point to bear in mind when a tumor of such appearance is encountered is the necessity of exploring the intestinal tract, particularly the pylorus, for the primary tumor. The removal of these secondary tumors is usually simple, and if they are encountered at the operating table, they may be removed to relieve pelvic discomfort even though a cure of the malignancy is limited.

Today when oophorectomy is common in connection with carcinoma of the breasts, it is surprising how frequently carcinoma is found in the ovaries. Warren and Witham report ovarian metastases in 9 per cent of 162 cases of mammary carcinoma. Rarely, breast cancer in the ovaries will take the histologic form of the Krukenberg tumor, but in most instances the adenocarcinoma of the breast is reproduced in the ovarian metastases. These metastatic sites in the ovary are seldom solitary but only one of multiple metastases.

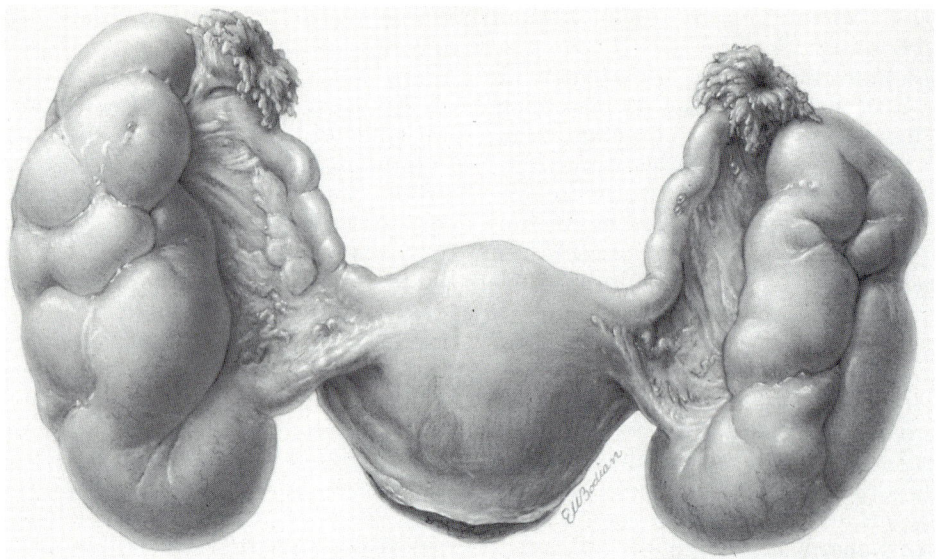

Fig. 38-21. Bilateral Krukenberg tumor secondary to carcinoma of the stomach.

SARCOMA

Sarcoma of the ovary is rare but may occur at any age. In the early stages the solid tumor may resemble the fibroma. Later, when it breaks through the capsule and becomes obviously malignant, it is difficult to distinguish it at the operating table from carcinoma. Sarcoma is much less apt to be bilateral than is carcinoma. The treatment is hysterectomy, with double salpingo-oophorectomy; the prognosis is poor.

TERATOMAS

Teratomas of the ovary are distinguished from dermoid cysts in that their elements are derived from all three germ layers. They are solid or semisolid. Teratomas may make their clinical appearance at any age, and a large proportion of them occur in children. Upon opening them, the presence of bone or cartilage usually indicates their identity. True teratomas are very malignant and recur in spite of radical surgery. Their response to irradiation is also poor. However, there are some less malignant tumors that should be classified as teratomas. Among these are the tumors that contain thyroid tissue. Small bits of thyroid tissue are not uncommon in dermoids, but in rare instances dermoids are found to contain large masses of thyroid tissue. From 5 to 10 per cent of struma ovarii are malignant, whereas only 1 to 3 per cent of cystic teratomas contain malignant tissue.

DYSGERMINOMAS

Dysgerminomas are rare ovarian tumors that were thought by Meyer to arise from undifferentiated gonads. They account for 1 to 5 per cent of all malignant ovarian tumors. Figure 38-22 shows a typical microscopic picture. They are solid growths, but, like other very cellular tumors, they frequently have softened areas due to degeneration. When small, they are well-encapsulated; the larger ones break through the capsule and show undoubted gross evidence of malignancy. Although on section they have a yellowish color, they may be very difficult to distinguish from other cellular ovarian tumors. One important clinical fact is that these tumors frequently occur in young women, while the mixed type of dysgerminoma, which contains malignant germ-cell elements, may occur in pseudohermaphrodites. The extremes of age in our laboratory reported by Novak are 6 to 38 years. Dysgerminomas always should be suspected when an ovarian tumor is discovered in a young, sexually underdeveloped woman. Since they so frequently occur during childhood, the question of surgical castration becomes a serious one.

Some tumors are of a rather low-grade malignancy, while others have been encountered that are highly malignant, particularly those tumors with admixed germ-cell elements. A unilateral salpingo-oophorectomy is probably permissible in very young women, when the *pure* tumor is small, although the Mayo group (Thoeny *et al.*) reports that of 14 patients who underwent conservative surgery, recurrence occurred in 6 cases (43%). Similarly, Pedowitz's experience in 70 cases followed for 5 years with a 27.1 per cent cure rate would warn the gynecologist of the seriousness of this ovarian tumor.

If there is evidence of breaking through of the capsule, hysterectomy and bilateral salpingo-oophorectomy are indicated, regardless of age. Although these tumors are generally quite radiosensitive, a 5-year survival rate of 35 per cent (Felmus and Pedowitz) suggests rapid spread of this tumor before symptoms are evident.

The widely divergent opinions concerning the conservative vs. the radical treatment of this tumor is related to the reported 5-year cure rates, which vary from 27 per cent (Pedowitz) to 86 per cent (Asadourian and Taylor). In an exhaustive study by de Lima from the Ovarian Tumor Registry in our laboratory, which includes 105 cases treated more than 5 years, the 5-year survival rate in the pure form was 73.4 per cent but only 27.3 per cent in the mixed tumors. Since the frequency of mixed tumors has been reported as high as 21 per cent (Santesson), one of the most important indications for radical treatment, including hysterectomy, adnexectomy, and postoperative irradiation, includes those tumors with an admixture of germ-cell elements. In view of the variable predictions for this tumor, our approach to this problem is to treat the patient conservatively when the

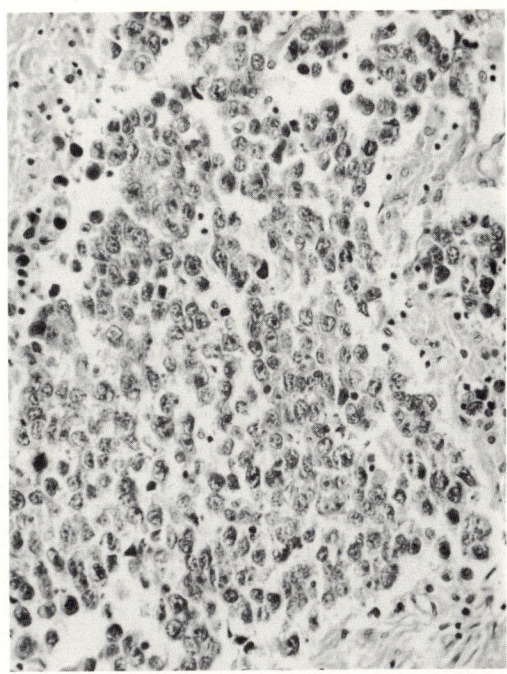

FIG. 38-22. Typical cellular structure of dysgerminoma.

tumor is small, unilateral, and well encapsulated, where biopsy of the opposite ovary is negative for metastases, and where the tumor is of the pure type. In all other instances, complete pelvic surgery and irradiation are indicated.

FUNCTIONING TUMORS OF THE OVARY

Feminizing Group

Granulosa cell carcinoma, thecoma, and luteoma comprise a group of functioning ovarian tumors that have a feminizing influence. The commonest of these three tumors is the granulosa cell tumor, and although the literature of the past several years has given much publicity to these tumors, they must be considered as relatively rare. They may produce precocious puberty in less than 5 per cent of such cases, including growth of breasts, growth of pelvic and axillary hair, development of the external genitalia and the uterus beyond the age of the child, and menstruation. When the tumor appears during the years of normal menstrual life, there is no change in the secondary sexual characteristics that already have developed completely, but often the menstrual cycle is disturbed in the form of excessive menstruation or long periods of amenorrhea. However, in some instances the menstrual cycle is unchanged. Postmenopausally, the tumors are often, though not always, associated with bleeding, and in some instances this bleeding is periodic, simulating normal menstruation. The postmenopausal uterus also grows and resumes a size comparable with that of a woman in her active menstrual life.

The effect of excessive estrogen on the endometrium usually creates the typical Swiss-cheese pattern of hyperplasia, both in menstruating and postmenopausal women. In some of the luteinized tumors progesterone as well as estrogen is secreted, and the effect on the endometrium is the formation of a decidua-like picture. When endometrial curettings show decidua-like changes without chorionic villi, the possibility of a luteinized feminizing tumor as well as the possibility of a tubal pregnancy must be considered. Mansell and Hertog noted a 15 per cent incidence of endometrial cancer associated primarily with thecomas, but Norris and Taylor have recently reported an incidence of 9 per cent for endometrial carcinoma and 22 per cent for varying degrees of adenomatous hyperplasia, although endometrial tissue was available for only one third of the patients in their study.

Granulosa cell tumors are usually of moderate size, but occasionally they have been reported of such size as almost to fill the abdomen (Plate 12, *top*). We have encountered tumors of microscopic size in routine histologic examination of the ovaries; the histories of the patients suggest that even these very small tumors are endocrinologically active. Although these tumors are usually solid, they are not as firm as fibromas. Often the tumors have a spongy feel as a result of the numerous cavities and areas of degeneration (Fig. 38-23). The tumor usually breaks through the capsule at a late stage in its development; however, some of the largest tumors are still perfectly encapsulated. On section, the

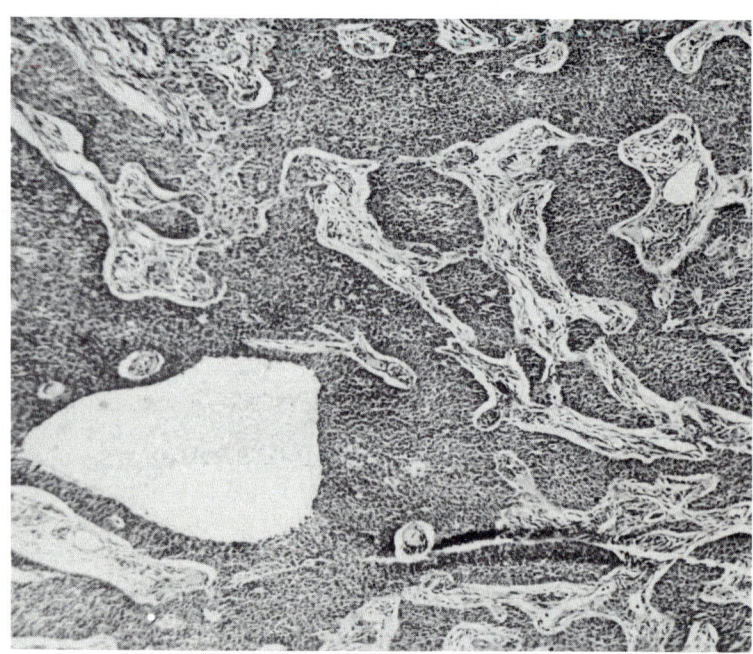

Fig. 38-23. Typical granulosa cell ovarian tumor.

granulosa cell tumors are generally grayish yellow in color and quite vascular.

The closely related theca cell tumors are generally firmer because of the presence of more fibrous tissue. Functionally, they cannot be distinguished from the true granulosa cell tumors. Many tumors contain both granulosa and theca components; in fact, many authors believe that all such tumors are in reality granulosa-thecomas.

Luteomas are considered by Novak and others to be simply granulosa cell tumors in which a certain amount of luteinization of the granulosa cells has taken place. The endometrium may show progesterone effect, although this is not always true. Grossly, the tumors can scarcely be distinguished from the granulosa tumors, but on section they have a more definite yellow color.

This entire group of feminizing tumors is to be regarded as malignant, although the experience of the majority of authors would indicate that they are not as malignant as most ovarian cancers. The 5-year cure rate is relatively high (68%, Kottmeier), but 11 per cent of Kottmeier's cases recurred 5 years or more following treatment. In the past few years we have seen recurrences 13, 16, and 20 years after the removal of the original tumor. A comparison of the recurrent tumor sections with those on file in our laboratory of the original growths indicates that the tumors were recurrences of the original ones removed. Furthermore, in one case in which the uterus had been left in at the first operation, the recurrence caused postmenopausal bleeding. In general, we believe that a complete pelvic operation should be done when the tumor is recognized at the operating table. Since the grade of malignancy is relatively low in many of these tumors, unilateral salpingo-oophorectomy is sometimes justifiable if the tumor occurs in a young girl. In a review of 203 patients with granulosa-thecoma tumors from the Armed Forces Institute of Pathology, Norris and Taylor noted that capsular and lymphatic invasion by the neoplasm were the primary features associated with persistence of the tumor, but that the type of treatment, the degree of cellular atypism, and mitotic activity were not.

Masculinizing Group

Arrhenoblastomas occur much less frequently than the feminizing tumors and are really among the rarest of ovarian neoplasms. Histologically, they are usually a combination of tubules and interstitial cells (Fig. 38-24). Those tumors in which the interstitial cells predominate usually produce the most marked masculinizing tumors. Arrhenoblastomas have been reported as occurring from the ages of 10 to 60 but are commonest in the decade of 20 to 30. Clinically, the patients first show signs of defeminization. The breasts atrophy, amenorrhea sets in, and there is a loss of subcutaneous fat, changing the body contour from the feminine to the masculine type. Later, true masculinization begins with the growth of an excessive amount of hair, hypertrophy of the clitoris, and a deepening of the voice. Urinary 17-ketosteroid levels are usually elevated above 15-20 mg./24 hr., which do not suppress completely with cortisone. The finding of an ovarian tumor in a woman with these remarkable changes should immediately cause one to suspect an arrhenoblastoma. At operation arrhenoblastomas are usually rather small, but tumors the size of grapefruit have been described. They are generally quite solid, although areas of degeneration may soften them in places. Even the larger tumors are well encapsulated. In spite of this, some of these tumors have proved to be malignant. However, like the granulosa cell tumors, they are in general less malignant than most ovarian cancers. One must be cautious in forming an opinion regarding the degree of malignancy, because so little time has elapsed since this rare tumor was recognized as a pathologic entity. Generally, total hysterectomy and bilateral adnexectomy should be done, but, as in granulosa cell tumors, when a small encapsulated tumor is found in a young individual, a unilateral salpingo-oophorectomy is permissible.

Adrenal tumors of the ovary are ex-

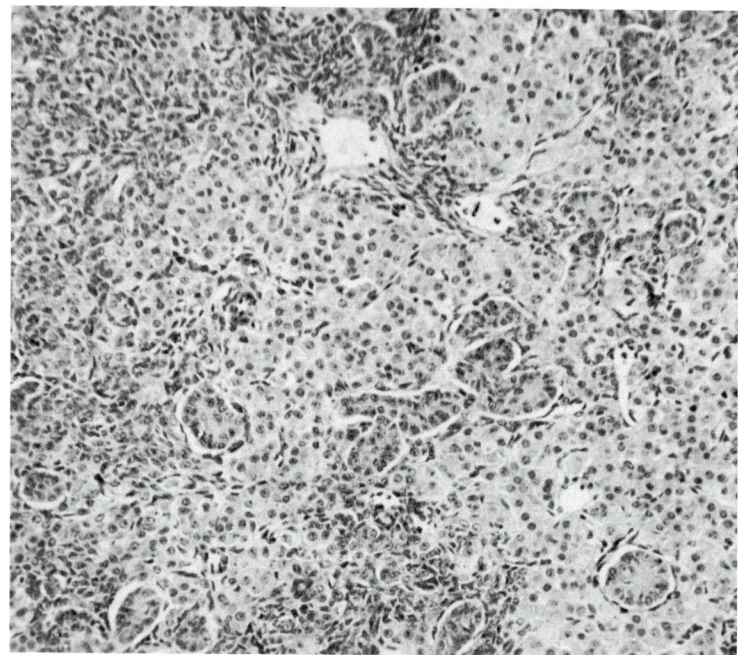

FIG. 38-24. Arrhenoblastoma, showing sections of tubules and lighter-staining interstitial cells.

tremely rare; a few have been reported that are histologically similar to adrenal cortex and are associated with masculinization.

GYNANDROBLASTOMA

In 1930 Robert Meyer suggested this name for a tumor composed of cells which were compatible with granulosa cell tumor and also arrhenoblastoma. The patient had evidence of masculinization and at the same time hypertrophy of the uterus. Since then several tumors have been described which resemble Meyer's histologically or clinically but few that satisfied both histologic and clinical requirements. The origin of these tumors is as uncertain as their contradictory hormonal manifestations. These tumors are mentioned briefly in this *Operative Gynecology* with the hope of alerting operating gynecologists so that with increased material for histologic, hormonal, and clinical study eventually a better understanding of these rare tumors may be forthcoming.

PAROVARIAN CYSTS

Parovarian cysts (Fig. 38-25) are not uncommonly encountered in gynecologic surgery. They arise from the vestigial remnant of the tubules of the wolffian body. In the mesosalpinx between the tube and hilum of the ovary, often one can see with good illumination the vestigial remnant of the main wolffian duct which runs more or less parallel with the tube and then curves inward and downward toward the uterus. It descends in the broad ligament parallel with the cervix and finally terminates at variable levels in the anterolateral portion of the vagina. The upper end of the wolffian duct may be dilated into cysts of Morgagni which lie near the fimbriated end of the tube. These cysts seldom give rise to clinical symptoms, but on rare occasions we have seen such a cyst twisted on its pedicle, causing acute pain and necessitating laparotomy. Coming off the main wolffian duct at right angles are several small ducts (the parovarium) within the broad ligament. From these, or from the main duct, cysts may arise which vary

Fig. 38-25. Typical parovarian cyst, thin-walled with prominent blood vessels in the wall.

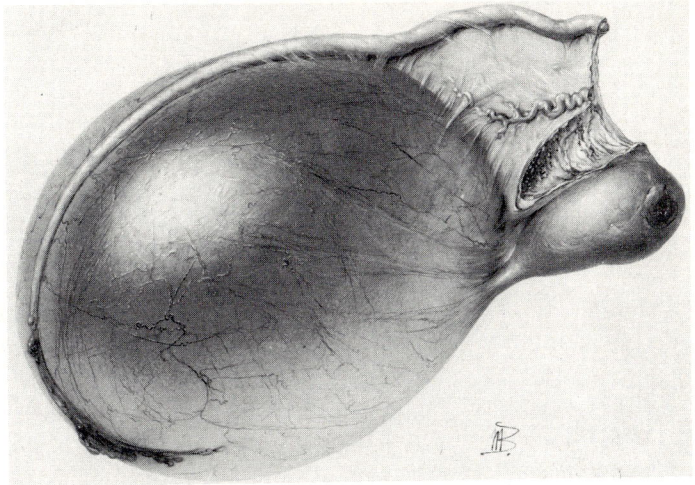

in size from 1 or 2 cm. to an enormous size, filling the abdomen like a huge ovarian cyst. The very large cysts are rare. The parovarium cyst is usually thin-walled (Plate 12, *bottom*) and easily identified by its position within the leaves of the broad ligament, with the tube lying stretched over it. To identify it further, the ovary is found intact or flattened out on the side of the cyst. Parovarian cysts are usually unilocular and filled with clear straw-colored fluid. Very rarely do they have a papillary tendency, and we have encountered malignancy on only one occasion.

BILATERAL POLYCYSTIC OVARIES: STEIN-LEVENTHAL SYNDROME

Polycystic ovaries have been recognized clinically for many years, but it remained for Stein and Leventhal in 1935 to correlate this ovarian picture with a clinical syndrome. The ovaries are usually enlarged from 2 to 3 times normal size, but in some cases the enlargement is very slight. The ovaries are smooth, lacking the wrinkled appearance of normal ovaries; they are whitish in color, due to the thickened fibrotic capsule and contain multiple follicular cysts (thecalutein cysts) (Fig. 38-26). At first there was considerable skepticism about the existence of this syndrome, but increased experience has convinced most gynecologists that it is a clinical entity and does respond to therapy. The symptom most commonly present is secondary amenorrhea. After puberty the periods may be quite regular for a time, or there may be periods of menometrorrhagia. Then the menstrual intervals become lengthened, and the flow becomes scantier. Long periods of amenorrhea usually develop eventually. Since there is failure of ovulation, sterility is inevitable as long as the ovarian condition remains unchanged. Basal temperature charts and endometrial biopsies confirm the lack of ovulation. Hirsutism may be present in 25 per cent of the cases. Instead of amenorrhea, menometrorrhagia may be present. Obesity, underdevelopment of the breasts, and acne may be part of the picture. In short, the picture is that of a sexually unattractive girl with an abnormal menstrual pattern.

The basal metabolic rate is usually normal. The 17-ketosteroids are slightly elevated in 25 per cent of the cases. The basal temperature does not show the rise noted with ovulation and should be recorded for a period of time for comparison after treatment. Endometrial biopsies show no evidence of ovulation.

The ovarian enlargement cannot be determined satisfactorily in many cases by bimanual examination. Stein reports

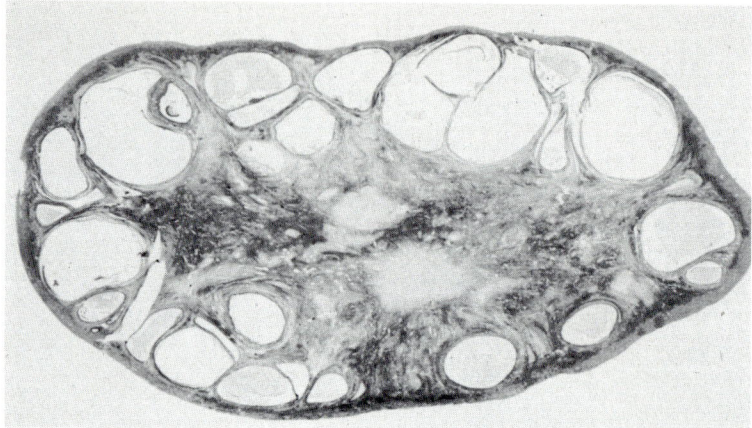

Fig. 38-26. Typical follicular cystic ovary from a woman with Stein-Leventhal syndrome.

that in over one half of his cases the bimanual examination failed to demonstrate enlarged ovaries when they were actually present. Obesity may be responsible for this in many cases, although Stein states that not over 15 per cent of the women in his cases were classified as obese. To determine the size of the ovaries Stein advocates gynecography and especially pneumoroentgenography. In our clinic we have preferred culdoscopy or laparoscopy, perhaps because we are more experienced with these procedures than with pneumoroentgenography, but they do have the advantage of allowing one to determine the absence of a corpus luteum, which is important for a diagnosis of this syndrome.

Treatment

Until recently Stein and his associates believed that there was no therapy for this condition except surgery. Stein practices wedge resection of the ovaries, removing approximately 50 per cent of the ovarian cortex and medulla. The edges of the remaining ovarian tissue are then approximated with fine catgut (Fig. 38-27). Other unsuccessful surgical procedures that have been used include splitting of the ovary, decapsulation, and multiple punctures. The purpose of these procedures is stated to be decompression of the ovaries to permit ovulation. Such procedures do not alter the fundamental physiology of the ovary. The wedge-shaped resection is merely a quantitative removal of part of the abnormally functioning ovarian tissue, which decreases the production of androgens and estrogens by the stimulated ovarian stroma (leutinized theca). The reduction of plasma androgen level (lowered 17-ketosteroid level) thus releases the suppressive influence of such hormones on the hypothalamus. The release of follicle-stimulating hormone (FSH) and luteinizing hormone (LH) from the anterior pituitary results in cyclic ovulation. If there are no other infertility factors present, pregnancy will occur in 75 to 85 per cent of the cases.

It is probably best to consider Stein's results, because one can be sure that his cases have been selected with great adherence to the proper criteria. A return to normal menstrual cycle was the rule, and of 62 married patients, 88.7 per cent became pregnant. One cannot help wondering what the percentage of pregnancies would have been without therapy. For example, we have had the opportunity of observing a woman with this syndrome over a number of years without surgical treatment. Observation and biopsy of the ovaries were possible in the course of an appendectomy. Histologic examination of the ovary confirmed the diagnosis. After 15 years of marriage and

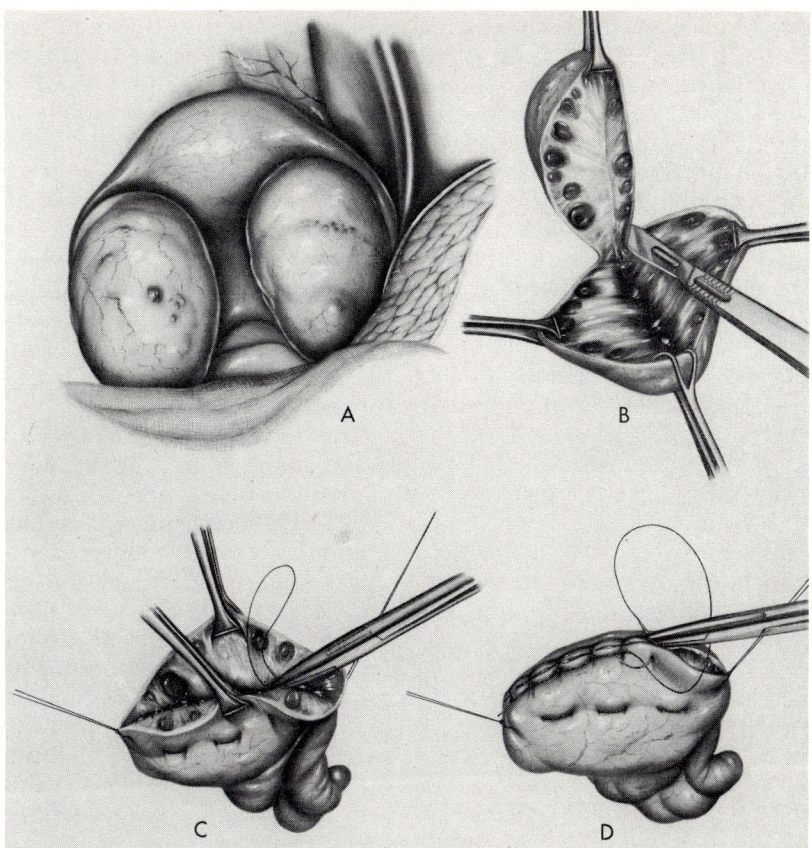

Fig. 38-27. (A) Large polycystic ovaries, nearly equal to the size of uterine fundus, with thickened, white, fibrotic capsule through which several follicular cysts may be seen. (B) Wedge resection of Stein ovary, removing nearly one half of the ovarian tissue, with the resection including the medullary portion of the ovary. Note the thickened capsule and the multiple theca-lutein cysts. (C) Double layer closure of wedged ovary with a continous horizontal mattress suture of No. 000 chromic catgut as the initial layer approximating the medulla of the ovary. (D) Continuous locking suture to approximate the cortex and ovarian capsule.

several years after all attempts at therapy had been given up, she became pregnant and had a normal child. Such instances refute Stein's premise that ovulation never occurs in these patients and support instead the views of others that gonadotropin release (FSH and LH) may occur in sufficient amounts to stimulate ovulation spontaneously, although admittedly this must be infrequent in the untreated patient. Stein also reports that 89.3 per cent of 75 patients operated on had normal menstrual function restored. Growth of the hypoplastic uterus was noted by these authors after surgical treatment, but hirsutism was not usually affected favorably.

The pathophysiology of this entity is therefore hormonal in nature and may result from an inbalance of the FSH and LH gonadotropin release mechanism in the hypothalamus. Ingersoll and McArthur demonstrated an increased amount of LH in the urine of such patients, which explains the histologic picture of excessive theca cell stimulation and luteinization in the ovary with increased androgen and occasionally increased estrogen excretion. The reduction of adrenal androgen by cortisone therapy is frequently sufficient to trigger ovulation in such patients without surgery.

However, a more effective method of medical treatment has recently been demonstrated by Kistner and others with the use of clomiphene citrate. This compound is known to enhance the release of FSH and LH and will produce ovulation effectively in such patients by the use of 50-100 mg./day for 5 days each month. One complication must be continuously observed, namely, the hyperstimulation of these cystic ovaries, which reportedly have ruptured, with intra-abdominal hemorrhage. The other disadvantage of the use of clomiphene is the fact that the syndrome usually recurs if the medication is not continued each month.

Our personal results with wedge resection in carefully chosen cases of Stein-Leventhal syndrome have been most gratifying. We have had the satisfaction very recently of seeing one of our treated cases request sterilization after her 3rd cesarean section.

TREATMENT OF OVARIAN CANCER

General Considerations

Since the first edition of this textbook there has been little progress in the early diagnosis and treatment of ovarian cancer. Carcinoma of the ovary is currently the 4th leading cause of death from malignancy in women, exceeded only by carcinoma of the breast, large bowel, and cervix uteri. In the State of New York and in Ontario the ovarian cancer death rate has exceeded the rate for cancer of the cervix. The overall 5-year survival rate reported in the literature during the past 5 years varies from 18 to 37 per cent. It is important to recall that this lethal disease accounts for 8 to 15 per cent of all genital malignancies after the age of 45, and that 15 per cent of all ovarian tumors are frankly malignant. Since the development of ovarian cancer is both insidious and clinically silent, the early detection of this disease is usually accidental and can only be improved by the routine gynecologic examination of asymptomatic women. The use of prophylactic ovarian ablation against ovarian cancer is discussed in Chapter 8 on Myomata Uteri and would seem advisable in the menopausal and postmenopausal patient undergoing pelvic surgery.

The most common symptoms of ovarian cancer include abdominal enlargement, abdominal pain, and abnormal bleeding. Approximately 10 per cent of our patients with ovarian cancer have been totally asymptomatic and were detected on routine pelvic examination. In Morton's series, 11 of 69 patients with ovarian cancer (16%) were totally missed until the abdomen was opened for some other indication.

The differential diagnosis of ovarian enlargement is one of the most difficult of all gynecologic problems. Distinguishing between ovarian enlargement due to a neoplasm or an enlargement due to a physiologic ovarian cyst requires experience and skill in clinical judgment. Retention or physiologic cysts will usually regress spontaneously and are usually seen in young patients where immediate removal without clinical observation would be contraindicated. Such retention cysts, usually thin-walled, are often easily compressible, but at times they are tense. A thicker-walled, semisolid cyst is more frequently neoplastic and is particularly suspicious where the surface is irregular and the tumor adherent. The more firm the tumor, the more likely it is to be a benign fibroma. Nodularity of the cul-de-sac or uterosacral ligaments in the presence of a suspicious adnexal mass must be differentiated from endometriosis but is also one of the hallmarks of ovarian cancer. In addition, the patient's age is an important factor in evaluating ovarian tumors since the highest incidence of ovarian cancer occurs between the ages of 55 and 65. During early adulthood, physiologic cysts of the ovary are quite common while malignant tumors, although occasionally present, are infrequent. In contrast, cystic enlargement of the ovary in a menopausal or postmenopausal patient cannot be considered to be a physiologic event but must be approached as a malignancy until proven to be benign. In the young female, such an ovarian cyst of greater than 6 cm.

would be followed conservatively at monthly intervals, and if it should not regress within 2 months, a laparotomy is indicated. In the older female, however, any clinically suspicious ovarian enlargement should be investigated surgically without delay. When considerable doubt exists regarding the nature of the ovarian tumor, culdoscopy or colpotomy may be helpful in making the decision. Cul-de-sac aspiration as advocated by Graham may be helpful in detecting early ovarian cancers where there is adnexal pathology.

The prognosis of ovarian cancer is based on three main factors: (1) the clinical stage of the disease, (2) the histologic type, and (3) the cellular differentiation. As previously stated, approximately 85 per cent of the malignant ovarian tumors consist of three histologic types: serous cystadenocarcinoma, mucinous cystadenocarcinoma, and solid adenocarcinoma. The more undifferentiated the cell type, the more infrequent is the cure.

Clinical Staging

In the past, comparisons of methods of therapy of ovarian cancer have been difficult due to lack of uniformity in precise staging of ovarian cancer. Clinical staging requires an accurate evaluation of the extent of the tumor growth at the time of exploratory laparatomy and prior to treatment of the disease. Consequently, cases that are not operated or are treated initially with irradiation cannot be accurately staged.

There have been many clinical classifications of ovarian tumors in the past. Heyman (1930) developed a classification according to the adequacy of the surgical removal of the disease. This was later adopted by the Iowa group but unfortunately includes group III, characterized as "recurrence after surgery or irradiation," which contradicts one of the primary purposes of staging of the tumor prior to treatment. Numerous additional classifications have been proposed, and a comparison of the more frequently quoted classifications is included in Table 38-1. In 1965 the International Federation of Gynecology and Obstetrics adopted clinical staging, which, if uniformly adopted in the future, will standardize the staging of ovarian cancer in future reports. On comparison of Munnell and Taylor's classification with the F.I.G.O. classification (Table 38-2), one will note that the F.I.G.O. classification is staged lower than the Munnell and Taylor method.

Primary Surgery

The surgical approach to the treatment of ovarian cancer remains the most effective method available at the present time. While the extent of the surgery depends on the spread of the tumor and the clinical stage of the disease, the most effective treatment includes hysterectomy, bilateral salpingo-oophorectomy and omentectomy. A total hysterectomy is preferred to subtotal, but in some instances when the tumors are fixed and the operation difficult, it is wise to do the lesser operation rather than to increase the operative risk by removing the cervix. In such cases when the neoplasm has infiltrated surrounding structures so that the operation is obviously incomplete anyway, the removal of the cervix does not influence the ultimate prognosis.

Inasmuch as the omentum is the most common site for implantations and metastases of ovarian cancer, Pemberton was an early advocate of omentectomy as a routine procedure in all cases of ovarian malignancy. Not only is omentectomy advisable in reducing the incidence of recurrent ascites, but it is beneficial in Stage I ovarian cancers for histologic study to evaluate the possibility of microscopic spread of the disease to the upper abdomen. Such histologic confirmation immediately changes the classification from a Stage I lesion to a Stage III lesion (F.I.G.O.) and provides a more accurate assessment of the extent of the disease. Munnell noted an improvement in his 5-year cure rate in advanced cases from 11 per cent to 27 per cent by this procedure. Removing the uterus and the opposite adnexa is important because of the rapid spread of the tumor to the opposite ovary as well as the lymphatics of the broad ligament, fallopian tube, and uterine wall.

TABLE 38-1. CLASSIFICATION OF CANCER OF THE OVARY BY CLINICAL EXTENT*

HEYMAN (KEETTEL)	RUTLEDGE AND BURNS	KOTTMEIER (F.I.G.O.)	MUNNELL AND TAYLOR
I. Surgical removal of entire primary (intact).	IA. One ovary involved. IB. Both ovaries involved.	I. Growth limited to the ovaries. Ia. Growth limited to one ovary, no ascites. Ib. Growth limited to both ovaries, no ascites. Ic. Growth limited to one or both ovaries, ascites present with malignant cells in the fluid.	I. One ovary involved.
IIA. Entire removal but with spill. IIB. Complete removal with questionable remaining pelvic metastases.	IIA. Ovaries removed but pelvic metastases. IIB. Pelvic metastases with or without oophorectomy.	II. Growth involving one or both ovaries with pelvic extension. IIa. Extension and/or metastases to the uterus and/or tubes only. IIb. Extension to other pelvic tissues.	II. Both ovaries involved.
III. Recurrence after surgery or irradiation.	IIIA. Abdominal metastases, primary removed. IIIB. Metastases outside peritoneal cavity.	III. Growth involving one or both ovaries with widespread intraperitoneal metastases to the abdomen.	III. Extension to any pelvic tissue.
IV. Inoperable.	IVA. Inoperable, biopsy only. IVB. No operation.	IV. Growth involving one or both ovaries with distant metastases outside the peritoneal cavity. Special category: Unexplored cases which are thought to be ovarian carcinoma.	IV. Abdominal extension.

*Munnell, E. W.: The changing prognosis and treatment in cancer of the ovary. A report of 235 patients with primary ovarian carcinoma, 1952–1961. Amer. J. Obstet. Gynec., *100*:791, 1968.

The most recent report of Munnell (1968) compares the current treatment of 235 patients of primary ovarian carcinoma between 1952 and 1961 with the original reports of 348 previous cases treated during 1921–51. The improved 5-year cure rate of 40 per cent was the principal result of aggressive maximum surgery utilized in the later group of patients as well as the use of postoperative radiotherapy.

The inoperability rate for ovarian cancer varies from one clinic to another, depending on the surgical experience of the operator and his enthusiasm for technically difficult surgery. Even though it is impossible to remove both ovaries and the uterus because of the extent of the disease, it is important to remove the bulk of the tumor where possible in an effort to reduce the patient's symptoms,

TABLE 38-2. COMPARISON OF CLASSIFICATIONS OF OVARIAN CANCER ACCORDING TO CLINICAL EXTENT OF DISEASE*

CLINICAL EXTENT	MUNNELL AND TAYLOR CLASSIFICATION	(F.I.G.O.) INTERNATIONAL CLASSIFICATION†
One ovary involved	I	Ia
Both ovaries involved	II	Ib
One or both ovaries involved as well as other pelvic organs or peritoneum	III	II
Ovary(ies) involved plus upper abdominal organs or peritoneum	IV	III

* Munnell, E. W.: *Ibid.*
† F.I.G.O. Ic omitted as well as F.I.G.O. breakdown of II into IIa and IIb.

particularly recurrent ascites, as well as to improve the response of the patient to additional therapy, including irradiation and/or chemotherapy.

IRRADIATION THERAPY

There is current interest in preoperative irradiation which stems from a report of Long, Johnson, and Sala (1967), who obtained 8-year survivals in 8 patients with extensive inoperable ovarian cancer; these patients received 5,000 rads tumor dose after an exploratory laparotomy and then had definitive pelvic surgery sometime later. Currently this program is under clinical trial for Stage II and III ovarian carcinomas by Vaeth and Buschke at the San Francisco Medical Center.

Recent advances in supervoltage irradiation therapy have improved the effectiveness of this method of treatment of ovarian cancer. Although there are conflicting reports in the literature concerning this subject, the greatest value of adjunct irradiation appears to be in the treatment of residual tumor confined to the pelvis (F.I.G.O., Stage IIb, or Munnell and Taylor, Stage III). Although Latour and Davis were unconvinced of the value of postoperative irradiation in advanced ovarian carcinoma, their technic of treatment included orthovoltage (220 Kv) with a tumor dose of only 3,000 rads to the pelvis. Similarly, MacKay and Sellers found no statistical difference in survival rates after complete or incomplete operation with cobalt or x-ray therapy as compared to surgery alone. Once again, the irradiation dosage is not included in their report. However, Kottmeier's experience at the Radiumhemmet has shown a definite improvement of the 5-year survival rate for ovarian carcinoma from 6.8 per cent without irradiation to 23.2 per cent survival with irradiation. The experience at Memorial Hospital as reported by Kaufman demonstrates a definite prolongation of life in irradiated patients with Stage III and Stage IV disease. Perhaps the most impressive evaluation of the effect of postoperative irradiation on ovarian carcinoma is included in Munnell's recent report of 235 cases of ovarian cancer between 1952 and 1961 from Columbia-Presbyterian Hospital. In comparing this recent series with the cases from two previous series of 1922–43 and 1945–51, there was a 5-year survival rate of 40 per cent in the recent series as compared to a 27.5 per cent and 29 per cent cure in the previous reports. There was essentially a similar distribution of cases by clinical staging among the three periods of study, and only the last series of cases received x-ray therapy routinely. Prior to 1952 only about half of the cases received x-ray therapy, while following 1952, 76 per cent received postoperative radiotherapy. The use of postoperative irradiation therapy for advanced cancer with dissemination in the upper abdomen will result in few 5-year cures. Because of the fact that one can treat the abdomen with only 3,000 rads without injury to the bowel and kidney, such treatment can be considered only palliative. In addition, postsurgical irradiation is not without complication. In the Memorial series, 49 per cent of the irradiated group subsequently developed intestinal obstruction, whereas obstruction occurred in only 11 per cent of the patients who did not receive irradiation.

The use of radioactive istopes, primarily radioactive gold in the peritoneal cavity, has improved the cure rates of Stage I ovarian cancer in Keettel's series and is reportedly useful in decreasing recurrent ascites. However, this modality of therapy is not useful with large and resectable masses of tumor and is not without complications—within our own clinic we have seen several instances of pocketing of the radioactive isotopes among loops of bowel with rather marked injury to the bowel wall (Fig. 38-28) or proctitis—and is not widely used.

CHEMOTHERAPY

The primary purpose of chemotherapy in the treatment of ovarian cancer must be considered palliative at the present time rather than a primary treatment. The degree of palliation depends on the type of the tumor and the extent of the disease. In addition to the use of chemotherapy in those cases that are unsuitable for surgery and irradiation, it is more frequently used as an adjunct to partial surgery where residual tumor is left in the abdomen and pelvis. In addition, it is currently being used simultaneously with irradiation therapy because of the radiomimetic effect of the drug, which causes increased tissue sensitivity to irradiation. The alkylating agents appear to be the most effective in this respect. Finally, prophylactic chemotherapy has been utilized in recent years to prevent tumor recurrence after apparently complete tumor removal or intraperitoneal spill of the tumor contents at the time of surgery.

Four major categories of chemotherapeutic agents, based on their common cytotoxic effects, are used in the treatment of gynecologic malignancies:

1. Alkylating agents
    Mechlorethamine (nitrogen mustard)
    Triethylenethiophosphoramide (Thiotepa or TSPA)
    Chlorambucil (Leukeran)
    Cyclophosphamide (Cytoxan, Endoxan)
    L-Phenylalanine mustard (Medphalan, L-sarcolysin, PAM, Alkeran)
2. Antimetabolites
    a. Folic acid analogues
        Amethopterin (methotrexate)
        Aminopterin
    b. Pyrimidine and purine analogues
        5-Fluorouracil
        6-Mercaptopurine
3. Antibiotics
    Dactinomycin (actinomycin D)
4. Plant alkaloids
    Vinblastine
    Vincristine

The alkylating agents derive their name from their ability to disrupt the DNA molecule by binding an alkyl group to a receptor substance, which leads to disruption of the DNA strands and crosslinking. The antimetabolites interfere with the normal metabolic activity of a cell by inhibiting or competing with enzyme systems. The antibiotics and plant alkaloids respectively act pri-

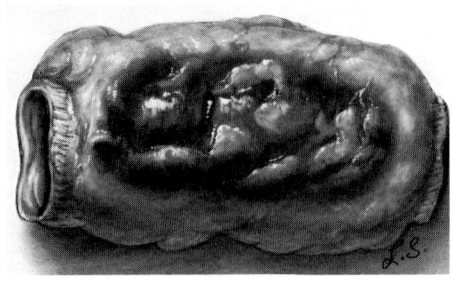

FIG. 38-28. Gangrenous section of transverse colon caused by pocketing of radioactive gold.

marily on the DNA molecule and arrest mitosis.

The most frequently used chemotherapeutic agents for the treatment of ovarian cancer are the alkylating agents and antimetabolites. The initial use of systemic alkylating agents for ovarian carcinoma was first demonstrated in 1952 by Rundles and Barton. Since 1959 the long-acting alkylating agents, parenteral thiotepa (thiophosphoramide) and oral chlorambucil (Leukeran) have been shown to produce a 30 to 70 per cent temporary ovarian cancer response. Although Kaufman concluded that there is probably no single preferable alkylating agent, the recent reports from M. D. Anderson Hospital by Rutledge and Burns with the use of phenylalanine mustard (PAM) have been most encouraging. When used either parenterally or orally, experience with PAM in 213 advanced ovarian cancers at the M. D. Anderson Hospital has revealed a 50 per cent response in the control of ascites, reduction of tumor mass, and symptomatic relief. Of special interest was the response of 13 patients with inoperable ovarian cancer who were treated with PAM and later explored for evaluation of the status of the disease. In each of these patients no residual tumor was found, and chemotherapy was discontinued. Two of these cases in whom the disease later recurred, 26 and 38 months, respectively, after the agent was discontinued, have again responded to the agent. This drug has been used in 213 cases both alone and in combination with x-ray therapy. Of the 50 per cent responders, there was either a 50 per cent regression in the measurable size of the tumor or a 50 per cent reduction in the serous effusion. Although Masterson and Nelson observed tumor regression in 140 (50%) of 280 patients treated with chlorambucil for 6 months or longer, this response was only temporary, for in time all of the cases showed recurrent disease. In addition, there was a 5 per cent incidence of serious toxicity resulting from utilizing 0.2 mg./kg./day.

Recently, the *combined* use of thiotepa and methotrexate has been reported by Greenspan from Mt. Sinai Hospital. In a series of 103 patients with ovarian carcinoma with advanced disease, 96 patients received 2 or more courses of methotrexate and thiotepa. Therapy was maintained for as long as $4\frac{1}{2}$ years, and the treatment was usually initiated 1 week after laparotomy. A loading dose of thiotepa consisted of 15 mg./q.i.d., and an average daily dose of methotrexate ranged from 5 mg. to 12 mg., administered orally in divided 2.5 mg. dosages until stomatitis appeared. The aim was gradually to produce toxic manifestations and yet avoid severe hematopoietic depression by abruptly stopping the drug at the first sign of toxicity. Maintenance thiotepa dosage of 15 mg. I.M. once per week was continued on the 3rd week after the initial treatment. There was gradual increase in the methotrexate and thiotepa dosages as tolerated. Of all adequately treated cases, 73 per cent showed significant objective tumor regression. Rapid objective regression for 6 months or longer was induced in two thirds of all the patients treated. This response was particularly noted among most of the postoperative Stage IV serous cystadenocarcinoma patients.

In considering the palliative use of chemotherapeutic agents for the treatment of advanced ovarian cancer, there are some general considerations which must be stated. In using such severely cytotoxic agents, one must be thoroughly versed in the natural history of the disease because the odds of prolonging life comfortably must be weighed against any ill effects of the complications of the treatment, namely, severe bone-marrow depression with resultant infection and possible death; severe gastrointestinal toxicity ranging from stomatitis to metabolic complications from diarrhea; alopecia, particularly with Cytoxan, and neuropathies. At present there are few 5-year survivals with chemotherapeutic agents, and therefore one must expect a recurrence of the disease.

Chemotherapy should be supervised by individuals properly trained in the use of these agents. Finally, one must maintain the dignity of the individual at the end-stage of the disease process. It may be considered inhumane for every patient with metastatic ovarian cancer to be given a "trial" of a toxic chemotherapeutic drug at the very terminal stage of the disease. A 3-month palliation period is not necessarily advantageous to the patient, particularly if, in addition to the discomfort of the disease, the physician produces a negative nitrogen balance in the patient, a partial or pancytopenia, or a disintegration of the gastrointestinal mucosa. Physicians must recognize man's right to live and die peacefully; otherwise life-preserving treatment may become a scientific weapon for the prolongation of agony.

SPECIAL CONSIDERATIONS

Intraperitoneal Spillage of Malignant Ovarian Cysts. While there is much confusion about the implications of intraperitoneal spillage at the time of surgery of ovarian cancer, there is evidence in Munnell's recent study that this accident produces no adverse effects in Stages I and II (F.I.G.O. Ia and Ib). Accidental rupture of malignant cysts does occur rather frequently, as reported in Grogan's study of 124 patients: in this group there was abdominal spillage in 12.9 per cent. Of the 16 cases reported, 9 patients were from Stage I lesions while 7 patients included Stage III and IV tumors. The probability of seeding metastases and so compromising life expectancy was not supported in Grade 1, Stage I lesions. In the advanced lesions, no disadvantage of this accident could be statistically documented. Similarly, Turner *et al.* noted 11.2 per cent with accidental rupture of an ovarian cyst at the time of surgical removal, and 9 of the 19 patients were reported living 5 to 11 years following laparotomy. Such reports verify our clinical experience that the recurrence of ovarian cancer in the pelvis is directly related to the cellular type and histologic grade of the tumor as well as the clinical stage of the disease at the time of treatment.

The Second-Look Operation. The second-look procedure was initiated at the University of Minneapolis in 1948 in patients who originally had cancers of the stomach, rectum, or colon with metastases to the regional lymph nodes. It was later extended to evaluate other tumors, including ovarian malignancies, approximately 6 months after the original operation. Of 14 patients who were re-explored for persistent ovarian carcinoma, Gilbertsen and Wangensteen noted that 3 of 14 patients survived for 38, 45, and 147 months following the 2nd operative procedure. This procedure is specifically valuable in patients who are inoperable at the time of initial laparotomy and who respond well to either irradiation or chemotherapy or a combination of both. A second look following such therapy is frequently rewarding, and surgical removal of the tumor is then possible.

PROGNOSIS IN OVARIAN CARCINOMA

Since publication of the first edition of this textbook there has been little progress in the "cure" of ovarian carcinoma. Improvement in the cure rate of this disease has not kept pace with advancements in the control of malignancy of the other organs of the reproductive tract. Analyzing the data from reports on ovarian cancer during the past quarter century identifies two main factors responsible for this dilemma:

1. Lack of a clinical method for the diagnosis of the early, silent malignant ovarian tumor.
2. The fact that more than two thirds of the cases of ovarian carcinoma are in the advanced clinical stage (F.I.G.O. II to III) before symptoms appear, and the diagnosis is confirmed.

Therefore, of all the factors relating to the prognosis for ovarian carcinoma, the anatomical extent of the tumor at the time of the initiation of treatment is by far the most important. Histologic type and cellular differentiation of the tumor weigh heavily in the response of the tumor to the various modalities of therapy. In all reports there is still a borderline group of ovarian tumors, approximately

10 to 15 per cent, concerning which there is some doubt as to whether the tumors are malignant, semimalignant, or frankly benign. Such variables produce inconsistent statistics for clinical comparison of the various programs of therapy.

In comparing the current 5-year survival rates based on clinical stage of the disease, the recent report from the Columbia-Presbyterian Hospital group (Munnell) is perhaps the most encouraging data available (Table 38-3).

TABLE 38-3. THE 5-YEAR SURVIVAL RATES IN OVARIAN CARCINOMA (1922–1961)*

CLINICAL STAGE†	5-YEAR SURVIVAL (%)		
	1922–1943	1944–1951	1952–1961
I (Ia)	59	77	84
II (Ib)	80	27	68
III (II)	20	13	31
IV (III)	5	2	13
All stages	28	31	42

* Munnell, E. W.: The changing prognosis and treatment in cancer of the ovary. A report of 235 patients with primary ovarian carcinoma, 1952–1961. Amer. J. Obstet. Gynec., *100*:790, 1968.
† F.I.G.O. classification stage in parentheses.

At the international level, Saxen and Hakama have analyzed the data on ovarian cancer from the United States, Norway, England, and Finland. The overall survival rate among the countries compared for all stages of ovarian cancer is quite similar, varying between 25 and 35 per cent. However, there has been some recent improvement in the survival rate from the United States Teaching Hospitals in the "localized" disease, which is now 70 to 80 per cent. As might be expected, the greater the percentage of localization, the better is the survival rate.

Finally, concerning the different types of treatment and the 5-year survival rate for ovarian cancer, there still seems to be no unanimity of opinion. Nevertheless, interest in the use of surgery and irradiation is increasing, with some upward trend in the improvement of the survival rate, as has been pointed out in this chapter.

TECHNICAL POINTS IN OVARIAN SURGERY

In most instances the removal of a benign ovarian cyst is among the simplest of surgical procedures. In some instances the mesovarium constitutes the pedicle of the cyst, and simply clamping, cutting, and ligating this pedicle are the entire operation. In more instances, however, cysts that require removal have grown to such size as to make it impractical to remove the cyst without the tube. The operation then becomes a salpingo-oophorocystectomy, and the first step is usually clamping, cutting, and suturing the infundibulopelvic ligament. Clamping, cutting, and suturing the remainder of the broad ligament frees the cyst up to the uterine cornu. The tube and the utero-ovarian ligament are excised from the uterine cornu with a small wedge of myometrium. This wound in the uterine cornu is closed with a figure-of-eight suture and covered over with a fold of the round and the broad ligaments. When possible, the rough stump of the infundibulopelvic ligament may be inverted by a purse string placed carefully in the peritoneum, being watchful not to injure the ovarian vessels.

When the cyst is complicated by adhesions due to pelvic infection or endometriosis, its removal may be difficult. Great care must be exercised in dissecting the cyst free from loops of bowel. When the adhesions are dense and the bowel wall intimately blended with the cyst wall, one should bear in mind the possibility of getting out of a difficult situation by splitting the layers of the cyst wall and leaving bits of the outer cyst wall on the bowel. The outer coat is without epithelial lining, and no harm is done by leaving bits of it on the intestine except where the tumor is malignant.

The removal of malignant tumors may be extremely difficult when, by invasion, they are adherent to surrounding structures. It is not the best surgical judgment to abandon the job of removing a malignant ovarian neoplasm simply because it is impossible to remove it cleanly. There are too many 5-year cures observed after incomplete removal followed by irradiation, to make this justifiable. Hence, except in cases where the intra-abdominal extension is very advanced, it is usually well to persist in the radical removal of the pelvic organs. Cutting through carcinomatous tissue causes bleeding, but such bleeding is seldom dangerous. Although such surgery is not clean-cut and is more sanguineous than one would choose, such bleeding usually can be controlled by the use of sutures or the temporary use of packs. Rarely, a cigarette drain with a raw gauze end may be required to control the bleeding.

The question of using a trocar to evacuate a large cyst, rather than making a greatly lengthened abdominal incision, often arises. In general, it is preferable to remove a large cyst intact, even though there is every indication from the external appearance of the cyst that it is benign, for there is always the possibility of malignant papillomata within the cyst. However, exceptions must be made. An enormous cyst, filling a greatly distended abdomen, may be evacuated when it appears to be entirely benign externally. Even when a cyst is of small size but adherent, puncture may be necessary in order to permit safe dissection under sight of the cyst wall from other structures which would be unsafe if carried out blindly. In evacuating a cyst one must attempt to avoid spilling any of the cyst contents; the area about the trocar should be protected with moist gauze.

When one anticipates a difficult dissection of an adherent ovarian tumor, often much time may be saved by preoperative ureteral catheterization. By constantly being able to locate the ureters by palpation the surgeon can proceed more rapidly, and the danger of injury to the ureters is greatly diminished.

Retention cysts of the follicular or corpus luteum variety and occasionally very small neoplastic cysts, such as dermoids, may be resected, leaving a reasonable part of an ovary. This procedure is particularly desirable when one is dealing with the sole remaining ovary in a young woman. In dealing with ovarian endometriosis, resection of the invaded portion of the ovary is often desirable. In general, the authors have no great enthusiasm for resection of a portion of an ovary, but occasionally it becomes the procedure of choice. The technic of resection is illustrated in Figure 38-2. The ovary is held in position for resection by 2 Allis clips, and the cyst is either shelled out with the scalpel handle or cut out. The wound is closed with a lock stitch of No. 0 or No. 00 catgut on an atraumatic round needle. This stitch is hemostatic and also nicely approximates the edges of the wound.

Parovarian cysts, when large, are usually removed with the tube and the ovary. When small, they can be enucleated from between the leaves of the broad ligament without damage to the blood supply of the tube or the ovary (Fig. 38-29). Closure of the opening in the broad ligament constitutes peritonization. Many large parovarian cysts develop entirely between the leaves of the broad ligament without forming a pedicle. In dissecting such cysts free one must bear in mind the presence of the ureters and avoid injuring them.

CARCINOMA OF THE FALLOPIAN TUBE

General Considerations

Primary carcinoma of the fallopian tube is the rarest tumor of the female reproductive tract, varying in frequency from 0.16 to 1.6 per cent, with an average incidence of 0.3 per cent. Historically, the first documented case of carcinoma of the tube was reported by Orthmann in 1888, and since that time this tumor has been reported sporadically in very small series due to its infrequent occurrence. A review of the German and English literature by Sedlis included 694 cases through 1960. More recently, the English literature includes at least 125 additional new cases through 1966. One of the largest series reported was by Hanton and co-workers, who reviewed 27 cases from the Mayo Clinic during a 20-year period ending in 1963.

Because of its rarity and other factors which will be discussed in this chapter, the diagnosis is seldom made preoperatively. Indeed, the diagnosis is often missed even at the operating table, where the operator removes a tube which he believes to be a simple hydrosalpinx. Cures are rare, chiefly because of the difficulties of early diagnosis. The senior author has cured only one case of primary tubal cancer. In that case a 5-cm. adnexal mass was palpated on the left side of the pelvis in an entirely asymptomatic postmenopausal woman. After a negative barium enema it was assumed that the mass was due to an ovarian enlargement, and the patient was explored abdominally. The left ovary was entirely normal, and the enlargement, which was adherent to the sigmoid, was due to a primary tubal carcinoma. A block dissection of a segment of the sigmoid, together with a total hysterectomy and a double salpingo-oophorectomy, was done. Microscopic examination of the removed sigmoid showed infiltration with malignant cells. Obviously, hysterectomy and double salpingo-oophorectomy alone would not have cured the patient, who is now clinically well 15 years after surgery with no evidence of recurrence.

From these introductory remarks one might conclude that the lesion at the time of surgery is more commonly in the advanced stage. However, the cure rate reported in the literature has improved recently, and it is possible that with some of the newer diagnostic procedures, which will be discussed in this chapter, earlier diagnoses may be made with an improvement in the prognosis of this disease.

Pathology

Grossly, a primary tubal carcinoma may appear identical with a free floating hydrosalpinx. Indeed, it often is a tube

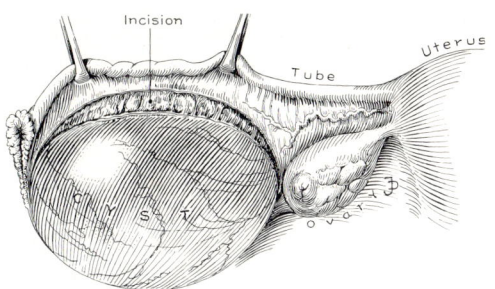

FIG. 38-29. Small parovarian cyst removed from broad ligament without disturbing the tube or the ovary.

distended with thin fluid, which is in fact a hydrosalpinx. The fact that it is free from adhesions might make one sufficiently suspicious to have the tube opened for inspection in the operating room. Papillary projections will be seen growing from the wall of the tube, distended with blood-tinged thin fluid. The wall of the tube may be so thinned that it is susceptible to rupture at even a gentle touch. On the other hand, we have seen tubes distended with grumous carcinomatous material with a thickened wall resembling pyosalpinx. On transecting such a tube the friable carcinomatous material may suggest inspissated pus.

Microscopically, the tumor is of the adenomatous type and usually papillary in architecture (Fig. 38-30). The papillary growth may outgrow its blood supply, causing sloughing of necrotic cells into the lumen.

Diagnostic Difficulties

The lesion occurs almost entirely in women over 40 and most often postmenopausally, although Ross, Ward, and Lindsay reported 2 cases in which the patients were 18 years of age. Hayden and Potter found the average age to be 48. The commonest presenting complaint is the appearance of a thin blood-tinged, watery discharge between periods or, more frequently, occurring postmenopausally. Occasionally, the initial complaint may be abdominal pain or distention, but these symptoms usually signify advanced disease. However, some relatively early cases have given rise to

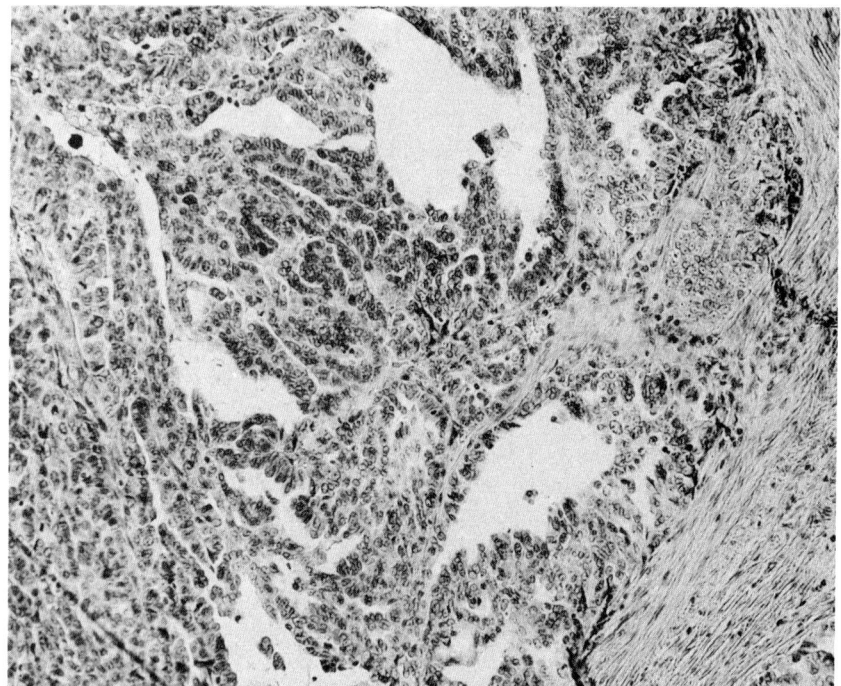

FIG. 38-30. Primary papillary carcinoma of the fallopian tube.

pain, apparently due to tubal distention. Often there may be no symptoms when the adnexal enlargement is discovered on routine pelvic examination.

Unless a mass is discovered on routine pelvic checkup, the problem resolves itself into the investigation of a woman at or beyond the menopause with scanty abnormal bleeding. A unilateral palpable mass may be felt, but in many instances no mass can be felt even under anesthesia. A vaginal and cervical cytologic smear should be taken, and a diagnostic curettage and cervical biopsy should be done. The curetted and biopsied tissue fails to explain the bleeding, but one is not relieved of the responsibility of further investigation. Such cases should always give concern, for they may indicate ovarian malignancy; in fact, percentagewise they are more apt to represent ovarian malignancy than tubal.

The cytologic report may be negative, positive, or suspicious of malignancy. Since many of these lesions occur in postmenopausal women, many of whom have occluded or almost occluded cervical canals, it is obvious that the vaginal smears may be negative, even though malignant cells are shed through the tubal lumen into the uterine cavity. In fact, Hayden and Potter report negative smears in the 5 cases in their series in which cytology was done. In 1947 Isbell et al. reported what is probably the first positive smear associated with primary tubal cancer. Brewer and Guderian have reported 2 cases of primary tubal cancer and one of tubal cancer secondary to carcinoma of the pancreas with positive vaginal smears. Fidler and Lock have reported 3 positive vaginal smears in 4 cases of tubal malignancy, and several other isolated cases with positive vaginal smears have been reported by Song, Frankel, and others. The cells found in the smear usually suggest adenocarcinoma.

These results indicate that when curettage and cervical biopsy fail to explain the abnormal bleeding and the smear is positive, neoplasm of the ovary or the tube should be suspected. This statement is valid even though the adnexa are not palpably enlarged. A single positive smear, not substantiated by curettage and biopsy, should always be repeated. When persistently positive, one should, of course, bear in mind the possibility of a minute missed cervical or endometrial lesion and continue his search for it. Failing to locate the malignancy in the uterus, cul-de-sac aspiration for cytologic examination of the fluid might reveal malignant cells from an ovary or tube. Also, culdoscopy could reveal a nonpalpable ovarian or tubal growth.

TREATMENT

The treatment of carcinoma of the tube is total hysterectomy and double salpingo-oophorectomy with as wide an excision of the involved tube as possible. If the lesion is adherent to the broad ligament, the latter structure, including the parametrium, should be excised as widely as possible. The tumor is bilateral in approximately 15 per cent of the cases, varying between 5 and 26 per cent. If the tube is found to be adherent to the bowel, it should be removed in a block dissection with the pelvic organs. Ross, who reported 9 cases with 1 full year survival, concluded that irradiation did not increase the survival rate. Although there is little doubt of the correctness of this statement, it would seem justifiable to use irradiation therapy postoperatively, especially if the residual tumor appeared to be localized.

Since the diagnosis is extremely difficult to make preoperatively in most cases, the therapeutic problem usually resolves itself into the advisability of surgery for an adnexal mass. The answer to this is identical with that of ovarian tumors. The abdomen should be explored. With a persistently positive vaginal smear, tubal carcinoma should always be kept in mind, and abdominal exploration is at times justifiable when the above-mentioned diagnostic procedures have been done. Although the prognosis is generally poor because of late diagnosis, Hayden and Potter report a 27 per cent 5-year salvage rate. Many of the cases which survive are those in which an early tubal malignancy is discovered incidental to operation for other obvious pelvic lesions.

A most favorable 5-year survival rate of 44 per cent has been reported recently from the Mayo Clinic, where there was no correlation of its cure rate with either postoperative irradiation or chemotherapy. An inadequate number of cases has been treated to date with chemotherapy for proper evaluation of the effectiveness of such drugs, but an occasional response to 5-fluorouracil has been reported. Erez and co-workers from Baylor have proposed a classification of primary carcinoma of the fallopian tube by anatomical staging that would permit a more accurate prognosis of the disease based on the anatomic spread of the lesion at the time of diagnosis and treatment. As is true for the treatment for ovarian carcinoma, omentectomy is useful in the treatment of carcinoma of the tube in eliminating the most common site of spread of the tumor to the upper abdomen as well as a diagnostic aid in identifying microscopic spread of the tumor into the upper abdomen. When such advanced lesions are diagnosed, there is essentially no method of therapy that is effective in controlling the continued spread of the disease, although many clinics are currently utilizing a combination of irradiation and chemotherapy, with only temporary remission of the tumor.

BIBLIOGRAPHY

Asadourian, L. A., and Taylor, H. B.: Dysgerminoma. An analysis of 105 cases. Obstet. Gynec., 33:370, 1969.

Brenner, F.: Das Oophoroma folliculare. Frankfurt Z. Path., No. 1, p. 150, 1907.

Brody, S.: Clinical aspects of dysgerminoma of the ovary. Acta Radiol. (Stockholm), 56: 209, 1961.

Cron, R., Cowan I. I., Gorthey, R. L., and Karioris, F. G.: Surgery and radioactive gold treatment in carcinoma of the ovary. Amer. J. Obstet. Gynec., 70:910, 1955.

Cullingworth, C. J.: Fibroma of both ovaries. Trans. Obstet. Soc. (London), 21:276, 1879.

de Lima, O. L.: Disgerminoma do ovário. Contribuicao para o seu estudo anatomoclinico. Docente-Livre na Regência da Cadeira de clinica Ginecológica da Escola Paulista de Medicina. São Paulo, 1966.

Dockerty, M. B., Pratt, J. H., and Decker, D. G.: Primary adenocarcinoma of the rectovaginal septum probably arising from endometriosis: Report of 2 cases. Cancer, 7:893, 1954.

Ewing, J. Neoplastic Diseases. ed. 3. Philadelphia, W. B. Saunders, 1928.

Falk, H. C., and Bunkin, I. A.: Management of ovarian tumors complicating pregnancy. Amer. J. Obstet. Gynec., 54:82, 1947.

Felmus, L. B., and Pedowitz, P.: Clinical malignancy of endocrine tumors of ovary and dysgerminoma. Obstet. Gynec., 29:344, 1967.

Fisher, E. R.: "Pseudomucinous" cystadenomas: A misnomer. Obstet. Gynec., 4:616, 1954.

Gilbertsen, V. A., and Wangensteen, O. H.: A summary of 13 years experience with the second look program. Surg. Gynec. Obstet., 114:438, 1962.

Gonzalez-Angulo, A., Kaufman, R. H., Braungardt, C. D., Chapman, S. C., and Hinshaw, A. J.: Adenocarcinoma of thyroid arising in struma ovarii (malignant struma ovarii): Report of 2 cases and review of the literature. Obstet. Gynec., 21:567, 1963.

Gottschalk, S.: Ein neuer Typus einer klein cystischen bösartigen Eierstockgeschwulst. Arch. Gynäk., 59:676, 1899.

Graham, J. B., Graham, R. M., and Schueller, E. F.: Pre-clinical detection of ovarian cancer. Cancer, 17:1414, 1964.

Greenspan, E. M.: Thio-TEPA and methotrexate chemotherapy of advanced ovarian carcinoma. J. Mount Sinai Hosp., 35:52, 1968.

Grogan, R. H.: Accidental rupture of malignant ovarian cysts during surgical removal. Obstet. Gynec., 30:716, 1967.

Haas, R. L.: Pregnancy and adnexal cysts. Amer. J. Obstet. Gynec., 58:283, 1949.

Hodari, A. A., and Hodgkinson, C. P.: Lymphangiogram of Meigs' syndrome. Report of a case. Obstet. Gynec., 32:477, 1968.

Ingersoll, F. M., and McArthur, J. W.: Longitudinal studies of gonadotrophin excretion in Stein-Leventhal syndrome. Amer. J. Obstet. Gynec., 77:795, 1959.

International Federation of Gynecology and Obstetrics: Classification and staging of malignant tumors in the female pelvis. J. Int. Fed. Obstet. Gynec., 3:209, 1965.

Julian, C. G., and Woodruff, J. D.: The role of chemotherapy in the treatment of primary ovarian malignancy. Obstet. Gynce. Surv., 24:1307, 1969.

Kaufman, R. J.: Management of advanced ovarian carcinoma. Med. Clin. N. Amer., 50:845, 1966.

Keettel, W. C., Fox, M. R., Longnecker, D. S., and Latourette, H. B.: Prophylactic use of radioactive gold in the treatment of primary ovarian cancer. Amer. J. Obstet. Gynec., 94:766, 1966.

Kelley, R. R., and Scully, R. E.: Cancer developing in dermoid cysts of the ovary. A report of 8 cases including a carcinoid and a leiomyosarcoma. Cancer, 14:989, 1961.

Kistner, R. W.: Further observations on effects of clomiphene citrate in anovulatory females. Amer. J. Obstet. Gynec., 92:380, 1965.

Kottmeier, H. L.: Modern trends in the treatment of patients with semi-malignant and malignant ovarian tumors. In M. D. Anderson Hospital and Tumor Institute, Houston, Texas: Carcinoma of the Uterine Cervix, Endometrium and Ovary. p. 285. Chicago, Year Book Medical Publishers, 1962.

Latour, J. P. A., and Davis, B. A.: A critical assessment of the value of x-ray therapy in primary ovarian carcinoma. Amer. J. Obstet. Gynec., 74:968, 1957.

Long, M. E., and Taylor, H. C., Jr.: Endometrioid carcinoma of the ovary. Amer. J. Obstet. Gynec., 90:936, 1964.

Long, R. T. L., Johnson, R. E., and Sala, J. M.: Variations in survival among patients with carcinoma of the ovary. Cancer, 20:1195, 1967.

Long, R. T. L., and Sala, J. M.: Radical pelvic surgery combined with radiotherapy in the treatment locally of advanced ovarian carcinoma. Surg. Gynec. Obstet., 117:202, 1963.

Lusi, A.: Metastatic ovarian tumors. In Gentil, F., and Junqueira, A. (eds.): Ovarian Cancer. p. 87. New York, Springer-Verlag, 1968.

MacKay, E. N., and Sellers, A. H.: Ovarian cancer at the Ontario Cancer Foundation Clinics, 1938-1958. Canad. Med. Assoc. J., 96:299, 1967.

Malkasian, G. D., Symmonds, R. E., and Dockerty, M. B.: Malignant ovarian teratomas: Report of 31 cases. Obstet. Gynec., 25:810, 1965.

Malloy, J. J., Dockerty, M. B., Welsh, J. S.,

and Hunt, A. B.: Papillary ovarian tumors. Amer. J. Obstet. Gynec., 93:867, 1965.

Mansell, H., and Hertig, A. T.: Granulosa-theca cell tumors and endometrial carcinoma. Obstet. Gynec., 6:385, 1955.

Masterson, J. G., and Nelson, J. H., Jr.: Role of chemotherapy in the treatment of gynecologic malignancy. Amer. J. Obstet. Gynec., 93:1102, 1965.

Mathieu, A., and Holman, A.: Tumors incident to and complicating pregnancy and labor. Northwest Med., 30:529, 1931.

Meigs, J. V.: Pelvic tumors other than fibromas of the ovary with ascites and hydrothorax. Obstet. Gynec., 3:471, 1954.

Meigs, J. V., and Cass, J. W.: Fibroma of the ovary with ascites and hydrothorax, with a report of 7 cases. Amer. J. Obstet. Gynec., 33:249, 1937.

Meyer, R.: Handbuch der spezielle pathologische Anatomic und Histologie. F. Henke and O. Lubarsch. vol. vii/3. Berlin, Julius Springer, 1930.

———: Zur Histogenese und Einteilung der Ovarialkystome, Mschr. Geburtsh. Gynäk., 44:302, 1916.

———: Quoted by Novak, E.: Gynecological and Obstetrical Pathology. Philadelphia, W. B. Saunders, 1940.

Morton, D. G.: Ovarian carcinoma. Amer. J. Obstet. Gynec., 95:359, 1966.

Munnell, E. W.: The changing prognosis and treatment in cancer of the ovary. A report of 235 patients with primary ovarian carcinoma, 1952-1961. Amer. J. Obstet. Gynec., 100:790, 1968.

Munnell, E. W., and Taylor, H. C., Jr.: Ovarian carcinoma. Amer. J. Obstet. Gynec., 58:943, 1949.

Norris, H. J., and Taylor, H. B.: Prognosis of granulosa-theca tumors of the ovary. Cancer, 21:255, 1968.

Novak, E.: Granulosa cell ovarian tumors as cause of precocious puberty, with report of 3 cases. Amer. J. Obstet. Gynec., 26:505, 1933.

Novak, E., and Te Linde, R. W.: Pathological anatomy of the corpus luteum (abscess, cyst, hematoma and neoplasm). Bull. Johns Hopkins Hosp., 34:289, 1923.

Novak, E. R., and Woodruff, J. D.: Gynecologic and Obstetric Pathology. ed. 6. Philadelphia, W. B. Saunders, 1967.

Pedowitz, P.: Dysgerminoma. Amer. J. Obstet. Gynec., 86:693, 1963.

Pedowitz, P., Felmus, L. B., and Grayzel, D. M.: Dysgerminoma of ovary. Amer. J. Obstet. Gynec., 70:1284, 1955.

Pemberton, F. A.: Carcinoma of the ovary. Amer. J. Obstet. Gynec., 40:751, 1940.

Peterson, W. F.: Malignant degeneration of benign cystic teratomas of ovary: Collective review of literature. Obstet. Gynec. Survey, 12:793, 1957.

Rundles, R. W., and Barton, W. B.: Triethylene melamime in the treatment of neoplastic disease. Blood, 7:483, 1952.

Rutledge, F., and Burns, B., Jr.: Chemotherapy in ovarian tumors. In Gentil, F., and Junqueira, A. C. (Eds.): Ovarian Cancer. p. 226. New York, Springer-Verlag, 1968.

Santesson, L.: Clinical and pathological survey of ovarian tumors treated at Radiumhemmet. I. Dysgerminoma. Acta Radiol. (Stockholm), 28:644, 1947.

Santesson, L., and Kottmeier, H. L.: General classification of ovarian tumors. In Gentil, F., and Junqueira, A. C.: Ovarian Cancer. New York, Springer-Verlag, 1968.

Saxen, E. A., and Hakama, M.: End Results Studies on Cancer of the Ovary. Nat. Cancer Inst. Monograph 15:135, 1964.

Schiller, W.: Zur Histogenese der Brennerschen Ovarialtumoren. Arch. Gynäk., 157:65, 1934.

Shanks, H. G.: Pseudomyxoma peritonei. J. Obstet. Gynaec. Brit Comm., 68:212, 1961.

Spiegelberg, O.: Fibrom des Eierstockes von enormer and Grosse, Mschr. Geburtsh., 28:415, 1866.

Stein, I. F.: Diagnosis and treatment of bilateral polycystic ovaries in the Stein-Leventhal syndrome. Int. J. Fertil., 3: 20, 1958.

Stein, I. F., and Leventhal, M. L.: Amenorrhea associated with bilateral polycystic ovaries. Amer. J. Obstet. Gynec., 29:181, 1935.

Tait, L.: On the occurrence of pleural effusion in association with disease of the abdomen. Med. Chir. Soc. Trans., 75:109, 1891.

Te Linde, R. W.: Granulosa cell tumors of the ovary and their relation to postmenopausal bleeding. Amer. J. Obstet. Gynec., 20:552, 1930.

Thoeny, R. H., Dockerty, M. B., Hunt, A. B., and Childs, D. S., Jr.: A study of ovarian dysgerminoma with emphasis on the role of radiation therapy. Surg. Gynec. Obstet., 113:692, 1961.

Thompson, J. D.: Primary ovarian adenoacanthoma. Obstet. Gynec., 9:403, 1957.

Trace, R. J., Kealy, E. C., and McCall, M. L.: An investigation of ovarian tissue and urinary 17-ketosteroids in patients with bilateral polycystic ovaries. Amer. J. Obstet. Gynec., 79:310, 1960.

Turner, J. C., Jr., Remine, W. H., and Dockerty, M. B.: Clinical pathologic study of 172 patients with primary carcinoma of the ovary. Surg. Gynec. Obstet., 109:198, 1959.

Vaeth, J. M., and Buschke, F. J.: The role of preoperative irradiation in the treatment of carcinoma of the ovary. Amer. J. Roentgen., 105:614, 1969.

Von Kahlden, C.: Cited by Marcus, C. C., and Marcus, S. L.: Struma ovarii (a report of 7 cases and review of subject). Amer. J. Obstet. Gynec., 81:752, 1961.

Warren, S., and Witham, E. M.: Studies on tumor metastases: Distribution of metastasis in cancer of the breast. Surg. Gynec. Obstet., 57:81, 1933.

Woodruff, J. D., Bie, L. S., and Sherman, R. J.: Mucinous tumors of the ovary. Obstet. Gynec., 16:699, 1960.

Woodruff, J. D., and Markley, R. L.: Struma ovarii. Obstet. Gynec., 9:707, 1957.

Carcinoma of Fallopian Tube

Brewer, J. I., and Guderian, A. M.: Diagnosis of uterine tube carcinoma by vaginal cytology. Obstet. Gynec., 8:664, 1956.

Cron, R. S., and Claude, J. L.: Primary papillary carcinoma of the uterine tube. Obstet. Gynec., 13:734, 1959.

Erez, S., Kaplan, A. L., and Wall, J. A.: Clinical staging of carcinoma of the uterine tube. Obstet. Gynec., 30:547, 1967.

Fidler, H. K., and Lock, D. R.: Carcinoma of the fallopian tube detected by cervical smear. Amer. J. Obstet. Gynec., 67:1103, 1954.

Fogh, I.: Primary carcinoma of the fallopian tube. Cancer, 23:1332, 1969.

Frankel, A. N.: Primary carcinoma of the fallopian tube. Amer. J. Obstet. Gynec., 72:131, 1956.

Hanton, E. M., Malkasian, G. E., Dahlin, D. C., and Pratt, J. H.: Primary carcinoma of the fallopian tube. Amer. J. Obstet. Gynec., 94:832, 1966.

Hayden, G. E., and Potter, E. L.: Primary carcinoma of the fallopian tube with report of 12 new cases. Amer. J. Obstet. Gynec., 79:24, 1960.

Isbell, N. P., et al.: A correlation between vaginal smear and tissue diagnosis in 1045 operated gynecologic cases. Amer. J. Obstet. Gynec., 54:576, 1947.

Lofgren, R., and Dockerty, M. B.: Primary carcinoma of the fallopian tube. Surg. Gynec. Obstet., 82:199, 1964.

McQueeney, A. J., Carswell, B. L., and Sheenan, W. J.: Malignant mixed müllerian tumor primary in uterine tube: Review of the literature and report of an additional case. Obstet. Gynec., 23:338, 1964.

Mitchell, R. M., and Mohler, R. W.: Primary carcinoma of the fallopian tube. Amer. J. Obstet. Gynec., 50:283, 1945.

Momtazee, S., and Kempson, R. L.: Primary adenocarcinoma of the fallopian tube. Obstet. Gynec., 32:649, 1968.

Orthmann, E. G.: Cited by Doran, A. H. G.: Primary cancer of the fallopian tube. J. Obstet. Gynaec. Brit. Emp., 2:381, 1902.

Picton, F. C. R. Primary cancer of fallopian tubes. Report of 3 cases, 2 with survival of 5 years. J. Obstet. Gynaec. Brit. Comm., 66:663, 1959.

Randall, C. L.: The significance of increased menstrual bleeding in women over 40. New York J. Med., 48:1635, 1943.

Rhu, H. S.: Primary carcinoma of the tube. Obstet. Gynec., 9:355, 1957.

Ross, W. M.: Primary tumors of the fallopian tube. Canad. Med. Assoc. J., 96:328, 1967.

Ross, W. M., Ward, C. V., and Lindsay, C. C.: Primary carcinoma of the fallopian tube: A report of 8 cases. Amer. J. Obstet. Gynec., 83:425, 1962.

Sedlis, A.: Primary carcinoma of the fallopian tube. Obstet. Gynec. Survey, 16:209, 1961.

Song, Y. S.: Cytologic diagnosis of carcinoma of the fallopian tube. Amer. J. Obstet. Gynec., 70:29, 1955.

Index

Index

Abdomen, bearing-down pain, 472-473
  closing of, 132-137
  distention of, 80-82
  drainage through, 256
  examination of, 17-18
  extra-uterine, infection, 448-452
    pregnancy, 336-340
  and fibroids, 150
  fluid in. See Ascites
  intestinal obstruction, 345-347
  opening, 125-132
    for fistula closure, 610, 611
    for myomectomy, 180-188
  preparation of, for surgery, 26-27, 138
  in Wertheim hysterectomy, 751-752
Abortion, 425-454
  and cervix, 388
  and fibroids, 151
  habitual, 437-444
    definition, 426
    double uterus, 285
  incomplete, diagnosis, 327
    treatment, 444-448
  induced, definition, 426
  infected, extra-uterine, 448-452
    treatment, 446-448
  instruments for, 28
  laws concerning, 426-428
  missed, definition, 426
  and myoma, 182
  septic, 257, 261-262, 263
  spontaneous, definition, 426
  therapeutic, 426-437
    indications for, 427-430
    perforating, 453-454
    and sterilization, 376
    technic, 431-437
  tubal, 317, 324
  uninfected, treatment, 444-448
  and uterus retrodisplacement, 473-474
Abscess, abdominal, from septic abortion, 450-452
  appendiceal, 366-367
  pelvic, 82
  perirectal, fistula from, 646
  tubo-ovarian rupture, 242-244
Acanthosis, 792
Acid, definition, 110
  excretion of, 111-112
Acid-base, balance, 112-114
  metabolism, 110-114
Acidosis, 113-114
  metabolic, 114, 257, 258
  respiratory, 113-114
  in shock, 74
Actinomycin D, for gynecologic malignancies, 846-848
Adenoacanthoma, 221, 792
Adenocarcinoma, of Bartholin's gland, 697
  of cervix, 735, 765
  cytology, 790-791
  endometrial, 792
  of vulva, 667-668
Adenomyoma, 192
Adenomyosis, 192-196
  of round ligament, 202
ADH, 102
Adhesions, from fibroids, 160, 162
  peritubal, 324
  small bowel, 344-347
Adnexa, tumors of, 817-853
Adnexectomy. See Salpingo-oophorectomy
Adrenal gland deficiency, 298
Adson clamp, illus., 31
Age, and carcinoma, of cervix, 718
  of vulva, 682
  and cervical dysplasia, 713-714
  and fibroids, 146-148
  and endometrial cancer, 789
  and leukoplakia vulvae, 676
  and myomectomy, 182
  old, and blood flow, 87
    and septic shock, 257
    and vaginal prolapse, 519
    and wound dehiscence, 139
  and oophorectomy, 821
  and pelvic TB, 264
  and pessary use, 531
  and surgery, 22-23
Airway, maintenance of, 54
  emergency, 59-62
  obstruction of, 57-60
    acidosis, 113
Aldridge, A. H., modification Goebell-Frangenheim-Stoeckel operation, 557-558
  operation for incontinence, 550
Alexander-Adams suspension of uterus, 474
Alkaloids, plant, for gynecologic malignancies, 846-848
Alkalosis, 113-114
  metabolic, 114
  respiratory, 258
Alkeran, for gynecologic malignancies, 846-848
Alkylating agents, for gynecologic malignancies, 846-848
17-Alpha-hydroxyprogesterone caproate, for recurrent carcinoma, 805-807
Ambulation, early, 87, 89
Amenorrhea, 418
  with pelvic TB, 264
  in Stein-Leventhal syndrome, 839
American Medical Association, abortion policy, 427
Amethopterin, for gynecologic malignancies, 846-848
Aminopterin, for gynecologic malignancies, 846-848
Amniocentesis, 436
Amputation, of cervix, 401-408
  high, technic, 405-406
  history of, 6
  low, technic, 403-405
  Schröder technic, 407

859

860 Index

Anastomosis, of bowel, end-to-end, technic, 350-355
  side-to-side, technic, 351, 354, 356-357
  ureteroileal, 620-622
  uretero-intestinal, 612-620
  ureterosigmoid, 775-778
  ureteroureteral, 272
    technic, 276-277
Androgenicity, 297
Androgens, for endometriosis, 218
Anemia, and anesthesia, 48
  secondary, 25
Anesthesia, 36-55
  for aspiration of uterus, 435
  with cervical cautery, 397-399
  complications, 49-51
  for culdoscopy, 312
  for curettage, 413-414, 420-421
  general, 40-42
  history, 3
  positions for, 39-40
  post-anesthetic period, 52-55
  preparation for, 36-39
  service, 36
  spinal, 42-46
    continuous, 46
    headache, 44
    technic, 45-46
  for vulvectomy, 684
Anesthesiologists, 36
Anesthetic, choice of, 37, 46-47
  spinal, 44, 45
  overdose, 50
Anomaly, rectovaginal fistula, 655-660
  of uterus, 281
  of vagina, 457-466
  treatment of, 10
Antibiotics, appendiceal abscess, 366-367
  for gynecologic malignancies, 846-848
  in septic shock, 259-260
  with vulvectomy, 694
Anticoagulant therapy, 89-90
  for thrombophlebitis, 90
Antidiuretic hormone, 102
Antigen-antibody reaction, and infertility, 298
Antihistamines, before anesthesia, 39
Antimetabolites, for gynecologic malignancies, 846-848
Antisepsis, development of, 3-4
Anus, fissures of, 361-362
  formation of, technic, 657-659
  sphincter, anomaly of, 656-657
    severing, 642, 651
  surgery of, 359-362
Apocrine gland carcinoma, and Paget's disease, 680, 681
Appendectomy, 235, 237
  with gynecologic surgery, 364-365
  with peritonitis, 365-367

during pregnancy, 369
  technic, 369-372
Appendicitis, 364-372
  differential diagnosis, 364, 367-368
  and salpingitis, 234-235, 237
Appendix, through culdoscope, 314
  endometriosis of, 203
  and gynecology, 364-372
  mucocele of, 821, 822
  retrocecal, 369-370
Arachnoiditis, adhesive, prevention, 43
Aramine, 73, 93
  for septic shock, 260, 262
Arias-Stella reaction, 327, 329
Armamentarium, with illus., 27-34
Arrest, cardiac, 62-64
Arrhenoblastomas, 837-838
Ascites, from cystadenoma, 822
  with fibroids, 150
  Meigs's syndrome, 828-829
  with ovarian carcinoma, 843, 845
  in tuberculosis, 265-266
Asepsis, development of, 3-4
Asphyxia, 57-62
  under anesthesia, 37
  postoperative, 53
Aspiration, of gastric contents, 65
  of uterus, 446
    curette for, illus., 435
    for therapeutic abortion, 431, 435
Asthma, anesthesia during, 47
Ataractic drug, before anesthesia, 38
Atelectasis, postoperative, 76-78
Atherosclerosis, and estrogen therapy, 119
Atlee, Washington, 1
Atropine, before anesthesia, 38, 78
Azospermia, 297-298

Babcock clamp, illus., 34
Bacitracin solution, 138
Backache, and uterus retrodisplacement, 472-473
Bacteremia, gram-negative, 256-263
Bacteria, in wound, 137
Bacteriuria, 85
Bag-mask ventilation, 42, 61
Balance, potassium, 107-110
  sodium, 104-107
  See also Electrolyte studies and Fluid
Baldy-Webster suspension of uterus, 474
Barbiturates, before anesthesia, 38
Bard-Parker knife, illus., 592

Bartholin's gland, carcinoma, 697-698
  cysts, 671-673
  in gonorrhea, 231-232, 233
Basal body temperature, 294, 295
Base, definition, 110
Basset operation, 683, 685-693, 698
Bastiaanse, van Bouwdijk, 8
BBT, 294, 295
Betadine, 27
Betatron, 742, 747
Biopsy, of cervix, 719, 736-737
  during pregnancy, 766
  clamp for, illus., 30
  with culdoscope, 320
  endometrial, 415, 795, 796, 801
  of leukoplakic areas, 396
  of melanoma, 696
  of vulva, 682, 683
Bishydroxycoumarin, 89
Bladder, calculus, 587, 589
  carcinoma of, 771
  catheterization of, 17
  drainage of, 590-591
    suprapubic, 83-85, 568, 584, 590, 679
  endometriosis of, 201, 203
  and fibroids, 149
  herniation of, 535
  in hysterectomy, 159, 177, 178
  and irradiation therapy, 744-745, 756
  surgery of, ileal loop substitution, 620-622
    Marshall-Marchetti-Krantz operation, 565-570
    peritoneum advancement, 478
    postoperative care, 82-83
    for stress incontinence, 553-555
    ureter implantation, 272, 277-280
    for urethrocele and vesical sphicter plication, 544-547
    Watkins transposition of uterus, 487, 488
Bleeding, after abortion, 434-435
  curettage for, 413
  dysfunctional, 417-423
    endometrial carcinoma, 794-795
  in ectopic pregnancy, 325
  from fibroids, 148-150
  functional, 195
    vaginal hysterectomy for, 179-180
  after hysterectomy, 177-179
  peritoneal, 326-332
    with interstitial pregnancy, 335
  postmenopausal, 148, 149
  and carcinosarcoma, 815
  during pregnancy, 444-445
  See also Hemorrhage and Menstruation

Index 861

Block, paracervical, 46
  spinal, 44-45
Block-Aid Monitor, 41
Blocking agent(s), adrenergic, 73-74
  neuromuscular, 41
Blood, coagulation, 86
  counts, 19
  gases in, 59
  pooling in muscles, 87
  pressure, monitoring, 68-71
    in shock, 326
  transfusion, in tubo-ovarian rupture, 243
  urea nitrogen level, monitoring, 79
  vessels, and estrogen therapy, 119
  volume, and anesthesia, 48, 49-50
    insufficient, 71
    in intraperitoneal bleeding, 330
    replacement of, 25, 72, 74
  studies, 19
Body, basal temperature, 294, 295
Boivin, Marie Anne, 6
Bonney forceps, illus., 31
Bowel. See Intestines
Breasts, in arrhenoblastoma, 837
  carcinoma of, and of endometrium, 794
    metastasis from, 833
  examination of, 17
  in Stein-Leventhal syndrome, 839
Breathing, arrested, 54-62
  postanesthesia, 53-54
  postoperative, 78
Brenner tumor, 827-828
Bricker, E. M., ileal loop bladder substitution, 620-622
Broders, A. C., classification of carcinoma, 790
Broedel, Max, 5
Bronchopneumonia, postoperative, 76-78
Bronchus, occulusion of, 76-77
Brunschwig, Alexander, exenteration, 9, 771
Buffering, of hydrogen ions, 110-112
Burnam, Curtis, 5
Burnham, Walter, 2

Calcium, requirements, 114
Calculus, of bladder, 587, 589
  in fistula, 610
Calorie, requirements, 97
Cancer, cauterization as prophylaxis against, 399
  of cervix, epidemiology, 701-706
    and endometrium, incidence, 789

radioresistant, 771-772
  treatment, 6-7
endometrial, with fibroids, 144
epidermoid, of Bartholin's gland, 697-698
  and leukoplakia, 676
obstructing large bowel, 348-349
in situ, 389
See also Carcinoma and Sarcoma
Cannula, Rubin's, illus., 30
Carbohydrate metabolism, and endometrial cancer, 794
Carcinoma, and abortion, 429
  of Bartholin's gland, 697-698
  of cervix, classification, 724, 732-736
    epidermoid, 734-735
    fistula from, 585-586
    hysterectomy for, 737, 738-741
    invasive, 732-767
      diagnosis and treatment, 736-745
    irradiation for, 737, 741-750
      fistulas from, 599-600, 608, 610
      rectovaginal, 646
    microinvasive, 724-729
      Wertheim hysterectomy, 726-729
    in pregnancy, 765-767
    in situ, 708-729
      biopsy, 717
      diagnosis, 719-722
      and invasive, 715-719
      and leukoplakia, 395
      microscopy, 708-713
      in pregnancy, 766
      recurrence, 724-725
      treatment, 723-724
        hysterectomy for, 179-180
    urinary diversion for, 611-612
  of corpus uteri, 789-807
  endometrial, 789-807
    classification, Broders', 790-792
      international, 796
    diagnosis, 795-796
      by curettage, 415
    and other, 794
    prognosis, 790
    recurrent, remissions, 805-807
    treatment, 804-807
      chemotherapy, 805-807
    in situ, 791, 793
    symptoms, 794, 795
    treatment, 797-807
      for Stage I, 801-802
      for Stage II, 802
      for Stage III, 802-803
      for Stage IV, 803
  endometrioid, 221

from estrogens, 118-119
fallopian tube, 805-853
gynecologic, chemotherapy, 846-848
incipient, 715
ovarian, classification, 831
  granulosa cell, 835-836
  metastatic, 833
  primary, cystic, 831-833
    solid, 829-831
  prognosis, 848-849
  treatment, 842-849
    chemotherapy, 846-848
    irradiation, 845-846
    surgery, 842-849
      second-look, 848
    technics, 849-850
  in situ, 9
See also Carcinoma, of cervix, endometrial, ovarian, etc.
of urethra, 581-583
  meatus, 572
of uterus, fundus of, 792-793
  squamous cell, 792
of vulva, basal cell, 695-696
  invasive, 682-695
    treatment, 683-693
  in situ, 681-682
Carcinosarcoma, of uterus, 811, 815-816
Caruncle, of urethra, 572-573
Castration, 423
  with hysterectomy, 817
See also Oophorectomy
Catheter, Foley, 79, 83-85, 280
  postoperative, 568
  silicone, 84
  subclavian, for CVP monitoring, 69-71
  ureteral, 4, 279
    with fistula, 27, 274-275
  for urethrogram, illus., 578
Catheterization, of bladder, in examination, 17
  before surgery, 26
  of ureter, 252-254, 271-272
Cauterization, of cervical polyp, 395
  of cervix, 303, 396-400
    technic, 399-400
    equipment, 397-398
  of Skene's glands, 233
Cecum, endometriosis of, 203
  volvulus of, 350
Cell(s), of adenocarcinoma, 790-791
  blood, and thrombosis, 86
  Brenner tumor, 828
  of carcinoma, of cervix, 732-736
    in situ, 708-713
    endometrium, in situ, 806-807
    fallopian tube, 852
    of vulva, basal, 695-696
      in situ, 682
  of carcinosarcoma of uterus, 815

Cell(s)—(Cont.)
  cystadenocarcinoma of ovary, 832
  cystadenoma, 823
  dermoid cyst, 825
  of dysgerminoma, 835
  fluid in, 98
  granulosa, 836
  of ovarian cyst, 820
  of sarcoma of uterus, 812-813
Cellulitis, pelvic, 82
  after exenteration, 785
  with vaginal hysterectomy, 180
Central venous pressure, 68-71, 74, 103
Cerclage, of cervix, 441-444
Cervicitis, 388-392
  acute, and curettage, 413
  chronic, treatment, 390-392
Cervix, amputation of, 401-408
  in Le Fort operation, 513-516
  in Manchester operation, 482-487
  Schröder technic, 407
  in Spalding-Richardson operation, 505, 509-511
  in Watkins operation, 487, 488
  biopsy, with curettage, 415
  block anesthesia of, 46
  cancer of, diagnosis, 702-705
    epidemiology, 701-706
    etiology, 705-706
    and fibroids, 153
    incidence, 789
    radioresistant, 771-772
    treatment, 6-7
  carcinoma of, and of endometrium, 794
    invasive, 732-767
      hysterectomy for, 737, 738-741
      irradiation, 737, 741-750
      irradiation fistula, 599-600, 608, 610
      rectovaginal, 646
    microinvasive, 724-729
      Wertheim hysterectomy, 726-729
    in pregnancy, 765-767
    in situ, 389, 708-729
      diagnosis, 719-722
      and invasive, 715-719
      treatment, 723-724
    urinary diversion for, 611-612
  cauterization, 303, 395, 396-400
  conization of, 400-401
  dilatation of, 410-412
    for curettage, 414
  dysplasia of, 713-715
  epithelium, cells of, 708-713
  in hysterectomy, 801
    total, 173
  incompetent, and abortion, 440-444
  and infertility, 295

  lacerations of, 388
  leukoplakia of, 395-396
  myoma of, 189-190
    hysterectomy for, 175-177
  nonmalignant lesions, 387-408
  perforation of, 453
  polyps of, 393-396
  and prolapsed uterus, 480
  pseudo-erosion, 387-388
  sarcoma of, 811, 812
  as site of pregnancy, 341
    treatment, 814-815
  stricture of, 392-393
  Sturmdorf tracheloplasty, 406-407
  trachelorraphy, 407-408
  tuberculosis of, 736
Cesarean section, and appendectomy, 369
  following perineal repair, 643
  and sterilization, 376-377, 378-379
Chemotherapy, antituberculous, 266
  for gynecologic malignancies, 846-848, 853
Chest, fluid, in Meigs's syndrome, 828-829
Childbearing, and Manchester operation, 483-484
  and myomectomy, 181
Childbirth, and cystocele, 535
  and enterocele, 636
  fistulas from, 585
    vesicourethrovaginal, 607
  and incontinence, 543
  lacerations from, 388, 641-646
  and rectocele, 625
  and ruptured appendix, 367
  and urethrocele, 534
Chlorambucil, for gynecologic malignancies, 846-848
Chloride, requirements, 114
Chloroform, as anesthetic, 3
Chloromycetin, for peritonitis, 367
  for septic shock, 260, 262
Chlorpromazine, 74
  before anesthesia, 39
  for septic shock, 261, 262
Chocolate cyst, 201, 203, 215
Choriocarcinoma, 329
Circulation, monitoring of, during anesthesia, 52
Circumcision, and cervical cancer, 705-706
Clamp(s), illustrations, 29, 30, 31, 32, 34
  Jacob's, illus., 411
Clark, John G., 7, 739
Clay, Charles, 2
Climacteric, female, 118
Clitoris, carcinoma of, 687
Clomiphene citrate, 423
  for hypothalamus dysfunction, 294

  for Stein-Leventhal syndrome, 842
Clostridium welchii, 256, 258, 260
Coagulation, of blood, 86
Cobalt 60, 742
Coelomic epithelium, 209
Coffey, Robert C., implantation of ureters, 614-618
  procedure, 242
Coitus, and cervical cancer, 705-706
  See also Dyspareunia
Coliform bacilli, in incision, 138
Collins, C. G., diagnosis of cancer, 683
  vulvectomy, 695
Colpocleisis, 519
  history of, 8
  for prolapse following hysterectomy, 520-522
Colporrhaphy, anterior, technic, 504-505, 506-507
Colposcopy, for diagnosis, 721, 722-723
  during pregnancy, 766
Colpostat, Silverstone spring, 747
Colpotomy, drainage via, 451
  instruments for, 28
  posterior, technic, 237-238
  of tubal pregnancy, 329-330
Colostomy, bag, 348
  after irradiation, 744
  for large bowel obstruction, 349
  in pelvic exenteration, 783-784
  for rectovaginal fistula, 600, 655
  before Rizzoli operation, 659
Compression, cardiac, 56, 62-64
Condylomata acuminata, of vulva, 669-671
Conization, of cervix, 400-401, 402, 719
  for diagnosis, 721-722, 725, 737
  during pregnancy, 766
  therapeutic, 723-724
Constipation, and fibroids, 150
  and hemorrhoids, 361
  voluntary, for rectovaginal fistula, 648
Cor pulmonale, 92
Cordonnier, J. J., 616
Cordonnier-Leadbetter, ureterosigmoid anastomosis, technic, 617-620
Corps ronds, 682
Corpus luteum, and abortion, 439
  cyst, 819-820
  failure, 294-295
  formation, absence of, 420
  hematoma, 200, 316-318
Corticosteroids, for septic shock, 74, 260, 262
Coumadin, 90
Cricothyreotomy, 60
Cuff salpingostomy, 305-307
Cul-de-sac, abscess, 237-238

bleeding into, 326
  drainage through, 254, 255
  enterocele through, 635-640
Culdocentesis, 326
Culdoplasty, 524-526, 528
  posterior, technic, 500, 502
Culdoscope, 311, 313
Culdoscopy, 311-322
  complications, 321-322
  for endometriosis, 217
  indications, 316-320
  position, 40
  of tubes, 301-302, 329
Cullen, Thomas S., 8
  sign of, 326
Curettage, endocervical, 719
  for diagnosis, 737
  of uterus, 412-416
    for dysfunctional bleeding, 420-423
    instruments for, 28
    technic, 414-416
    for therapeutic abortion, technic, 431-434
Curette, illus., 29, 415
CVP. See Pressure, central venous
Cyanosis, 58
  during anesthesia, 52
Cyclophosphamide, for gynecologic malignancies, 846-848
Cyst, Bartholin's gland, 671-673
  of corpus luteum, 819, 820
  endometrial, 198-201, 203, 205
  of ovary, 216
  ovarian, 318
    benign, removal, 849
    dermoid, 824-826
      carcinoma in, 831, 833
    evacuation, 850
    follicular, 818-819
    neoplastic, 820-826
    retention, 818-819
    spillage from, 848
    rupture of, 818
    Stein-Leventhal syndrome, 839-842
  parovarian, 838-839
    removal, 850
  of Skene's ducts, 574-575
  suburethral, 576-577
  thecalutein, 839
  of vulva, 671-674
Cystadenocarcinoma, mucinous, 831
  serous, 831
Cystadenoma, mucinous, 820-822
  serous, 822-824
Cystitis, with cystocele, 535
  and diverticula of urethra, 579
  and incontinence, 543
Cystocele, 534-541
  of cervix, and hemiamputation, 407
  definition, 535
  in Heaney hysterectomy, 492

and prolapsed uterus, 480
  Watkins operation, 485-489 490-491
and prolapsed vagina, 519, 520, 625
repair of, and amputation of cervix, 405
  technic, 536-539
  with vaginal hysterectomy, 539-541
Cystomas, benign and malignant, 831
  ovarian, 824
Cystometrogram, 553
Cystoscope, Kelly, 4
  examination by, 587, 588-589
  before irradiation therapy, 745
Cystotomy, vaginal, 604
Cystourethrocele, 504
  and incontinence, 543
  repair, with sling operation, 558
Cytology, of adenocarcinoma, 790-791
  Brenner tumor, 828
  carcinoma of cervix, 732-736
  carcinoma of fallopian tube, 851-852
  carcinoma in situ, of endometrium, 806-807
  of cervical pathology, 708-719
  cystadenocarcinoma of ovary, 832
  of dermoid cyst, 825
  discovery of, 9
  of dysgerminoma, 835
  granulosa tumor, 836
  of ovarian cysts, 820
  of sarcoma of uterus, 812-813
  of serous cystadenoma, 823
Cytoxan, for gynecologic malignancies, 846-848

Dactinomycin, for gynecologic malignancies, 846-848
Davis, Hugh J., colposcopy, 722-723
Death, sudden, prevention of, 43
Decidua, of pregnancy, 327
Defecation, painful, in endometriosis, 214
Dehiscence, of wound, 138-141
Dehydration, before surgery, 22
Delalutin, for recurrent carcinoma, 805-807
Demerol, before anesthesia, 38-39
Deming, C. L., 549
Dextran, 72, 73, 74, 90
Diabetes mellitus, and endometrial cancer, 793-794
  and Wertheim hysterectomy, 764
Diaphragm, in Wertheim hysterectomy, 751

Diarrhea, potassium loss through, 109
  water loss, 100
Diathermy, for gonorrhea, 236
  for septic abortion, 452
Dibenzyline, for endotoxic shock, 257
  for septic shock, 261
Dicoumarol, 89, 90
Diet, and abortion, 438-439
  postoperative, 80
  preoperative, 25, 38
Diethylstilbestrol, for endometriosis, 218
Digitalization, preoperative, 25-26
Dilatation, of cervix, 410-412
  after cauterization, 399
  for stenosis, 392-393
  and curettage, 410-423
    for diagnosis, 327
    of carcinoma, 795, 796, 801
    in infertility, 299, 303
    instruments for, 28
    before Manchester operation, 484
    for septic abortion, 262, 263
    for therapeutic abortion, 431-434
    before Watkins operation, 488
Dilator(s), cervical, illus., 399
  Goodell, illus., 413
  Hegar, illus., 411
Diseases, abortion need in, 428-430
  inflammatory, pelvic, 230-267
Dissector, blunt, illus., 33
Distention, abdominal, 345
  postoperative, 80-82
Diverticulitis, 349
Diverticulum, Meckel's, 347
  of urethra, 577-581
Donald, A., Manchester operation, 9
  operation for prolapsus uteri, 482-487
Dose rate probe detector, 749-750
Dosimeter, 749
  illus., 750
Dosimetry, of irradiation therapy, 749-750
Douching, of artificial vagina, 464
  after cauterization, 399
  after conization of cervix, 401
  for gonorrhea, 233, 236
  with pessaries, 531
  for septic abortion, 452
Drainage, of abdomen, 450-452
  through abdomen, 256
  of bladder, after fistula repair, 590-591
  suprapubic, 568, 584, 679
  in hysterectomy, 173

Drainage—(Cont.)
  Wertheim, 763-764
  from incision, 141
    infected, 138
  of pelvis, 131
  for salpingitis, 253-256
  of vulvectomy, 691, 694
Drug, before anesthesia, 38, 51
  for cardiac arrest, 63, 64
Ducts, Skene's, cysts of, 574-575
Dysgerminoma, of ovary, 834-835
Dysmenorrhea, with adenomyosis, 194
  and cervical stenosis, 392-393
  with endometriosis, 214
  and fibroids, 150
  neurectomy for, 225-226
  ovarian sympathectomy for, 229
  with pelvic TB, 264
Dyspareunia, 155
  after 50, 626
  with endometriosis, 214, 215
  and leukoplakia, 676
  from pelvic infection, 238
  See also Coitus
Dysplasia, and carcinoma in situ, 713-715

ECF. See Fluid, extracellular
Ectopic pregnancy. See Pregnancy
Ectoplasia of cervix, 387-388
Edema, of legs, with fibroids, 150
Electrocardiogram, for cardiac arrest, 63
Electrolyte studies, routine, 19
Embolectomy, pulmonary, 92
Embolism, air, during anesthesia, 51
  prevention, 89
  pulmonary, 91-93
Emmett, T. A., 4
  trachelorrhaphy, 407-408
Endarteritis, ischemic, after irradiation, 744
Endocervix, curettage, 415
  polyp from, 394-396
Endometriosis, 192-221, 317
  definition, 8, 192
  extra-uterine, 196-221
  histology, 203-214
  malignancy of, 220-221
  sites of, 197-203
  symptoms, 214-215
  treatment, 217-220
    culdoscopy, 319
    presacral neurectomy, 225
    surgery, 218-220
    Wertheim hysterectomy, 764
Endometritis, and curettage, 413
Endometrium, and abortion, 439
  biopsy, and ovulation, 294
  cancer of, 789-807
  ectopic, 196
  of ectopic pregnancy, 327-329

  hyperplasia of, 419-423
    and cancer, 792-793
    Swiss-cheese, 836
  sarcoma of, 811, 812
  tuberculosis of, 265
Endosalpingitis, 450
Endotoxin, 257
Endoxan, for gynecologic malignancies, 846-848
Enema, barium, before irradiation therapy, 745
  postoperative, 81
  preoperative, 25
Enovid, for dysfunctional bleeding, 421
  for endometriosis, 218
Enteritis, regional, 347
Enterocele, 635-640
  in cul-de-sac, 500, 502
  repair, Moschowitz technic, 637, 638-369
    with vaginal hysterectomy, 639-640
  Spalding-Richardson operation, 505
  with vaginal prolapse, 519, 520
Enterostomy, 355, 358
  for fistula, 348
Epidemiology, of cancer of cervix, 701-706
  of gonorrhea, 320
Epidermidization, 716
  of cervix, 389-390, 394, 710, 712
Epinephrine, for cardiac arrest, 63
Episiotomy, 641
Epispadias, 548
Epithelium, cervical, cells of, 708-712
  dysplastic, 713-715
Ergotrate, in abortion, 454
Escherichia coli, 258, 260, 262
  sulfasuxidine for, 645
Estes, W. L., Jr., 307-308
Estrogen(s), administration of, 118-121
  and cervical dysplasia, 713, 714
  deficiency, and leukoplakia, 675-678
  causing dysfunctional bleeding, 417
  for dysfunctional bleeding, 421
  for endometriosis, 218-219
  and endometrium, 792
  excessive, 836
  and fibroids, 143
Estrone, implantation of, 121
Ether, discovery of, 3
Ethisterone, for dysfunctional bleeding, 421
Evisceration, of wound, 138-141
Examination, gynecologic, 17-19
  under anesthesia, 26
  annual, 817
  laboratory, 19-21
    normal values, 20-21
  preanesthetic, 37

Exenteration, pelvic, 771-787
  anterior, 785
  cure rate, 786
  procedure, 773-787
  for recurrent carcinoma, 805
Exercise, leg, preventing thrombosis, 89
Explosion, in anesthetics, 42
Exsanguination, cardiac arrest from, 66

Falk, H. C., 244
Fallopian tube, carcinoma of, 850-853
Fascia, stripper, illus., 555
  of uterus, 481
Fascia lata, of ox, for suspension, 521-523
  sling, 551, 552, 553
  strip, technic, 554-565
Feces, Mikulicz sigmoidostomy, 652-653, 655
Femur, necrosis, and irradiation, 745
Ferguson forceps, illus., 34
Fertility. See Infertility
Fetus, in abdominal pregnancy, 339-340
  and appendicitis, 367, 368-369
  death of, 325
  potential malformation, and abortion, 430
  and sterilization, 377
Fever, in septic shock, 259
Fibrillation, treatment of, 63-64
Fibrin, formation of, 86
Fibroids, uterine, 143-190
  and abortion, 440
  degeneration of, 144-145, 149, 150
  pedunculated, removal, 186, 187, 188
  sarcomatous change, 811-813
  treatment, 813-815
  treatment of, 151-156
  myectomy, 180-188
  See also Myoma(ta)
Fibrolipoma, of uterus, 144
Fibroma, of ovary, 826-829
  of vulva, 665
Fibromyoma, of vulva, 665
Figure-of-eight sutures, 134
Finney, J. M. T., 15
Fissure, anal, 361-362
Fistula, anal, 361-362
  intestinal, 347-348
  after irradiation, 744-745
  rectovaginal, 646-660
    congenital, 655-660
    diagnosis and treatment, 648-655
    large, closure, 649-650, 652-653
      Latzko technic, 651-652, 654

Index 865

small, closure, 648-651
ureteral, 272, 274
ureterocervicovaginal, 273
uretero-intestinal, Coffey technic, 615, 616-617, 618
ureterovaginal, 273, 274
urinary, after exenteration, 785
 after hysterectomy, 740-741, 764, 765
vesicourethrovaginal, operation, 604-605
 involving sphincter, operation for, 606-608
vesicovaginal, diagnosis and treatment, 586-591
 etiology, 585-586
 history of, 2-3, 584-585
 with hysterectomy, 153
 instruments, 591-593
 Latzko operation, 608-610
 and rectovaginal, operation for, 599-600
 simple, closure, 594-598
 small closure, 592-595
 transabdominal closure, 610-611
 and urethrovaginal, 584-622
Floor, pelvic, muscles, 482
Fluid, balance, 97-104
 extracellular, 98, 106
 hydrogen ions in, 110
 and sodium, 104
 replacement, 72, 74, 259
 requirements, 97
 postoperative, 79
 See also Water
Fluoroscopy of uterus, 299-301
5-Fluorouracil, for gynecologic malignancies, 846-848
Flushing, of lungs, with oxygen, 53
Focus, of infection, removal, 261-262, 263
Folic acid analogs, for gynecologic malignancies, 846-848
Food. *See* Diet
Forceps, illus., 30, 31, 32, 34
 ureteral stone, illus., 416
 for vesicovaginal fistula, illus., 592, 593
Form, vaginal, 463-465
Fothergill, W. E., operation, for prolapsus uteri, 482-487
Frangenheim (Cöln), 549
Frank, Robert, artificial vagina, 458-459
Freund, W. A., 738
Fulguration, of condylomata acuminata, 671
 of endometrial cysts, 219
 urethral caruncle, 573-574
 urethral prolapse, 573-574
 vesicovaginal fistula, 591

Gametes, defective, 438-439

Gantrisin, for urinary infection, 568
Gas gangrene, 256
Gases, blood, 59
Gilliam suspension of uterus, 242, 474
 technic, 475-478
 and vaginal repair, 512-513
Gloves, rubber, 5-6
Goebell, R., 549
Goebell-Frangenheim-Stoeckel operation, 544, 550
 results, 569-570
 technic, 555-565
Gonococcus, resistant, 230
Gonorrhea, 230-256
 and Bartholin's gland cysts, 671
 cervicitis from, 388
 and condylomata acuminata, 669
Goodell dilator, illus., 413
Goodsell's law, of fistula, 361-362
Gram's smear, 231
Green, T. H., Jr., 739
Gridiron incision, 131-132
 closure, 136
Gusberg curette, 415
Gynandroblastoma, 838
Gynecology, and intestinal tract, 344-362
 operative, history, 1-10

Halban's disease, 420
Hammock, peritoneal, 526
Harkin, Dwight E., 656
Headache, postspinal-anesthesia, 44
Heaney clamp, illus., 31
Heaney, N. Sproat, vaginal hysterectomy, 490, 492-500
Heart, arrest, 62-64
 compression, external, 62-64
 internal, 64
 disease of, and abortion, 428-429
 and anesthesia, 47-48
 in exsanguination, 66
 monitoring of, 52, 68-75
 "myoma," 147
Heat cradle, for thrombophlebitis, 90
Hegar dilators, illus., 411
Hematocolpos, with imperforate hymen, 461
Hematoma, follicular, 819
 after vulvectomy, 694
 and wound healing, 139
Hematometra, surgery for, 282, 283
Hematoperitoneum, 326, 327
Hematosalpinx, 282
Hematuria, in endometriosis, 215
Hemiamputation, of cervix, 407

Hemorrhage, after abortion, 434-435
 during anesthesia, 50
 cardiac arrest from, 66
 from cystadenoma, mucinous, 821
 serous, 822
 with interstitial pregnancy, 335
 from ovarian cyst, 819
 posthysterectomy, 177-179
 postoperative, 55
 shock from, 71-75
 surgical control, 75-76
 with tubal pregnancy, 330-331
 after vulvectomy, 694
Hemorrhoids, 359-361
 with rectocele, 626
Heparin, 89, 90
Hernia, 344-347
 vaginal. *See* Rectocele, Enterocele, Cystocele
 after vulvectomy, 694
Heyman, applicator for radium, illus., 798
 capsules of radium, 801
 cautery cone, 723-724
Hidradenoma, of vulva, 666-669
Higgins, Charles C., 615
Hirsutism, Stein-Leventhal syndrome, 839
History, of pelvic surgery, 1-10
 taking of, 15-17
Homans' sign, 88
Hormones, and dysfunctional bleeding, 421-423
 and endometriosis, 196, 217, 218, 219, 220
Horns, of uterus, 281-292
Hospitals, and sterilization, 374-375
Hovelacque, hypogastric plexus of, 225
Hunner, Guy, 396-397
Hunner's ulcer, 554
Hydrocortisone, enemas, 744
Hydrogen ion, conversion to pH, 115
 in metabolism, 110, 111-112
Hydronephrosis, 273-274, 279, 588
 and fibroids, 147
Hydrosalpinx, 238, 318
Hydrothorax, Meigs's syndrome, 828-829
Hydroureter, 588
 and fibroids, 147
Hydroxyprogesterone caproate, 440
Hykinone, 89
Hymen, imperforate, 461
Hypercarbia, 57, 58
Hyperestrogenism, 420
Hyperkalemia, 108, 109
Hyperplasia, endometrial, 419-423
 and cancer, 792, 793, 795

Index

Hypertension, and abortion, 428
 and endometrial cancer, 793-794
 pulmonary, 92
Hyperventialtion, during anesthesia, 52
 in septic shock, 258
Hypospadias, deforming urethra, 563
Hypotension, and anesthesia, 37, 43-44, 49-51, 55
 surgical, 51
Hypothalamic-pituitary-ovarian dysfunction, 420
Hypothalamus, dysfunction, 294
Hypoventilation, 57-62
 during anesthesia, 52
Hypovolemia, before surgery, 22
Hypoxemia, 55-58
 postoperative, 53-54
Hypoxia, from spinal anesthesia, 43
Hysterectomy, abdominal, for abortion, 436-437
 development of, 10
 for fibroids, 152-154
   Richardson technic, 163-173
   modfications, 172-175
   subtotal, 156-163
 for carcinoma of corpus uteri, 803-804
 for cervical disease, 396
 and cervicitis, 391-392
 complications, hemorrhage, 177-179
   rectovaginal fistula, 646
   ureter injury, 270-272, 274
   vaginal prolapse, 518-526, 528
   vesicovaginal fistula, 608-609
 for dermoid cyst, 826
 for dysfunctional bleeding, 423
 for endometrial cancer, 798-803
 for endometriosis, 218
 first, 2
 for interstitial pregnancy, 336-338
 for pelvic TB, 266
 for salpingitis, 239-242
 and salpingo-oophorectomy, for arrhenoblastoma, 837
   for carcinoma, of fallopian tube, 853
     ovarian, 831, 843-845
   for cystadenoma, 822
   for cystoma, 824
   for dysgerminomas, 835
 for septic shock, 262
 and sterilization, 378-389
 for therapeutic abortion, 431
 total, and adnexectomy, for carcinosarcoma, 816
   for sarcoma of uterus, 813-815
   cervical myoma, 175-177

 for tubal pregnancy, 331
 for tubo-ovarian abscess rupture, 242-244
 vaginal, for carcinoma in situ of cervix, 723
   development, 8
   for endometrial cancer, 800-801
   enterocele following, 636
   enterocele repair with, 637, 639-640
   for myomata, 179-180
   for prolapsed uterus, 479, 489-490, 492-500
   for retrodisplacement of uterus, 474, 475
 Wertheim, modified, 726-729
   and pregnancy, 767
   radical, 750-765
     complications, 764-765
Hysteropexy, 479
Hysterorrhaphy, 479
Hysterosalpinography, 299-301

Ileum, endometriosis of, 203
 loop, as bladder substitute, 612, 613, 620-622, 775
Ileus, adynamic, 346
 postoperative, 80-82
 after tubo-ovarian rupture, 243
Ilopan, postoperative, 80
Implantation, of ovary in uterus, 307-308
 of tube into uterus, 303-305
 of ureter, into bladder, 272
   technic, 277-280
   into ileium, 612, 613
   into sigmoid, 612-620
Implants, from cystadenoma, 822
Incisions, of abdomen, 125-132
 closing of, 132-137
 secondary, 140-141
 for appendectomy, 366-367
 for vulvectomy, 685, 686, 687
 breakdown, 693-694
 See also Wound
Incontinence, and fistula, 587
 rectal, 641-642
 of urine, stress, 540-544
   fascia lata sling operations, 555-570
   Goebell-Frangenheim-Stoekel operation, 555-565
   Marshall-Marchetti-Krantz operation, 551, 565-570
   not curable by plication, 548-570
 treatment, 10
 urgency, 543, 554
Induction, of anesthesia, 40
Induration, ligneus, 238
Infarction, pulmonary, 92
Infection, of cervix, 388-392

 chronic, following abortion, 452
 with cystocele, 535
 focus of, removal, 261-262, 263
 gonorrheal, 230-256
 urinary tract, postoperative, 83-85, 567-568
 and uterine curettage, 413
Infertility, 293-308
 culdoscopic investigation of, 320
 dilatation for, 410-411
 in endometriosis, 215
 from genital TB, 263, 264
 male factors, 296-298
 and surgery, 308-309
Inflation, artificial, 59-62
Inhalation, foreign matter, 65
Injection, hypertonic, for abortion, 436
Injury, of ureters, 270-280
Insemination, artificial, 298
Instruments, for abortion, 28
 for colpotomy, 28
 for dilatation and curettage, 28
 for pelvic surgery, 27
   illustrations, 29-34
   radical, 28-29
 for radium insertion, 28
 for Rubin's test, 28
 for vaginal procedures, 27-28
Insufflation, tubal, 296, 298-299, 302
Intensive care unit, 53
Intestines, anastomosis of, technics, 350-357
 fistula, 347-348
 and gynecology, 344-362
 injury to, 255, 346
   in abortions, 453-454
 obstruction of, after exenteration, 785-786
 of large, 348-358
 of small, 344-347
 in Wertheim hysterectomy, 751
Intubation, intestinal, 346-347
 tracheal, 41-42
   before culdoscopy, 312
Irradiation, of adenocarcinoma, of cervix, 765
 of carcinoma, of cervix, 737, 741-750
   complications, 743-745
   dosimetry, 749-750
   results, 741-745
   technic, 745-749
 endometrial, 798-803
   recurrent, 804-805
 of fallopian tube, 853
 ovarian, 845-846
 of urethra, 582-583
 for carcinosarcoma, of uterus, 816
 for endometriosis, 217
 of fibroids, 151-152
 fistula from, 347, 599-600

Index 867

rectovaginal, 646
vesicovaginal, 608, 610
incomplete, 771
nuclear, 742
during pregnancy, 767
of sarcoma of uterus, 814
sterilization, 378
Irving sterilization, 378, 381-382
Isoniazin, for pelvic TB, 266
Isoproterenol, 73
for endotoxic shock, 258, 261
Isuprel, 73, 74
for endotoxic shock, 258, 261, 262

Jacob's clamp, illus., 29, 411
Jewett, H. J., 615-616
Jones, Georgeanna, 421-423
Howard, 10

Kalchman, G. C., 336
Kegel, A. H., perineal exercises, 547
Kelly, Howard A., 4, 5, 6
side-to-side amputation of uterus, 160, 163
plication operation, 541-542, 551, 552
results, 568-570
needle holder, illus., 33
Kidney, disease of, and abortion, 429
function of, 101, 111-112
sodium regulation, 104
and ureter damage, 272-279
and vesicovaginal fistula, 613-614
in Wertheim hysterectomy, 751
Knife, for vesicovaginal fistula, illus., 592
Koontz, fascia lata of ox, 522-523
Krantz, K. E., 551
Kraurosis, of vulva, 674-675
Krukenberg tumor, 833, 834

Labia majora, leukoplakia of, 687
Labia minora, cysts of, 674
Labor. See Childbirth
Laboratory determinations, normal values, 20-21
gynecological pathological, first, 8
Lacerations, of cervix, 388
perineal, 641-646
Lahey thyroid clamp, illus., 32
Laparoscopy, for ectopic pregnancy, 329
of tubes, 301-302
Laparotomy, and drainage for salpingitis, 253-256
enterocele repair during, 638-639
and gonorrheal infection, 236

pack, 127-128
pelvic, instruments for, 27
scar from, endometriosis of, 202
for tubal pregnancy, 330-335
Laryngospasm, 58
Latzko operation, rectovaginal fistula, 651-652, 654
vesicovaginal fistula, 608-610
Laws, abortion, 426-428
sterilization, 374-375
Leadbetter, uterosigmoid anastomosis, 775-778
Le Fort operation, ventral fixation of uterus, 513-516, 517-518
Leiomyomatosis, intravenous, 145
Leucocytosis, bowel obstruction, 345
Leukeran, for gynecologic malignancies, 846-848
Leukoplakia, and carcinoma, 683
of cervix, 395-396
precancerous, 676
of vulva, 675-679, 687
Leventhal, M.L., 839
Levin tube, 81
Lewis Recording Cystometer, 553
Lidocaine, for fibrillation, 63, 64
hyperbaric, 44
Ligaments, broad, and uterus, 481, 482, 483
round, endometriosis of, 202
and uterus, 481, 482, 483
uterosacral, 471, 481, 482, 483
shortening, technic, 478-479
Ligation, hypogastric artery, 75-76
of ureter, accidental, 270, 273
vena cava, 93
Ligneous induration, 238
Linea alba, 125-126
Lipiodol, 299, 300, 302
Lipoma, of vulva, 665
Lister, Joseph Lord, 4
Lithopedion, 325
Liver, and exenteration, 773
in Wertheim hysterectomy, 751
Lock suture, 135
Long, Crawford, 3
Löwenberg test, 88
Lungs, disease of, and abortion, 429
and anesthesia, 47
embolism, 91-93
endometriosis in, 197
foreign matter in, 65
infarction, 92
postoperative complications, 75-79
"shock," 65-66
before surgery, 22
water loss from, 100
Luteoma, of ovary, 835, 837
Lymph nodes, and endometrial

cancer, 797
Lymphadenectomy, of groin, 690
for carcinoma of vulva, 684
pelvic, in exenteration, 778-780
in Wertheim hysterectomy, 752-758
Lymphatics, and endometriosis, 209
inguinal, 688
para-aortic, and exenteration, 773
metastases into, 805
in Wertheim hysterectomy, 751
of vulva, 683-685
Lymphedema, following vulvectomy, 694
Lymphocyst, in Wertheim hysterectomy, 763-764

Magnesium, requirements, 114
Malformations. See Anomalies
Malignancy, and abortion, 429
of arrhenoblastomas, 837
of cervicitis, 390
at cervix, 817
of leukoplakis, 395
of polyp, 394
of cystadenoma, mucinous, 821
serous, 822-823
of dysgerminomas, 834
in endometriosis, 220-221
of feminizing tumors, 837
gynecologic, chemotherapy, 846-848
of hidradenoma, 667-668
of ovarian tumors, 817
solid, 829
of Paget's disease, 681
papillomatous tumors, 831
Manchester operation, prolapsed uterus, 9, 482-487
and amputation of cervix, 405
enterocele repair with, 637
Marchetti test, 551, 554
Marshall, C. M., incision of, 685-686
V.F., 551
Marshall-Marchetti-Krantz operation, 551, 565-570
Marsupialization, of cyst, 672-673
Martin, Franklin, 615
Martzloff, K. H., 732-733, 737
Masterson, J. G., 739
Mattress sutures, 134-135
Maylard, A. E., incision, 128-131
McBurney incision, 366
McDowell, Ephraim, 1
McGraw, Theodore, 738
McIndoe, Archibald, construction of vagina, 460-466
Mechlorethamine, for gynecologic malignancies, 846-848
Meckel's diverticulum, 347
Medication, preanesthetic, 38

Medphalan, for gynecologic malignancies, 846-848
Medroxyprogesterone acetate, 295, 439
Meigs, J. V., 739
Meigs's syndrome, 828-829
Melanoma, of vulva, 696-697
Meltzer, R. M., 336
Menarche, dysfunctional bleeding, 418
Menge pessary, 531
Menopause, 118-121
  dysfunctional bleeding, 418
  and endometrial cancer, 789-790
  and fibroids, 148, 149
  kraurosis of vulva, 674-675
  and ovary ablation, 154-155
  premature, 219
  suspension of uterus following, 474
Menorrhagia, 418
  with adenomyosis, 194
  in endometriosis, 215
  and fibroids, 148-149
  with pelvic TB, 264
Menstruation, cessation of, 118-121
  culdoscopy of, 320
  in ectopic pregnancy, 325-326
  and fibroids, 148-150
  and ovarian cysts, 818-820
  patient's history, 16
  and pelvic TB, 264
  preservation of, 181
  retrograde, 8, 206-215
    experimental, 210-212
  and uterus retrodisplacement, 473
Meperidine, before anesthesia, 38-39
6-Mercaptopurine, for gynecologic malignancies, 846-848
Mersilene tape, 475, 551
  for vaginal suspension, 524-426, 528
Mesentery, in Wertheim hysterectomy, 751
Metabolism, acid-base, 110-114
  fluid, 97
Metaphen, 27
Metaplasia, squamous, 389-390, 394
  of cervix, 712
  of endometrium, 792
Metaraminol, 73, 93
  for septic shock, 260, 262
Methyltestosterone, for endometriosis, 218
Metrorrhagia, in endometriosis, 215
Meyer, Robert, 838
Mikulicz sigmoidostomy, 652-653 655
Miller, Norman, 8, 550
  paradoxical operation, 642

Miller-Abbott tube, 346-347
Mittelschmerz, neurectomy for, 225
Mitzenbaum scissors, illus., 759
Mole, definition, 114
  hydatidiform, 329
    aspiration of, 435
Monkeys, endometriosis in, 209-212
Morcellation, of uterus, 493
Morphine, before anesthesia, 38-39
Mortality, from abortions, 425
  from anesthesia, 37
Moschowitz, Alexis V., enterocele repair, 637, 738-639
Mouth-to-mouth ventilation, 60-61
Mucin, in ovarian cyst, 821
Mucocele, of appendix, 821, 822
Mucous plugs, 76-77, 78
Mucus, cervical, and fertility, 295
Müllerian mucosa, 207
Munnell, E. W., 844-845, 849
Muscles, at Maylard incision, 128-131
  at midline incision, 125-127
  of pelvic floor, 482, 624
  relaxants of, 41
  of uterus, 471
Myelitis, prevention, 43
Myoma, and abortion, 440
  cervical, removal, 189-190
  heart, 147
  pedunculated, removal, 186-188
  uteri, 143-190
    asymptomatic, 145-148
    hysterectomy for, 156-163
    postmenopausal growth, 146
    sarcomatous, 811-813
    treatment, 813-815
Myomectomy, abdominal, 180-188
  first, 1-2
  indications, 182-183
  vaginal, 186-190
Myometrium, fibroids in, 143

Nabothian cysts, 399
Nabothian follicle, 389
Narcotic drug, before anesthesia, 38
Navel. See Unbilicus
Necrosis, aseptic, of femur, and irradiation, 745
Needle holder, illus., 33, 592
Neisseria gonorrhoeae, 231
  and urethral diverticula, 577
Nembutal, before anesthesia, 38
Neomycin, discovery of, 8
Neo-synephrine, in conization, 721
Neothalidine, before hysterectomy, 750
Nephrostomy, bilateral, 273, 274

Nerve(s), pelvic autonomic, 227, 228
  presacral, resection of, 225-229
Neurectomy, presacral, 225-229
  for endometriosis, 219
Neuromuscular stimulator, 41
Nitrofurazone, suppository, 25
Nitrogen mustard, for gynecologic malignancies, 846-848
Nitrous oxide, early use, 3
Norethindrone, for dysfunctional bleeding, 421
  for endometriosis, 218
Norethynodrel, for dysfunctional bleeding, 421
  for endometriosis, 218
Norlutin, for dysfunctional bleeding, 421
Novak, E., 208-209
Nutrition, deficient, and abortion, 438-439

Obesity, and anesthesia, 48
  and endometrial cancer, 793-794
  and Wertheim hysterectomy, 764
  and wound healing, 139
Obstruction, abdominal, 81-82, 344-347
Ochsner, clamp, illus., 31
Ohkawa, K., 739
Oligomenorrhea, with pelvic TB, 264
Olshausen suspension of uterus, 474
Omentectomy, for carcinoma, of fallopian tube, 853
  of ovary, 831, 843
  for sarcoma of uterus, 814-815
Omentum, metastases into, 831, 843
  in Wertheim hysterectomy, 751
Oophorectomy, for Brenner tumor, 828
  and carcinoma of breast, 833
  for corpus luteum cyst, 820
  for cystadenoma, mucinous, 821
  for cystoma, ovarian, 824
  earliest, 1
  for fibroma, 827
  and hysterectomy, 154-156, 170
    for dermoid cyst, 826
  and salpingectomy, 247-251
  for salpingitis, 239-242
Operating room, fire prevention, 42
  housekeeping technics, 137
Operations. See Surgery
Osteitis, pubis, postoperative, 569
Osteoporosis, and estrogen therapy, 120
Osmole, definition, 115

Index 869

Ovary(ies), carcinoma of, classification, 831
cystic, 831-833
diagnosis, 842
and of endometrium, 794
metastatic, 833
prognosis, 848-849
solid, 829-831
treatment, 842-849
chemotherapy, 846-848
irradiation, 845-846
surgery, 843-845
second-look, 848
technics, 849-850
culdoscopy of, 314-315, 319-320
cyst(s), dermoid, 824-826
endometrial, 216
neoplastic, 820-826
parovarian, 838-839
retention, 818-819
rupture, 818
spillage from, 848
cystadenoma, mucinous, 820-822
serous, 822-824
cystoma, 824
denervation, 229
and dysfunctional bleeding, 417-418
dysgerminoma of, 834-835
endometriosis of, 198-201
and estrogen activity 154-155
fibromas of, 826-829
gynandroblastoma, 838
and hysterectomy for benign disease, 154-156
implantation, in uterus, 307-308
pregnancy in, 340-341
sarcoma of, 834
Stein-Leventhal syndrome, 839-842
teratoma of, 834
tuberculosis of, 265-266
tumors of, 817-850
classification, 843-845
functioning, feminizing, 835-837
masculinizing, 837-838
pathology, 818
solid, benign, 826-829
torsion of pedicle, 817-818
Ovoids, rubber, for radium, 747, 801
illus., 748
Ovulation, detection of, 293-294
with dysfunctional bleeding, 420
lack, Stein-Leventhal syndrome, 839-842
Ox, fascia lata of, for suspension, 521-523, 551
Oxygen, inhalation of, 62, 63
Oxygenation, after anesthesia, 54-55
monitoring of, 52

Oxytocin, with abortions, 431, 432, 434, 435, 436, 437, 445, 454

Pack, laparotomy, 127, 128
Paget's disease, of vulva, 679-681
Pain, in ectopic pregnancy, 325
in endometriosis, 214
and fibroids, 150
Panculdoscope, 312, 322
Panhysterectomy. See Hysterectomy, total
Papanicolaou smear, 18, 148, 736
for carcinoma in situ, 719-721
for endometrial carcinoma, 795
false-negative, 721
during pregnancy, 766
screening, 701-705
and vulvar carcinoma, 682
Papillomata, of cystadenoma, 822, 823
of vulva, 669-671
Paquelin cautery, 397
Paregoric, preoperative, 350
Parry-Jones, E., incision of, 685-686
Patient, age of, and surgery, 22
for anesthesia, 46-48
position of, 39-40
permission from, 181, 241-242
physical status, 36-37
preoperative care, 15-34
emotional, 23-24
physical, 25
Pelvis, drainage of, 131
examination of, 18
under anesthesia, 327
for ectopic pregnancy, 326
in infertility, 299
exenteration of, 771-787
floor of, anatomy, 482, 624-625
inflammatory disease of, 230-267
and abdominal pregnancy, 337
and ectopic pregnancy, 323
tuberculosis, 263-267
surgery of, 1-10
instruments for, 28-29
in Wertheim hysterectomy, 751-752, 758-764
Penicillin, for abortion, 447, 450, 454
for gonorrhea, 232-233
for peritonitis, 367
for salpingitis, 235
for septic shock, 260, 262
for sarcoma of uterus, 814
Pentothal Sodium, for cervical cauterization, 398
for conization of cervix, 401
for curettage, 413-414
Perforation of uterus, in curettage, 416-417
Perineometer, 547

Perineum, Kegel exercises, 547
lacerations, 641-646
repair, 626
layer, 645-647, 648
of vaginal outlet, 626-629
Warren flap, 643-645
Peritoneoscopy, 311
Peritoneum, of bladder, advancement, 478
closure, in exenteration, 783-785
in endometriosis, 198-199
incision of, 126, 127
Peritonitis, from abortion, 448-452
acute, 234-236
from appendicitis, 365-367
tuberculous, 264-265
Perspiration, water loss, 100
Pessary(ies), 527-531
for cystocele, 535-536
for elderly, 519
for prolapse, 513
Smith-Hodge, 472, 473, 474
Pfannenstiel incision, 128-129
closure, 136
pH, conversion to hydrogen-ion concentration, 115
Phenothiazine, before anesthesia, 39
Phenoxybenzamine, for endotoxic shock, 257, 261
L-Phenylalanine mustard, for gynecologic malignancies, 846-848
Phlebothrombosis, 88, 91
Phlegmasia alba dolens, 88
Phlegmasia cerulea dolens, 90
Phosphorus, requirement, 114
Pituitary growth hormone, and endometrial cancer, 794
Placenta, in abdominal pregnancy, 340
curettage of, 416
forceps, illus., 30
Plasma expander, 72, 74
Plication, vesical sphincter, and urethrocele operation, 544-547
Pneumonitis, postoperative, 76-78
Podophyllin in benzoin, for condylomata acuminata, 670
Polymenorrhea, with pelvic TB, 264
Polyps, cervical 393-396, 712
endometrial, 414, 416
Pomeroy technic, for sterilization, 378-381
Pontocaine, 44
Potassium, balance, 107-110
Pregnancy, abdominal, 336-340
diagnosis, 337, 339-340
secondary, 337
after amputation of cervix, 401
anesthesia during, 45, 48
appendicitis during, 367-369
cervical, 341

Pregnancy—(Cont.)
  cervical carcinoma during, 765-767
  and culdoscopy, 322
  ectopic, 323-341
    diagnosis, 326-330
      by culdoscopy, 316-319
    pathophysiology, 324-325
    ruptured, 72
    test, 330
  and endometriosis, 196, 206, 216
  and fibroids, 146-147, 150-151
  hemorrhoids during, 359-360
  interstitial, 335-336
  and myomectomy, 181
  ovarian, 340-341
  pessary use during, 529
  and suspension of uterus, 474
  tubal, symptoms, 325-326
    treatment, 330-335
  uterine and extra-uterine, 341
  following Watkins transposition operation, 487
Pregnandiol excretion, 295
Prematurity, and appendicitis, 367
Presacral neurectomy, 225-229
Pressure, central venous, monitoring, 68-71, 74, 103
Price, P. B., 550
Proctosigmoidoscopy, before irradiation therapy, 745
Progesterone, and abortion, 439-440
  and dysfunctional bleeding, 417
  and endometrium, 792
  substitution therapy, 421-423
Progestogens for recurrent endometrial cancer, 805
Prolapse, urethral, 573-574
  of uterus, 479-518
    Manchester operation, 482-487
    vaginal hysterectomy for, 489-490, 492-500
    vaginal, 518-526, 528
    colpocleisis, 520-522
    Grant-Ward operation, 521-523
    mersilene strap suspension, 524-526, 528
    Williams-Richardson suspension 524, 525
Promethazine, before anesthesia, 39
Prostatism, female, 544
Prostigmin, postoperative, 80
Prothrombin time, 89
Provera, 295, 439, 440
Pruritis, and carcinoma of vulva, 683
  and leukoplakia, 676
  neurectomy for, 225
  and Paget's disease, 681

Pseudo-erosion of cervix, 387-388
Pseudomyxoma peritonei, 821-822
Psychiatry, in gynecology, 15
Psychosis, and abortion, 429-430
  and sterilization, 376
Puberty, precocious, 835-836
Pulse, monitoring of, during anesthesia, 52
Purine analogues, for gynecologic malignancies, 846-848
Pyelitis, postoperative, 273
Pyelogram, before irradiation therapy, 745
  unilateral kidney, 613, 614
Pyelostomy, 274
Pyometra, from cervical adhesions, 393
  and endometrial carcinoma, 795-796
  surgery for, 283-284
Pyosalpinx, 238
  surgery for, 285
Pyrimidine analogues, for gynecologic malignancies, 846-848
Pyuria, 85

Race, and abdominal pregnancy, 336
  and ectopic pregnancy, 323
  and fibroids, 143, 154
Rad, 749
Radiation therapy, 745-750. See Irradiation
Radium, castration by, 423
  for endometrial cancer, 798-803
  intracavitary, 745-750
    instruments for, 28
    Heyman applicator, illus., 798
  for sarcoma of uterus, 814
  therapy, 5, 741
Radiumhemmet, 741, 798
Recovery room, 53
"Rectal stalk," 759
Rectocele, 624-640
  and prolapsed uterus, 480
  and prolapsed vagina, 519, 520
  repair of, 632-635
    with vaginal outlet, 627-632
Rectovaginal fistula, See Fistula
Rectum, adhesion to uterus, 162
  in anterior exenteration, 785
  carcinoma of, 771
  endometriosis of, 203
  examination of, 18
  fistula into vagina, 646-660
  injury to, 646
  and irradiation of pelvis, 744, 745
  laceration of, 643-646
    of sphincter, 641
  surgery of, 359-362

Reis, Emil, 7
Relaxants, of muscle, 41
Respiration, during anesthesia, 41, 51-52
  in shock, 65-66
  water loss, 100
Resectoscope, and incontenence, 543, 544
Resuscitation, cardiopulmonary, 55-66
Resuscitators, 61-62
Retardation, mental, and sterilization, 376
Retractor, Edebohls', illus., 33
Retrocession, of uterus, 471
Retrodisplacement, of uterus, 469-479
Rheomacrodex, 73
Richardson, Edward, H., abdominal hysterectomy, 163-173
  modifications, 172-175
  uterine prolapse operation, 505, 508-512
Ring pessary, 531
Rizzoli, F., operation for absence of anus, 657, 659-660
Robb, Hunter, 6
Roentgen unit, 741, 749
Rubella, and abortion, 430
Rubin's cannula, illus., 30
Rubin's test, 296, 298-299, 302
  instruments for, 28
Rupture, tubal, 325

Salpincolysis, 303
Salpingectomy for chronic salpingitis, 239-242
  cysts following, 819
  interstitial pregnancy following, 335-336
  technic, 245-247
  for tubal pregnancy, 332-334
  See also Tube
Salpingitis, acute, 234-238
  and curettage, 413
  diagnosis, 234-235
  treatment, 235-236
  and appendicitis, differential diagnosis, 364
  chronic, 238-242
    and ectopic pregnancy, 323-324
    surgery for, 238-242, 244-251
    drainage at laparotomy, 253-256
  with fibroids, 154
Salpingo-oophorectomy, for carcinoma of corpus uteri, 803-804
  for endometrial cancer, 801
  for endometriosis, 218-219
  with hysterectomy, 170
    for sarcoma of uterus, 813-815

for Meigs's syndrome, 829
for ovarian tumor, 513
for pelvic TB, 266
for septic shock, 262
and tubal pregnancy, 336-338
Salpingostomy, 305-308
Salpix, 299, 300
for urethrogram, 579
Sampson, J. A., 206-215
L-Sarcolysin, for gynecologic malignancies, 846-848
Sarcoma, botryoides, 814
of cervix, 811, 812, 814-415
in myoma, 144-145
of ovary, 834
of uterus, 811-816
Scar, endometriosis of, 202
Schauta-Amreich operation, 739
Schiller test, 719, 721, 724
Schröder, amputation of cervix, 407
Schuchardt incision, 588-589
Scissors, bladder, illus., 593
Scopolamine, before anesthesia, 38
Screening, for cervical cancer, 701-705, 720-721
Sebaceous cysts, of vulva, 673-674
Seconal, before anesthesia, 38
Secretion, from breasts, 17
Sedation, preoperative, 25
Semen, quality of, 297
Septum, uterine, 281, 282-284, 290
Shaving, of patient, 26
Shaw, Wilfred, 551
Shirodkar-Barter cerclage operation, 441-444
Shock, and anesthesia, 48
from ectopic pregnancy, 326
hemorrhagic, 71-75
hypovolemic, 50
anesthesia during, 43
lungs in, 65-66
postoperative, 71-75
septic, 256-263, 448
after tubo-ovarian rupture, 243
treatment, 259-263
Sigmoid, endometriosis of, 203
ureters anastomosed to, 612-620, 775-778
volvulus, 349-350
Sigmoidostomy, Mikulicz, in rectovaginal fistula repair, 652-653, 655
Silastic Cystocath, 84
Silastic tubing, 276
in ureters, 776-777
Silk sutures, 134-135
Silver wire sutures, 141
Silvertone spring colpostat, 747
Simpson, Sir J. Y., 7
Sims, J. Marian, 2-3
Sims-Huhner test, 296

Singley pickup forceps, illus., 32
Sintrom, 90
Skene's ducts, cysts of, 574-575
in gonorrhea, 231-233
Skin, graft, for vagina, 461-463
and intestinal fistula, 348
necrosis of, following vulvectomy, 693-694
papillomata of, 669
sodium loss through, 106
water loss through, 100
Sling operation, fascia lata, for urinary incontinence, 555-570
Smear, cervical, cytology of, 795
vaginal, irrigational, 704
Papanicolaou, 119
screening, 701-705, 719
and fallopian tube malignancy, 853
Smith-Hodge pessary, 527, 529, 530
Sodium, balance, 104-107
Sodium para-aminosalicylic acid, for pelvic TB, 266
Sodium warfarin, 90
Soporifics, 3
Sound, uterine, illus., 411
Sovak, F. W., cuff salpingostomy, 305-307
Spalding-Richardson operation, 505, 508-512
enterocele repair with, 638
Speculum, Sims's, 3
Sperm, adequacy of, 296
Sphincter, vesical, absence of, 548
plication, 541-542, 543-547
Spina bifida, and incontinence, 548
Spine, anesthesia via, 42-46
Squier, J. B., 549
Staphylococcus aureus, infection from, 137-138
Stein, I. F., 839, 840-841
Stein-Leventhal syndrome, 319-320, 420, 839-842
Stenosis, of cervix, 392-393, 410
Sterility, and fibroids, 146-147, 150
myomectomy for, 182
pessary to relieve, 529
and uterus retrodisplacement, 473
See also Infertility
Sterilization, 374-382
and abortion, 436
hospital committee on, 375
indications for, 375-377
methods, 378-382
Irving technic, 378, 381-382
Pomeroy technic, 378-381
puerperal, 377
with Watkins operation, 487, 489
Stilbestrol, for dysfunctional bleeding, 421

Stocking, elastic, 90
Stoeckel, W., 549
Stomach, full, and anesthesia, 49
Stone forceps, illus., 32
Strassman, Paul, 10
Strassman operation on septum, 282
Streptomycin, for abortion, 447, 450, 454
for gonorrhea, 236
for pelvic TB, 266
for septic shock, 260, 262
Stricture, of cervix, 392-393
Stroma cells, 327-329
Struma ovarii, 826
Sturmdorf tracheloplasty, technic, 406-407
Suction, gastric, 80
Suicide, and pregnancy, 430
Sulfasoxisole, for urinary infection, 568
Sulfasuxidine, discovery of, 8
for perineal repair, 643, 645
Surgery, for fibroids, 151, 152-154
indications for, 15
injuring ureters, 270-280
instruments for, 27-34
opening abdomen, 125-132
pelvic, evaluation for, 22
history, 1-10
postoperative care, 68, 80
preoperative care, 15-34
preparation of patient, 23-25, 26-27
pulmonary complications, 75-79
pulmonary embolectomy, 92
for thrombophlebitis, 90-91
urinary tract infection, 83-85
Suspension, of uterus, 474-479
Gilliam technic, 475-478
of vaginal vault, Te Linde-Mattingly technic, 500-504
Sutures, closing abdomen, 134
in repair of vaginal fistulas, 589, 591
skin, 135
tension, 133
Sweat, sodium loss in, 106
Sweat-gland tumor, of vulva, 666-669
Sympathectomy, ovarian, 229

Tait, Robert Lawson, 4
Tar cyst, 201
Taussig, F. J., leukoplakis, 675-676, 684
Tears. *See* Lacerations
Technic, anastomosis, of bowel, end-to-end, closed, 350, 354-355
open, 350-353
side-to-side, 351, 354, 356-357
ureteroureteral, 276-277

872 Index

Technic—(Cont.)
  anus, formation of, 657-659
  appendectomy, 369-372
  bladder, advancement of peritoneum, 478
    repair of, 177, 178
    substitution, Bricker's ileal loop, 620-622
  cervix, amputation, high, 405-406
    low, 403-405
    carcinoma of, irradiation, 745-749
    cauterization of, 399-400
    conization of, 400-401, 402
    dilatation of, 411-412
  Coffey II ureterosigmoid anastomosis, 616-617, 618
  colpocleisis, 520-522
  colporrhaphy, 504-505, 506-507
  colpotomy, 237-238
  Cordonnier-Leadbetter, ureterosigmoid anastomosis, 617-620
  culdoscopy, 312
  cystocele repair, 536-539
    with vaginal hysterectomy, 539-541
  dilatation and curettage, for abortion, 431-434
  enterocele repair, 638, 639
  fascia lata strip, 554-565
  Frank artificial vagina, 458-459
  Gilliam suspension of uterus, 475-478
  Goebell-Frangenheim-Stoekel operation, 555-565
    Aldridge modification, 557-558
    transected sling modification, 563-565
  Grant-Ward operation, 521-523
  Heaney vaginal hysterectomy, 490, 492-500
  hemorrhoid excision, 360
  hysterectomy, for carcinoma of corpus uteri, 803-804
    subtotal abdominal, 156-163
    total, for cervical myoma, 175-177
      Richardson, 163-173
      modifications, 172-175
  hysterosalpinography, 300
  Irving sterilization, 381-382
  Latzko, rectovaginal fistula, 651-652, 654
    vesicovaginal fistula, 608-610
  Le Fort operation, 513-516
    Goodall-Power modification, 514, 517-518
  Manchester operation, 484-487
  McIndoe construction of vagina, 460-466
  Moschowitz repair of enterocele, 637, 638-639
  myomectomy, abdominal, 183-188
    vaginal, 186-190
  neurectomy, presacral, 227-229
  ovarian surgery, 849-450
  perineum, repair of, layer, 645-647, 648
    and vaginal outlet, 626-629
  Pomeroy sterilization, 378-381
  rectocele, repair of, 632-635
    and vaginal outlet, 627-632
  rectovaginal fistula, closure, 648-651, 652-653
  Rizzoli operation for absence of anus, 659-660
  salpingectomy, 245-247
    with tubal pregnancy, 332-334
  salpingo-oophorectomy, 247-251
    including interestitial pregnancy, 336-338
  Shirodkar-Barter cerclage operation, 441-444
  Spalding-Richardson operation, 508-512
  spinal anesthesia, 45-46
  Sturmdorf tracheloplasty, 406-407
  Te Linde-Mattingly vaginal vault suspension, 500-504
  trachelorraphy, 408
  tube, conservation of, 334
    implantation into uterus, 303-305
  ureter, implantation of, 277-280
  ureterostomy, 253-254
  urethra, restoration of, and urinary continence, 600-604
  urethrocele and vesical sphincter plication, 544-547
  uterus, bisection operation, 249-252
    curettage of, 414-416
    double, 287-292
  uterosacral ligaments, shortening, 478-479
  vagina, lengthening of, 466-468
    suspension, to abdominal wall, 524, 526-527
      mersilene tape, 524-526, 528
  vesicourethrovaginal fistula operation, 604-605
    involving sphincter, 606-608
  vesicovaginal fistula closure, and rectovaginal fistula, 599-600
    simple, 594-598
    small, 592-595
    transabdominal, 610-611
  vulvectomy and lymphadenectomy, 685-693
  Warren flap repair of perineum, 643-645
  Watkins transposition operation, 488-491
  Wertheim hysterectomy, 751-765
    modified, 726-729
  Wharton operation, 459-461
  Williams-Richardson vaginal suspension, 524, 525
Te Linde-Mattingly suspension of vaginal vault, 500-504
Temperature, basal body, 439
Tension sutures, 133, 140
Teratoma, of ovary, 834
Testis, varicocele of, 296-297
Testosterone, for leukoplakis, 676-677
Tetracaine, hyperbaric, 44
Tetracycline, for gonorrhea, 233, 236
THAM, 74
  during resuscitation, 63
Thecalutein cysts, 839
Thecoma, of ovary, 835, 837
Therapy, estrogen replacement, 118-121
  of infected wound, 138
  irradiation, development of, 5
Thiotepa, for gynecologic malignancies, 846-848
Thorazine, 74
  for septic shock, 261, 262
Thrombectomy, 90-91
Thrombin, deposition, 86
Thromboembolism, 85
Thrombophlebitis, 85-91
  treatment, 89, 90-91
  following vulvectomy, 694
  following Wertheim hysterectomy, 764
Thrombosis, prophylaxis, 88-89
  silent, 91
  venous, 85-91
Thrombus, red and white, 86
Thyroid, and abortion, 438, 439
  in ovarian teratomas, 826
Trachea, intubation. See Tube, tracheal
Tracheloplasty, Sturmdorf, 406-407
Trachelorrhaphy, of cervix, 407-408
Tracheotomy, 60
Triethylenethiophosphoramide, for gynecologic malignancies, 846-848
Trigonitis, and incontinence, 543
Trocar, for culdoscopy, 311
Tromexan, 90
Trophoblast, 324
Tube(s), fallopian, conservation of, 334
  through culdoscope, 314-317
  gonorrheal infection, acute, 234-238
    chronic, 238-242
  and infertility, 295-296
  insufflated, 302

Index 873

pregnancy in, 323
rupture, 325
in septic abortion, 449
surgery of, 308-309
excision, 244-245
technics, 245-247, 247-251
for tubal pregnancy, 332-334
implanted into uterus, 303-305
and sterilization, 380-382
tuberculosis of, 265-266
Levin, 81
Miller-Abbott, 346-347
pharyngeal, for airway, 59-60
rectal, 81
tracheal, 41-42, 48, 53, 63, 65
for airway, 54, 59-60
tracheostomy, 60
Tuberculosis, anesthesia during, 47
of cervix, 736
female genital, 263-267
culdoscopy for, 320
of intestinal fistula, 348
Tubo-ovarian abscess, rupture, 242-244
Tuboplasty, 303-309
Tumor(s), adnexal, 817-853
Brenner, 827-828
culdoscopic investigation, 320
Krukenberg, 833, 834
mixed mesodermal, 815-816
obstructing large bowel, 348-349
ovarian, 817-850
classification, 843-845
feminizing, 835-837
masculinizing, 837-838
pathology of, 818
pedicle, torsion of, 817, 818
solid, 826-829
of uterus, benign, 143-190
of vulva, 665-671
Tympanites, postoperative, 80-81

Uchida sterilization, 379
Ulcer, "rodent," 695-696
Umbilicus, "blue," 326
endometriosis of, 202
Unconsciousness, and asphyxia, 58
Urecholine, postoperative, 568
Uremia, from ligated ureters, 273
Ureter(s), anstomosis, to ileum loop, 612-613, 620-622
to sigmoid, 612-620, 775-778
Coffey II technic, 616-617, 618
Cordonnier-Leadbetter technic, 617-720
catheterization, 271-272
identification and intubation of, 251-254, 271

implantation of, 591
in bladder, 272, 765
technic, 277-280
injury of, 270-280
and irradiation of pelvis, 744-745, 746
ligation of, 79, 270, 273
valves, defective, 549
in Wertheim hysterectomy, 726, 763
Ureteral stone forceps, illus., 416
Ureterostomy, cutaneous, 611-612
technic, 253, 254
Ureteroureteral anastomosis, 272
technic, 276-277
Urethra, anomalies, 548
carcinoma of, 581-583
caruncle of, 572-573
and construction of vagina, 462
cyst under, 576-577
diverticulum of, 577-581
in Heaney hysterectomy, 492
prolapse of, 573-574
reconstruction of, 549-551, 600-604
and stress incontinence, 553
surgical conditions, 572-583
Urethritis, and incontinence, 543
Urethrocele, 534-547
definition, 534
and incontinence, 543
and vesical sphincter plication, 544-547
Urethrogram, 578
apparatus, illus., 579
Urethropexy, retropubic, 554
Urethrovaginal fistula. See Fistula
Urine, diversion of, 600, 611-622
in exenteration, 774-778, 783-784
incontinence of, treatment, 10, 600-604
stress, 534, 540-544
choice of operation, 551-555
Marshall-Marchetti-Krantz operation, 551, 565-570
not curable by plication, 548-570
sling operations, 555-570
vesical sphincter plication, 544-547
with vulvectomy, 691
output, monitoring, 73, 74
postoperative, 79, 82-83
in vagina, 274
water loss through, 99-100
Urograms, 274, 275, 279
Urography, intravenous, 588
Uterus, adenomyosis, 192-196
amputation, in subtotal hysterectomy, 159, 160
anatomy of, 470-471
anomaly of, and abortion, 440
congenital absence, 457

aspiration of, for therapeutic abortion, 431, 435
bicornuate, 10 281-292
anastomosis, 283-284, 287-292
surgery of, 281-292
bisection operation, technic, 249-252
bleeding, dysfunctional, 417-423
in endometriosis, 215
and estrogen therapy, 120-121
carcinoma of, 833
curettage of, 412-416
therapeutic, 420-423
descent of, and cystocele, 534
with relaxed vaginal outlet, 625
endometriosis of surface, 200-202
evacuation of, instrumental, 446-448
medical, 445
injection of, for therapeutic abortion, 431
interstitial pregnancy, 335-336
resection for, 336-338
malpositions of, 469-531
myomata of, 143-190
myomectomy, abdominal, 183-188
vaginal, 186-190
ovary implanted in, 307-308
packing of, for therapeutic abortion, 431, 432, 434-435
perforation of, in curettage, 416-417
by dilator, 412
infected, 447
pessary for, 527-531
during pregnancy, 452-454
preservation of, 242, 331-332
prolapse of, 479-518
anatomic considerations, 480-482, 483
and enterocele, 636
history of surgery, 9
Manchester operation, 482-487
Spalding-Richardson operation, 505, 508-512
vaginal hysterectomy for, 489-490, 492-500
replacement, manual, 529-530
retrodisplacement of, 469-479
rudimentary, 282
sarcoma of, 811-816
septate, 282-292
surgery of, history of, 1-2
suspension of, 474-479
Gilliam technic, 475-478
and vaginal repair, 512-513
history of, 469-470
transposition operation, 485-489, 490-491

874 Index

Uterus—(Cont.)
  tube implanted, technic, 303-305
  ventral fixation, 513-518
  See also Hysterectomy

Vagina, absence of, 10, 457-466
    partial, 466-468
  anatomy of, 624-625
  artificial, 457
    form for, 461, 463-465
    Frank nonsurgical, 458-459
    McIndoe operation, 460-466
    Wharton operation, 459-461
  bleeding from, after hysterectomy, 177-179
  discharge from, after cauterization, 398-399
  endometrial carcinoma in, 804
  endometriosis of, 202
  eversion of, 520
  fistulas into, 584-622
    from rectum, 646-660
    See also Fistula
    in hysterectomy, 173-174
  hysterectomy through, 179-180
    for sterilization, 379
  Le Fort operation, 513-516
    Goodall-Power modification, 514, 517-518
  myectomy via, 186-190
  outlet, relaxed, 624-640
  prolapse following hysterectomy, 518-526, 528
    colpocleisis, 520-522
    Grant-Ward technic, 521-523
    mersilene strap repair, 524-526, 528
    Williams-Richardson suspension, 524, 525
  repair, with Gilliam suspension, 512-513
    of outlet and perineum, 626-629
    and rectocele, 627-632
    of rectocele, 632-634, 634-635
  smear from, irrigational, 704
    Papanicolaou, 119, 701-705
  Spalding-Richardson operation, 508-512
  surgery of, instruments for, 27-28
  suspension of, in Wertheim hysterectomy, 728

  urine in, 274
  vault, Te Linde-Mattingly suspension, 500-504
Vaginitis, and curettage, 413
  and pessaries, 529
van Bouwdijk-Bastiaanse, M. A., 737
Varicocele, and infertility, 296-297
Vasodilators, for septic shock, 73-74, 261, 262
Vasopressors, for cardiac arrest, 63, 64
  for shock, 73, 260
Vein(s), subclavian, catheter in, 70
  thrombosis in, 87-88
  varicose, 88
Vena cava, ligation of, 93
Venous pressure. See Pressure
Ventilation, artificial, after anesthesia, 54
  methods, 60-62
  monitoring of, 51-52
Ventrofixation, 479, 480
Vesicovaginal fistula. See Fistula
Vinblastine, for gynecologic malignancies, 846-848
Vincristine, for gynecologic malignancies, 846-848
Vistaril, before anesthesia, 38
Vital signs, monitoring, 51-52, 68
Voiding, from fistula, 586
  mechanism of, 82
Volsellum, illus., 34
Volvolus, diagnosis of, 350
Vomiting, during anesthesia, 49
  bowel obstruction, 345
  water loss, 100
Vulva, carcinoma, basal cell, 695-696
    in situ, 681-682
  cysts of, 671-674
    sebaceous, 673-674
  kraurosis, 674-675
  leukoplakia of, 675-679
  melanoma of, 696-697
  Paget's disease, 679-681
  surgical conditions, 665-698
  tumors of, 665-671
Vulvectomy, for carcinoma in situ, 682
  conservative, 677-679
  for leukoplakia, 677-679
  for Paget's disease, 681
  partial, 665-669

  total, and lymphadenectomy, for carcinoma, 685-693
    complications, 693-694
    results, 694-695
  for melanoma, 696-697

Warren, J. Collins, repair perineal laceration, 8, 643-645
Water, in body, 98-104
  intoxication, 102
Watkins, Thomas J., operation for cystocele and prolapse, 485-489, 440-491
Way, S., 684, 789
  incision of, 685-687
  vulvectomy, 694, 695
Weight, atomic, body minerals, 115
Wells, Horace, 3
  Sir Thomas Spencer, 4
Wertheim, E., 7
  clamp, illus., 32
  hysterectomy, modified, 726-729
    radical, 737, 739, 750-765
      complications, 764-765
      lymphadenectomy, 752-758
      pelvic dissection, 758-764
      pelvic exploration, 751-752
      and pregnancy, 767
      and ureters, 270-271, 274
Wharton, L. R., construction of vagina, 459-461
Wilkins, Lawson, 10
Williams, J. Whitridge, 4
Winsbury-White, H. P., 615
Wolffian ducts, cysts of, 674
  parovarian, 838-839
Wound, healing of, 138-141
  infection, 137-138
Wynn's solution, 138

X-ray, therapeutic, 745-750
  for sarcoma of uterus, 814
Xylocaine, 44
  for fibrillation, 63

Younge biopsy punch, 719
  illus., 737

Zygote, 324